MRI-Arthroscopy Correlations

Stephen F. Brockmeier
Editor

MRI-Arthroscopy Correlations

A Case-Based Atlas of the Knee,
Shoulder, Elbow and Hip

Section Editors
Stephen F. Brockmeier
John J. Christoforetti
Larry D. Field
Mark D. Miller
Michael J. O'Brien
Felix H. Savoie, III

With 522 Figures

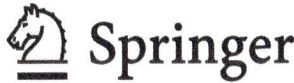 Springer

Editor
Stephen F. Brockmeier, MD
Associate Professor
Department of Orthopedic Surgery
University of Virginia
Charlottesville, VA, USA

ISBN 978-1-4939-4539-9   ISBN 978-1-4939-2645-9   (eBook)
DOI 10.1007/978-1-4939-2645-9

Springer New York Heidelberg Dordrecht London
© Springer Science+Business Media New York 2015
Softcover reprint of the hardcover 1st edition 2015

Printed on acid-free paper

Springer Science+Business Media LLC New York is part of Springer Science+Business Media (www.springer.com)

To my wife Kristin, whom I love and admire more than anyone in this world
To my children, who keep me grounded, entertained, and provide a reason
for my being
To my mentors, past and present, who have afforded me guidance, inspiration,
and humility

Preface

The advent of magnetic resonance imaging scanning and the development of arthroscopic surgical techniques are the two principal events responsible for revolutionizing Sports Medicine to where it is today. The confluence of these two entities spans two specialties, Orthopedic Surgery and Radiology, and allows for increasingly accurate diagnosis of pathology and advanced treatment options to aid in optimizing patient outcomes and recovery.

This text, *MRI-Arthroscopy Correlations*, represents a microcosm of daily patient care. By aligning the MRI findings associated with the spectrum of problems seen in the most commonly treated joints in sports medicine with the diagnostic findings seen during arthroscopy of the same joint in the same patient, the reader is able to correlate this pathology and apply these findings to the clinic, the radiology reading room, or the operating suite. At our institution, we have found this type of interactive correlation to be an exceedingly effective tool for education and continued learning, an impetus for interdisciplinary research collaboration, and a critical part of our approach to optimum patient care. Furthermore, we have found this case-based correlation between MRI imaging and arthroscopic findings and treatment to be a well-received and effective method for teaching and discussion at meetings and instructional courses.

We have organized this book into four parts highlighting the four major joints in which MRI and arthroscopy are most commonly used in Sports Medicine: knee, shoulder, elbow, and hip. Each of the part editors, Dr. Mark D. Miller (knee), Dr. Felix H. "Buddy" Savoie III, Dr. Larry D. Field, Dr. Michael J. O'Brien (elbow), Dr. John J. Christoforetti (hip), and myself (shoulder), are nationally recognized experts, teachers, and pioneers in their respective areas of sports medicine and have covered the gamut of topics in each of their parts. Chapters are formatted to present an overview of the specific disease entity first, followed by selected cases chosen by the chapter authors that best illustrate common or noteworthy disease entities or pathology with an emphasis on the parallel MRI imaging and arthroscopic findings.

I want to thank Drs. Miller, Savoie, Field, O'Brien, and Christoforetti for their tremendous contributions to this book, and I also want to thank the many contributing authors for volunteering their time, expertise, and cases to make this book successful.

We hope you find this book interesting and educational and that it fosters similar collaboration in your practices and institutions.

Charlottesville, VA, USA   Stephen F. Brockmeier

Contents

Contributors

Elaine J. Ahillen, MD Department of Orthopedic Surgery, TRIA Orthopedic Center, Bloomington, MN, USA

Mark W. Anderson, MD Department of Radiology and Medical Imaging, University of Virginia, Charlottesville, VA, USA

Asheesh Bedi, MD Department of Orthopedic Surgery, University of Michigan School of Medicine, Ann Arbor, MI, USA

Jonathan P. Braman, MD Department of Orthopedic Surgery, University of Minnesota Medical School, Minneapolis, MN, USA

Karen K. Briggs, MPH Steadman Philippon Research Institute, Vail, CO, USA

Stephen F. Brockmeier, MD Department of Orthopedic Surgery, University of Virginia, Charlottesville, VA, USA

M. Tyrrell Burrus, MD Department of Orthopedic Surgery, University of Virginia Health System, Charlottesville, VA, USA

Brian Busconi, MD Department of Orthopedics, UMass Memorial Medical Center, Worcester, MA, USA

J.W. Thomas Byrd, MD Department of Orthopedics and Rehabilitation, Vanderbilt University School of Medicine, Nashville, TN, USA

Jonathan Capelle, MD Department of Orthopedics, Mississippi Sports Medicine and Orthopedic Center, Jackson, MS, USA

Austin W. Chen, MD Department of Orthopedic Surgery, University of Illinois Hospital at Chicago, Chicago, IL, USA

E. Michael Chester, MD Department of Radiology, Duke University Medical Center, Durham, NC, USA

John J. Christoforetti, MD Department of Orthopedic Surgery, Sports Medicine Division, Allegheny Health Network, West Penn Hospital, Pittsburgh, PA, USA

Austin J. Crow, MD Department of Orthopedic Surgery, University of Virginia Hospital, Charlottesville, VA, USA

Healthy J. Desai, MD Department of Orthopedics, Ridgecrest Regional Hospital, Ridgecrest, Ridgecrest, CA, USA

Department of Orthopedics, Long Beach Memorial Medical Center, Long Beach, CA, USA

David R. Diduch, MD, MS Department of Orthopedic Surgery, University of Virginia Health System, Charlottesville, VA, USA

Benjamin G. Domb, MD American Hip Institute, Westmont, IL, USA

Adventist Hinsdale Hospital, Hinsdale, IL, USA

Brian C. Domby, MD Department of Orthopedics, Sports Medicine, University of Colorado Hospital, Boulder, Boulder, CO, USA

Kevin F. Dunne, BS American Hip Institute, Westmont, IL, USA

Rami Joseph Elkhechen, MD Orthopedic Care Specialists of North Palm Beach, North Palm Beach, FL, USA

Gregory C. Fanelli, MD GHS Orthopedics, Danville, PA, USA

Fernando Portilho Ferro, MD Department of Orthopedic Surgery, Hospital de Acidentados, Goiânia, Brazil

David Paul Fessell, MD Department of Radiology, University of Michigan School of Medicine, Ann Arbor, MI, USA

Larry D. Field, MD Mississippi Sports Medicine and Orthopedic Center, Jackson, MS, USA

Jason W. Folk, MD Department of Orthopedic Surgery and Sports Medicine, Greenville Health System—Steadman Hawkins Clinic of the Carolinas, University of South Carolina School of Medicine, Greenville, SC, USA

Seth C. Gamradt, MD Keck Medical Center of USC, University of Southern California, Los Angeles, CA, USA

Michael B. Gerhardt, MD Institute for Sports Science, Cedars-Sinai Medical Center, Santa Monica, CA, USA

Steven A. Giuseffi, MD Department of Orthopedic Surgery, Mississippi Sports Medicine and Orthopedic Center, Jackson, MS, USA

Justin W. Griffin, MD Department of Orthopedic Surgery, University of Virginia Health System, Charlottesville, VA, USA

Lawrence V. Gulotta, MD Department of Sports Medicine and Shoulder Service, Hospital for Special Surgery, New York, NY, USA

F. Winston Gwathmey, MD Department of Orthopedic Surgery, University of Virginia Health System, Charlottesville, VA, USA

Wendell M.R. Heard, MD Department of Orthopedic Surgery, Division of Sports Medicine, Tulane University School of Medicine, Tulane Medical Center, New Orleans, LA, USA

E. Rhett Hobgood, MD Mississippi Sports Medicine and Orthopedic Center, Jackson, MS, USA

Evan W. James, BS Steadman Philippon Research Institute, Center for Outcomes-Based Orthopedic Research, Vail, CO, USA

Shawn Evette Johnson, MD Department of Sports Medicine, Ochsner Clinic, Jefferson, LA, USA

Abdurrahman Kandil, MD Department of Orthopedics, University of Virginia Medical Center, Charlottesville, VA, USA

Scott T. King, DO Orthopedic and Spine Specialists, York, PA, USA

Gabrielle Konin, MD Department of Radiology and Imaging, Hospital for Special Surgery, New York, NY, USA

Peter R. Kurzweil, MD Department of Orthopedics, Long Beach Memorial Medical Center, Long Beach, CA, USA

Chris M. LaPrade, BA Department of Biomedical Engineering, Steadman Philippon Research Institute, Vail, CO, USA

Robert F. LaPrade, MD, PhD The Steadman Clinic, Vail, CO, USA

William James Malone, DO Musculoskeletal Radiology Division, Department of Radiology, Geisinger Medical Center, Danville, PA, USA

Eric C. McCarty, MD Department of Orthopedics, University of Colorado School of Medicine, Boulder, CO, USA

Department of Integrative Physiology, University of Colorado, Boulder, CO, USA

Department of Orthopedics, Sports Medicine, University of Colorado Hospital, Boulder, CO, USA

Department of Athletics, University of Colorado, Boulder, CO, USA

Benjamin S. Miller, MD Mississippi Sports Medicine and Orthopedic Center, Jackson, MS, USA

Mark D. Miller, MD Department of Orthopedic Surgery, University of Virginia Health System, Charlottesville, VA, USA

Department of Orthopedic Surgery, Head Team Physician, James Madison University, Charlottesville, VA, USA

Ryan A. Mlynarek, MD Department of Orthopedic Surgery, University of Michigan School of Medicine, Ann Arbor, MI, USA

Julie A. Neumann, MD Department of Orthopedic Surgery, Duke University Medical Center, Durham, NC, USA

Michael J. O'Brien, MD Department of Orthopedic Surgery, Division of Sports Medicine, Tulane University School of Medicine, Tulane Medical Center, New Orleans, LA, USA

Patrick M. O'Brien, MD Mississippi Sports Medicine and Orthopedic Center, Jackson, MS, USA

Michael P. Palmer, MD 88th Medical Group, Surgical Operations Squadron, Wright Patterson Air Force Base, Wright Patterson AFB, OH, USA

Marc J. Philippon, MD The Steadman Clinic and Steadman Philippon Research Institute, Vail, CO, USA

John M. Redmond, MD American Hip Institute, Westmont, IL, USA

Craig M. Roberto, DO Williamsville, NY, USA

James R. Ross, MD Department of Orthopedic Surgery, Broward Orthopedic Specialists, Fort Lauderdale, FL, USA

Gary Salvador, MS, PA-C Sports Medicine North, Peabody, MA, USA

Felix H. Savoie III, MD Department of Orthopedic Surgery, Tulane University School of Medicine, Tulane Medical Center, New Orleans, LA, USA

David L. Schub, MD Department of Orthopedic Surgery, Kaiser Permanente Hospital—San Diego, San Diego, CA, USA

Jesse Seamon, MD Department of Orthopedic Surgery, Saint Louis University Hospital, St. Louis, MO, USA

Kathryne J. Stabile, MD, MS Department of Orthopedic Surgery, Duke University Medical Center, Durham, NC, USA

James S. Starman, MD Department of Orthopedic Surgery, University of Virginia Hospital, Charlottesville, VA, USA

Misty Suri, MD Department of Sports Medicine, Ochsner Clinic, Jefferson, LA, USA

Robert Z. Tashjian, MD Department of Orthopedic Surgery, University of Utah, Salt Lake City, UT, USA

Dean C. Taylor, MD Department of Orthopedic Surgery, Duke University Medical Center, Durham, NC, USA

Stephen R. Thompson, MD, MEd, FRCSC Department of Orthopedics, Eastern Maine Medical Center, Bangor, ME, USA

Marc Tompkins, MD Department of Orthopedic Surgery, University of Minnesota Medical School, Minneapolis, MN, USA

Joshua A. Tuck, DO, MS Department of Orthopedic Surgery, LECOM Wellness Center, LECOM Orthopedic and Sports Medicine, Lake Erie College of Osteopathic Medicine, Erie, PA, USA

Bastian Uribe-Echevarria Marbach, MD Institute for Orthopedic Sports Medicine and Rehabilitation, University of Iowa Hospitals and Clinics, Iowa City, IA, USA

Wade C. VanSice, MD, MPH Department of Orthopedic Surgery, Tulane University School of Medicine, Tulane Medical Center, New Orleans, LA, USA

Ryan J. Warth, MD Department of Orthopedic Surgery, University of Texas Health Sciences Center, Houston, TX, USA

Brian C. Werner, MD Department of Orthopedic Surgery, University of Virginia, Charlottesville, VA, USA

Bryan Whitfield, MD Department of Orthopedic Surgery and Sports Medicine, Greenville Health System—Steadman Hawkins Clinic of the Carolinas, Greenville, SC, USA

Phillip Williams, MD Department of Orthopedic Surgery, Hospital for Special Surgery, New York, NY, USA

Richard B. Williams, MD Department of Orthopedics, Sports Medicine, University of Colorado Hospital, Boulder, CO, USA

Jeffrey B. Witty, MD Acadiana Orthopaedic Center at Lafayette General, Lafayette, LA, USA

Brian R. Wolf, MD, MS Department of Orthopedics and Rehabilitation, University of Iowa, Iowa City, IA, USA

Bojan Zoric, MD Sports Medicine North, Peabody, MA, USA

About the Editors

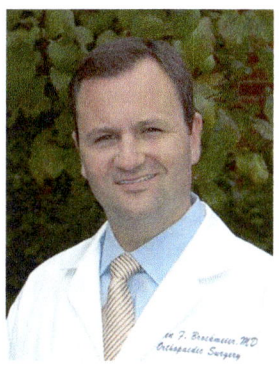

Dr. Stephen F. Brockmeier is a board-certified Orthopedic Surgeon with a sub-specialty certification in Sports Medicine. He joined the University of Virginia Department of Orthopaedic Surgery in 2010, where he is currently an Associate Professor and specializes in Sports Medicine and Shoulder Reconstructive Surgery. His primary areas of clinical and research interest are in arthroscopic and reconstructive surgery of the knee and shoulder with a specific focus on sports injuries of the upper extremity. He serves as a team physician for the University of Virginia Athletics as well as for James Madison University and is the fellowship director for the University of Virginia Sports Medicine Fellowship program.

Prior to joining the UVA faculty, Dr. Brockmeier completed undergraduate studies at the University of Virginia and medical school and Orthopedic residency training at Georgetown University, followed by a fellowship in sports medicine and shoulder surgery at the Hospital for Special Surgery in New York where he trained with Dr. Russell Warren, Dr. David Altchek, and many other leaders in the Sports Medicine field. He then spent 3 years in practice in Charlotte, North Carolina, specializing in sports medicine, arthroscopy, and shoulder surgery. While in Charlotte, he served as a team physician for the Charlotte Bobcats.

Dr. Brockmeier is actively involved on the national level in a number of societies including the American Orthopaedic Society for Sports Medicine (AOSSM), where he currently serves on the Council of Delegates and the Education Committee. He is a member of the American Shoulder and Elbow Society (ASES) and serves on the Editorial Board for *Techniques in Shoulder and Elbow* Surgery and *The Orthopaedic Journal of Sports Medicine*.

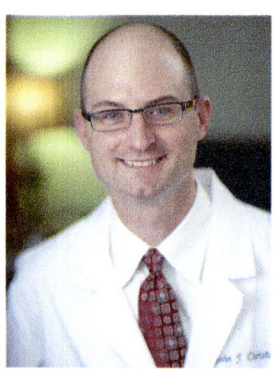

John J. Christoforetti is an Assistant Professor at Drexel University School of Medicine in clinical practice at the Allegheny Health Network in Pittsburgh, Pennsylvania, USA. He serves as a consultant for hip injury to the Pittsburgh Pirates, Pittsburgh Riverhounds, Robert Morris University, and the US Olympic Regional Medical Center. He is faculty-at-large for the American Hip Institute in Chicago, Illinois. Dr. Christoforetti specializes in arthroscopy of the hip, shoulder, and knee.

Dr. Christoforetti's educational process began as an undergraduate at the University of Notre Dame and continued at Georgetown University School of Medicine followed by orthopedic residency at Georgetown University Hospital. In 2004, he conducted basic scientific research at the National Institutes of Health cartilage and mesenchymal stem cell laboratory under the mentorship of Rocky Tuan, Ph.D. In 2006, he studied hip preservation surgery with Jeffrey Mast, M.D., and Michael Karch, M.D., through an AO North America Surgical Preceptorship in Mammoth Lakes, California. He completed his formal training with the Steadman-Hawkins Clinic faculty in the Carolinas with director Dr. Richard J Hawkins and in Vail, Colorado, with Dr. Marc J Philippon.

In 2008, Dr. Christoforetti and coauthors received the Aircast Award for Clinical Science from the American Orthopaedic Society for Sports Medicine for his pioneering radiographic survey of femoroacetabular impingement findings in professional baseball pitchers. He is currently a Master Instructor of Hip Arthroscopy for the Arthroscopy Association of North America and Editorial Board member for the Journal of Arthroscopic and Related Surgery. He is director of the Center for Athletic Hip Injury at the Allegheny Health Network and coordinates multidisciplinary evaluation of non-arthritic hip disorders. His research interests include clinical outcomes in joint preservation surgery, healthcare innovation, and basic biomechanical and applied investigations into the tissues and motion patterns of the human hip.

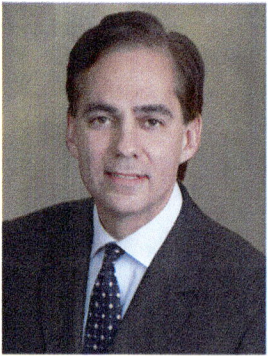

Larry D. Field is an orthopedic sports medicine surgeon specializing in shoulder and elbow surgery and serves as a program director for the ACGME accredited Sports Medicine and Arthroscopy Fellowship Program at the Mississippi Sports Medicine Center in Jackson, Mississippi. He completed his orthopedic surgical training at the University of Mississippi with additional fellowship training in Interlaken, Switzerland, with Dr. Bruno Noesberger and with Professor Ulrich Holz in Stuttgart, Germany. Dr. Field also completed a sports medicine fellowship training program at the Hospital for Special Surgery in New York. Dr. Field is active in clinical research related to shoulder and elbow disorders and has written and edited several books on these conditions. In addition, Dr. Field has published over 150 peer-reviewed scientific papers, review articles, and book chapters on shoulder and elbow related topics and lectures nationally and internationally regarding shoulder and elbow problems. Dr. Field is actively involved in a number of professional orthopedic organizations and societies including ISAKOS, AOSSM, ASES, AOA, AAOS, and AANA where he currently serves on the Board of Directors. Dr. Field also participates as an editorial board member for the *Journal of Shoulder and Elbow Surgery* and *Techniques in Shoulder and Elbow Surgery*.

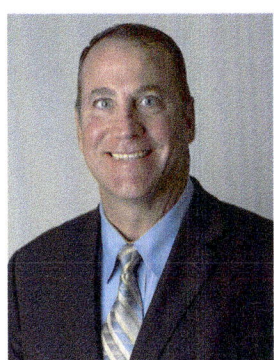

Dr. Mark D. Miller is the Head of the Division of Sports Medicine and the S. Ward Casscells Professor of Orthopaedic Surgery at the University of Virginia. He is a Distinguished Graduate of the Air Force Academy and the Uniformed Services University F. Edward Hebert' School of Medicine. Dr. Miller is a highly decorated retired Colonel in the US Air Force and former team physician for the US Air Force Academy. He currently serves as team physician for James Madison University in Harrisonburg, Virginia. Dr. Miller has over 25 orthopedic text-books that he has written and/or edited including the "best selling" Review of Orthopaedics (now in its 7th Edition) and is the author of over 200 peer-reviewed articles. He is the Founder/Director of the popular Miller Review Course and is a highly sought-after speaker.

Dr. Miller has been very active in several professional societies including the American Orthopaedic Society for Sports Medicine (AOSSM) and is the former chair for three different committees in that society. He was an American Orthopaedic Association North American Traveling Fellow and both a Traveling Fellow and a Godfather for the AOSSM Traveling Fellowship program. Dr. Miller has been named as a "Top Doctor" for numerous regional, national, and international programs. Although widely known for his expertise in knee surgery, Dr. Miller is also an accomplished shoulder surgeon and sports medicine specialist. He is married to his wife, Ann, and has four grown children and two grandchildren.

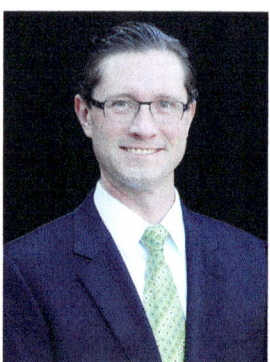

Dr. Michael J. O'Brien received his medical degree from the Tulane University School of Medicine in 2003. After completing his Orthopaedic Surgery residency at the University of Maryland and a Shoulder and Elbow Reconstruction fellowship at the Rothman Institute at Thomas Jefferson University in Philadelphia, he returned to New Orleans in 2009 to become Assistant Professor of Clinical Orthopaedics at Tulane. He is certified by the American Board of Orthopaedic Surgery and is an active member of the American Shoulder and Elbow Society (ASES), Arthroscopy Association of North America (AANA), Southern Orthopaedic Association (SOA), Louisiana Orthopaedic Association (LOA), and the American Academy of Orthopaedic Surgeons (AAOS). Dr. O'Brien serves on the AANA Research and Technology Committees, Tulane eCW Steering Committee, and Tulane Quality Directors Committee. He is the Louisiana Councilor to the SOA and is also Tulane's newest member of the Association of American Medical Colleges Council of Faculty and Academic Societies. He has over 25 articles and book chapters to his credit and lectures locally, nationally, and internationally. His interests include arthroscopy of the shoulder and elbow, rotator cuff disease, shoulder and elbow reconstruction including total shoulder replacements and total elbow replacements, sports medicine, ligament reconstruction of the knee, and fracture care in both adults and children. He practices at the Tulane Institute of Sports Medicine in uptown New Orleans, where he is a team physician for the New Orleans VooDoo of the Arena Football League, Loyola University New Orleans, and Tulane University.

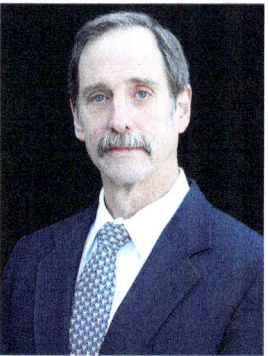

Dr. Felix H. Savoie III is an internationally recognized expert in the areas of Shoulder and Elbow Surgery and Sports Medicine. He is ABOS certified in Orthopaedic Surgery and Sports Medicine. A 1982 graduate of the Louisiana State University School of Medicine in New Orleans, he completed his internship and residency at the University of Mississippi Medical Center in Jackson. After completing an AO fellowship in Switzerland and Hand and Microvascular Surgery and Arthroscopy fellowships in the United States, he returned to Jackson to enter private practice and as an Assistant Professor of Orthopaedic Surgery at the University of Mississippi. While he continues as a Clinical Associate Professor there, he came to the Tulane University School of Medicine in 2007 after Hurricane Katrina to take on the mantle of Professor of Clinical Orthopaedics, Chief of the Division of Sports Medicine, and Director of the Tulane Institute of Sports Medicine, and a year later was named Vice-Chairman of the Department of Orthopaedics.

He is currently Vice President of a the American Shoulder and Elbow Surgeons, a Past President and Trustee of the Arthroscopy Association of North America, a past member of the NCAA Committee on Competitive Safeguards and Medical Aspects of Sports, and a member of the Louisiana High School Sports Association Sports Medicine Advisory Committee. Dr. Savoie also serves on the Editorial and Review Boards of several peer-reviewed journals, and in various capacities in numerous international, national, regional, and local societies.

Dr. Savoie is the author of over 100 peer-reviewed journal articles and 72 book chapters and editor of six textbooks. He is in great demand as a speaker, presenting over 1,600 lectures throughout the United States and over 20 other countries. He has been a frequent contributor to VuMedi and Audio-Digest Orthopaedics, helping to expand medical instruction to the Internet, and has participated in several broadcasts of live surgical procedures around the world.

He is a strong advocate of research, with multiple ongoing projects. His interests lie in every facet of orthopedics, from work on the cellular level, to improvements in surgical instruments and techniques, and increasing safety on the field of play.

MR Imaging for the Orthopedic Surgeon

Mark W. Anderson

Introduction

Magnetic resonance imaging (MRI) is a powerful diagnostic tool that has become a mainstay in orthopedic imaging. Its ability to provide a detailed depiction of normal and pathologic tissue is unparalleled, and with recent improvements in both hardware and software, the diagnostic information made available to the clinician continues to improve. The goal of this chapter is to provide an overview of MRI for the orthopedic surgeon leading to a practical understanding of how it works and when it is most useful in the workup of an orthopedic patient by addressing these questions:

- What is MRI and how does it work?
- Why does the MR image look the way it does?
- What should normal musculoskeletal tissues look like on MR images?
- What do common types of musculoskeletal pathology look like on MR images?
- When is MRI most useful, and when should a different imaging modality be chosen?
- What is on the horizon for MR imaging?

Hopefully, this basic introduction will provide enough information for you to begin looking at MR images yourself, but if you would like a more detailed information, several general references are provided [1–5].

What Is MRI and How Does It Work?

At its core, MRI is unlike any other imaging modality. The machine looks something like a computed tomography (CT) scanner since the patient is placed on a gantry that is posi-

tioned within a tube-like bore of the machine, but unlike CT, no X-rays are used. The basic components of an MR unit are a large magnet and a source of radio waves. Hydrogen atoms are very abundant throughout the body, and since they contain an unpaired electron, they react like small bar magnets within a magnetic field. As such, when the body is placed within the scanner, hydrogen protons tend to line up parallel with the magnetic field. When energy is then pulsed into the body in the form of radio waves, some of the protons will absorb this energy and "flip" into a higher-energy state. When the pulse is turned off, these protons will relax back to a lower-energy state and release energy in the form of radio waves which are detected by the machine and then used to create the MR image (Fig. 1.1).

Most MR imaging units use a superconducting magnet that is made up of wires coiled around the open bore of the machine. These wires are supercooled with cryogens such as liquid helium to reduce electrical resistance and as such, the machine is *always* "on," and anyone working in the magnetic field must be careful to not bring any ferromagnetic objects into the scanning room since these can become lethal missiles if they are pulled into the magnet's bore.

The field strength of clinical MR machines range from 0.2 Tesla (T) to 3 T, with most operating at 1.5 or 3 T. Typically, the higher the field strength, the better the images, and although that is not always the case, lower-field-strength units are not able to produce very high-resolution images, even with an optimized technique. Because a certain percentage of patients are too claustrophobic to tolerate the rather small bore of a standard machine, some MR units are designed with a larger bore (known as an "open" magnet), and smaller "extremity" scanners are also available in which only the affected extremity is placed within the machine. A major drawback of this type of machine is that it cannot be used to image more central joints such as the shoulder or hip.

In addition to placing the patient within the large "body" coil that surrounds the bore of the machine, smaller "surface" coils that conform more closely to the size of the body part

M.W. Anderson, MD (✉)
Department of Radiology and Medical Imaging, University of Virginia, Charlottesville, VA, USA
e-mail: Mwa3a@hscmail.mcc.virginia.edu

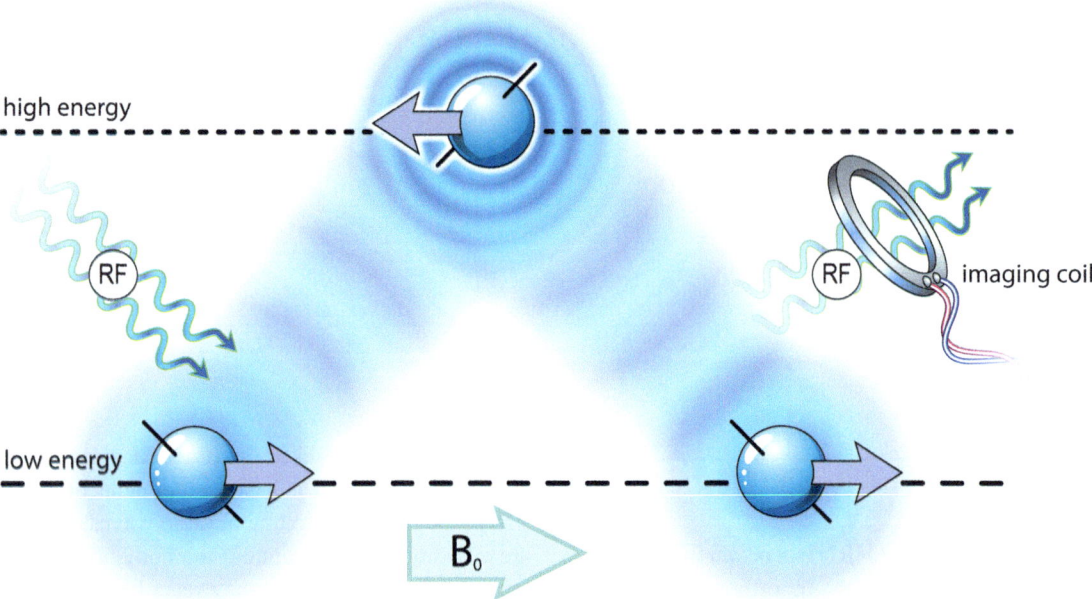

Fig. 1.1 Magnetic resonance. A hydrogen proton absorbs radiofrequency energy and flips into a higher-energy state. As the radiofrequency is turned off, the proton relaxes back to a lower-energy state and releases energy in the form of radio waves which are detected and used to create MR image (B_0 = direction of the main magnetic field)

Fig. 1.2 Surface coil. In preparation for an MRI of the wrist, the patient's hand is placed into the surface coil (*inset*) which is then placed into the bore of the magnet during scanning

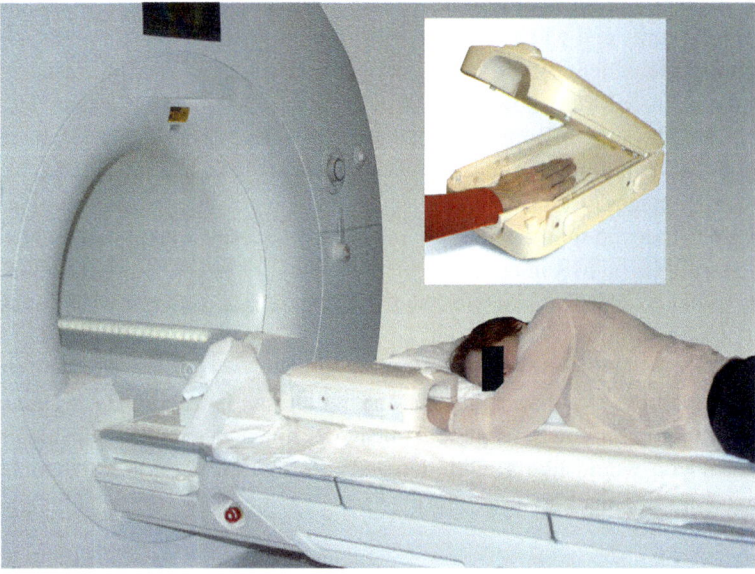

being imaged are used for most MSK MR imaging examinations (Fig. 1.2). These are critical for producing high-resolution images since they can be positioned very close to the tissues of interest and maximize the amount of signal detected.

Because of the nature and configuration of the machine, two patient-related factors should be considered before ordering an MR imaging study. First, because of the large magnetic field involved, patients must be screened for certain implants such as a pacemaker or some types of intracranial aneurysm clips as well as for a history of metal fragments within the eyes. These may be affected by the magnetic field and cause potentially fatal injuries.

Also, because of the relatively small bore of many machines, some patients will be too claustrophobic to complete the examination. Possible solutions include performing the exam with a larger "open-bore" magnet or "extremity" scanner or by administering sedatives either before or during the study.

Why Does the Image Look the Way It Does?

T1 and T2

Protons are influenced by the local molecular environment of the tissue in which they reside. As a result, protons in one type of tissue will behave differently from protons within a different tissue, and these differences provide the basis for the superb soft tissue contrast observed on MR images. The manner in which protons within a given tissue react during an MR scan is described by two characteristics known as "T1" and "T2" that are unique to each type of tissue. By changing the way in which the parameters for a given scan are set up, the images produced may emphasize differences in these values resulting in what are called "T1-weighted" (T1W) or "T2-weighted" (T2W) images, respectively. By comparing the appearances of a tissue on T1W and T2W images, the type of tissue present can often be deduced based on its signal characteristics.

For example, the signal intensity of fluid is quite low on a T1-weighted (T1W) image and very bright on a T2-weighted (T2W) image (Fig. 1.3a, b). This is why each MR examination is composed of several imaging "sequences" that are obtained with different scanning parameters, and a basic understanding of the most common pulse sequences used in musculoskeletal (MSK) imaging is important.

Pulse Sequences

When performing an MR imaging study, several different "sequences" are obtained with each sequence displaying the tissues in a different way. The most common sequences used in MSK imaging are T1, T2, proton density, inversion recovery, and gradient echo. It is not critical to know the details of how each sequence is performed, but it is helpful to know what the normal appearances of various tissues are on each. (See the next section on Normal Musculoskeletal Tissues and Table 1.1.)

Gadolinium Contrast Agents

Gadolinium-based contrast agents are commonly used in MR imaging studies. This agent produces increased signal intensity on T1W images and can be administered intravenously (analogous to iodinated contrast with CT scanning) or as a dilute solution that is directly injected into a joint to perform an MR arthrogram. (The latter is considered an "off-label" use by the Food and Drug administration, but it is a routine procedure in most practices.)

Intravenous

Any tissue that contains increased vascularity will take up intravenous gadolinium and demonstrate bright enhancement on T1W images (Fig. 1.4a). Typical situations in which intravenous gadolinium is used include suspected infection in the soft tissue or bone, evaluation of a soft tissue mass, or in a postoperative tumor case.

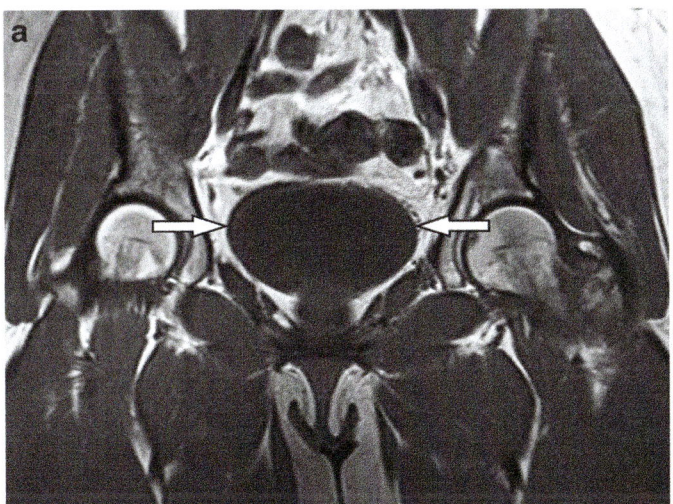
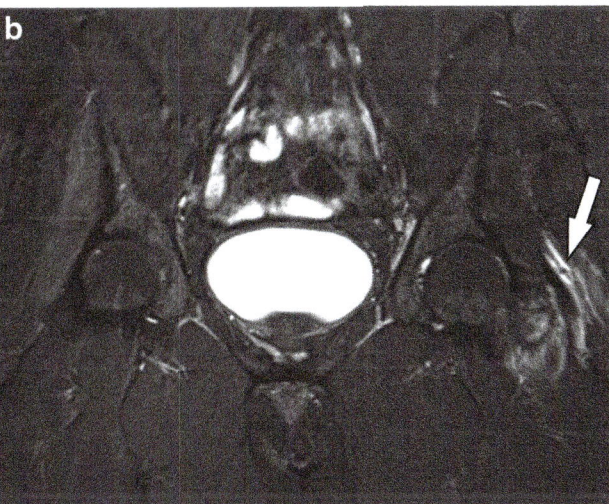
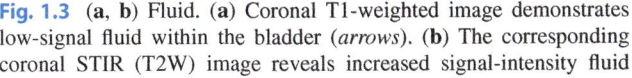

Fig. 1.3 (**a, b**) Fluid. (**a**) Coronal T1-weighted image demonstrates low-signal fluid within the bladder (*arrows*). (**b**) The corresponding coronal STIR (T2W) image reveals increased signal-intensity fluid within the bladder as well as tearing of the left gluteus medius/minimus tendons along the greater trochanter (*arrow*)

Table 1.1 Tissue appearance by MR pulse sequence

	Fat	Fluid	Fibrocartilage	Hyaline cartilage	Tendons, ligaments	Yellow marrow	Red marrow
T1	Bright	Dark	Dark	Intermed	Dark	Bright	Intermed
T2	Bright	Bright	Dark	Intermed-dark	Dark	Bright	Bright
Proton density	Bright	Intermed	Dark	Intermed	Dark	Bright	Intermed-bright
Inversion recovery (STIR) *Also fat-sat T2*	Dark	Bright	Dark	Dark	Dark	Dark	Bright
Gradient echo	Variable	Variable	Dark	Usually bright	Intermed-dark	Variable	Variable

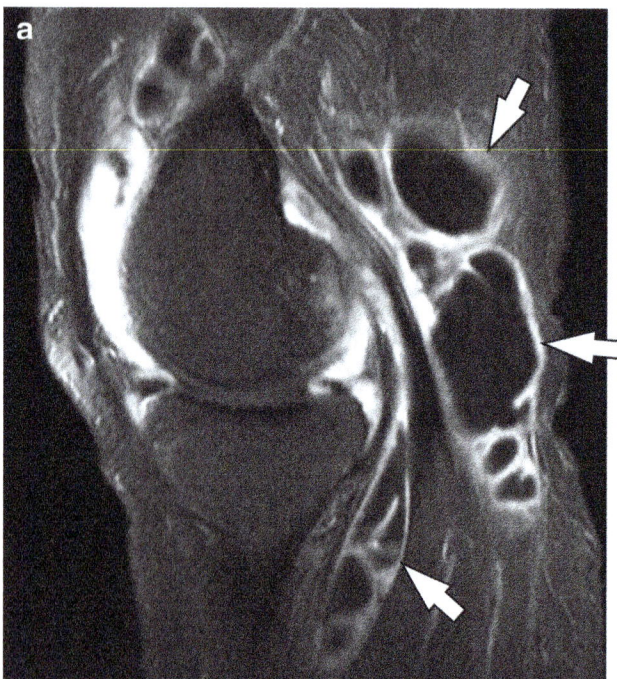 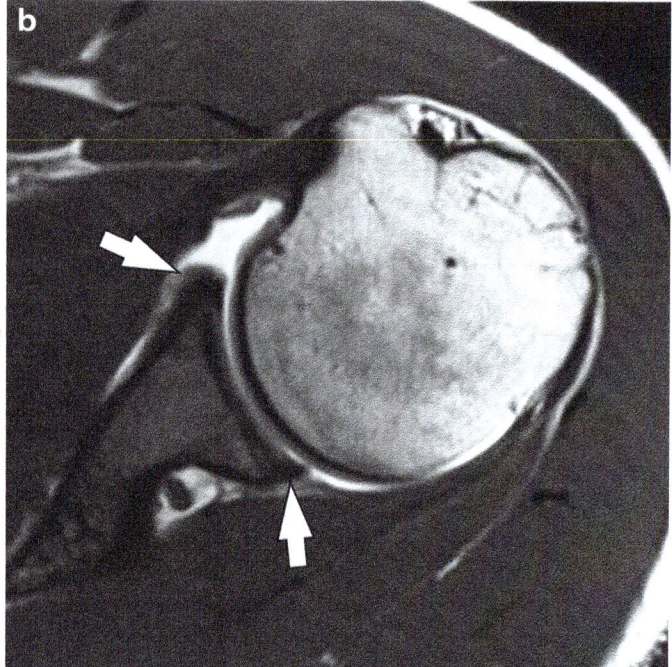

Fig. 1.4 (**a, b**) Gadolinium contrast. (**a**) Sagittal T1-weighted image with fat saturation obtained after the intravenous injection of gadolinium contrast material reveals pronounced synovial thickening and enhancement throughout the joint and a multilocular popliteal (Baker's) cyst (*arrows*). Note the central areas of nonenhancing fluid within the cyst. (**b**) Axial T1-weighted image from an MR arthrogram showing high-signal-intensity gadolinium distending the joint and outlining the glenoid labrum (*arrows*)

Intra-articular (MR Arthrography)

Many intra-articular structures become more conspicuous when a joint is distended with fluid, and while this can be accomplished with simple saline, a dilute gadolinium solution is typically used combined with T1W imaging (Fig. 1.4b). This is most commonly performed in the shoulder and hip but can be used in any joint to better assess articular cartilage or other structures such as a previously repaired meniscus or labrum.

Fat Saturation

Another technique that is commonly used in MSK examinations is the application of "fat saturation" during scanning. This refers to techniques that turn the typically bright signal intensity of fat dark, and a fat-saturated sequence is usually easy to recognize since most of the image will be quite dark overall. This technique can be advantageous for a number of reasons.

Since most types of pathology result in increased fluid content in the affected tissues, these areas will be bright on a T2W image, and by darkening the normally high-signal-intensity fat, the areas of pathology will become much more conspicuous than if fat saturation is not used (Fig. 1.5a, b). Additionally, when gadolinium contrast is administered intravenously, any tissues that have increased vascularity will take up the contrast and brighten on T1W images and once again, if fat saturation is applied, any areas of enhancement will be much easier to identify (Fig. 1.4a).

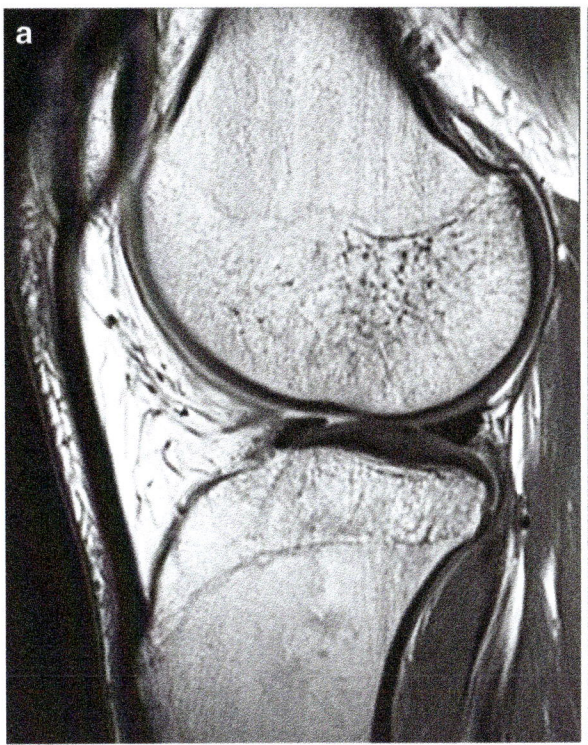
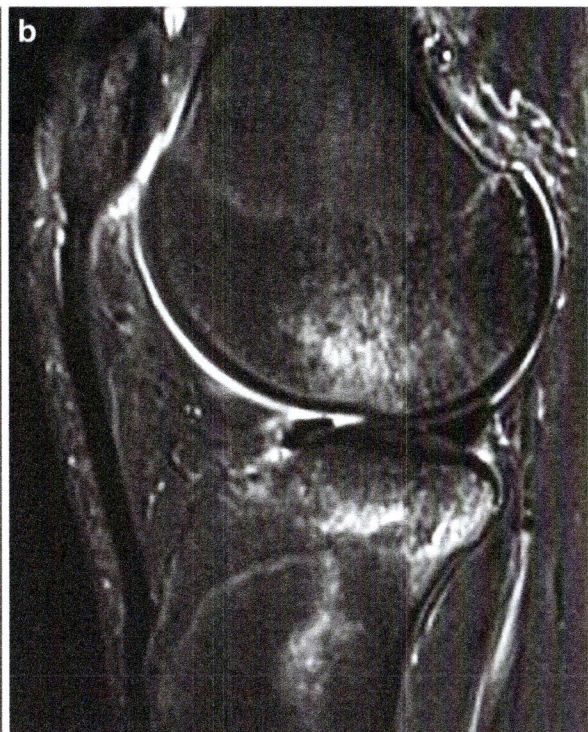

Fig. 1.5 (**a, b**) Bone marrow contusions. (**a**) The marrow within the distal femur and proximal tibia appears normal on this sagittal proton-density-weighted image; however, a corresponding sagittal STIR image (**b**) in which the fat is suppressed reveals prominent high-signal-intensity edema/hemorrhage at the sites of bone marrow injury

What Should Normal Musculoskeletal Tissues Look Like on MRI? (Table 1.1)

Fluid

As mentioned previously, fluid displays a characteristic appearance on MR images. On a T1W sequence, the signal intensity of fluid will be homogeneously low (lower than skeletal muscle), while on a T2W image, it becomes very bright (Fig. 1.3a, b). As such, if you can identify a structure that is known to be fluid filled such as the bladder or thecal sac, you can determine whether you are viewing a T1W or T2W image based on whether the fluid is dark (T1) or bright (T2). Also, since most types of pathology result in increased fluid content within the affected tissues, these will be most easily detected on a fat-saturated T2W sequence since the fluid will be very conspicuous against the dark background of suppressed fat.

Fibrocartilage

Fibrocartilaginous structures such as the menisci in the knee or the glenoid labrum demonstrate low signal intensity on all sequences (Fig. 1.6).

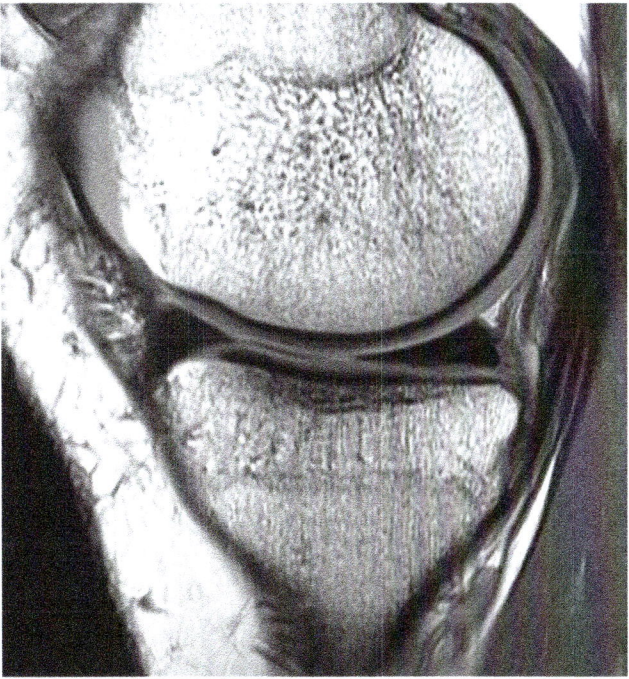

Fig. 1.6 Normal meniscus. Sagittal proton-density-weighted image shows diffusely low signal intensity within the anterior and posterior horns of a normal medial meniscus, a characteristic appearance of fibrocartilage. Note the small areas of intermediate signal intensity within the meniscal substance compatible with mild mucoid degeneration

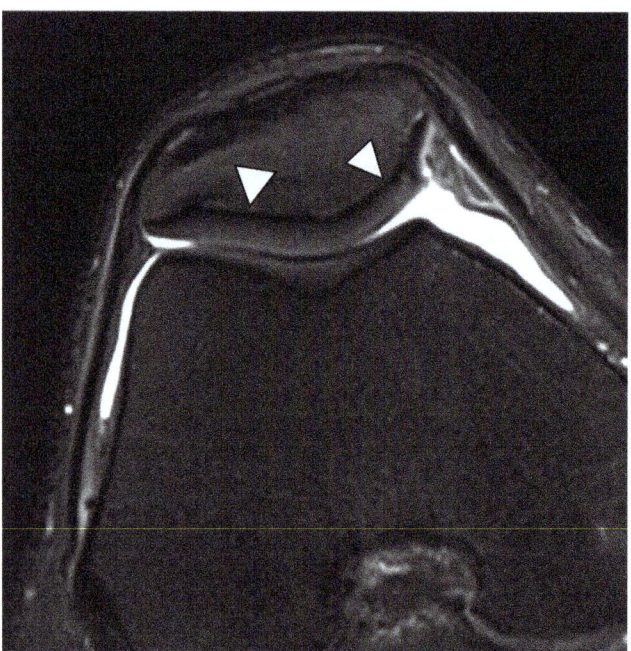

Fig. 1.7 Normal articular cartilage. This axial fat-saturated T2-weighted image through the patellofemoral joint provides good contrast between the high-signal-intensity joint fluid, intermediate-signal-intensity hyaline cartilage, and thin, low-signal-intensity subchondral plate (*arrowheads*)

Hyaline Cartilage

The MR appearance of hyaline articular cartilage is variable and depends upon which imaging sequence is used. The most important thing when evaluating articular cartilage is to use a sequence that provides excellent contrast between cartilage and joint fluid. The common techniques for doing this include proton density or fat-saturated T2W (or STIR) sequences in which the articular cartilage is of lower signal intensity than adjacent joint fluid (Fig. 1.7).

Tendons/Ligaments

In general, tendons and ligaments demonstrate diffusely low signal intensity on all pulse sequences with a few exceptions such as the distal quadriceps tendon and the anterior cruciate ligament which normally display a somewhat striated appearance (Fig. 1.8a, b).

Muscle

Skeletal muscle demonstrates a distinctive appearance on MR images. It is of intermediate to low signal intensity on both T1W and T2W images but is most easily recognized by the bright fatty striations that course through the normal muscle. These are most easily recognized on a T1W image (Fig. 1.9).

Bone/Marrow

Normal Marrow

The long bones and vertebrae contain varying amounts of both yellow (fatty) and red (hematopoietic) marrow. In childhood, red marrow tends to predominate at most sites, but with increasing age, conversion to yellow marrow occurs throughout the skeleton so that in the adult red marrow is typically found only in the axial skeleton and proximal portions of the humeri and femurs. In the older patient, even these sites tend to convert to fatty marrow.

Yellow marrow is recognized on MR imaging by its bright signal intensity on T1W images and its low signal intensity on fat-saturated sequences. Because of its increased cellularity, red marrow appears as a hazy, low-signal-intensity tissue on T1W images that appears relatively bright on fat-saturated T2W images. Unfortunately, most types of marrow pathology such as injury, tumor, or infection will produce similar signal characteristics, so it is important to know how to differentiate these entities.

Findings that suggest the presence of normal red marrow rather than tumor include (1) signal intensity that is equal to or brighter than skeletal muscle on T1W images (because of the presence of fat intermingled with hematopoietic cells within the red marrow) and (2) a metaphyseal distribution that typically, though not always, stops at the level of the old physis (Fig. 1.10a, b).

What Do Common Types of Musculoskeletal Pathology Look Like on MRI?

Fibrocartilage

The normal meniscus of the knee appears as a smoothly marginated low-signal-intensity triangle when cut in cross section on MR images, as do the glenoid and acetabular labra. With advancing age, increasing intrasubstance degeneration will produce intermediate signal intensity within the meniscus or labrum on T1W and T2W images that is not as bright as fluid. A true tear is diagnosed when abnormal signal intensity is seen to extend to one of its articular surfaces (Fig. 1.11).

Hyaline Cartilage

Morphologic abnormalities of articular cartilage will be best demonstrated on pulse sequences that provide good soft tissue contrast between joint fluid, cartilage, and the subchondral bone. Cartilage fibrillation, fissures, and focal defects will be outlined by high-signal-intensity fluid (Fig. 1.12). Linear fluid-like high signal intensity at the bone/cartilage

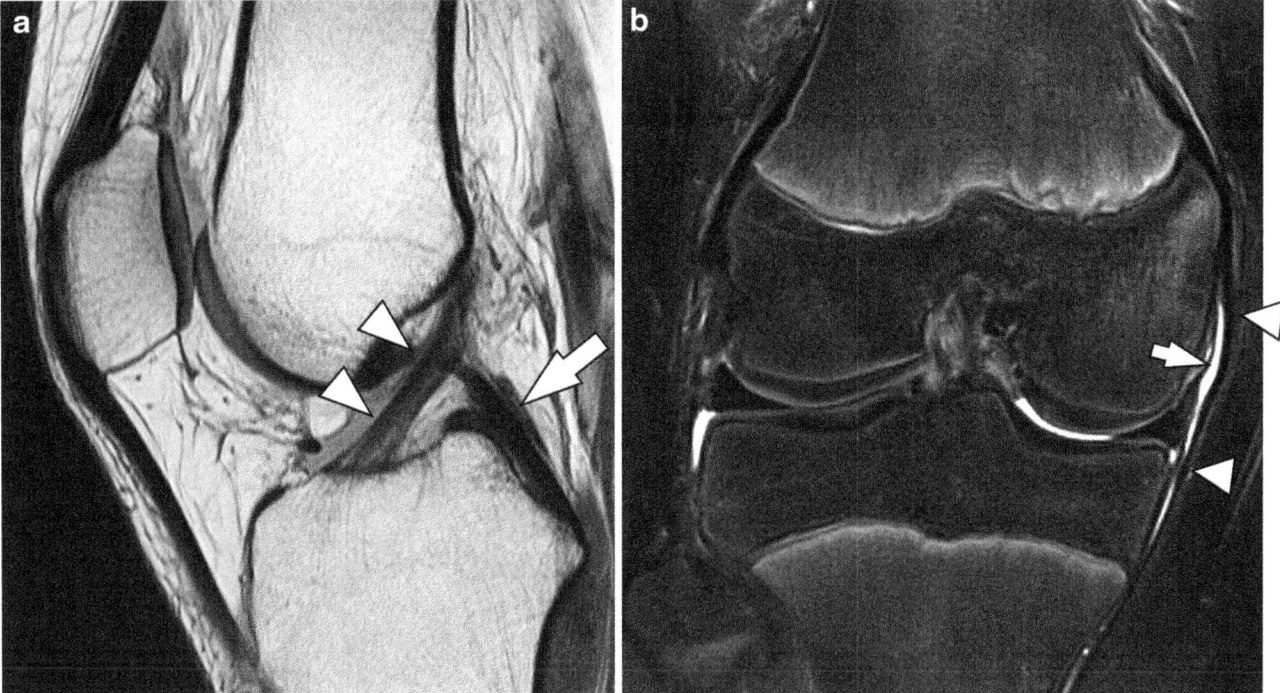

Fig. 1.8 (**a, b**) Normal tendon/ligament. (**a**) Sagittal proton-density-weighted image demonstrates normal low signal intensity within the quadriceps and patellar tendons. Note also the mildly striated appearance of the anterior cruciate ligament (*arrowheads*) as compared with the more homogeneously dark posterior cruciate ligament (*arrow*), a normal finding. (**b**) Coronal fat-saturated T2-weighted image shows the low-signal-intensity medial collateral ligament (*arrowheads*) and high-signal-intensity fluid in the underlying MCL bursa (*arrow*)

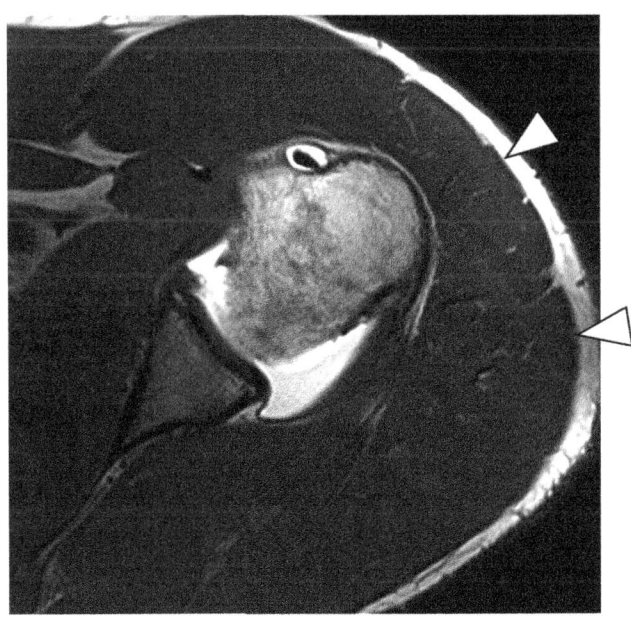

Fig. 1.9 Normal muscle. Axial T1-weighted image displays the normal "marbled" appearance of the muscles of the shoulder that results from their characteristic high-signal-intensity fatty striations. This is most pronounced within the posterolateral deltoid muscle (*arrowheads*)

interface indicates chondral delamination which may not be evident at arthroscopy (Fig. 1.13a, b). Newer MR imaging techniques that assess the composition of hyaline cartilage will be mentioned at the end of the chapter.

Ligaments and Tendons

When evaluating a ligament or tendon, the "magic-angle" artifact may mimic ligament or tendon pathology. This artifact occurs within a highly ordered collagen-based structure such as a ligament or tendon when it is oriented approximately 55° to the main magnetic field. With certain MR pulse sequences (T1, proton density, gradient echo), intermediate signal intensity will be seen within the tendon or ligament and may mimic pathology. This can be recognized as artifactual by looking at the structure on a corresponding T2W sequence, since the spurious signal intensity disappears on these images, and the structure demonstrates its normally low signal intensity (Fig. 1.14a, b).

True ligamentous injury ranges from a sprain or stretching of the ligament to a partial or complete tear. A sprain usually results in soft tissue edema, recognized by its increased signal

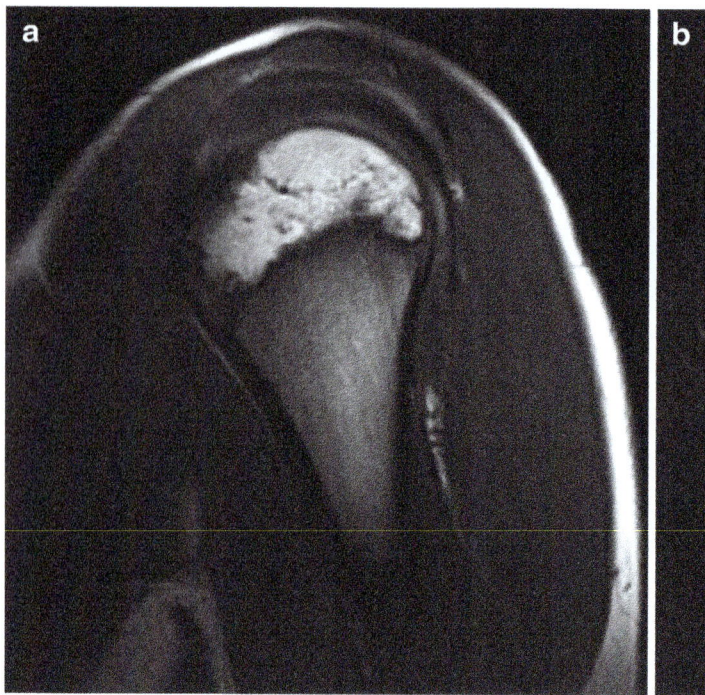
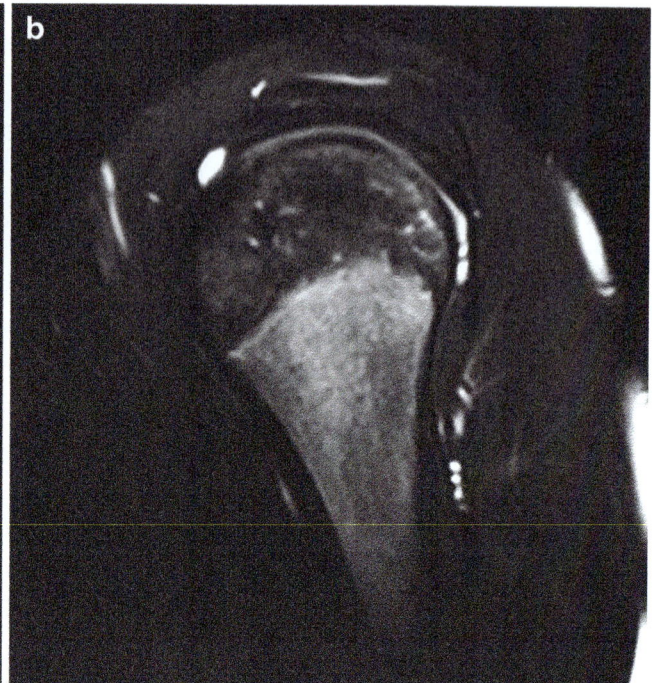

Fig. 1.10 (**a**, **b**) Normal marrow. Sagittal T1-weighted (**a**) and fat-saturated T2-weighted (**b**) images display normal hematopoietic (*red*) marrow within the proximal humeral shaft and normal fatty (*yellow*) marrow within the epiphysis. Note that the fatty marrow demonstrates increased signal intensity on the T1-weighted image and is suppressed (*dark*) in **b**, paralleling subcutaneous fat, while the *red marrow* demonstrates increased signal intensity on that image due to its higher fluid content

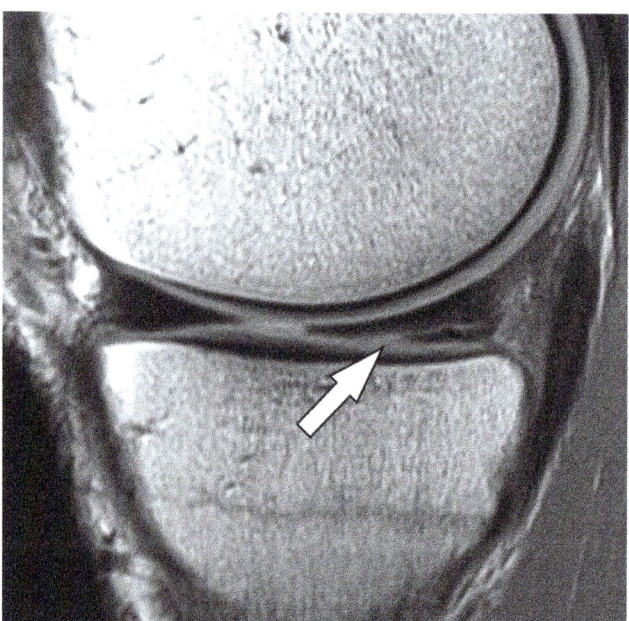

Fig. 1.11 Meniscal tear. This saggital proton density image reveals a horizontal tear of the posterior horn of the medial meniscus extending to its inferior articular surface (*arrow*)

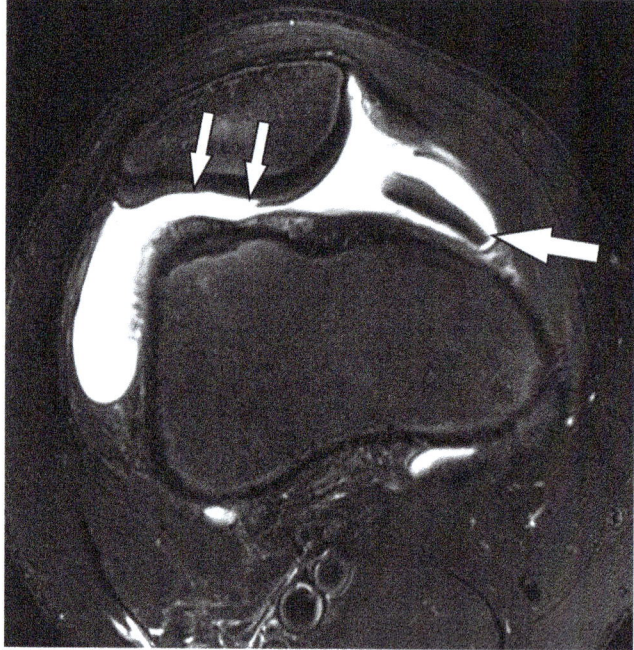

Fig. 1.12 Cartilage injury. Axial fat-saturated T2-weighted image shows mild lateral subluxation of the patella, a partial thickness cartilage defect along its lateral facet (*small arrows*), and the displaced chondral fragment surrounded by high-signal-intensity joint fluid in the lateral patellofemoral recess (*large arrow*)

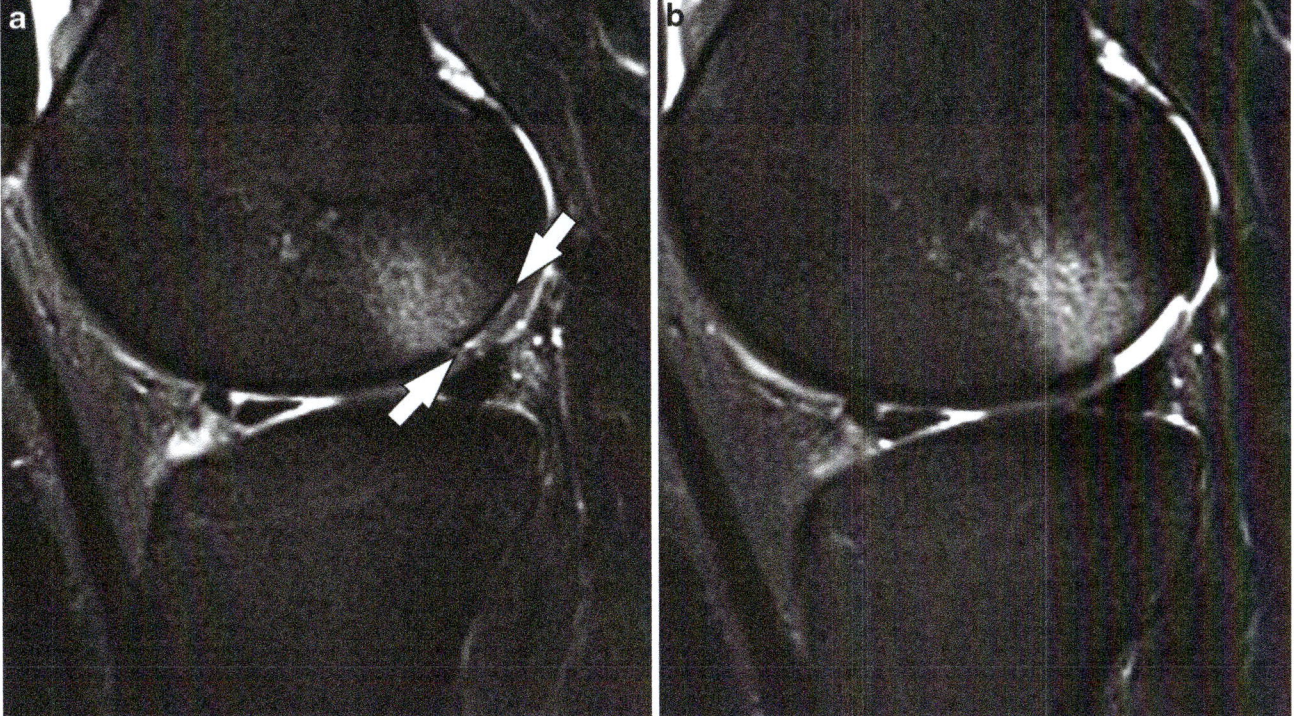

Fig. 1.13 (**a, b**) Cartilage injury. (**a**) Sagittal STIR image reveals a focal subchondral bone contusion as well as partial delamination of the overlying cartilage (*arrows*) in this college basketball player who sustained a knee injury. (**b**) Follow-up sagittal STIR image obtained 2 weeks later reveals interval loss of the articular cartilage at the site of the delamination

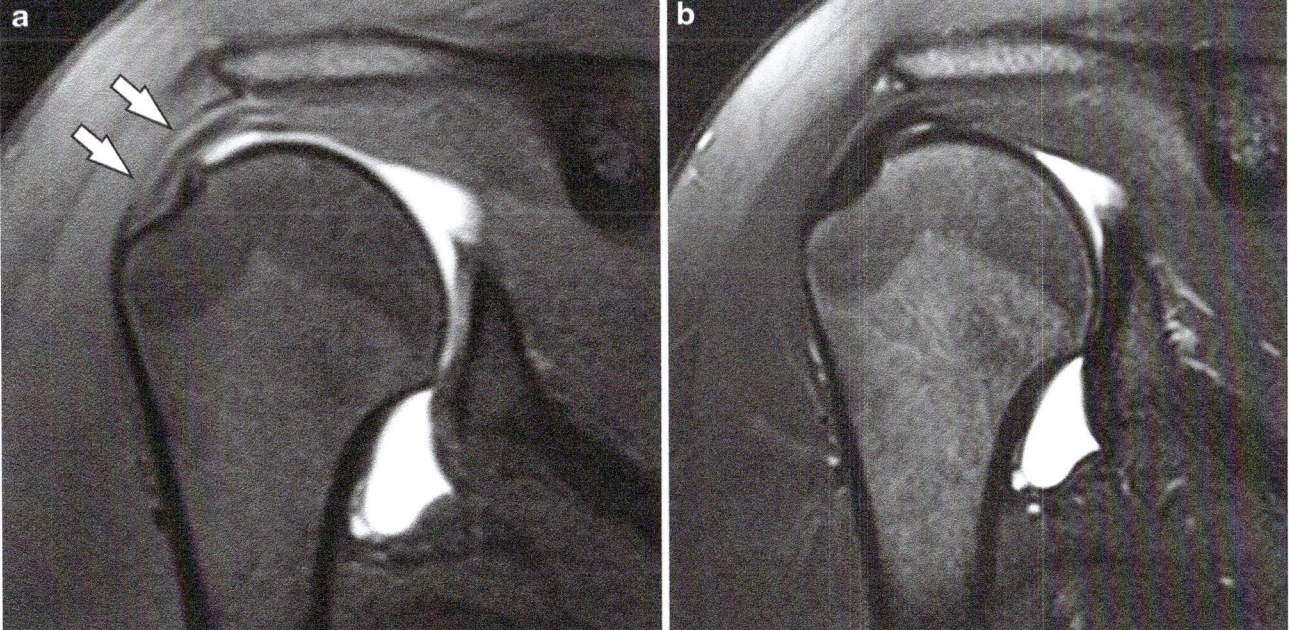

Fig. 1.14 (**a, b**) Magic-angle artifact. (**a**) Oblique-coronal fat-saturated T1-weighted image from an MR arthrogram reveals intermediate signal intensity within the distal infraspinatus tendon (*arrows*). (**b**) This artifactual signal intensity disappears, and the tendon demonstrates its normal low signal intensity on a corresponding fat-saturated T2-weighted image

Fig. 1.15 (**a**, **b**) Ligament injury. (**a**) Sagittal proton-density-weighted image demonstrates complete rupture of the anterior cruciate ligament with no intact fibers identified. (**b**) A coronal fat-saturated T2-weighted image in a different patient reveals a complete tear of the proximal medial collateral ligament (*arrow*)

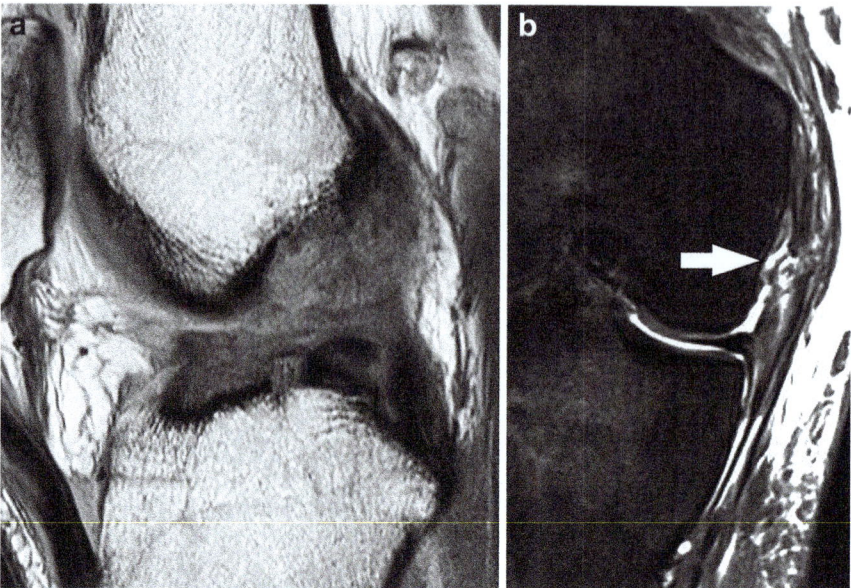

intensity on T2W images, adjacent to an otherwise normal ligament. A partial tear results in disruption of some of its fibers, whereas a complete tear is diagnosed when all fibers are disrupted (Fig. 1.15a, b). Again these types of pathology will be best demonstrated on T2W images due to the increased fluid content of the injured tissues.

Mucoid degeneration within a tendon is recognized as intermediate intrasubstance signal intensity on all sequences and is termed "tendinosis" rather than "tendinitis" since it does not involve an inflammatory infiltrate. A partial tendon tear is diagnosed when some of its fibers are shown to be disrupted, typically on T2W images (Fig. 1.16a, b). A complete tendon tear is usually easily diagnosed with MR imaging.

Muscle

Injury

Acute injury to skeletal muscle will result in high-signal-intensity fluid and/or hemorrhage within the affected tissues. A grade 1 injury (strain) demonstrates feathery, edema-like signal intensity between otherwise intact muscle fibers. A grade 2 injury (partial tear) shows interstitial fluid as well as a variable degree of muscle fiber disruption, while a grade 3 injury (complete tear) displays complete fiber disruption at the site of the tear (Fig. 1.17a, b).

Atrophy

A variety of etiologies such as prior trauma, denervation, chronic ischemia, or diabetes may result in muscle atrophy. This is easily recognized on MR imaging studies by the high-signal-intensity fat replacing the normally dark skeletal muscle fibers on T1W images (Fig. 1.18).

Bone Injury

MR imaging is an extremely powerful tool for evaluating osseous trauma. Injuries to bone lie along a spectrum that ranges from a contusion (medullary hemorrhage and trabecular fractures) to a complete fracture. Radiographs are a good initial screening tool in the case of a suspected fracture but are quite insensitive for demonstrating most types of bone injuries. Because MR imaging is able to directly display posttraumatic abnormalities within trabecular bone and the medullary cavity, it is exquisitely sensitive for detecting radiographically occult injuries.

A bone contusion will appear as abnormal ill-defined signal intensity within the medullary portion of the bone on MR images. These are most conspicuous on fat-saturated T2W or STIR images since the associated edema and hemorrhage will appear very bright against a dark background of low-signal-intensity fat (Fig. 1.19a). T1W images are less sensitive but may show an area of ill-defined low signal intensity against the bright marrow fat. The detection of a periarticular contusion may explain the patient's symptoms and avoid an unnecessary arthroscopy if there is no evidence of internal derangement otherwise.

A fracture is diagnosed when a linear focus of abnormal signal is seen within the marrow edema on either T1W or fat-saturated T2W images (Fig. 1.19b). Unless the fracture extends to involve the cortex, it is often undetectable with radiographs (and even CT) but is readily apparent on MR images. As a result, MR imaging is extremely useful for evaluating a patient in which there is a strong suspicion of fracture but negative radiographs, and this can be especially helpful when evaluating an elderly patient who presents emergently with hip pain, and a decision must be made to either admit them for stabilization or discharge them home.

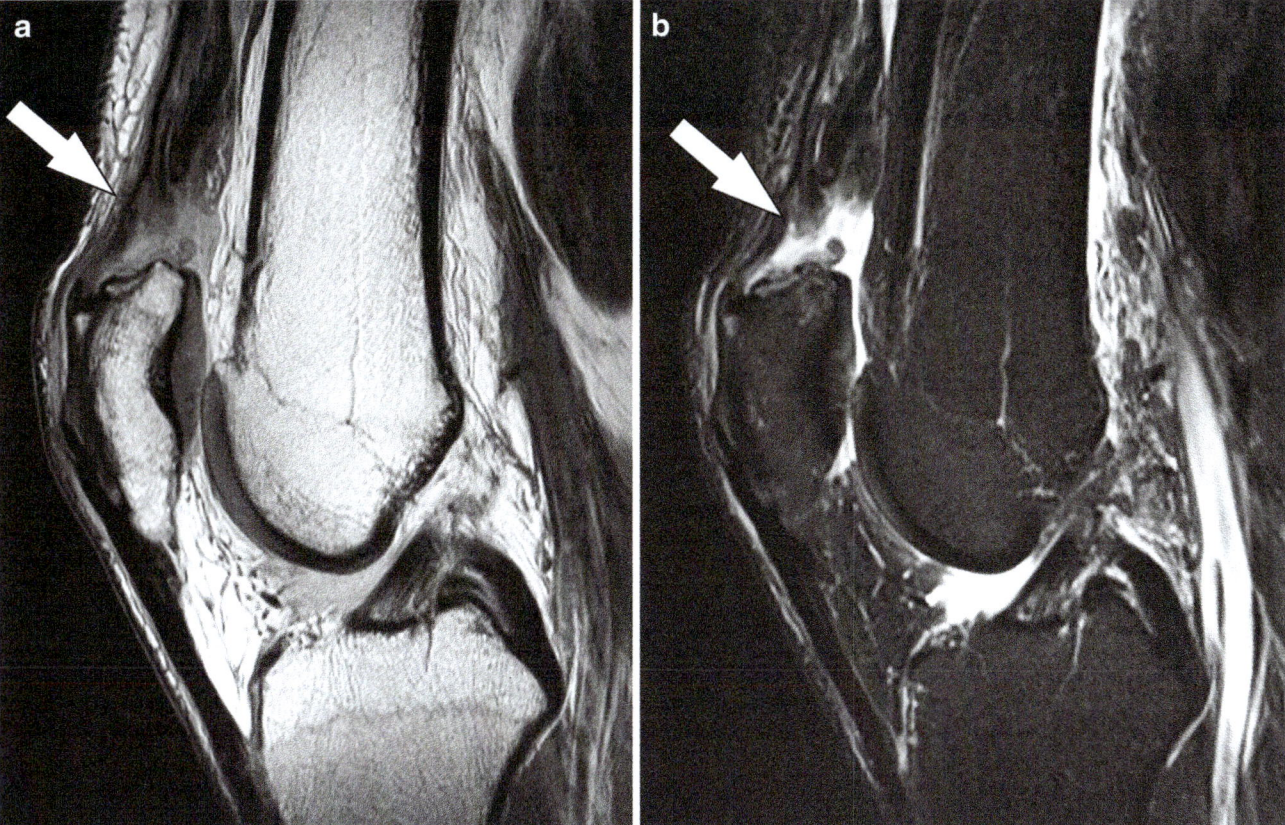

Fig. 1.16 (**a, b**) Tendon injury. Sagittal proton density (**a**) and sagittal STIR (**b**) images demonstrate a high-grade, near-complete tear of the distal quadriceps tendon (*arrows*)

Infection

Infectious conditions of the musculoskeletal system may involve the soft tissues or bone. It can be very difficult to determine the extent of involvement on a clinical exam, and while other imaging modalities may be helpful in this scenario, MR imaging often plays an important role in the workup of these patients.

Soft tissue infections include cellulitis, fasciitis, myositis, and abscess. Cellulitis demonstrates diffuse edema-like signal, best seen on fat-saturated T2W images, infiltrating the subcutaneous fat but not deeper tissues (Fig. 1.20a, b). This appearance is nonspecific and could be related to venous or lymphatic obstruction or simple subcutaneous edema as seen in low-protein states and other conditions. Infectious fasciitis results in fluid tracking along deep fascial planes, often with edema-like signal intensity in the adjacent muscles, and pyomyositis produces focal intramuscular abscesses that are identified by their typical appearance of low signal on T1W images, high signal on T2W images, and nonenhancing fluid surrounded by a bright, peripherally enhancing wall on post-gadolinium fat-saturated T1W images (Fig. 1.21a–c).

The diagnosis of osteomyelitis can be challenging on MR images since other entities such as traumatic contusion, chronic stress reaction, or the painful bone marrow edema syndrome can produce similar MR imaging abnormalities within the marrow. The appearance of the marrow on T1W images is most helpful for differentiating these conditions since confluent low signal intensity (as dark as the adjacent muscle) is typically seen in osteomyelitis, whereas other entities often produce only a hazy, feathery type of signal abnormality. Other findings suggesting osteomyelitis include cortical destruction (loss of the dark cortical margin on T1W and T2W images), an adjacent abscess or a cutaneous sinus tract extending to the abnormal bone, or direct continuity of the bone with a skin ulcer (Fig. 1.22a–c).

Tumor

Bone

MR imaging is extremely sensitive for detecting primary and secondary tumors of the bone given its ability to directly display the neoplastic tissue within the bone marrow.

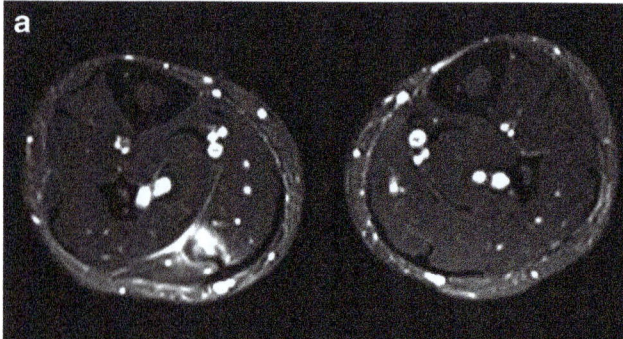

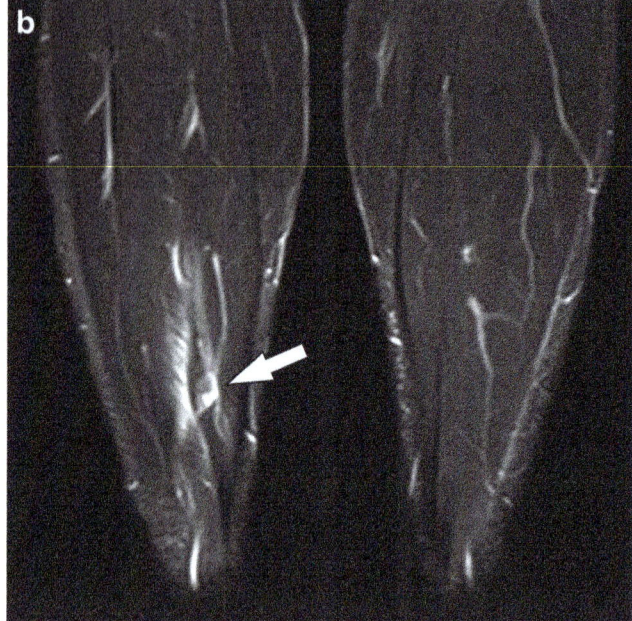

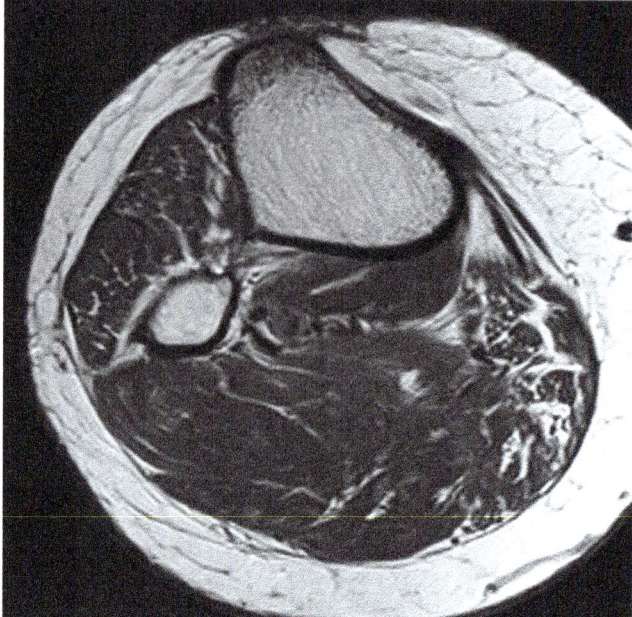

Fig. 1.18 Muscle atrophy. Axial T1-weighted image demonstrates increased fat content in a portion of the medial head of the gastrocnemius muscle indicating segmental fatty atrophy

Fig. 1.17 (**a**, **b**) Muscle injury. Axial (**a**) and coronal (**b**) STIR images of the lower legs reveal a partial tear of the right soleus muscle at its musculotendinous junction with high-signal-intensity edema/hemorrhage and within the muscle as well as partial disruption of the tendon (*arrow*)

This is unlike radiographs and CT and radionuclide bone scans that rely on secondary changes within the bone for tumor detection. Most tumors demonstrate low signal intensity on T1W images and some degree of increased signal on T2W images, with the exception of blastic lesions which will be dark on all sequences due to their sclerotic nature. Despite its exceptional sensitivity, the MR appearance of most primary bone tumors is relatively nonspecific, and conventional radiographs typically provide the most reliable information regarding tumor type and degree of aggressiveness. The primary role for MR imaging in these cases is to assess the local stage of the tumor given its exquisite depiction of the intraosseous and extraosseous extent of the lesion (Fig. 1.23a–c).

Soft Tissue

In the case of soft tissue masses, MR imaging provides a specific diagnosis in a large percentage of cases. A benign lipoma is easily recognized because of its homogeneous fat signal

intensity on all pulse sequences (Fig. 1.24a–c). Similarly, simple cysts, fibrous lesions, vascular malformations, hematomas, and pigmented villonodular synovitis demonstrate specific MR imaging findings that allow for a confident diagnosis.

When Is MRI Most Useful and When Should a Different Modality Be Chosen?

From the previous discussion, it is clear that MR imaging is a powerful tool for evaluating many types of orthopedic pathology. Even so, conventional radiographs should be initially obtained for most indications since they provide a relatively rapid and cost-effective screening tool. MR imaging is often the next modality of choice, but may not be possible due to the presence of a pacemaker or other contraindication. Additionally, it may not be the study of choice in certain clinical scenarios. Table 1.2 provides suggested imaging algorithms for different types of orthopedic pathology.

What Is on the Horizon for MR Imaging?

3D Imaging

Several new techniques allow for acquiring a volume of MR imaging data at one time, rather than by acquiring a series of single slices. The data can then be used to create extremely thin slices such that the resulting voxels are isometric (measure the same in all three dimensions), thereby making it

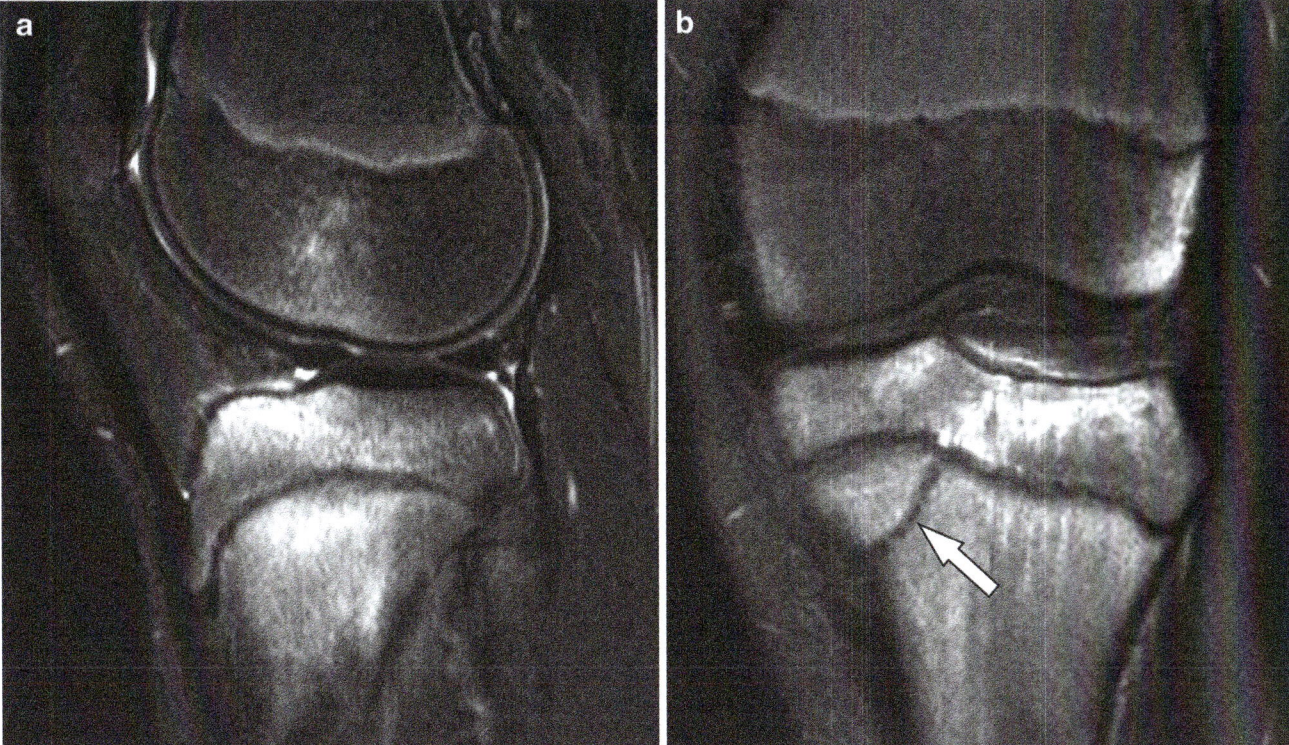

Fig. 1.19 (**a, b**) Bone injury. (**a**) Sagittal STIR image of the knee in a 13-year-old male who sustained a hyperextension injury demonstrates extensive, ill-defined high signal intensity within the proximal tibia and femoral condyle consistent with areas of marrow contusion. (**b**) Coronal fat-saturated T2-weighted image shows an associated metaphyseal fracture (*arrow*)

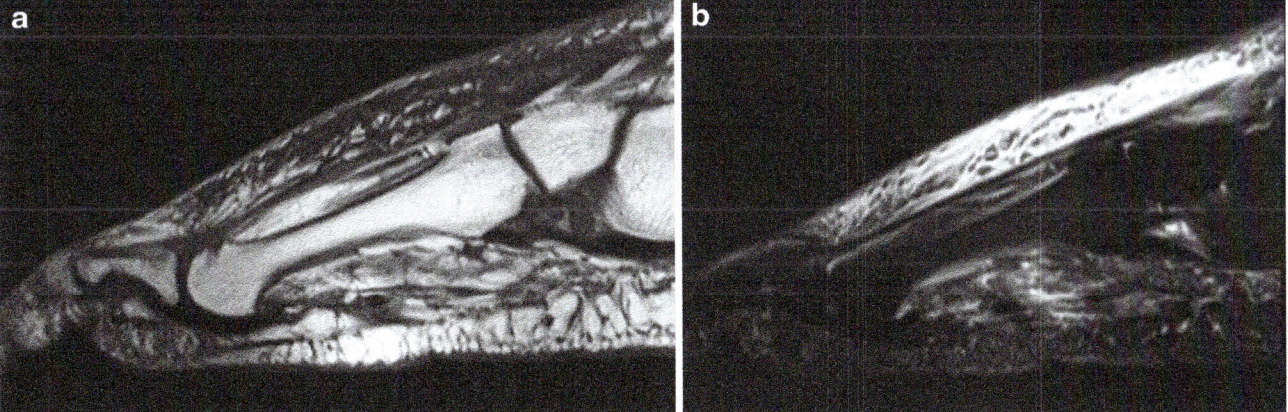

Fig. 1.20 (**a, b**) Cellulitis. Sagittal T1 (**a**) and sagittal (**b**) STIR images reveal extensive edema infiltrating the dorsal subcutaneous fat in this patient with clinically apparent cellulitis

possible to create reconstructed images of identical resolution in virtually any plane from one dataset. This will result in tremendous time savings given the need to obtain only one 3D acquisition rather than multiple sequences and should allow for improved diagnostic capabilities. These techniques should become more common in routine clinical practice in the near future.

Cartilage Imaging

In addition to evaluating morphologic abnormalities of the articular cartilage, several new MR imaging techniques (T2-mapping, dGEMRIC, T1-rho, diffusion-weighted imaging) are designed to look at its components such as glycosaminoglycans, water content, and collagen network.

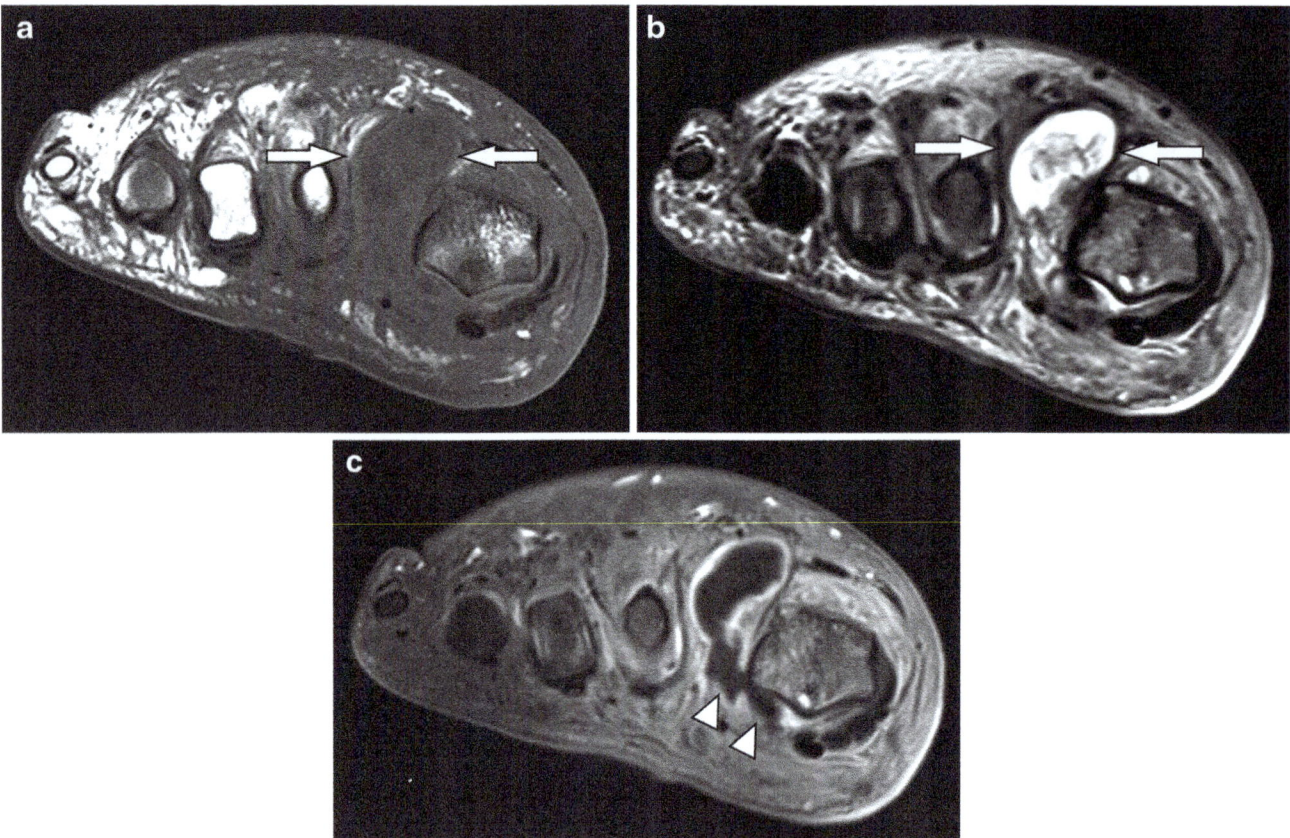

Fig. 1.21 (**a–c**) Abscess. Short-axis T1 (**a**) and STIR (**b**) images demonstrate extensive soft tissue edema within the forefoot as well as a focal abscess between the first and second metatarsals (*arrows*). (**c**) Short-axis fat-saturated T1-weighted image after the intravenous administration of gadolinium contrast material. Note how the extension of the abscess to the first metatarsal phalangeal joint is more conspicuous on this post-contrast image (*arrowheads*)

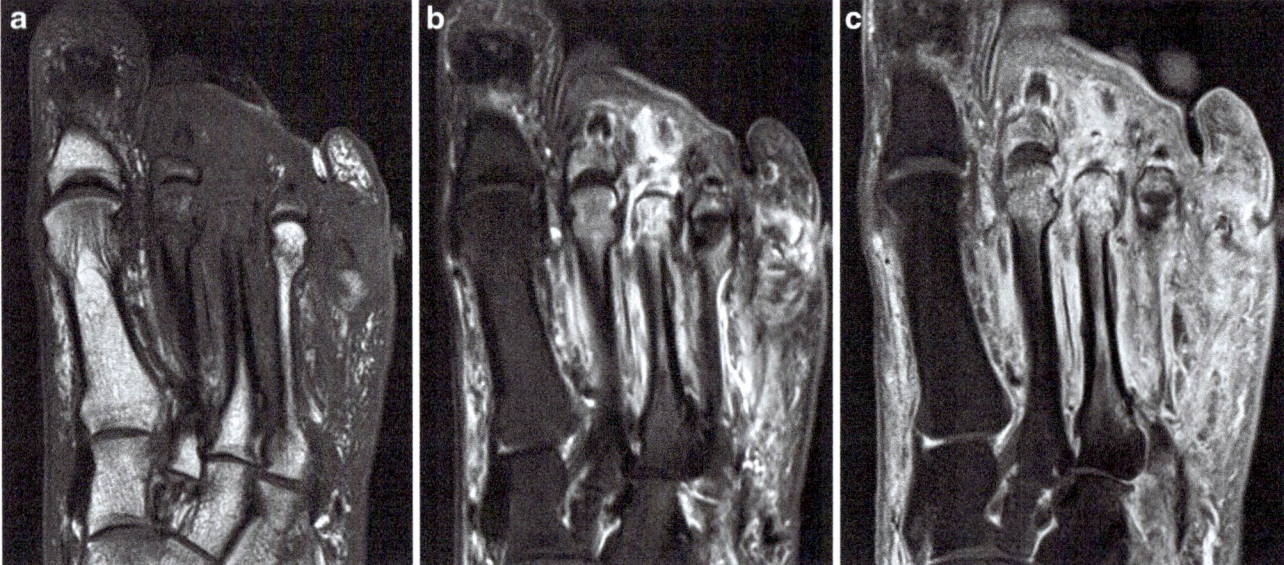

Fig. 1.22 (**a–c**) Osteomyelitis. Long-axis T1-weighted (**a**), fat-saturated T2-weighted (**b**), and post-gadolinium fat-saturated T1-weighted (**c**) images reveal extensive, confluent abnormal signal intensity and enhancement in the distal second and third metatarsals consistent with osteomyelitis

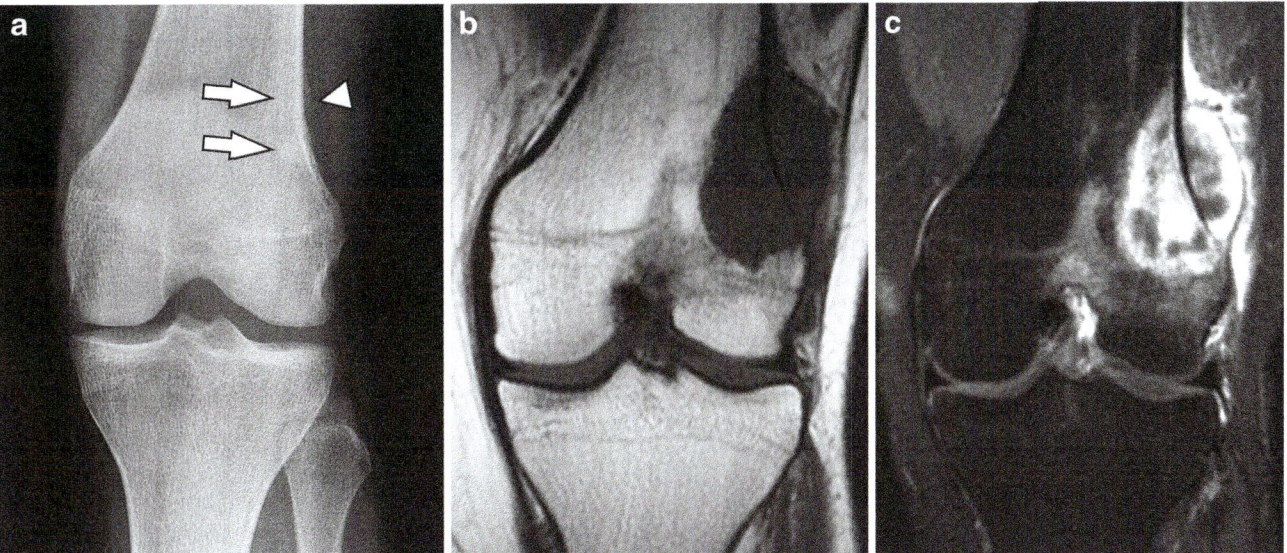

Fig. 1.23 (**a–c**) Bone tumor. (**a**) Frontal view of the knee demonstrates faint endosteal sclerosis (*arrows*) and ill-defined periosteal reaction (*arrowhead*) along the lateral metaphysis of the distal femur. Coronal T1 (**b**) and STIR (**c**) images reveal a large osseous neoplasm with a prominent extraosseous component, shown to be an osteosarcoma on biopsy

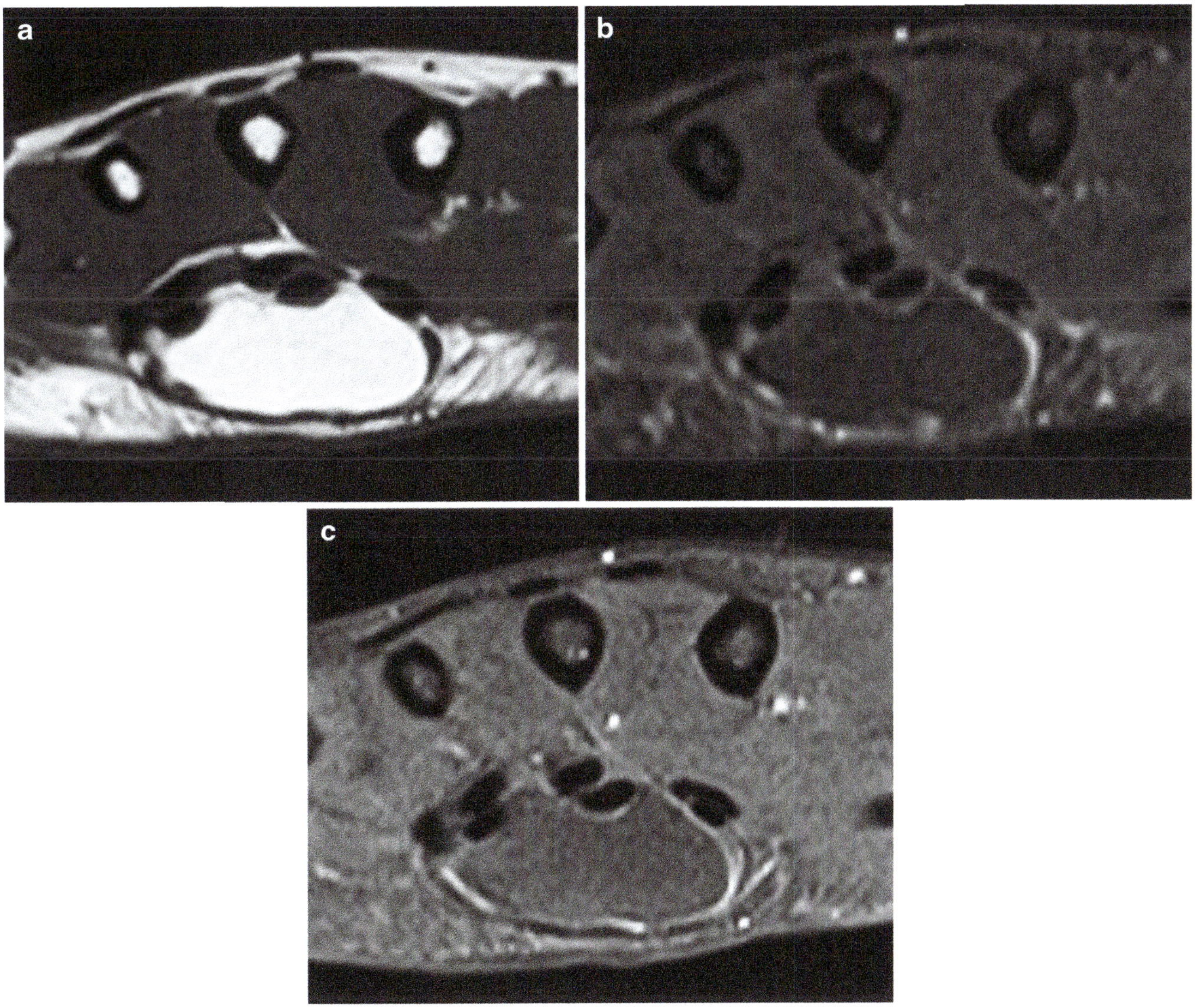

Fig. 1.24 (**a–c**) Soft tissue tumor. Axial T1 (**a**), STIR (**b**), and post-gadolinium fat-saturated T1-weighted (**c**) images of the hand depict a smoothly marginated mass demonstrating homogeneous fatty signal intensity superficial to the flexor tendons at the level of the mid-palm, compatible with a benign lipoma

Table 1.2 Imaging algorithms

Indication		Primary modality	Secondary modality	Other options
Acute injury	Bone	Radiography	MRI	CT
				Bone scan
	Soft tissue	Radiography	MRI	Ultrasound
Stress injury	Bone	Radiography	MRI	Bone scan
Cartilage		MRI	MR arthrography	CT arthrography
Infection	Bone	Radiography	MRI	Bone scan
	Soft tissue	MRI	Ultrasound	Radiography (if gas-forming infection suspected)
Tumor	Bone	Radiography	MRI local staging	CT—distant spread or site of primary
	Soft tissue	Radiography	MRI	Ultrasound

Currently, these are too cumbersome to be used in routine clinical practice, and further clinical studies will be needed before they are more widely used.

References

1. Helms CA, Major NM, Anderson MW, Kaplan PA, Dussault R. Musculoskeletal MRI. 2nd ed. Philadelphia, PA: Saunders; 2009. p. 1–19. Chapter 1, Basic principles of musculoskeletal MRI.

2. Westbrook C. MRI in practice. 4th ed. West Sussex: Wiley; 2011.

3. Jacobs MA, Ibrahim TS, Ouwerkerk R. MR imaging: brief overview and emerging applications. Radiographics. 2007;27: 1213–29.

4. Bitar R, Leung G, Perng R, et al. MR pulse sequences: what every radiologist wants to know but is afraid to ask. Radiographics. 2006;26:513–37.

5. Crema MD, Roemer FW, Marra MD, et al. Articular cartilage in the knee: current MR imaging techniques and applications in clinical practice and research. Radiographics. 2011;31:37–62.

Part I

The Knee

Section Editor: Mark D. Miller

Diagnostic Knee Arthroscopy and Arthroscopic Anatomy

2

M. Tyrrell Burrus and Mark D. Miller

Overview and Brief History

Since 1918, when Kenji Takagi used a cystoscope to evaluate tuberculous knees, there have been significant improvements in knee arthroscopic equipment and techniques [1]. Digital high-definition cameras, the fiber-optic light source, smaller but more durable arthroscopic instrumentation, advances in anesthesia medicine, and our understanding of a sterile operative field have made knee arthroscopy into a powerful tool for orthopedic surgeons. Although it was initially met with skepticism, knee arthroscopy has become an extremely common orthopedic procedure in the United States. Of the almost one million performed in 2006, 99 % of those were carried out in the outpatient setting [2]. These numbers represent a 49 % increase in case volume from 1996 to 2006. This boom in the number of arthroscopic procedures appears to be justified as it is now the gold standard for treating many types of intra-articular knee pathology. Compared to open techniques, knee arthroscopy provides many real advantages such as smaller incisions, no violation of the extensor mechanism, decreased recovery time, decreased risk of neurovascular injuries and infections, decreased operative time, and decreased blood loss.

When considering performing an arthroscopic procedure, the surgeon must perform a thorough history and physical, review the preoperative imaging, and develop a surgical plan. This plan does not only include the actual procedure itself, but it should include the appropriate anesthesia option, operating room setup, patient positioning, and portal placement. This chapter will discuss all of these topics with the goal of providing orthopedic surgeons with a useful tool for safely treating knee musculoskeletal disorders.

Anesthesia Options

As with most orthopedic surgical procedures, a variety or combination of anesthetic modalities can be utilized. Some form of general anesthesia, often a laryngeal mask airway (LMA), is used to provide patient relaxation as manipulation of the limb is always necessary. For more lengthy and complicated arthroscopic procedures such as anterior cruciate ligament (ACL) or medial patellofemoral ligament (MPFL) reconstructions, regional anesthesia is provided by the anesthesia block team prior to the procedure. Most regional blocks must cover both the sciatic and femoral nerve distributions to be successful [3]. Depending on surgeon preference, local anesthesia is injected around the portal locations, either prior to incision or at the completion of the procedure [4]. While not commonly performed in the United States, low-dose spinal anesthesia is an option even for ambulatory surgery [5].

Setup and Positioning

Prior to the patient entering the room, the surgeon must communicate with the operating room and anesthesia staff regarding the most logical and efficient room setup. A room of adequate size must be available to accommodate the additional arthroscopic equipment, and the anesthesia team and scrub nurse must have sufficient room at either ends of the bed. Traditionally, the arthroscopic stack and equipment is positioned on the contralateral side of the bed from where the surgeon will stand and will contain the monitor, fluid

M.T. Burrus, MD (✉)
Department of Orthopedic Surgery, University of Virginia Health System, Charlottesville, VA, USA
e-mail: Mtb3u@hscmail.mcc.virginia.edu

M.D. Miller, MD
Department of Orthopedic Surgery, University of Virginia Health System, Charlottesville, VA, USA

Department of Orthopedic Surgery, Head Team Physician, James Madison University, Charlottesville, VA, USA
e-mail: Mdm3p@hccmail.mcc.virginia.edu

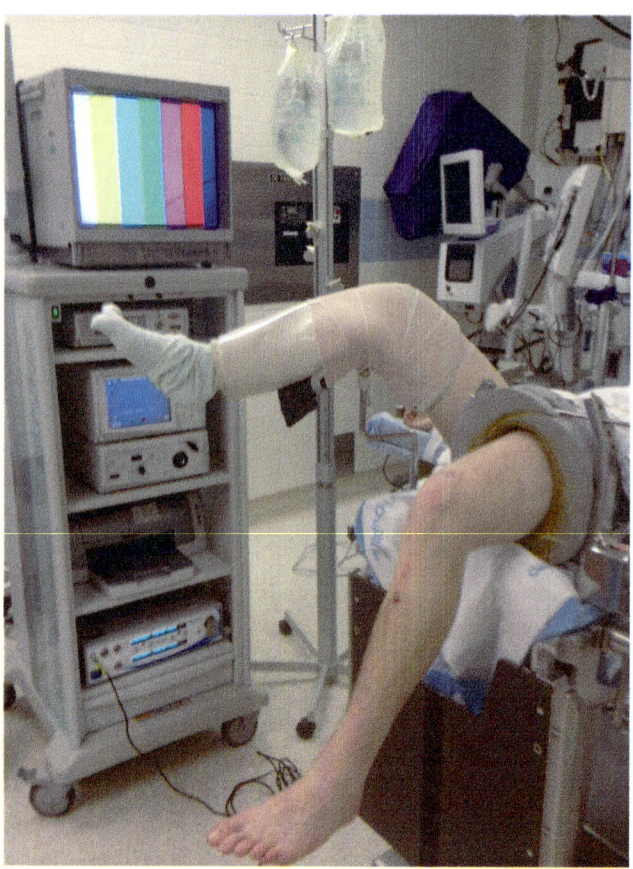

Fig. 2.1 Patient positioning using a well leg holder with the contralateral hip abducted and flexed and placed in a well-padded leg holder. The end of the table has been completely flexed out of the operative field. Also notice the placement of the arthroscopic tower and accessories on the contralateral side of the operative extremity

counterforce to improve visualization of knee compartments. An adjustable side post is commonly used and should be placed at a level that allows the leg to be abducted with sufficient room for the surgeon to stand inside the medial aspect of the leg. Conversely, a well leg holder can be used with the distal aspect of the table dropped and the contralateral hip abducted, flexed, and placed in a well-padded leg holder (Fig. 2.1). More involved procedures might require additional table attachments but must be placed with care to not block access to the knee during instrument passage. Most surgeons use a non-sterile tourniquet inflated to 250 mm of mercury which must be placed high enough on the operative thigh for adequate exposure of the knee.

Pertinent Knee Anatomy and Portal Location

Prior to choosing the appropriate portal location, the surgeon should draw out the pertinent knee anatomy using a sterile marking pen. These structures should be outlined with the knee in 60°–90° of flexion as this is how the knee will look when the incisions are made, and flexion tightens the overlying soft tissues and makes the underlying structures more prominent and easier to palpate. Knowledge of local neurovascular structures is imperative, especially for the more posterior portals. In general, the patella, patellar tendon, medial and lateral tibial joint lines, and medial and lateral femoral condyles are outlined with marker.

Primary Portals

The two primary portals, anterolateral and anteromedial, are the workhorse portals of knee arthroscopy (Fig. 2.2a–c). They do not place any significant neurovascular structures at risk, are easy to identify, and facilitate a wide variety of procedures: diagnostic arthroscopy, medial and lateral meniscectomies, shaving chondroplasty, most microfracture techniques, removal of loose bodies, and all-inside meniscal repair as well as many others. Most surgeons create 1 cm longitudinal incisions which allow for more superior-inferior mobility of instruments versus transverse incisions which allow for more medial-lateral instrument mobility.

Anterolateral Portal
Almost universally, the anterolateral portal is the first portal created and functions as the primary viewing portal. An incision is made distal to the inferior edge of the patella in line with the lateral border of the patella. As further reference, it should be just lateral to the patellar tendon and 1 cm superior to the tibial joint line. These landmarks should place the incision in a soft spot.

pump (if desired) and arthroscopic fluid bags, arthroscopic shaver housing, electrocautery unit, and high-definition printer (Fig. 2.1). A Mayo stand will be brought in from this side, and the shaver, electrocautery device, camera, and tubing will be placed here. Prior to draping the patient, ensuring that everything is set up, including placing the shaver pedal at the surgeon's feet, will ensure a more efficient operation and help to minimize surgeon frustration.

Every knee arthroscopic procedure can be performed with the patient supine on the operating room table. If additional lateral or medial posterior knee access is needed, a bump under the ipsilateral or contralateral hip, respectively, should be considered. If intraoperative fluoroscopy is planned, the patient will need to be moved to the distal end of the bed to accommodate a lateral radiograph. Proximal and distal patient positioning is also important if a well leg holder is used as the bed needs to break just proximal to the knee.

Depending on surgeon preference, a table attachment should be placed on the side rails to provide an immobile

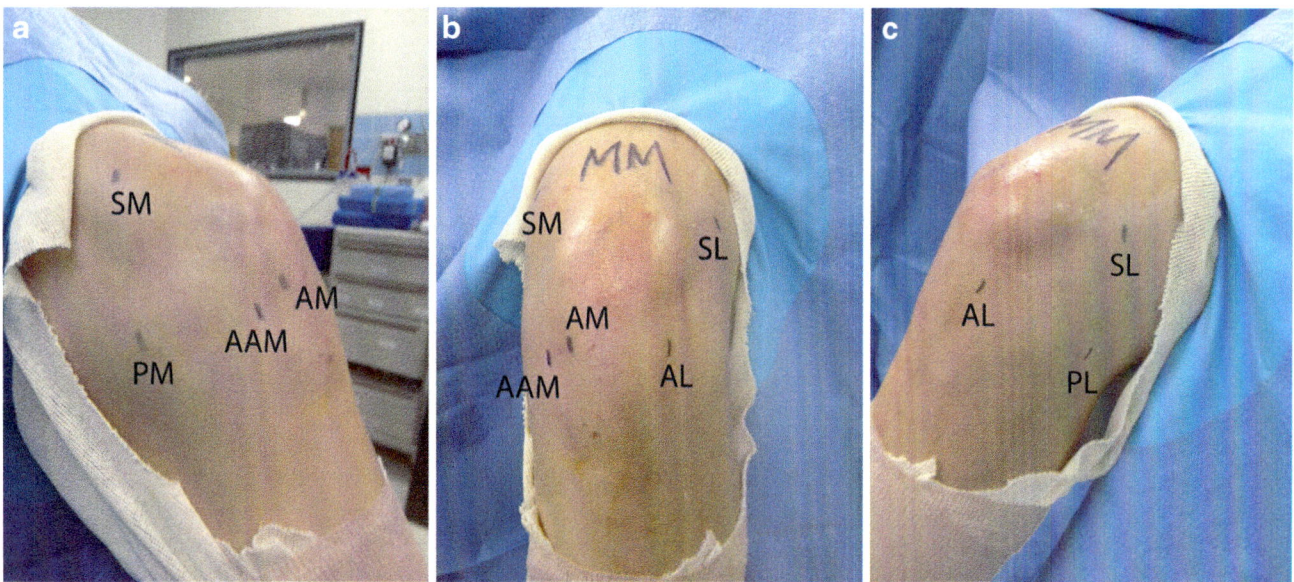

Fig. 2.2 (**a**)–(**c**) The locations of commonly used primary and secondary arthroscopic portals are drawn on the patient's knee. *AM* anteromedial, *AL* anterolateral, *AAM* accessory anteromedial, *SM* superomedial, *SL* superolateral, *PM* posteromedial, *PL* posterolateral

Anteromedial Portal

In almost all arthroscopic procedures, this is the second portal created and, unlike the anterolateral, is often made under direct visualization. The location is essentially a mirror image of the anterolateral flipped to the other side of the patellar tendon: 1 cm distal to the inferior border of the patella in line with the medial border of the patella, just medial to the patellar tendon, and it often falls 1 cm proximal to the medial tibial plateau. However, this basic location should be altered to accommodate the pathology. For a tear of the posterior horn of the medial meniscus, a biter and shaver must be able to slide under the medial femoral condyle which may require a slightly more inferior portal. Conversely, a lateral meniscus tear necessitates a slightly more superior portal in order to slide over the elevated tibial spines. This portal is initially localized with an 18 gauge spinal needle which can be advanced all the way into the involved compartment to determine if this portal location will permit the desired procedure. Then a #11 scalpel pierces the capsule, and a straight hemostat develops the path into the joint. Most arthroscopic instrumentation will be used through this portal.

Secondary Portals

The secondary portals listed below are not created for every knee arthroscopy but rather are used in particular circumstances when the primary portals do not provide adequate access (Fig. 2.2a–c).

Accessory Anteromedial Portal

With the advent of a more anatomic ACL reconstruction and a concurrent departure from transtibial technique, this portal was created to assist in localizing the entry point of the femoral tunnel [6]. Located medial and slightly inferior to the standard anteromedial portal, a spinal needle is inserted in the proposed location and should slide just anterior to the medial femoral condyle and come to rest in the location where the surgeon plans to drill the femoral ACL tunnel. With the knee in hyperflexion, this is the angle in which the tunnel will be drilled and the graft passed and secured. While passing instrumentation in and out of this portal, great care must be taken to avoid iatrogenic damage to the medial femoral condyle.

Posteromedial Portal

This portal is approximately 2½ cm distal and 2½ cm posterior to the medial epicondyle. With the knee flexed to 90°, this location is approximately 1–2 cm above the joint line. Utilizing the modified Gillquist maneuver or view, this and the posterolateral portals are more accurately localized. In this maneuver, the arthroscopic sheath and the blunt obturator are placed in the contralateral anterior portal and are slid along the ipsilateral condyle in the notch until it "pops" into the posterior knee. This can also be gently performed under direct visualization with the scope still in place, which may be a safer technique. Once the arthroscope is in the correct location, the overhead lights can be turned off so that the arthroscopic light will transilluminate the proposed portal location (Fig. 2.3a). Some surgeons recommend using a 70° scope for this maneuver. An

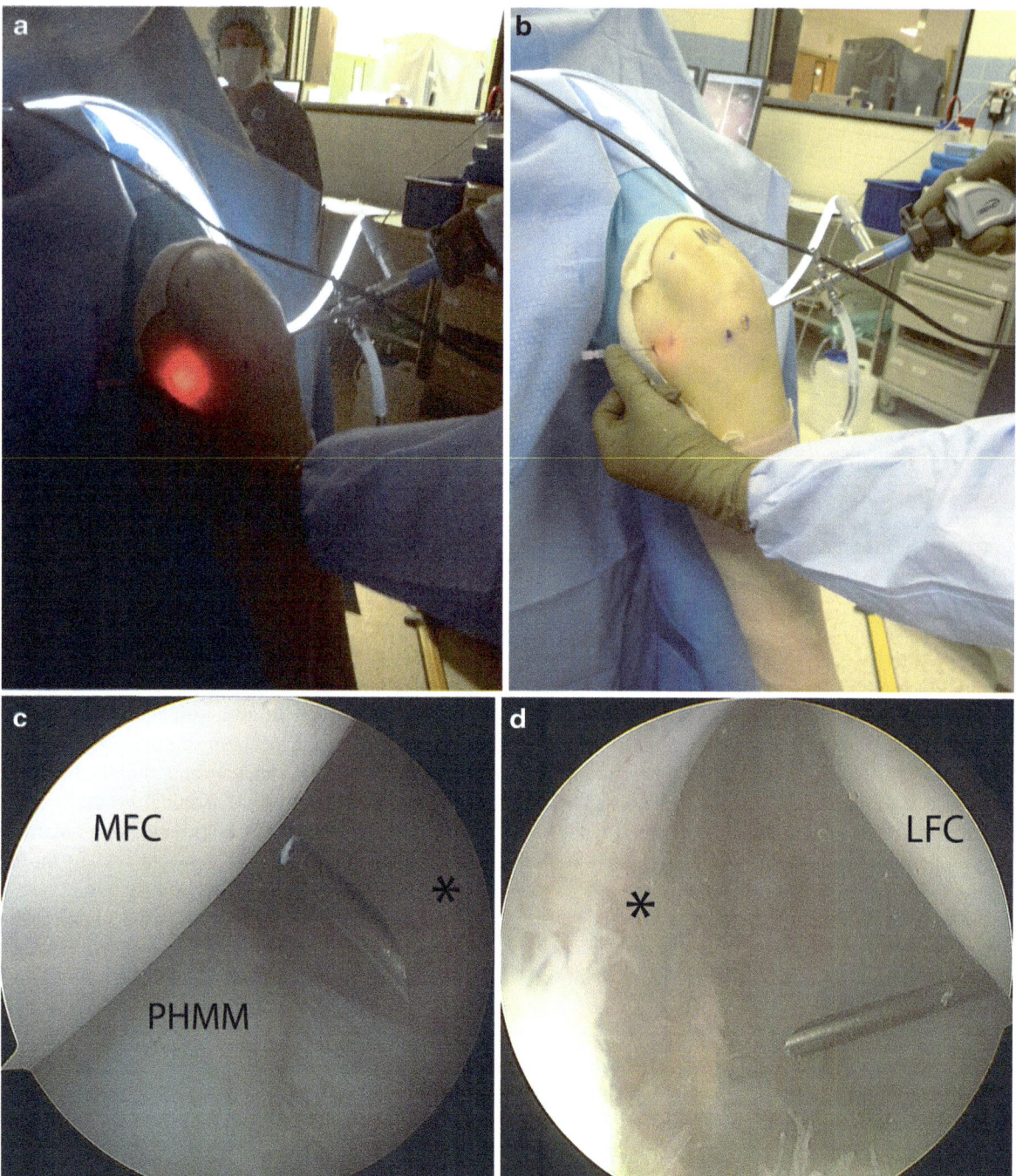

Fig. 2.3 (**a**) After performing the modified Gillquist maneuver to place the arthroscope in the posterior knee, the overhead lights are turned off so that the posteromedial portal location is transilluminated. (**b**) An 18 gauge spinal needle is placed at this location and confirmed arthroscopically. Note that the arthroscope is in the anterolateral portal. (**c**) In the posterior knee, the 18 gauge needle is seen very easily, and this trajec-tory can be used to address posteromedial pathology. (**d**) This same technique should also be used to establish the posterolateral portal, but the arthroscope is placed in the anteromedial portal. *MFC* medial femoral condyle, *LFC* lateral femoral condyle, *PHMM* posterior horn of the medial meniscus, *Asterisk* posterior knee capsule

additional benefit of transillumination is that overlying neuro-vascular structures can be visualized as dark lines running in a superior-inferior direction. An 18 gauge spinal needle assures the correct location (Fig. 2.3b, c), which is followed by the "nick and spread" method to avoid injuring the saphenous nerve and long saphenous vein [7]. McGinnis et al. found that

the soft spots on the posteromedial aspect of the knee and 1 cm superior to this location were safe portals, but 1 cm inferior was always directly in the path of the saphenous nerve [8]. This portal provides access to posteromedial structures such as the posterior horn of the medial meniscus and the posterior cruciate ligament (PCL) [9].

Posterolateral Portal

As a general rule of thumb, this portal is located just anterior to the biceps tendon (thus anterior to the common peroneal nerve) and just posterior to the iliotibial (IT) band. As described above, the Gillquist maneuver with a spinal needle allows for accurate localization of this portal with the knee in flexion [7] (Fig. 2.3d). In 90° of flexion in a cadaveric model, the common peroneal nerve was noted to travel approximately 25 mm posterior to the portal location, compared to 20 mm with the knee in extension [10].

Superomedial Portal

This portal is located 2–3 cm proximal to the superior pole of the patella just medial to the quadriceps tendon and is made in extension after being localized with a spinal needle. It is commonly used for arthroscopic fluid inflow and outflow, although more advanced arthroscopic tubing and instrumentation have minimized the necessity of an extra portal solely for this use.

Superolateral Portal

This portal is essentially a mirror image of the superomedial portal. It can also be used for arthroscopic fluid inflow and outflow and to observe patellar tracking and to perform an arthroscopic lateral retinacular release.

Transpatellar Portal

For this portal, a vertical incision is made 1 cm distal to the inferior pole of the patella in the middle third of the tendon. This is a less commonly used portal but can be very useful for viewing or grasping loose bodies or meniscal fragments. Avoid this portal if a bone-patellar tendon-bone ACL autograft is planned as some minor damage to the patellar tendon is unavoidable.

Proximal Superomedial Portal

Located 4 cm proximal to the medial pole of the patella, this portal allows for assessment of patellar tracking as well as visualization of the anterior horns of both menisci and the tibial attachment of the ACL [11].

Far Lateral/Medial Portal

Additional accessory portals may be created as needed as long as careful attention is paid to surrounding neurovascular structures. These portals can be utilized to access areas of the knee not well visualized by the other portals mentioned above.

Diagnostic Knee Arthroscopy

In the following paragraphs, the basics of the diagnostic knee arthroscopy are described. During the procedure, it is imperative that the surgeon be thorough and inspects the knee in a methodical and systematic way. Directing all attention at the pathology seen on preoperative magnetic resonance imaging (MRI) and not conducting an exhaustive diagnostic arthroscopy may result in residual pathology causing a clinical failure of the surgery. During the initial diagnostic arthroscopy, the surgeon may choose to treat the pathology as it is encountered versus returning to the involved compartment after completing the complete diagnostic arthroscopy. While either approach is correct, the knee must be wholly investigated by the completion of the procedure.

With the knee flexed and landmarks drawn, the anterolateral portal is created with a #11 blade inserted to a depth sufficient to incise the joint capsule. The blade should be directed toward the intercondylar notch as to not damage the lateral femoral articular cartilage. As with any portals around the joint line, it is wise to insert the knife with the blade facing superior and to extend the portal incision proximally as to not blindly cut down onto the meniscus. Following the scalpel, the trocar and sheath are introduced into the joint and slid into the suprapatellar pouch as the knee is brought into extension. Forcing the trocar into the joint should be avoided, as the articular cartilage can be easily damaged by plunging.

Once the sheath is nestled in the suprapatellar pouch, the trocar is removed, the 30° white-balanced arthroscopic camera with the fiber-optic light source is inserted, and the appropriate tubing (arthroscopic fluid inflow and outflow) is attached. Depending on the expected pathology and surgeon preference, arthroscopic fluid can be pressurized by gravity alone or by an inflow pump set usually to 60 mm of mercury. Once the setup is completed, the patellofemoral articular surfaces and joint tracking are inspected, and any chondromalacia is noted (Fig. 2.4a, b). Loose bodies or synovitis can be found here, and then the inspection should proceed into the lateral gutter or recess. Loss bodies tend to collect here, and gentle palpation over the skin can dislodge them into the camera's view. The camera is then brought up and over the lateral femoral condyle, across the trochlear groove into the medial gutter or recess, and then the knee is slowly flexed while observing for femoral condylar articular cartilage damage or a plica.

With the knee slightly flexed, the arthroscope can be directed into the medial compartment. A valgus stress is applied with assistance of a post, well leg holder, or assistant in order to open up this compartment and allow evaluation of its posterior aspect (Fig. 2.5). Additionally, flexing and extending the knee bring different sections of the medial femoral condyle into view, and knee extension followed by knee flexion can assist in gaining access to the posterior horn of the meniscus. Prior to inspection of this compartment, most surgeons create the anteromedial portal which is used to insert instruments to better evaluate any intra-articular pathology. Through this portal, an arthroscopic probe is inserted and used to define the characteristics of meniscal

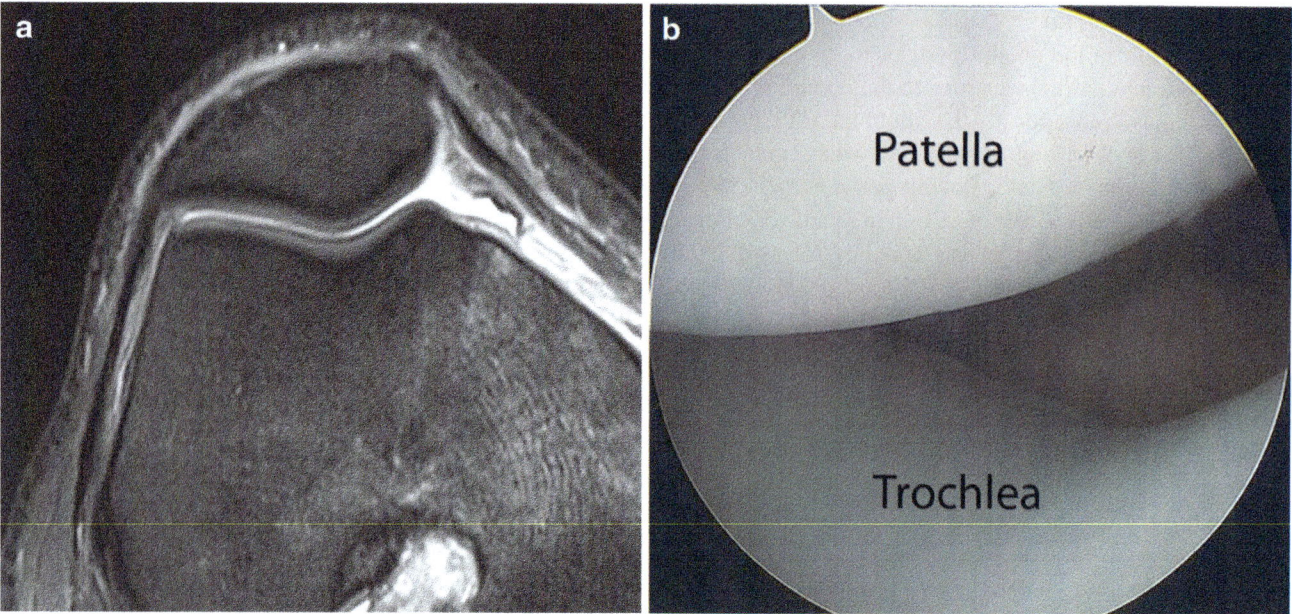

Fig. 2.4 (**a**) An axial T2-weighted MRI image shows healthy cartilage of the patella and femoral trochlea as well as the congruence of the two. (**b**) Viewed from the anterolateral portal, the patellofemoral articulation is well visualized

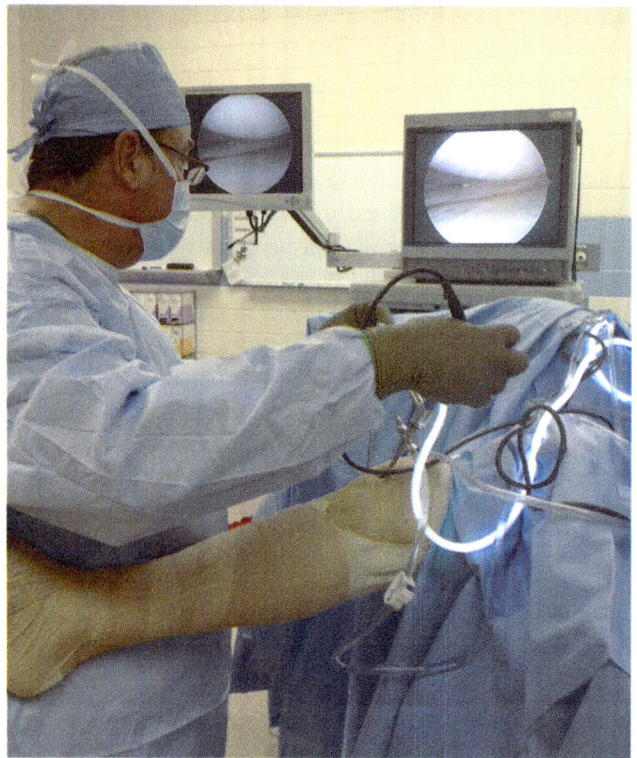

Fig. 2.5 To perform an arthroscopic evaluation of the medial compartment, a valgus stress is applied across the knee by using the leg holder or post and the hip of the surgeon. Alternatively, an assistant can apply this force

tears and cartilage damage (Fig. 2.6a–c). A normal meniscus should have a smooth articular margin although some undulation at the inner edge is not unexpected. The probe characterizes a meniscal tear by noting meniscal displacement, depth of the tear, or the presence of fragments flipped above or below the joint line. Additionally, the probe should be slid along the articular cartilage to delineate any areas of softening or fissuring. If any pathology is identified, then an arthroscopic shaver, curette, awl, or other instruments may be used through this anterolateral portal.

After the medial compartment is inspected, the arthroscope and probe are swung into the intercondylar notch which is best evaluated with the knee in flexion. The tension on the ACL and PCL can be estimated by tugging on them with the probe (Fig. 2.7a–d). By extending the knee, ACL notch impingement can be assessed.

After the notch is inspected, the arthroscopic instrumentation needs to be carried up and over the ligamentum mucosum. Note that some surgeons will perform a limited debridement of the ligamentum mucosum and of the fat pad, whereas others will work around it secondary to concerns of postoperative pain and hemarthrosis. With the knee flexed to 90°, the instruments should be placed just lateral to the ACL in preparation for the "figure of four" position, at which point they will slide nicely into the lateral compartment as the varus stress is applied (Fig. 2.8). The varus force can be increased by applying an inferiorly

Fig. 2.6 (**a, b**) Coronal and sagittal T1-weighted MRI imaging allows for evaluation of the medial compartment articular surfaces and the meniscus. Note that the meniscus appears *triangular-shaped* when the imaging cut is orthogonal to the meniscus. In other words, the body appears *triangular* on coronal imaging, and the anterior and posterior horns appear *triangular* on sagittal imaging. (**c**) Viewed from the anterolateral portal while a valgus forced is applied across the knee, the medial compartment including the meniscus and articular cartilage can be inspected with the arthroscope. *Block arrow* body of medial meniscus, *dashed arrow* anterior horn of the medial meniscus, *solid arrow* posterior horn of the medial meniscus, *MFC* medial femoral condyle, *MTP* medial tibial plateau, *Asterisk* medial meniscus

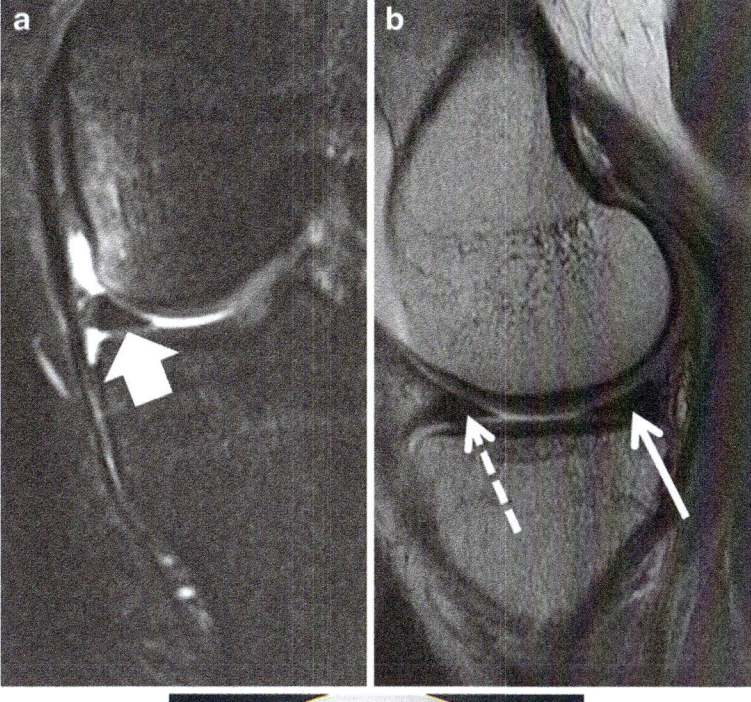

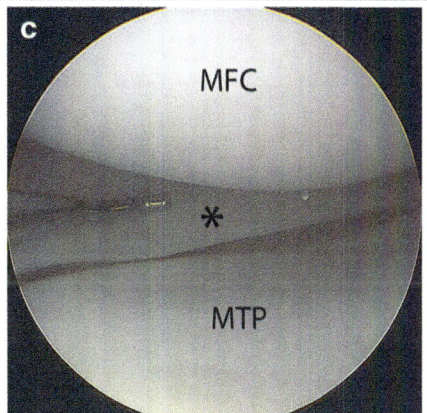

directed force over the distal femur while lifting the foot superiorly. This portion of the procedure can be quite cumbersome for surgeons unfamiliar with knee arthroscopy, as the plane of hand movements is perpendicular to the plane viewed on the monitor. In addition to meniscal tears and cartilage damage, diagnostic arthroscopy in the lateral compartment includes evaluation of the popliteus tendon and hiatus (Fig. 2.9a, b).

It should be noted that although the anterolateral portal is most commonly the viewing portal, the surgeon should not hesitate to view through the anteromedial portal and place instruments through the anterolateral portal. Examples of when this would be appropriate:

- When performing an ACL reconstruction with an accessory anteromedial portal, viewing through the anteromedial portal allows the surgeon to correctly place the femoral tunnel starting point.
- When debriding a tear of the anterior horn of the medial meniscus, working through the anterolateral portal provides arthroscopic biters with an improved angle to the meniscus.
- For high-grade chondromalacia of the lateral femoral condyle, placing the microfracture awl through the anterolateral portal facilitates orthogonal perforation of the subchondral bone relative to the articular surface.

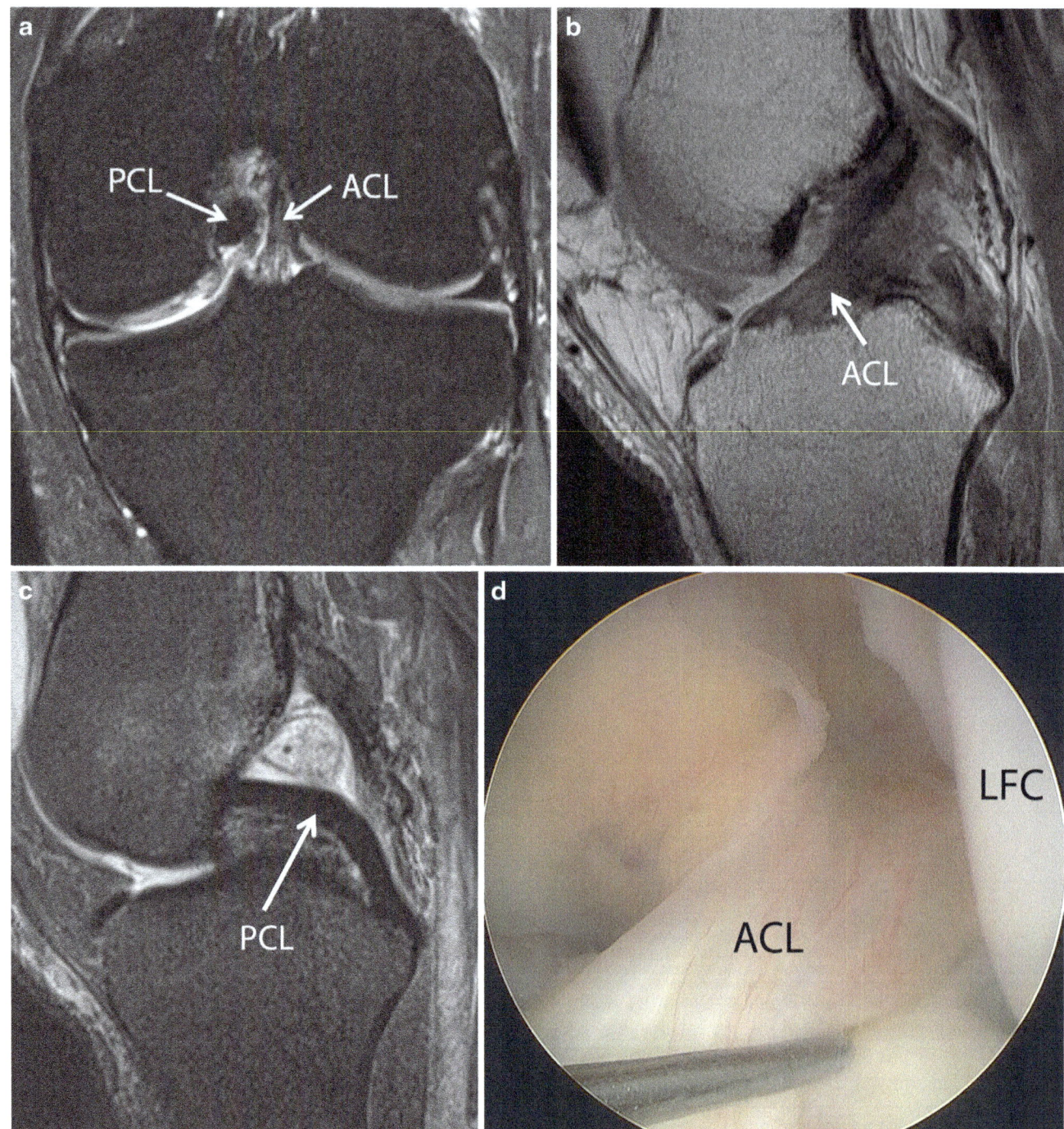

Fig. 2.7 (**a**) Coronal T2-weighted MRI image showing the intercondy-lar notch with the ACL and PCL. (**b**) Sagittal T1-weighted image of the ACL with its normal striated appearance. (**c**) Sagittal T2-weighted image showing the more well-defined PCL. (**d**) Arthroscopic image of the notch with the probe around the ACL. *ACL* anterior cruciate liga-ment, *PCL* posterior cruciate ligament, *LFC* lateral femoral condyle

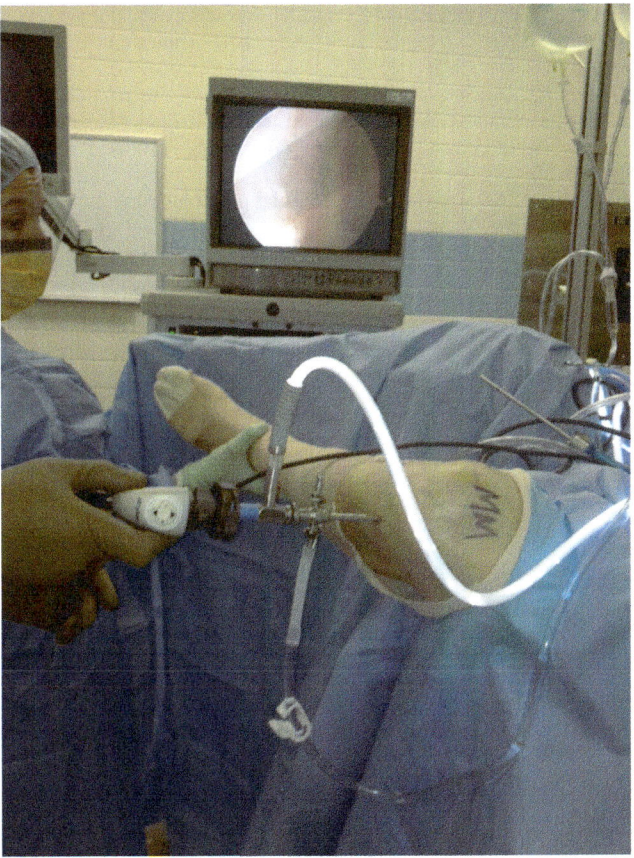

Fig. 2.8 To perform an arthroscopic evaluation of the lateral compartment, a varus force is applied by placing the leg in the "figure of four" position. Note that the camera must be turned 90° relative to the floor in order to provide the appropriate horizontal images on the monitor

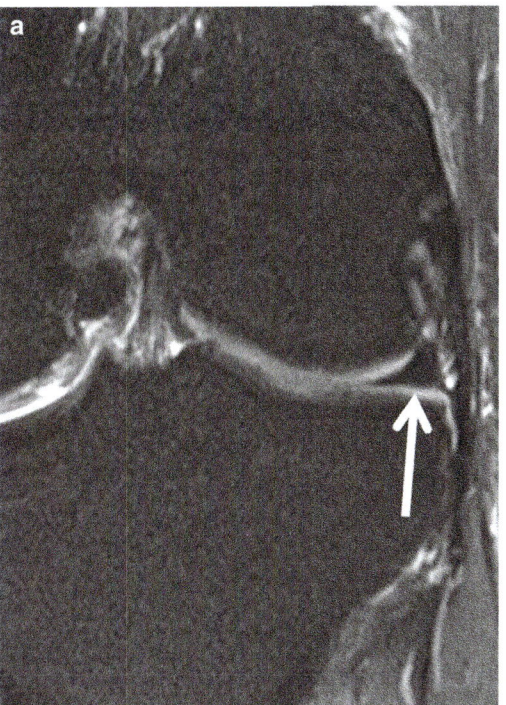

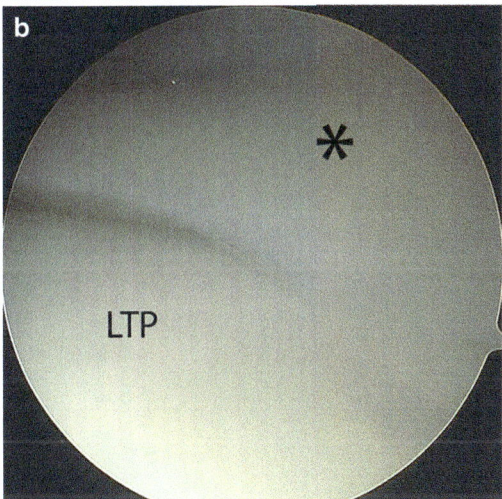

Fig. 2.9 (**a**) Coronal T2-weighted MRI imaging showing the body of the lateral meniscus. (**b**) Arthroscopy allows for evaluation of the lateral compartment articular surfaces and the meniscus

Summary

Due to its expanding indications and continued evolution, today's orthopedic surgeon must possess the ability to perform a basic knee arthroscopy. For a variety of intra-articular knee processes, arthroscopic treatment has become the gold standard when compared to its antiquated open counterpart. However, the surgeon must have a strong understanding of knee anatomy relative to arthroscopic portal locations to minimize iatrogenic neurovascular injuries. With appropriate patient selection and proper surgical technique, knee arthroscopy can provide patients with substantial pain relief and a meaningful return of their knee function.

References

1. Jackson RW. A history of arthroscopy. Arthroscopy. 2010;26: 91–103.
2. Kim S, Bosque J, Meehan JP, Jamali A, Marder R. Increase in outpatient knee arthroscopy in the United States: a comparison of national surveys of ambulatory surgery, 1996 and 2006. J Bone Joint Surg Am. 2011;93:994–1000.
3. Montes FR, Zarate E, Grueso R, Giraldo JC, Venegas MP, Gomez A, Rincon JD, Hernadez M, Cabrera M. Comparison of spinal anesthesia with combined sciatic-femoral nerve block for outpatient knee arthroscopy. J Clin Anesth. 2008;20:415–20.
4. Shaukat Y, Malik E, El-Khateeb H, Koeweiden E. The role of local anaesthesia in knee arthroscopy. J Orthop. 2013;10:193–5.
5. Krul-Sterk A, Klip H, Kuizenga K, Schiere S. Drugs used for spinal anaesthesia in patients undergoing ambulatory knee arthroscopy: a

survey of Dutch anaesthesiologists. Eur J Anaesthesiol. 2009; 26:82–3.

6. Tompkins M, Milewski MD, Brockmeier SF, Gaskin CM, Hart JM, Miller MD. Anatomic femoral tunnel drilling in anterior cruciate ligament reconstruction: use of an accessory medial portal versus traditional transtibial drilling. Am J Sports Med. 2012;40:1313–21.

7. Kramer DE, Bahk MS, Cascio BM, Cosgarea AJ. Posterior knee arthroscopy: anatomy, technique, application. J Bone Joint Surg Am. 2006;88 Suppl 4:110–21.

8. McGinnis MD, Gonzalez R, Nyland J, Caborn DN. The posteromedial knee arthroscopy portal: a cadaveric study defining a safety zone for portal placement. Arthroscopy. 2011;27:1090–5.

9. Gold DL, Schaner PJ, Sapega AA. The posteromedial portal in knee arthroscopy: an analysis of diagnostic and surgical utility. Arthroscopy. 1995;11:139–45.

10. Ahn JH, Lee SH, Jung HJ, Koo KH, Kim SH. The relationship of neural structures to arthroscopic posterior portals according to knee positioning. Knee Surg Sports Traumatol Arthrosc. 2011;19: 646–52.

11. Schreiber SN. Proximal superomedial portal in arthroscopy of the knee. Arthroscopy. 1991;7:246–51.

Meniscus Tear MRI Correlation

Healthy J. Desai and Peter R. Kurzweil

Introduction

Knee arthroscopy has become the most common orthopedic procedure performed in the United States [1]. The knee was the first joint to be examined arthroscopically, and many principles of arthroscopy of other joints were originally developed for the knee. Knee arthroscopy became popular in the United States in the 1980s, and substantial progress has been made over the past few decades.

Since the introduction of magnetic resonance imaging (MRI) in the 1980s, MRI equipment and techniques have evolved substantially to provide an accurate delineation of anatomy and pathology of the human knee. MRI is now widely accepted as a critical tool for clinical decision-making and surgical planning in many patients with signs and symptoms of internal derangement of the knee [2–4]. MRI is often an integral tool when diagnosing knee disorders and has proven useful to improve surgical planning [5, 6].

Successful repair of menisci depends on tear location and pattern. Longitudinal and some oblique tears are reparable, whereas radial, horizontal, and complex tears generally are not. Vascularity is also important for outcome of the repair. Repairs of tears are most successful when they are located in the vascularized periphery of the meniscus, preferably with a peripheral rim that is less than 4 mm wide [7, 8].

H.J. Desai, MD (✉)
Department of Orthopedics, Ridgecrest Regional Hospital, Ridgecrest, CA, USA

Department of Orthopedics, Long Beach Memorial Medical Center, Long Beach, CA, USA
e-mail: info@dr-healthy.com

P.R. Kurzweil, MD
Department of Orthopedics, Long Beach Memorial Medical Center, Long Beach, CA, USA
e-mail: Pkurzweil@aol.com

Prior studies evaluating the meniscus tear pattern and location by MRI have had mixed results in predicting the reparability of meniscus tears [9, 10]. In this chapter, we will explore the association between the MRI and arthroscopic appearance of the different types of meniscal tears.

Normal Meniscus

The menisci are comprised of fibrocartilages that are C-shaped structures which occupy the peripheral articular space between the femur and tibia. They are divided into the anterior horn, body, and posterior horn. In cross section, menisci are triangular or wedge shaped, being thickest peripherally and tapering to a point at their central free edges. This triangular appearance is seen on cross-sectional sagittal and coronal MRIs. Sagittal images through the body and coronal images through the anterior and posterior horns show a bow tie appearance (Fig. 3.1a–f).

The medial meniscus is larger, more oblong, and normally has a larger posterior horn than anterior horn in cross section. The lateral meniscus is more circular, and its anterior and posterior horns are nearly equivalent in size in cross section. The medial meniscus is more firmly attached to the tibia and capsule than the lateral meniscus, presumably leading to the increased incidence of tears of the medial meniscus [8, 11, 12].

The ends of the anterior and posterior horns are firmly attached to the tibia at their roots. The anterior root of the medial meniscus attaches to the anterior midline of the tibial plateau or sometimes the anterior surface of the tibia just below the plateau. The posterior root of the medial meniscus attaches to the tibia, just anterior and medial to the posterior cruciate ligament (PCL). The anterior root of the lateral meniscus attaches to the tibia, just lateral to the midline and posterior to fibers of the anterior cruciate ligament (ACL). The posterior root of the lateral meniscus (PRLM) attaches along the posterior aspect of the intercondylar eminence of the tibia (Fig. 3.2a–c) [8, 12–14].

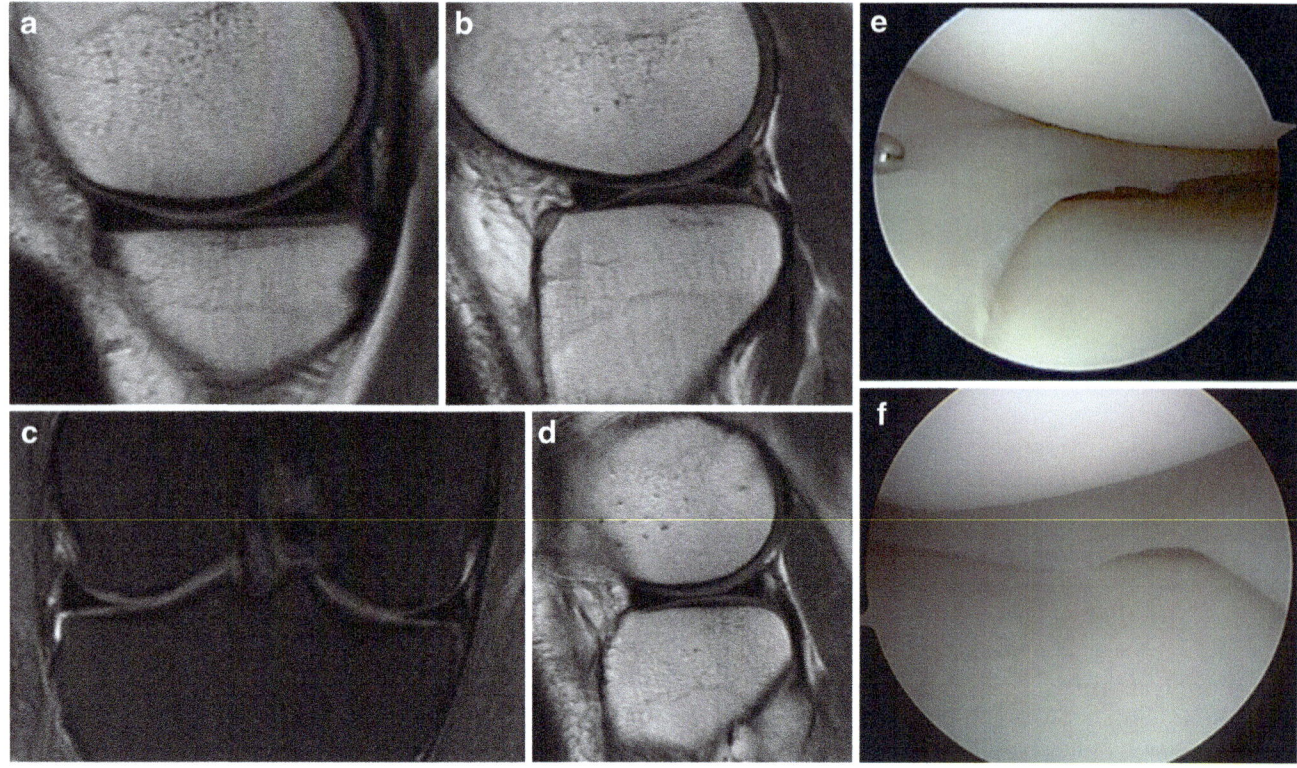

Fig. 3.1 Normal menisci. Sagittal proton density (PD) images through normal medial (**a**) and lateral (**b**) menisci in cross section demonstrate the normal appearance of the anterior and posterior horns as *black triangles*. (**c**) Mid-coronal fat-suppressed T2 image demonstrates the normal *triangular* appearance of the bodies of both menisci. (**d**) Far sagittal image of the lateral meniscus cuts through the edge shows the bow tie appearance. Arthroscopic images of the normal medial (**e**) and lateral (**f**) menisci demonstrate the smooth surfaces and edges

MRI of Meniscal Tears: Criteria and Accuracy

Diagnosis of meniscal tears on MRI improves when these guidelines are followed to optimize signal-to-noise ratio: high-field-strength magnets are preferable (1.5 T and stronger); a high-resolution surface coil should be used; the field of view should only encompass the necessary structures and routinely be 16 cm or less; image slices should not be too thick (3–4 mm); and the matrix size should be at least 256×192 or higher [15]. Some authors have suggested that many tears are best seen on sequences with a low echo time, namely, T1-weighted and proton density sequences [15]. However, it is the authors' experience that tears are often better seen on the T2 images. This is probably related to fluid being more pronounced on the T2 sequences and subsequently accentuates fluid-filled defects in the meniscal tear.

A normal meniscus is low signal on all sequences. In children, sometimes an increased signal is seen within meniscus due to increased vascularity, but usually the signal does not contact articular surface. It is important to know the age of the patient when interpreting the MRI. Otherwise, the increased vascularity in children has sometimes led to false-

positive reading of a meniscus tear. Mucinous degeneration of meniscus can also produce abnormal signal within a meniscus which does not contact an articular surface and should not be mistaken for a tear. This has also been described as grade 2 signal [12, 16, 17] (Fig. 3.3).

The most common criterion for diagnosing meniscus tear on MRI is an increased signal extending in a line or band to the articular surface. Another finding is the abnormal size or shape of the meniscus, which would indicate damaged surfaces [12, 16, 17]. Studies by Kaplan and colleagues [18] and De Smet and coworkers [19] showed that the abnormal signal must unequivocally contact the surface of the meniscus. Although it may seem easy to read a meniscus as torn from an MRI, it is actually sometimes difficult to interpret whether the abnormal signal comes close to or actually touches the surface.

To provide a greater degree of accuracy, De Smet advocated the "two-slice-touch rule." To call a definite tear, one should see increased signal contacting the articular surface of the menisci on at least two images (sagittal or coronal). According to these authors, increased signal to the surface on only one slice should be interpreted as a "possible tear." Cases of only one abnormal slice correlated to tears at

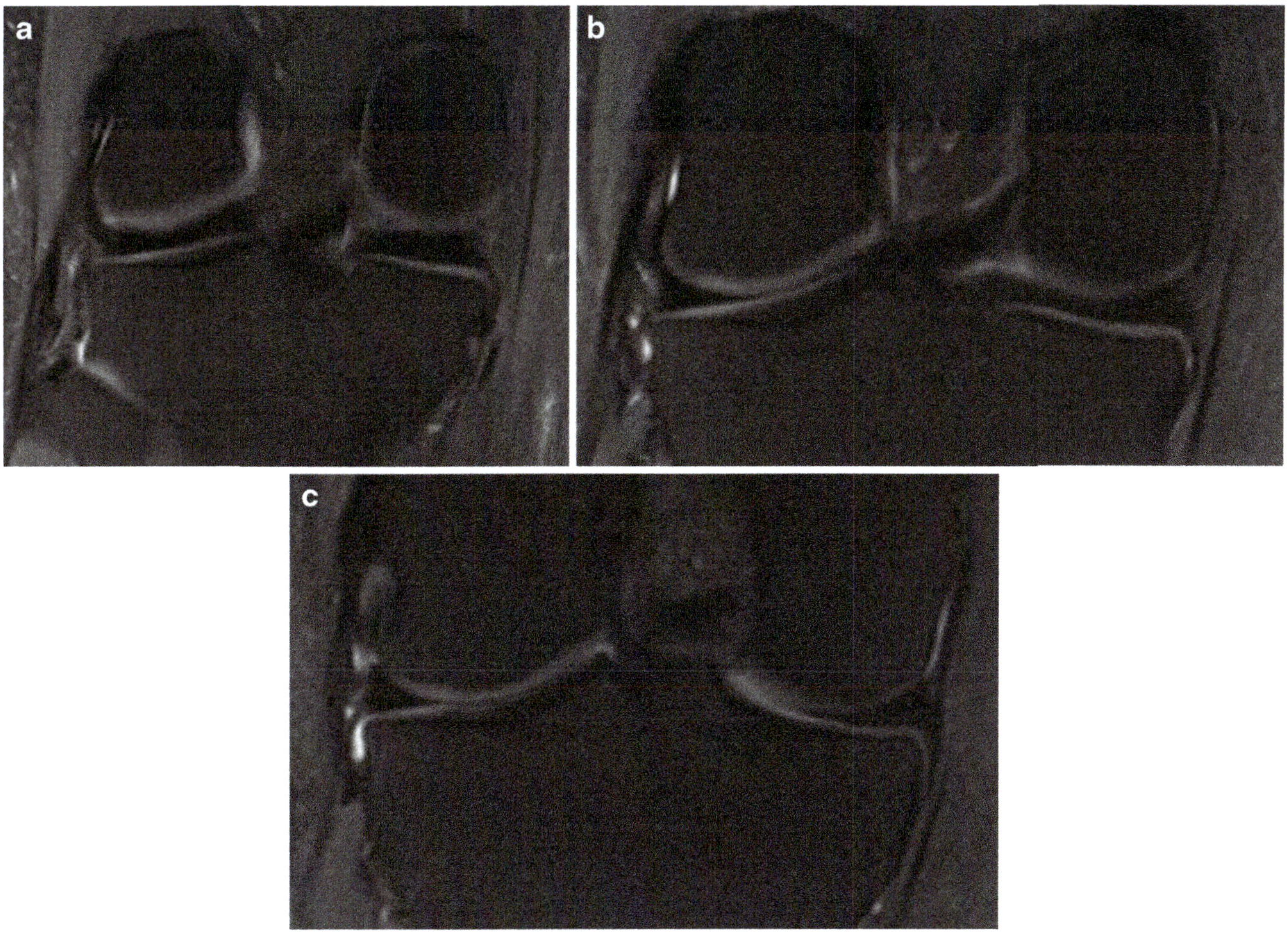

Fig. 3.2 (**a**)–(**c**) Normal posterior meniscal roots. Fat-suppressed T2 coronal images from posterior (**a**) to anterior (**c**) show the posterior horns of the menisci inserting into the tibia at the root ligament attachments alongside the posterior cruciate ligament

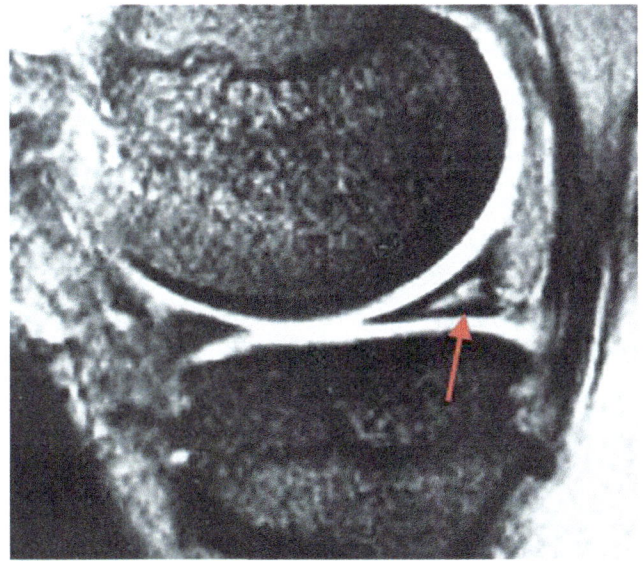

Fig. 3.3 Sagittal fat-suppressed T2 image of a 14-year-old patient showing a grade 2 signal in the posterior horn of the medial meniscus (PHMM). Note that signal does not contact articular surface

arthroscopy 55 % of the time for the medial meniscus and 30 % for the lateral [19] and only 43 and 18 % in a follow-up study 13 years later [20].

Accuracy of diagnosing meniscus tear with these criteria has been good. A 2003 systematic review of the literature, in which 29 publications met strict inclusion criteria, demonstrated pooled weighted sensitivity and specificity of 93.3 % and 88.4 % for the medial meniscus and 79.3 % and 95.7 % for the lateral meniscus, respectively [21]. Subsequent studies show improvement in these numbers [20, 22].

Most meniscal tears are visible and best seen on sagittal images. This is because most tears occur in the posterior horns [12]. However, one study showed that some tears are better seen or only seen on coronal images [23]. More recently, few reports suggest very thin axial images through the menisci to improve accuracy and tear description [24]. Fortunately, the MRI scan includes images in all three planes, and all three should be looked at carefully. Specific tear orientations vary and may only be clear in one of the three planes.

Patterns of Meniscal Tears

Whether a torn meniscus is reparable depends on the type or pattern of tear, its location, and the quality of the meniscal tissue. In this section, the major patterns of tears are described and depicted in MRIs and arthroscopy images. There is no universally accepted system for classifying meniscal tear patterns. A classification system developed by the International Society of Arthroscopy, Knee Surgery, and Orthopedic Sports Medicine [25, 26] is used here, and associated names when they are in common use are provided. These patterns include longitudinal-vertical, bucket handle, horizontal, radial, vertical flap, horizontal flap, and complex [25, 26].

Longitudinal Tears: Case 1 (Fig. 3.4a–d)

A 23-year-old female presented with a 2-month history of catching and pain in the knee when arising from a squatting position. Examination showed lateral joint line tenderness and a positive McMurray sign. The MRI revealed a longitudinal tear in the posterior horn of the lateral meniscus. Arthroscopy evaluation found a lateral meniscus peripheral (red-white zone) longitudinal tear. The patient underwent an all-inside lateral meniscus repair.

Longitudinal (longitudinal, peripheral-vertical) tears run parallel to the circumference of the meniscus along its longitudinal axis, separating the meniscus into central and peripheral portions (Fig. 3.4a–d). They may contact articular

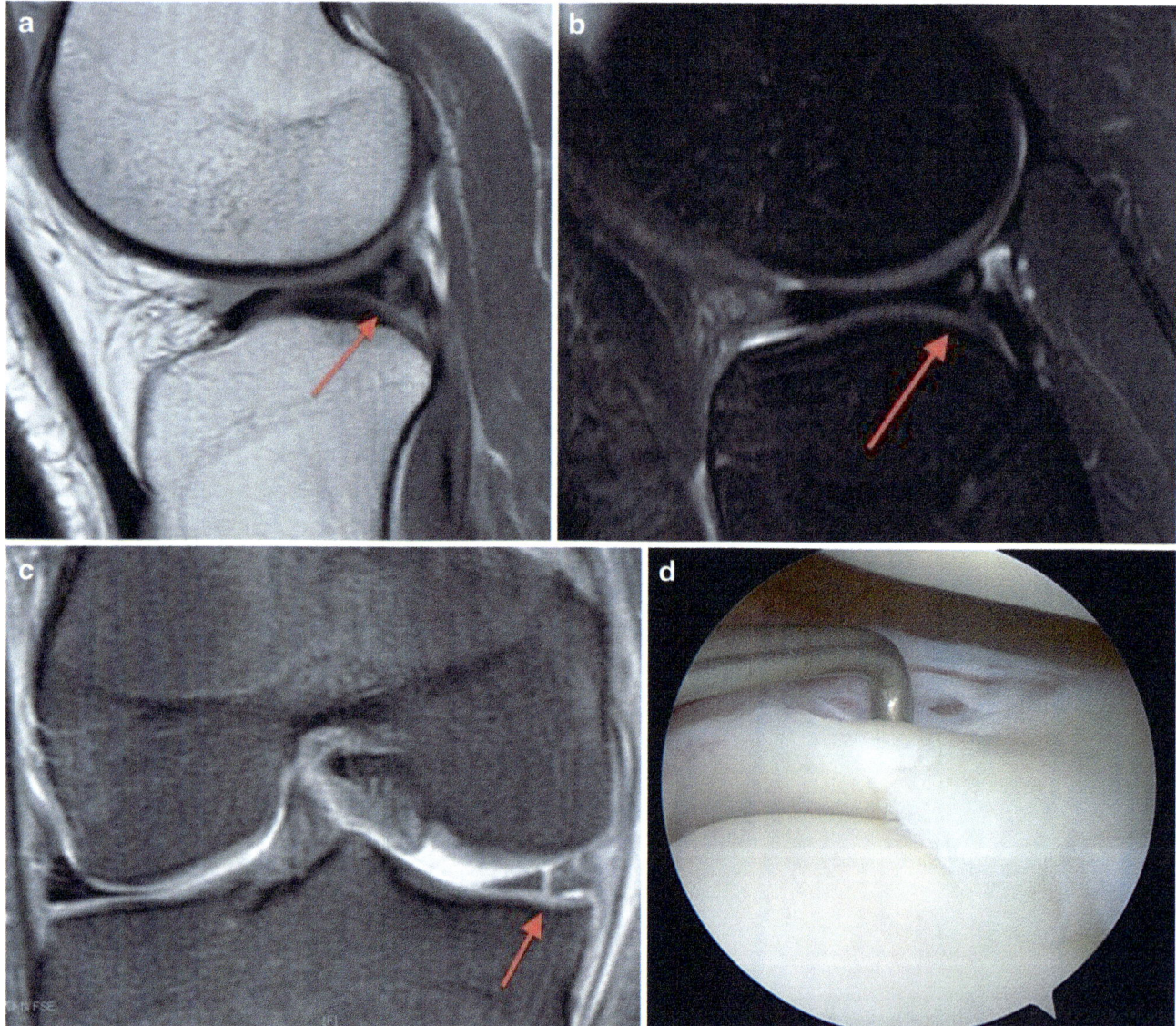

Fig. 3.4 Longitudinal-vertical tear. Sagittal PD (**a**) and fat-suppressed T2 (**b**) images show a longitudinal tear (*arrow*) in the posterior horn of the lateral meniscus (PHLM). (**c**) Coronal fat-suppressed T2 image showing the longitudinal tear. (**d**) Arthroscopic image of the same patient shows a probe in the longitudinal PHLM tear

surfaces of the meniscus. Longitudinal tears usually are the result of a specific injury, typically accompanying ACL tears, and usually start in the posterior horn [11, 12]. These lesions frequently occur in the periphery of the meniscus and are often amenable to repair.

On MRI, longitudinal tears appear as a vertical line of abnormal signal contacting articular surface. They maintain a relatively constant distance from the periphery of the meniscus [17].

Bucket-Handle Tears: Case 2 (Fig. 3.5a–d)

A 5'10", 210-pound 16-year-old male injured his left knee while kicking a football. He presented after a few months with symptoms of instability. Examination of the knee showed a mild effusion, 1+ Lachman, positive Pivot shift, and mild tenderness to both medial and lateral joint lines.

The MRI showed complete ACL tear with displaced bucket handle medial meniscus tear.

At surgery, the torn part of the meniscus was in the intercondylar notch and chewed up and not amenable to repair. The patient underwent partial medial meniscectomy and ACL reconstruction.

If a horizontal tear involves a long segment of the meniscus, the central fragment may displace centrally from the peripheral portion of the meniscus [17, 27]. Viewed from above, it resembles the handle on a bucket. The fragment commonly displaces into the intercondylar notch, although it may predominantly displace anteriorly [16]. If it displaces anteriorly, a portion of the displaced fragment may be visible in the intercondylar notch.

Bucket handle tears (BHT) often cause pain and mechanical symptoms, such as locking, catching, and giving way [16]. They are more frequent in the medial meniscus than the lateral and often occur in conjunction with ACL tears [27–29].

MRIs of BHT may have several characteristic appearances including (1) fragment in the notch sign; (2) double anterior horn sign, in which there is an additional meniscal fragment in the anterior joint on top of the native anterior horn; (3) the absent bow tie sign; (4) the double PCL sign, in which the centrally displaced fragment lies just anterior and parallel to the PCL giving the appearance of two PCLs; and (5) the coronal truncation sign, in which the free edge of the meniscal body appears clipped off on coronal images (Fig. 3.5a–d) [30–32].

Horizontal Tears: Case 3 (Fig. 3.6a–d)

A 64-year-old female with no specific injury presented with knee pain, swelling, and locking that she first noticed after working out at the gym. Exam showed a mild effusion and medial joint line tenderness.

Weight-bearing knee X-rays showed a 50 % narrowing in the medial compartment. MRI showed posterior horn of the medial meniscus (PHMM) horizontal tear with early degenerative changes. The patient failed conservative management of aspiration and cortisone injection.

Arthroscopy revealed a horizontal tear of PHMM, and a partial medial meniscectomy was performed.

Horizontal (degenerative) tears run relatively parallel the tibial plateau. Most horizontal tears extend to the inferior articular surface. These tears are usually degenerative in nature and usually not associated with a discrete injury [12, 16]. These tears may occur in the posterior horn, body, or anterior horn.

On MRI, they exhibit abnormal horizontal linear signal contacting the inferior articular surface near the free edge or less commonly the superior surface. They divide the meniscus into superior and inferior halves (Fig. 3.6a–d) [11, 12].

Radial Tears: Case 4 (Fig. 3.7a–c)

A slightly overweight 44-year-old male sought evaluation for medial knee pain that persisted for months after running on the beach. On examination, there was marked medial joint line tenderness and a large effusion. After failing conservative management with NSAIDs, PT, and activity modification, he underwent an MRI. This scan showed a radial MMT. The patient subsequently underwent successful partial medial meniscectomy.

Radial tears comprise approximately 15 % of tears in some surgical series [33, 34]. They are vertically oriented but extend perpendicular to the longitudinal axis of the meniscus. Radial tears start at the free edge of the meniscus and may extend through part of its circumference or all the way to the peripheral margin [17]. These tears commonly occur at the center of the posterior horn of the medial meniscus or at the junction of the anterior horn and body of the lateral meniscus [12].

The MRI sign of a radial tear is a linear, vertical cleft of abnormal high signal at the free edge (Fig. 3.7a–c). For radial tears that are oriented obliquely, one may observe the marching cleft sign, because the location of the vertical cleft of abnormal high signal shifts position from one image to the next [12, 33]. Radial tears are often filled with joint fluid and stand out more on fat-suppressed T2-weighted images [34]. Axial images can be especially helpful in identifying some radial tears and giving a realistic appreciation of their depth [12]. Radial tears are exceptions to the two-slice-touch rule since tear can lie between image slices in one plane.

Vertical Flap Tears: Case 5 (Fig. 3.8a–c)

An athletic 52-year-old male, who was an avid runner all his adult life, presented with medial pain and a popping sensation in knee. There was no history of a specific knee injury.

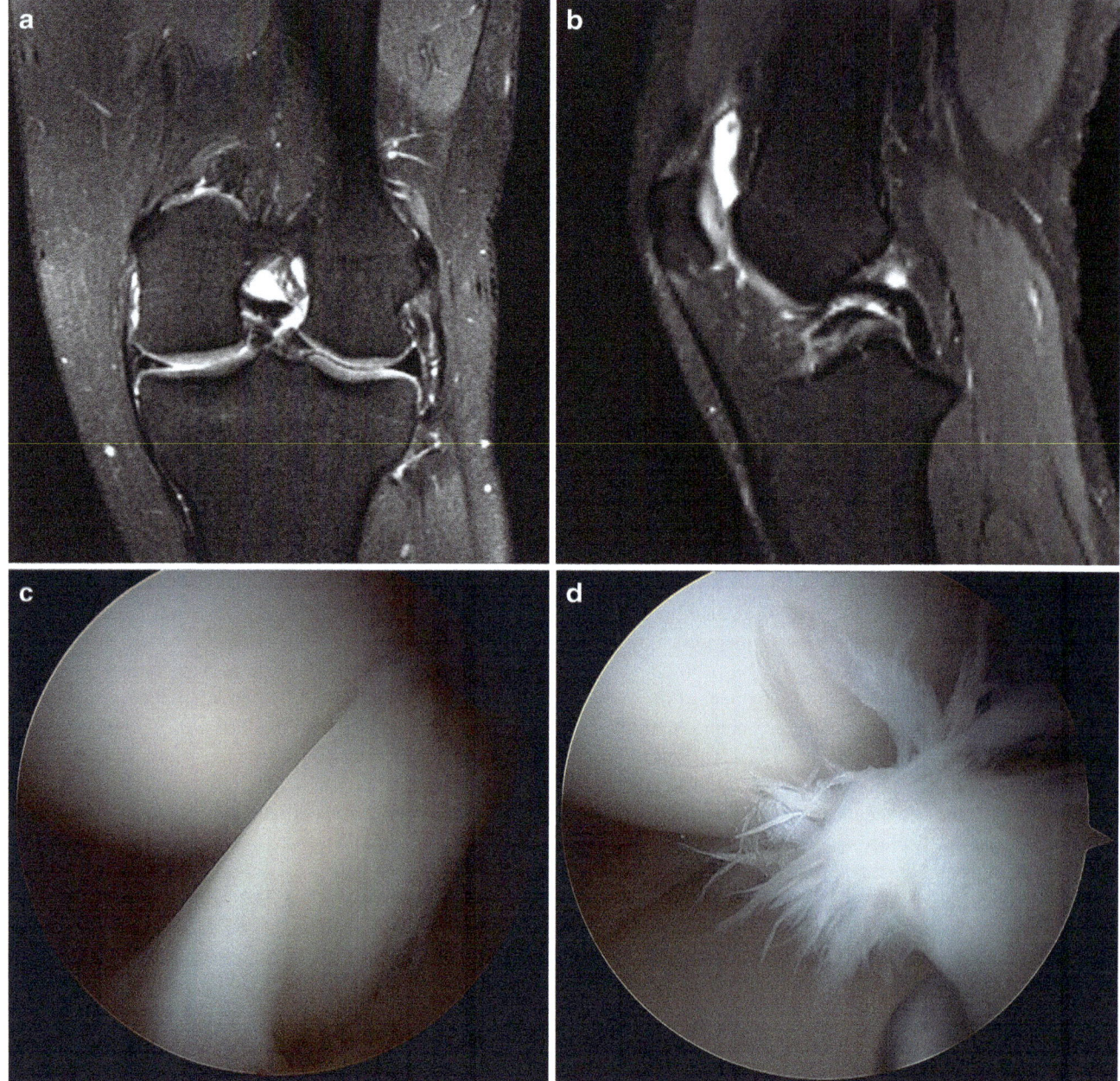

Fig. 3.5 Displaced bucket-handle tear. (**a**) Coronal fat-suppressed T2 image shows truncation of the body of the medial meniscus with fragment displaced into the notch. (**b**) Sagittal fat-suppressed T2 image shows the double PCL sign, representing the displaced meniscal fragment lying below the PCL. (**c**, **d**) Arthroscopic image demonstrates meniscal fragment displaced into the notch

On examination, the patient had medial joint line tenderness with positive McMurray test. The MRI revealed a vertical flap (oblique) tear of the medial meniscus. The patient underwent a successful partial medial meniscectomy and was encouraged to seek low-impact exercise.

Vertical flap (oblique, flap, parrot's beak) tears are unstable tears and occur in younger patients. They are usually due to an acute injury [16]. They resemble radial tears: they typically begin as a vertical tear at the free edge of the meniscus and extend radially; however, they change their radial orientation and turn to run parallel to the meniscus [16]. The unstable portion of meniscus separated by this tear resembles a parrot's beak.

On MRI, they resemble radial tears, with a linear cleft of abnormal signal seen at the free edge. However, the tear

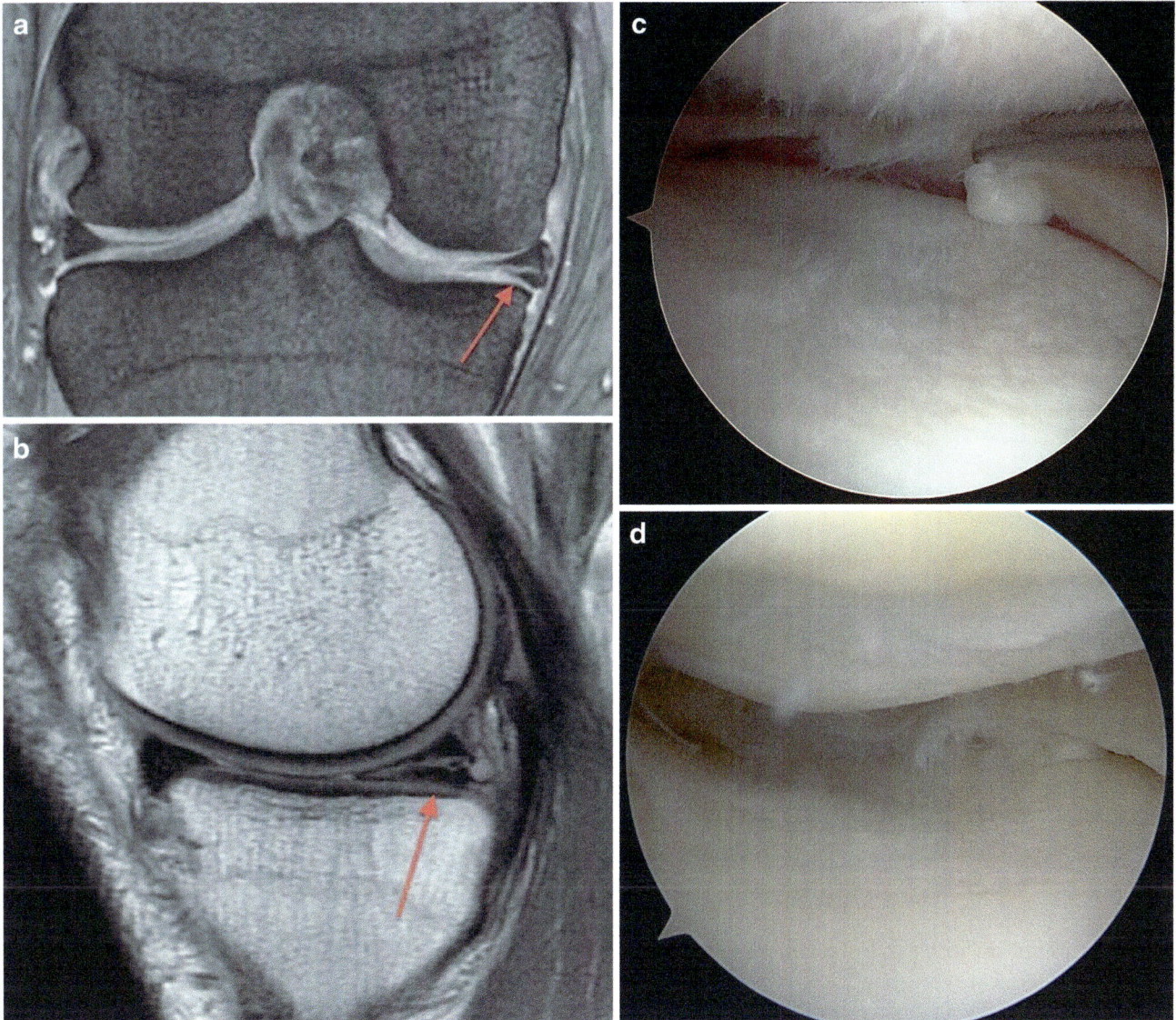

Fig. 3.6 Horizontal tear. Sagittal (**a**) and coronal (**b**) PD images show a horizontal tear (*arrow*). (**c**) Arthroscopic image in the same patient showing the horizontal PHMM tear. (**d**) Arthroscopic image of another patient showing horizontal PHMM tear

changes plane of orientation over its course. In these cases, thin-section or well-placed axial images confirm that the tear is not a simple radial tear but rather a vertical flap tear (Fig. 3.8a–c).

Horizontal Flap Tears: Case 6 (Fig. 3.9a–d)

A moderately overweight 56-year-old female tripped and fell, landing on her knee. She presented with diffuse pain and swelling and reported catching and locking of the knee. She failed to improve with conservative management over 2 months. An MRI revealed a horizontal flap tear of the medial meniscus. Arthroscopy showed a displaced unstable flap tear of the medial meniscus, and this portion was resected. This resolved her symptoms.

Horizontal flap tears are horizontal tears involving a short portion of the meniscus in which the torn segment is unstable and displaced peripherally [25, 32, 35] (Fig. 3.9a–d). These tears often cause mechanical symptoms [36].

MRI shows truncation or a horizontal tear [37]; sometimes, the displaced flap may not be obvious. When these tears occur in the body of the meniscus, the unstable fragment may displace into the superior recess underlying the medial collateral ligament or less commonly the inferior recess; similar displacement of tears of the lateral meniscal

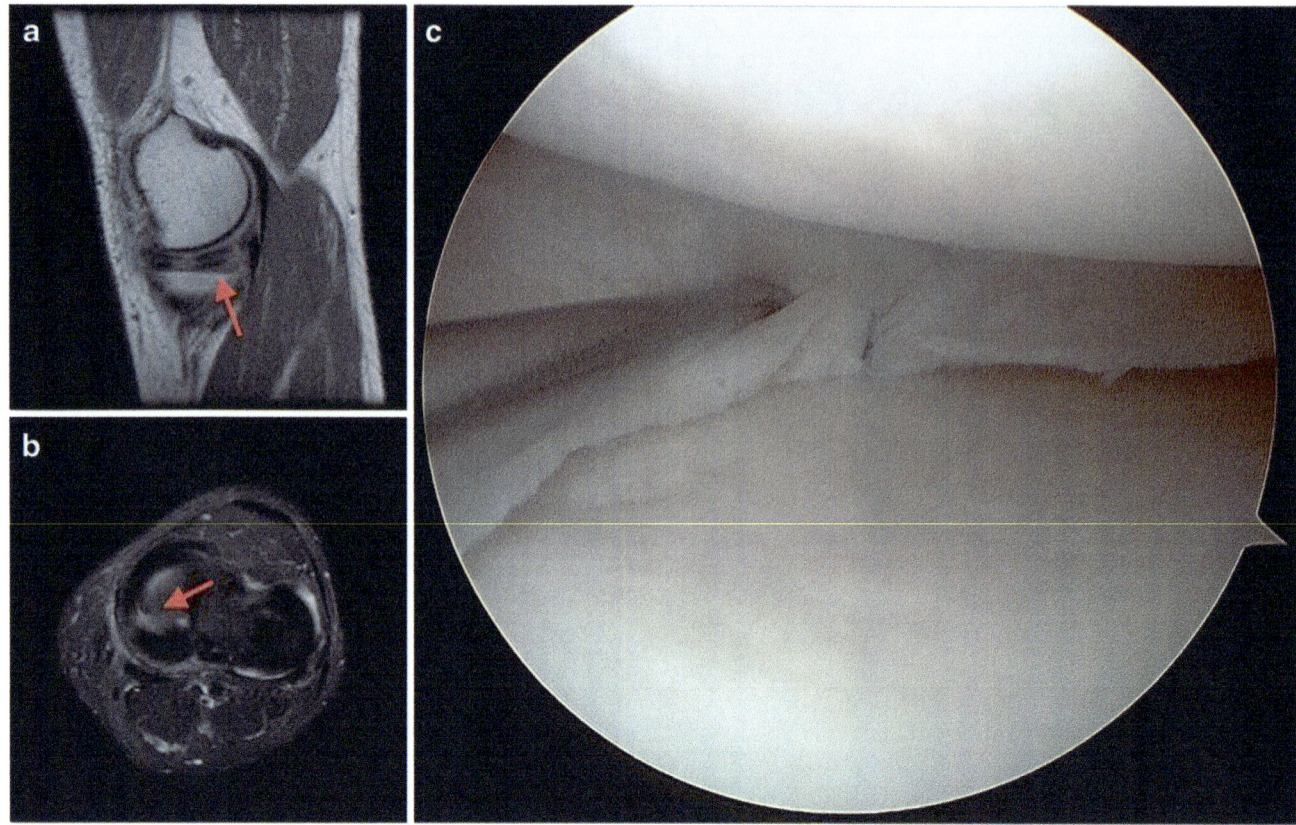

Fig. 3.7 Radial tear. Sagittal PD (**a**) and fat-suppressed axial T2 (**b**) images show a radial tear (*arrows*). (**c**) Arthroscopic image in the same patient demonstrates this radial tear

body is less common [37]. Fragments lying in the medial inferior recess are difficult to see at routine arthroscopy and only become evident when one slides a probe under the inferior surface of the peripheral meniscus [35]. Similarly, posterior horn lateral meniscus (PHLM) horizontal flap tears may displace into the posterior notch or the popliteal hiatus [36, 37].

Complex Tears: Case 7 (Fig. 3.10a–d)

An athletic 60-year-old male sought treatment for pain and catching in the knee that had been worsening for the last 3 months and was exacerbated by jogging. An MRI revealed a complex tear of the PHMM. At arthroscopy, a complex tear of the PHMM was found. The patient underwent a partial medial meniscectomy with resolution of symptoms.

Complex meniscal tears are often multi-planar. These tend to be degenerative tears, often in older patients, and are typically not amenable to repair. On MRI, there is significant disruption of meniscal architecture, and there are multiple lines of abnormal signal in both coronal and sagittal planes (Fig. 3.10a–d) [12, 25].

Root Tear: Case 8 (Fig. 3.11a–d)

A healthy, active 47-year-old male presented with a sudden onset knee pain and swelling which began while playing tennis. He noted it started after twisting his knee while serving. Examination showed medial joint line tenderness, a small effusion, and a positive McMurray. An MRI revealed a posterior root tear of the medial meniscus. During arthroscopy, a partial posterior root tear of the medial meniscus was found along with grade 2 degenerative changes of the articular cartilage. The unstable portion of the meniscus was trimmed, and by 4 months the patient reports resolution of symptoms and returns to all activities.

Meniscal root tears are not part of the ISAKOS classification of meniscal tears [25]. These tears were typically thought to be difficult to see at arthroscopy [11, 38] and have been frequently overlooked on MRI [39]; however, a better understanding of its appearance on MRI will improve the radiologic diagnosis [40].

Most root tears are radial tears and are located posteriorly [40]. Posterior root tears of the medial meniscus are more commonly degenerative and typically occur in patients

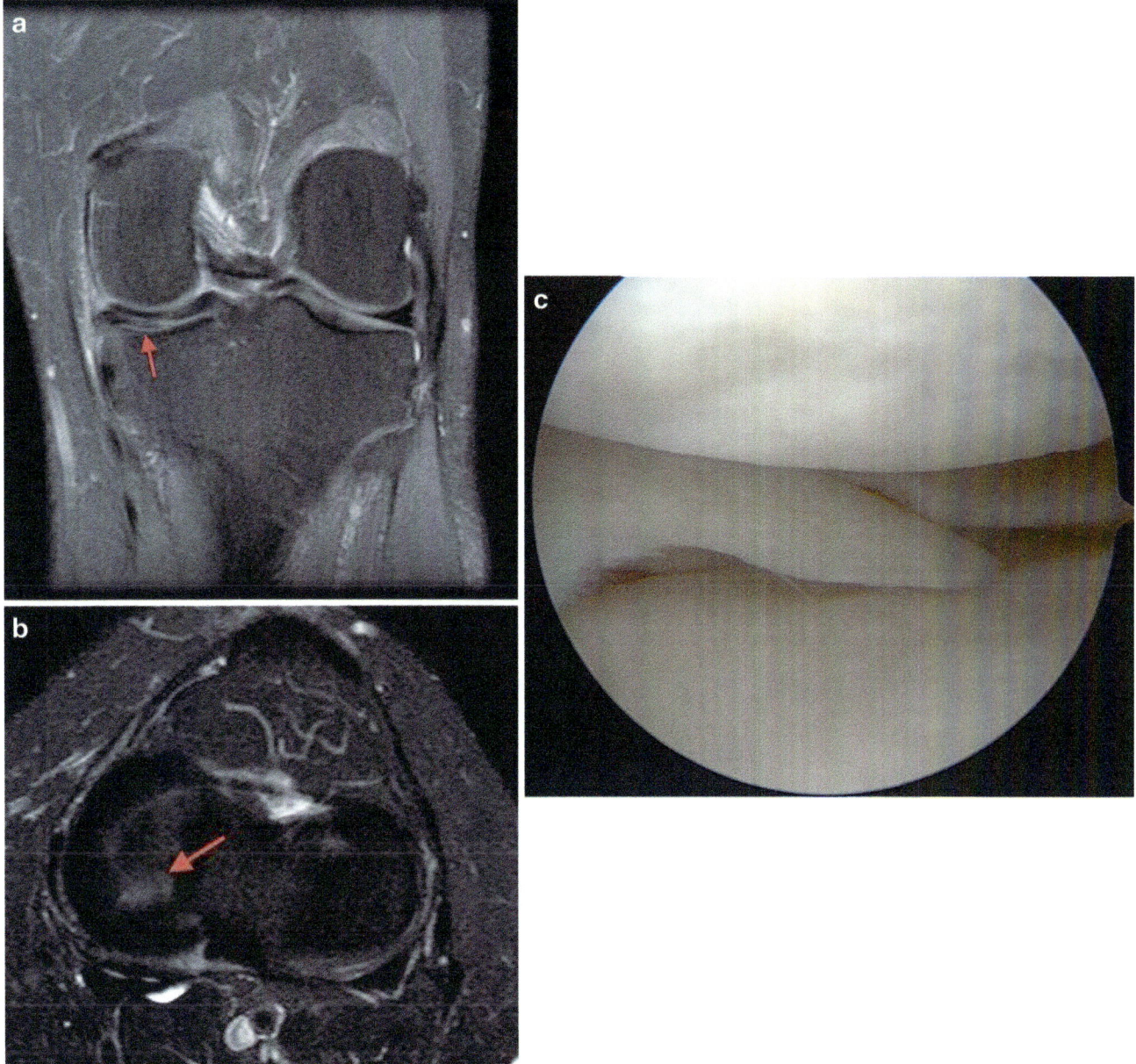

Fig. 3.8 Vertical flap (oblique) tear. (**a**) Coronal fat-suppressed T2 image shows radial component of the tear. (**b**) Axial fat-suppressed T2 image shows in detail the shape of the tear (*arrow*). (**c**) Arthroscopic image of the same patient demonstrates this vertical flap tear

older than 40, whereas posterior root tears of the lateral meniscus often are associated with ACL tears in younger patients [26, 38, 41].

On MRI, one must inspect both the coronal and sagittal images, carefully following the roots to their insertion. Because fluid dissects into many radial root tears, fluid-sensitive sequences are often the most helpful [11]. Radial root tears demonstrate a fluid cleft on coronal images and often exhibit a ghost meniscus on consecutive sagittal images, in which the posterior root is the normal black signal on one image and essentially invisible on the next (Fig. 3.11a–d) [12].

PRLM tears may show more abnormal signal than the typical cleft and ghost meniscus [26]. An increased signal in the PRLM may indicate a tear in patients younger than age 30 or who have a concomitant ACL tear; it may indicate synovitis and fraying in patients older than age 40 with degenerative changes and no injury [12].

The other cardinal sign of root tears, particularly of the posterior root of the medial meniscus, is extrusion [39]. Extrusion is defined as extension of the body of the meniscus more than 3 mm beyond the edge of the tibial plateau on a mid-coronal MRI (Fig. 3.12). However, extrusion is

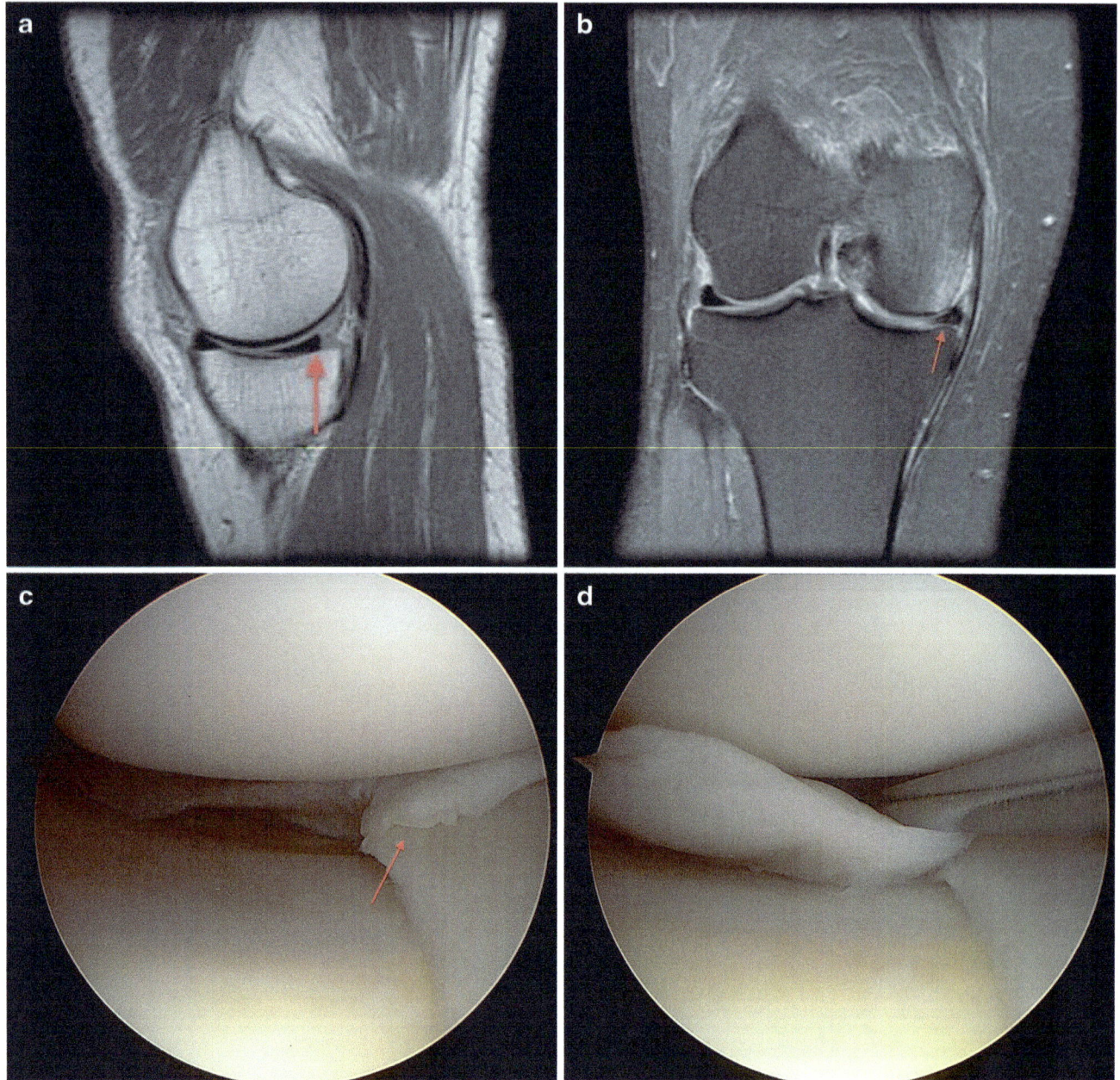

Fig. 3.9 Horizontal flap tear. (**a**) Sagittal PD image demonstrates a truncated, irregular appearance to the PHMM (*arrow*). (**b**) Coronal fat-suppressed T2 image shows truncated and abnormal medial meniscus (*arrow*). (**c**, **d**) Arthroscopic images demonstrate the displaced flap extending peripherally (*arrow*, **c**) followed by probing of the flap (**d**)

not a specific sign. Extrusion is also common in high-grade radial tears elsewhere in the meniscus, complex tears, and extensive chondrosis [42–44]. Extrusion is also seen with arthritis, particularly when standing X-rays demonstrate joint space narrowing of the affected compartment.

Secondary MRI Signs of Meniscal Tears

There are many secondary signs of a meniscus tear that can be noted on MRI. In patients with acute injuries, the presence of a tibial bone contusion directly underneath

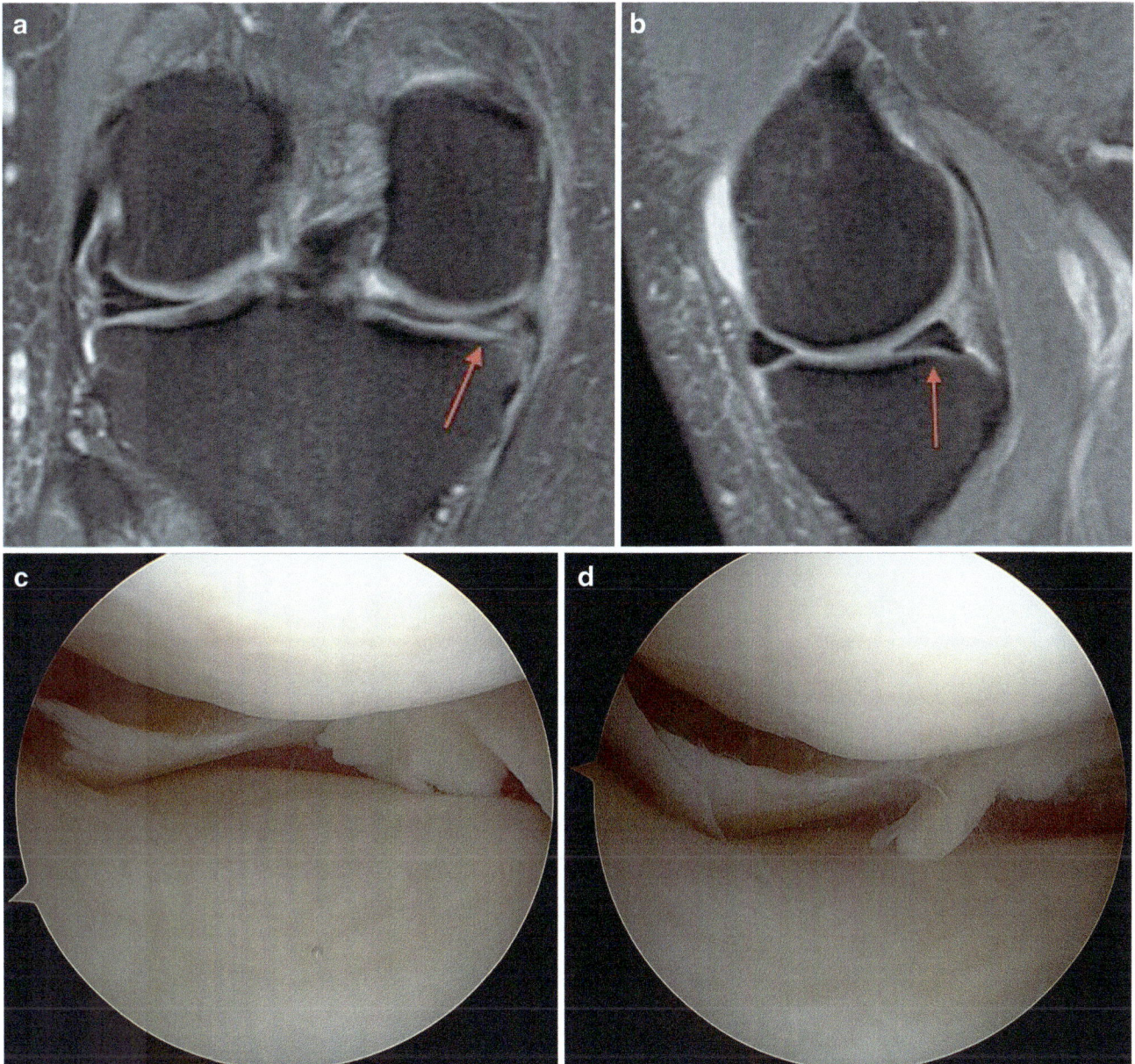

Fig. 3.10 Complex tear. (**a, b**) Coronal and sagittal fat-suppressed T2 images show horizontal and vertical components to this complex tear of the PHMM (*arrows*). (**c, d**) Arthroscopic image of this complex tear

the meniscus suggests an overlying meniscus tear [12] (Fig. 3.12). In a 1999 study, Kaplan and coworkers [45] found an MRI evidence of menisco-capsular separation or peripheral posterior horn meniscal tears overlying medial tibial contusions in 24 of 25 patients with ACL tears.

A parameniscal cyst is a contained fluid collection immediately adjacent to the peripheral rim of a meniscus. These cysts may indicate underlying meniscus tears, with joint fluid seeping through the tear to form cyst (Fig. 3.13a–d) [46].

Transverse Meniscal Ligament

Most menisci have a transverse meniscal ligament (geniculate ligament) attaching the anterior horns of the two menisci to each other. Where the transverse ligament attaches to the anterior horn of lateral meniscus, there may be a line of increased signal that may be confused for a meniscus tear. Recognizing the location and following the transverse ligament away from this site on sequential sagittal images help one not to mistake this normal attachment for a tear (Fig. 3.14a, b) [12].

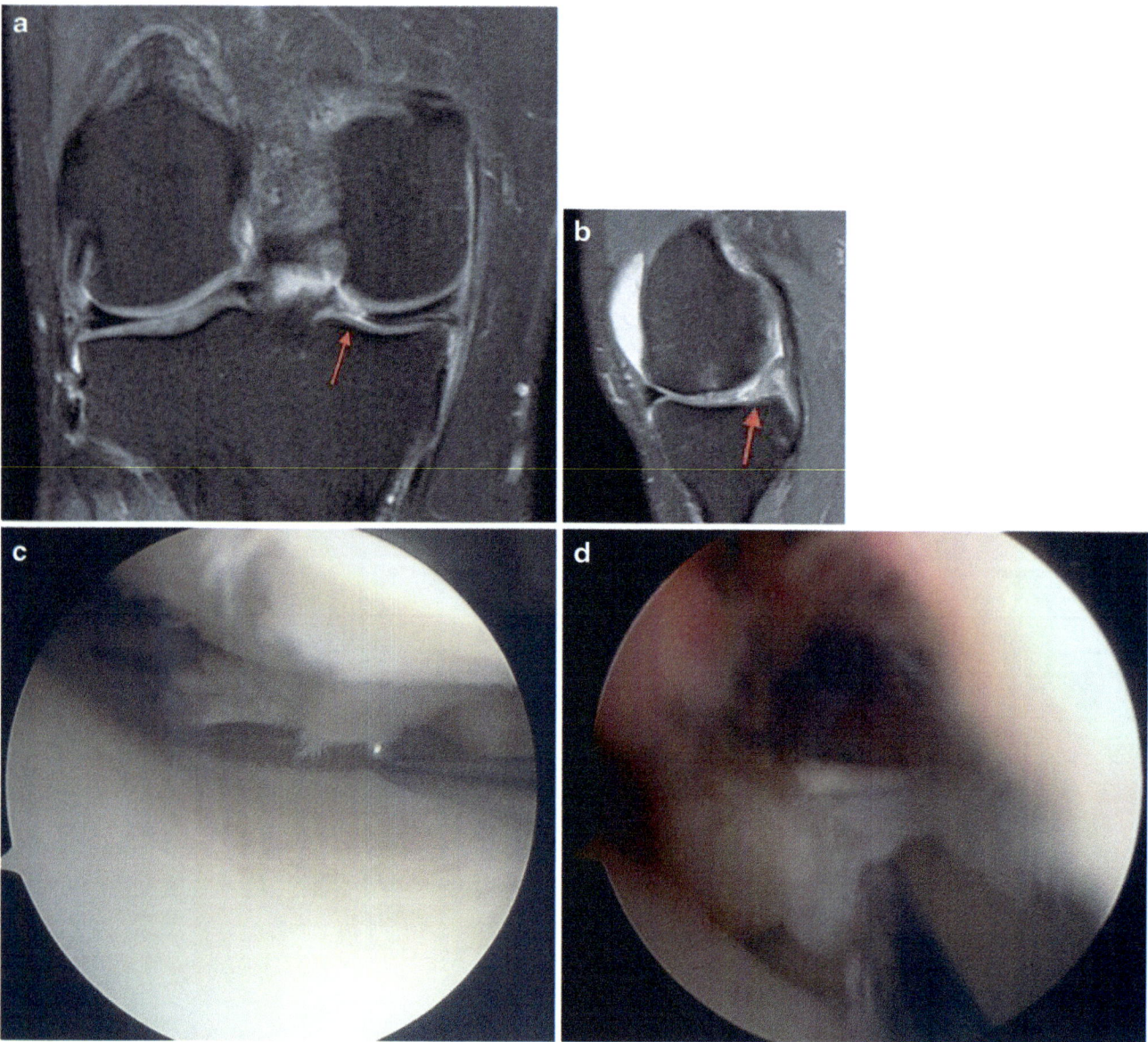

Fig. 3.11 Posterior root tear. (**a**) Coronal fat-suppressed T2 image demonstrates a radial tear of the root of the PHMM (*arrow*). (**b**) Sagittal fat-suppressed T2 image shows the ghost (absent) meniscus sign (*arrow*). (**c, d**) Arthroscopic image shows a probe adjacent to the root tear

Discoid Menisci

A discoid meniscus is elongated and thicker than a typical meniscus and extends farther toward the center of the joint than expected. Discoid menisci are more common in Japanese and Korean than Western populations and may be complete, like a slab; incomplete, in which they are enlarged but still somewhat triangular; or the rare Wrisberg variant, in which the dominant attachment is the meniscofemoral ligaments in lieu of a substantial tibial attachment [47]. Discoid menisci are approximately ten times more common laterally than medially [48, 49].

The simplest method to diagnose a discoid meniscus on MRI is to measure the shortest transverse width of the meniscal body on coronal images; when this is greater than 14 mm, the meniscus is characterized as discoid (Fig. 3.15a–c) [50]. On sagittal sequences, three or more "bow ties" also suggest a discoid meniscus [49]. The literature remains inconclusive as to whether MRI accuracy for tears of discoid meniscus is reduced relative to that in nondiscoid menisci. Although abnormal signal contacting the surface and morphologic irregularity has been highly predictive of tear for some [51], accuracy has been diminished in other studies [12, 48].

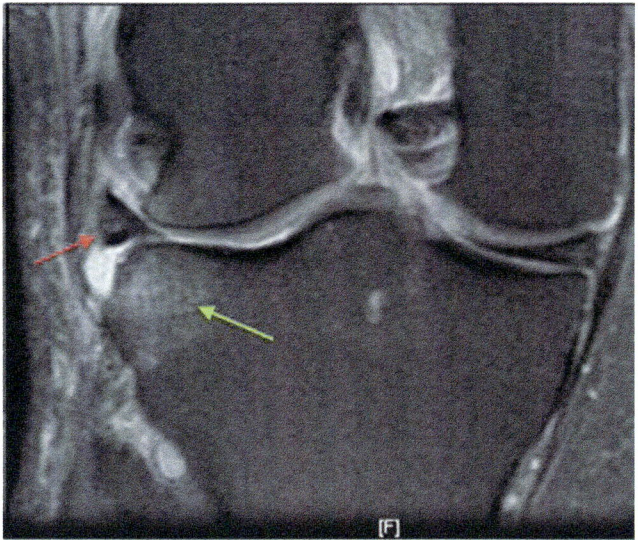

Fig. 3.12 Extruded meniscus. Coronal fat-suppressed T2 image shows extruded lateral meniscus (*red arrow*) along with underlying tibial bone contusion (*green arrow*)

Summary

There are multiple treatment options for meniscus tears. The treatment and outcome depend on multiple factors like tear pattern, displacement, and stability. The descriptions and images of meniscal tears on MRIs and the accompanying arthroscopy images will help physicians better recognize meniscus tears at imaging.

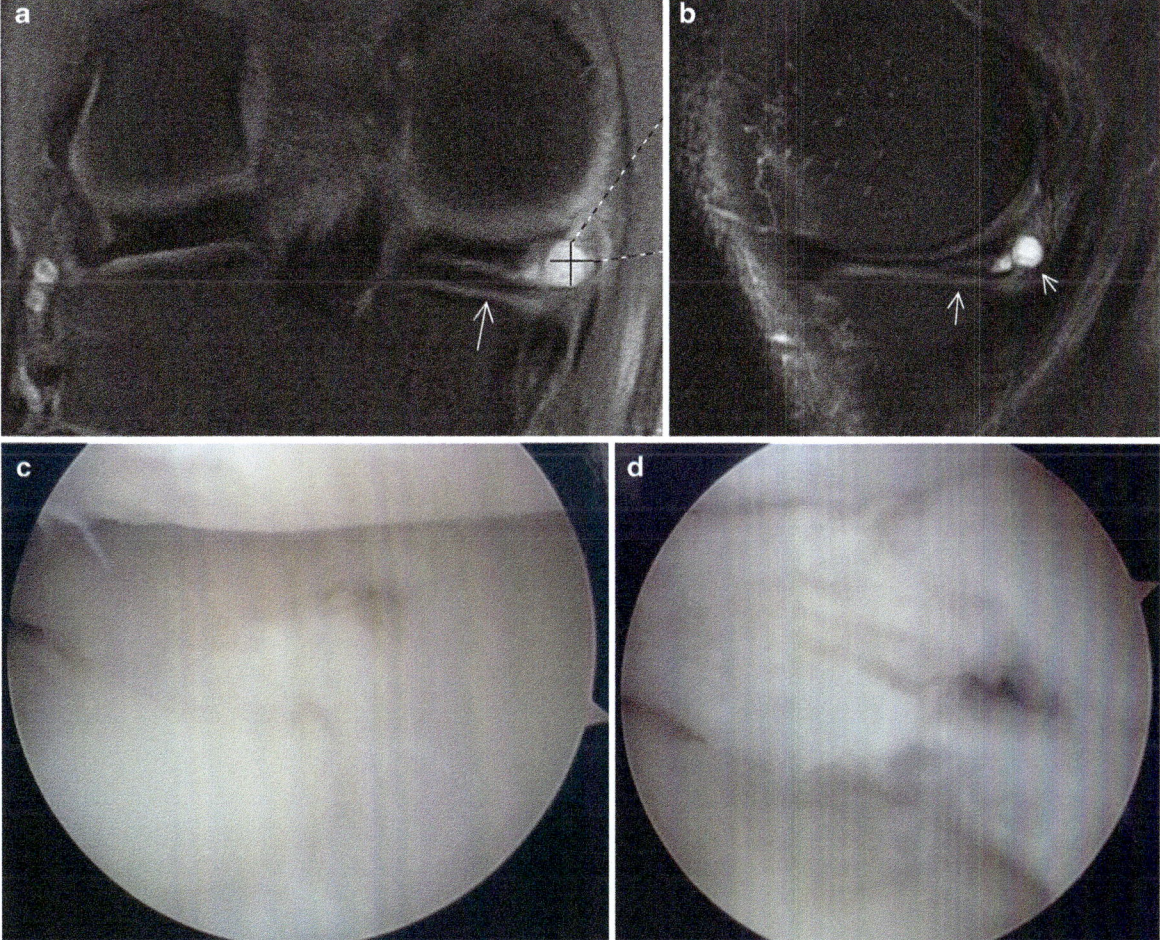

Fig. 3.13 Secondary sign: parameniscal cyst. Coronal fat-suppressed T2 (**a**) and sagittal fat-suppressed T2 (**b**) images demonstrate a horizontal tear of the PHMM (*solid* and *long arrow*) along with a high signal fluid collection (*dotted line* and *small arrow*) adjacent to the periphery of the meniscus, consistent with a parameniscal cyst. (**c**) Arthroscopic image showing the tear. (**d**) Arthroscopy picture after partial meniscectomy showing opening of the parameniscal cyst

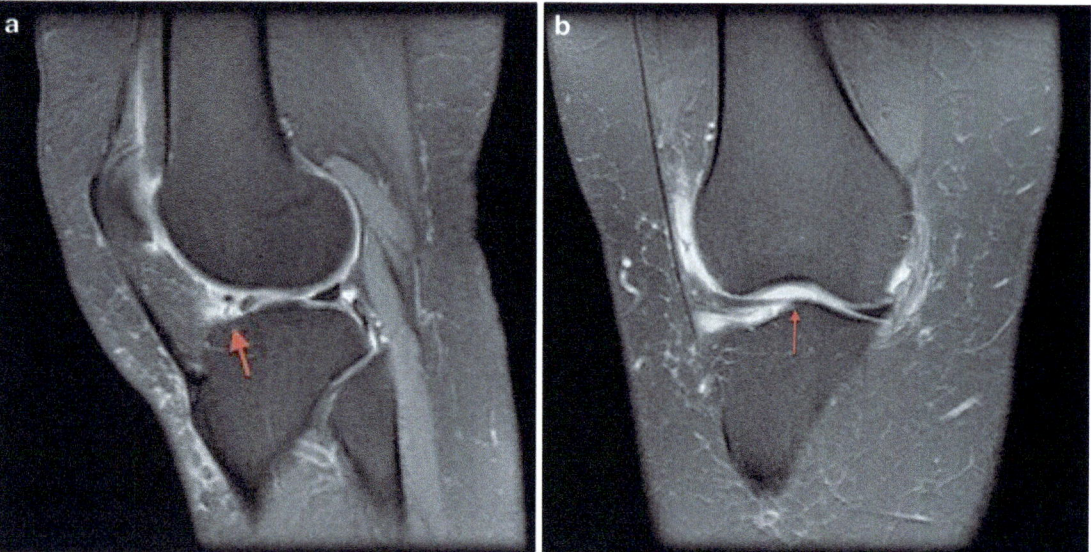

Fig. 3.14 (**a**, **b**) Sagittal and coronal fat-suppressed T2 images show the transverse meniscal ligament (*arrows*) which can sometimes be confused for lateral meniscus anterior horn tear

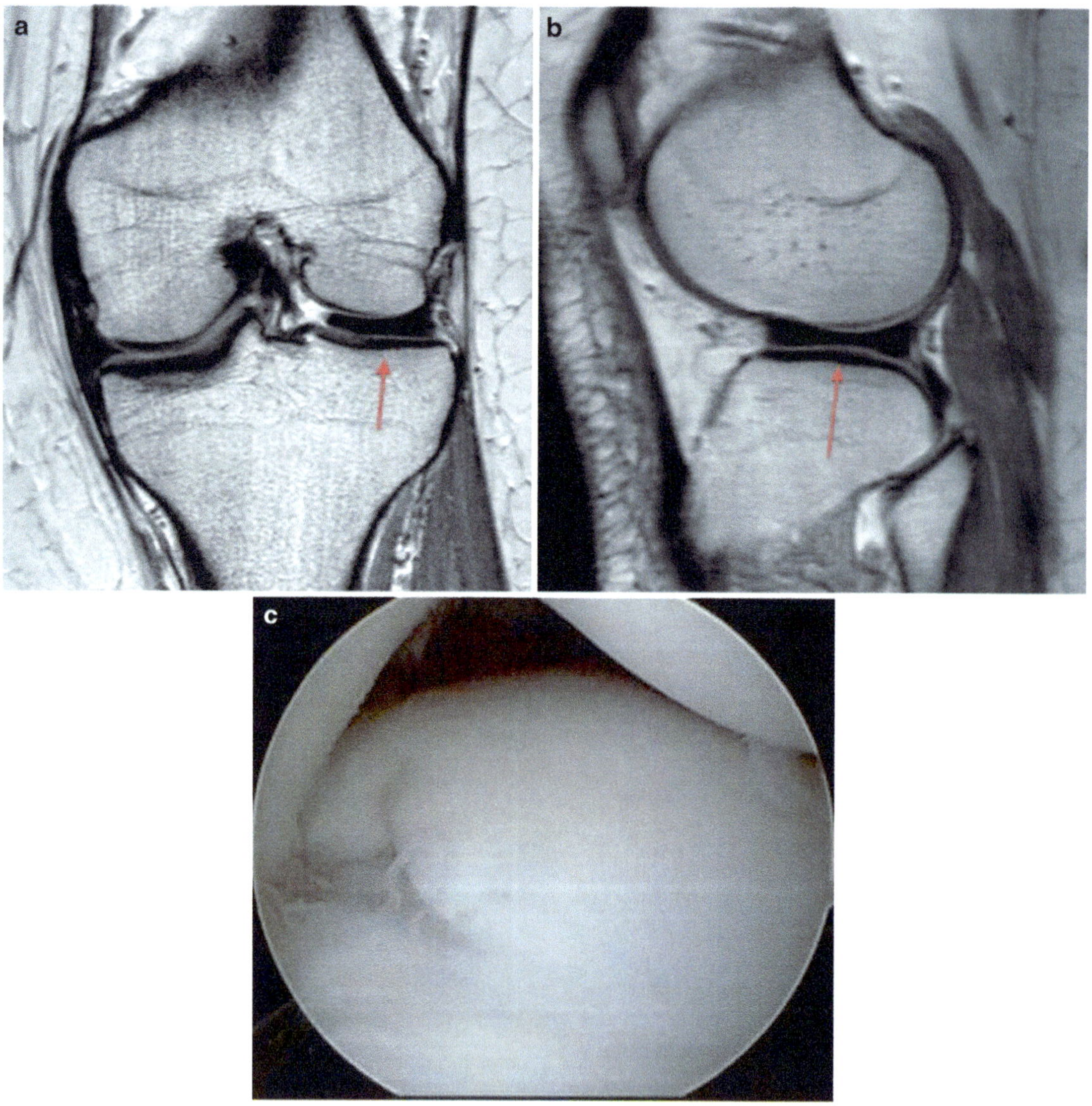

Fig. 3.15 Discoid menisci. Mid-coronal PD (**a**) and sagittal PD (**b**) images of a complete discoid lateral meniscus (type I) demonstrate the body of the lateral meniscus to be larger than typical (*arrows*). (**c**) Arthroscopic image shows to cover nearly the entire lateral tibial plateau

References

1. Higuchi H, Kimura M, Shirakura K, et al. Factors affecting long-term results after arthroscopic partial meniscectomy. Clin Orthop Relat Res. 2000;377:161–8.
2. Weinstabl R, Muellner T, Vecsei V, et al. Economic considerations for the diagnosis and therapy of meniscal lesions: can magnetic resonance imaging help reduce the expense? World J Surg. 1997;21(4):363–8.
3. McNally EG, Nasser KN, Dawson S, et al. Role of magnetic resonance imaging in the clinical management of the acutely locked knee. Skelet Radiol. 2002;31(10):570–3.
4. Elvenes J, Jerome CP, Reikeras O, et al. Magnetic resonance imaging as a screening procedure to avoid arthroscopy for meniscal tears. Arch Orthop Trauma Surg. 2000;120(1–2):14–6.
5. Feller JA, Webster KE. Clinical value of magnetic resonance imaging of the knee. ANZ J Surg. 2001;71(9):534–7.
6. Yan R, Wang H, Yang Z, et al. Predicted probability of meniscus tears: comparing history and physical examination with MRI. Swiss Med Wkly. 2011;141(w13314):1–7.
7. Tenuta JJ, Arciero RA. Arthroscopic evaluation of meniscal repairs. Factors that effect healing. Am J Sports Med. 1994;22(6):797–802.
8. Rath E, Richmond JC. The menisci: basic science and advances in treatment. Br J Sports Med. 2000;34(4):252–7.
9. Jee WH, McCauley TR, Kim JM, et al. Meniscal tear configurations: categorization with MR imaging. AJR Am J Roentgenol. 2003;180(1):93–7.
10. Nourissat G, Beaufils P, Charrois O, et al. Magnetic resonance imaging as a tool to predict reparability of longitudinal full-thickness meniscus lesions. Knee Surg Sports Traumatol Arthrosc. 2008;16(5):482–6.
11. Rosas HG, De Smet AA. Magnetic resonance imaging of the meniscus. Top Magn Reson Imaging. 2009;20(3):151–73.
12. De Smet AA. How I diagnose meniscal tears on knee MRI. AJR Am J Roentgenol. 2012;199(3):481–99.
13. Brody JM, Hulstyn MJ, Fleming BC, et al. The meniscal roots: gross anatomic correlation with 3-T MRI findings. AJR Am J Roentgenol. 2007;188(5):W446–50.
14. Kohn D, Moreno B. Meniscus insertion anatomy as a basis for meniscus replacement: a morphological cadaveric study. Arthroscopy. 1995;11(1):96–103.
15. Fox MG. MR imaging of the meniscus: review, current trends, and clinical implications. Magn Reson Imaging Clin N Am. 2007;15(1):103–23.
16. Huysse WC, Verstraete KL, Verdonk PC, et al. Meniscus imaging. Semin Musculoskelet Radiol. 2008;12(4):318–33.
17. Anderson MW. MR imaging of the meniscus. Radiol Clin N Am. 2002;40(5):1081–94.
18. Kaplan PA, Nelson NL, Garvin KL, et al. MR of the knee: the significance of high signal in the meniscus that does not clearly extend to the surface. AJR Am J Roentgenol. 1991;156(2):333–6.
19. De Smet AA, Norris MA, Yandow DR, et al. MR diagnosis of meniscal tears of the knee: importance of high signal in the meniscus that extends to the surface. AJR Am J Roentgenol. 1993; 161(1):101–7.
20. De Smet AA, Tuite MJ. Use of the "two-slice-touch" rule for the MRI diagnosis of meniscal tears. AJR Am J Roentgenol. 2006;187(4):911–4.
21. Oei EH, Nikken JJ, Verstijnen AC, et al. MR imaging of the menisci and cruciate ligaments: a systematic review. Radiology. 2003; 226(3):837–48.
22. Sampson MJ, Jackson MP, Moran CJ, et al. Three Tesla MRI for the diagnosis of meniscal and anterior cruciate ligament pathology: a comparison to arthroscopic findings. Clin Radiol. 2008;63(10): 1106–11.
23. Magee T, Williams D. Detection of meniscal tears and marrow lesions using coronal MRI. AJR Am J Roentgenol. 2004; 183(5):1469–73.
24. Gokalp G, Nas OF, Demirag B, et al. Contribution of thin-slice (1 mm) axial proton density MR images for identification and classification of meniscal tears: correlative study with arthroscopy. Br J Radiol. 2012;85:e871–8.
25. Anderson AF, Irrgang JJ, Dunn W, et al. Interobserver reliability of the International Society of Arthroscopy, Knee Surgery and Orthopaedic Sports Medicine (ISAKOS) classification of meniscal tears. Am J Sports Med. 2011;39(5):926–32.
26. De Smet AA, Blankenbaker DG, Kijowski R, et al. MR diagnosis of posterior root tears of the lateral meniscus using arthroscopy as the reference standard. AJR Am J Roentgenol. 2009;192(2):480–6.
27. Rao N, Patel Y, Opsha O, et al. Use of the V-sign in the diagnosis of bucket-handle meniscal tear of the knee. Skelet Radiol. 2012; 41(3):293–7.
28. Sparacia G, Barbiera F, Bartolotta TV, et al. Pitfalls and limitations of magnetic resonance imaging in bucket-handle tears of knee menisci. Radiol Med. 2002;104(3):150–6.
29. Magee TH, Hinson GW. MRI of meniscal bucket-handle tears. Skelet Radiol. 1998;27(9):495–9.
30. Dorsay TA, Helms CA. Bucket-handle meniscal tears of the knee: sensitivity and specificity of MRI signs. Skelet Radiol. 2003; 32(5):266–72.
31. Ververidis AN, Verettas DA, Kazakos KJ, et al. Meniscal bucket handle tears: a retrospective study of arthroscopy and the relation to MRI. Knee Surg Sports Traumatol Arthrosc. 2006;14(4):343–9.
32. Ruff C, Weingardt JP, Russ PD, et al. MR imaging patterns of displaced meniscus injuries of the knee. AJR Am J Roentgenol. 1998;170(1):63–7.
33. Harper KW, Helms CA, Lambert III HS, et al. Radial meniscal tears: significance, incidence, and MR appearance. AJR Am J Roentgenol. 2005;185(6):1429–34.
34. Magee T, Shapiro M, Williams D. MR accuracy and arthroscopic incidence of meniscal radial tears. Skelet Radiol. 2002;31(12):686–9.
35. Lecas LK, Helms CA, Kosarek FJ, et al. Inferiorly displaced flap tears of the medial meniscus: MR appearance and clinical significance. AJR Am J Roentgenol. 2000;174(1):161–4.
36. Vande Berg BC, Malghem J, Poilvache P, et al. Meniscal tears with fragments displaced in notch and recesses of knee: MR imaging with arthroscopic comparison. Radiology. 2005; 234(3):842–50.
37. McKnight A, Southgate J, Price A, et al. Meniscal tears with displaced fragments: common patterns on magnetic resonance imaging. Skelet Radiol. 2010;39(3):279–83.
38. Brody JM, Lin HM, Hulstyn MJ, et al. Lateral meniscus root tear and meniscus extrusion with anterior cruciate ligament tear. Radiology. 2006;239(3):805–10.
39. Ozkoc G, Circi E, Gonc U, et al. Radial tears in the root of the posterior horn of the medial meniscus. Knee Surg Sports Traumatol Arthrosc. 2008;16(9):849–54.
40. Lee YG, Shim JC, Choi YS, et al. Magnetic resonance imaging findings of surgically proven medial meniscus root tear: tear configuration and associated knee abnormalities. J Comput Assist Tomogr. 2008;32(3):452–7.
41. Koenig JH, Ranawat AS, Umans HR, et al. Meniscal root tears: diagnosis and treatment. Arthroscopy. 2009;25(9):1025–32.
42. Choi CJ, Choi YJ, Lee JJ, et al. Magnetic resonance imaging evidence of meniscal extrusion in medial meniscus posterior root tear. Arthroscopy. 2010;26(12):1602–6.

43. Lerer DB, Umans HR, Hu MX, et al. The role of meniscal root pathology and radial meniscal tear in medial meniscal extrusion. Skelet Radiol. 2004;33(10):569–74.

44. Costa CR, Morrison WB, Carrino JA. Medial meniscus extrusion on knee MRI: is extent associated with severity of degeneration or type of tear? AJR Am J Roentgenol. 2004; 183(1):17–23.

45. Kaplan PA, Gehl RH, Dussault RG, et al. Bone contusions of the posterior lip of the medial tibial plateau (contrecoup injury) and associated internal derangements of the knee at MR imaging. Radiology. 1999;211(3):747–53.

46. De Smet AA, Graf BK, del Rio AM. Association of parameniscal cysts with underlying meniscal tears as identified on MRI and arthroscopy. AJR Am J Roentgenol. 2011;196(2):W180–6.

47. Kim YG, Ihn JC, Park SK, et al. An arthroscopic analysis of lateral meniscal variants and a comparison with MRI findings. Knee Surg Sports Traumatol Arthrosc. 2006;14(1):20–6.

48. Ryu KN, Kim IS, Kim EJ, et al. MR imaging of tears of discoid lateral menisci. AJR Am J Roentgenol. 1998;171(4):963–7.

49. Rohren EM, Kosarek FJ, Helms CA. Discoid lateral meniscus and the frequency of meniscal tears. Skelet Radiol. 2001;30(6):316–20.

50. Araki Y, Yamamoto H, Nakamura H, et al. MR diagnosis of discoid lateral menisci of the knee. Eur J Radiol. 1994; 18(2):92–5.

51. Yoo WJ, Lee K, Moon HJ, et al. Meniscal morphologic changes on magnetic resonance imaging are associated with symptomatic discoid lateral meniscal tear in children. Arthroscopy. 2012; 28(3):330–6.

Chondral Lesions

Brian C. Domby, Richard B. Williams, and Eric C. McCarty

Introduction

Articular cartilage damage is a common cause of disability in the knee. Damage to the articular cartilage can span from isolated chondral defects to diffuse cartilage loss and osteoarthritis. Articular cartilage is composed of type II (hyaline) cartilage. Cartilage is avascular and lacks ability to heal on its own. Extension of the lesion through the subchondral plate can stimulate bleeding, infiltration of marrow cells, and a fibrocartilaginous healing response. However, this fibrocartilage is predominately type I collagen and has inferior wear characteristics to organized type II hyaline cartilage [1]. Lesions that do not penetrate to subchondral plate lack a healing response unless something is done to stimulate healing [2].

The most commonly used classification system for articular cartilage injury is the Outerbridge classification. Grade 0 is normal cartilage. Grade I is softening and swelling of the cartilage. Grade II is partial-thickness defect with fissures that do not extend to subchondral bone. Grade III is fissures that extend to subchondral bone. Grade IV is exposed subchondral bone.

Patients with articular cartilage lesions often present with activity-related pain and swelling. This pain is typically isolated to a compartment of the knee and they may also have mechanical symptoms. They may walk with an antalgic gait and have an effusion. Tenderness along the joint line or in the affected compartment is typically present. Concomitant malalignment of the limb and ligamentous instability may also be present and must be addressed if present [2]. Patellar instability is a common cause of patellar articular cartilage injury.

Imaging of the knee should include anteroposterior weight-bearing, Rosenberg (45° flexion posteroanterior), lateral, and axial view of the patella (Merchant or Skyline). Full-length standing hip-to-ankle images should be acquired to quantify malalignment [2]. Advanced imaging with magnetic resonance imaging (MRI) should be done to evaluate the articular cartilage and subchondral bone and to assess for concomitant meniscus and ligamentous injuries or deficiencies. However, the accuracy of MRI in predicting the size of the lesion has been questioned and has been found to underestimate the size of the lesion [3, 4].

Nonoperative treatment options for articular cartilage defects in the knee include weight loss, physical therapy, exercise, bracing, injections (corticosteroid and viscosupplementation), activity modification, and anti-inflammatories.

Operative treatment is considered if nonoperative treatment measures fail. Techniques can be divided into conventional and advanced techniques. Conventional techniques include debridement (chondroplasty) and marrow-stimulating techniques. Marrow-stimulating techniques include abrasion chondroplasty, drilling, and microfracture. These techniques penetrate the subchondral plate and invoke a bleeding response and extravasation of bone marrow elements to form a clot in the defect. This clot remodels to a fibrocartilaginous tissue which has inferior wear characteristics to normal type II hyaline cartilage [2, 5].

Advanced cartilage repair techniques can be divided into cartilage restoration procedures and cartilage replacement. Cartilage restoration procedures include autologous chondrocyte implantation (ACI), matrix-associated ACI (MACI), and juvenile allogeneic cartilage (DeNovo). Cartilage replacement techniques include osteochondral autograft

B.C. Domby, MD (✉) • R.B. Williams, MD
Department of Orthopedics, Sports Medicine, University
of Colorado Hospital, Boulder, CO, USA
e-mail: bdomby@gmail.com; Richard.williams@ucdenver.edu

E.C. McCarty, MD
Department of Orthopedics, Sports Medicine, University
of Colorado Hospital, Boulder, CO, USA

Department of Orthopedics, University of Colorado School
of Medicine, Boulder, CO, USA

Department of Integrative Physiology, University of Colorado,
Boulder, CO, USA

Department of Athletics, University of Colorado,
Boulder, CO, USA
e-mail: Eric.mccarty@ucdenver.edu

transfer and osteochondral allograft transfer. The type of cartilage procedure chosen depends on many factors including the size of the lesion, condition of the underlying bone, location of the lesion, prior procedures performed, and expectations of the patient.

This chapter will utilize a case-based format to demonstrate the correlation between MRI and arthroscopy for articular cartilage lesions of the knee. Diagnosis and management of each patient will be discussed for each case. Seven cases will be presented, including:

1. Grade II and IV femoral condyle lesion treated with microfracture
2. Grade IV femoral condyle lesion treated with osteochondral autograft transplantation (OATS)/mosaicplasty
3. Nontraditional, unstable osteochondritis dissecans (OCD) of the knee treated with arthroscopic fixation
4. Traditional, unstable osteochondritis dissecans (OCD) of the knee treated with open fixation
5. Grade II–III femoral condyle lesion after failed chondroplasty treated with osteochondral allograft
6. Grade IV femoral condyle lesion with deficient bone treated with osteochondral allograft
7. Grade IV patella lesion treated with ACI

Case 1: Grade II and IV Femoral Condyle Lesion Treated with Microfracture

History/Exam

A 19-year-old male collegiate football player reported to the orthopedic clinic reporting a one-week history of right knee pain and swelling. The pain was located along the medial and lateral joint line. He did not recall any specific traumatic events. Symptoms worsened as the season progressed, as did the swelling. He had occasional clicking in association with the pain. He denied any catching, locking, or instability.

On physical examination the right knee was found to have intact skin without any erythema or warmth. There was a moderate-sized effusion. There was tenderness along the medial and lateral joint line. McMurray test was mildly positive. The knee was stable to varus and valgus stress. Lachman's, anterior drawer, and posterior drawer were negative.

Imaging

Magnetic resonance imaging was obtained to further evaluate the meniscus and chondral surfaces. A full complement of images was obtained. The technique used included fat-suppressed, fast T2-weighted images acquired axially, sagittally, and coronally, as well as T1-weighted sagittal images.

A full-thickness chondral defect measuring 8 mm involving the posterior weight-bearing aspect of the lateral femoral condyle was identified. There was mild bone marrow edema associated with the chondral defect, demonstrated in Fig. 4.1a–c. The medial meniscus and lateral meniscus were intact. All ligamentous structures were intact. Of note, the medial femoral condyle had increased signal on T2 images. However, the chondral surfaces of the medial compartment were intact.

The patient had continued symptoms at the end of the season, particularly lateral joint line pain and swelling. Given the MRI findings of a full-thickness chondral defect involving the lateral femoral condyle, surgical treatment was discussed. After reviewing the risks and benefits, the patient elected to pursue a diagnostic arthroscopy and likely microfracture of the chondral defect.

Arthroscopy

The patient was taken to the operating room and placed in the supine position. A standard diagnostic arthroscopy of the right knee was performed. Multiple small chondral loose bodies were identified, measuring <2 mm, demonstrated in Fig. 4.2a, b. A small, focal grade IV chondral defect was identified involving the lateral femoral condyle. It measured 4 mm in size and was surrounded by an approximate 4 mm rim of mild grade II chondral changes, seen in Fig. 4.2c. Finally, there was a small horizontal cleavage tear involving the lateral meniscus, which was flipped into the femoral notch, demonstrated in Fig. 4.3a, b. These arthroscopic findings of the chondral defect correlated nicely with the MRI findings.

The small chondral loose bodies were removed with a 4.0 mm arthroscopic shaver without difficulty. The horizontal cleavage tear involving the lateral meniscus was addressed with a partial meniscectomy using the arthroscopic biters and shaver, shown in Fig. 4.3c. Finally, the chondral defect of the lateral femoral condyle was addressed. The cartilage defect was debrided down to the subchondral bone. Care was taken to maintain stable shoulders around the defect. A microfracture awl was then used to penetrate the subchondral bone. The arthroscopic fluid flow was turned off, and bleeding from the microfracture holes was confirmed, seen in Fig. 4.4a, b.

Case 2: Grade IV Femoral Condyle Lesion Treated with Osteochondral Autograft Transplantation (OATS)/Mosaicplasty

History/Exam

A 33-year-old male presented with a 6-month history of waxing and waning left knee pain. He initially experienced pain when he hyperextended his knee while

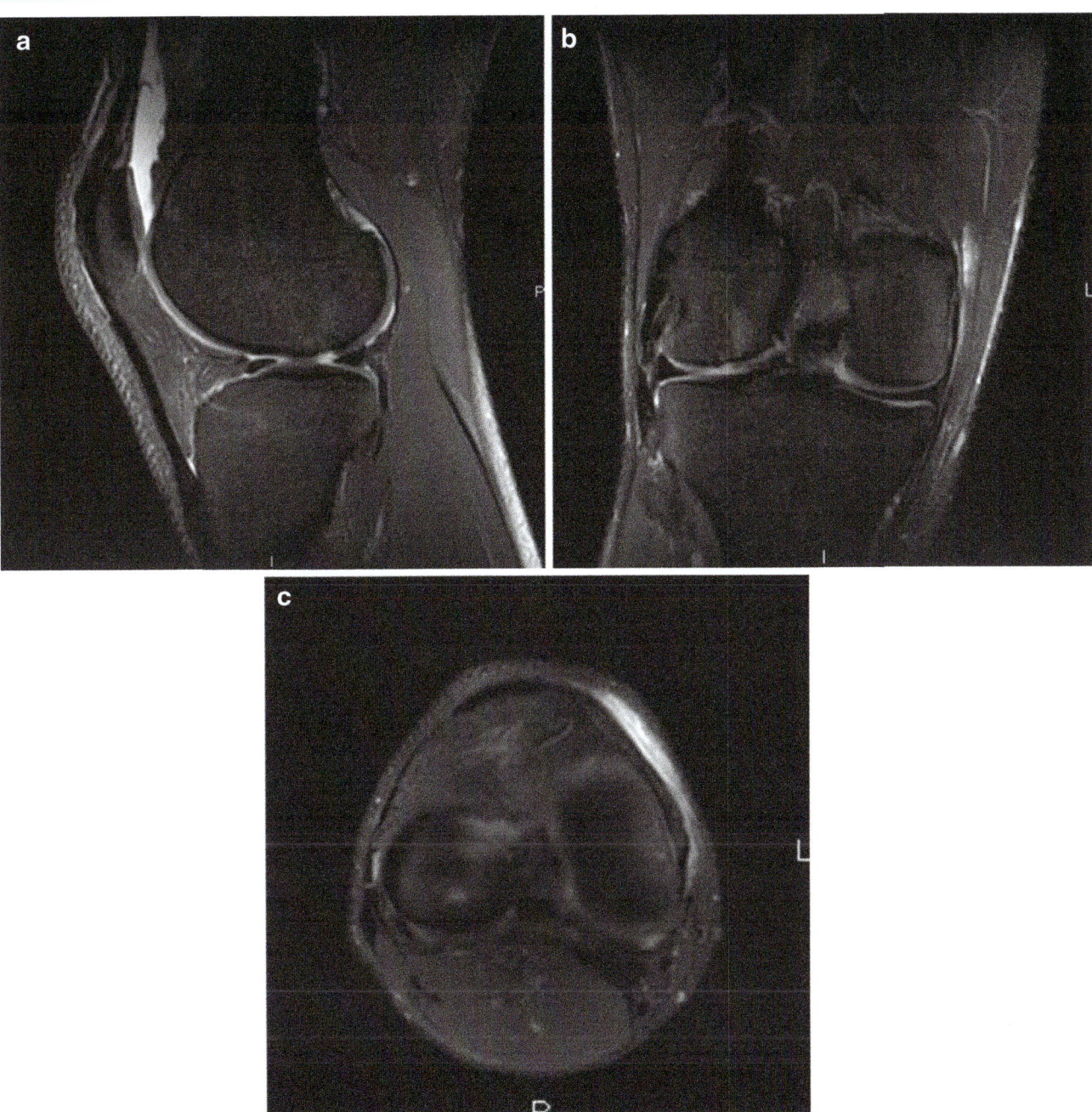

Fig. 4.1 (**a**)–(**c**) Select sagittal, coronal, and axial T2 images from a 3-T MRI of the right knee without contrast. A contained grade IV lesion measuring approximately 8 mm involving the lateral femoral condyle. There is a small amount of signal within the underlying bone without any cyst formation or bone loss

removing an engine block from an automobile. He felt a pop in his knee and developed laterally based pain and an effusion within hours of the injury. He treated the knee conservatively and had a resolution of his pain and effusion. However, as these symptoms resolved, he began to develop a sense of instability. One instability event leads to another hyperextension event with sharp lateral pain and effusion development. His lateral pain, effusions, and instability have continued since the second hyperextension injury.

On physical examination the left knee was found to have intact skin with no erythema or warmth. There was a moderate-sized effusion. The knee was tender along the lateral joint line. Active range of motion was noted to be 15°–90° of flexion. Passively, the knee's range of motion improved to 10°–100°. Pain was recreated laterally with deep flexion. McMurray testing produced a lateral catch and pain. The knee was stable to varus and valgus stress. The Lachman's, anterior drawer, and posterior drawer were negative. The remainder of the extremity was neurovascularly intact.

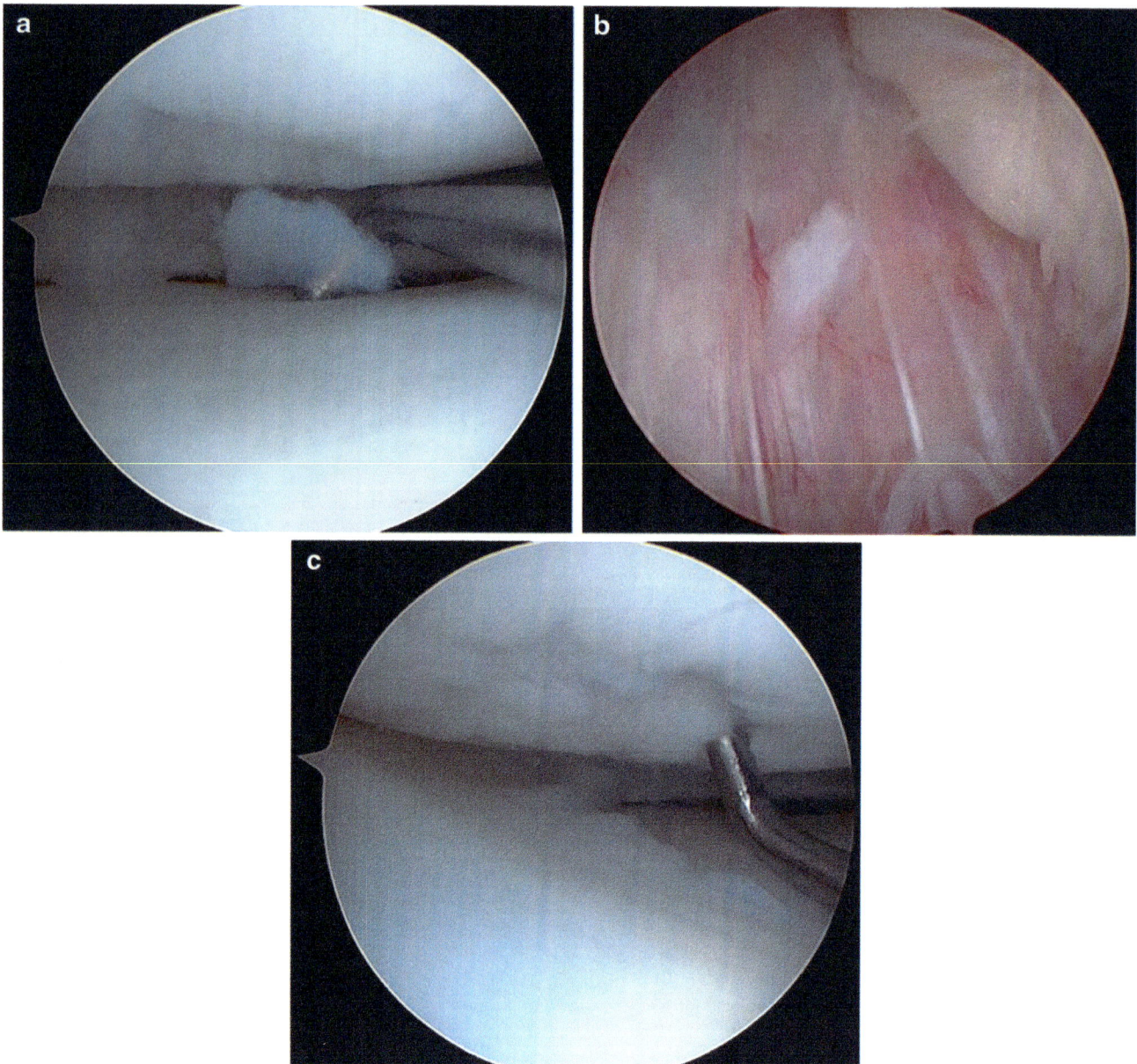

Fig. 4.2 (a)–(c) Two arthroscopic views demonstrating loose chondral pieces measuring 2–4 mm. A chondral defect involving the lateral femoral condyle measuring approximately 8 mm

Imaging

Plain radiographs of the left knee demonstrated well-maintained joint spaces on the AP and Rosenberg views. No lucencies were identified on AP or lateral views, as shown in Fig. 4.5a, b.

Magnetic resonance imaging was obtained to further evaluate the meniscus and chondral surfaces. A full complement of images was obtained. The technique used included fat-suppressed, fast T2-weighted images acquired axially, sagittally, and coronally, as well as T1-weighted sagittal images.

The MRI demonstrated bone marrow edema involving the posterolateral femoral condyle. The cartilage overlying this area of bony edema had a notable signal abnormality on T2 images. There was a linear band of signal intensity at the interface between the cartilage and subchondral bone, which was suggestive of a delamination or flap. The area of delamination measured approximately 1.4 cm in the anterior to posterior dimension. A small joint effusion was present, demonstrated in Fig. 4.6a, b. The remainder of the MRI was normal.

Given the patient's continued lateral pain and effusion, arthroscopy and possible cartilage procedure were discussed.

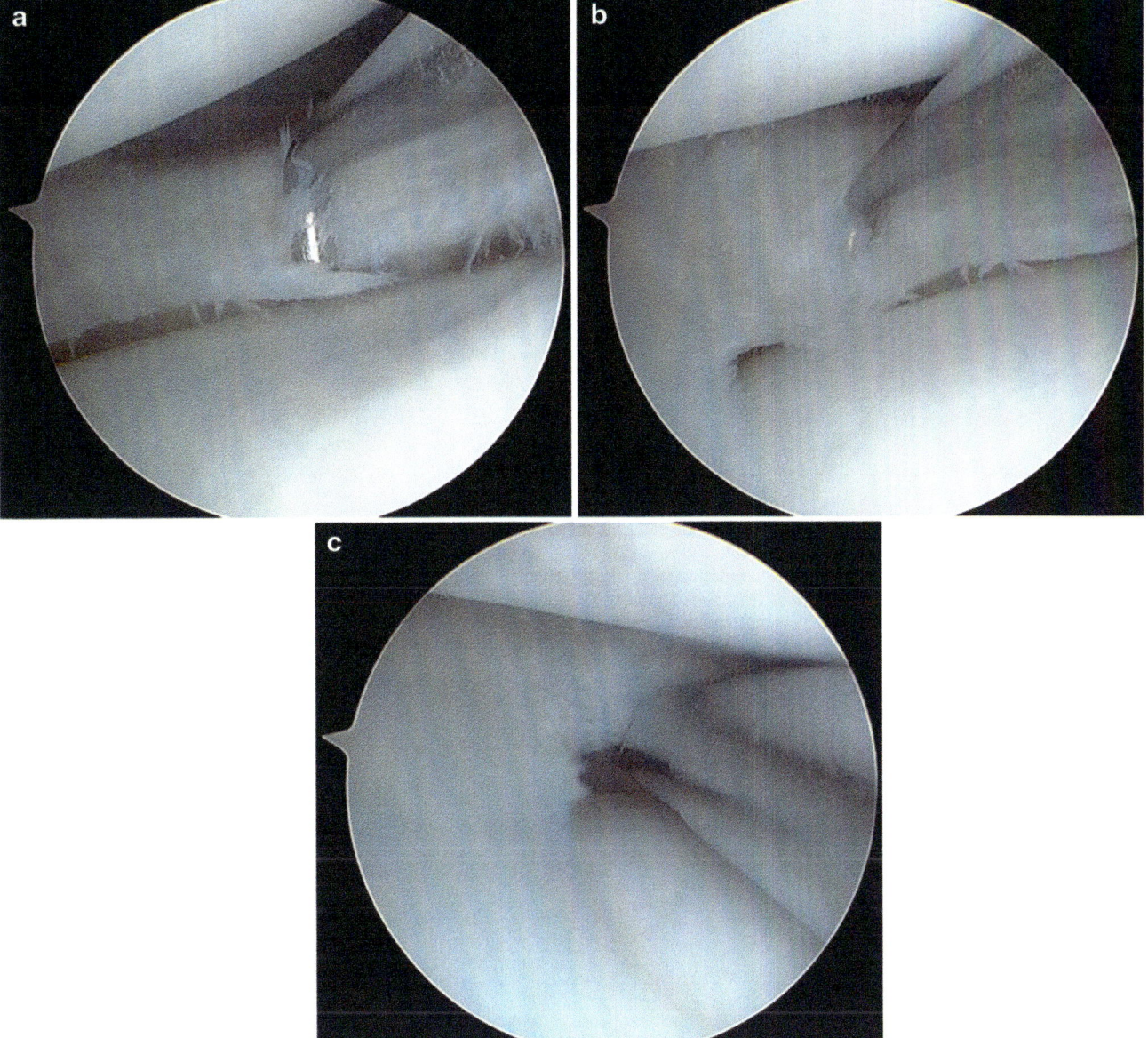

Fig. 4.3 (**a**)–(**c**) Two arthroscopic views depicting the horizontal cleavage tear involving the lateral meniscus. There was an unstable flap component that could be displaced into the joint with an arthroscopic probe. The tear was debrided with a 4.0 mm arthroscopic shaver

After reviewing the risks and benefits of surgery, the patient decided to proceed with surgery.

Arthroscopy

The patient was taken to the operating room and placed in the supine position. A standard diagnostic arthroscopy of the right knee was performed. A grade IV chondral defect with an overlying flap of cartilage was found involving the lateral femoral condyle with the knee flexed to 45°. It measured 9 mm in the medial to lateral dimension and 15 mm in the anterior to posterior dimension. It was slightly narrower at its most anterior portion, demonstrated in Fig. 4.7a, b. This correlated to the MRI images.

The defect was debrided down to the subchondral bone with an arthroscopic shaver and sized with the osteochondral autograft transplantation system, as shown in Fig. 4.8a–c. It was decided to use the superomedial aspect of the trochlea as the donor sight for the osteochondral autograft. Two donor plugs were harvested from this region, measuring 10×14 mm and 6×14 mm, respectively. The transplant site was then prepared by removing a 10×12 mm and 6×12 mm core of bone. The 10×4 mm donor plug was then placed into the corresponding hole followed by the 6×14 mm donor plug, demonstrated in Fig. 4.9a–c.

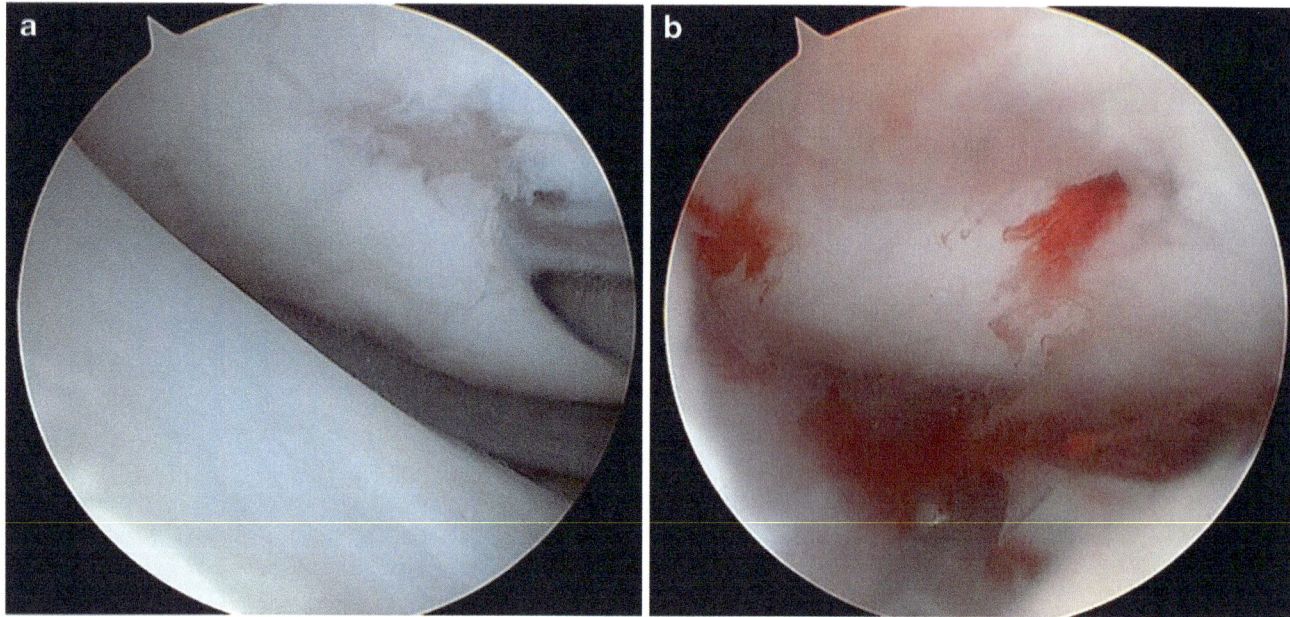

Fig. 4.4 (**a, b**) Arthroscopic views of the chondral lesion after debridement to stable shoulders showed that the area of grade IV changes was 4 mm with a surrounding 4 mm ring of grade II changes. An arthroscopic awl was used to perform a microfracture. When flow was turned off, there was bleeding from the microfracture holes

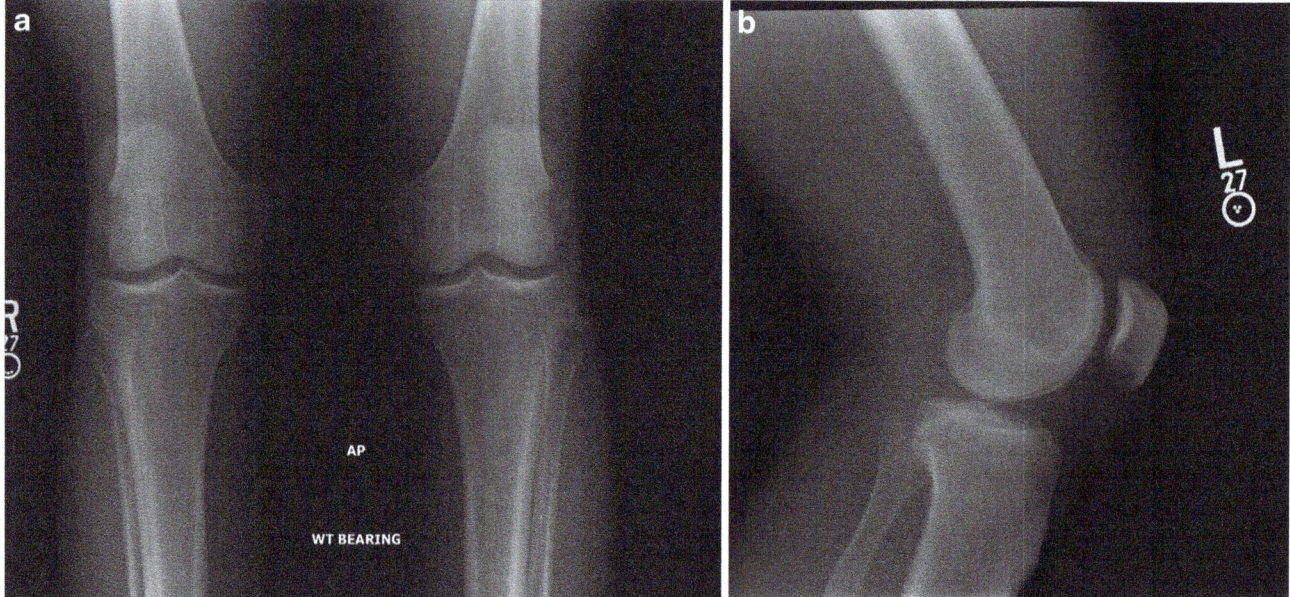

Fig. 4.5 (**a, b**) AP and lateral views of the left knee showing well-maintained joint spaces with no lucencies

Discussion for Microfracture and OATS/Mosaicplasty

Cartilage lesions are evident on both T1 and T2 MR sequencing. These lesions can appear as cartilage thinning, fissuring, or full-thickness defects. The full-thickness defects are easily identified on T2 imaging, as the defect will fill with joint fluid. This shows up as a bright white signal within the cartilage defect extending to the black layer of the subchondral bone. Depending on how long the defect has been present, its size, and the overall limb alignment, the underlying bone may have white signal within it on T2-weighted images signifying bony edema.

During arthroscopy, cartilage lesions will present in many different ways. The Outerbridge classification helps to define the severity of these defects. Grade I chondral changes

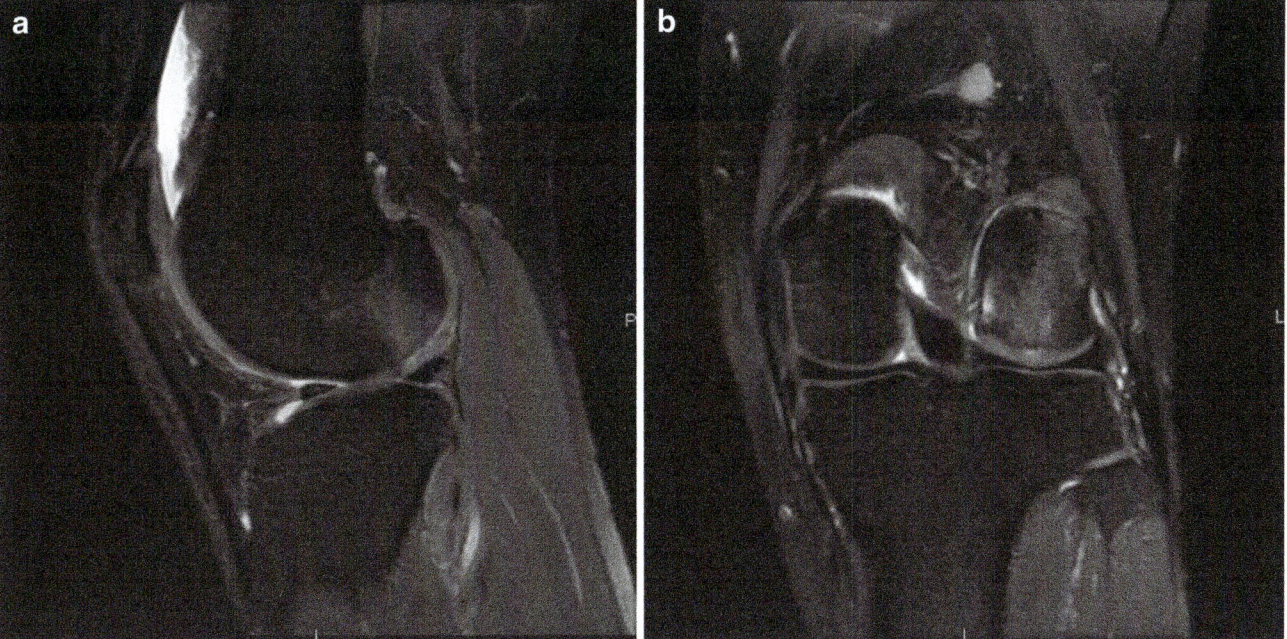

Fig. 4.6 (**a**, **b**) Select sagittal and coronal T2 views of the left knee with a 3-T MRI without contrast. They demonstrate a chondral lesion involving the posterior portion of the lateral femoral condyle. There is fluid signal between the cartilage and underlying subchondral bone, suggesting a flap-type configuration to the chondral lesion. The lesion measures 15 mm in the AP dimension and 9 mm in the medial to lateral dimension. There is also signal within the bone without cyst formation or bone loss

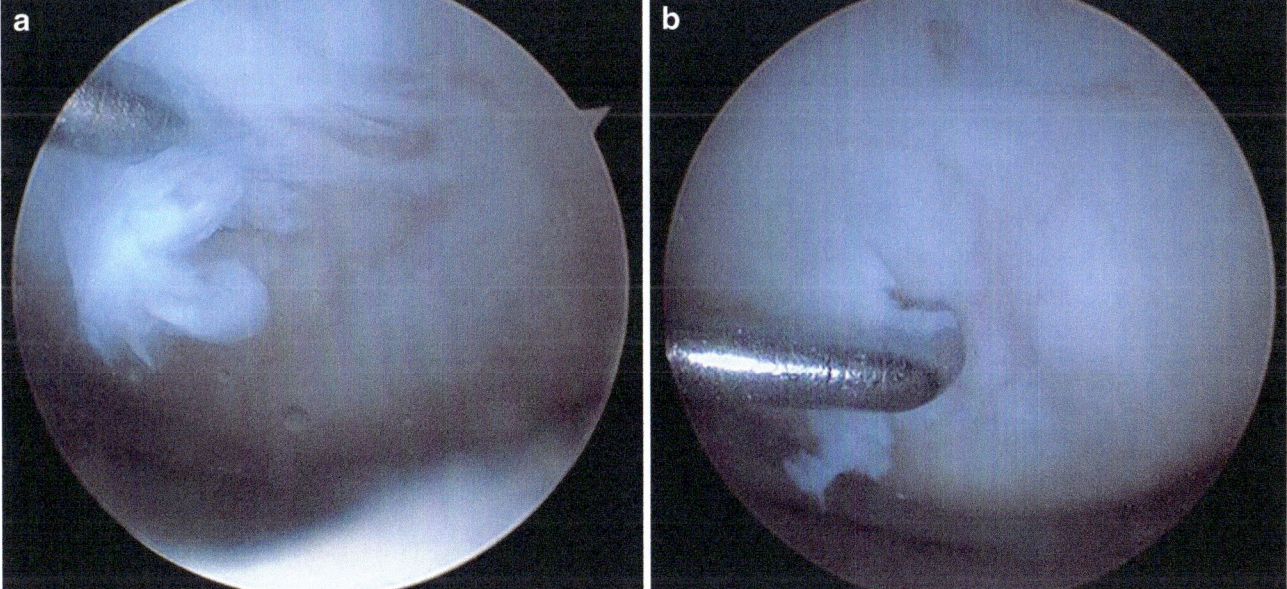

Fig. 4.7 (**a**, **b**) Arthroscopic views showing a large flap lesion of the posterior portion of the lateral femoral condyle with the knee flexed to 45°

present as cartilage softening and/or blistering. Grade II chondral changes appear as mild thinning of the cartilage and possible fissuring. The fissures do not extend down to the subchondral bone. Grade III chondral changes present as cartilage thinning and fissuring that extends all the way to the subchondral bone. Finally, grade IV changes appear as full-thickness cartilage defects that extend to the subchondral bone.

In treating these chondral lesions, grade I changes are typically left alone. Grade II changes are debrided to stable transitions between the normal and thinned cartilage. Grade III and grade IV chondral defects require more aggressive treatment.

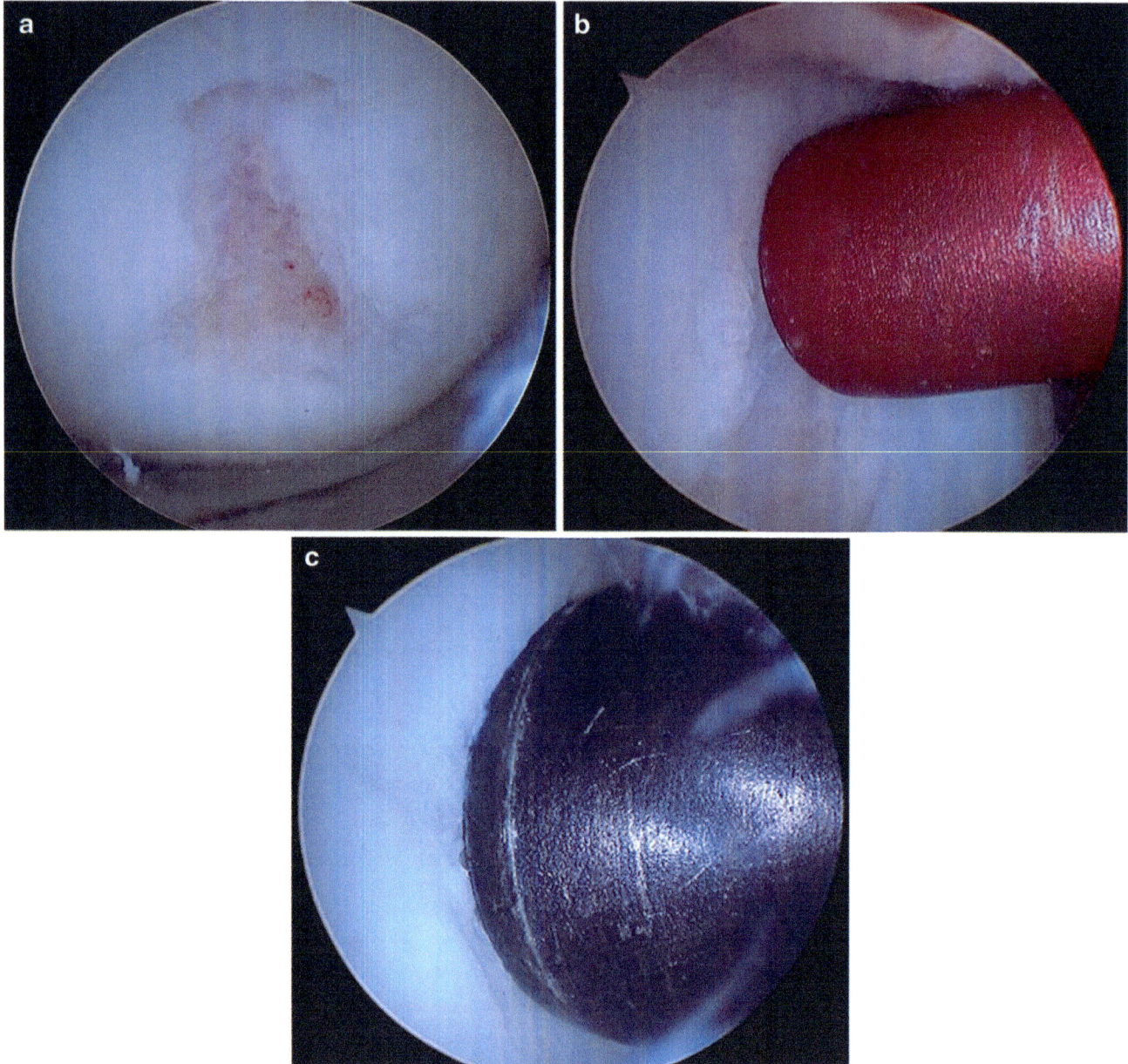

Fig. 4.8 (**a**)–(**c**) Arthroscopic view of the lesion after debridement. The two components of the lesion measured 6 mm and 10 mm in diameter, respectively

The treatment begins with debriding the lesions back to a stable cartilage shoulder. The calcified cartilage layer is then removed, exposing the subchondral bone. Further decisions on treatment are then made depending on the relative size of the lesion.

Microfracture and other bone marrow-stimulating techniques work well for lesions less than 2 cm². Short-term results are good. However, the longevity of the fibrocartilage that fills in the cartilage defect is questionable in long-term studies secondary to the fibrocartilage's inferior biomechanical properties compared to hyaline cartilage.

OATS is reserved for lesions that are typically less than 10 mm² or a stacked lesion, as seen in Case 2. Mosaicplasty can be used for larger lesions. The benefit of these procedures is that the cartilage defect is being filled with hyaline cartilage, with only a small band of fibrocartilage forming between the donor plug and surrounding cartilage. The disadvantage of these procedures is the morbidity of taking the donor plug from a non-weight-bearing portion of the knee. Another disadvantage of mosaicplasty is that it is likely that more fibrocartilage will fill in between the various plugs.

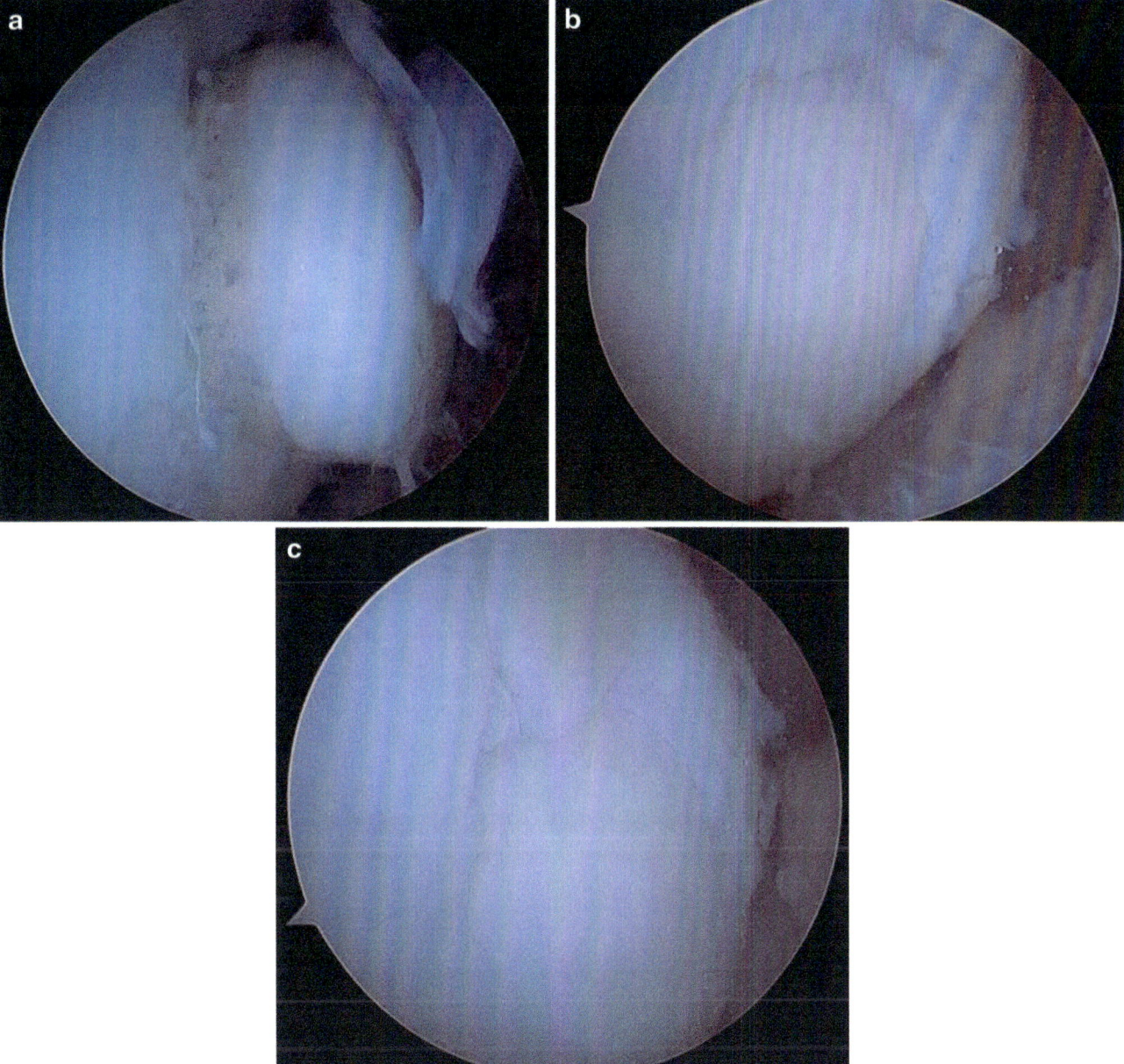

Fig. 4.9 (a)–(c) Arthroscopic views of the 10×14 mm plug being advanced into its receiving site until it was flush. Final arthroscopic view of the final two plugs in place at their receiving sites

Case 3: Nontraditional, Unstable Osteochondritis Dissecans (OCD) of the Knee Treated with Arthroscopic Fixation

History/Exam

A 13-year-old female presented to the orthopedic clinic after a 3-week history of right knee pain. This began as she increased her activity from softball to playing for three separate basketball teams. The pain was localized to the deep, lateral portion of the knee. It was aggravated by knee flexion and impact from running and jumping. There was associated swelling since the pain began, along with clicking and catching. She stated that the knee gave out on average of two times per day. She found that ice helped with the symptoms, but NSAIDS were not helpful. Of interest, the patient's older sister had a history of osteochondritis dissecans.

On exam, the right knee had intact skin. There was a small effusion. The knee was tender to palpation along both the medial and lateral joint lines. The knee was stable to varus and valgus stress. The Lachman's, anterior drawer, and posterior drawer test results were negative. McMurray and Wilson test results were also negative.

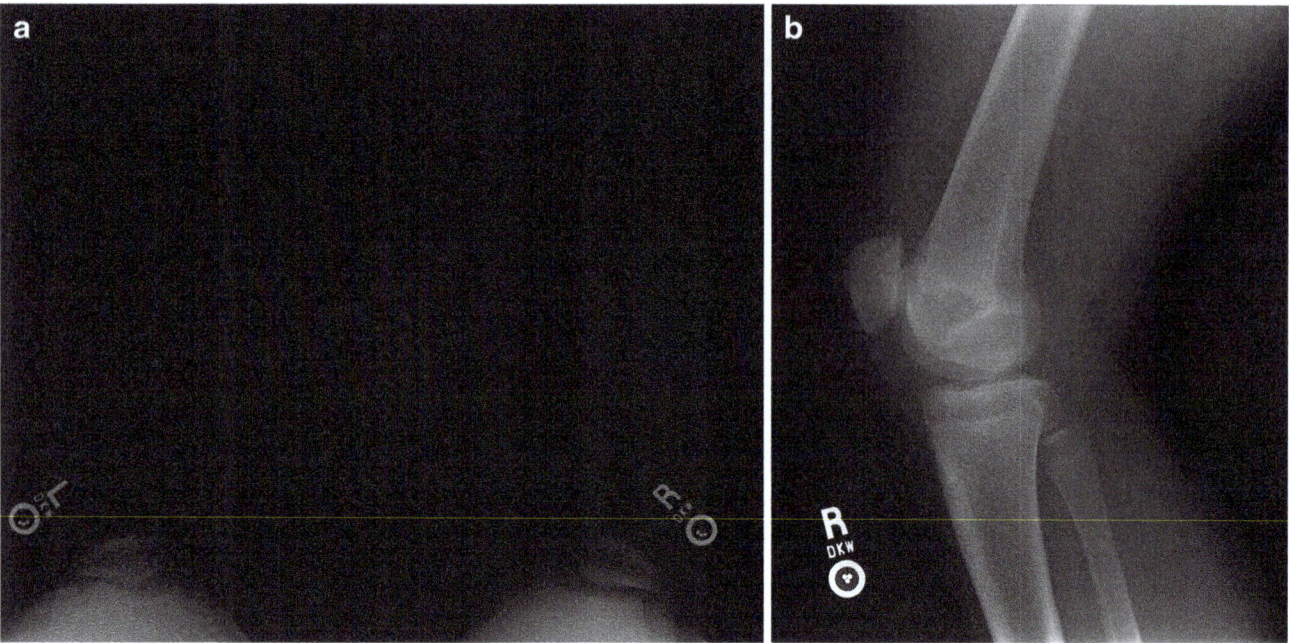

Fig. 4.10 (a, b) Merchant and lateral views of the right knee showing a lucency at the lateral trochlea

Imaging

Plain radiographs of the right knee demonstrated well-maintained joint spaces on the AP and Rosenberg views. There were no identified lucencies on these two views. On the Merchant view, a lucency was identified over the lateral trochlea. A suggestion of this lucency was also seen on the lateral, as shown in Fig. 4.10a, b.

Magnetic resonance imaging was obtained to further evaluate the meniscus and chondral surfaces. A full complement of images was obtained. The technique used included fat-suppressed, fast T2-weighted images acquired axially, sagittally, and coronally, as well as T1-weighted sagittal images.

A 16×19 mm osteochondral lesion was noted in the superior aspect of the lateral trochlea. There was a fragmented and sclerotic fragment overlying the osteochondral lesion. Fluid extended deep to the fragment, and there was subjacent marrow edema, all seen in Fig. 4.11a–c. The chondral surfaces of the patella, medial compartment, and lateral compartment were found to be intact. The medial meniscus and lateral meniscus were normal. All ligamentous structures were intact.

The MRI identified an unstable osteochondritis dissecans lesion of the superior portion of the lateral trochlea. After discussing the risks and benefits of surgical treatment of the osteochondral lesion, the patient and her family wished to proceed with osteochondral fixation.

Arthroscopy

The patient was taken to the operating room and placed in the supine position. A standard diagnostic right knee arthroscopy was performed. A 12 mm loose chondral piece was identified at the superolateral aspect of the trochlea. It was tethered at its most superior portion by a thin piece of cartilage, and there was exposed bone underneath, as seen in Fig. 4.12a–c. The fragment reduced easily into its donor site. The decision was made to proceed with fragment fixation. The base of the donor site was curetted through an accessory portal lateral to the patella and bone marrow stimulation was performed, as shown in Fig. 4.13a–c. The fragment was reduced and held in place with a spinal needle. Another accessory portal was made next to the superolateral aspect of the patella. A guide wire was placed into the fragment. This was drilled by hand using a 1.7 mm drill bit. A 2 mm cannulated screw was then advanced to fix the fragment, demonstrated in Fig. 4.14a, b. Two additional cannulated screws were placed to form a triangular pattern of fixation, as shown in Fig. 4.14c. The fragment was stable following fixation. The screw heads were buried just below the articular cartilage. The knee was then debrided of any loose debris. The patient's weight-bearing status was not limited since the OCD lesion did not involve a weight-bearing portion of the knee. The postoperative plane was to remove the screws at 12 weeks.

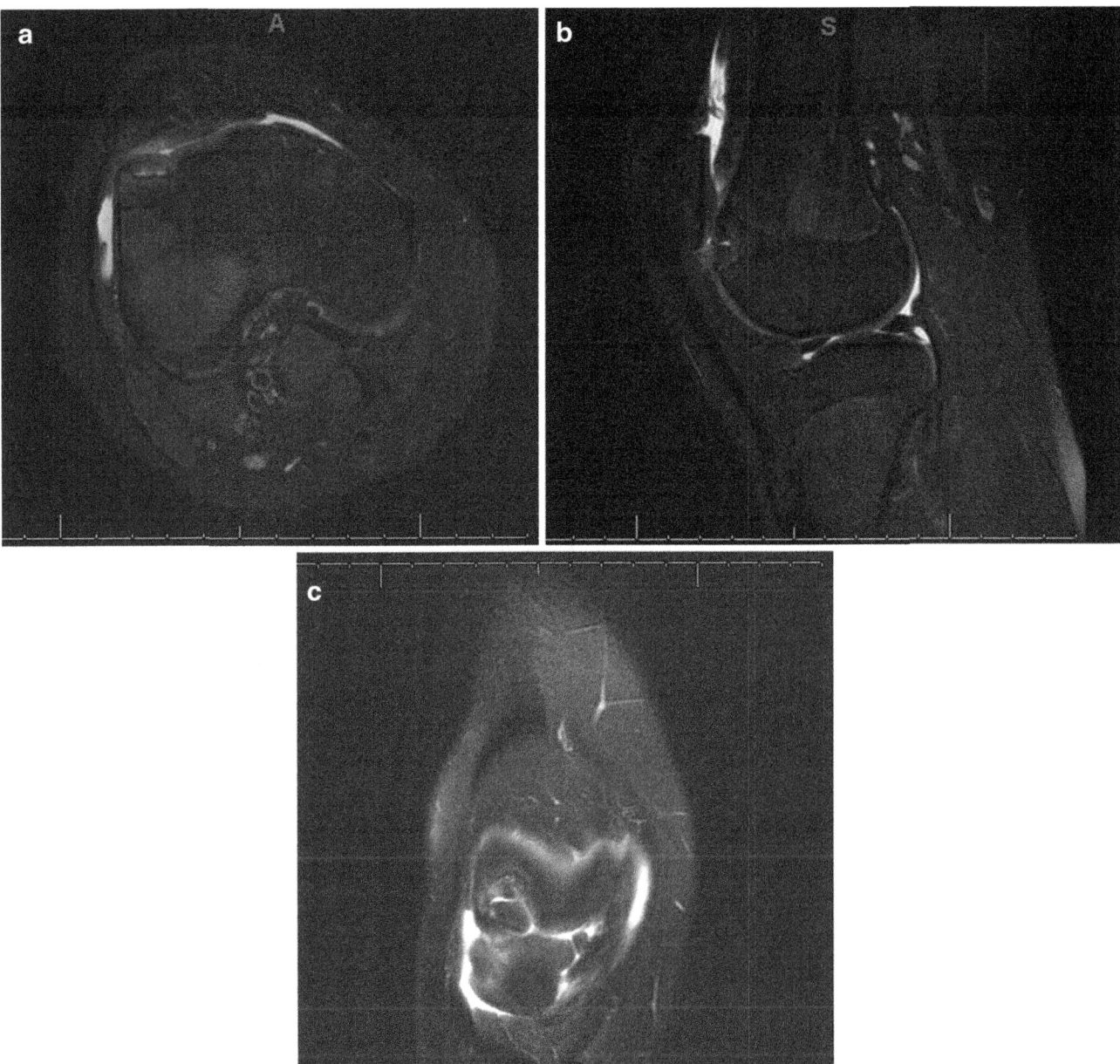

Fig. 4.11 (a)–(c) Select axial, sagittal, and coronal T2 views of the right knee from a noncontrast 3-T MRI. They demonstrate an unstable OCD lesion of the lateral trochlea which is fragmented and measures 16×19 mm

Case 4: Traditional, Unstable Osteochondritis Dissecans (OCD) of the Knee Treated with Open Fixation

History/Exam

A 15-year-old male presented with a several-month history of left knee pain. The pain started insidiously, without any history of trauma. The pain was described as being deep within the knee. The pain was aggravated by high-impact activities and deep knee flexion. He noted swelling and tightness within the knee since the pain began. He also stated that there was an associated catching sensation within the knee.

On exam, the left knee had intact skin with no erythema or warmth. There was a moderate-sized effusion. There was tenderness just to the medial side of the patellar tendon. The knee was stable to varus and valgus stress. The Lachman's, anterior drawer, and posterior drawer were negative. Medially based pain was reproduced with McMurray and Wilson testing. The remainder of the extremity was neurovascularly intact.

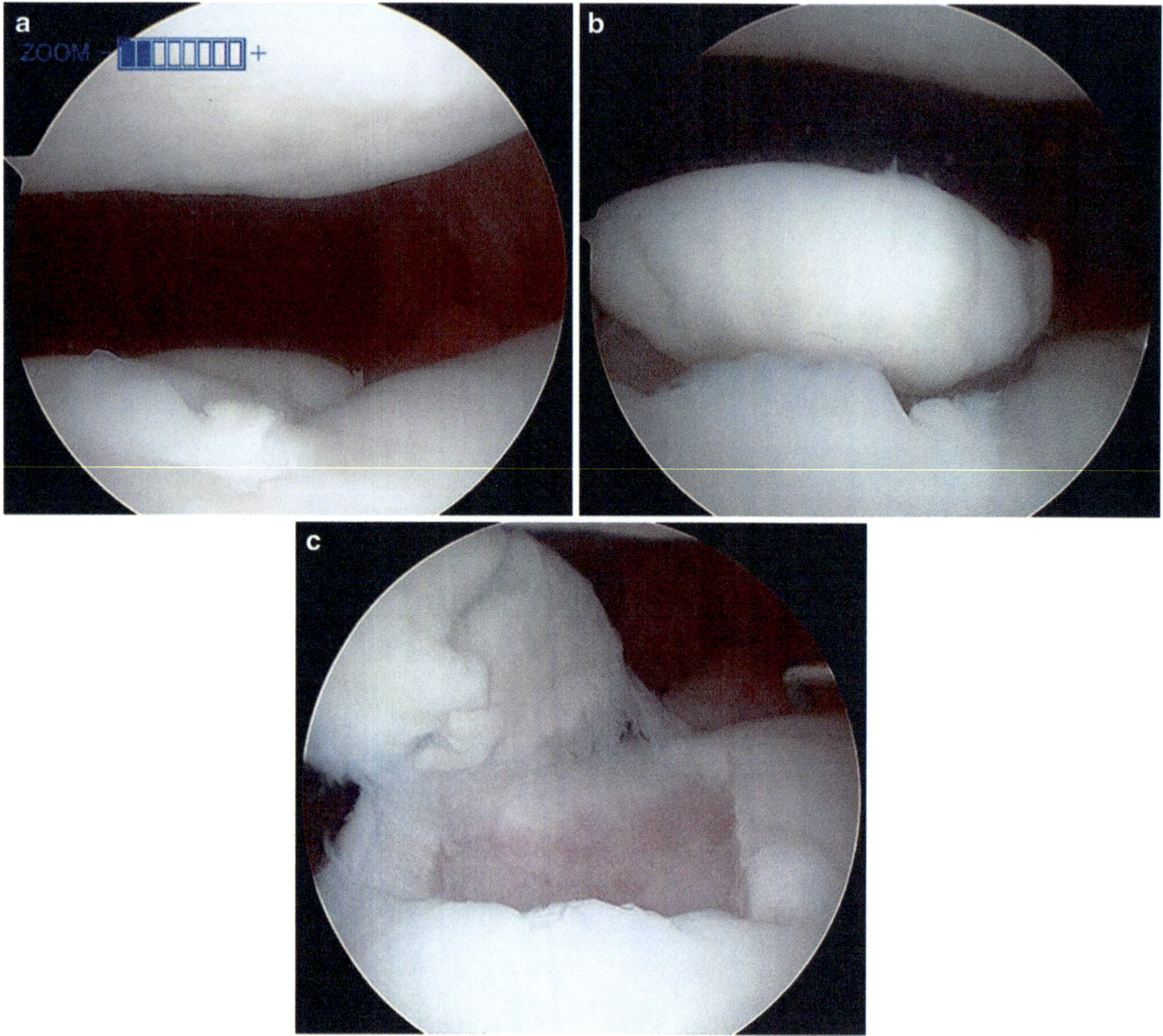

Fig. 4.12 (**a**)–(**c**) Arthroscopic views showing the unstable OCD lesion of the superior aspect of the lateral trochlea. It is a large flap connected by a small superior strip of intact cartilage. There are two bone fragments attached to the flap of cartilage

Imaging

The patient presented with magnetic resonance imaging already obtained. Additional magnetic resonance imaging was obtained to further evaluate the meniscus and chondral surfaces. A full complement of images was obtained. The technique used included fat-suppressed, fast T2-weighted images acquired axially, sagittally, and coronally, as well as T1-weighted sagittal images.

The MRI demonstrated a large focus of osteochondritis dissecans involving the posterolateral aspect of the medial femoral condyle. The lesion was fragmented into two separate pieces. There was a fluid signal on T2 imaging between the cartilage lesion and the underlying bone, demonstrated in Fig. 4.15a, b. The two fragments had a combined measurement of 34 × 22 mm. The T1 images showed a disruption in the cartilage surface with an irregularity of the underlying bone, shown in Fig. 4.15c. The remaining portions of the MRI were normal.

The MRI suggested that the OCD lesion was unstable. The unstable lesion was discussed at length with the patient and his parents. They elected to proceed with surgical fixation of the lesion after reviewing the risks and benefits.

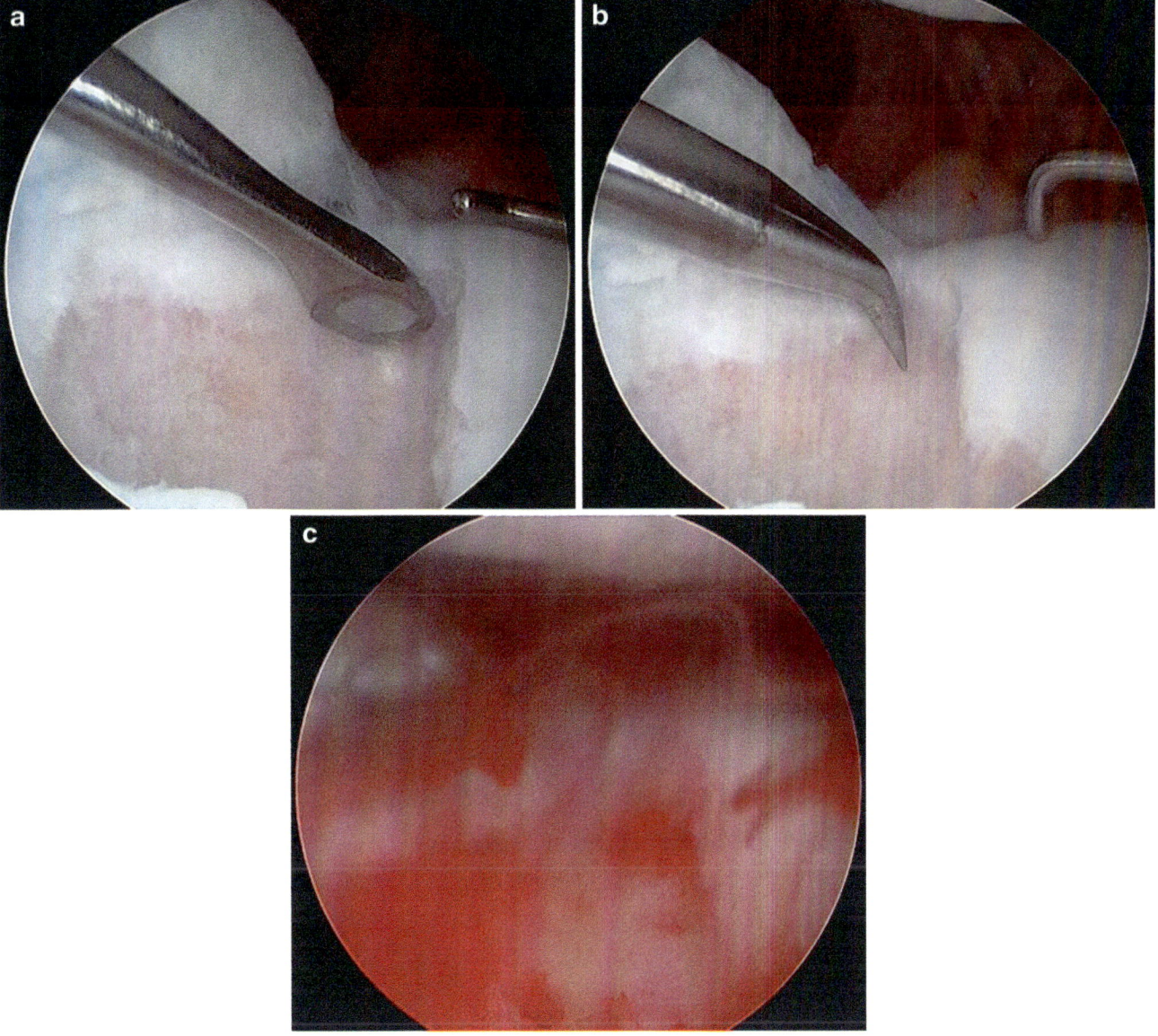

Fig. 4.13 (**a**)–(**c**) Arthroscopic views of the underlying bone being debrided and microfractured with an arthroscopic awl. Bone bleeding was stimulated by the microfracture

Arthroscopy

The patient was taken to the operating room and placed in the supine position. A standard diagnostic right knee arthroscopy was performed. Upon entering the medial compartment, a large fissure was identified involving the lateral portion of the medial femoral condyle, demonstrated in Fig. 4.16a. The fissure extended in a near circumferential pattern, with the only attachment being anterior, and extended down to the bone when probed, shown in Fig. 4.16b, c. When the flap was lifted, there was a large bony defect that measured 35×20 cm; see Fig. 4.16d. The missing bone was attached to the cartilage flap as two large fragments. The remainder of the knee was found to be normal.

A medial parapatellar arthrotomy was then made to access the medial femoral condyle and the OCD lesion was identified, seen in Fig. 4.17a. The bony bed of the OCD lesion was cleared of all fibrous tissue. The chondral flap, with its attached bone, was reduced into the bony bed. Three 2.0 mm screws were then used to stabilize the OCD lesion. The screw heads were buried just below the articular cartilage, demonstrated in Fig. 4.17b. The knee was then taken through a range of motion smoothly and the incisions were closed in a layered fashion.

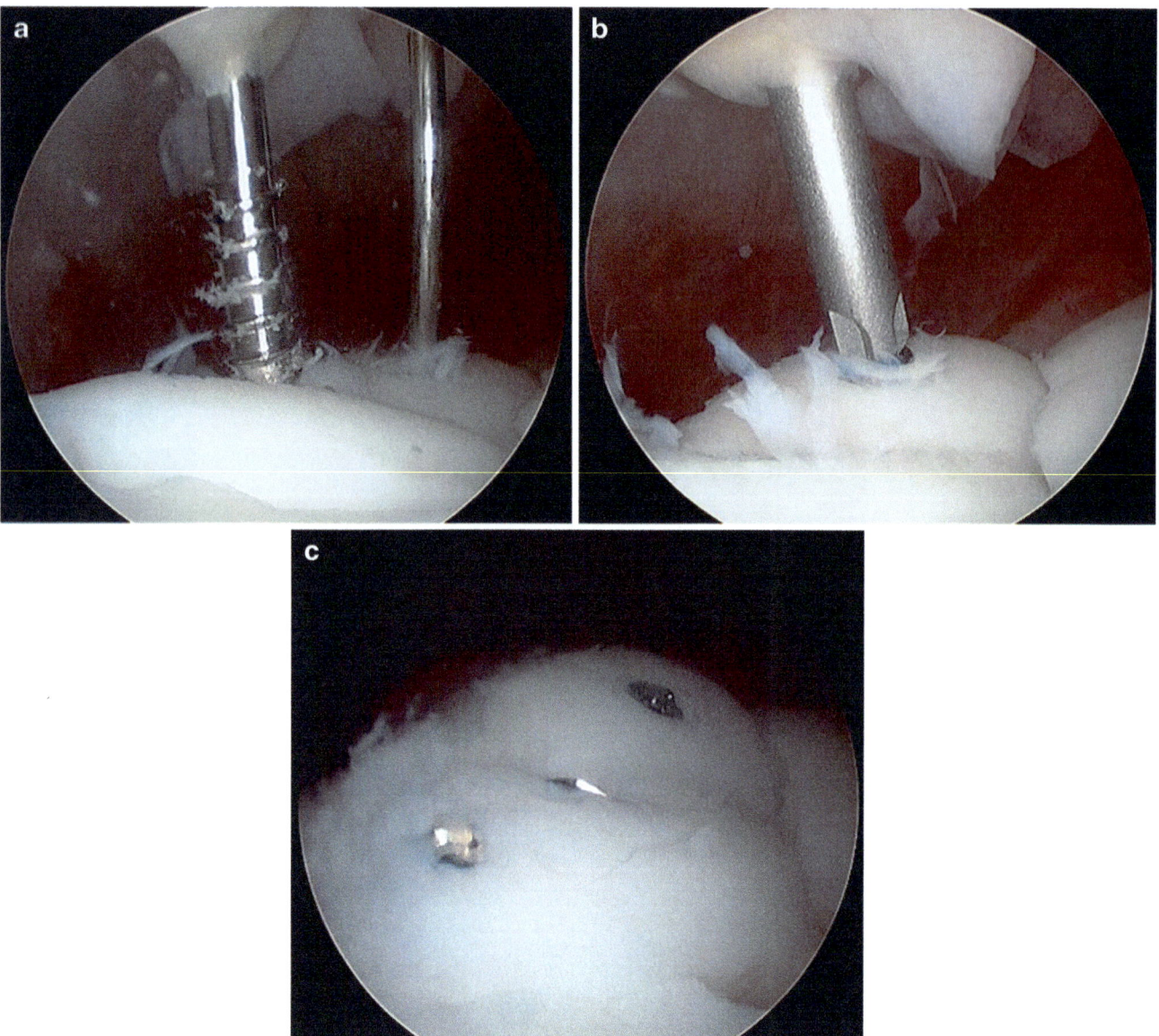

Fig. 4.14 (**a**)–(**c**) Arthroscopic images of the OCD lesion being stabilized with a spinal needle as a cannulated screw is advanced over a K-wire. The final fixation was achieved with three 2.0 mm cannulated screws

Discussion for Osteochondritis Dissecans (OCD)

Osteochondritis dissecans lesions of the knee are commonly seen in adolescents. They typically involve the posterolateral portion of the medial femoral condyle, as seen in Case 4. However, they can involve other portions of the knee, like the superolateral trochlea as seen in Case 3. The treatment algorithm in adolescents depends on the state of the physis and the stability of the lesion. The stability of the lesion is most easily assessed with an MRI. These lesions are evident on both T1 and T2 sequencing. On T1 sequencing, the cartilage may appear normal in a stable lesion. However, the underlying bone will have an irregular surface as this is both a cartilage and bone issue. The T2 images are more telling as to the stability of the lesion. In both Case 3 and Case 4, the OCD lesion was unstable. This was evident by the white signal of the joint fluid interposed between the OCD lesion and underlying bone. The MRI findings correlate nicely with the findings at arthroscopy. Lesions greater than 5 mm are best addressed with open reduction and internal fixation when the lesion is amenable, while an attempt at arthroscopic reduction and fixation can be made with lesions less than 5 mm. When possible, it is important to attempt fixation of the OCD lesion, as it preserves the patient's native hyaline cartilage and bone. Successful fixation will maintain joint congruence, eliminate mechanical symptoms, and relieve pain.

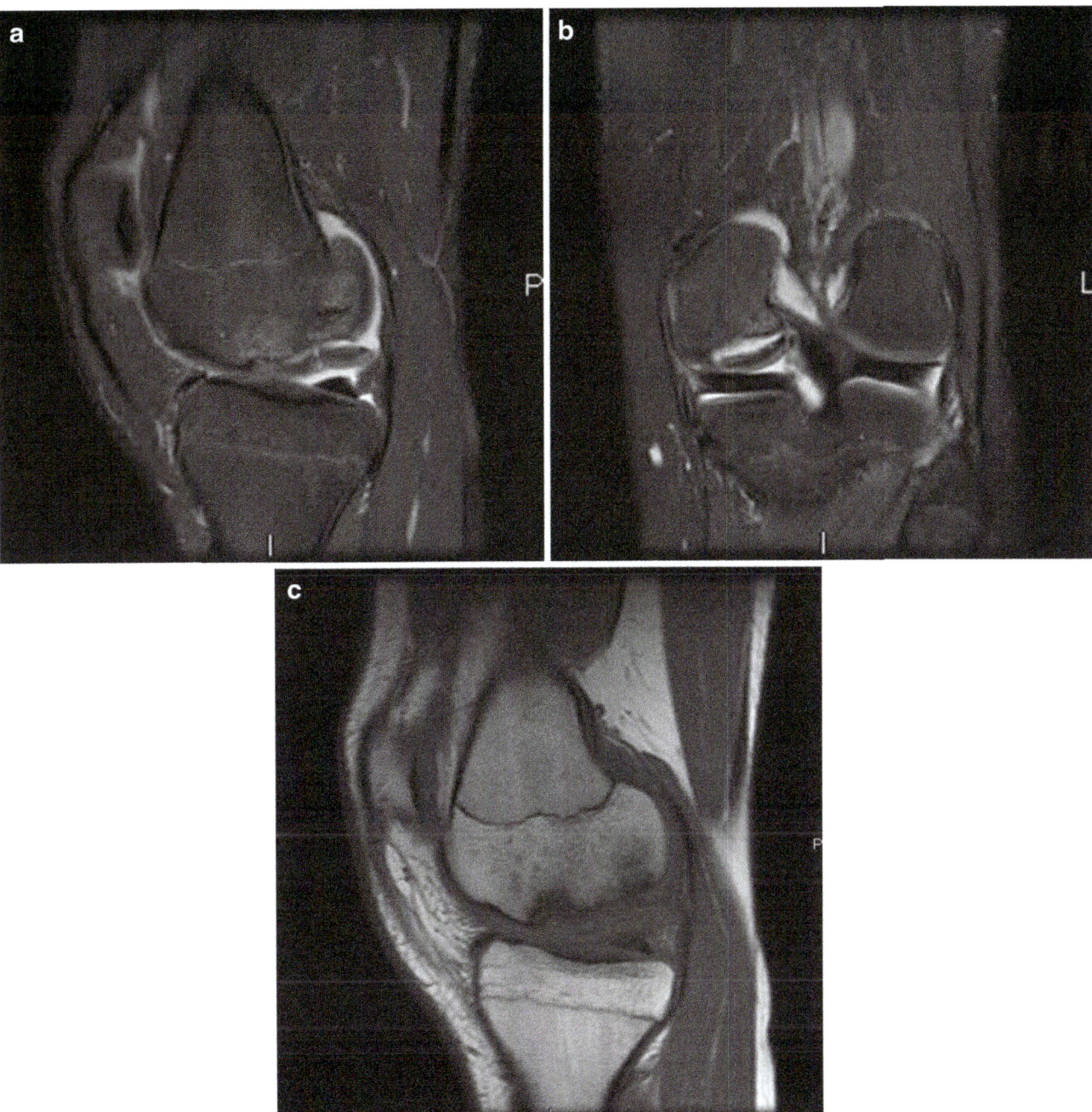

Fig. 4.15 (a)–(c) Select sagittal and coronal T2 images from a 3-T MRI of the left knee show an unstable, fragmented OCD lesion involving the posterior aspect of the medial femoral condyle. The lesion measures 34 × 22 mm. A select sagittal T1 image demonstrates irregularity of the underlying bone

Case 5: Grade II–III Femoral Condyle Lesion After Failed Chondroplasty Treated with Osteochondral Allograft

History/Exam

A 42-year-old male presented for evaluation of persistent right medial knee pain. The patient underwent ACL reconstruction 1 year previously and chondroplasty of the medial femoral condyle. He has no complaints of instability or mechanical symptoms. He is very active and desires to continue to cycle, ski, and hike. He is unable to run without significant medial knee pain. He has had only minimal relief with a medial compartment unloader brace.

On physical exam, he walks with an antalgic gait and has neutral alignment. He has good symmetric quadriceps mass, full range of motion, and no effusion. He has a stable

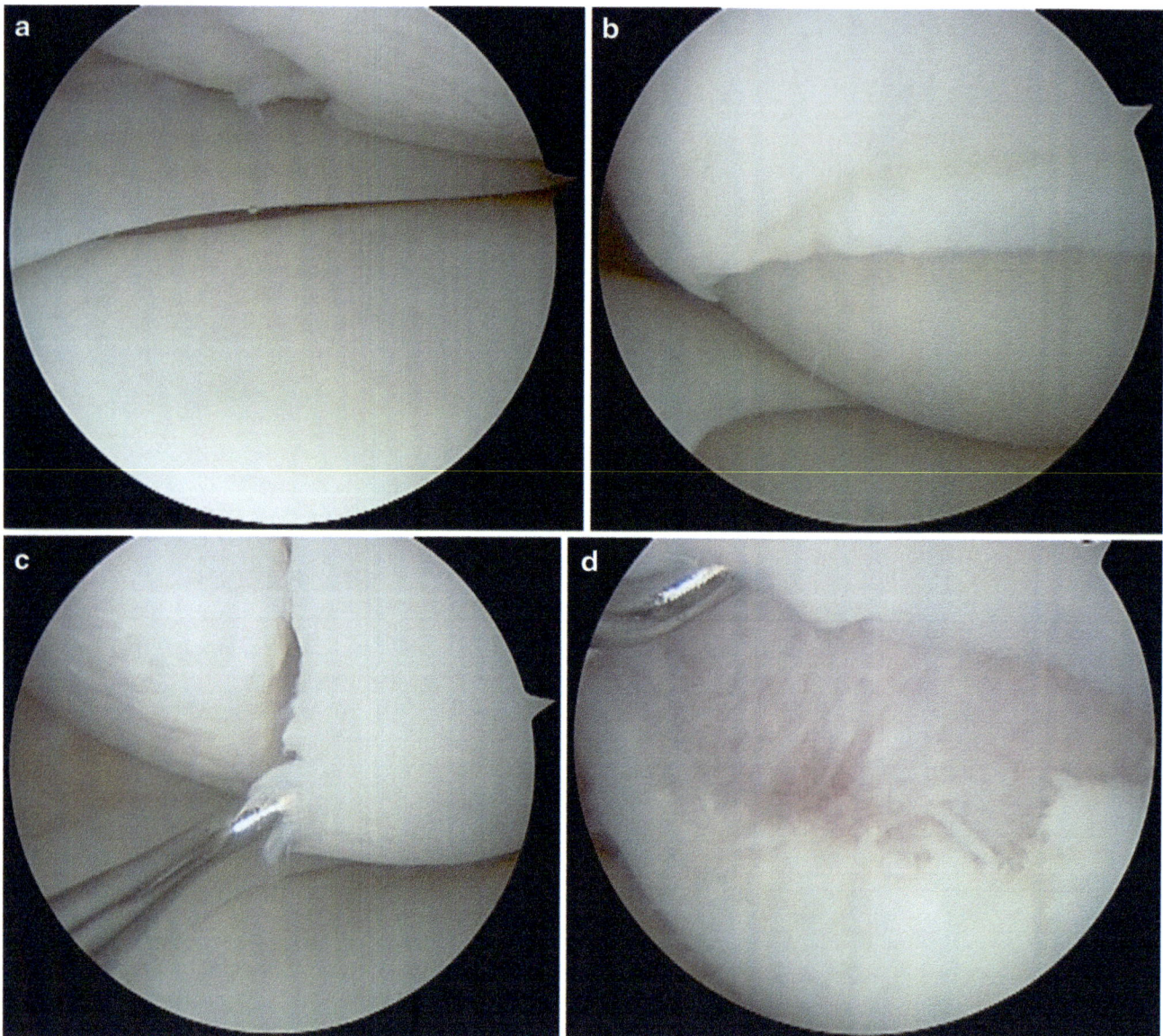

Fig. 4.16 (**a**)–(**d**) Arthroscopic views of the posterior portion of the medial femoral condyle. It was near circumferential with only a small flap of cartilage holding the lesion in place. The underlying bone had a thin layer of fibrous tissue over it. The lesion measured 35×20 mm

Lachman's and does not pivot. He has mild tenderness along the medial joint line and tenderness over the medial femoral condyle. Exam otherwise is normal.

Plane radiographs showed good tunnel position and no degenerative changes. A full-length alignment film showed neutral alignment. Advanced imaging with MRI was obtained to evaluate the cartilage lesion on the medial femoral condyle.

Imaging

MRI without contrast of the right knee was obtained on a 3-T magnet. Standard sequences obtained were axial proton-

density (PD) fat saturation, coronal T1 and T2, and sagittal T1 and T2. A contained grade II–III cartilage lesion is seen on the medial femoral condyle and measures approximately 13×14 mm (Fig. 4.18a–f). There is underlying subchondral edema without any cysts (Fig. 4.18b–e).

Arthroscopy

The patient failed to improve despite nonoperative treatment including extensive physical therapy and bracing. Diagnostic arthroscopy was discussed for planning for staged cartilage restoration procedure. Risks and benefits were reviewed. He elected to proceed.

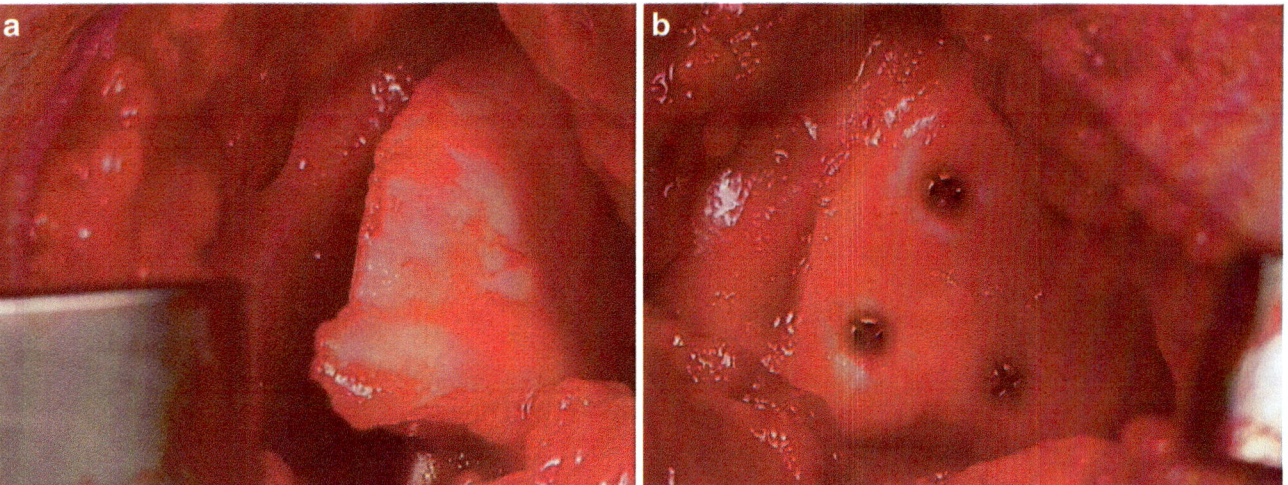

Fig. 4.17 (**a, b**) A medial parapatellar arthrotomy was made to expose the lesion. The bone bed was prepared and the lesion was fixed with three 2.0 mm screws

Examination under anesthesia was normal. Arthroscopic pictures are shown in Fig. 4.19a–c. A standard diagnostic arthroscopy revealed an intact ACL and normal lateral compartment and patellofemoral compartment. Evaluation of the medial compartment revealed a normal meniscus and an 18×18 mm round high-grade cartilage defect in the central weight-bearing portion of his medial femoral condyle. This was probed and there was fibrocartilage in the base but was soft and subchondral bone could be probed through multiple fissures. His tibial cartilage was normal.

Given the size of the lesion, normal surrounding cartilage, normal menisci, and that he failed to improve after chondroplasty, further cartilage restorative procedures were discussed. He elected to proceed with an osteochondral allograft to the medial femoral condyle and underwent osteochondral allografting to the medial femoral condyle 4 months later (Fig. 4.20a–c).

Discussion

This patient's findings on magnetic resonance imaging on a 3-T magnet were subtle other than the subchondral edema seen in the medial femoral condyle. However, this was nearly a 4 cm² lesion that had filled with fibrocartilage and had multiple fissures to subchondral bone. Diagnostic arthroscopy proved to be very helpful in this case to better understand the extent of this lesion. He responded well to an osteochondral allograft to the medial femoral condyle and had significant improvement in his medial knee pain. A high tibial osteotomy was not indicated based on his alignment.

Case 6: Grade IV Femoral Condyle Lesion with Deficient Bone Treated with Osteochondral Allograft

History/Physical

A 20-year-old male university club soccer player presented for evaluation of acute lateral knee pain and swelling that happened while playing soccer. He denies any trauma. He is unable to fully extend his knee and unable to bear weight secondary to pain. He did report some previous mild lateral knee pain but has always been able to play through the discomfort. He denies history of swelling or mechanical symptoms.

On physical exam he had a moderate effusion and lacks 15° of extension. He had tenderness along the lateral joint line but none medially. Ligamentous exam was stable. He demonstrated significant pain with attempted weight bearing. He has neutral appearing alignment.

Imaging

Plane films of the knee showed a well-delineated focal defect in the center of the lateral femoral condyle with irregularity and deficiency of the subchondral bone. Given his symptoms and radiographic findings, an MRI of the knee was ordered to further evaluate the extent of the lesion.

MRI without contrast of the right knee was obtained on a 3-T magnet. Sequences obtained were axial proton-density

(PD) fat saturation, coronal T1 and T2, and sagittal T1 and T2. A large grade IV osteochondral defect with deficient subchondral bone is seen on the lateral femoral condyle (Fig. 4.21a, b). The lesion is large but is contained. There is underlying edema within the bone and cystic changes. These findings are appreciated on both the coronal and sagittal T2 sequences seen in Fig. 4.21a, b. The cruciate and collateral ligaments are intact. Medial and lateral menisci are normal appearing. Cartilage in the medial and patellofemoral compartments is unremarkable.

Arthroscopy

Given the patient's symptoms and imaging findings, the decision was made to proceed with diagnostic arthroscopy, debridement, and removal of loose bodies. It was planned that he would undergo subsequent osteochondral allografting at a later date. He underwent sizing radiographs and was placed on a list for a lateral femoral condyle osteochondral allograft.

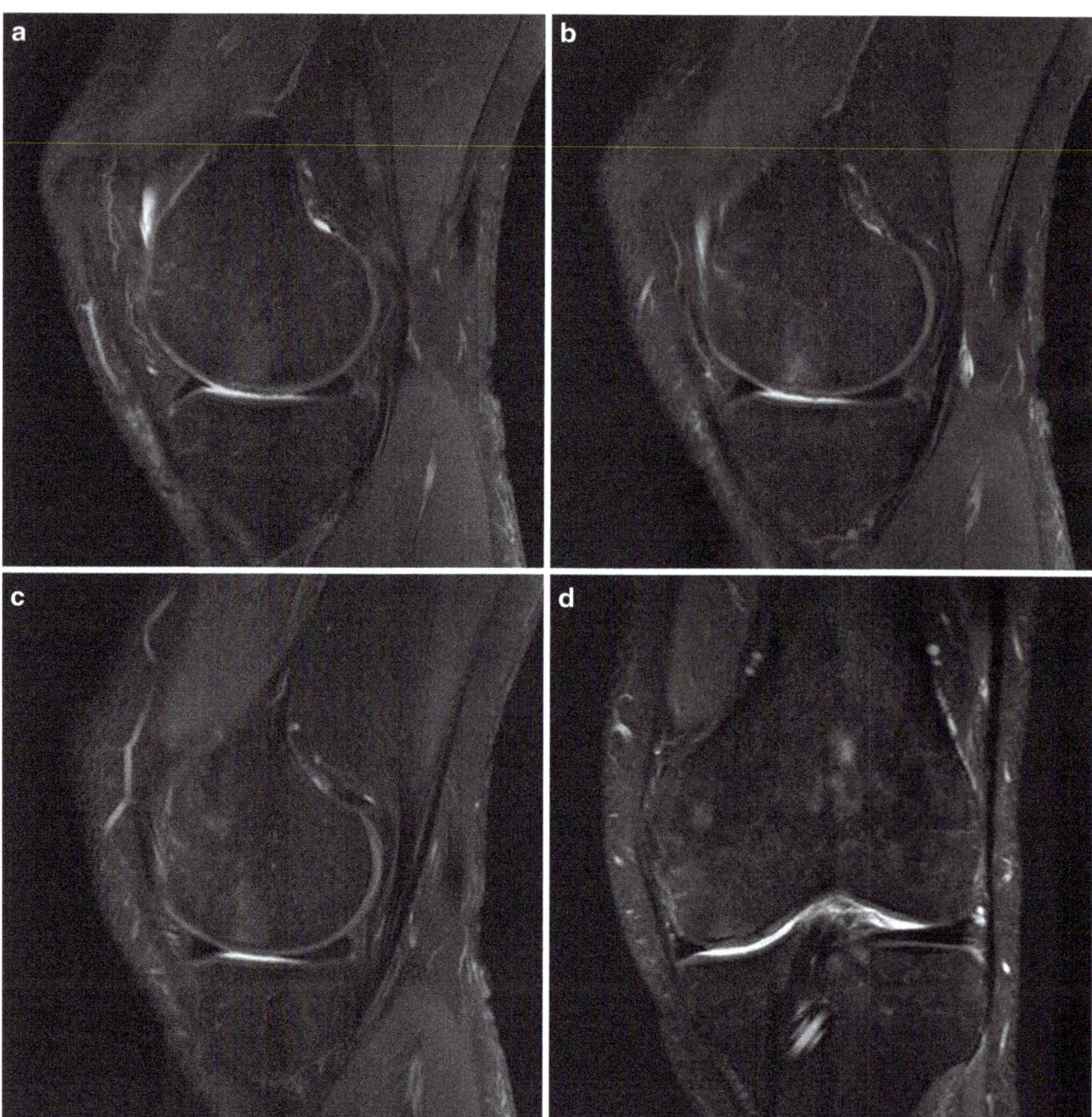

Fig. 4.18 (**a**)–(**f**) Select sagittal and coronal images from a 3-T MRI without contrast of the right knee. A contained grade II–III cartilage lesion is seen on the medial femoral condyle and measures approximately 13×14 mm. There is underlying subchondral edema without any cysts or deficient bone

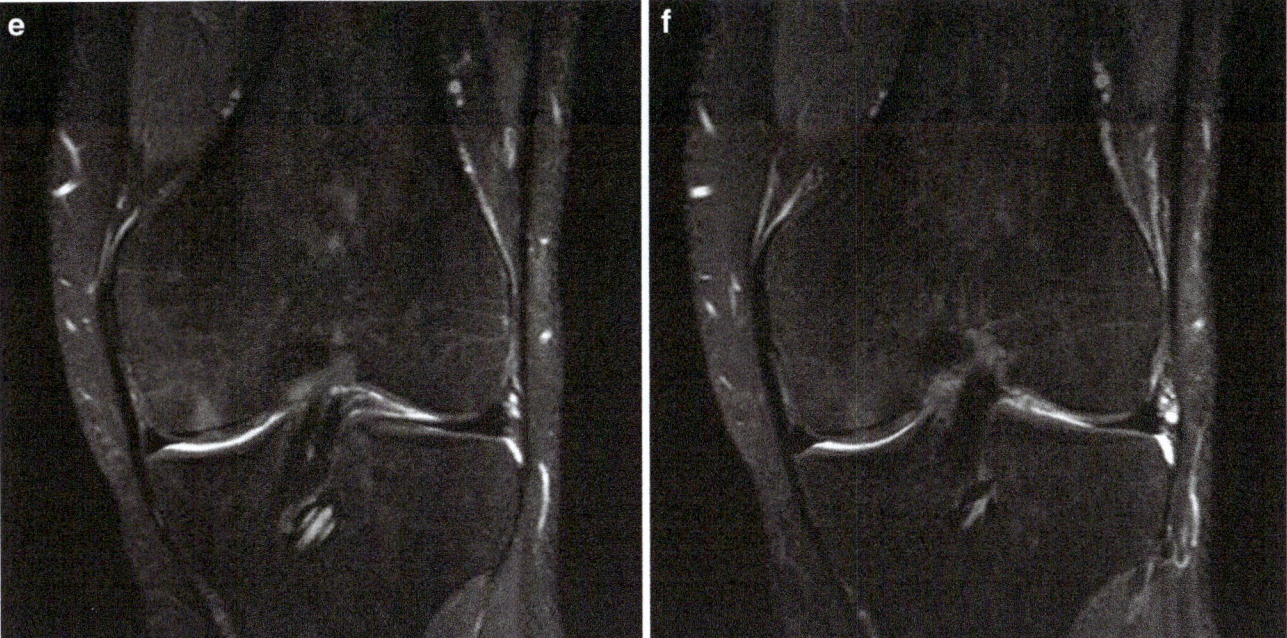

Fig. 4.18 (continued)

Diagnostic arthroscopy revealed normal medial and patellofemoral compartments. Evaluation of the lateral compartment revealed a focal osteochondral defect of the femoral condyle with deficient subchondral bone (Fig. 4.22a–c). Surrounding cartilage was normal and cartilage on the tibial plateau was normal. There was some fraying of the lateral meniscus. Multiple osteochondral loose bodies were encountered and removed. He underwent debridement of some fraying of the body of the lateral meniscus. Postoperatively, he was placed in a lateral compartment unloader brace while he awaited an osteochondral allograft. The patient returned to the operating room 5 months later and underwent osteochondral allografting to the lateral femoral condyle (Fig. 4.23a, b).

Discussion

This patient's MRI findings correlated well with his findings at arthroscopy. The MRI showed a contained full-thickness cartilage defect with deficient subchondral bone in the medial femoral condyle. Given the size of the lesion and deficient subchondral bone, it was felt that an osteochondral allograft was most appropriate. He did not have a malalignment so an osteotomy was not indicated. He underwent debridement of some fraying of the body of the lateral meniscus, but was not meniscus deficient, so meniscus transplant was not indicated.

Case 7: Grade IV Patella Defect Treated with ACI

History/Exam

A 23-year-old male presented for evaluation of his right knee. He has previously undergone right knee patellar stabilization, removal of loose bodies, and a "cartilage procedure" by an outside surgeon. This was done for patellar instability secondary to a traumatic event 6 years previously. He is no longer having instability but has had continued right knee pain, with recurrent effusions. He is unable to run for long distances because of pain and complains of "clicking and popping" when ascending and descending stairs.

On physical exam, he has a well-healed surgical incision on the right knee at the medial aspect of the patella. He has full range of motion and a moderate effusion. Evaluation of the patellofemoral joint reveals 1–2 quadrant medial and lateral patellar glide with a good medial checkrein. He has patellofemoral crepitus, a positive patellar grind test, and a negative J sign. He is tender at the medial patella facet. He has excellent quadriceps tone and recruitment. He has no joint line tenderness and a negative McMurray's. Ligamentous examination and alignment is normal.

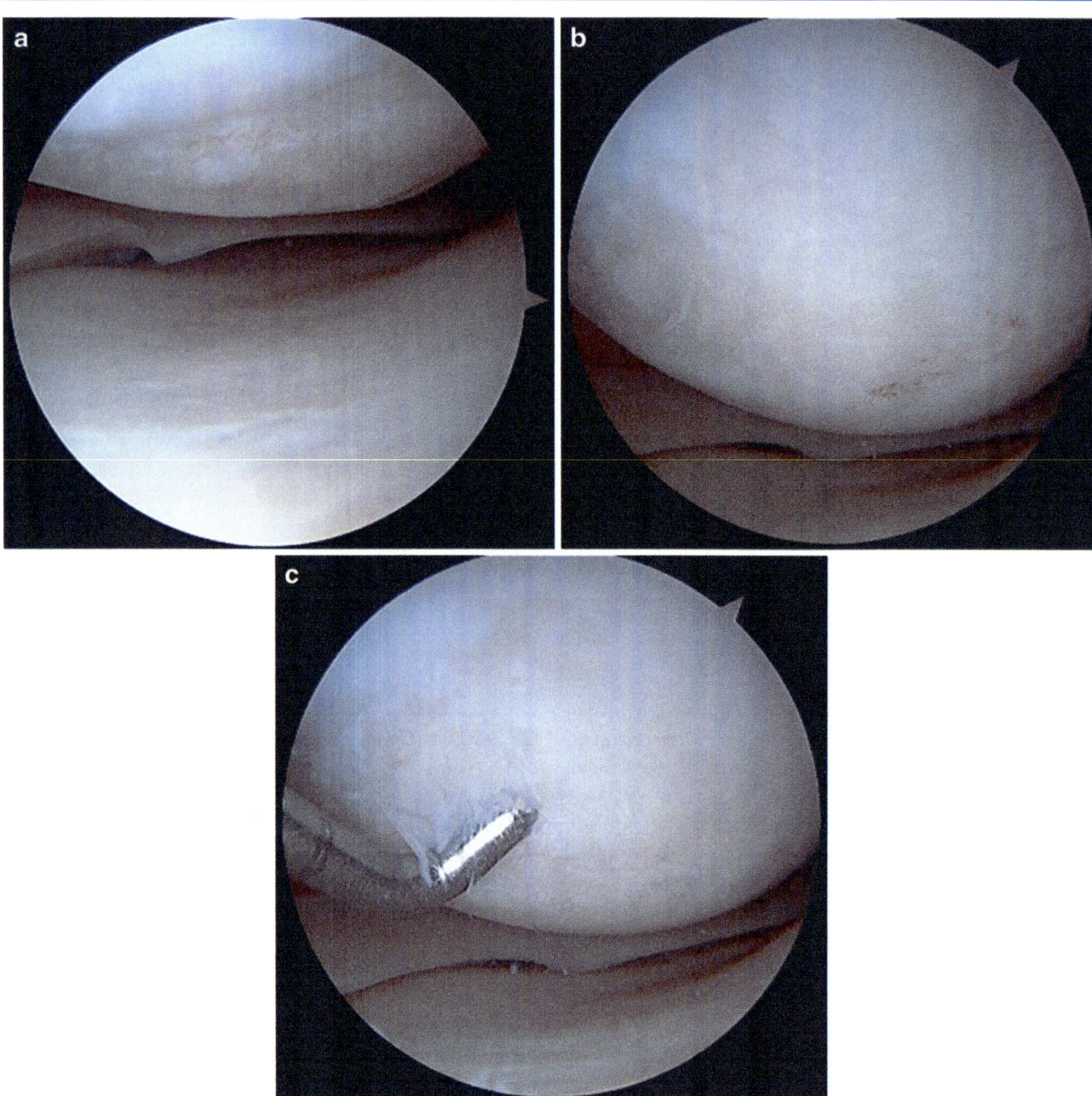

Fig. 4.19 (**a**)–(**c**) Arthroscopic images of the medial compartment show an 18×18 mm round lesion in the central weight-bearing portion of his medial femoral condyle filled in with fibrocartilage. The sub-chondral bone could be probed through multiple fissures. His tibial cartilage was normal

Imaging

Plain radiography demonstrated fragmentation on merchant view at the medial border of the patella and irregularity in the subchondral bone on the medial facet. There was no other significant pathology. MRI without contrast was obtained to further evaluate the extent of the chondral and bone loss on the patella.

The sequence of images obtained included axial proton-density (PD) fat saturation, coronal T1 and T2, and sagittal T1 and T2. These images were obtained on a 3-T magnet. Select axial PD and sagittal T2 sequence images are shown in Figs. 4.24a–d and 4.25a–d. The MRI demonstrates full-thickness chondral loss extending from medial patella facet past the patellar apex. There is underlying cystic changes and bone edema. The size of the lesion measures approximately

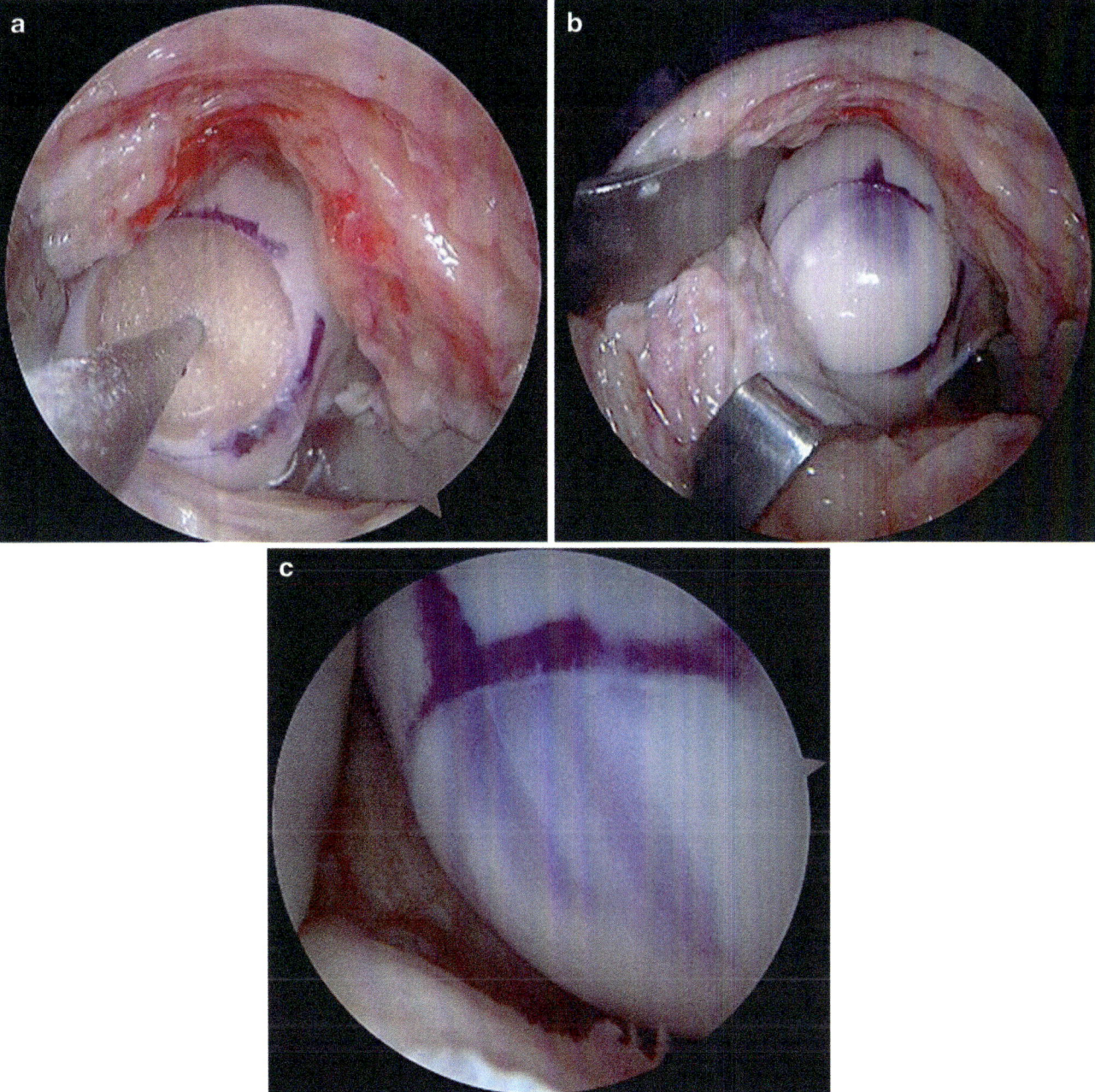

Fig. 4.20 Open (**a**, **b**) and arthroscopic (**c**) images at the time of osteochondral allografting of the lesion on the femoral condyle. The recipient socket is shown (**a**). (**b**) and (**c**) show the osteochondral plug after implantation

1.8×2 cm. The lesion is not contained medially. The tibial tubercle–trochlea groove (TT–TG) distance was normal.

Arthroscopy

Given the cartilage defect seen on MRI consistent with the patient's clinical examination, risks and benefits of operative intervention were discussed with the patient. Diagnostic arthroscopy, debridement, and cartilage biopsy were discussed to better understand the extent of the lesion for planning for potential staged cartilage restoration. Risks and benefits were reviewed. He elected to proceed.

Diagnostic arthroscopy showed centrally tracking patella and advanced cartilage wear in the patellofemoral compartment. He had a grade IV lesion noted of the patella. This was best characterized through the superolateral portal with a 70° scope. This was a full-thickness lesion that extended off the

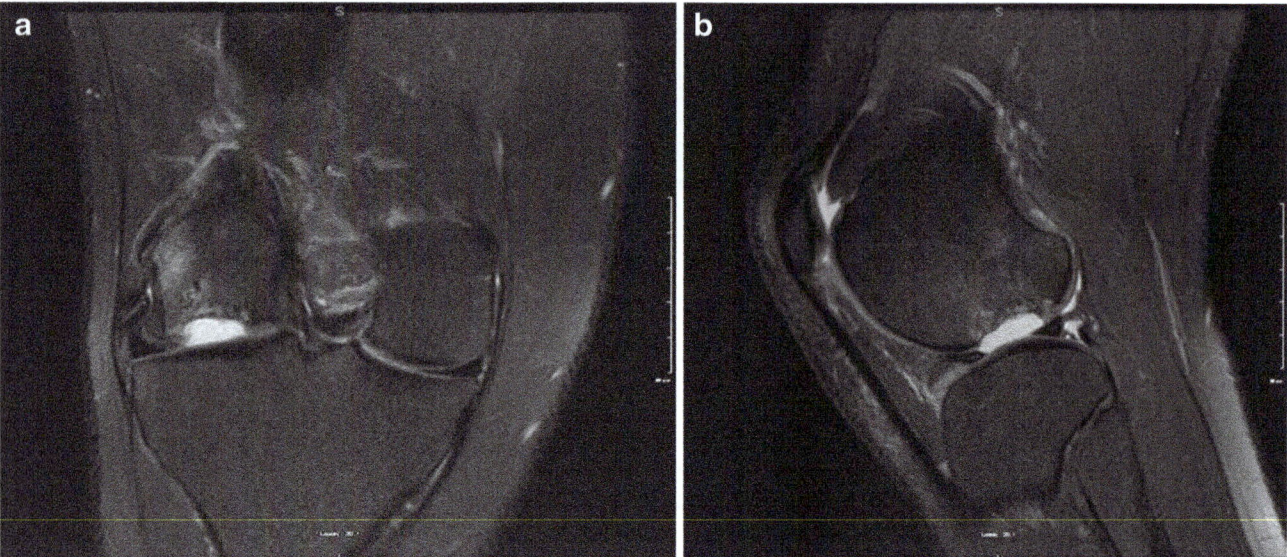

Fig. 4.21 Select coronal (**a**) and sagittal (**b**) 3-T MRI images show a large grade IV osteochondral defect with deficient subchondral bone which is seen on the lateral femoral condyle. The lesion is large but is contained. There is underlying edema within the bone and cystic changes

medial patellar facet into the patellar apex. There was some chondral delamination extending laterally from the apex (Fig. 4.26a–c). The lesion was debrided back to a stable rim and measured to be 17×20 mm. The medial trochlea had some grade I and II changes. Multiple small loose bodies were removed. Three "tic-tac"-sized cartilage biopsies were obtained from the notch for staged autologous chondrocyte implantation (ACI) procedure.

The patient returned to the operating room 8 weeks later and underwent autologous chondrocyte implantation (ACI). Figure 4.27a–c shows the lesion before and after ACI with a collagen patch.

Discussion

This patient developed a large grade IV lesion of the medial patellar facet following a patellar dislocation. He underwent stabilization by another surgeon with what appears to have been a soft tissue repair and removal of loose bodies. His symptoms persisted despite nonoperative management. His lesion was well characterized by the 3-T MRI. It can be appreciated on MRI that the lesion is grade IV, uncontained medially, and involves nearly the entire medial half of the patella which is what was found at arthroscopy. However, after debridement to stable vertical walls, the lesion was larger than initially measured on MRI. He did have subchon-dral edema with some cystic changes; however, he did not have any gross bony deficiency. His TT–TG distance was normal and he had no recurrent evidence of instability, so he was not felt to be indicated for patellar realignment or medial patellofemoral ligament (MPFL) reconstruction.

Conclusions

Cartilage injuries to the knee are well-established causes of pain, effusions, and mechanical symptoms. Diagnosing cartilage lesions within the knee can be difficult due to ligamentous and meniscal injuries present in a similar manner. Establishing a correct diagnosis is based on a careful history, physical exam, and appropriate imaging. The imaging modality of choice for properly diagnosing cartilage lesions is magnetic residence imaging (MRI). The MRI is also useful in diagnosing other injuries. Responsive cartilage lesions and unstable OCD lesions are best addressed with surgical intervention. The correct procedure is determined by patient age, weight, limb alignment, ligamentous and meniscal integrity, relative size of the lesion, and involvement of the underlying bone. Surgical options vary from simple debridement, microfracture, osteochondral autograft transplantation (OATS)/mosaicplasty, allograft transplantation, cartilage restoration with ACI- or DeNovo-type procedures, or internal fixation.

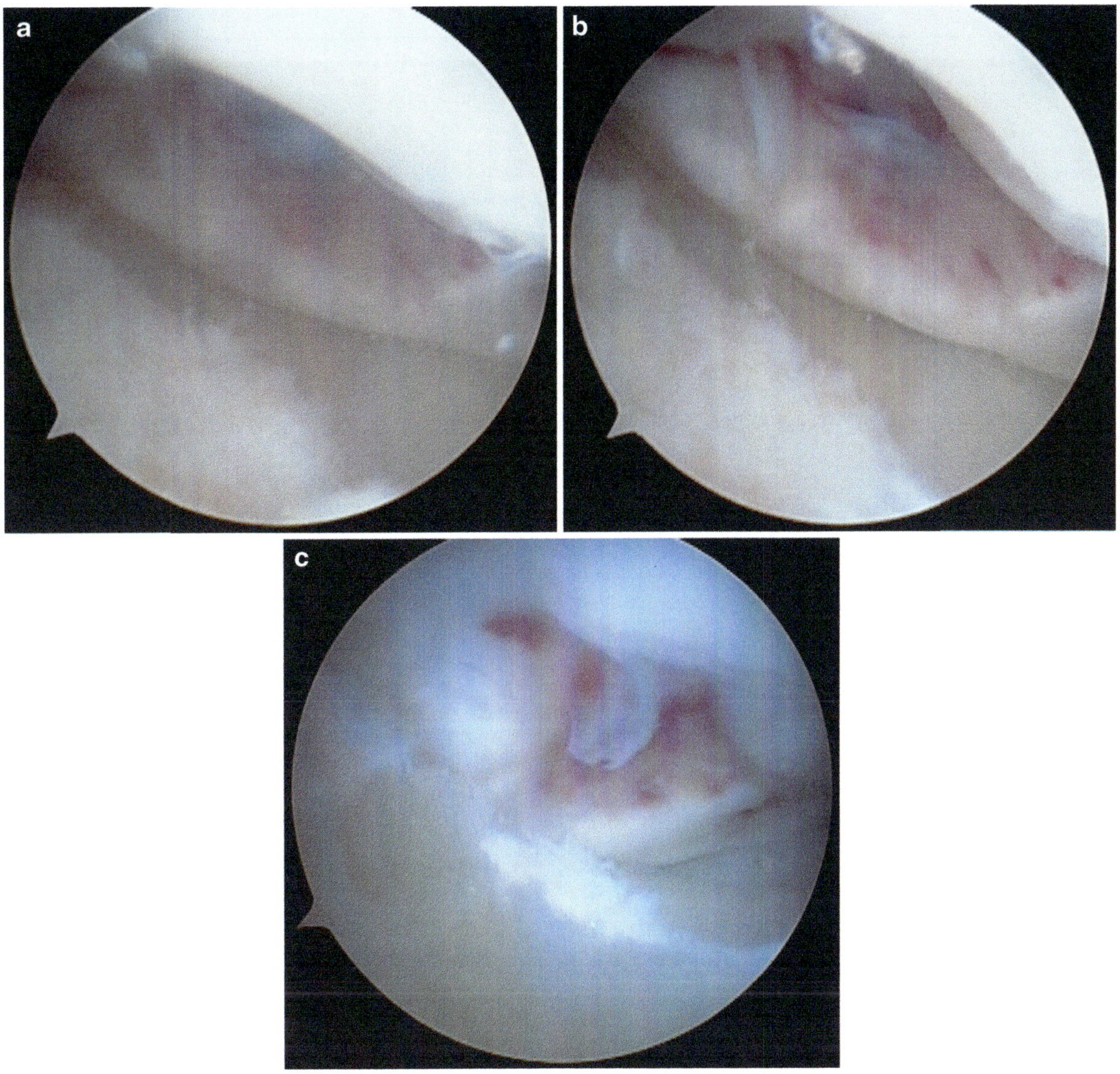

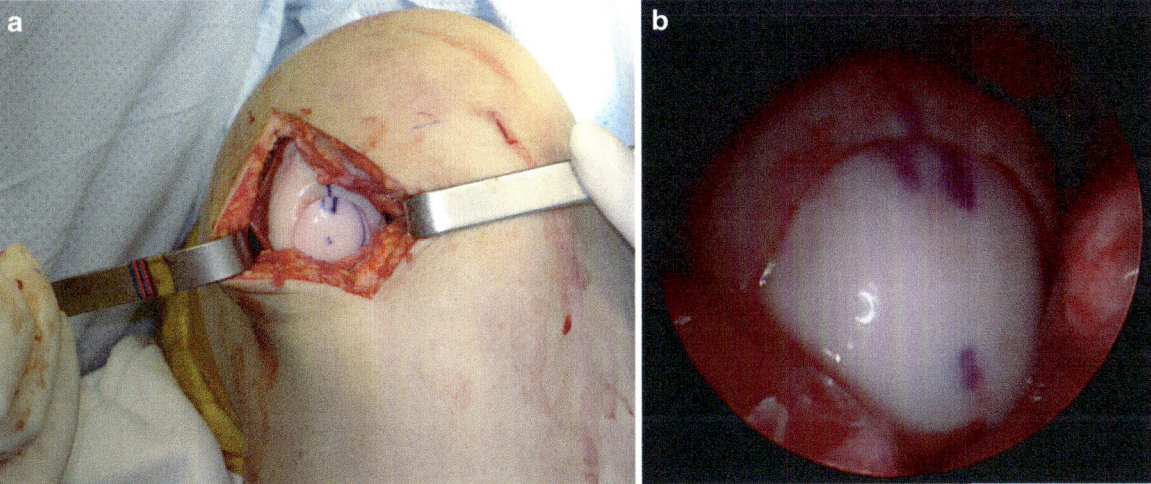

Fig. 4.22 (**a**)–(**c**) Arthroscopic images of the lateral compartment show a focal osteochondral defect of the femoral condyle with deficient subchondral bone. Surrounding cartilage is normal and cartilage on the tibial plateau is normal. There is some fraying of the body of the lateral meniscus

Fig. 4.23 (**a**, **b**) Open pictures at the time of osteochondral allografting through a lateral parapatellar arthrotomy demonstrating the allograft in place in the lateral femoral condyle

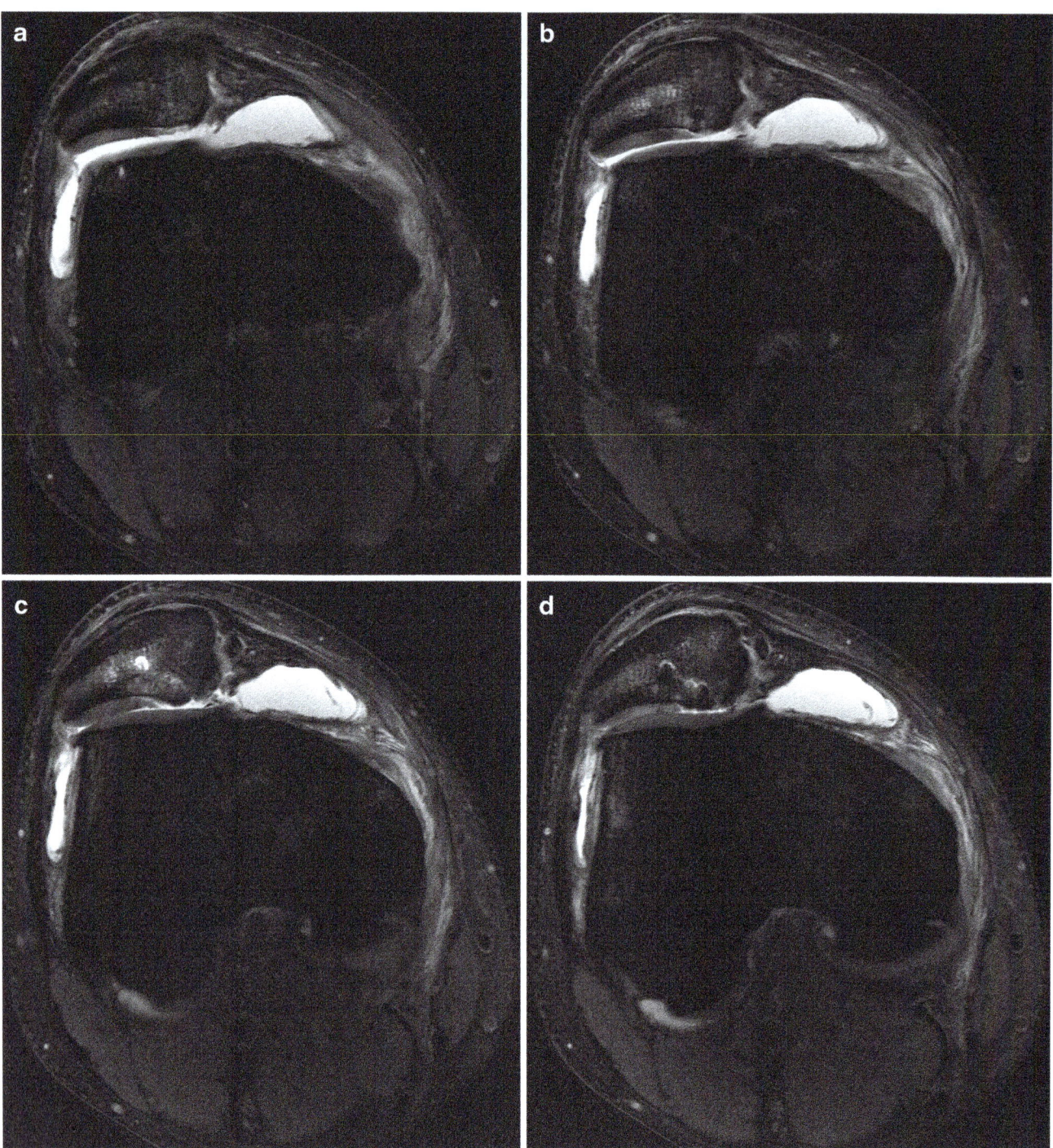

Fig. 4.24 (**a**)–(**d**) Axial PD fat-saturation images from 3-T magnet show full-thickness chondral loss extending from medial patella facet past the patellar apex (**c**). There is underlying cystic changes and bone edema (**c**, **d**). The size of the lesion measures approximately 1.8 × 2 cm. The lesion is not contained medially

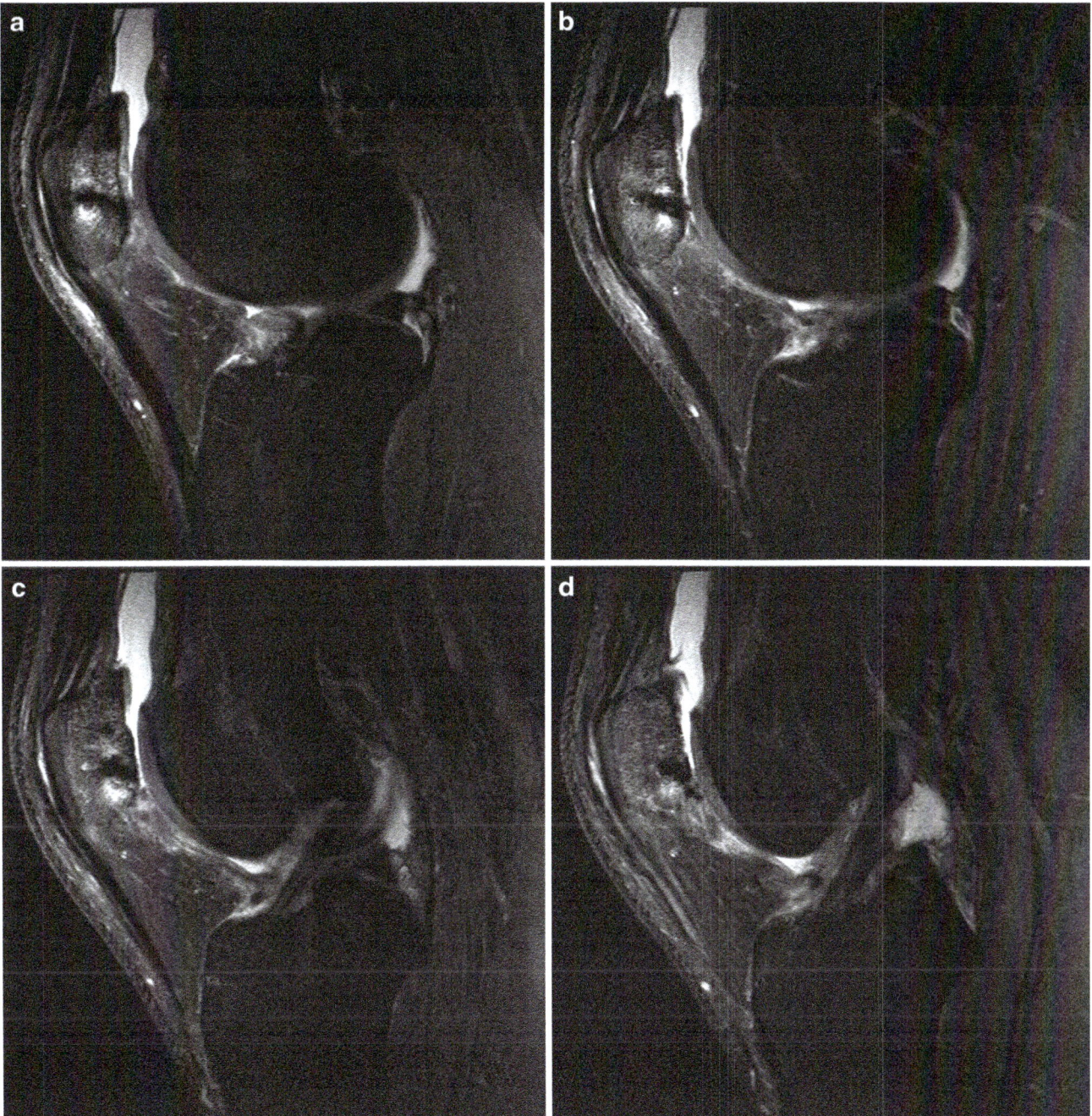

Fig. 4.25 (**a**)–(**d**) Sagittal T2 images from 3-T magnet show full-thickness chondral loss on the inferior two-thirds of the patella with underlying edema and some cystic changes

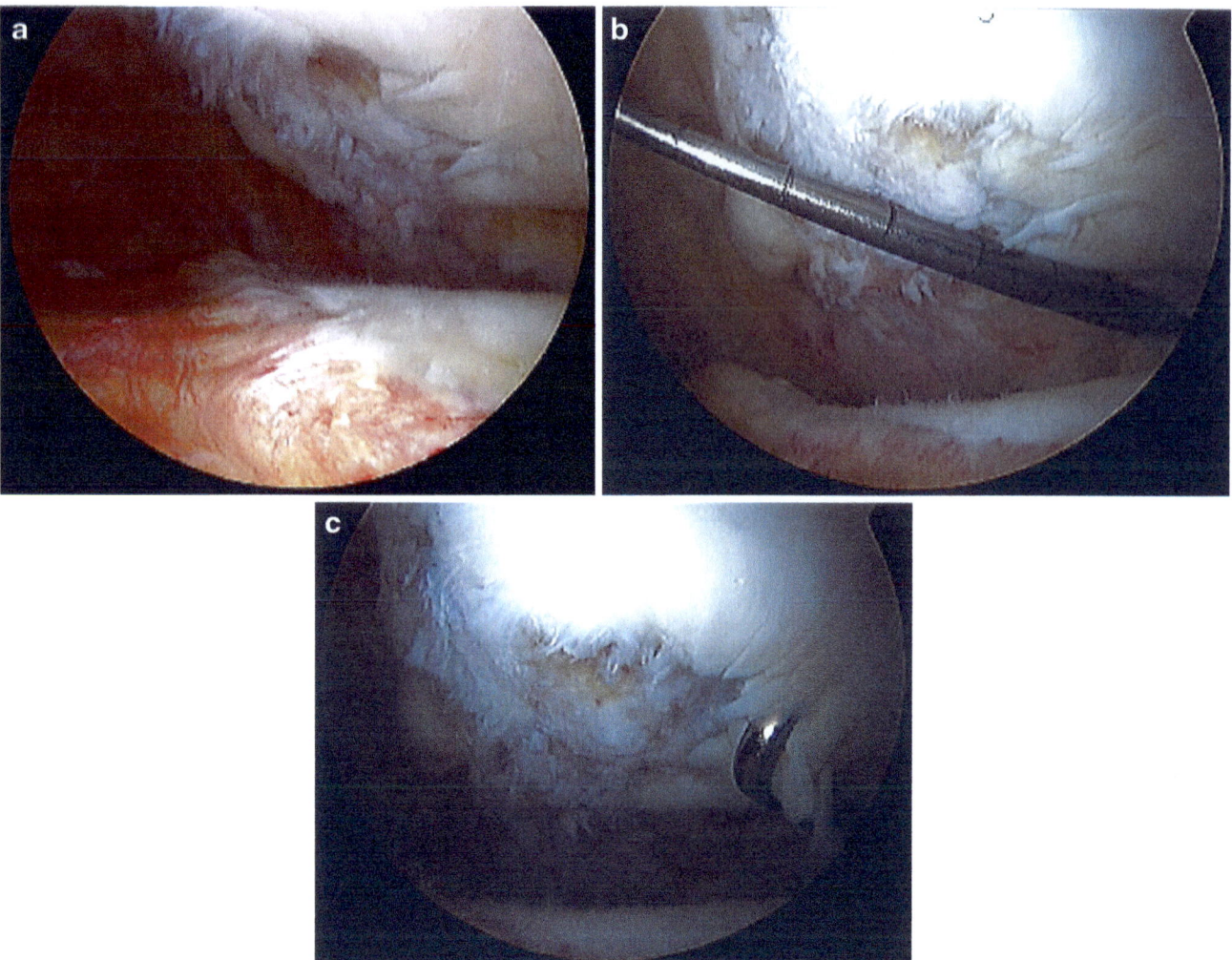

Fig. 4.26 (a)–(c) Arthroscopic images with a 70° scope from a superolateral portal show a grade IV lesion extending from the medial patellar facet into the patellar apex. There was some chondral delamination extending laterally from the apex (c)

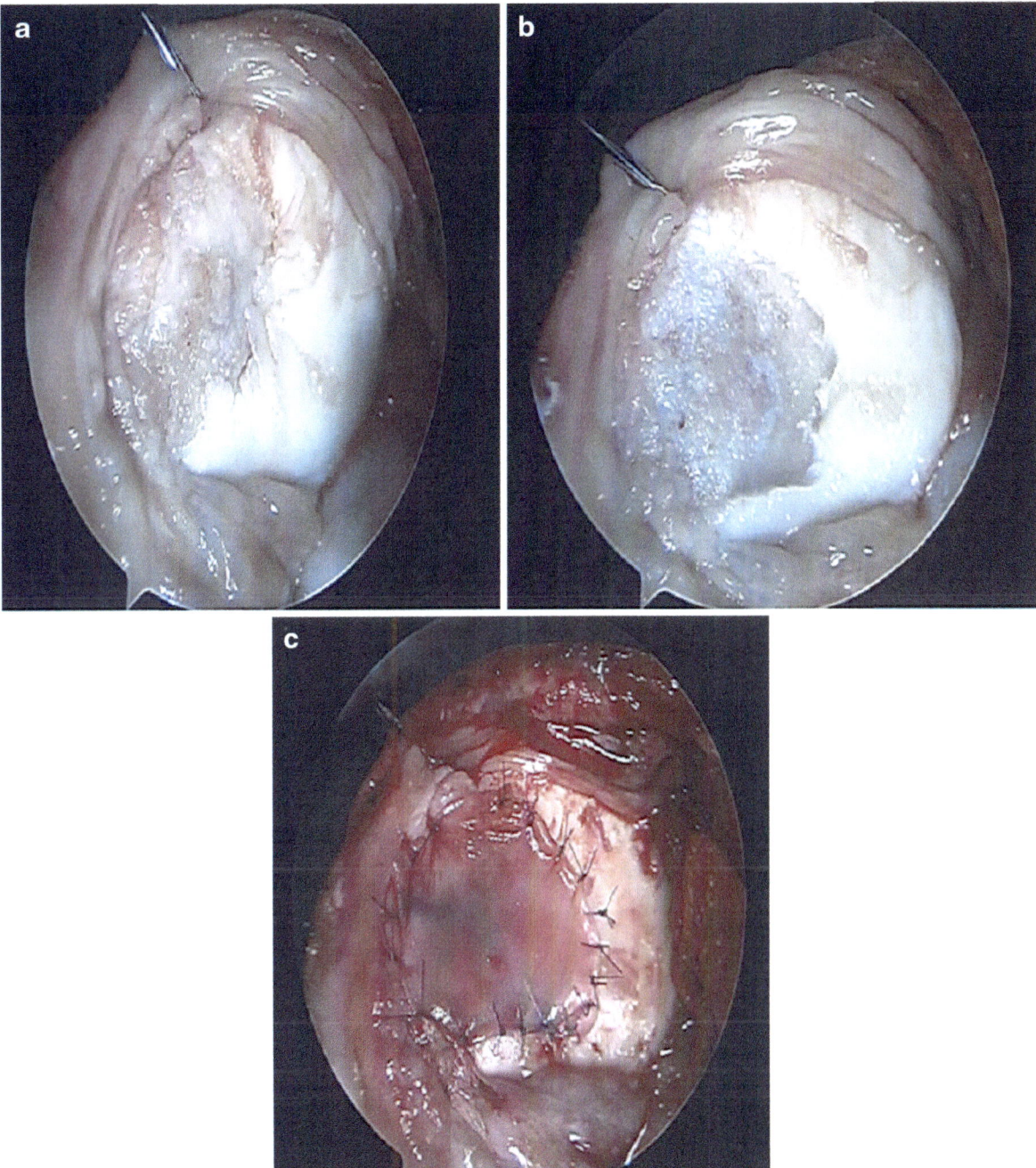

Fig. 4.27 (**a**)–(**c**) Open pictures at the times of autologous chondrocyte implantation (ACI). The lesion was debrided to stable margins and through the calcified cartilage layer (**b**). A collagen patch was sized and sutured into position with 6-0 vicryl (**c**). The lesion was not contained medially (**b**) so the patch was sutured to soft tissue medially (**c**)

References

1. Nehrer S, Spector M, Minas T. Histologic analysis of tissue after failed cartilage repair procedures. Clin Orthop Relat Res. 1999;365:149–62.

2. Alford JW, Cole BJ. Cartilage restoration, Part 1: Basic science, historical perspective, patient evaluation, and treatment options. Am J Sports Med. 2005;33(2):295–306.

3. Gomoll AH, Yoshioka H, Watanabe A, Dunn JC, Minas T. Preoperative management of cartilage defects by MRI underestimates lesion size. Cartilage. 2011;2(4):389–93.

4. Campbell A, Knopp M, Kolovich G, Wei W, Jia G, Siston R, Flanigan D. Preoperative MRI underestimates articular cartilage defect size compared with findings at arthroscopic knee surgery. Am J Sports Med. 2013;41:590.

5. Alford JW, Cole BJ. Cartilage restoration, Part 2: Techniques, outcomes, and future directions. Am J Sports Med. 2005;33(3): 443–60.

Anterior Cruciate Ligament Injury and Reconstruction

Justin W. Griffin and Mark D. Miller

Introduction

Anterior cruciate ligament (ACL) tears are a common knee injury, especially in young and physically active individuals. The ACL has been perhaps the most studied ligament in the human body in the last decade. Its importance to knee function has been demonstrated by the substantial functional impairment and decreased performance experienced after ACL injury [1]. This is especially true in the high-level athlete performing cutting, pivoting, and kicking activities [2]. The ACL confers stability to the knee by resisting both rotational and translational forces, thereby facilitating the normal kinematics of the knee [3–5]. Anatomic, hormonal, environmental, and biomechanical factors appear to influence the incidence of ACL injuries with females having a four- to six-fold increase in rate of ACL injury compared to men [3].

The clinical diagnosis of an ACL injury can be challenging, and concomitant pathology is important to recognize. The classic history for an ACL tear is a noncontact pivoting injury resulting in immediate swelling after hearing a "pop." The patient is typically unable to return to play because of pain and difficulty with pivoting and cutting. The key physical examination maneuver to diagnose an ACL injury is the Lachman, performed in 20–30° of knee flexion. Perceived side-to-side difference should be assessed and determination of an "end point" of translation noted. The pivot shift is also helpful, but the maneuver is sometimes difficult to perform in the clinic because of guarding by the patient. Least reliable is the anterior drawer, performed at 90° knee flexion, as hamstring spasticity and difficulty with motion can mask an injury.

Plain radiography is often the first study ordered to rule out other abnormalities and may demonstrate a Segond fracture, which is pathognomonic for ACL injury. Magnetic resonance imaging (MRI) remains the imaging technique of choice for patients with suspected ACL tear where the diagnosis is in question. MRI is also useful in identifying concomitant knee pathology. Arthroscopy remains the gold standard for diagnosing ACL rupture and meniscal tear in a patient with persistent symptoms.

ACL reconstruction has evolved considerably over the past 30 years. Advances have largely centered on an understanding of the anatomy of footprint of the ACL. Recent studies have identified the importance of anatomic ACL reconstruction to restore the ACL to its native dimensions, insertion sites, and collagen orientation to confer ideal rotational and translational stability [2, 6–8]. The anatomy of the ACL consists of two distinct bundles; the anteromedial and posterolateral, representing intracapsular structures supplied predominately by the middle geniculate artery.

Treatment for ACL injuries includes operative reconstruction or nonoperative rehabilitation. The age and level of activity of the patient must be considered prior to making any recommendations. The primary candidates for ACL reconstruction are active patients with functional instability. Current evidence suggests that ACL deficiency can lead to chondral damage as well as meniscal tears and that reconstruction leads to long-term functional and cost benefits in the right patient though some studies suggest increased arthrosis on later follow-up [5, 9].

Standard management protocol includes early active range of motion to regain full knee range of motion with closed chain weight bearing exercises prior to surgical reconstruction. After the pathology is characterized by diagnostic arthroscopy, treatment options depend upon the patient, injury, and surgeon preferences. Concomitant pathology,

J.W. Griffin, MD (✉)
Department of Orthopedic Surgery, University of Virginia Health System, Charlottesville, VA, USA
e-mail: griffin@virginia.edu

M.D. Miller, MD
Department of Orthopedic Surgery, University of Virginia Health System, Charlottesville, VA, USA

Department of Orthopedic Surgery, Head Team Physician, James Madison University, Charlottesville, VA, USA
e-mail: Mdm3p@hccmail.mcc.virginia.edu

including meniscal tears, chondral defects, or other ligamentous injuries, can be addressed in the same setting.

This chapter will utilize a case-based format to demonstrate the correlation between MRI and arthroscopy for pathology and review the diagnosis and management of each patient. Three cases will be presented, including a complete ACL rupture requiring reconstruction, a partial ACL injury and a bony avulsion injury of the tibial insertion of the ACL.

Case 1: ACL Rupture

History/Exam

An 18-year-old rugby player presented to our orthopedic clinic 1 week following a tackling injury where another player's head collided with his knee during play. A patella dislocation was reduced on the field and a large effusion was evident immediately. One week later, he reported a resolving effusion as well as feeling of instability with attempted return to play. He had sought advice from his trainer and team physical therapist concerning his symptoms and presented to our orthopedic clinic for further evaluation.

On physical examination, the patient was found to have a moderate effusion with obvious lack of end point with Lachman examination. Lateral joint line tenderness was notable with a positive McMurray's. A pivot shift was noticeably positive in the office. No varus or valgus opening or asymmetry with the contralateral knee was noted on examination. The patient was otherwise neurovascularly intact and without symptoms in his contralateral knee. He had pain and difficulty with straight leg raise without a palpable patella tendon defect. Given the patient's examination and desire to return to competitive play, advanced imaging was obtained to evaluate for additional pathology.

Imaging

Plain radiographs were obtained demonstrating no bony avulsions or other associated injuries. There was no evidence of arthritic changes or areas of significant cartilage loss. Magnetic resonance imaging was obtained to further evaluate the patient's ACL, menisci, and other soft tissue structures, given his persistent symptoms. A complete sequence of images was obtained, including coronal fat-saturated T1 and T2 sequences, sagittal T1 and fat-saturated T2, and axial T1 and T2 sequences. Sagittal T2-weighted images are demonstrated in Fig. 5.1a, and coronal T2-weighted images are demonstrated in Fig. 5.1b.

A complete midsubstance ACL tear was present as shown in Fig. 5.2a, b. Acute hemarthrosis was present with

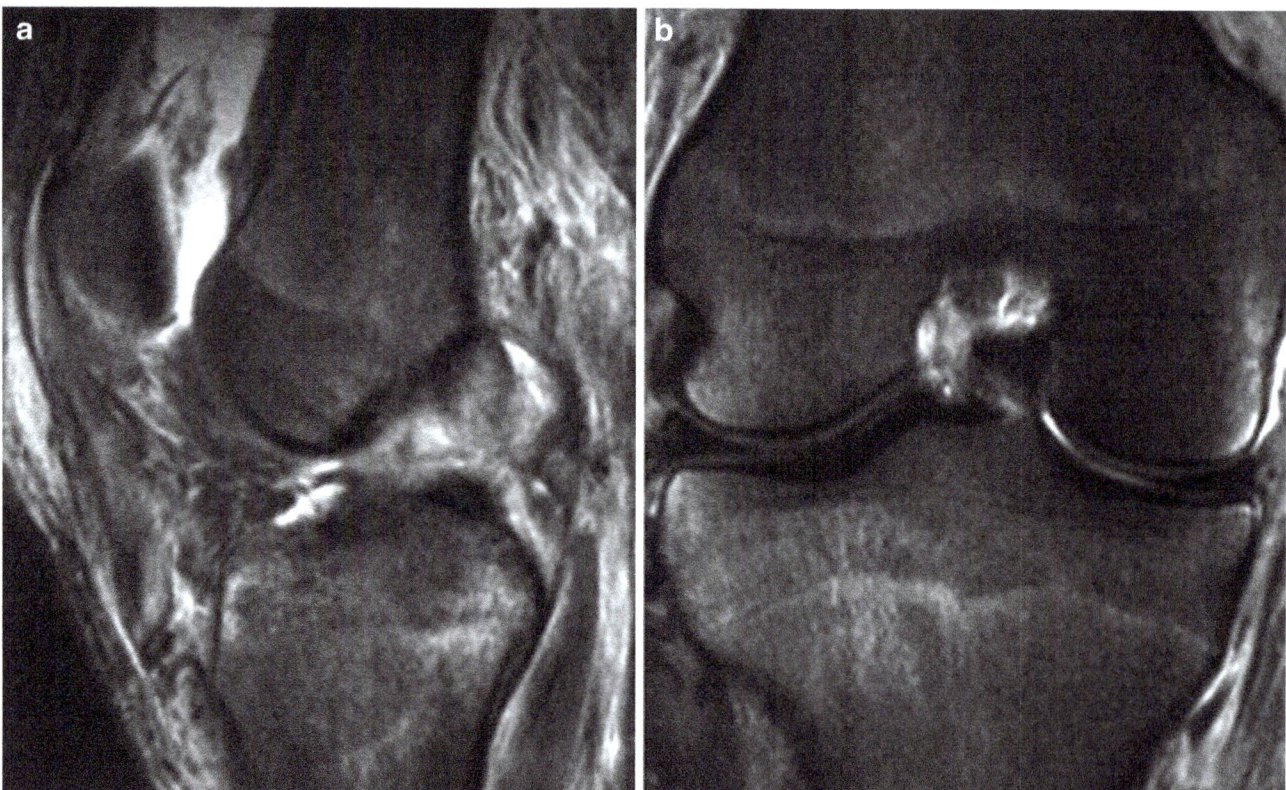

Fig. 5.1 (**a**, **b**) T2 sagittal image is shown demonstrating absence of the ACL as well as the typical bone bruise pattern. Coronal T2-weighted image demonstrates the "empty notch sign"

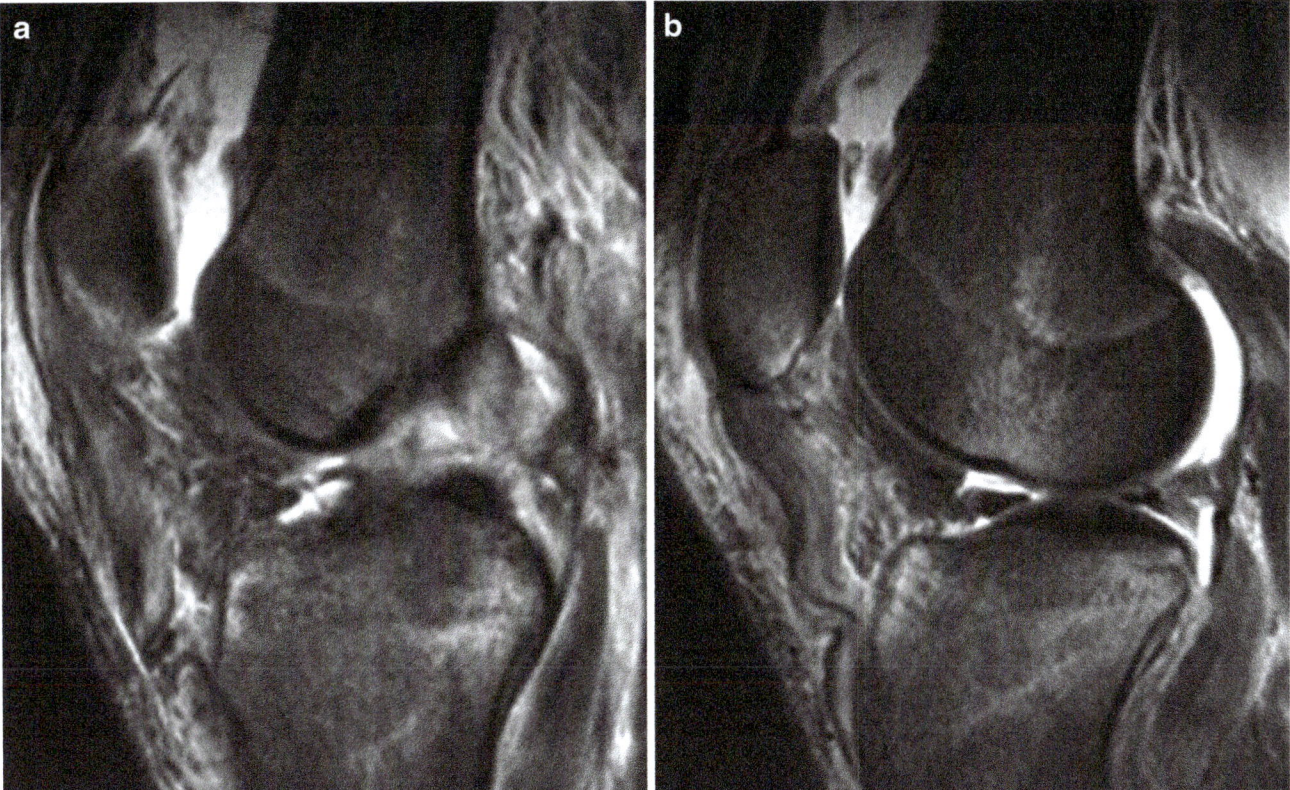

Fig. 5.2 T2 sagittal imaging demonstrates edema within the substance of the ACL with complete disruption (**a**). Partial tearing of the patella tendon is seen at this level (**b**)

a typical bone contusion pattern present as shown in Fig. 5.3. The ACL is seen as an edematous mass without the typically taught fibers. The lateral meniscus visualized best on the sagittal T2-weighted image (Fig. 5.3) showed no meniscal tear. The medial meniscus was intact as was the MCL. No posterior cruciate ligament or articular cartilage pathology was present. The patella tendon was partially disrupted with a wavy appearance to a portion of its fibers (Fig. 5.2b).

MRI allowed for confirmation of ACL tear as well as diagnosis of a patella tendon disruption of uncertain severity. This was consistent with the patient's clinical examination; therefore, risks and benefits of operative intervention were discussed with the patient. He elected to proceed with possible patella tendon repair and planned reconstruction of the ACL given his age and hopes to continue to compete at a collegiate level.

Arthroscopy

The patient was taken to the operating room and placed supine with a post placed in the appropriate position. Given recent evidence suggesting graft size is an important factor in ACL reconstruction failure, we typically prep in the other

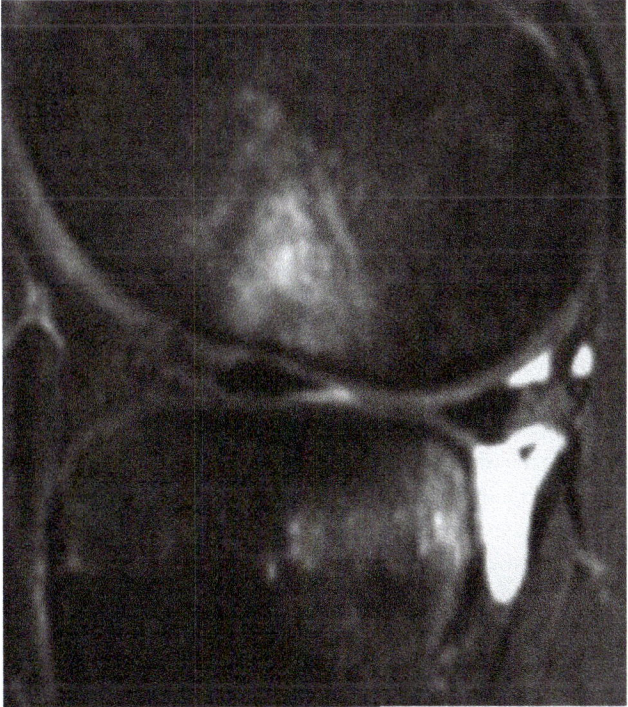

Fig. 5.3 The typical bone bruise pattern is shown on T2-weighted imaging about the lateral femoral condyle and posterolateral tibial plateau. Additionally, the tibia is noted to be translated forward relative to the posterior aspect of the distal femur producing an "anterior drawer" on imaging

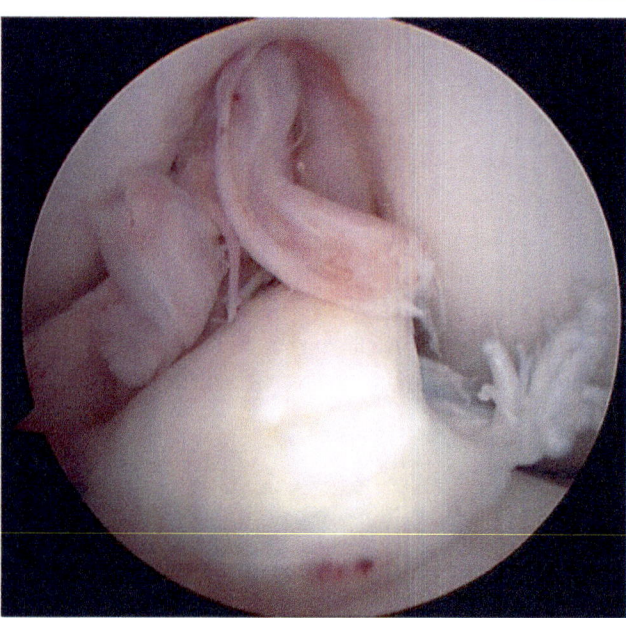

Fig. 5.4 Arthroscopic visualization of the intercondylar notch reveals a complete tear of the ACL with fibrous proliferation and remaining stump on the tibial side

lower extremity when utilizing hamstring graft to reserve the ability to take contralateral graft if needed. The hamstring tendon graft was harvested in the usual fashion. The graft was prepared on the back table, and a standard diagnostic arthroscopy of the knee was completed. The ACL was completely absent with a remaining stump seen demonstrated in Fig. 5.4 with no intact fibers remaining. The articular cartilage and medial meniscus were found to be intact. This correlated well with the findings on MRI.

Following diagnostic arthroscopy, the tibial footprint and ACL over the top position in the back of the notch were debrided using arthroscopic baskets and shaver. Next, the appropriate position off the back of the posterolateral notch was chosen for guide pin placement (Fig. 5.5a). An offset guide can be used here to retain 1–2 mm of posterior wall following drilling. We like to use an accessory medial (AM) portal for separate femoral tunnel drilling to allow more horizontal, anatomic femoral tunnel drilling with the knee in hyperflexion (Fig. 5.5b) [8].

Once the femoral tunnel is drilled to the appropriate depth, a commercially available tibial guide is used to place a guide wire for the tibial tunnel using intra-articular landmarks. Once the tibial tunnel is prepared, a Beath needle is used to pass the graft utilizing suture (Fig. 5.5c), and it is fixed on the femoral side with an interference screw. Once the femoral side is fixed, the knee is cycled through the complete ROM, and the graft is tensioned and the tibial side fixed. The final graft was inspected and noted to have excellent tension in Fig. 5.5d. Finally, the patella tendon was repaired using a Krackow suture technique as shown in Fig. 5.6a, b.

Discussion

MRI demonstrated a complete ACL tear. Several direct MRI signs suggest complete disruption of the ACL in this case. The ACL is discontinuous and does not have the turgor of a normal ACL (Fig. 5.1a). This is best examined on MRI in the sagittal plane where the fibers seen on the T2-weighted image as no longer taught. In the acute setting, the ACL appears as an edematous mass, producing the so-called empty notch sign where fluid rather than ACL fills the intercondylar notch (Fig. 5.1b).

The indirect signs of an ACL injury on MRI are also seen here including the typical hemarthrosis, though this is a largely nonspecific finding. Additionally, the characteristic bone bruise pattern is noted about the lateral femoral condyle and posterolateral tibial plateau due to the prior pivoting event (Fig. 5.3). Often an anterior drawer can be seen where the tibia sits slightly more anterior to a line drawn parallel to the posterior aspect of the distal femur (Fig. 5.3). A Segond fracture which is noticeable on X-ray can also be seen on MRI as shown in the T1 image in Fig. 5.7. The PCL may also appear buckled in some cases.

Case 2: Partial ACL Rupture

History/Exam

A 20-year-old female collegiate soccer player sustained a noncontact injury to her left knee during play. She was seen on the sidelines and noted to have a sizeable effusion and pain with knee range of motion and was unable to return to play. She was subsequently seen in our sports medicine clinic several days later and exhibited an ongoing effusion.

Physical examination of the knee demonstrated no opening with varus or valgus stress. A pivot shift was not possible in the office due to her pain and swelling. She did however have a 2+ Lachman's on her symptomatic side as compared to her asymptomatic side. Patellar apprehension testing was negative as was McMurray's provocative maneuvers. Given the patient's desire to continue to play collegiate soccer and her examination, advanced imaging was obtained to confirm suspected ACL injury and evaluate for additional pathology.

Imaging

Initial plain radiography was unremarkable for any bony abnormality. Given the persistent symptoms, concerning examination and effusion, MRI without contrast was obtained. A complete sequence of images was obtained, including sagittal gradient, STIR, proton density, coronal gradient and fat-saturated T2, and axial fat-saturated T2

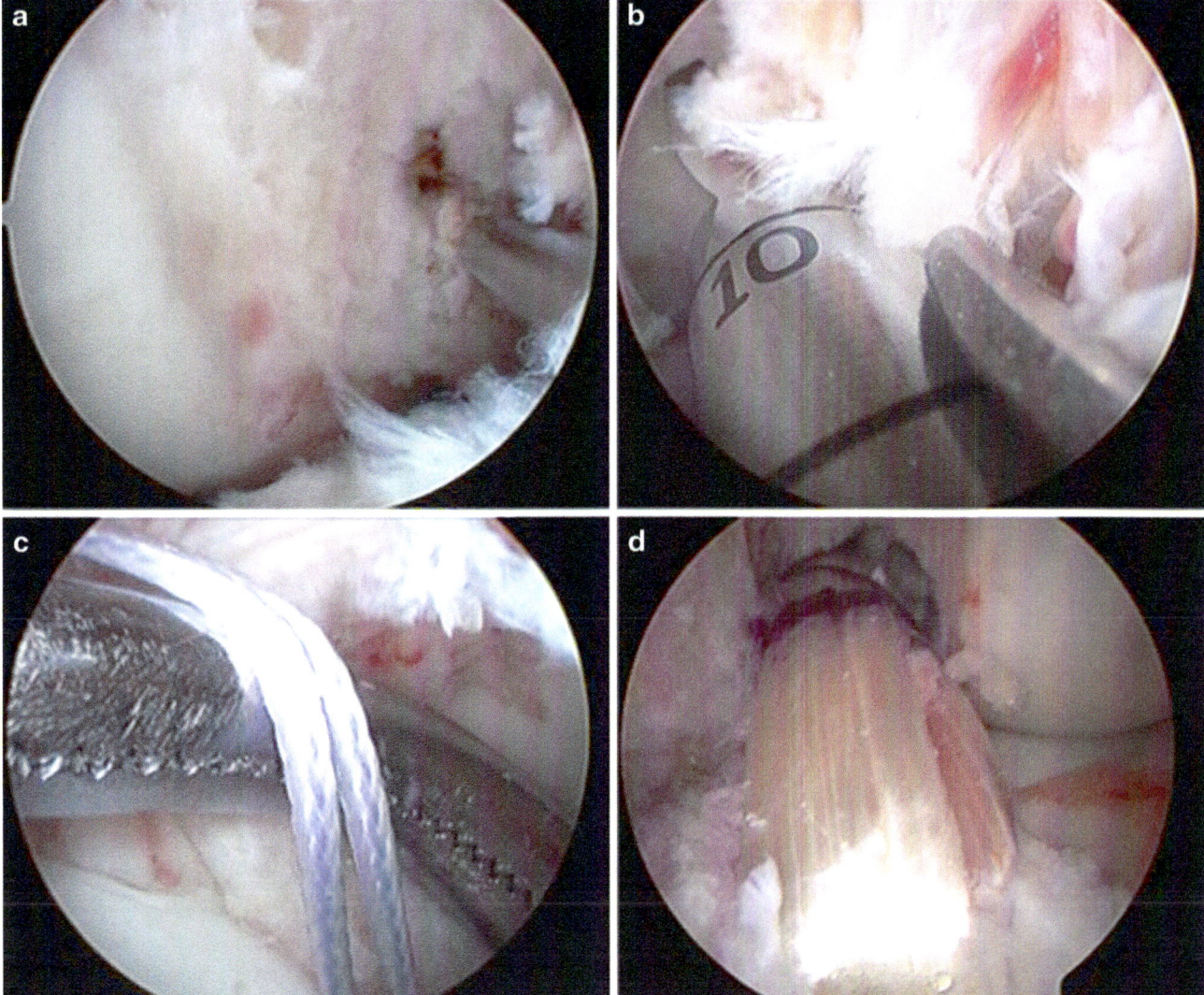

Fig. 5.5 ACL reconstruction steps are shown with placement of a guide pin in the anatomic position utilizing an accessory inferomedial portal (AM portal) (**a**). Femoral tunnel drilling is performed with a skid in place in hyperflexion to protect the femoral condyle (**b**). Both needle and suture are passed through the tunnel to allow for graft shuttling (**c**). The autograft is fixed with interference screw fixation (**d**)

without contrast. Coronal T2-weighted images and sagittal images are demonstrated in Fig. 5.8a, b.

The sagittal images showed no abnormality in the medial and lateral meniscus with a normal cartilage layer throughout. The ACL visualized in the sagittal plane T2 weighted revealed increased signal evident within the substance of the ACL with some remaining continuity (Fig. 5.8a). The PCL, LCL, and MCL were all intact with no focal abnormalities. In the coronal plane, the more medial portion of the ACL attachment to the tibial spine was noted to have increased edema and possible midsubstance tearing (Fig. 5.9a, b). No significant bony edema was seen in the STIR sequences.

The patient's history, physical exam, and MRI were consistent with an ACL tear though MRI imaging was not convincing of a complete ACL injury. A lengthy discussion was had with the patient and her family, trainer, and coach regarding the risks and benefits of watchful waiting versus early arthroscopic exploration and possible reconstruction. They elected to undergo arthroscopy as opposed to attempted early rehabilitation, with a plan to address her ACL with reconstruction if found to be compromised.

Arthroscopy

On the day of surgery following a preoperative nerve block, the patient was taken to the operating room and placed supine upon the operating room table and positioned for ACL reconstruction given our suspicion of ACL injury. Examination under anesthesia was performed as previously described.

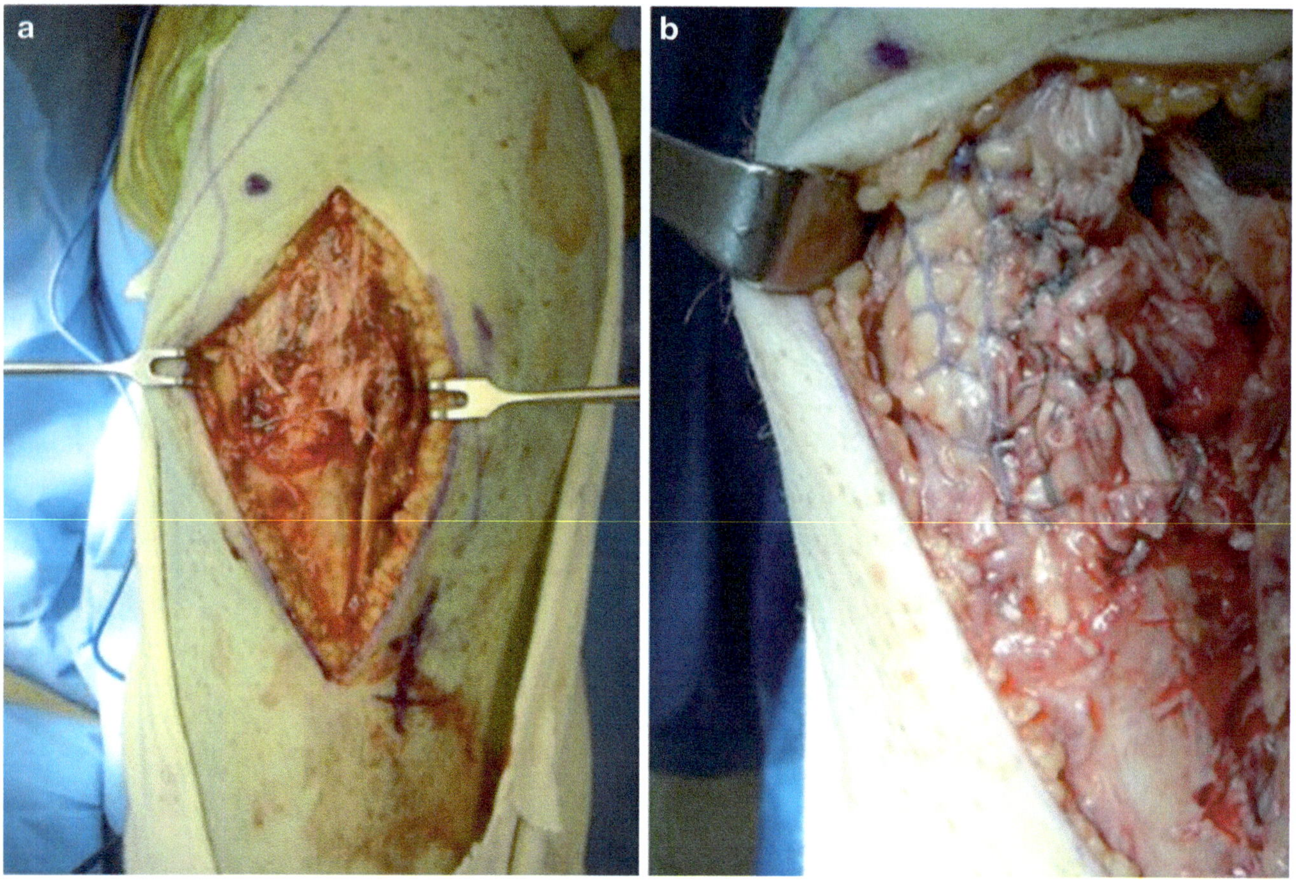

Fig. 5.6 Intraoperative photo demonstrates a partial patella tendon rupture (**a**). This is repaired primarily utilizing Krackow suture technique (**b**)

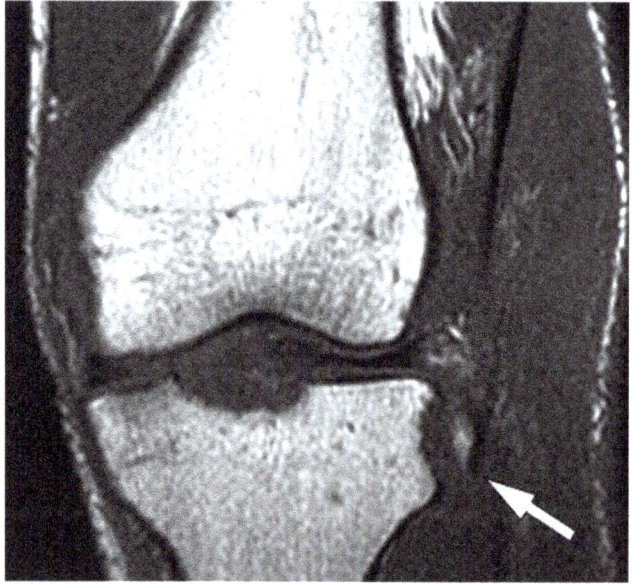

Fig. 5.7 T1-weighted coronal image demonstrates a Segond fracture

If the examination is unclear, a diagnostic arthroscopy is always performed before harvesting graft. Again under anesthesia, a Lachman was performed which showed side-to-side difference with a soft end point. A nonsterile tourniquet was placed around the operative extremity. Standard inferolateral and inferomedial portals were made and a diagnostic arthroscopy completed to establish whether her ACL was in fact torn. We evaluated the patellofemoral joint, medial and lateral gutters, and compartments to assess for any meniscal disease, loose bodies, or cartilage injury of which none were found.

Visualization of the notch of the ACL demonstrated a partial ACL injury as shown in Figs. 5.9a, b and 5.10a, b. The posterolateral bundle of the ACL appeared intact and taught. The anteromedial bundle however was not intact, and a residual stump was present on the tibial side from the prior attachment. The rest of the diagnostic scope was unremarkable for chondral damage or meniscal injury. Given the patient's expectations preoperatively and her current activity as a collegiate soccer player, decision was made to perform arthroscopic-assisted ACL reconstruction.

Although several graft options are available, autograft is a common graft option and has been demonstrated to lead to lower failure rates than allograft options in young patients [10]. In this case bone patella bone and hamstring autograft are reasonable options for this young athlete. With a combination of arthroscopic punch, motorized shaver, and electrocautery as needed, the ACL footprint was debrided. After debriding the

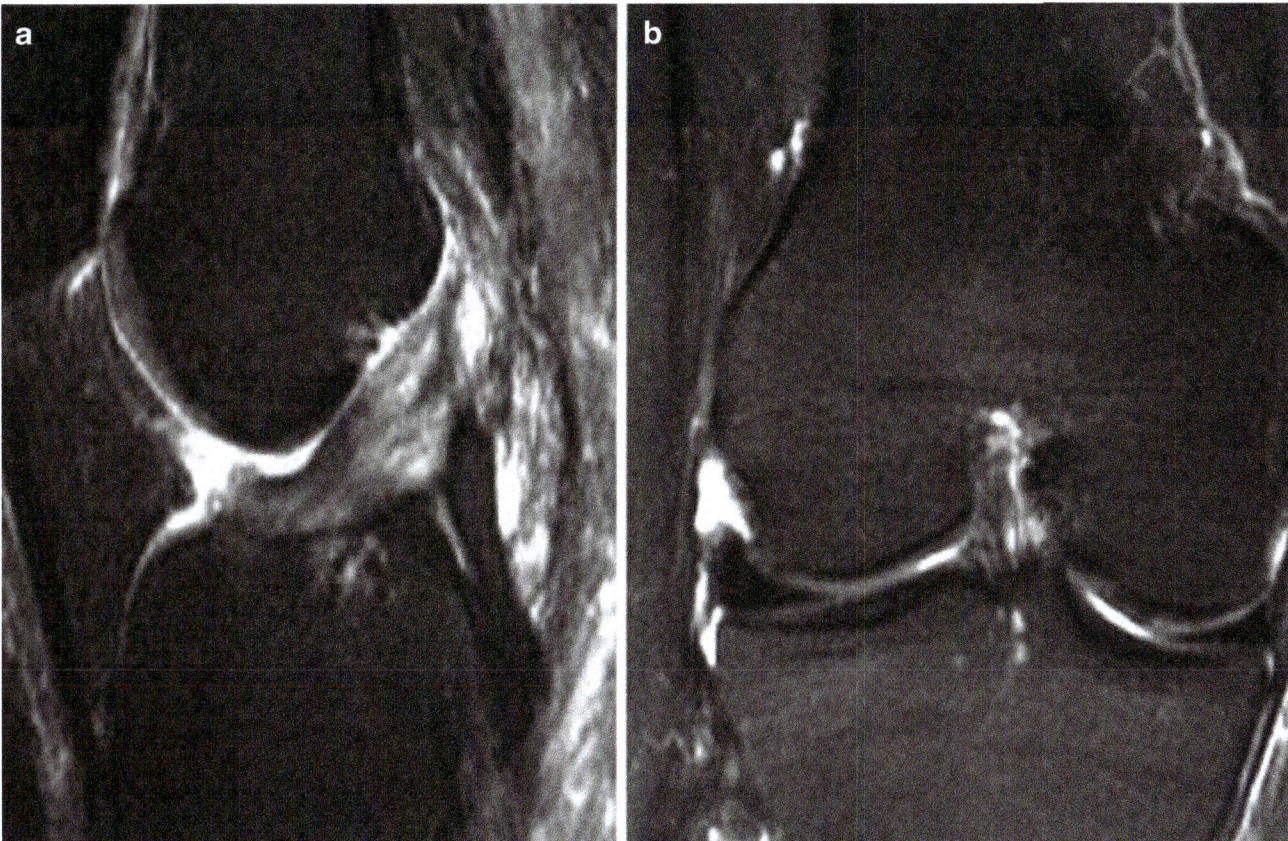

Fig. 5.8 Sagittal MRI demonstrates edema within the ACL with remaining intact fibers (**a**). The coronal plane imaging is shown which reveals increased fluid and potential disruption in the anteromedial aspect of the tibial footprint (**b**)

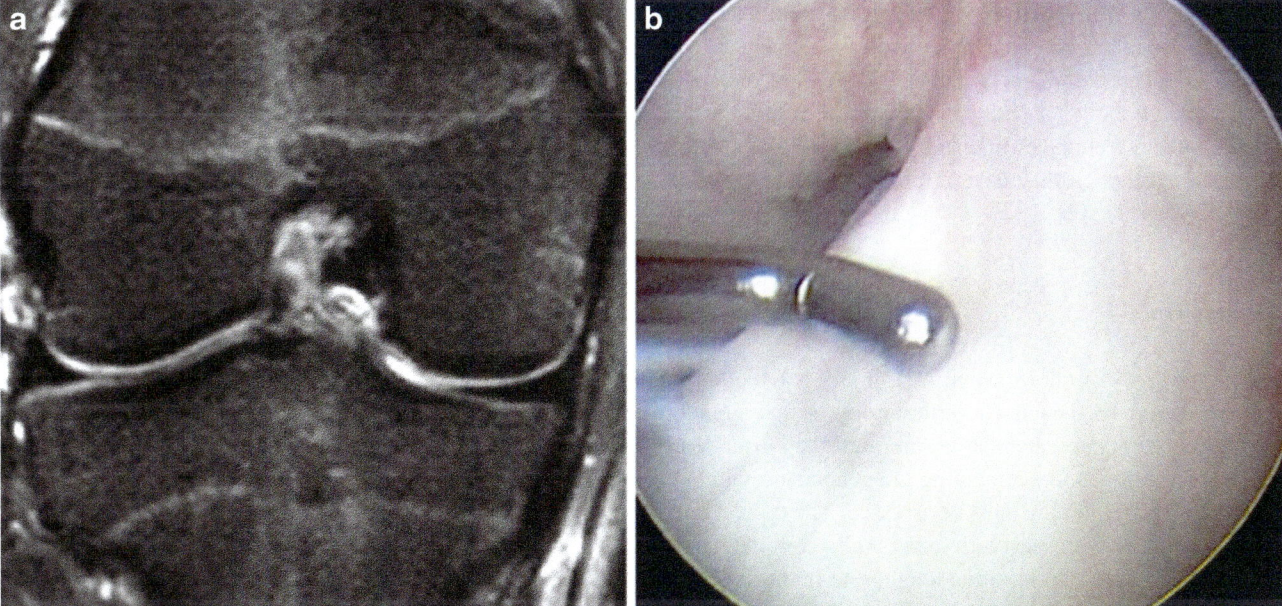

Fig. 5.9 A partial empty intercondylar notch is shown on coronal T2-weighted MRI (**a**). A partially intact ACL is shown on arthroscopy (**b**)

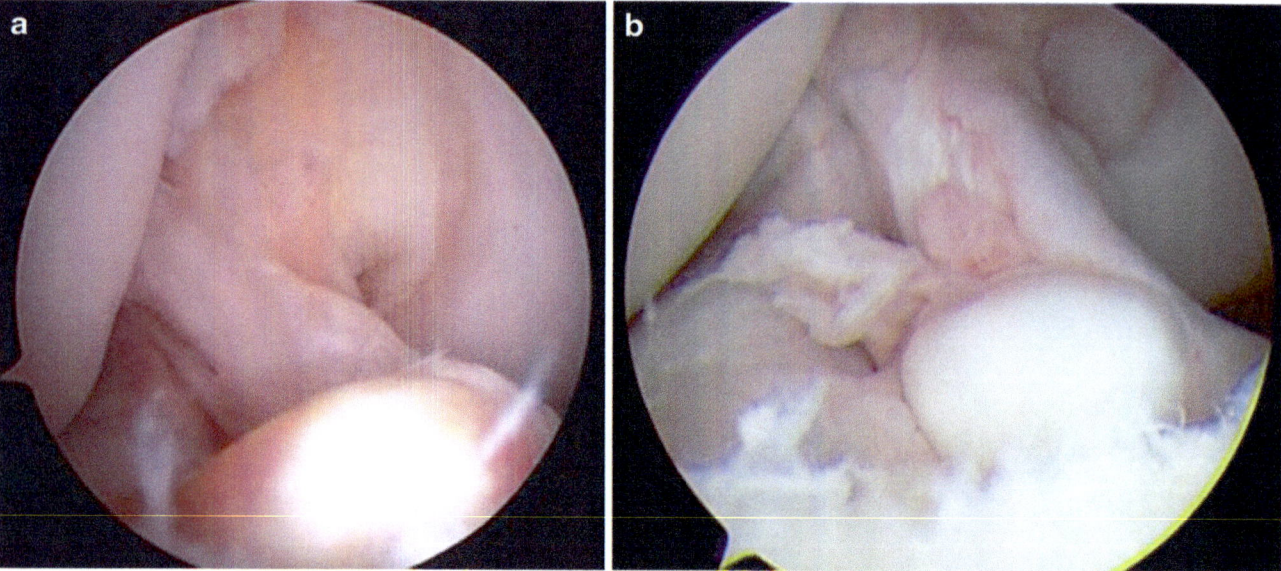

Fig. 5.10 Arthroscopic visualization of the notch demonstrates intact posterolateral bundle (**a**) with obviously less caliber than a typical ACL. The remaining stump of likely the anteromedial bundle of the ACL is seen as a cyclops lesion on the tibial side (**b**) with some remaining intact fibers shown

ruptured ACL fibers, tunnels are drilled in the tibia and femur for the prepared grafts after sizing (Fig. 5.11a–d). In our hands, grafts are subsequently fixed utilizing interference screw fixation. We prefer to place the tibial tunnel in the posteromedial aspect of the ACL footprint and the femoral tunnel in the 10–10:30 position for the right knee leaving 2 mm of posterior wall in a more horizontal graft orientation. We performed a single-bundle technique utilizing an accessory inferomedial portal for guide wire placement and independent femoral drilling to allow for more anatomic graft placement [7, 8] (Fig. 5.11d). This portal is approximately 3–4 cm medial to the patellar tendon though should be localized under arthroscopy. Double-bundle techniques and individual-bundle techniques are described though they have not been widely adopted by most surgeons [11, 12].

Discussion

MRI is the study of choice when ACL injury is uncertain or exam is equivocal. Diagnostic arthroscopy in this situation may be necessary to establish an absolute diagnosis. With partial ACL injuries, the remaining fibers appear taught and the percentage remaining must be assessed. The typical bone contusion pattern present with most ACL complete tears (72 % in complete tears) is often not present in the setting of a partial ACL injury (12 % incidence) [13]. The final determination is whether the knee is stable or unstable with only the remaining ACL fibers. This discussion should be undertaken with the patient, family, and athletic trainer.

With appropriate indications and proper surgical technique, ACL reconstruction outcomes after partial ACL injury are very good overall. However, many surgeons choose to treat partial injuries nonoperatively in the less-active patient without overt knee instability. Comparative studies looking at hamstring and patella tendon autograft have yielded equivalent results [10]. Athletes can often return to play at 4 months postoperatively. Controversy remains regarding the technique for ACL reconstruction and the ideal graft choice; however, most literature suggests equivalent outcomes between autograft choices [10].

Case 3: Bony ACL Avulsion Injury

History/Exam

A 35-year-old male presented to our sports medicine clinic with pain in his left knee that began approximately 4 days prior. The patient reported that while coaching his daughter's basketball team, his knee gave way when he was running down the court. He had immediate pain and swelling and was able to bear weight but unable to continue coaching that day. He was seen at a local clinic where he was given crutches and a soft brace. An aspiration performed by the clinic improved his pain tremendously. Prior to this injury, he had one prior knee arthroscopy of which he does not remember the details. He had tried nonsteroidal anti-inflammatories, muscle relaxants, physical therapy, and stretching prior to presentation without relief.

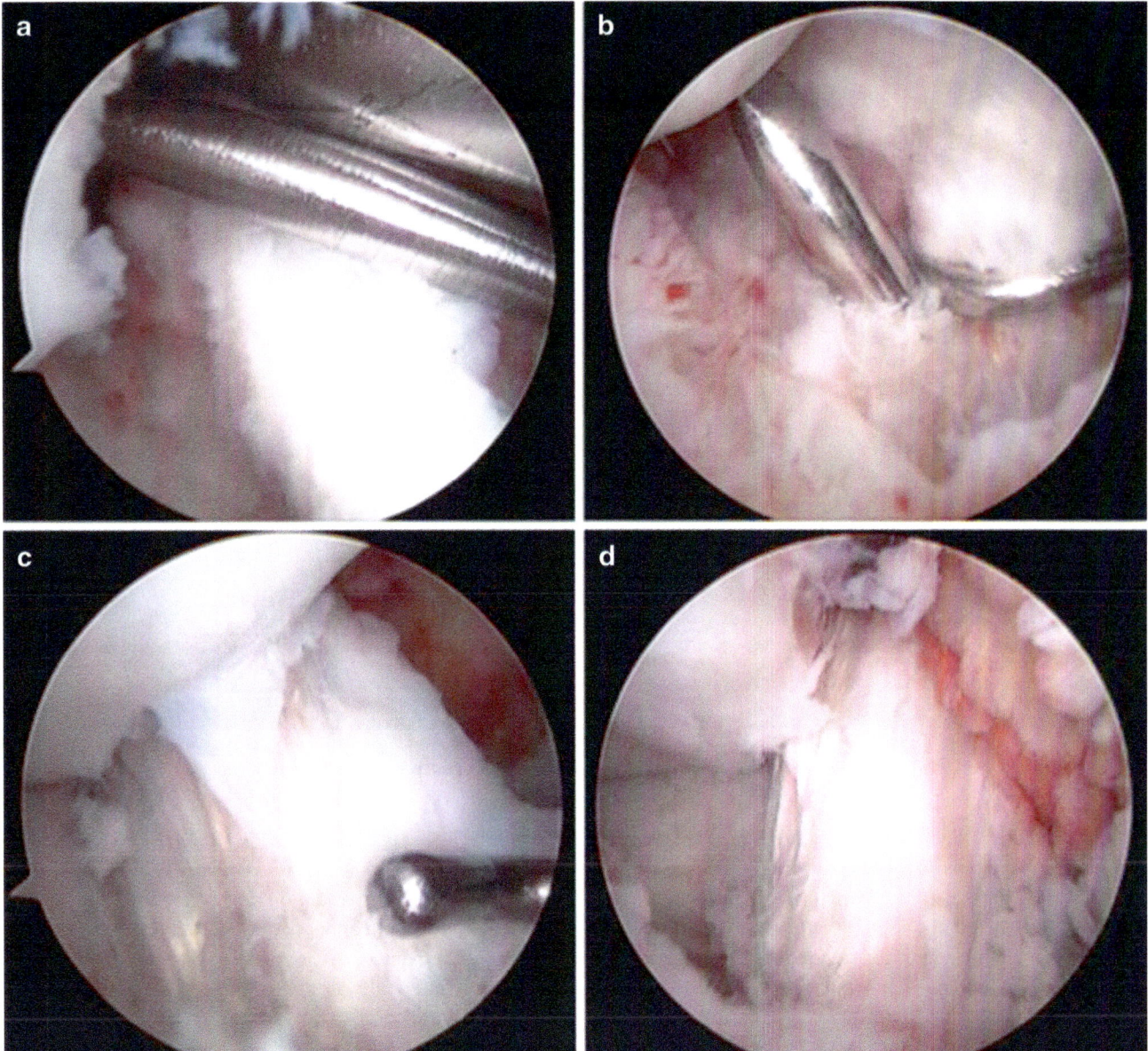

Fig. 5.11 Following complete debridement of the remaining ACL, a guide pin is placed through an accessory AM portal on the femoral side (**a**) and later the tibial side (**b**). Final graft is taught and well fixed (**c**, **d**)

On physical examination, he was noted to have pain with range of motion and a moderate effusion. Range of motion was noted to be limited compared to the contralateral side. He lacked approximately 10° extension, with flexion up to 90° with significant effort. Additionally, lateral joint line tenderness was present and McMurray's exam was positive in the clinic. Lachman's was grossly positive with no firm end point and a pivot shift was reproducible. There was no opening with varus or valgus stress and a negative posterior drawer.

Given the acute nature of his injury as well as difficulty with range of motion, decision was made to evaluate further

with MRI. Additionally, the brace was discontinued at this time with instructions to work on aggressive range of motion with formal physical therapy. The initial radiographs obtained at the outside clinic revealed a bony abnormality not fully appreciated about the tibial spine.

Imaging

Radiographs obtained at the outside hospital suggested a possible injury about the tibial spine. There was no evidence of arthritic changes in the medial and lateral compartments.

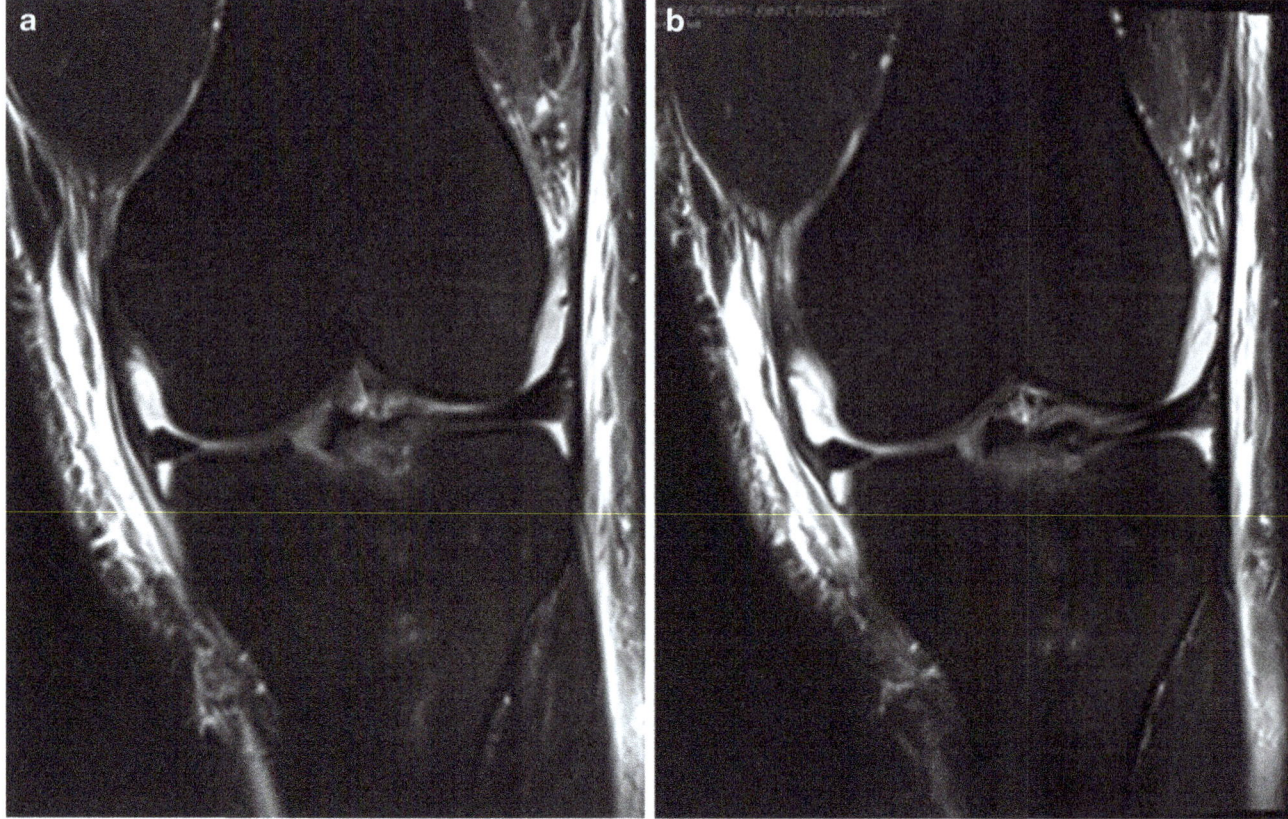

Fig. 5.12 Coronal MRI STIR imaging reveals increased signal in the proximal tibial eminence at the ACL attachment (**a**, **b**)

MRI without contrast was obtained to further evaluate the patient's soft tissue anatomy. A complete sequence of images was obtained, including sagittal gradient, STIR, proton density, coronal gradient and fat-saturated T2, and axial fat-saturated T2 without contrast. Coronal fat-saturated T2-weighted images are demonstrated in Fig. 5.12a, b, and sagittal stir images are demonstrated in Fig. 5.13a, b.

The sagittal images (Fig. 5.13a, b) demonstrate normal medial meniscus with an anterior horn root insertion of the lateral meniscus avulsed with a bone fragment along with the adjacent ACL. A focal radial tear of the posterior horn of the lateral meniscus can be seen on the sagittal STIR image as well. Increased signal is evident within the substance of the ACL with avulsion of the anterior tibial spine noted in coronal T2-weighted image (Fig. 5.12a, b). The PCL, LCL, and MCL were all intact with no focal abnormalities. Mild focal thickening and edema are present within the patella tendon possibly from chronic patella tendinitis.

In addition to the bony avulsion of the ACL and the anterior horn of the lateral meniscus, a very minimally depressed lateral tibial plateau fracture is seen at the posterior aspect of the plateau. Typical lipohemarthrosis is seen within the joint. The patient's history, physical exam, and MRI were consistent with an ACL tear. His symptoms were persistent with

consistent sense of instability with any activity and stair climbing. Surgical intervention was offered, with a plan to address his ACL with either fixation depending on the size of the bony fragment or ACL reconstruction with hamstring autograft. Additionally, arthroscopy would allow for evaluation of his lateral meniscus.

Arthroscopy

The patient was taken to the operating room and placed supine upon the operating room table with a post placed in the appropriate position as well as the leg holder appropriately positioned. Once the patient was asleep, an exam under anesthesia was performed as we always do prior to any knee arthroscopy. A pivot shift was reproducible in the operating room. Both extremities were prepped in as we typically do when considering hamstring reconstruction to allow for contralateral harvest if needed to supplement a small graft. A tourniquet was placed nonsterile around the operative extremity. Standard inferolateral and inferomedial portals were made and a diagnostic arthroscopy completed. Of note, arthroscopy was performed first in this situation given the uncharacteristic findings on MRI.

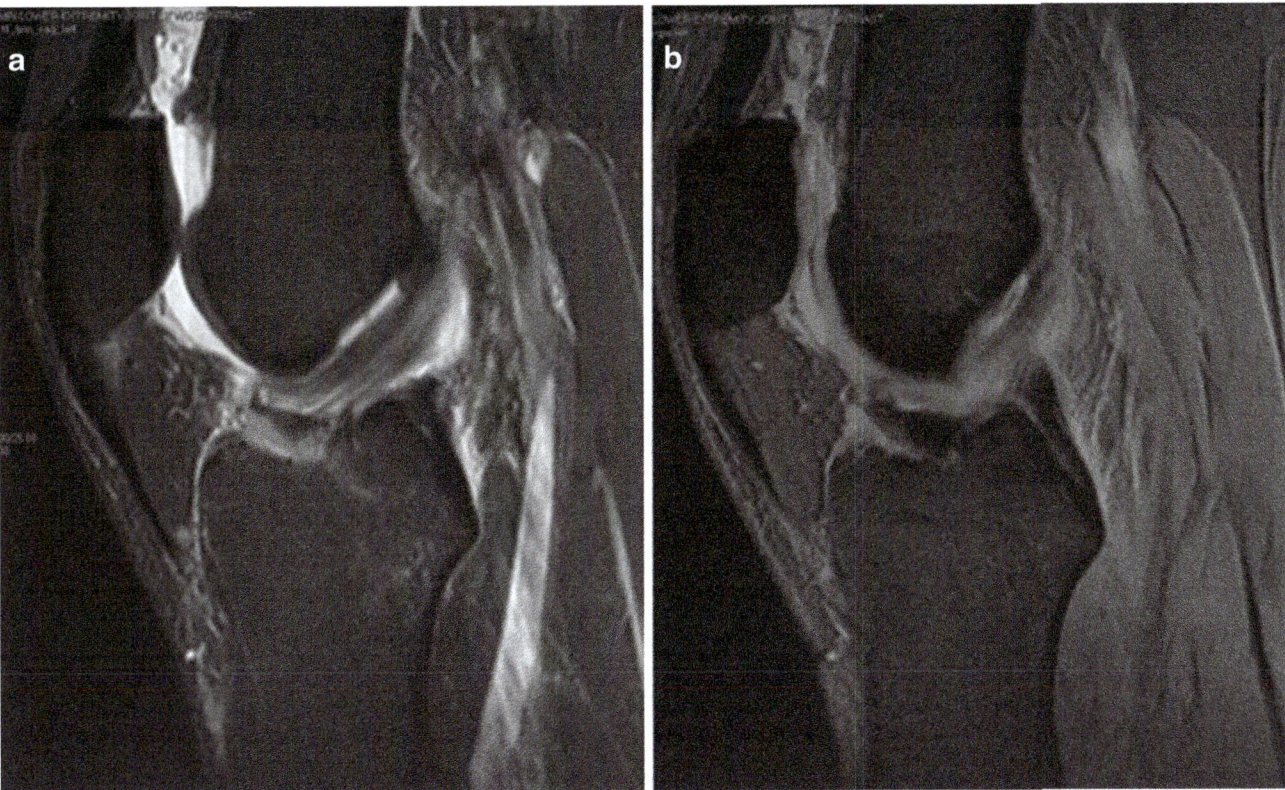

Fig. 5.13 ACL fibers appear taught attached to the elevated tibial eminence (**a**). The bony attachment of the ACL is elevated anteriorly with little remaining posterior cortical attachment (**b**)

Following evacuation of bloody effusion, we were able to visualize the joint, which had no evidence of chondromalacia. No loose bodies were noted on arthroscopy. The camera was brought into the notch where the ACL was seen to be intact throughout its midsubstance Fig. 5.14a. However, when the scope was brought more anterior and inferior, the entire tibial eminence of the ACL was noted to have pulled off with an associated bleeding bony bed (Fig. 5.14a, b). This bed was covered with a layer of fibrous tissue deposited over the previous weeks leading up to surgery. Examination of the medial compartment revealed no medial meniscus tear. The knee was then brought into the figure-of-four position, and the arthroscope was brought into the lateral compartment where the anterior horn of the lateral meniscus was displaced and attached to the bony tibial eminence piece.

We prepared the bony bed of the meniscus and ACL tibial attachment using an arthroscopic shaver to remove the underlying fibrinous material. A burr was utilized to aid in the reduction of the bony fragment (Fig. 5.14b, c) to allow for slight recession of the fragment. The ACL fully attached to the bony fragment was then reduced to its native position with an arthroscopic probe. Guide pins for screw fixation were placed medial and lateral to the patella tendon in a con-

verging fashion (Fig. 5.14d). We confirmed this reduction under fluoroscopy and direct visualization. We were pleased with the length of our pins and subsequently predrilled and tapped. Two partially threaded 6.5 mm screws and washers were placed over guide wire (Fig. 5.15a–d) with excellent reduction confirmed under arthroscopy and fluoroscopy with final radiographs taken postoperatively (Fig. 5.16a, b).

Following fixation, the ACL was once again examined and was taught. The lateral meniscus was once again examined, and the posterior lateral meniscus tear was found to have healed needing no further intervention. The arthroscope was removed and a Lachman test was performed with a firm end point noted. The patient was placed in an IROM set from 0 to 90 to begin range of motion immediately with protected weight bearing for 2 weeks.

Discussion

MRI is the imaging of choice for possible ACL avulsion injuries. While CT may help with establishing the amount of bone avulsed off the tibial eminence, MRI allows for simultaneous diagnosis of other concomitant knee pathology,

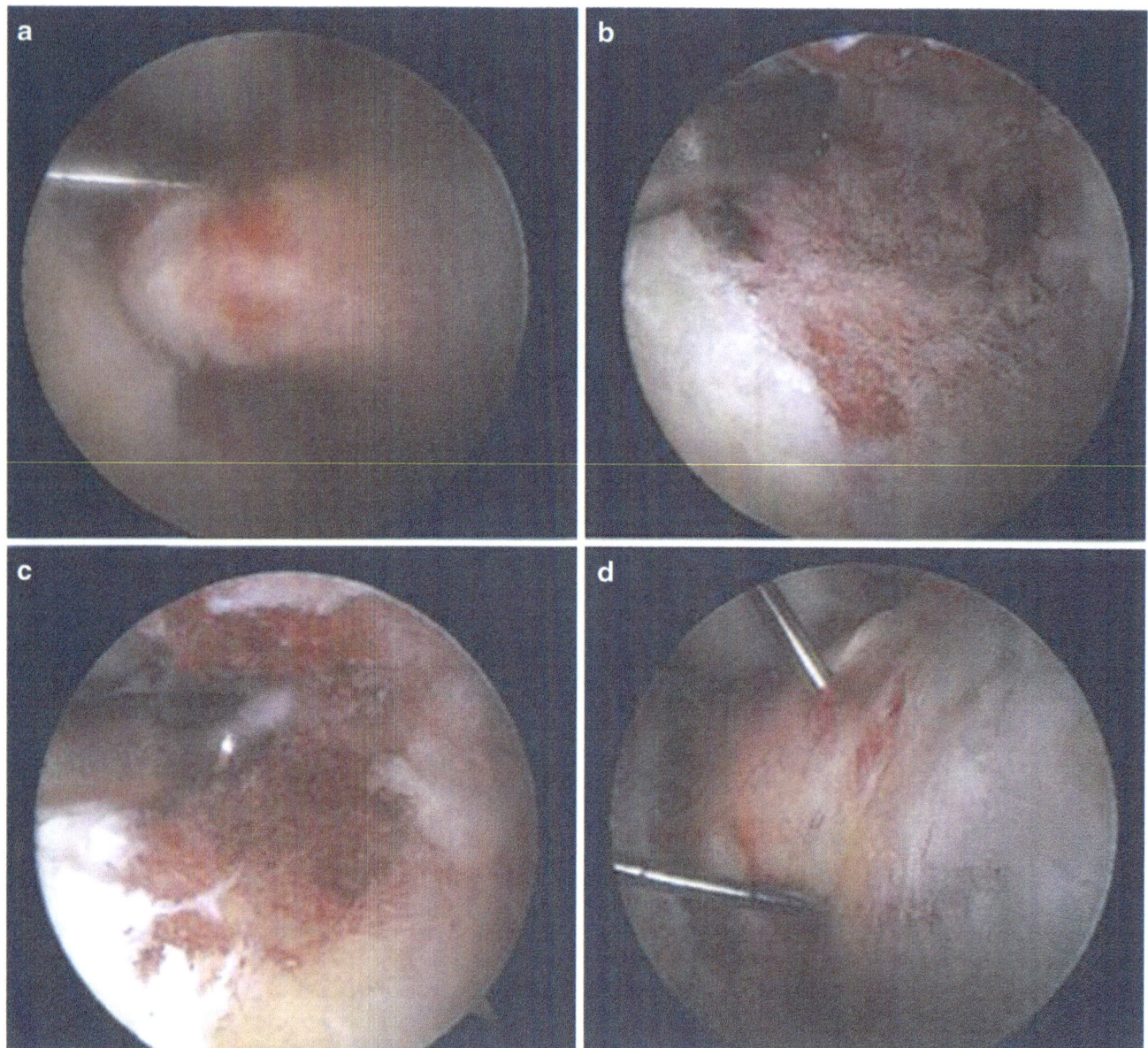

Fig. 5.14 Bloody effusion is noted on arthroscopy due to the acuity of the fracture. The ACL remains completely attached to a large tibial eminence avulsion and is being pulled down with an arthroscopic probe with attached anterior horn of the lateral meniscus (**a**). The bed beneath the elevated ACL is covered with fibrous tissue (**b**). An arthroscopic burr is used to debride the overlying tissue and recess the bony bed (**c**). Once reduction is achieved, two guide wires are placed medial and lateral to the patella tendon to hold the reduction (**d**)

which in this case included lateral meniscal pathology. MRI is estimated to have a sensitivity and specificity over 90 % for detecting ACL injury in the setting of bony avulsion injury. MRI is the preferred modality for evaluating the other soft tissue structures of the knee that may be causing symptoms.

Tibial eminence fractures are well described in the orthopedic literature [14]. Anatomically, they represent avulsion injuries to the insertion of the anterior cruciate ligament (ACL) on the tibia and are considered the childhood equivalent of an ACL tear. Tibial avulsion injuries of the ACL are less common in the adult patient though they do occur [15]. Management of these injuries can include nonsurgical or surgical options. Nonoperative modalities include therapy, range of motion, and strengthening programs with appropriate utilization of nonsteroidal anti-inflammatory agents (NSAIDS). Surgical options include ACL reconstruction with allograft or autograft or fixation in the setting of a large bony fragment.

Meyers and McKeever described a classification of these injuries dividing them into three types [16]. Type I describes a nondisplaced or minimally displaced eminence fracture,

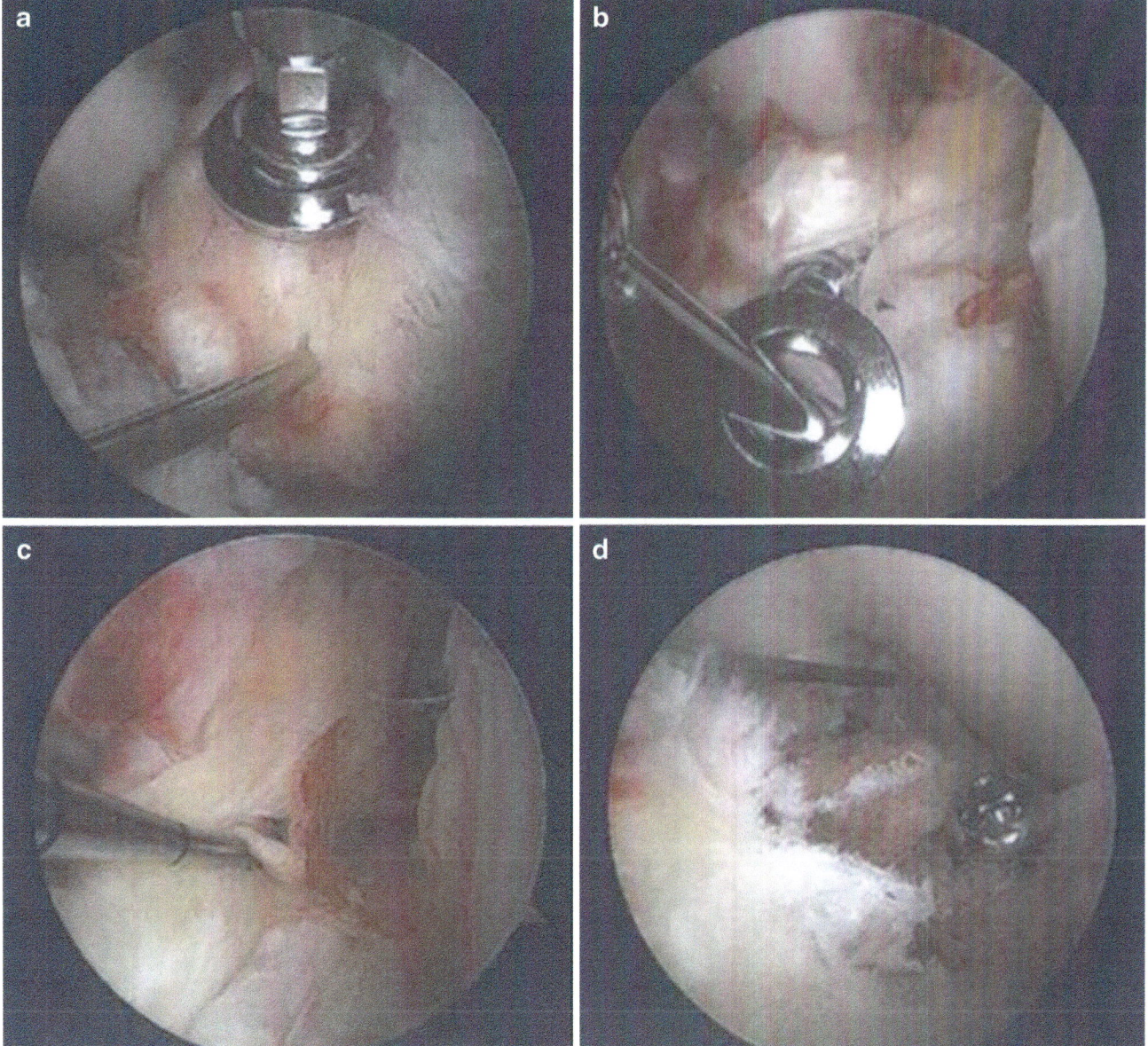

Fig. 5.15 Two partially threaded 6.5 mm screws are placed over guide wire along with washers (**a, b, c**). Excellent reduction is achieved with no notch impingement noted on full extension (**d**)

which can be treated nonoperatively. In type II, the anterior third is displaced proximally with up to one half of the attachment off though the posterior attachment is still present. Type III fractures represent complete displacement. Immobilization in extension can be pursued for type I and some type II injuries with most type III injuries requiring fixation. Regardless of the treatment method, residual laxity may be present after tibial eminence avulsion injuries. Arthroscopy and MRI for damage to other attached soft tissue structures allow for accurate reduction and treatment of these injuries [17]. Fixation can be achieved with sutures or hardware [17–22]. Outcomes for different fixation methods do not appear to differ [20].

Conclusions

ACL injuries are a common reason for knee surgery in young and healthy patients. The clinical diagnosis of ACL tear is straightforward, though coexistent pathology is frequently present and must be recognized for surgical and rehabilitation planning. A careful history, physical examination including provocative maneuvers, and imaging as dictated from the exam are key in establishing an appropriate diagnosis. Magnetic resonance imaging (MRI) remains the imaging technique of choice for patients with suspected ACL tear. MRI is also useful in identifying concomitant

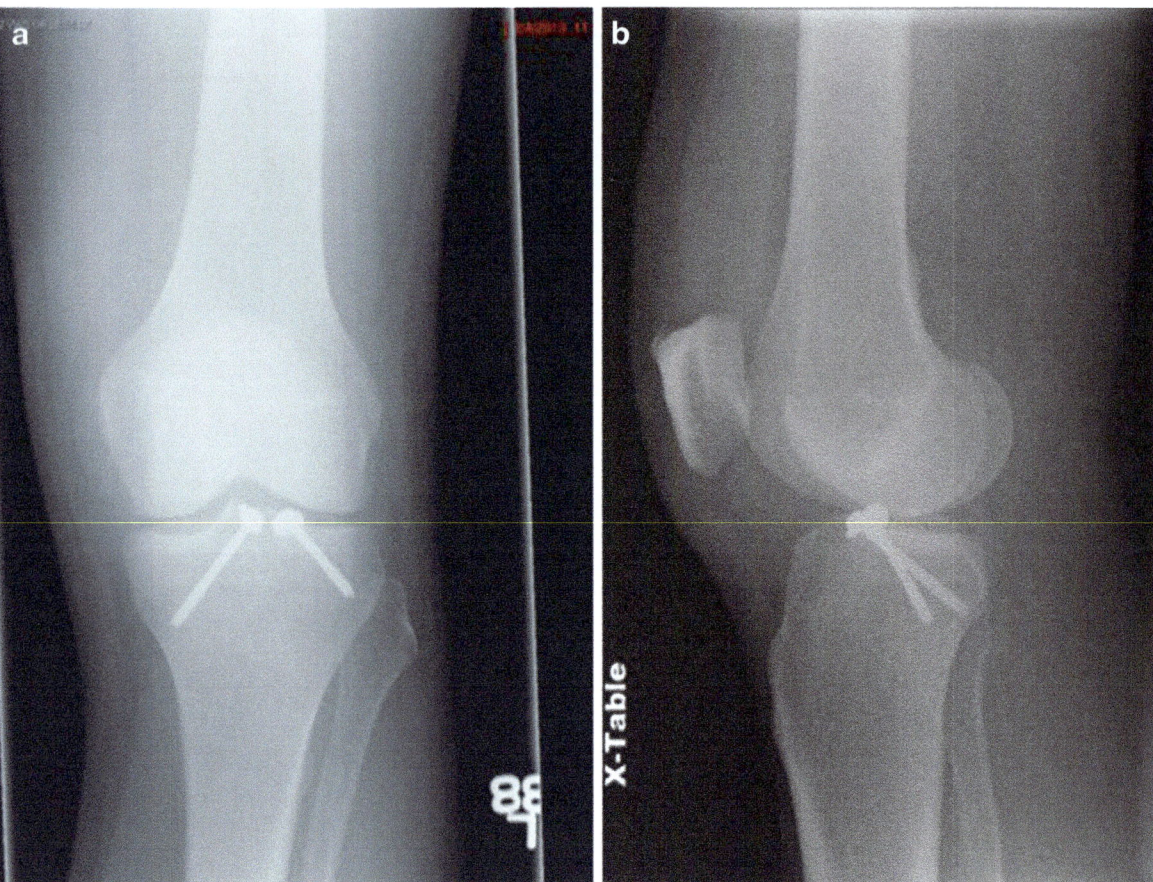

Fig. 5.16 Postoperative radiographs demonstrate divergent screw fixation with reduction of the tibial eminence (**a, b**)

knee pathology that may change staging of intervention. Surgical intervention can be pursued in the carefully chosen active patient, and the approach must be individualized. Lower demand patients may be better managed with nonoperative care. Treatment options are few including autograft, allograft, and double-bundle reconstruction though some extra-articular techniques are still used in some centers. Techniques for improving ACL reconstruction are under constant analysis and development.

References

1. Lyman S, Koulouvaris P, Sherman S, Do H, Mandl LA, Marx RG. Epidemiology of anterior cruciate ligament reconstruction: trends, readmissions, and subsequent knee surgery. J Bone Joint Surg Am. 2009;91(10):2321–8.
2. Fu FH, Bennett CH, Ma CB, Menetrey J, Lattermann C. Current trends in anterior cruciate ligament reconstruction. Part II. Operative procedures and clinical correlations. Am J Sports Med. 2000; 28(1):124–30.
3. Boden BP, Sheehan FT, Torg JS, Hewett TE. Noncontact anterior cruciate ligament injuries: mechanisms and risk factors. J Am Acad Orthop Surg. 2010;18(9):520–7.
4. Daniel DM, Stone ML, Dobson BE, Fithian DC, Rossman DJ, Kaufman KR. Fate of the ACL-injured patient. A prospective outcome study. Am J Sports Med. 1994;22(5):632–44.
5. Drogset JO, Grontvedt T, Robak OR, Molster A, Viset AT, Engebretsen L. A sixteen-year follow-up of three operative techniques for the treatment of acute ruptures of the anterior cruciate ligament. J Bone Joint Surg Am. 2006;88(5):944–52.
6. Duffee A, Magnussen RA, Pedroza AD, Flanigan DC, MOON Group, Kaeding CC. Transtibial ACL femoral tunnel preparation increases odds of repeat ipsilateral knee surgery. J Bone Joint Surg Am. 2013;95(22):2035–42.
7. Golish SR, Baumfeld JA, Schoderbek RJ, Miller MD. The effect of femoral tunnel starting position on tunnel length in anterior cruciate ligament reconstruction: a cadaveric study. Arthroscopy. 2007; 23(11):1187–92.
8. Tompkins M, Milewski MD, Brockmeier SF, Gaskin CM, Hart JM, Miller MD. Anatomic femoral tunnel drilling in anterior cruciate ligament reconstruction: use of an accessory medial portal versus traditional transtibial drilling. Am J Sports Med. 2012;40(6): 1313–21.
9. Ajuied A, Wong F, Smith C, Norris M, Earnshaw P, Back D, et al. Anterior cruciate ligament injury and radiologic progression of knee osteoarthritis: a systematic review and meta-analysis. Am J Sports Med. 2014;42(9):2242–52.
10. Foster TE, Wolfe BL, Ryan S, Silvestri L, Kaye EK. Does the graft source really matter in the outcome of patients undergoing anterior cruciate ligament reconstruction? An evaluation of autograft versus

allograft reconstruction results: a systematic review. Am J Sports Med. 2010;38(1):189–99.

11. Chen JL, Allen CR, Stephens TE, Haas AK, Huston LJ, Wright RW, et al. Differences in mechanisms of failure, intraoperative findings, and surgical characteristics between single- and multiple-revision ACL reconstructions: a MARS cohort study. Am J Sports Med. 2013;41(7):1571–8.

12. Iriuchishima T, Horaguchi T, Kubomura T, Morimoto Y, Fu FH. Evaluation of the intercondylar roof impingement after anatomical double-bundle anterior cruciate ligament reconstruction using 3D-CT. Knee Surg Sports Traumatol Arthrosc. 2011;19(4):674–9.

13. Zeiss J, Paley K, Murray K, Saddemi SR. Comparison of bone contusion seen by MRI in partial and complete tears of the anterior cruciate ligament. J Comput Assist Tomogr. 1995;19(5):773–6.

14. Ando T, Nishihara K. Arthroscopic internal fixation of fractures of the intercondylar eminence of the tibia. Arthroscopy. 1996;12(5):616–22.

15. Kendall NS, Hsu SY, Chan KM. Fracture of the tibial spine in adults and children. A review of 31 cases. J Bone Joint Surg Br. 1992;74(6):848–52.

16. Meyers MH, McKeever FM. Fracture of the intercondylar eminence of the tibia. J Bone Joint Surg Am. 1970;52(8):1677–84.

17. Bonin N, Jeunet L, Obert L, Dejour D. Adult tibial eminence fracture fixation: arthroscopic procedure using K-wire folded fixation. Knee Surg Sports Traumatol Arthrosc. 2007;15(7):857–62.

18. Kobayashi S, Terayama K. Arthroscopic reduction and fixation of a completely displaced fracture of the intercondylar eminence of the tibia. Arthroscopy. 1994;10(2):231–5.

19. Kogan MG, Marks P, Amendola A. Technique for arthroscopic suture fixation of displaced tibial intercondylar eminence fractures. Arthroscopy. 1997;13(3):301–6.

20. Hunter RE, Willis JA. Arthroscopic fixation of avulsion fractures of the tibial eminence: technique and outcome. Arthroscopy. 2004;20(2):113–21.

21. Matthews DE, Geissler WB. Arthroscopic suture fixation of displaced tibial eminence fractures. Arthroscopy. 1994;10(4):418–23.

22. Yang SW, Lu YC, Teng HP, Wong CY. Arthroscopic reduction and suture fixation of displaced tibial intercondylar eminence fractures in adults. Arch Orthop Trauma Surg. 2005;125(4):272–6.

Posterior Cruciate Ligament

6

Gregory C. Fanelli and William James Malone

Anatomy and Biomechanics

The posterior cruciate ligament plays an integral role in knee joint stability. It is the primary restraint to posterior translation of the proximal tibia and is a secondary restraint to varus, valgus, and external rotation forces [1]. Posterior knee structures including the posteromedial and posterolateral capsule; MCL; LCL; and arcuate, meniscofemoral, and fabellofibular ligaments provide the primary restraint from 0° to 30° [2–5]. The PCL provides increasing resistance to posterior translation from 30° to 90° of knee flexion, and at 90° of knee flexion, the posterior cruciate ligament provides 95 % of the total restraining force for the straight posterior drawer [2, 6].

Injury Mechanism

The goal of the evolving techniques in PCL reconstruction is to restore the normal kinematics and in situ forces of the knee. The incidence of PCL injuries has been reported to be from 1 % to 40 % in acute knee injuries [7–13]. This incidence is dependent on the patient population reported, with PCL tears occurring more frequently in trauma patients than in athletic injury patients [10–12]. PCL tears may result from a variety of injuries. A thorough history of the mechanism of injury can allow for increased suspicion for PCL tear as well as associated ligamentous injuries.

The majority of PCL injuries occur from a posteriorly directed force on the proximal tibia. These most often result from "dashboard" injuries with the knee in a flexed position or a fall onto a flexed knee with the foot in a plantar flexed position. The most common mechanism for isolated PCL tears is forced hyperflexion of the knee [14]. These injuries commonly result in partial tears of the PCL with the PMB remaining intact. Injury patterns involving hyperextension, forced varus or valgus, and knee dislocations are associated with PCL tears plus other ligament injuries [10–12, 15].

History and Physical Examination

PCL disruptions can be interstitial disruptions, bony avulsions from the tibia or femur, or insertional disruptions. PCL injuries range from isolated partial tears to PCL injuries associated with multi-ligament injuries. As injury severity varies, so does the patients presenting complaint. Patients with PCL injuries may present with minimal symptoms with a history of a benign fall months ago to a severe MVA with acute hemarthrosis. Diagnosis begins with a through history including injury mechanism, time since injury, and initial and current symptoms. Patients may describe a direct force applied to the proximal tibia or an episode of forced hyperflexion. More severe injuries involving the PCL plus other ligaments occur with a history of hyperextension, forced varus or valgus, or knee dislocation.

Unlike patients with ACL injuries, patients with isolated PCL injuries rarely report feeling a "pop" or relate a sense of instability initially [16]. Acutely, patients may report stiffness, swelling, moderate pain in the back of the knee, or pain with deep knee flexion [17]. Many patients may not appreciate any disability initially but develop symptoms over time. Patients with chronic PCL tears may complain of anterior knee pain, difficulty in ambulating steps, pain with sprinting or deceleration, or instability [17]. Multi-ligament injuries involving the PCL are rarely asymptomatic. These patients usually have initial swelling of the knee followed by feelings of instability.

A through exam of the knee begins with assessment of the patient's overall alignment and gait. Subtle varus alignment

G.C. Fanelli, MD (✉)
GHS Orthopedics, Danville, PA, USA
e-mail: gregorycfanelli@gmail.com

W.J. Malone, DO
Musculoskeletal Radiology Division, Department of Radiology,
Geisinger Medical Center, Danville, PA, USA

S.F. Brockmeier (ed.), *MRI-Arthroscopy Correlations: A Case-Based Atlas of the Knee, Shoulder, Elbow and Hip*,
DOI 10.1007/978-1-4939-2645-9_6, © Springer Science+Business Media New York 2015

and varus recurvatum thrust during gait increase suspicion of posterolateral corner injury. In patients with multi-ligament injuries to the knee, careful neurovascular exam is important to evaluate vascular status as well as foot dorsiflexion and eversion for integrity of the peroneal nerve. Careful observation of the knee should include documentation of contusions or abrasions of the proximal tibia as well as popliteal ecchymosis.

Various physical examination tests have been described that detect PCL tears [8, 9, 18–25]. These tests include the posterior drawer test, the Godfrey test (posterior sag sign), the quadriceps active test, posterior tibial drop back, decreased tibial step off, full extension varus and valgus laxity, false-positive anterior drawer test, and positive pseudo-Lachman test. The basic function of each of these tests is to demonstrate posterior proximal tibial displacement relative to the distal femur with the knee flexed to 90°. This posterior tibial displacement can occur in a straight anteroposterior plane, or a rotational component also may be involved indicating posterolateral or posteromedial instability. It is important for all tests that one ensures that the tibia is not situated in a posteriorly displaced starting position.

Arthrometer Testing

A helpful adjunct to the physical examination is the use of the knee ligament arthrometer. We routinely use the KT-1000 knee ligament arthrometer for initial, preoperative, and postoperative evaluations in our patients with knee ligament injuries. When evaluating patients with PCL injuries, we place particular emphasis on the PCL screen, corrected anterior, and corrected posterior measurements [25].

Imaging Studies

Imaging studies include plain radiographs consisting of standing anteroposterior (AP) views of both knees and a tunnel view, a 30° flexion lateral view, and a 30° AP axial view of both patellas. Stress radiographs can provide additional diagnostic information to help grade PCL tears. Schulz et al. performed Telos device stress X-rays of 1041 consecutive patients with PCL injuries and found that posterior tibial displacement in excess of 8 mm was indicative of complete insufficiency of the PCL, and displacement exceeding 12 mm suggested additional injury of the secondary restraining structures of the knee [26].

Magnetic resonance imaging (MRI) has become the study of choice in acute PCL injuries. A large prospective study found that MRI was 99 % accurate in diagnosing the presence of PCL injury, confirmed by arthroscopy. MRI is useful as it can also assess menisci, articular surfaces, and other ligaments of the knee. However the accuracy of MRI in detecting chronic PCL deficiency has been questioned. Recent studies have demonstrated that the PCL can assume a normal appearance on MRI as early as 6 months following injury. This MRI change does not correlate with improvement in clinical examination [15, 27–29].

In the case of chronic PCL injuries, baseline and serial bone scans are used to monitor changes that may indicate the development of arthrosis mostly in the medial and patellofemoral compartments.

Arthroscopic Evaluation of the Posterior Cruciate Ligament

Examination under anesthesia allows thorough physical examination of the knee to detect multidirectional instability (especially occult posterolateral and posteromedial instability). Diagnostic arthroscopy allows visualization of the intra-articular pathology, including meniscal tears and articular cartilage injury or degeneration. The three-zone method of arthroscopic evaluation of the posterior cruciate ligament described by Fanelli et al. enables arthroscopic visualization of direct findings and indirect findings associated with posterior cruciate ligament injury and insufficiency [15].

Indications for surgical treatment of acute posterior cruciate ligament injuries include insertion site avulsions, a decrease in tibial step of 8 mm or greater, and PCL tears combined with other structural injuries. Indications for surgical treatment of chronic PCL injuries are when an isolated posterior cruciate ligament tear becomes symptomatic or when progressive functional instability develops.

Surgical timing is dependent upon vascular status, reduction stability, skin condition, systemic injuries, open versus closed knee injury, meniscus and articular surface injuries, other orthopedic injuries, and the collateral/capsular ligaments involved. Certain ACL/PCL/MCL injuries can be treated with brace treatment of the medial collateral ligament followed by arthroscopic combined ACL/PCL reconstruction 4–6 weeks after healing of the MCL. Other cases may require repair or reconstruction of the medial structures and must be assessed on an individual basis.

Combined ACL/PCL/posterolateral injuries are addressed as early as safely possible. ACL/PCL/posterolateral repair-reconstruction performed between 2 and 4 weeks post injury allows sealing of capsular tissues to permit an arthroscopic approach and still permits primary repair of injured posterolateral structures.

Open PCL-based multiple-ligament knee injuries/dislocations may require staged procedures. The collateral/capsular structures are repaired through irrigation and debridement, and the combined ACL/PCL reconstruction is performed at a later date after wound healing has occurred.

Care must be taken in all cases of delayed reconstruction to confirm that the tibiofemoral joint is reduced by serial anteroposterior and lateral radiographs.

The surgical timing guidelines outlined above should be considered in the context of the individual patient. Many patients with multiple-ligament injuries of the knee are severely injured multiple-trauma patients with multisystem injuries. Modifiers to the ideal timing protocols outlined above include the vascular status of the involved extremity, reduction stability, skin condition, open or closed injury, and other orthopedic and systemic injuries. These additional considerations may cause the knee ligament surgery to be performed earlier or later than desired. We have previously reported excellent results with delayed reconstruction in the PCL-based multiple-ligament injured knee [30–35].

Case 1

History/Physical Exam

A 16-year-old high school football player was injured during preseason practice session. The patient was tackled with the left foot planted and posterior and external rotation force applied to the proximal tibia. The patient presented several weeks after the injury with pain and functional instability of the affected knee.

Physical examination revealed symmetrical range of motion of both knees. The affected knee had negative tibial step offs and a grade 3 positive posterior drawer. The posterolateral drawer was positive, and the posteromedial drawer

was negative. The knee was stable to valgus stress, and there was positive varus laxity at zero and 30° of knee flexion with a firm end point. The Lachman test was negative, and the pivot shift was negative. The dial test was positive at both 30° and 90° of knee flexion.

Imaging Studies

Plain radiography did not demonstrate any significant pathology. Stress radiography of the knees obtained at 90° of knee flexion comparing the involved left knee to the normal right knee revealed increased posterior displacement of the left tibia compared to the right (Fig. 6.1a, b). Magnetic resonance imaging revealed full-thickness tear of the posterior cruciate ligament seen in the midportion of the ligament primarily extending to the insertion with no detachment of the insertion. There is edema and some tearing of the posterolateral capsular structures, although no gross disruption of the fibular collateral ligament or popliteus tendon. The remaining structures were intact (Fig. 6.2a, b).

Arthroscopy

The patient was taken to the operating room and positioned supine on the fully extended operating table. The examination of the left knee under anesthesia was in agreement with the physical examination outlined above. Arthroscopic examination of the left knee joint revealed the articular cartilage in all three compartments to be intact, medial and lateral

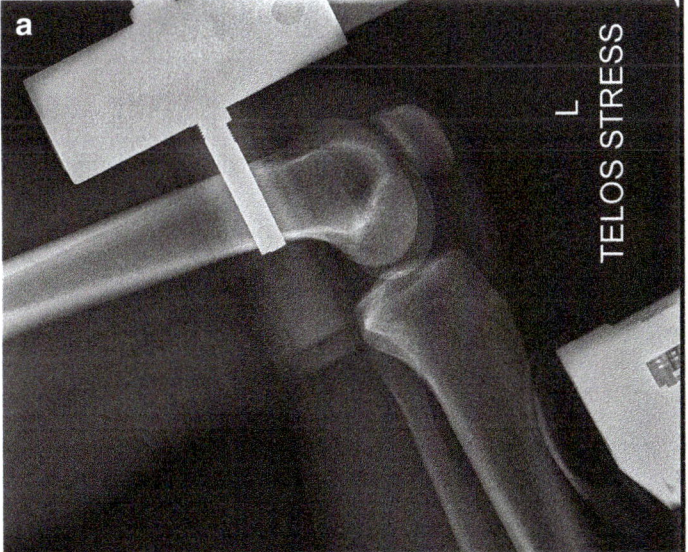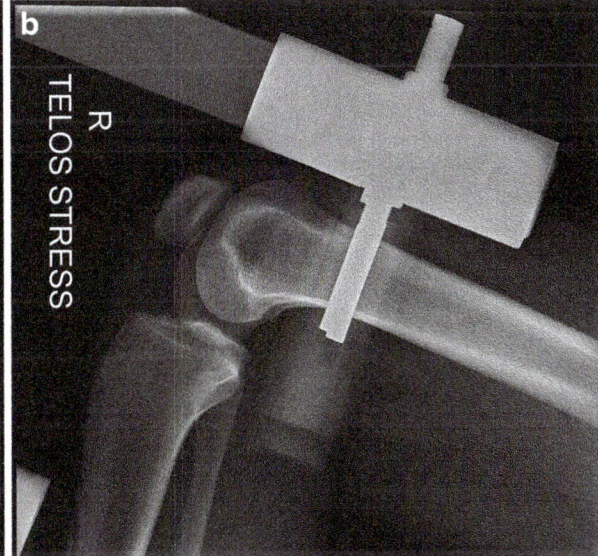

Fig. 6.1 Stress radiographic measurement of a posterior cruciate ligament and posterolateral corner of the injured knee. (**a**) Demonstrates posterior subluxation of the tibia relative to the femur at approximately 90° of knee flexion. (**b**) Demonstrates normal relationship of the femur and tibia in the patient's uninjured normal knee

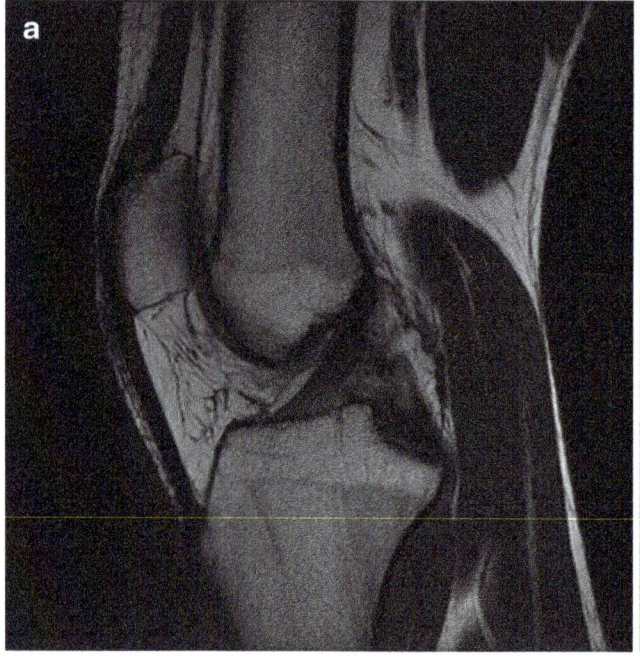
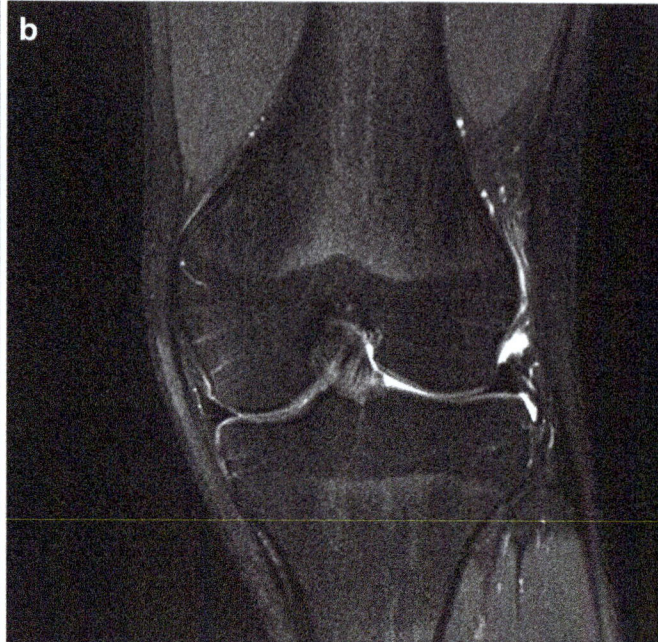

Fig. 6.2 (**a**) Magnetic resonance imaging revealed full-thickness tear of the posterior cruciate ligament seen in the midportion of the ligament primarily extending to the insertion with no detachment of the insertion. (**b**) MRI of the posterolateral corner revealed edema and some tearing of the posterolateral capsular structures, although no gross disruption of the fibular collateral ligament or popliteus tendon. The remaining structures were intact

menisci to be intact, lateral joint space opening (positive drive thru sign), zone 1–2 posterior cruciate ligament tear, and the anterior cruciate ligament to be intact but exhibiting the sloppy ACL sign consistent with PCL injury [15] (Fig. 6.3a, b).

Discussion and Surgical Reconstruction

The patient had a functionally unstable knee indicating the need for surgical reconstruction. Since this was a chronic injury with consistent soft tissue configuration, a single-stage combined posterior cruciate ligament and posterolateral reconstruction was performed. The arthroscopic findings were in agreement with the physical examination findings and the MRI findings of combined posterior cruciate ligament injury and posterolateral corner injury. Combined posterior cruciate ligament reconstruction and posterolateral reconstruction were performed. PCL reconstruction was a transtibial arthroscopic double-bundle reconstruction using Achilles tendon and tibialis anterior allograft tissue using mechanical graft tensioning, and the posterolateral reconstruction was a fibular head-based figure of eight reconstruction using semitendinosus allograft tissue combined with a posterolateral capsular shift procedure and peroneal nerve decompression and neurolysis [36–38] (Fig. 6.4a–d).

Case 2

History/Physical Exam

A 31-year-old man fell from a height of approximately 5 ft and upon landing twisted his left knee resulting in a left tibiofemoral knee dislocation that was reduced at the scene of the accident. Physical examination in the emergency department revealed neurovascular structures to be intact. Range of motion was restricted secondary to pain. The affected knee had negative tibial step offs and a grade 3 positive posterior drawer at 90° of knee flexion. The posterolateral drawer was positive, and the posteromedial drawer was negative. There was severe varus laxity at zero and 30° of knee flexion with no discernible end point. The Lachman test was positive, and the pivot shift was positive. The dial test was positive at both 30° and 90° of knee flexion. There was no valgus laxity with the medial side being the stable hinge.

Imaging Studies

Plain radiography demonstrated good reduction and alignment of the tibiofemoral and patellofemoral joint. Stress radiography of the knees was not obtained preoperatively due to the severe instability of the left knee.

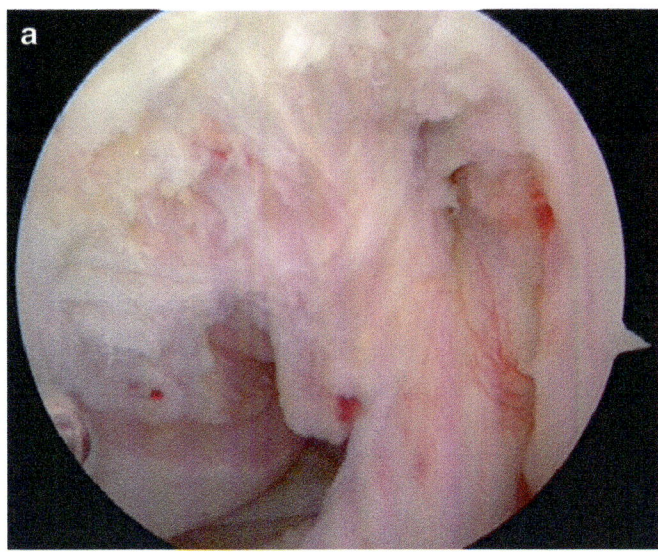 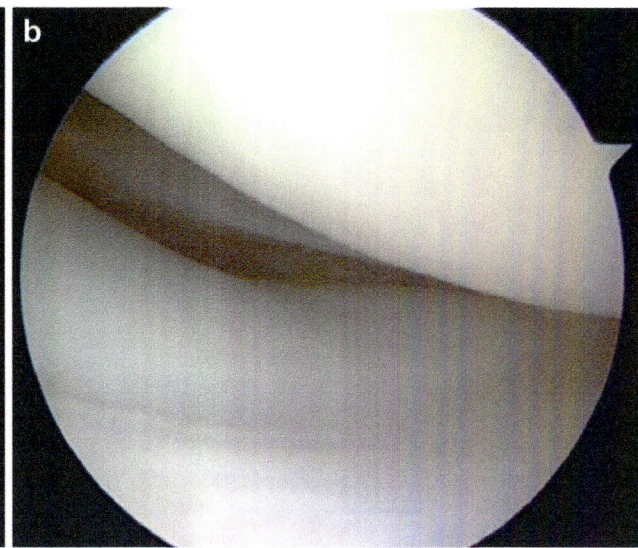

Fig. 6.3 Arthroscopic photographs of the posterior cruciate ligament tear and the posterolateral corner. (**a**) Arthroscopic evaluation of the PCL revealed a zone 1–2 posterior cruciate ligament tear, with the anterior cruciate ligament to be intact but exhibiting the sloppy ACL sign consistent with PCL injury. (**b**) Arthroscopic evaluation of the lateral compartment and posterolateral corner revealed lateral joint space opening in the figure four position with a positive drive thru sign consistent with posterolateral instability of the knee

Magnetic resonance imaging revealed full-thickness complete tears of the posterior and anterior cruciate ligaments (Fig. 6.5a, b). There was increased signal in the proximal medial collateral ligament just distal to its femoral attachment with associated periligamentous edema consistent with a moderate sprain. A tear of the meniscofemoral ligament was also noted. The posteromedial corner structures were intact, as well as the pes tendons.

The lateral and posterolateral structures were severely damaged (Fig. 6.6a, b). The conjoined tendon of the biceps femoris and the fibular collateral ligament were completely torn and retracted from their fibular attachments with surrounding edema. There was a near complete tear of the popliteus tendon from its femoral origin. There was a low-grade sprain of the popliteus at the myotendinous junction, with a sprain of the popliteal fibular ligament without complete disruption. There was a lateral capsular avulsion with the iliotibial band intact.

The extensor mechanism, patellofemoral stabilizers, and articular cartilage in the medial, lateral, and patellofemoral compartments were all intact. There was a bone bruise on the medial femoral condyle.

Treatment Decision

The patient had a severe left knee injury with gross instability and severe damage to the lateral and posterolateral structures. The decision was made to proceed with a two-stage

approach for surgical treatment of this PCL, ACL, and type C posterolateral multiple-ligament injured knee that was an acute tibiofemoral knee dislocation [39].

Discussion and Surgical Reconstruction

Stage 1 was repair and reconstruction of the lateral posterolateral side/corner structures approximately 10-day post injury when the skin and other soft tissues had stabilized (Fig. 6.7a, b). The patient had been immobilized in a brace locked in full extension with provisional preoperative mobilization. Stage 1 surgery consisted of peroneal nerve decompression and neurolysis, primary repair of all injured lateral and posterolateral structures, and posterolateral reconstruction with a fibular head-based figure of eight reconstruction using semitendinosus allograft tissue combined with a posterolateral capsular shift procedure [36–38]. Stage 2 was an arthroscopic combined posterior and anterior cruciate ligament reconstruction performed 4 weeks after the stage 1 procedure. Posterior cruciate ligament reconstruction was a transtibial arthroscopic single-bundle reconstruction using Achilles tendon allograft tissue, and the anterior cruciate ligament reconstruction was an arthroscopic transtibial femoral tunnel reconstruction using Achilles tendon allograft tissue and mechanical graft tensioning for both the PCL and ACL reconstructions [40, 41] (Fig. 6.8a, b).

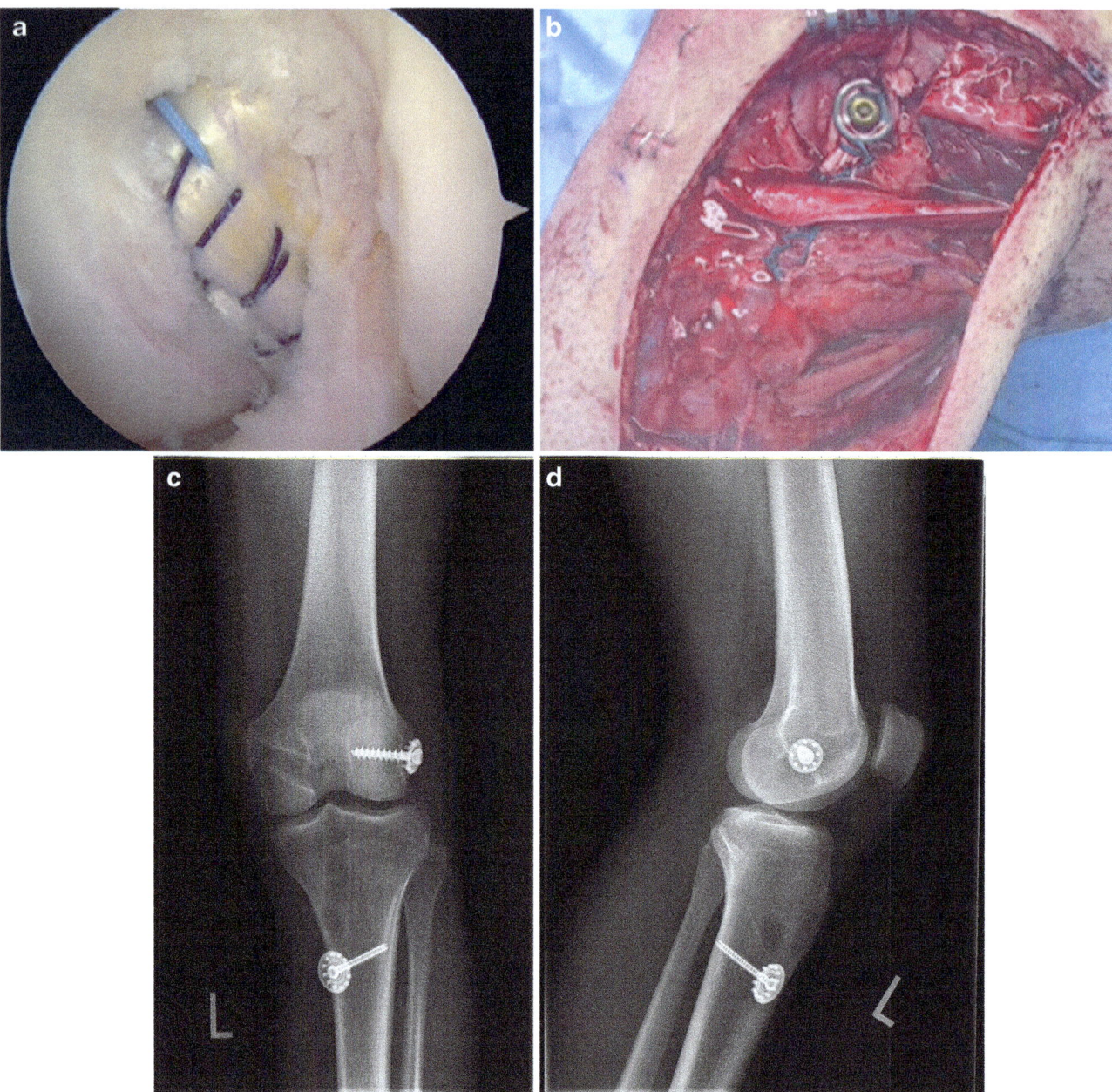

Fig. 6.4 Posterior cruciate ligament and posterolateral reconstruction of the knee. (**a**) Posterior cruciate ligament reconstruction was performed using a transtibial arthroscopic double-bundle reconstruction with an Achilles tendon allograft for the anterolateral bundle and tibialis anterior allograft for the posteromedial bundle. A mechanical graft-tensioning device was used for graft tensioning. (**b**) Posterolateral reconstruction was performed using a fibular head-based figure of eight reconstruction with a semitendinosus allograft tendon combined with a posterolateral capsular shift procedure. Peroneal nerve decompression and neurolysis is always performed, and the peroneal nerve is carefully protected throughout the procedure. (**c**, **d**) Postoperative anteroposterior and lateral radiographs of the posterior cruciate ligament and posterolateral reconstructed knee demonstrating tunnel and hardware position and orientation

Conclusions

Posterior cruciate ligament injuries may occur as an isolated injury or in combination with other ligaments in the multiple-ligament injured knee. A careful history, physical examination, vascular studies, MRI evaluation, and diagnostic arthroscopy used in combination are essential for an accurate diagnosis and for surgical planning. Caution must be exercised in chronic posterior cruciate ligament injuries since the MRI may demonstrate a normal-appearing posterior cruciate ligament even when there is significant laxity on clinical examination. Chronic posterolateral or posteromedial instability may also demonstrate significant patholaxity with a normal-appearing MRI. The combination

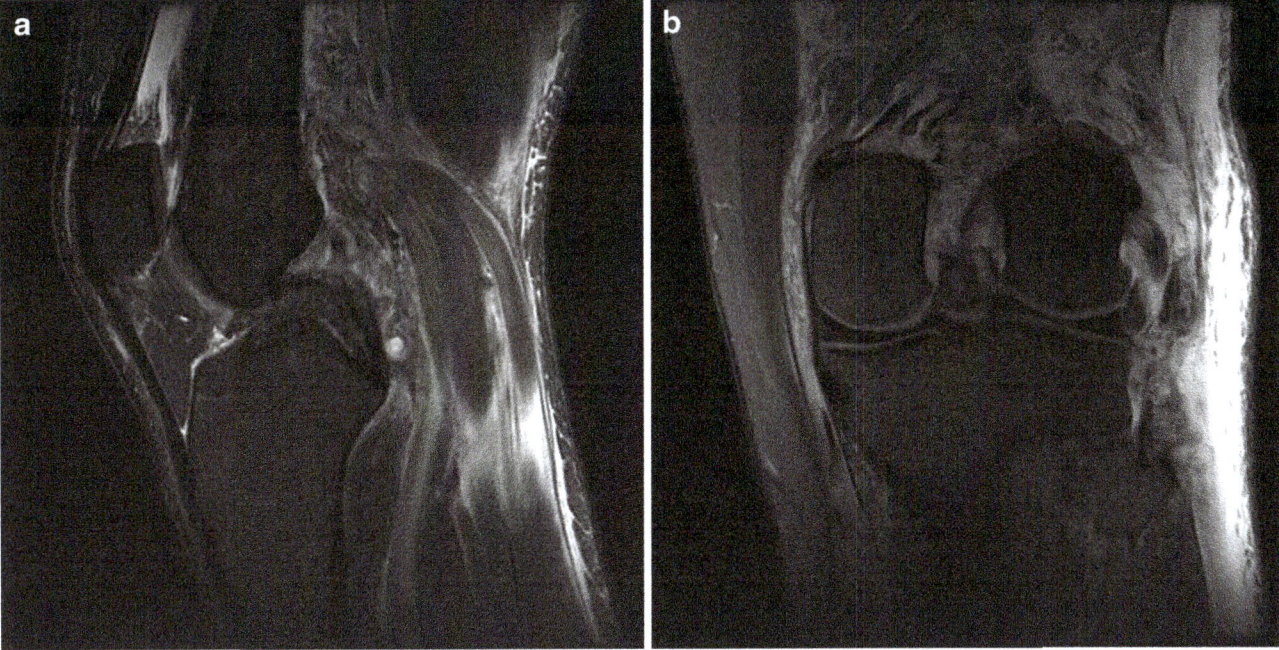

Fig. 6.5 Magnetic resonance imaging studies demonstrating injury to the posterior and anterior cruciate ligament and the posterolateral corner of the left knee. (**a**) Magnetic resonance imaging revealed full-thickness complete tears of the posterior and anterior cruciate ligaments consistent with the patient's mechanism of injury, history, and clinical examination. (**b**) MRI demonstrates increased signal in the proximal medial collateral ligament just distal to its femoral attachment with associated periligamentous edema consistent with a moderate sprain. A tear of the meniscofemoral ligament was also noted. The posteromedial corner structures

were intact, as well as the pes tendons. MRI demonstrates that the lateral and posterolateral structures were severely damaged. The conjoined tendon of the biceps femoris and the fibular collateral ligament were completely torn and retracted from their fibular attachments with surrounding edema. There was a near complete tear of the popliteus tendon from its femoral origin. There was a low-grade sprain of the popliteus at the myotendinous junction, with a sprain of the popliteal fibular ligament without complete disruption. There was a lateral capsular avulsion with the iliotibial band intact

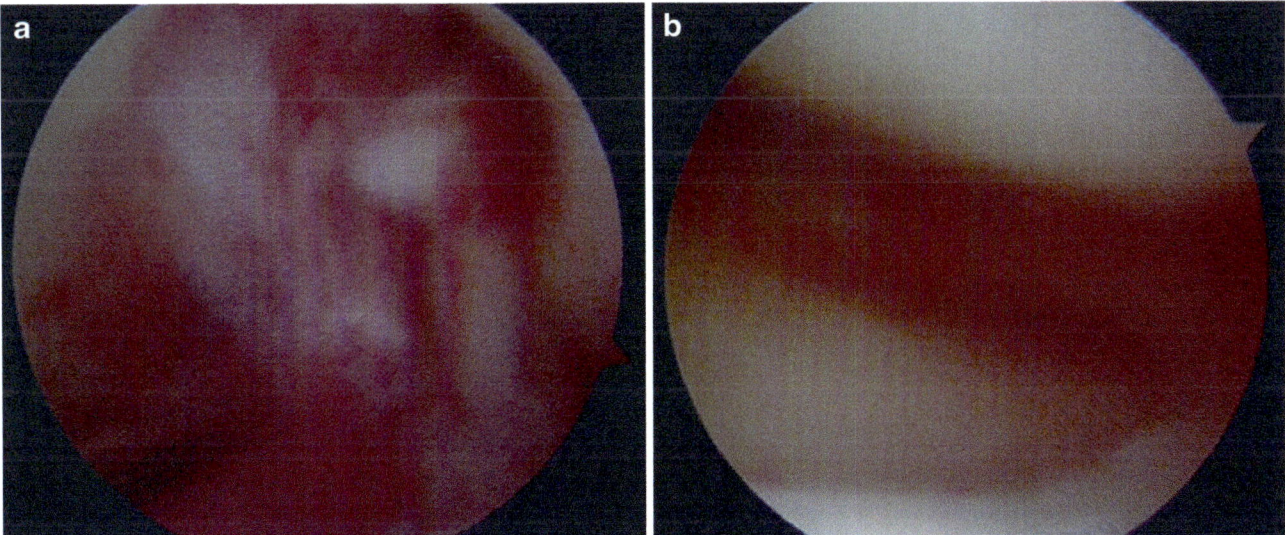

Fig. 6.6 Arthroscopic view of the injured posterior and anterior cruciate ligaments (**a**) and the injured posterolateral corner structures (**b**).

Note in **b** the drive thru sign with the knee in the figure four position and the position of the lateral meniscus relative to the femur and tibia

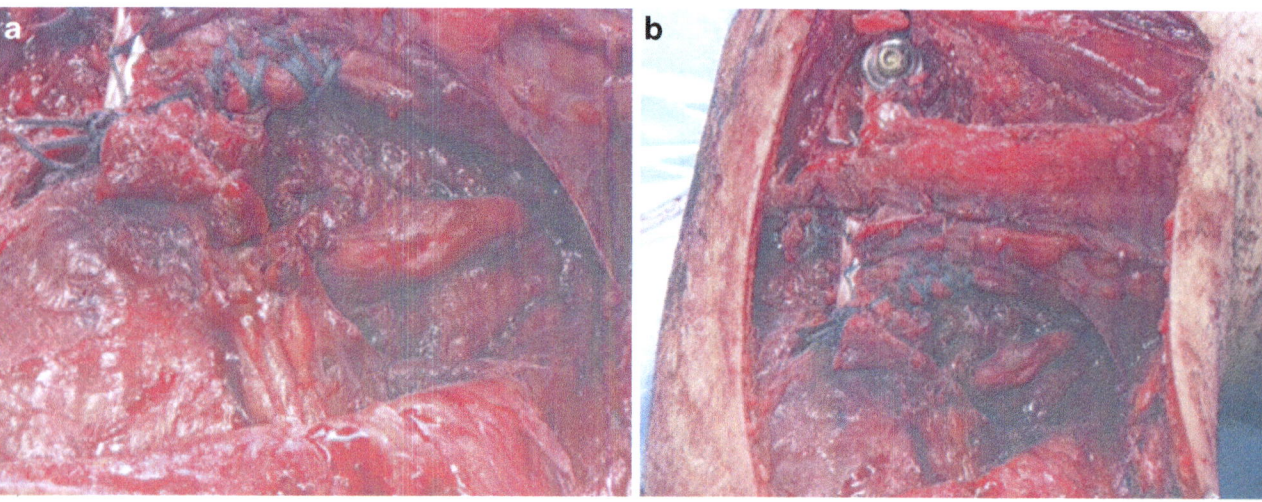

Fig. 6.7 Repair and reconstruction of the lateral side structures. (**a**) Peroneal nerve decompression and neurolysis and primary repair of injured lateral and posterolateral structures. (**b**) Posterolateral reconstruction performed using a fibular head-based figure of eight recon- struction with a semitendinosus allograft tendon combined primary repair of injured lateral and posterolateral structures. Peroneal nerve decompression and neurolysis is always performed, and the peroneal nerve is carefully protected throughout the procedure

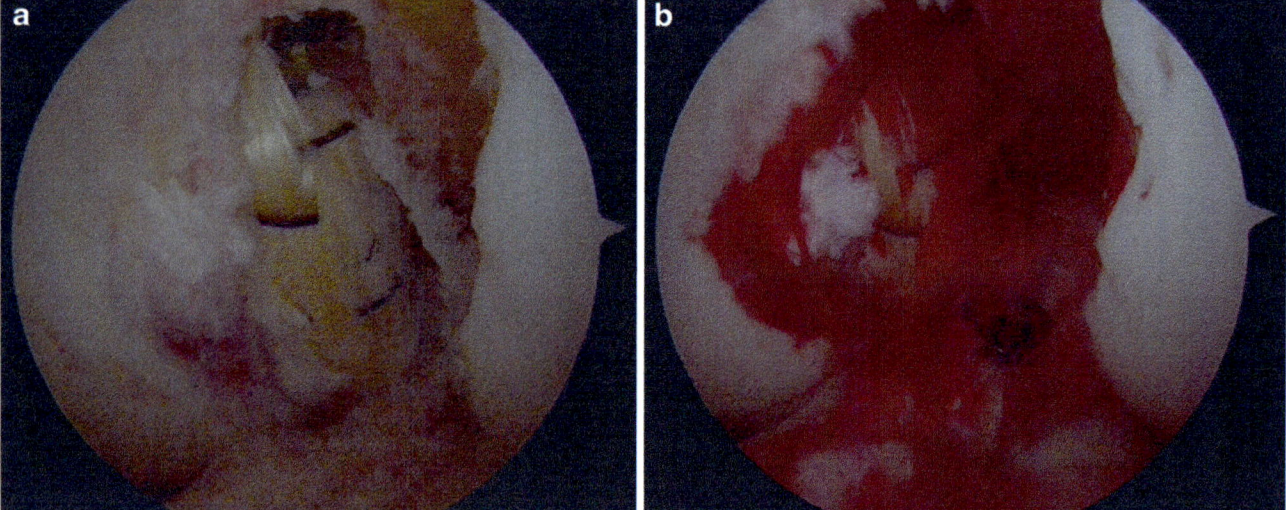

Fig. 6.8 Combined arthroscopic posterior and anterior cruciate ligament reconstruction. (**a**) Posterior cruciate ligament reconstruction performed using a transtibial arthroscopic single-bundle reconstruction using an Achilles tendon allograft to reconstruct the anterolateral bundle of the posterior cruciate ligament. (**b**) The anterior cruciate ligament reconstruction performed using the single-bundle arthroscopic transtibial femoral tunnel reconstruction with Achilles tendon allograft tissue and mechanical graft tensioning for both the PCL and ACL reconstructions

of history, physical examination, magnetic resonance imaging, and arthroscopic evaluation used in combination will maximize the probability for an accurate diagnosis in the posterior cruci- ate ligament injured knee.

References

1. Cooper DE, Warren RF, Warner JJ. The posterior cruciate ligament and posterolateral structures of the knee: anatomy, functions, and patterns of injury. Instr Course Lect. 1991;40:249–70.
2. Grood ES, Stowers SF, Noyes RF. Limits of movement in the human knee: effect of sectioning the posterior cruciate ligament and posterolateral structures. J Bone Joint Surg Am. 1988;70: 88–97.
3. Veltri DM, Deng X-H, Torzilli PA, et al. The role of the popliteo- fibular ligament in the stability of the human knee. A biomechanical study. Am J Sports Med. 1996;24:19–27.
4. Gupte CM, Bull AMJ, Thomas RD, Amis AA. The meniscofemoral ligaments: secondary restraints to posterior drawer. J Bone Joint Surg Br. 2003;85:765–73.
5. Ritchie JR, Bergfeld JA, Kambic H, Manning T. Isolated sectioning of the medial and posteromedial capsular ligaments in the posterior cruciate ligament-deficient knee: influence on posterior tibial trans- lation. Am J Sports Med. 1998;26:389–94.
6. Fox RJ, Harner CD, Sakane M, Carlin GJ, Woo SL. Determination of the in situ forces in the human posterior cruciate ligament using robotic technology. A cadaveric study. Am J Sports Med. 1998; 26:395–401.

7. Johnson JC, Bach BR. Current concepts review, posterior cruciate ligament. Am J Knee Surg. 1990;3:143–53.

8. Clancy WG, Shelbourne KD, Zoellner GB, Keene JS, Reider B, Rosenberg TD. Treatment of knee joint instability secondary to rupture of the posterior cruciate ligament. Report of new procedure. J Bone Joint Surg [Am]. 1983;65:310–22.

9. Degenhardt TC, Hughston JC. Chronic posterior cruciate instability: nonoperative management. Orthop Trans. 1981;5:486–7.

10. Fanelli GC. PCL injuries in trauma patients. Arthroscopy. 1993; 9:291–4.

11. Fanelli GC, Edson CJ. Posterior cruciate ligament injuries in trauma patients: Part II. Arthroscopy. 1995;11(5):526–9.

12. O'Donoghue DH. An analysis of end results of surgical treatment of major injuries to the ligaments of the knee. J Bone Joint Surg [Am]. 1955;37:1–13.

13. Parolie JM, Bergfeld JA. Long term results of nonoperative treatment of isolated posterior cruciate ligament injuries in the athlete. Am J Sports Med. 1986;14:35–8.

14. Fowler PJ, Messieh SS. Isolated posterior cruciate ligament injuries in athletes. Am J Sports Med. 1987;15:553–7.

15. Fanelli GC, Giannotti B, Edson CJ. Current concepts review. The posterior cruciate ligament: arthroscopic evaluation and treatment. Arthroscopy. 1994;10(6):673–88.

16. McAllister DR, Petrigliano FA. Diagnosis and treatment of posterior cruciate ligament injuries. Curr Sports Med Rep. 2007;6(5): 293–9.

17. Margheritini F, Mariani PP. Diagnostic evaluation of posterior cruciate ligament injuries. Knee Surg Sports Traumatol Arthrosc. 2003;11:282–8.

18. Schulz MS, Russe K, Weiler A, et al. Epidemiology of posterior cruciate ligament injuries. Arch Orthop Trauma Surg. 2003;123: 186–91.

19. Daniel DM, Stone ML, Barnett P, et al. Use of the quadriceps active test to diagnose PCL disruption and measure posterior laxity of the knee. J Bone Joint Surg [AM]. 1988;70:386–91.

20. Grood ES, Hefzy MS, Ledenfield TN. Factors affecting the region of most isometric femoral attachments. Am J Sports Med. 1989; 17:197–207.

21. Hughston JC, Baker CL, Norwood LA. Acute combined posterior cruciate and posterolateral instability of the knee. Am J Sports Med. 1983;12:204–8.

22. Jakob RP, Hassler H, Staubli HU. Experimental studies on the functional anatomy and the pathomechanism of the true and reversed pivot shift sign. Acta Orthop Scand. 1981;5(suppl):18–32.

23. Loss WC, Fox JM, Blazina ME, Del Pizzo W, Friedman MJ. Acute posterior cruciate ligament injuries. Am J Sports Med. 1981;9: 86–92.

24. Shelbourne KD, Benedict F, McCarrol JR, et al. Dynamic posterior shift test. Am J Sports Med. 1989;17:275–7.

25. Daniel DM, Akeson W, O'Conner J, editors. Knee ligaments—structure, function, injury, and repair. New York: Raven; 1990.

26. Schulz MS, Steenlage ES, Russe K, Strobel MJ. Distribution of posterior tibial displacement in knees with posterior cruciate ligament tears. J Bone Joint Surg Am. 2007;89:332–8.

27. Gross ML, Grover JS, Bassett LW, et al. Magnetic resonance imaging of the posterior cruciate ligament: clinical use to improve diagnostic accuracy. Am J Sports Med. 1992;20:732–7.

28. Boks SS, Vroegindeweij D, Koes BW, et al. Follow-up of posttraumatic ligamentous and meniscal knee lesions detected at MRI: systematic review. Radiology. 2006;238:863–71.

29. Servant CT, Ramos JP, Thomas NP. The accuracy of magnetic resonance imaging in diagnosing chronic posterior cruciate ligament injury. Knee. 2004;11:265–70.

30. Fanelli GC, Giannotti BF, Edson CJ. Arthroscopically assisted combined anterior and posterior cruciate ligament reconstruction. Arthroscopy. 1996;12(1):5–14.

31. Fanelli GC, Giannotti BF, Edson CJ. Arthroscopically assisted combined posterior cruciate ligament/posterior lateral complex reconstruction. Arthroscopy. 1996;12(5):521–30.

32. Fanelli G et al. Arthroscopically assisted combined anterior and posterior cruciate ligament reconstruction in the multiple ligament injured knee: 2- to 10-year follow-up. Arthroscopy. 2002;18(7): 703–14.

33. Fanelli GC, Edson CJ. Combined posterior cruciate ligament-posterolateral reconstructions with Achilles tendon allograft and biceps femoris tendon tenodesis: 2- to 10-year follow up. Arthroscopy. 2004;20:339–45.

34. Fanelli GC, Beck JD, Edson CJ. Current concepts review: the posterior cruciate ligament. J Knee Surg. 2010;23(2):61–72.

35. Fanelli GC, Beck JD, Edson CJ. Single compared to double bundle PCL reconstruction using allograft tissue. J Knee Surg. 2012; 25(1):59–64.

36. Fanelli GC, Beck JD, Edson CJ. Arthroscopic transtibial double bundle PCL reconstruction. J Knee Surg. 2010;23(2):89–94.

37. Fanelli GC, Beck JD, Edson CJ. Combined PCL ACL lateral and medial side injuries: treatment and results. Sports Med Arthroscopy Rev. 2011;19(2):120–30.

38. Fanelli GC, Edson CJ. Surgical treatment of combined PCL, ACL, medial, and lateral side injuries (global laxity): surgical technique and 2 to 18 year results. J Knee Surg. 2012;25(4):307–16.

39. Fanelli GC, Feldman DD. Management of combined anterior cruciate ligament/posterior cruciate ligament/posterolateral complex injuries of the knee. Oper Tech Sports Med. 1999;7(3):143–9 (Fanelli posterolateral instability classification system).

40. Fanelli GC. Surgical treatment of combined PCL ACL medial and lateral side injuries (global laxity): acute and chronic. In: Fanelli GC, editor. The multiple ligament injured knee. A practical guide to management. 2nd ed. New York: Springer; 2013. p. 281–301.

41. Fanelli GC. Mechanical graft tensioning in multiple ligament knee surgery. In: Fanelli GC, editor. The multiple ligament injured knee. A practical guide to management. 2nd ed. New York: Springer; 2013. p. 323–30.

Medial Collateral Ligament Injuries of the Knee

Jesse Seamon and Mark D. Miller

Introduction

The medial collateral ligament (MCL) is the most commonly injured knee ligament and is present either in isolation or in combination with other knee ligament injuries greater than 40 % of the time [1–4]. In general, these injuries occur due to a valgus stress across the knee joint, either from a direct blow to the lateral knee or from noncontact injuries that result in relative tibial external rotation and valgus forces across the knee joint [5]. While many lower-grade MCL injuries may occur in isolation, most high-grade injuries are accompanied by associated injury to the posteromedial corner (PMC), anterior cruciate ligament (ACL), or meniscus [3]. The posterior oblique ligament (POL) of the PMC and the ACL seem to be the most commonly associated injured structures with complete tears, present in greater than 99 % and 75 %, respectively, in a series of 93 surgically treated knees with grade III MCL tears in the series by Sims and Jacobson [6]. Although the MCL is the primary restraint to valgus stress across the medial side of the knee at all flexion angles, other structures contribute to this stability, namely, the posteromedial corner (PMC) of the knee which includes the posterior oblique ligament, oblique popliteal ligament (OPL), posterior horn of the medial meniscus, and the tendinous expansion of the semimembranosus insertion [4, 6–8]. Combined injury to the MCL and PMC results in both valgus and anteromedial rotatory instability (AMRI) of the knee [1, 4–6].

J. Seamon, MD (✉)
Department of Orthopedic Surgery, Saint Louis University Hospital, St. Louis, MO, USA
e-mail: Jseamon23@gmail.com

M.D. Miller, MD
Department of Orthopedic Surgery, University of Virginia Hospital, Charlottesville, VA, USA

Department of Orthopedic Surgery, Head Team Physician, James Madison University, Charlottesville, VA, USA
e-mail: Mdm3p@hccmail.mcc.virginia.edu

The MCL (also called tibial collateral ligament or TCL) is divided into both a superficial medial collateral ligament (sMCL) and deep medial collateral ligament (dMCL) component [2]. The sMCL originates along the posterior aspect of the medial femoral condyle in the region of the adductor tubercle [3, 4, 9]. A recent radiographic and cadaveric study has pinpointed this location to a region that is typically posterior to a tangential line drawn along the posterior femoral cortex and proximal to a line drawn tangential to Blumensaat's line [9]. The distal sMCL has two distinct limbs. The more proximal and posterior limb attaches to the semimembranosus tendon and blends with the posteromedial joint capsule [3]. The more distal and anterior limb attaches broadly on the proximal medial tibia deep to the pes anserine tendons and approximately 4.5–7 cm below the joint line [2–4]. The dMCL is continuous with the medial knee capsule and can be thought of as a thickening of the middle 1/3 of this region of the capsule [4]. It is intimately associated with the medial meniscus and consists of a meniscofemoral portion that runs from the distal femur to the medial meniscus and a meniscotibial portion that runs from the medial meniscus to the proximal tibia [2]. A bursal layer exists between the sMCL and dMCL [3]. The POL can appear to be continuous with the posterior portion of the sMCL but has a discrete origin on the adductor tubercle of the femur and spans posteriorly and inferiorly to blend with the semimembranosus and posterior tibia along the joint capsule [6]. The OPL runs from the posteromedial tibia and semimembranosus to the posterior lateral femoral condyle [4].

The anatomy of the medial side of the knee is complex, consisting of three distinct tissue layers and multiple structures in addition to the MCL that all contribute to valgus and rotatory stability of the knee [1–6, 10]. Classically, the anatomy of the knee has been defined in three layers, denoted roman numerals I–III as described by Warren and Marshall [10]. The anatomy of the medial side of the knee has also been described in thirds by Sims and Jacobson, with an anterior, middle, and posterior third, each consisting of three distinct layers [6].

The superficial layer (layer I) is comprised of the deep crural fascia. It is continuous with the medial patellar extensor retinaculum anteriorly and blends in distally with the sartorial fascia over the pes anserine and proximally with the fascia overlying the quadriceps [2, 3, 5]. Layer II consists of the sMCL, the medial patellofemoral ligament, the OPL, the POL, and the semimembranosus [1, 4]. Layer I and layer II merge anteriorly. Layer III is the deepest layer and consists of the capsule and dMCL [2]. Layer II and layer II merge posteriorly.

As stated above, the medial sided anatomy can be divided into anterior, middle, and posterior thirds [6]. The anterior third of the medial knee is the least clinically relevant and consists of the medial extensor retinaculum [1, 4, 6]. The middle third consists of the sMCL and the dMCL [5]. The posterior third represents the PMC with its associated ligamentous and tendinous structures [1, 4–6]. From a surgical standpoint, it is helpful to think of the anatomy in this way, since primary repair and reconstructive efforts are mostly divided into the middle and posterior third of the anatomy and functionally middle 1/3 injuries result in pure valgus instability in flexion, while posterior 1/3 injuries result in more AMBRI and valgus instability in extension.

The sMCL is the primary restraint to valgus stress at all flexion angles, while the PMC provides the primary restraint to tibial external rotation and an increasing contribution to valgus stability with knee extension [5, 7]. The tensile strength of the sMCL is similar to that of the ACL [4]. The dMCL may not play a major role in valgus stability, but seems to play a role in anchoring the medial meniscus and as a restraint to external tibial rotation [3]. The sMCL has been shown to experience maximum strain at the femoral origin, and this is the most common site of rupture followed by the tibial insertion and mid-substance tears [3, 4, 11].

History and physical exam still represent the most accurate method for the diagnosis of MCL injuries [1, 4–6]. The skin is carefully inspected for signs of bruising or the presence of abrasions. A thorough vascular exam should be performed, especially in the presence of a high-energy mechanism as many knee dislocations present with the knee already reduced [1]. Palpation should include the entire length of the MCL as well as the posteromedial knee to check for PMC tenderness [1]. Valgus stress test should be performed with the knee in 30° of flexion to best isolate the MCL and again in full extension to look for coexisting cruciate or PMC injuries [7]. The Slocum test should be performed. To do this, the anterior drawer test should be performed with the foot in external rotation to help elucidate the presence of PMC injuries as evidenced by anterior translation of the tibia while externally rotated [1, 4, 5]. A posterior drawer and the Lachman tests are performed to rule out cruciate injuries as well as varus stress tests to rule out lateral collateral ligament (LCL) injuries. The presence of knee effusion should also be noted. As with any extremity exam, comparison should be made to the contralateral limb.

Traditionally, MCL injuries are classified in a system of Grades I–III. Unfortunately, multiple classification systems have been described using this scale with different meanings for each grade and different physical exam criteria leading to multiple descriptions of Grade I–III injuries [4]. This is further complicated by the fact that the radiology grading system uses Grades I–III, and it is based on different criteria than the clinical classification [3]. In general, Grade I injuries are thought of as sprains with only a sparse number of disrupted fibers [2]. They are often low-energy, noncontact injuries resulting from valgus and external rotation forces across the medial side of the knee. On MRI, high signal is often seen superficial to the ligament only [3, 11]. On valgus stress test at 30° of knee flexion, no instability is appreciated, but pain is often present [2]. Grade II injuries are partial tears of the MCL and usually result from higher-energy mechanisms such as a direct blow to the lateral knee [2, 7]. MRI will reveal the presence of signal both superficial to and within the MCL at the site of injury [2, 3, 11]. On clinical exam, there is more diffuse tenderness along the MCL, and there may be some laxity with a valgus stress test at 30° of knee flexion but with a firm endpoint and less than 10 mm of joint space widening [7]. Grade III injuries represent complete disruption of the medial collateral ligament. On MRI the ligament will be completely ruptured, either in the midsubstance or from the insertion points on the medial femoral condyle or proximal tibia [3, 11]. Joint space widening is >10 mm with valgus stress test at 30° and no firm endpoint is usually felt [2, 7]. The presence of valgus laxity in full extension suggests concomitant injury to the posteromedial corner or collateral ligaments [7].

The MCL is well visualized on MRI. It is seen as a low-intensity signal band on all coronal imaging sequences. In general, the T2-weighted coronal sequence is most helpful for initial evaluation as the MCL is easily seen and edema is readily located around and within the ligament as a hyperintense signal [2, 3, 11]. Hyperintense signal within the ligament is representative of a tear on all sequences [3, 11]. Chronic MCL injuries are often seen as a thickened appearance of the ligament on MRI [3, 11]. The femoral and tibial insertion points are both readily seen on coronal plane imaging. The axial images serve to provide added information in regard to the PMC, especially T1-weighted images with intra-articular contrast [1]. MRI has an accuracy of 87 % in regard to detecting MCL injury [3]. MRI may not be necessary for clinical Grade I and Grade II injuries, but should be considered for Grade III injuries, or any injury associated with valgus laxity in full extension or with significant knee effusion or bruising around the knee [4].

Arthroscopic findings in MCL injuries are highly dependent on the degree of injury. Isolated sMCL injuries will not be directly visualized since only the deep portion of layer III is readily visible. Excessive medial opening of the knee with minimal valgus stress may be appreciated during arthroscopy in cases of sMCL injury [2]. Deep MCL injuries are readily apparent by examining the medial meniscus. If the dMCL is torn from the tibial attachment, the meniscus will appear elevated superiorly from the joint line; and if torn forms the femoral side, more apparent space can be observed above the meniscus [2]. The "meniscal rise" sign has been described by Sims and Jacobson and is liftoff of the medial meniscus relative to the tibia during valgus stress test at 30° of knee flexion [6]. In addition, in very high-energy tears, the proximal fibers of the medial meniscus may be visible through complete tears of the medial joint capsule or can even be flipped into the joint space. Lastly, posteromedial capsular hemorrhage may be present in up to 60 % of patients [6].

Treatment of Grade I and Grade II MCL injuries is with conservative measures [1, 3–5, 7]. Generally, a hinged IROM-type knee brace is utilized allowing for unrestricted sagittal plane motion to prevent stiffness. For most Grade I and Grade II injuries, healing is evident by 6 weeks and seen clinically as lack of medial sided pain and no sense of medial instability.

Treatment of Grade III MCL injuries is more controversial, with good results reported for both operative and nonoperative management. Many surgeons advocate for a trial of nonoperative management with a hinged brace for 6 weeks assuming that clinical exam and imaging have elucidated an isolated MCL injury. If instability persists after 6 weeks of bracing, then proceeding with surgical repair or reconstruction is usually considered [1, 4]. Acute surgical intervention may be considered for large bony avulsions, clear AMRI on physical exam, interposition of soft tissue such as the pes anserine in a tibial MCL avulsion injury, intra-articular ligament entrapment, or preexisting valgus knee alignment [1, 3–7]. MCL repair is undertaken if adequate tissue is present in the acute setting, in chronic insufficiency, or when inadequate tissue is present, augmentation or reconstruction with semitendinosus or gracilis autograft becomes necessary. A recent meta-analysis by Kovachevich et al. did not show any significant difference in outcomes between primary repair and reconstruction of the MCL in patients with multiligament knee injuries [12]. Equivalent biomechanical results have been shown for anatomic augmented repair and reconstruction [13].

Treatment of high-grade MCL injuries associated with ACL injuries or other multiligament knee injuries is also not universally agreed upon [1, 3–5, 7]. Reconstruction of the ACL combined with MCL repair/reconstruction can lead to significant knee stiffness. Many surgeons allow the MCL injury to heal with conservative measures in a hinged brace while continuing to work on regaining full knee ROM over a 6-week period. As with isolated MCL injuries, if valgus instability still persists after 6 weeks, then repair of the MCL should be strongly considered at the time of ACL reconstruction. This is followed by ACL reconstruction. There is no universally accepted treatment protocol for combined ACL and MCL injuries at this point [1, 3–5].

This chapter will utilize a case-based format to demonstrate the correlation between MRI and arthroscopy for MCL pathology and review the diagnosis and management of each patient. Two cases will be presented:

1. A Grade III MCL tear in a football player with ACL and PCL ruptures
2. A Grade III MCL tear in a football player with an ACL tear

Case 1

History

A twenty-year-old college football player presents to the office 48 h after sustaining an injury in practice. He was attempting to block another player when he was hit on the lateral side of the left knee and hear an audible pop.

Exam

On physical examination, the patient had a 1+ knee effusion. He was diffusely tender along the medial aspect of the left knee. 2+ posterior drawer and 1+ Lachman, 3+ laxity with valgus stress test at 30° of flexion, and 2+ valgus instability at full extension. Negative dial test and negative varus stress test. 2+ DP and PT pulses, intact motor function across the ankle with normal sensation.

Imaging

Valgus stress radiographs taken in full extension seen in Fig. 7.1a show significant medial joint space widening indicative of complete MCL rupture with concomitant collateral ligament injury. Figure 7.1b shows a lateral radiograph of the left knee showing significant posterior translation of the tibia relative to the femur with posteriorly directed force. Figure 7.1c shows a comparison view of the contralateral knee.

Figure 7.1d shows a T2-weighted coronal sequence MRI of the left knee demonstrating complete disruption of the sMCL from the tibial insertion. The dMCL is also ruptured from its tibial attachment with a residual wisp of ligament clearly visible on the medial tibia. The medial meniscus is extruded and elevated superiorly with the intact femoral portion of the dMCL. The tibial portion of the sMCL can be seen incarcerated in the joint inferior to the medial meniscus.

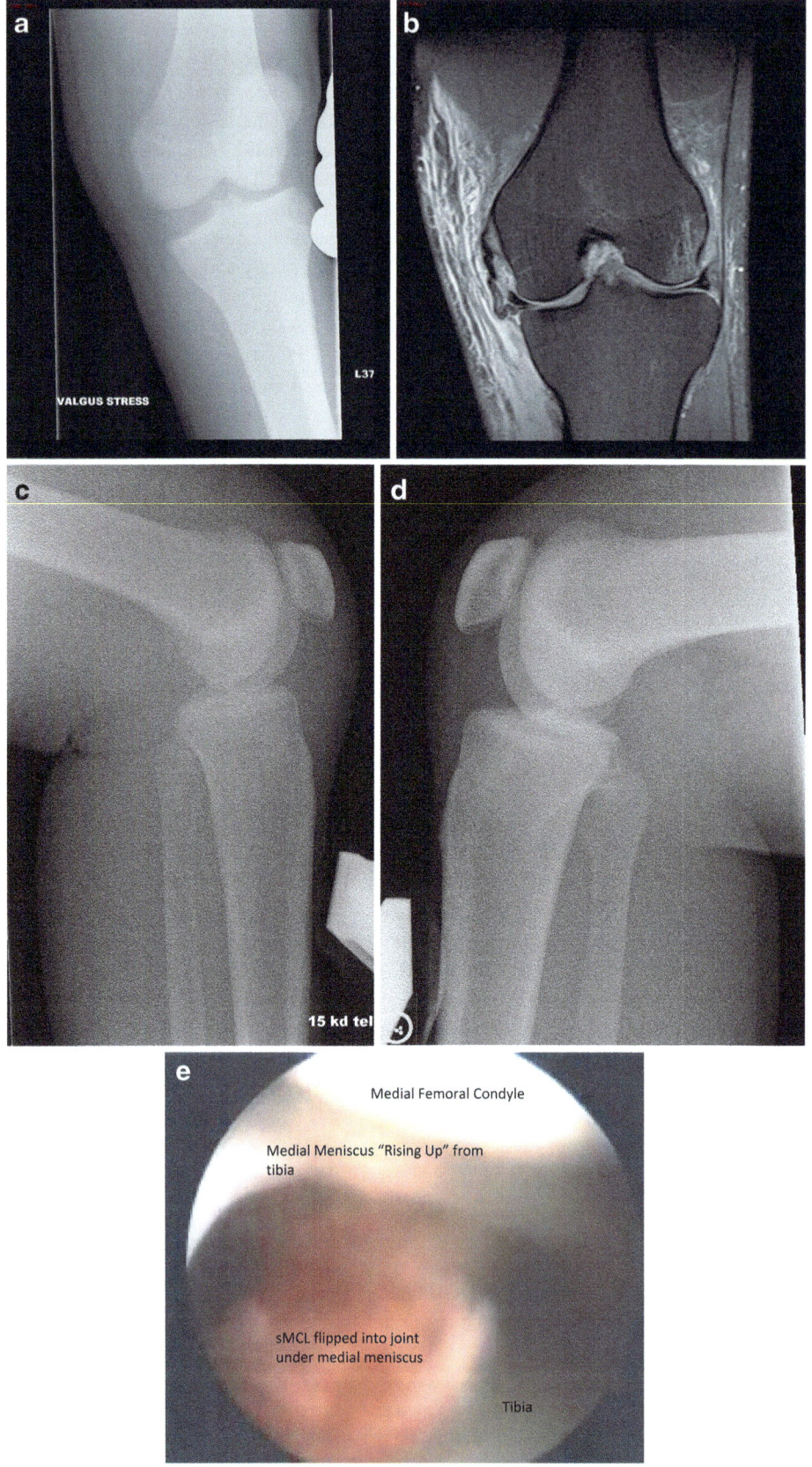

Fig. 7.1 (a) Valgus stress radiograph demonstrating medial compartment opening consistent with a complete MCL injury. (b) Coronal MRI demonstrating a distal MCL injury with displacement into the joint. (c) Stress radiograph demonstrating a PCL injury. Note posterior displacement of the tibia in relation to the femoral condyles. Compare with (d) which shows the contralateral normal side. (e) Arthroscopic view demonstrating displacement of the MCL into the knee. (f) Operative view showing superficial MCL (forceps) after extraction from the joint. (g) Deep repair of medial meniscus (distally) and deep MCL (proximally). Superficial MCL is in a right angle clamp proximally. HI. AP (h) and lateral radiographs (i) demonstrating MCL repair/reconstruction (and PCL inlay reconstruction)

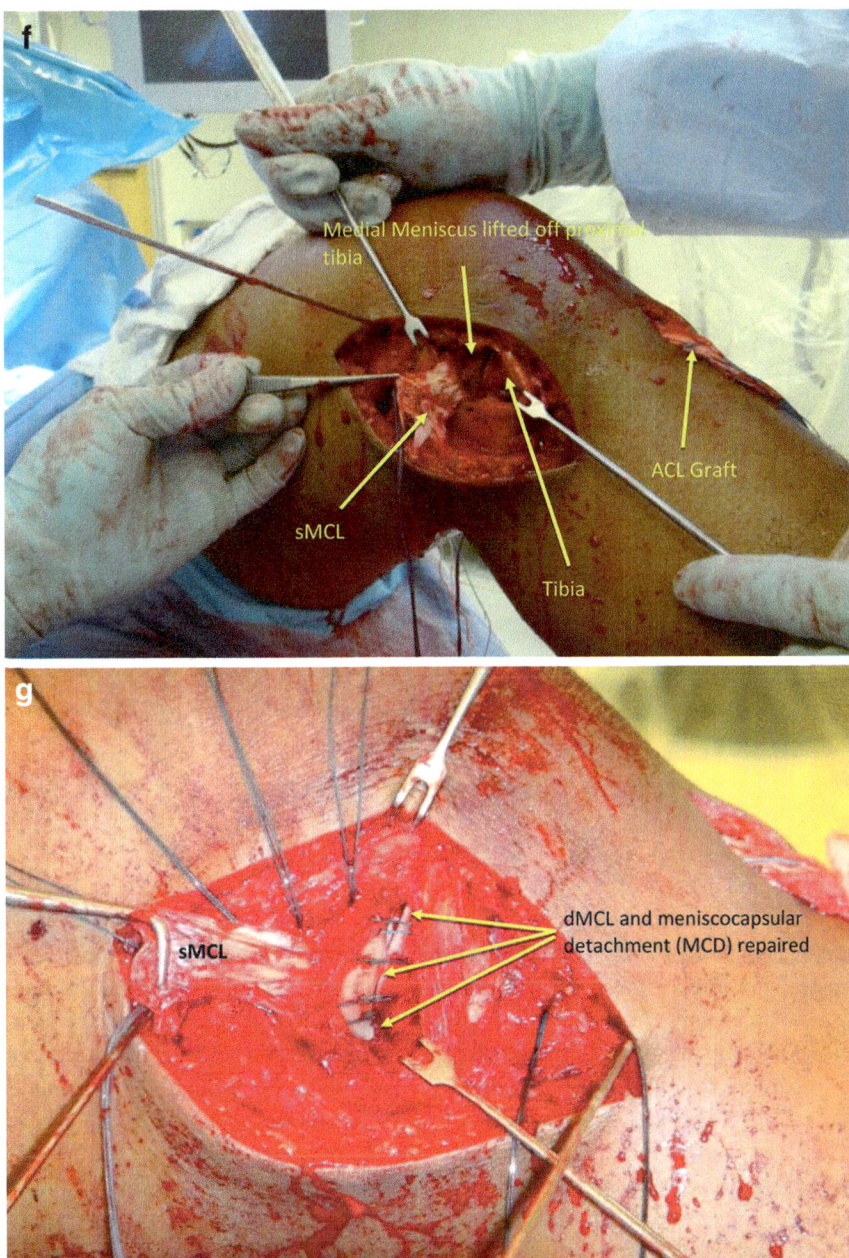

Fig. 7.1 (continued)

A bone bruise is also seen on the lateral femoral condyle. Additional MRI sequences (not shown) revealed a rupture of the ACL and PCL.

Arthroscopy

Arthroscopic exam confirmed the presence of an ACL and PCL rupture. Figure 7.1e shows an arthroscopic picture taken from the inferolateral portal looking into the medial compartment. A "meniscus rise" sign [6] is present due to complete rupture of the tibial portion of the dMCL. In addition, the tibial portion of the sMCL can be seen flipped into the joint underneath the medial meniscus.

The ACL was reconstructed arthroscopically with a semitendinosus and gracilis autograft from the ipsilateral side. The PCL was reconstructed using a posterior tibial inlay technique with bone-patellar tendon-bone (BPTB) autograft from the ipsilateral side.

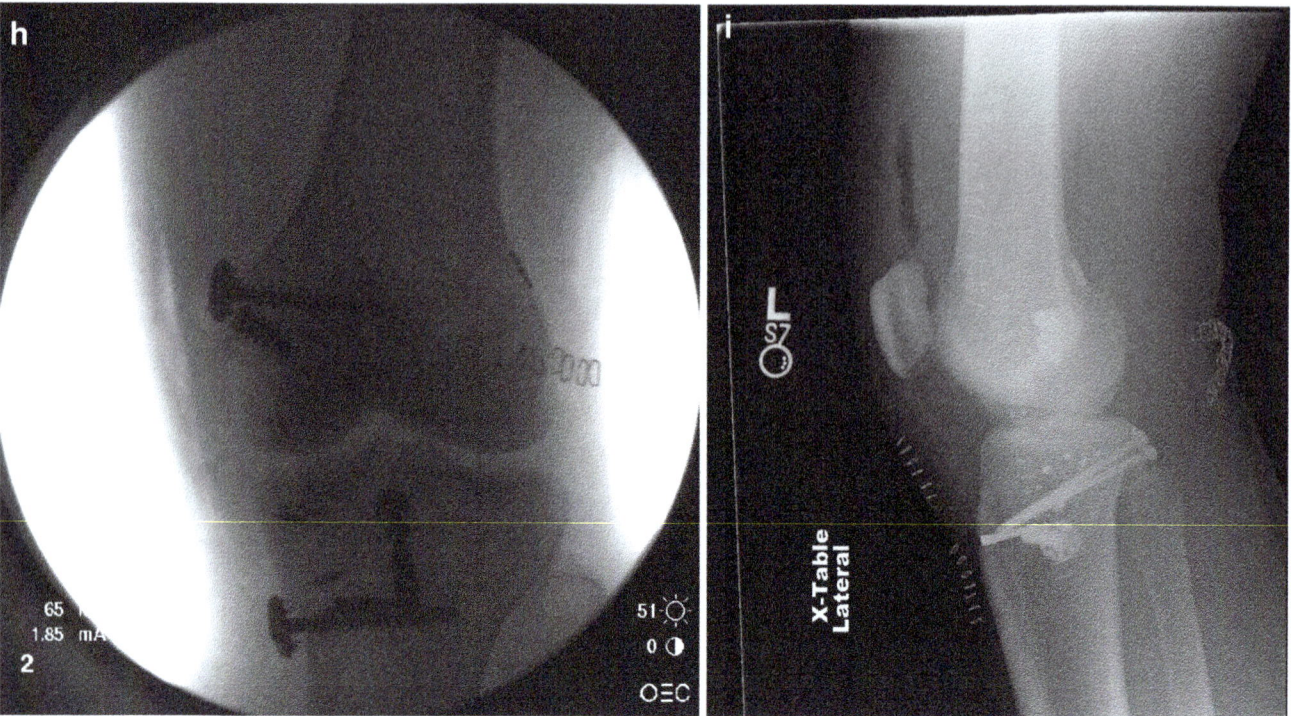

Fig. 7.1 (continued)

A separate medial incision centered just posterior to the midline of the knee joint was made running longitudinally from the adductor tubercle to a point 7–8 cm passed the joint line distally. As expected, the sMCL was completely ruptured from its tibial attachment and flipped into the joint between the medial tibial plateau and medial meniscus. The medial meniscus was separated from the overlying capsule along its posterior portion. The dMCL was still attached to the medial meniscus and avulsed from the proximal medial tibia. Figure 7.1f is an intraoperative photo showing the tibial portion of the sMCL after it has been freed from the knee joint. Though subtle, space can be seen beneath the medial meniscus with the tibial portion of the dMCL still attached and projecting posteromedially. Figure 7.1g shows the medial meniscus and tibial portion of the dMCL after repair with three suture anchors. The sMCL is flipped up proximally with sutures in it for planned repair. The semimembranosus tendon was intact, but in addition to the posteromedial meniscocapsular detachment (MCD), the POL was torn from the tibia, and it is expanded onto the semimembranosus. The meniscocapsular detachment and tibial portion of the dMCL were repaired primarily with three suture anchors along the medial tibial margin. The sMCL was then repaired primarily back to the tibial surface utilizing suture anchors. Tibial sided avulsion injuries heal less predictably than femoral sided avulsion injuries, so the decision was made to augment or repair with semitendinosus allograft, which we would also use to reconstruct the posteromedial corner, namely, the ruptured POL. The isometric point of the femoral origin of the sMCL was identified with fluoroscopic guidance by drawing an imaginary line tangential to the posterior femoral cortex and to Blumensaat's line horizontally. The MCL origin sits just proximal to the horizontal line and just posterior to the posterior femoral cortex line [9]. A guidewire was placed and the sMCL was attached both proximally and distally with a 6.5 mm screw and soft tissue washer construct. The sMCL is looped around the semimembranosus prior to attachment as has been described by Stannard [1].

Postoperative images are seen in Fig. 7.1h, i.

Discussion Points

- General imaging findings with MCL ruptures
- Anatomy of the superficial and deep MCL
- The role of the PMC in knee stability and techniques for reconstruction
- Allograft augmentation of the MCL and PMC in the setting of multiligament knee injuries

Case 2

History

The patient is a 20-year-old football wide receiver at the collegiate level. He sustained a noncontact external rotation, axial load, and valgus injury to his right knee after landing with a caught football at an awkward position. He presents to our surgery center 2 weeks after the injury.

Physical Exam

Moderate right knee effusion, bruising, and tenderness along the medial aspect of the right knee are noted. Marked valgus instability with both at 30° and at full extension. 2+ Lachman negative posterior drawer test, negative dial test at 30 and 90°. Negative varus stress test.

Imaging

MRI images are shown in Fig. 7.2a, b. Figure 7.2a shows a T2-weighted coronal image of the right knee. The sMCL is ruptured from the tibial attachment and mildly retracted; a portion of the pes anserine tendons can be seen interposed between the avulsed ligament and the proximal medial tibia. There is marked edema between anatomic layers II and III, and the tibial portion of the dMCL is not well visualized.

Arthroscopy

Figure 7.2b is an arthroscopic image of the medial compartment of the knee as seen through the inferolateral portal with the knee in 30° of flexion and valgus stress applied. The medial meniscus is seen to lift off the tibia with increased apparent space readily seen between the medial meniscus and the tibia. This is due to the tearing of the sMCL and at least a portion of the tibial portion of the dMCL.

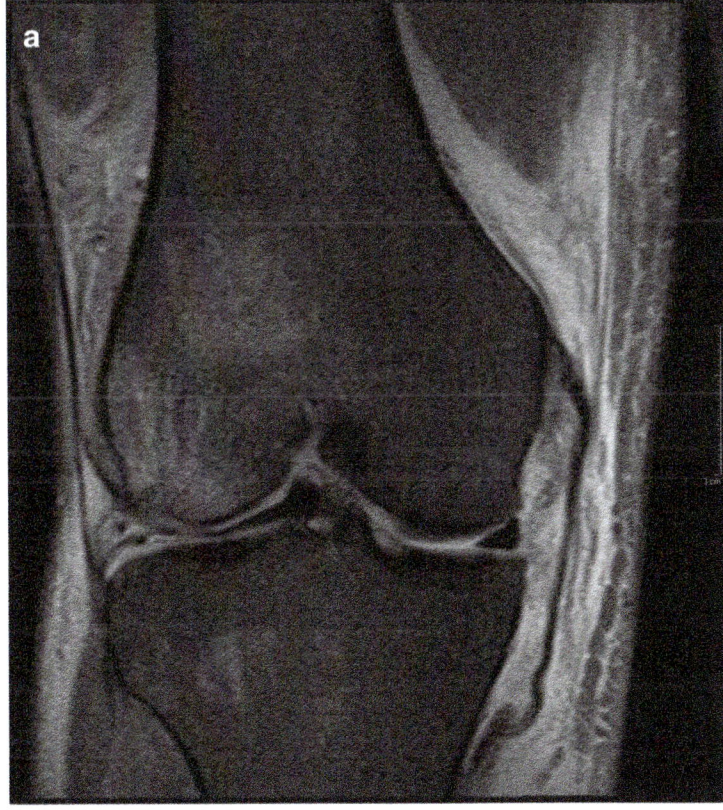
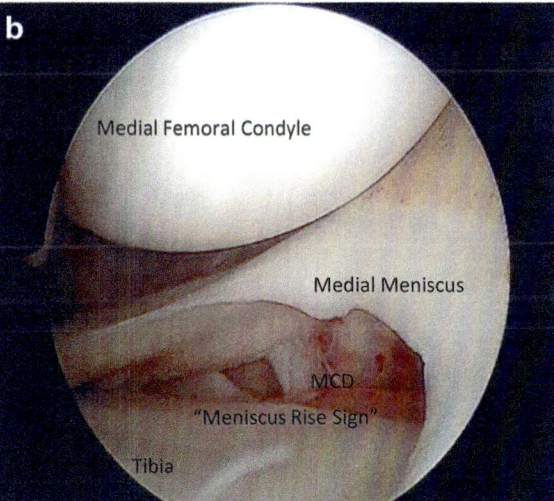

Fig. 7.2 (**a**) Coronal MRI demonstrating MCL distal injury and displacement over (superficial to) the pes insertion (Stener-like lesion). (**b**) Arthroscopic view demonstrating medial opening associated with a distal MCL injury. Note that the meniscus "stays" with the uninjured proximal (femoral) side. (**c, d**) Operative view demonstrating mobilization and repair of superficial MCL distally. (**e**) Another case demonstrating a more chronic distal MCL injury

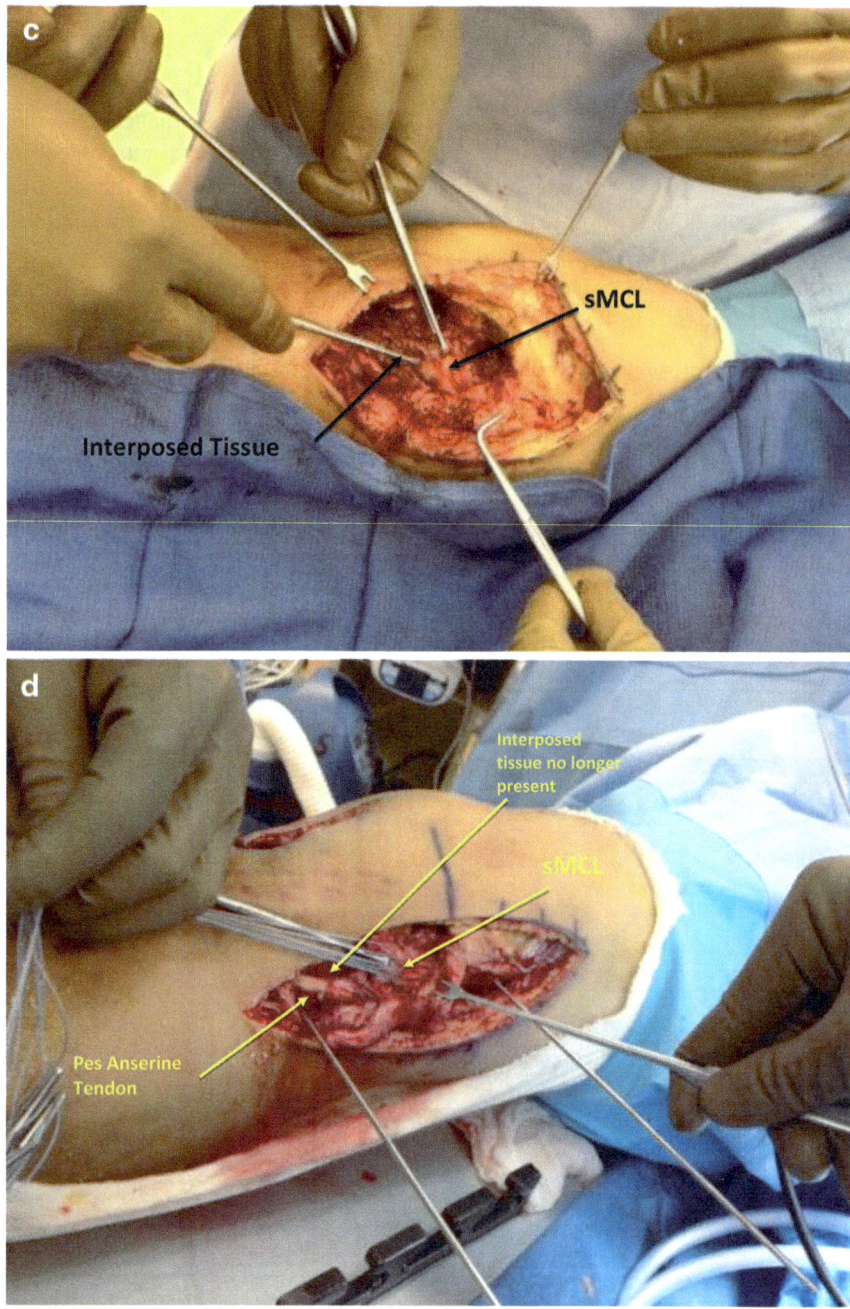

Fig. 7.2 (continued)

Surgical Details

The lateral meniscus was repaired with an inside out technique after reducing the bucket handle component and rasping the intact bleeding edge. The ACL was reconstructed with BPTB autograft.

A longitudinal incision was made along the medial aspect of the knee just posterior from the midline in the sagittal plane. The incision extended from just above the joint line to

a point approximately 5–7 cm below the joint line. Sharp dissection was carried down through the skin and SQ tissue, and the crural fascia comprising anatomic layer I was completely disrupted. The MCL was directly visualized and found to be completely detached from its tibial attachment and flipped back down on top of the gracilis and semitendinosus tendons and on top of the intact distal portion on anatomic layer I. This is seen in the intraoperative photo labeled Fig. 7.2c. The MCL was mobilized and flipped back further proximally.

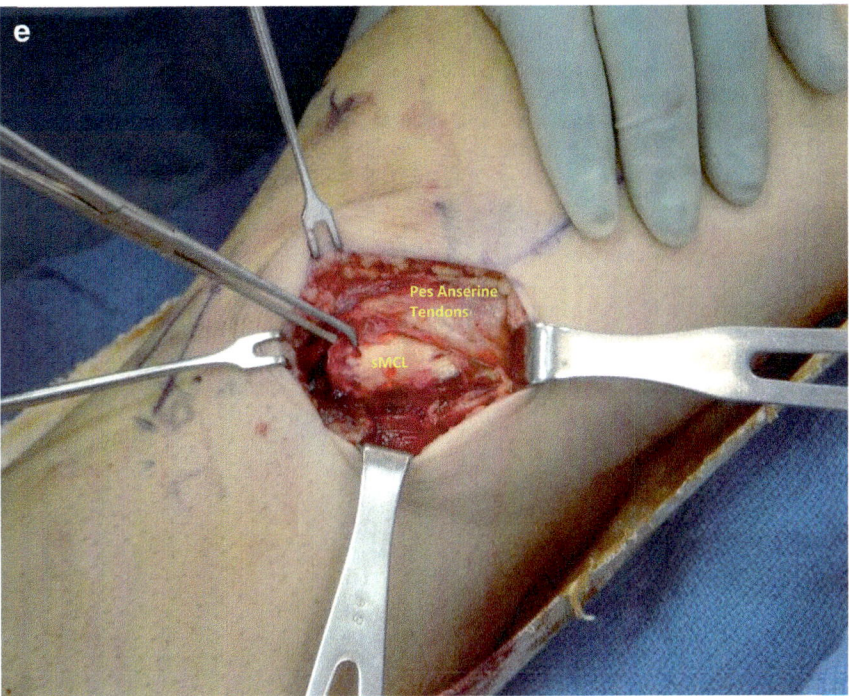

Fig. 7.2 (continued)

The anterior tibial portion of the dMCL was ruptured, and there was a meniscocapsular detachment propagating from this region posteriorly. The dMCL was repaired with double-loaded suture anchors along its anterior half; these sutures were also passed through the meniscocapsular separation to repair this as well. Figure 7.2d shows the sMCL just prior to reattachment with two anchors and with interposed soft tissue moved out of the way. Figure 7.2e is an intraoperative image taken from a different patient with a tibial avulsion of the sMCL but without interposed tissue between the sMCL and proximal tibia. The sMCL can be clearly seen passing beneath the pes anserine tendons, whereas in the prior photos, there is more extensive disruption with the sMCL sitting superficially to these structures. In this case, the sMCL was then repaired with two suture anchors in the proximal tibia deep to the pes anserine tendons.

While MRI and arthroscopy can provide valuable information in the diagnosis of these injuries, the gold standard remains a thorough history and appropriate physical exam.

The majority of isolated MCL injuries can be managed nonoperatively with a hinged brace and immediate knee motion. Surgical treatment is necessary when valgus stability is not restored after a 6–8-week trial of bracing or when AMBRI is present on exam. Certain acute conditions such as interposed tissue, large bony avulsions, or entrapped ligamentous tissue within the joint may necessitate surgical intervention as well. Treatment of Grade III MCL injuries associated with ACL ruptures is controversial, but there seems to be a trend toward nonoperative management of the MCL injury followed by delayed reconstruction of the ACL. Most Grade III MCL injuries associated with knee dislocations are managed with surgical repair.

Conclusions

Knee medial collateral ligament injuries represent the most common knee ligament injury in both athletes and the general population. The majority of patients present with medial sided knee pain and varying degrees of valgus instability depending on the degree of damage to the MCL and the associated PMC. A thorough understanding of the complex anatomy along the medial side of the knee is necessary to properly evaluate and treat this patient population.

References

1. Stannard JP. Medial and posteromedial instability of the knee: evaluation, treatment, and results. Sports Med Arthrosc Rev. 2010;18(4):263–8.
2. Milewski MD, Sanders TG, Miller MD. MRI-Arthroscopy correlation: the knee. J Bone Joint Surg Am. 2011;93:1735–45.
3. Schein A, Matcuk G, Patel D, Gottsegen CJ, Hartshorn T, Forrester D, White E. Structure and function, injury, pathology, and treatment of the medial collateral ligament of the knee. Emerg Radiol. 2012;19: 489–98.

4. Phisitkul P, James SL, Wolf BR, Amendola A. MCL injuries of the knee: current concepts review. Iowa Orthop J. 2006;26:77–90.

5. Jacobson KE, Chi FS. Evaluation and treatment of medial collateral ligament and medial-sided injuries of the knee. Sports Med Atrhosc Rev. 2006;14(2):58–66.

6. Sims WF, Jacobson KE. The posteromedial corner of the knee: medial-sided injury patterns revisited. Am J Sports Med. 2004;32(2): 337–45.

7. Azar MA. Evaluation and treatment of chronic medial collateral ligament injuries of the knee. Sports Med Arthrosc Rev. 2006; 14(2):84–90.

8. Maeseneer M, Shahabpour M, Pouders C. MRI spectrum of medial collateral ligament injuries and pitfalls in diagnosis. JBR-BTR. 2010;93:97–103.

9. Radiographic landmarks for locating the femoral origin of the superficial medial collateral ligament. Am J Sports Med. 2013;41(11): 2527–32.

10. Warren LF, Marshall JL. The supporting structures and layers of the medial side of the knee: an anatomical analysis. J Bone Joint Surg Am. 1979;61(1):56–62.

11. Farshad-Amaker NA, Potter HG. MRI of knee ligament injury and reconstruction. J Magn Reson Imaging. 2013;38: 757–73.

12. Kovachevich R, Shah JP, Arens AM, Stuart MJ, Dahm DL, Levy BA. Operative management of the medial collateral ligament in the multiligament injured knee: an evidence-based systematic review. Knee Surg Sports Traumatol Arthrosc. 2009;17:823–9.

13. Wijdicks CA, Michalski MP, Rasmussen MT, Goldsmith MT, Kennedy NI, Lind M, Engebretsen L, Laprade RF. Superficial medial collateral ligament anatomic augmented repair versus anatomic reconstruction: an in vitro biomechanical analysis. Am J Sports Med. 2013;41:2858–65.

The Posterolateral Corner of the Knee

8

Evan W. James, Chris M. LaPrade, and Robert F. LaPrade

Introduction

The posterolateral corner (PLC) of the knee is a commonly injured, yet largely misunderstood, region of the knee. Posterolateral corner injuries, including those to the fibular (lateral) collateral ligament (FCL), popliteus tendon, and popliteofibular ligament (PFL), are most commonly caused by twisting or hyperextension in an athlete, high-velocity trauma after a motor vehicle accident, or contact after a fall [1, 2]. The incidence of FCL, popliteus tendon, and PFL injuries is similar and reportedly occurs in approximately 9 % of all knee ligament injuries [3]. In a trauma setting, Fanelli et al. reported that PLC injuries were present in 27 % of all acute knee injuries and in 62 % of all posterior cruciate ligament (PCL) injuries [1]. LaPrade et al. reported that PLC injuries accounted for 16 % of all acute knee ligament injuries and 9 % of knee injuries presenting with hemarthrosis [3]. Other studies have also reported that 72–87 % of PLC injuries were combined ligament injuries with concurrent cruciate or collateral ligament tears [2–4]. In short, posterolateral corner injuries are common but often missed and should be considered as part of any standard diagnostic knee assessment.

The PLC contains numerous structures that together provide static and dynamic stability by resisting hyperextension, tibial external rotation, and varus gapping [5]. The three most important static stabilizers are the popliteus tendon, PFL, and FCL. Of the three primary static stabilizers, only the popliteus tendon courses intra-articularly and is directly visible during arthroscopy [6, 7]. The popliteus tendon, which originates from the popliteus muscle, attaches to the anterior fifth and proximal half of the popliteal sulcus after coursing anterolaterally around the lateral femoral condyle [6]. Other PLC structures such as the posterolateral joint capsule, coronary ligament, oblique popliteal ligament, fabellofibular ligament, and lateral meniscus posterior horn also contribute to static stability in the knee [5]. Contributors to dynamic stability include the popliteus muscle, iliotibial band, biceps femoris muscle, and lateral gastrocnemius tendon.

Biomechanical studies have elucidated the importance of correctly diagnosing and treating patients with PLC tears, especially when combined with anterior cruciate ligament (ACL) and PCL injury. Two studies have reported that complete sectioning of the FCL, PFL, and popliteus tendon resulted in significantly higher forces on both ACL and PCL reconstruction grafts [8, 9]. This may contribute to cruciate ligament graft failure if PLC injuries are not addressed concurrently. In addition, lateral knee instability after PLC injury results in two abnormal gait patterns: the "varus thrust gait" and the "quadriceps avoidance pattern" [5]. With a "varus thrust gait," the patient experiences increased adduction and lateral compartment liftoff, which contributes to medial compartment cartilage damage. With a "quadriceps avoidance pattern," the knee experiences a hyperextension thrust when the knee is ACL and PLC deficient. Tibiofemoral contact pressures are theorized to be increased as a result [5]. For these reasons, PLC injuries now are commonly reconstructed to minimize the risk of recurrent instability [10, 11], ACL or PCL graft failure [8, 9], and degenerative cartilage changes in the knee.

A thorough understanding of the quantitative anatomy of the primary posterolateral corner static stabilizers is essential for performing an anatomic-based posterolateral corner repair or reconstruction. The FCL attaches 1.4 mm proximally and 3.1 mm posteriorly to the lateral epicondyle [6].

E.W. James, BS (✉)
Steadman Philippon Research Institute, Center for Outcomes-Based Orthopedic Research, Vail, CO, USA
e-mail: ejames@sprivail.org

C.M. LaPrade, BA
Department of Biomedical Engineering, Steadman Philippon Research Institute, Vail, CO, USA
e-mail: claprade@sprivail.org

R.F. LaPrade, MD, PhD
The Steadman Clinic, Vail, CO, USA
e-mail: rlaprade@thesteadmanclinic.com

S.F. Brockmeier (ed.), *MRI-Arthroscopy Correlations: A Case-Based Atlas of the Knee, Shoulder, Elbow and Hip*, DOI 10.1007/978-1-4939-2645-9_8, © Springer Science+Business Media New York 2015

Distally, the FCL attaches 8.2 mm anteriorly to the anterior margin of the fibular head and 28.4 mm distally to the tip of the fibular styloid process. The PFL originates at the popliteus musculotendinous junction and is split into anterior and posterior divisions. The anterior and posterior portions both attach to the popliteus complex at the proximolateral musculotendinous junction. The distolateral attachments of the anterior and posterior division attach 2.8 mm and 1.6 mm distally to the apex of the fibular styloid process on its posteromedial downslope, respectively.

The purpose of this chapter is to illustrate correlations between magnetic resonance imaging (MRI) and arthroscopy in order to facilitate better diagnosis and treatment planning in patients with PLC and associated injuries. Three cases will be presented:

1. Grade III (complete) PLC tear, ACL tear, biceps femoris avulsion, and lateral meniscus posterior horn tear
2. ACL, FCL, PFL, and lateral meniscus tear
3. Chronic popliteus tendon and lateral meniscus tear

Case 1: Grade III (Complete) PLC Tear, ACL Tear, Biceps Femoris Avulsion, and Lateral Meniscus Posterior Horn Tear

History/Exam

A 31-year-old female presented to clinic 2 weeks after experiencing a right knee injury while playing softball. The injury occurred after a traumatic varus-directed force was applied to her knee during a collision with another player. She was unable to bear weight on her right side after the injury and presented to an urgent care clinic, where radiographs revealed an avulsion fracture of the fibula. She was referred to an orthopedic clinic for further evaluation.

On physical examination, the patient had widespread swelling in her right lower extremity and tenderness to palpation over the fibular head. Her range of motion was limited from 0° to 60° of knee flexion, compared to 0° to 135° of knee flexion in her contralateral uninjured knee. No end point was felt on varus stress testing at 0° and 20° of knee flexion or on the Lachman test. No valgus laxity was found at 0° or 20° of knee flexion.

Imaging

Right knee radiographs in the anteroposterior (AP), longstanding, lateral, Rosenberg, and sunrise views from the urgent care were reviewed. An avulsion fracture of the biceps femoris off of the fibular head was discovered.

A right knee MRI was ordered and reviewed, revealing an avulsion fracture of the biceps femoris off of the fibular head

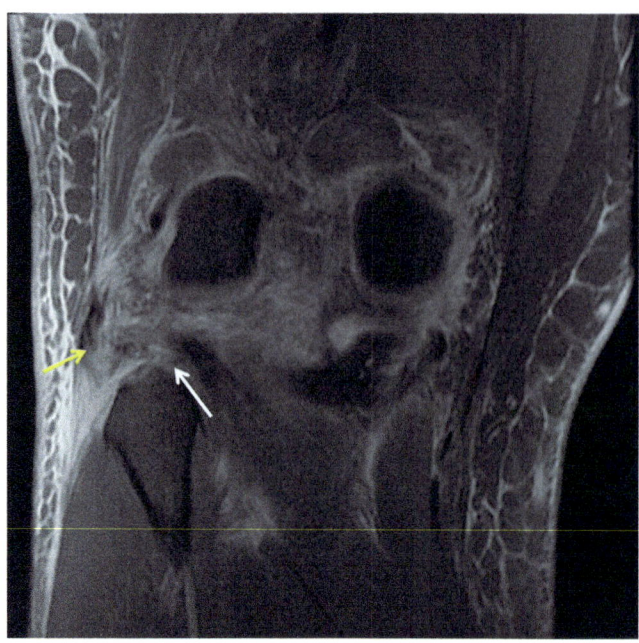

Fig. 8.1 A PD FS COR MRI indicating the presence of a PFL tear (*white arrow*) and an avulsion of the biceps femoris (*yellow arrow*)

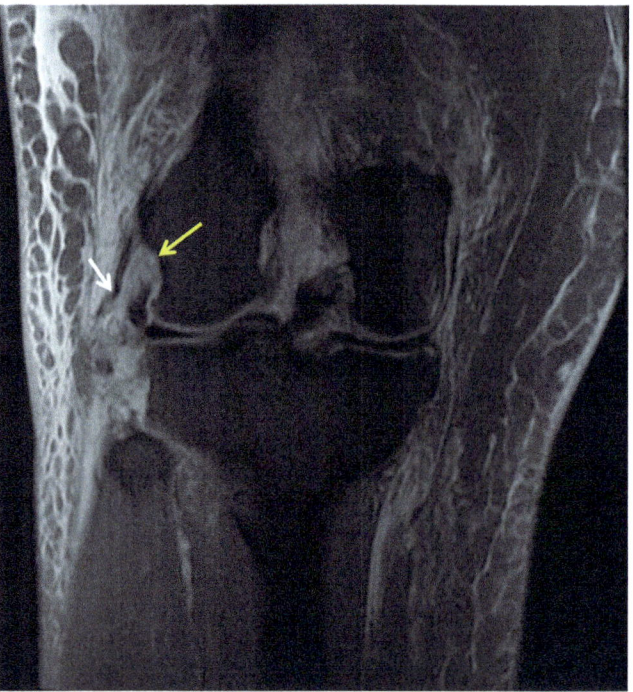

Fig. 8.2 A PD FS COR MRI indicating a popliteus tendon (*yellow arrow*) and FCL tear (*white arrow*)

(Fig. 8.1), a severe PLC knee injury with evidence of a grade III FCL tear and popliteus tendon disruption (Fig. 8.2), and a complete ACL tear. Her PCL and MCL appeared uninjured. In addition, evidence of possible peroneal nerve damage and a posterior horn tear of the lateral meniscus were noted (Fig. 8.3). The integrity of her knee articular cartilage was

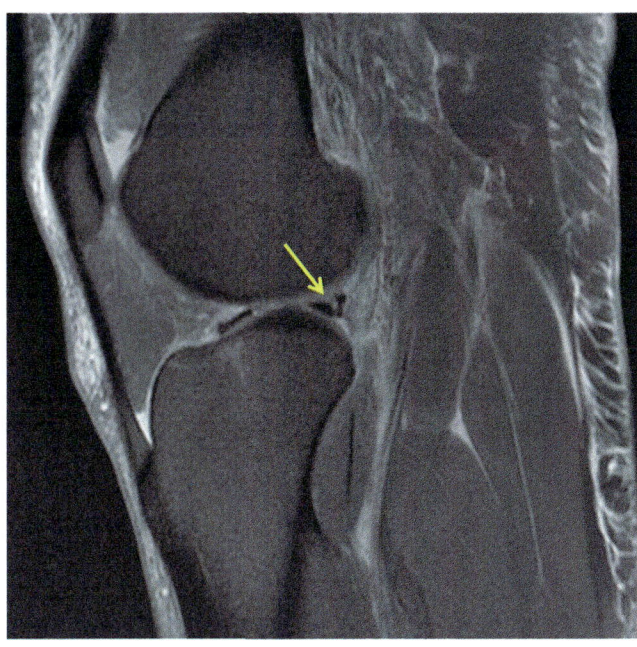

Fig. 8.3 A PD FS sagittal MRI indicating the presence of a posterior horn lateral meniscus vertical tear (*yellow arrow*)

indeterminable. However, a bone bruise to the medial compartment of the tibial plateau or medial femoral condyle, which has been reported to be a common secondary sign of a grade III PLC injury [4], was present in addition to the observed structural damage.

After discussing all treatment options, the patient elected to proceed with surgery immediately, including an ACL reconstruction and an anatomic-based PLC reconstruction. She also consented to undergo any additional repairs or reconstructions that were deemed necessary during the exam under anesthesia and arthroscopic evaluation.

Arthroscopy

The patient was induced under anesthesia. A preoperative Doppler ultrasound showed some mild superficial blood clots, so surgery proceeded without a tourniquet. During the examination under anesthesia, a side-to-side difference of 4 cm of increased heel height in her right lower extremity was found. There was mild stiffness in her right knee, but it could be flexed back to full flexion. The Lachman and pivot shift tests were both grades 2+. The varus stress test revealed grade 3+ varus gapping at 0° and 30° of flexion. Her posterolateral drawer was positive for posterolateral instability, and the dial test showed approximately 15° of increased external tibial rotation at 30° and 90° of knee flexion. Together, the exam under anesthesia was consistent with the diagnosis made on clinical exam and diagnostic imaging.

The posterolateral surgical approach was created by making a standard laterally based hockey stick incision that extended down to the iliotibial band. After dissection over the iliotibial band and the short and long heads of the biceps femoris, the lateral capsule, distal aspect of the iliotibial band, and biceps femoris were noted all to be completely torn off of their attachments to the tibia and fibula. Careful dissection was then performed to complete a peroneal nerve neurolysis. After the neurolysis was completed, the biceps femoris was released from its scarred-in position proximally. The fibular head and the location of the normal FCL attachment to the fibula were identified. The fibular head reconstruction tunnel was reamed and a passing stitch was placed. A periosteal elevator was used to locate the popliteal sulcus. The tibial tunnel was reamed to pass the popliteus tendon and popliteofibular ligament grafts anteriorly, and a passing stitch was placed through this tunnel.

Next, the iliotibial band was split and an incision was made through the lateral capsule. The popliteus tendon (Fig. 8.4a, b) and FCL were torn at their femoral attachment sites. Guide pins were placed beginning at the native anatomic footprints and directed proximomedially to avoid passing through the intercondylar notch. After verifying correct pin placement, tunnels were reamed over the guide pins to a diameter of 9 mm and a depth of 20 mm. A split Achilles tendon graft was prepared, and 9 × 20-mm bone plugs were passed into the tunnels using two passing sutures.

Next, the arthroscopic portion of the procedure was initiated by creating medial and lateral parapatellar arthroscopic portals. The patient's suprapatellar pouch was hemorrhaged and removed. While the patellar articular cartilage was normal, the medial aspect of the trochlea had a large full-thickness articular cartilage defect, which was not apparent on MRI. The lesion was 10 mm medial to lateral and approximately 20 mm proximal to distal. After trimming the edges with a curette, a microfracture procedure was performed.

The medial compartment was inspected next. There was no medial compartment "drive-through" sign. The medial meniscus and tibiofemoral articular cartilage were normal. The ACL was completely torn. A 10-mm closed socket tunnel was created between the native attachment of the anteromedial and posterolateral ACL bundles on the femur. The tibial ACL attachment site was identified and outlined.

Next, the lateral compartment was inspected. The lateral meniscus was torn at its attachment to the ligament of Wrisberg and separated away from its tibial attachment (Fig. 8.5a–c). The popliteus tendon was completely torn off of its femoral attachment. A "drive-through" sign was present in the lateral compartment (Fig. 8.6) [2]. The lateral meniscus was repaired with two vertical mattress sutures. The tibial ACL reconstruction tunnel was reamed using a cruciate ligament aiming device and a 10-mm reamer. Once

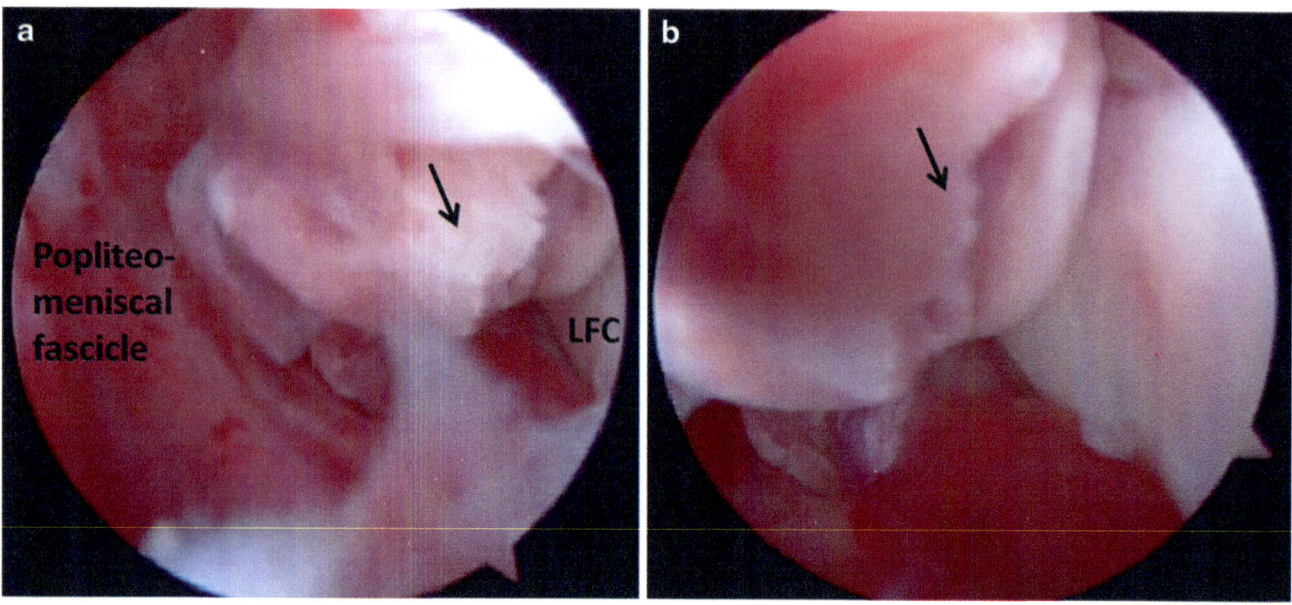

Fig. 8.4 (**a**, **b**) Arthroscopic images demonstrating the presence of a popliteus tendon tear, black arrow (right knee). *LFC* lateral femoral condyle

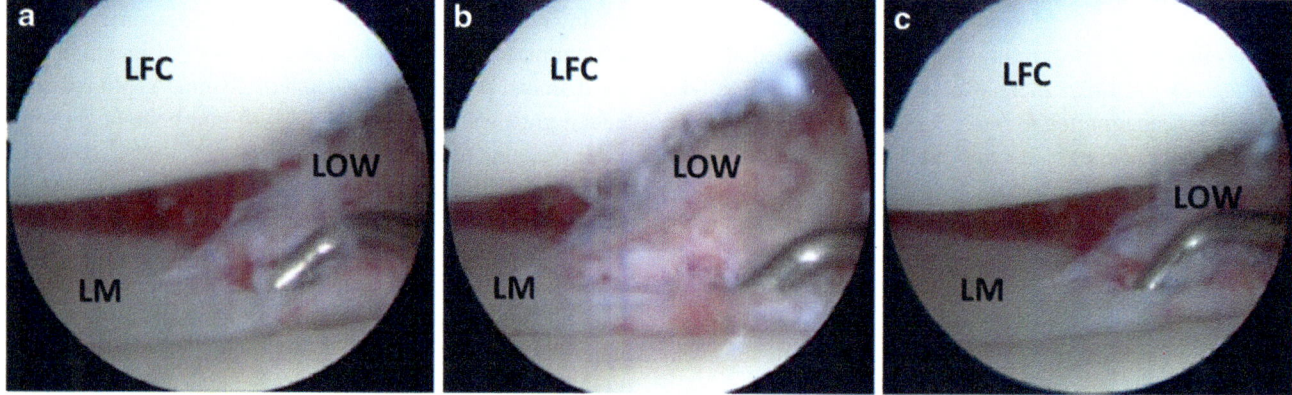

Fig. 8.5 (**a**, **b**, **c**) Arthroscopic images demonstrating a tear in the posterior horn of the lateral meniscus (probe) near the attachment of the ligament of Wrisberg (right knee). *LFC* lateral femoral condyle, *LM* lateral meniscus, *LOW* ligament of Wrisberg

the ACL graft was pulled into place, it was fixed with a titanium interference screw.

The FCL and popliteus tendon grafts were passed into their respective femoral tunnels and fixed with 7 × 20-mm titanium interference screws. The popliteus tendon graft was passed down to the popliteal hiatus, and the FCL graft was passed under the superficial layer of the iliotibial band. The avulsed biceps femoris was found, and it was passed through the biceps bursa to allow for a more anatomic position of the biceps femoris once it was repaired. Once properly positioned and tensioned, the FCL graft was fixed in the fibular head with a 7 × 23-mm bioabsorbable screw. Both the popliteus tendon and FCL grafts were pulled together anteriorly through the tibial reconstruction tunnel with a passing suture, and the grafts were cycled through knee flexion and extension to eliminate any slack. Both grafts were fixed at 20° of flexion. Stability of the grafted structures was confirmed using the dial test and posterolateral drawer test.

The lateral capsule was repaired using a suture anchor to openly repair the lateral meniscus. Two anchors were placed in the fibular head, and the biceps femoris was repaired while the knee was in full extension. Finally, the ACL was fixed in the tibial tunnel with a 9 × 20-mm interference screw, which eliminated her positive Lachman's test. The procedure was completed by closing the incisions in the lateral capsule, iliotibial band, and superficial skin.

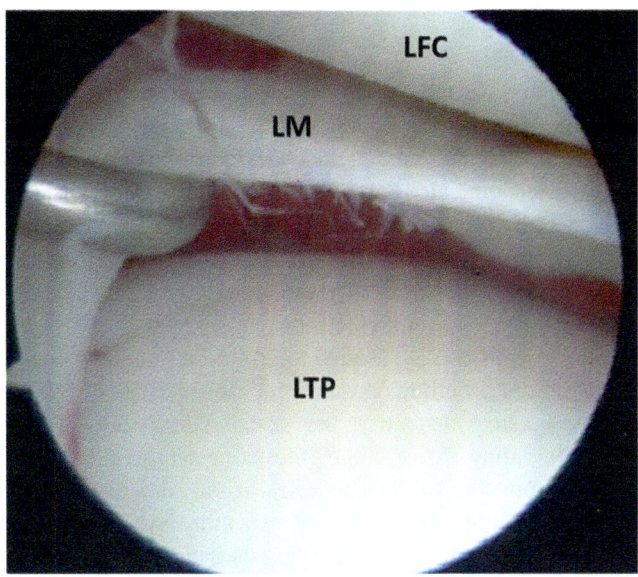

Fig. 8.6 Arthroscopic visualization of the lateral compartment indicates the presence of a "drive-through" sign, consistent with a posterolateral corner injury (right knee). *LFC* lateral femoral condyle, *LM* lateral meniscus, *LTP* lateral tibial plateau

Discussion

By combining elements of the patient's history, physical exam, diagnostic imaging, and arthroscopy, it is possible to formulate a comprehensive understanding of complex, combined posterolateral corner injuries. In this case, the correlation between diagnostic imaging on MRI and the intraoperative findings on arthroscopy helped to identify complex injury patterns and formulate an appropriate surgical treatment plan.

The MRI demonstrated an avulsion fracture of the biceps femoris. Diagnostic MRI was also helpful in evaluating the integrity of the cruciate and collateral ligaments. With regard to the PLC, the MRI was able to discern the presence of grade III popliteus tendon and FCL injuries, both later confirmed at arthroscopy. However, due to the extended and complex nature of injuries in this patient, the injury patterns of the posterior horn lateral meniscus, peroneal nerve, and articular cartilage of the patient were difficult to determine on MRI and required further examination. In addition, a large trochlear cartilage defect was not discovered until the time of arthroscopy and was not evident on MRI.

A total PLC reconstruction, such as with this patient, is often performed in combination with other repairs and reconstructions since the majority of PLC injuries are combined injuries. Therefore, open and arthroscopic procedures may both be required to complete the requisite repairs and reconstructions for each patient. For this reason, the findings on MRI must be confirmed both through open and arthroscopic examination. In this patient, many of the repairs or recon-

structions, such as the biceps femoris repair and the total PLC reconstruction, were completed through an open incision due to the extra-articular location of the structures. However, the reconstruction of the ACL and the examination of the posterior horn of the lateral meniscus, articular cartilage of the knee joint, and intra-articular popliteus tendon all required the use of arthroscopy. In cases with a wide variety of complex ligamentous, tendinous, or meniscal pathology, arthroscopy may be necessary in order to confirm the presence of articular cartilage damage or meniscal tears. Arthroscopy is also used to verify the presence of a lateral compartment "drive-through" sign, which has been described as a frequent indication of a grade III PLC corner injury [2]. The "drive-through" sign was seen in this patient, which was consistent with the MRI diagnosis of a grade III PLC injury. In addition, MRI diagnosis of the presence of bone bruises on the medial tibial plateau or medial femoral condyle may also increase suspicion of a PLC injury [4].

Case 2: ACL, FCL, Lateral Meniscus, and PFL Tear

History/Exam

A 40-year-old male presented to clinic 1 month after twisting and injuring his right knee while skiing and dropping off a 15-foot cliff. He experienced pain and swelling immediately after the injury and reported to an outside hospital where an MRI series and radiographs were obtained.

On physical exam, the patient had an obvious antalgic gait, favoring his right side. There was a moderate effusion of the right knee. Range of motion in the right knee revealed 5° of hyperextension and 120° of flexion with some pain secondary to swelling. The patient's contralateral knee exhibited 8° of hyperextension and 130° of flexion. He had a 2+ Lachman's test and negative posterior drawer test along with increased gapping with varus testing at 30° of knee flexion. There was no increased varus gapping at 0°. His knee was otherwise stable, with no increased gapping to valgus testing at 0° and 30° of knee flexion. The dial test demonstrated symmetric external tibial rotation at 30° and 90° of knee flexion. In light of the instability found on physical exam, imaging studies performed at an outside hospital were reviewed, and bilateral varus stress radiographs were obtained to assist with the diagnostic assessment.

Imaging

A full bilateral knee series was reviewed. Radiographs of the right knee demonstrated well-preserved medial and lateral tibiofemoral joint spaces and ruled out the presence of fractures. Varus stress radiographs demonstrated a side-to-side increase in varus gapping in the right knee compared to the left knee of 2.19 mm. An MRI performed at an outside hospital demonstrated a complete ACL midsubstance tear (Fig. 8.7), edema and discontinuity along the FCL, and a radial tear in the body of the lateral meniscus (Fig. 8.8a–c). Some changes were noted in the popliteofibular ligament, but a tear could not be definitively ruled in or out (Fig. 8.9). No articular cartilage pathology was noted.

After reviewing the results of the history, physical exam, and imaging, an ACL allograft reconstruction, FCL reconstruction, and lateral meniscus repair were recommended, and the patient elected to proceed with surgery.

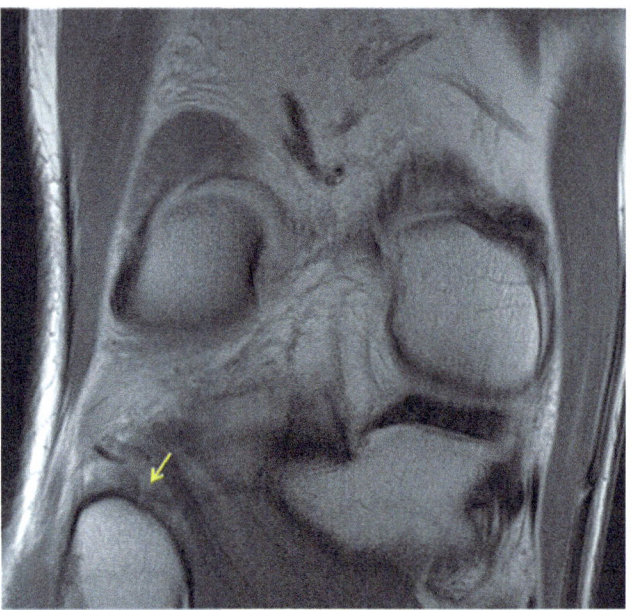

Fig. 8.7 A PD TSE FS sagittal MRI of a complete ACL tear

Arthroscopy

The patient was induced under general anesthesia, and an exam under anesthesia demonstrated a 2+ Lachman's and pivot shift test, 1+ varus gapping at 0° of knee flexion, and 3+ varus gapping at 30° of knee flexion. These findings correlated well with the findings on MRI and the results of the previous physical exam.

A standard lateral hockey stick incision was made and a posteriorly based skin flap was developed. A common peroneal neurolysis was performed to prevent a foot drop due to postoperative swelling. A small incision was made in the biceps bursa to identify the distal attachment of the FCL. Palpating through the interval between the lateral gastrocnemius and soleus muscles, it was determined that the popliteofibular ligament (PFL) was torn. A 6-mm tunnel was reamed into the lateral fibular head, and after placing a passing stitch in the distal FCL, the proximal FCL attachment was located through an incision made in the iliotibial band. A 6-mm tunnel was reamed over a guide pin at the proximal FCL footprint. Next, an incision was made over the anteromedial tibia, and a semitendinosus tendon autograft was harvested with an open hamstring harvester.

On arthroscopy, the lateral compartment demonstrated a "drive-through" sign, consistent with lateral ligament instability (Fig. 8.10) [2], and the ACL was completely torn and bulbous. There was some blistering on his articular cartilage on the medial femoral condyle, which is consistent with the bone bruising commonly associated with a PLC injury [4]. The posterior cruciate ligament (PCL) was intact. An 11×25-mm closed socket femoral tunnel was reamed midway between the anteromedial and posterolateral bundles of the ACL. A tibial tunnel was placed just adjacent to the lateral meniscus root.

The midsubstance of his lateral meniscus had a complete radial tear, which was repaired using an arthroscopically

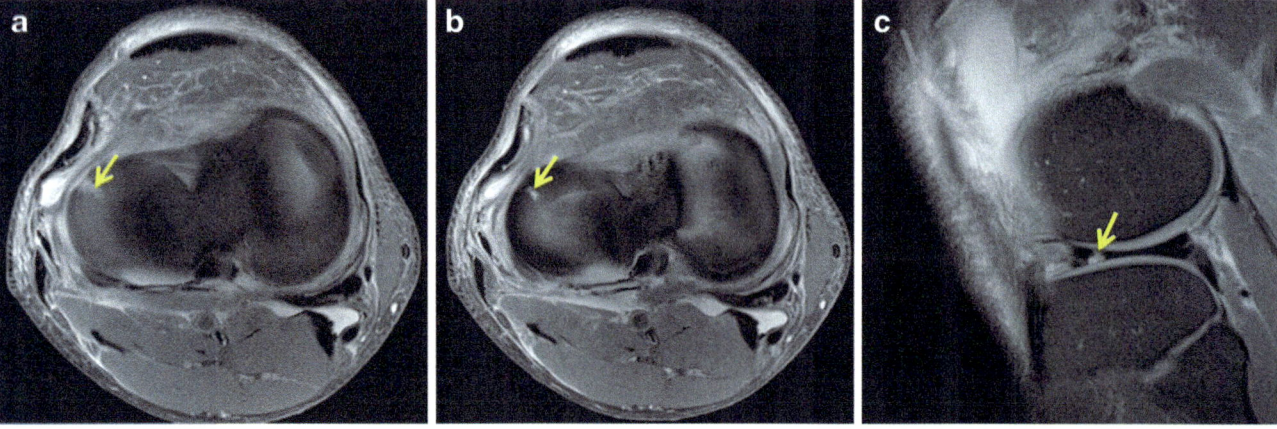

Fig. 8.8 A PD FS axial MRI of an anterior horn lateral meniscus partial thickness tear (**a**, **b**). A PD TSE FS sagittal MRI of a radial tear in the anterior horn of the lateral meniscus (**c**)

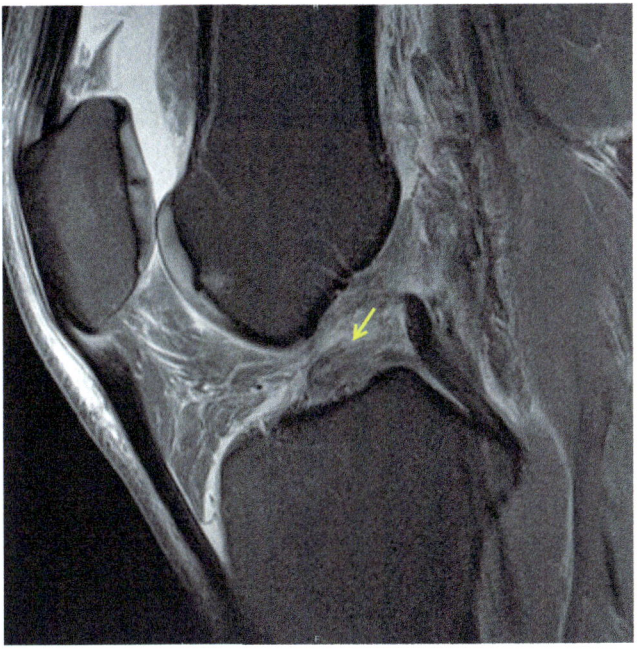

Fig. 8.9 A PD TSE sagittal MRI of a suspected PFL tear that was subsequently confirmed upon probing at the time of surgery

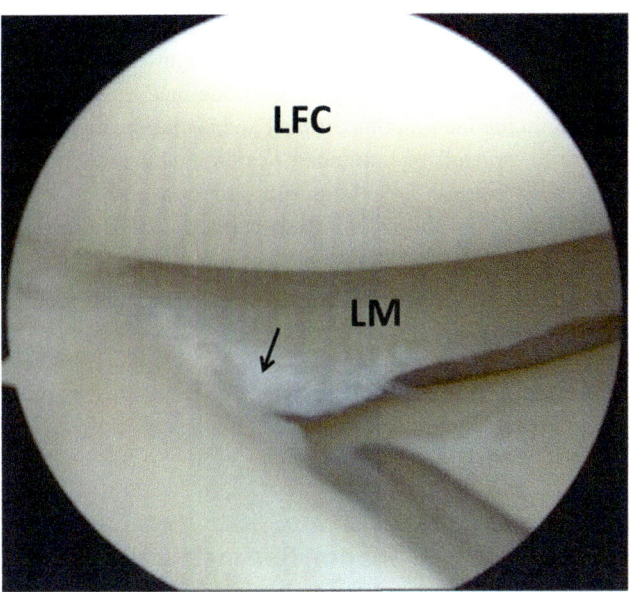

Fig. 8.11 Lateral meniscus radial tear (*black arrow*) (right knee). *LFC* lateral femoral condyle, *LM* lateral meniscus

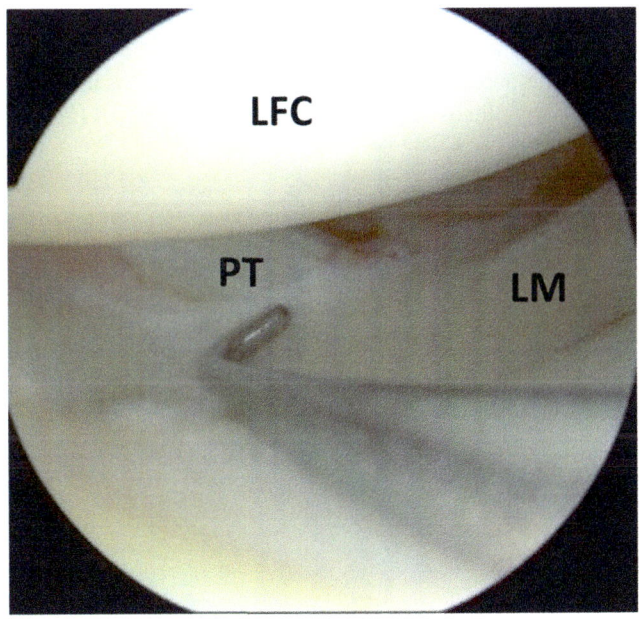

Fig. 8.10 "Drive-through" sign, lateral tibiofemoral compartment (right knee). *LFC* lateral femoral condyle, *LM* lateral meniscus, *PT* popliteus tendon

assisted repair technique with four vertical mattress sutures (Fig. 8.11). The torn margins of the meniscus were reapposed and demonstrated excellent stability.

A patellar tendon allograft was secured in the femoral tunnel using a 7×20-mm titanium interference screw. Next, the FCL graft was secured in the femur with a bioabsorbable

screw, shuttled under the superficial layer of the iliotibial band, and through to the fibular head. With a valgus reduction force, the varus gapping was eliminated and the graft was secured in place at 30° of flexion. To repair the PFL, a suture anchor was placed in the fibular head and the torn margins were reapposed with the knee in 60° of flexion and neutral rotation. Finally, the ACL graft was secured in the tibial tunnel with a 9×20-mm titanium screw.

Discussion

The use of MRI and varus stress radiography helped diagnose the presence of ACL and lateral meniscal tears, as well as injuries to the FCL and PFL of the posterolateral corner. An FCL and/or PFL tear appears as a linear increase in signal intensity on T2 MRI due to the presence of edema and/or tissue discontinuity. Even though it was not noted preoperatively for this patient, blistering of the articular cartilage presents as increased signal intensity at the bone-cartilage interface with or without bony edema. This presence of bone bruising to the medial tibial plateau, which was observed in this patient on arthroscopy, or to medial femoral condyle, may be an indicative of PLC injury on MRI [4]. Increased varus gapping on varus stress radiography is also indicative of an FCL injury [12]. Injuries to the FCL and PFL require the use of open surgery through a laterally based incision to reconstruct these ligaments that do not course intra-articularly.

Arthroscopy revealed the presence of a "drive-through" sign that is typically associated with PLC injuries. The lateral compartment "drive-through" sign is defined as increased gapping in the lateral compartment and is classically associated with isolated or combined posterolateral corner ligament injury [2]. While this sign is useful for assessing lateral compartment instability on arthroscopy, posterolateral corner FCL and PFL pathology must be confirmed through an open lateral incision. In addition, arthroscopy is helpful to verify and repair the meniscal tears that may lead to adverse outcomes if unrepaired. Reconstruction of the FCL and PFL and repair of a meniscus tear typically result in favorable outcomes after surgery and return to high levels of activity [13, 14].

Case 3: Popliteus Tendon Reconstruction and Lateral Meniscus Repair

History/Exam

A 20-year-old wrestler reported to clinic after a history of right knee pain for approximately 1 year. He first injured his knee during a wrestling match after experiencing excessive downward pressure on his right knee while in the figure four position [15]. At an outside institution, he was diagnosed with right knee proximal tibiofibular joint instability

and underwent a proximal posterior tibiofibular joint reconstruction. However, after rehabilitation, he continued to have right knee lateral-sided pain and lateral instability when he returned to full activity. He reported to clinic for a second opinion.

On physical examination, there was a normal gait pattern and lower extremity strength was intact. No effusion or edema in the right knee was seen and there was no quadriceps atrophy. Examination of the proximal tibiofibular joint showed no residual instability. His range of motion was symmetric at −3° to 135° of flexion with no pain or evidence of recurvatum in either knee. The right knee was stable to varus and valgus testing at 0° and 30° of knee flexion. However, there was a significant side-to-side increase in right knee external rotation on the dial test at 90° of flexion, which increased suspicion for a possible popliteus muscle or tendon injury.

Imaging

Radiographs were obtained, which showed a neutral mechanical axis and uniform preservation of joint spaces. Due to the positive dial test, an MRI was ordered to further evaluate the status of his popliteus muscle tendon complex. Results indicated proximal popliteus tendinosis and scarring (Fig. 8.12a, b).

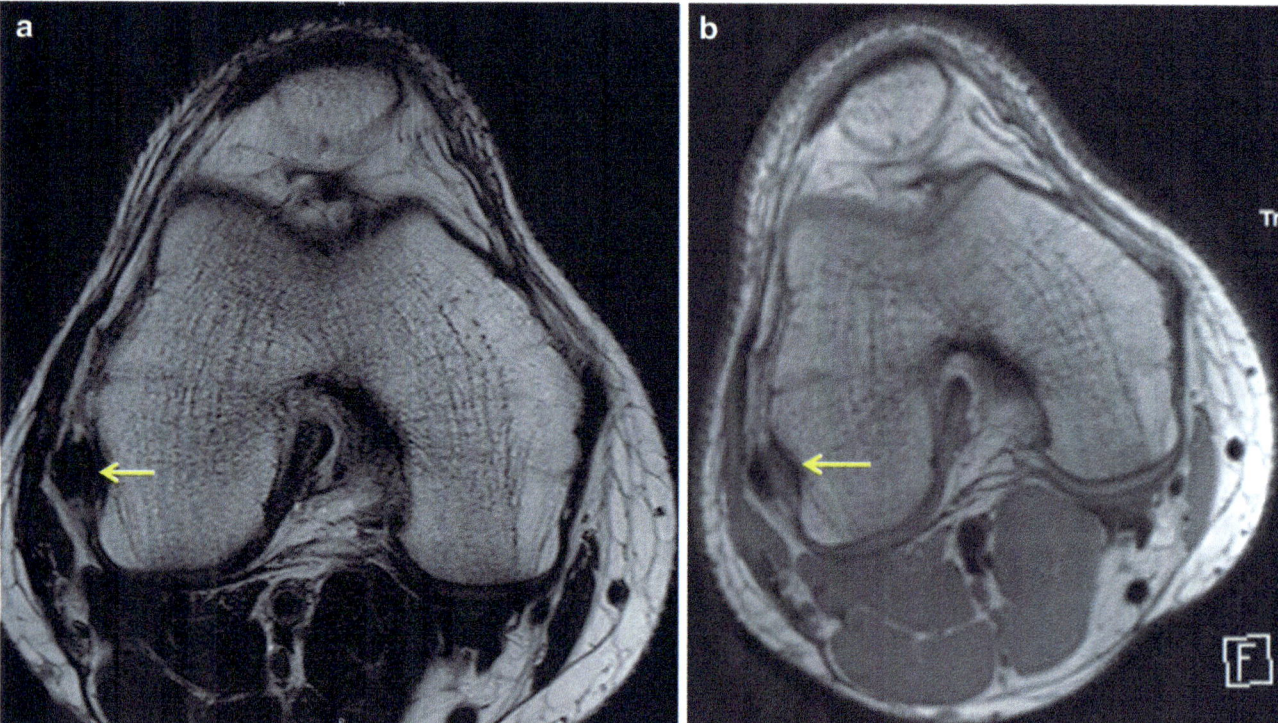

Fig. 8.12 A T2 TSE (**a**) and PD FS (**b**) axial MRI demonstrating a popliteus tendon tear (*yellow arrow*)

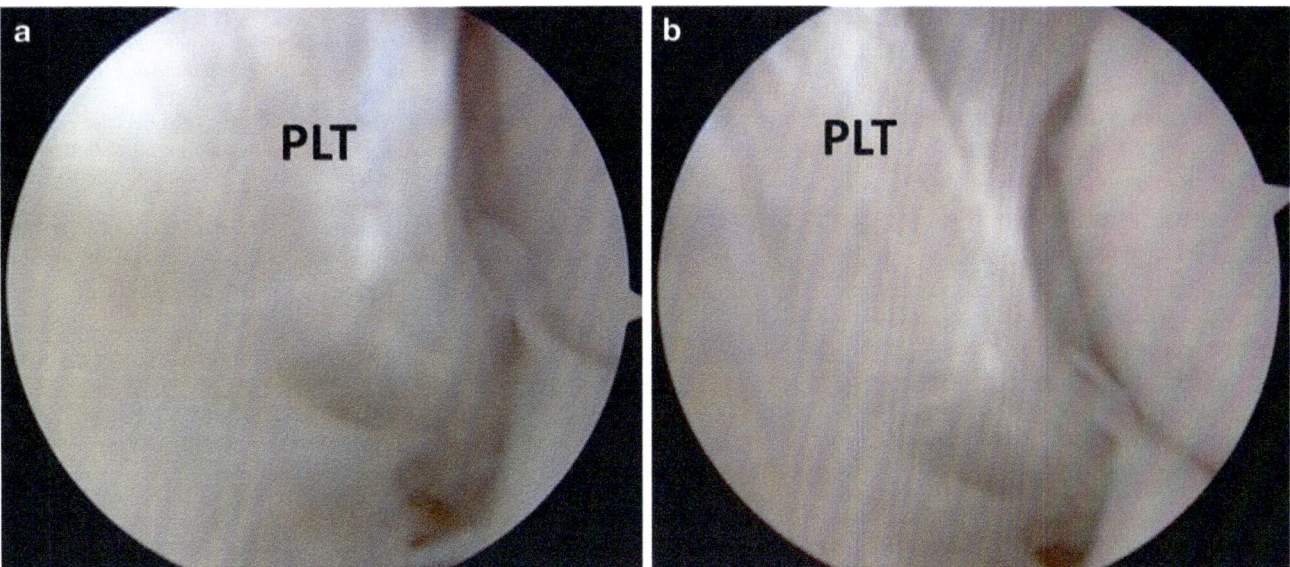

Fig. 8.13 (a, b) Second look arthroscopic image demonstrating a healed popliteus tendon reconstruction (lateral gutter, right knee). *PLT* popliteus tendon

No meniscus pathology was seen on MRI and all other knee ligaments and tendons appeared intact.

Arthroscopy

A lateral hockey stick incision was created and the superficial layer of the iliotibial band was identified. A peroneal neurolysis was performed, which released the nerve from a substantial amount of scar tissue encasements using careful sharp and blunt dissection. The interval between the lateral gastrocnemius and soleus muscles was expanded, and the musculotendinous junction of the popliteus was palpated. An arthrotomy incision was made to identify the popliteus tendon. It was in a posteriorly subluxed position and very loose and nonfunctional. A guide pin was placed at the native anatomic attachment site for the popliteus tendon and reamed to create a 6×25-mm closed socket tunnel. Next, the flat spot distal and medial to Gerdy's tubercle was identified, and a guide pin was placed and directed posteriorly toward the musculotendinous junction of the popliteus muscle. This was reamed with a 6-mm reamer.

On arthroscopic evaluation, his lateral meniscus was unstable and able to be pulled into the joint with probing. Six vertical mattress sutures were placed in the superior and inferior surfaces of the meniscus, and it was pulled back into the appropriate position.

Next, a semitendinosus autograft was harvested and tabularized for the popliteus tendon reconstruction. Using passing sutures, the semitendinosus autograft was passed into the femoral tunnel and secured with a bioabsorbable screw. The tibial graft insertion was secured with a bioabsorbable screw at 60° of flexion and in neutral tibial rotation. Second look arthroscopy revealed excellent healing of the popliteus tendon graft (Fig. 8.13a, b).

Discussion

Isolated popliteus tears appear as a linear increase in signal intensity and can be found anywhere from the popliteal sulcus on the lateral femoral condyle to the musculotendinous junction where the popliteus tendon joins with the popliteus muscle body. Isolated popliteus tears are rare with the majority seen in association with injury to the FCL and PFL. On arthroscopy, the popliteus tendon can be visualized in the lateral gutter and the integrity of the attachment to the femur verified. In the case of acute tears, the popliteus tendon is often located in an avulsed position along the lateral gutter. In chronic tears, the popliteus tendon becomes scarred to the lateral capsule, and the tibia must be externally rotated to verify the integrity of the femoral attachment of the popliteus tendon. If it is torn, it will be pulled away from the femur when the tibia is externally rotated. During open procedures, the popliteus tendon can also be visualized through an arthrotomy incision along the lateral capsule. When injured, repair or reconstruction of the popliteus tendon is imperative due to the risk of chronic instability [16].

In this case, a meniscal tear was missed on MRI but was discovered on arthroscopic probing. When a meniscus tear is present, meniscal repairs that focus on preserving the meniscal tissue are favored over partial or total meniscectomies due to unfavorable long-term outcomes and an increased risk of osteoarthritis that have been reported after meniscectomies [17, 18]. This case demonstrates the utility of MRI for the identification of rare isolated popliteus tendon injury, while reinforcing the importance of a thorough exam at the time of surgery to identify additional pathology, such as meniscal tears, that may not have been readily apparent on initial MRI evaluation.

References

1. Fanelli GC, Edson CJ. Posterior cruciate ligament injuries in trauma patients: Part II. Arthroscopy. 1995;11(5):526–9.
2. LaPrade RF, Terry GC. Injuries to the posterolateral aspect of the knee. Association of anatomic injury patterns with clinical instability. Am J Sports Med. 1997;25(4):433–8.
3. LaPrade RF, Wentorf FA, Fritts H, Gundry C, Hightower CD. A prospective magnetic resonance imaging study of the incidence of posterolateral and multiple ligament injuries in acute knee injuries presenting with a hemarthrosis. Arthroscopy. 2007;23(12):1341–7.
4. Geeslin AG, LaPrade RF. Location of bone bruises and other osseous injuries associated with acute grade III isolated and combined posterolateral knee injuries. Am J Sports Med. 2010;38(12): 2502–8.
5. Lunden JB, Bzdusek PJ, Monson JK, Malcomson KW, LaPrade RF. Current concepts in the recognition and treatment of posterolateral corner injuries of the knee. J Orthop Sports Phys Ther. 2010;40(8):502–16.
6. LaPrade RF, Ly TV, Wentorf FA, Engebretsen L. The posterolateral attachments of the knee: a qualitative and quantitative morphologic analysis of the fibular collateral ligament, popliteus tendon, popliteofibular ligament, and lateral gastrocnemius tendon. Am J Sports Med. 2003;31(6):854–60.
7. Sanchez 2nd AR, Sugalski MT, LaPrade RF. Anatomy and biomechanics of the lateral side of the knee. Sports Med Arthrosc. 2006;14(1):2–11.
8. LaPrade RF, Muench C, Wentorf F, Lewis JL. The effect of injury to the posterolateral structures of the knee on force in a posterior cruciate ligament graft: a biomechanical study. Am J Sports Med. 2002;30(2):233–8.
9. LaPrade RF, Resig S, Wentorf F, Lewis JL. The effects of grade III posterolateral knee complex injuries on anterior cruciate ligament graft force. A biomechanical analysis. Am J Sports Med. 1999;27(4):469–75.
10. Stannard JP, Brown SL, Farris RC, McGwin Jr G, Volgas DA. The posterolateral corner of the knee: repair versus reconstruction. Am J Sports Med. 2005;33(6):881–8.
11. Levy BA, Dajani KA, Morgan JA, Shah JP, Dahm DL, Stuart MJ. Repair versus reconstruction of the fibular collateral ligament and posterolateral corner in the multiligament-injured knee. Am J Sports Med. 2010;38(4):804–9.
12. LaPrade RF, Heikes C, Bakker AJ, Jakobsen RB. The reproducibility and repeatability of varus stress radiographs in the assessment of isolated fibular collateral ligament and grade-III posterolateral knee injuries. An in vitro biomechanical study. J Bone Joint Surg Am. 2008;90(10):2069–76.
13. LaPrade RF, Spiridonov SI, Coobs BR, Ruckert PR, Griffith CJ. Fibular collateral ligament anatomical reconstructions: a prospective outcomes study. Am J Sports Med. 2010;38(10):2005–11.
14. LaPrade RF, Johansen S, Agel J, Risberg MA, Moksnes H, Engebretsen L. Outcomes of an anatomic posterolateral knee reconstruction. J Bone Joint Surg Am. 2010;92(1):16–22.
15. LaPrade RF, Konowalchuk BK. Popliteomeniscal fascicle tears causing symptomatic lateral compartment knee pain: diagnosis by the figure-4 test and treatment by open repair. Am J Sports Med. 2005;33(8):1231–6.
16. LaPrade RF, Wozniczka JK, Stellmaker MP, Wijdicks CA. Analysis of the static function of the popliteus tendon and evaluation of an anatomic reconstruction: the "fifth ligament" of the knee. Am J Sports Med. 2010;38(3):543–9.
17. McDermott I. Meniscal tears, repairs and replacement: their relevance to osteoarthritis of the knee. Br J Sports Med. 2011;45(4): 292–7.
18. Pengas IP, Assiotis A, Nash W, Hatcher J, Banks J, McNicholas MJ. Total meniscectomy in adolescents: a 40-year follow-up. J Bone Joint Surg Br. 2012;94(12):1649–54.

Patellofemoral Disorders

9

James S. Starman, Austin J. Crow, and David R. Diduch

Introduction

Pathology involving the patellofemoral joint is a common complaint among patients seeking orthopedic evaluation, and due to the wide spectrum of potential causes, its management can be challenging for both patients and providers [1, 2]. Identifying specific causes of and potential interventions for patellofemoral disorders requires a solid understanding of the anatomic components which comprise this area of the knee. The osseous elements of the patellofemoral joint consist of the femoral trochlea and the patella. The relative position of the tibial tubercle and the rotatory orientation of the tibia and femur are also important, however, and can significantly affect overall patellofemoral function [3]. The primary soft tissue structures involved in patellofemoral disorders include the medial patellofemoral ligament (MPFL), the lateral patellar retinaculum, and the quadriceps muscle, specifically the vastus medialis oblique (VMO).

The first step in the diagnosis and treatment of patellofemoral disorders is a thorough history and clinical examination. Some patients report insidious onset of pain in the patellofemoral region without a discrete history of knee injury, while others report a history of one or more patellar dislocation events which may or may not require formal reduction. It is important to differentiate between complaints of pain alone versus those including instability and to define the differences between subjective and objective instability [4]. Pain symptoms are commonly exacerbated when the knee is in positions of deep flexion, such as going up- or downstairs, or when standing up from a seated position.

J.S. Starman, MD (✉) • A.J. Crow, MD
Department of Orthopedic Surgery, University of Virginia Hospital, Charlottesville, VA, USA
e-mail: Jstarman20@msn.com; Ajc9v@hscmail.mcc.virginia.edu

D.R. Diduch, MD, MS
Department of Orthopedic Surgery, University of Virginia Health System, Charlottesville, VA, USA
e-mail: Drd5c@hscmail.mcc.virginia.edu

Instability symptoms may be elicited by a variety of activities, including both sports and activities of daily living.

Physical examination of the knee begins with an assessment of the overall limb alignment, to look for evidence of varus or valgus knee orientation, rotational abnormalities of the femur or tibia, and the relative height of the patella in relation to the knee joint. Any evidence of muscular atrophy or asymmetry, specifically of the VMO, should be noted, along with the presence of any joint effusion. Next, a dynamic observation of the patellofemoral joint should be completed, documenting the tracking of the patella as the knee is actively brought through a flexion–extension arc. This may identify a pathologic "J" sign, reflecting lateral displacement of the patella at the extended knee position. The Q angle, measured as the angle of pull between the quadriceps mechanism and patellar tendon, should also be assessed. Provocative examination tests for the patellofemoral joint include evaluation of patellar tilt, which can identify problems with excessive tightness or laxity of the lateral retinaculum, and patellar apprehension, in which the examiner attempts to displace the patella laterally and looks for a reflexive tightening of the quadriceps muscle in the attempt to pull the patella back in the medial direction. Similarly, assessment of patellar glide can provide information about the overall laxity of the patellar restraints. Finally, the patellar grind test, in which the examiner depresses the patella against the trochlea while moving the knee through a flexion–extension arc, may provide evidence of chondromalacia within the patellofemoral joint.

The initial imaging of patellofemoral disorders consists of standard PA, lateral, and merchant views of the knee. If indicated, mechanical alignment films may also be obtained to assess for excess varus or valgus [3]. In the clinical setting of acute patellar dislocation, it is important to rule out the possibility of a displaced osteochondral fragment, which may occur either during dislocation or relocation of the patella. Lateral radiographs are essential in the assessment of trochlear morphology, and as described by Dejour, the crossing sign, supratrochlear spur, and double contour may

S.F. Brockmeier (ed.), *MRI-Arthroscopy Correlations: A Case-Based Atlas of the Knee, Shoulder, Elbow and Hip*,
DOI 10.1007/978-1-4939-2645-9_9, © Springer Science+Business Media New York 2015

indicate trochlear dysplasia [5]. Dejour's classification of trochlear dysplasia describes four types of morphology [5]. The lateral radiograph can also be assessed for evidence of patella alta or baja, using the Caton–Deschamps ratio or Insall–Salvati ratio [6]. Merchant views allow assessment of the patellar tilt and patellar subluxation, which may be abnormal in the setting of an excessively tight retinaculum [7].

Cross-sectional imaging is also an important tool in the radiographic assessment of patellofemoral disorders. The tibial tubercle–trochlear groove (TT-TG) distance measures the lateral offset of the tibial tubercle relative to the deepest portion of the trochlea, and a TT-TG greater than 20 mm is associated with patellar instability [4]. Magnetic resonance imaging (MRI) is useful in the evaluation of both chondral lesions and medial patellofemoral restraints. MRI has been found to be 85 % sensitive and 70 % specific for evaluation of MPFL ligament disruption and 83 % sensitive and 84 % specific for detecting grade II, III, or IV chondromalacia of the patella [8, 9].

For many patients with patellofemoral disorders, an initial nonoperative trial with rest, nonsteroidal anti-inflammatories, and physical therapy may be effective in relieving symptoms [10–12]. However, in patients with chronic instability or multiple dislocation events, and in those patients with significant chondral lesions, surgery may be indicated [13–19]. This chapter will utilize a case-based format to highlight the most common operative strategies used in the treatment of patellofemoral disorders, with correlations drawn between clinical, radiographic, and MRI findings and observations made at the time of surgery. Three cases will be presented, including:

1. Patellar maltracking requiring tibial tubercle osteotomy and MPFL reconstruction
2. Chronic patellar instability requiring trochleaplasty (bilateral)

3. Chronic patellar and trochlear cartilage defects requiring allograft cartilage transplantation with the particulated juvenile chondrocyte implantation technique

Case 1

History/Exam

A 40-year-old female presented to clinic for evaluation of long-standing left knee patella instability and pain, with 1 month of locking and catching when arising from a chair. The patient reported a history of a probable patellar dislocation which occurred in high school during an ice skating twisting injury. Her initial treatment at that time was with bracing for 1 month. Since then, the patient reported multiple subluxation episodes without a frank dislocation. Treatments consisting of rest, activity modification, NSAIDs, bracing, and therapy had not provided adequate relief, forcing her to give up certain activities such as jogging. On examination, there was a significant patellar grind, a crepitus, and a Q angle of 20. There was no significant joint effusion. On testing of the MPFL, there was a soft endpoint with lateral patellar translation and apprehension.

Imaging

Based on the patients' physical examination and history, plain radiographs and MRI were obtained for confirmation of the diagnosis and possible surgical planning. Initial imaging of the knee confirmed excessive lateral patellar tilt and subluxation, with moderate degenerative changes of the lateral patellar facet (Fig. 9.1a–c). A complete sequence of MRI imaging without contrast was obtained. Axial T2 magnetic

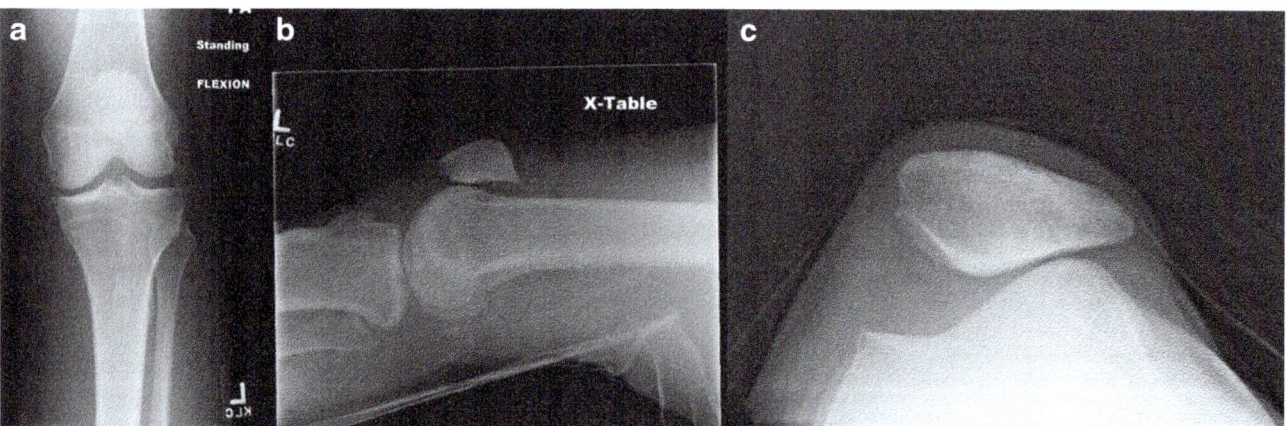

Fig. 9.1 (a–c) PA, lateral, and merchant views of the left knee, demonstrating excessive patellar tilt and subluxation, with moderate degenerative changes of the lateral patellar facet

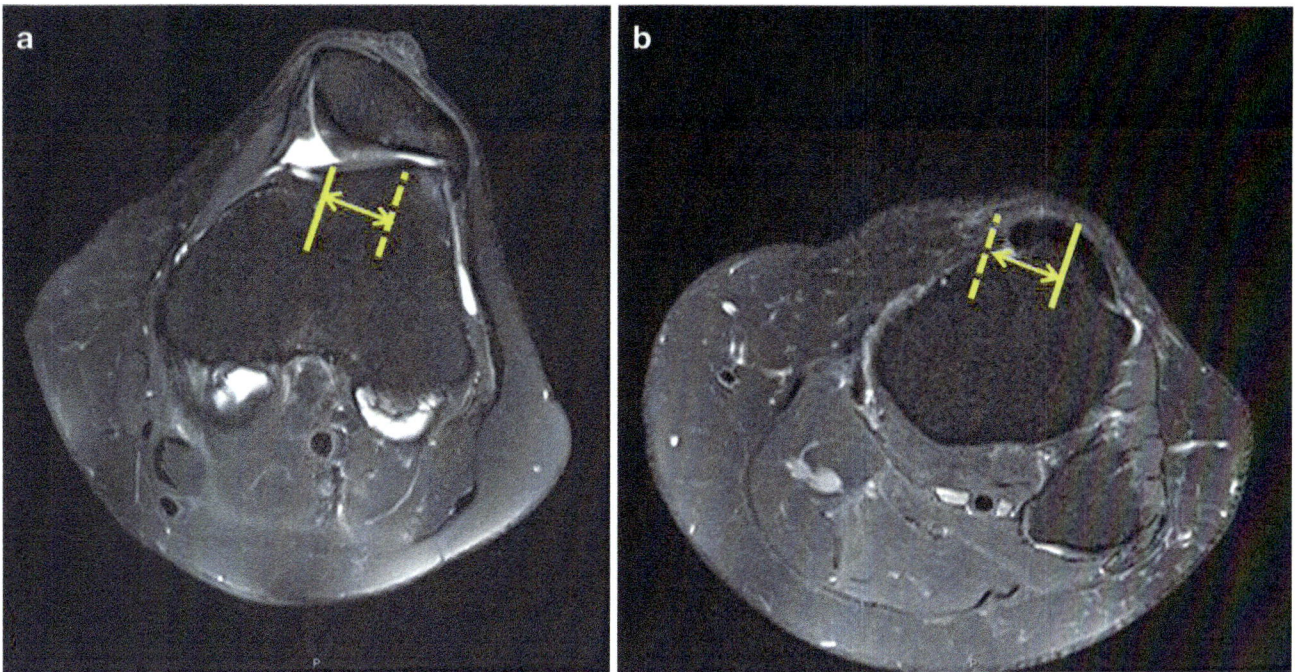

Fig. 9.2 (**a, b**) MRI demonstrating increased TT-TG distance and patellar malalignment. *Solid line* demonstrates trochlear groove in **a** and tibial tubercle in **b**. *Dashed lines* indicate the superimposed line of the opposing structure. The *arrow* represents the TT-TG distance

resonance imaging showed a TT-TG distance of 20 mm, with lateral patellar compression syndrome and extensive full-thickness cartilage loss throughout the lateral patellar facet and periphery of the lateral trochlea in a 10×15 mm area with subchondral marrow edema and cystic change (Fig. 9.2a, b). Even though there was no obvious tear identified involving the MPFL or patellar retinaculum, the degree of subluxation indicated MPFL attenuation or incompetence. The remaining structures of the knee appeared normal, although mild bursitis within the semimembranosus was identified.

Given the patients' findings of increased TT-TG distance, excessive patellar tilt and subluxation, and chondral wear of the lateral patellar facet, she was indicated for surgery consisting of anteromedialization osteotomy of the tibial tubercle, lateral retinacular release, MPFL reconstruction with hamstring autograft, and shaving chondroplasty of the patella.

Surgery

At the time of surgery, a diagnostic arthroscopy was performed, with confirmation of full-thickness cartilage loss on the lateral patellar facet and lateral trochlea. A shaving chondroplasty was performed, debriding the chondromalacia back to a stable rim (Fig. 9.3a, b). Next, the open portion of

the procedure was initiated. An 8 cm incision along the medial patellar edge extending to the level of the tibial tubercle was placed. An open lateral retinacular release was performed, with care taken to protect the superior lateral geniculate artery. This was able to correct the excessive lateral patellar tilt. Next, attention was turned to the tibial tubercle osteotomy. A 45° angle of osteotomy was chosen, and the distal periosteum of the osteotomy was left intact to serve as a hinge point. A correction of 1 cm of medialization and 7 mm of anteriorization was achieved to reduce the TT-TG to a desired 10 mm. Provisional clamps were placed, and tracking was checked prior to placement of two 4.5 mm bicortical screws (Fig. 9.4). The final step involved MPFL reconstruction to address the patella subluxation. Gracilis autograft was harvested in the standard fashion and prepared on the back table. The proximal medial border of the patella was dissected, and two parallel 3.2 mm tunnels were drilled from the medial border to the anterior mid-patella to allow a looped passage of the gracilis graft, leaving the free ends for attachment in the femur. Schottle's point was identified at the junction between Blumenstadt's line and the posterior femoral condyles, along the posterior cortical line of the femur [16] (Fig. 9.5). A guide pin was placed at the MPFL origin. Isometry was then checked with the graft around the guide pin by taking the knee through a full range of motion.

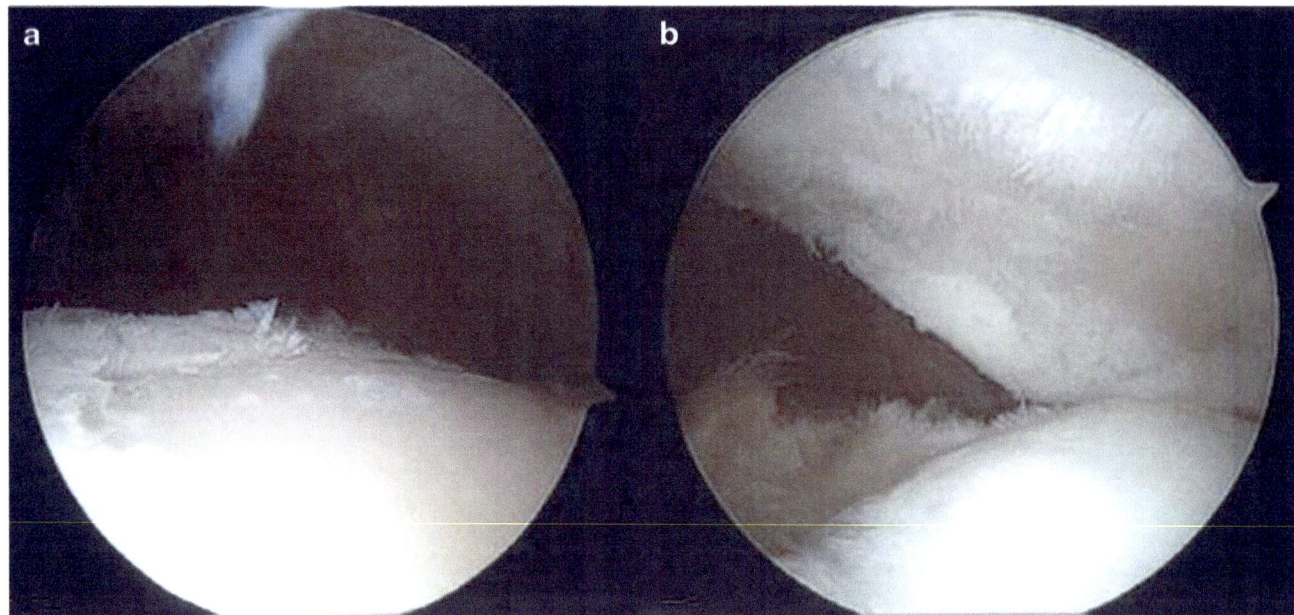

Fig. 9.3 Arthroscopic images showing full-thickness cartilage loss on both the lateral trochlea (**a**) and lateral patellar facet (**b**)

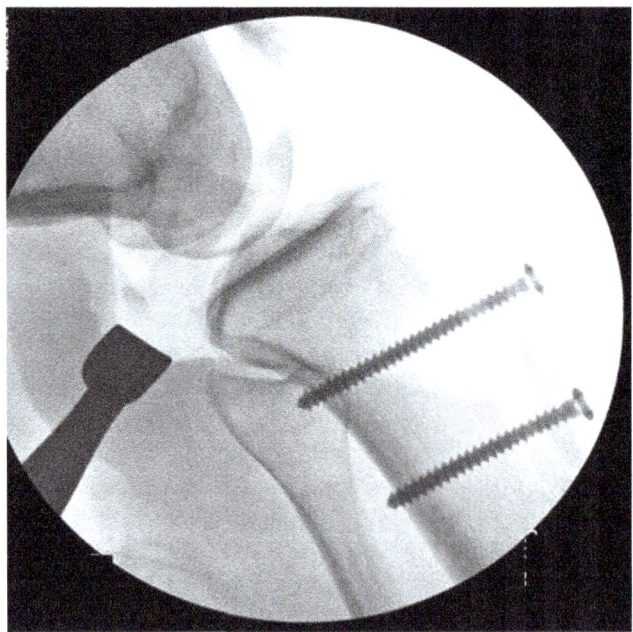

Fig. 9.4 Intraoperative fluoroscopy showing bicortical screw fixation of tibial tubercle osteotomy

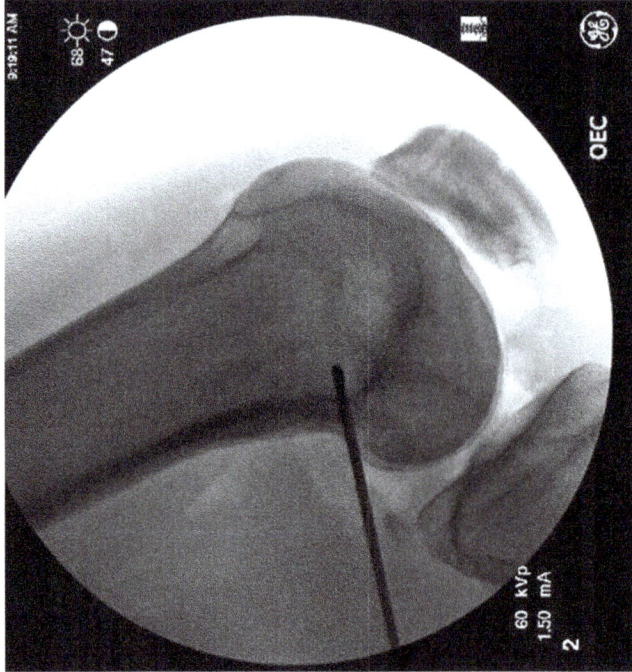

Fig. 9.5 Lateral intraoperative radiograph showing Schottle's point, the junction between Blumenstadt's line and the posterior femoral condyles, along the posterior cortical line of the femur

After verification, final graft passage and interference screw femoral fixation was completed with the knee at 45° of flexion so that the patella was fully seated within the trochlear groove during tensioning.

Postoperatively, the patient was initially restricted to 50 % weight bearing until the osteotomy was healed (Fig. 9.6a–c).

Flexion began at 0–60° and increased by 30° every 2 weeks in a hinged brace. She ultimately went on to heal uneventfully, although she continued to report occasional anterior knee pain and slight irritation related to the tibial tubercle screws, which required hardware removal at 15 months postoperative. Final radiographs prior to hardware removal are shown in Fig. 9.7a, b.

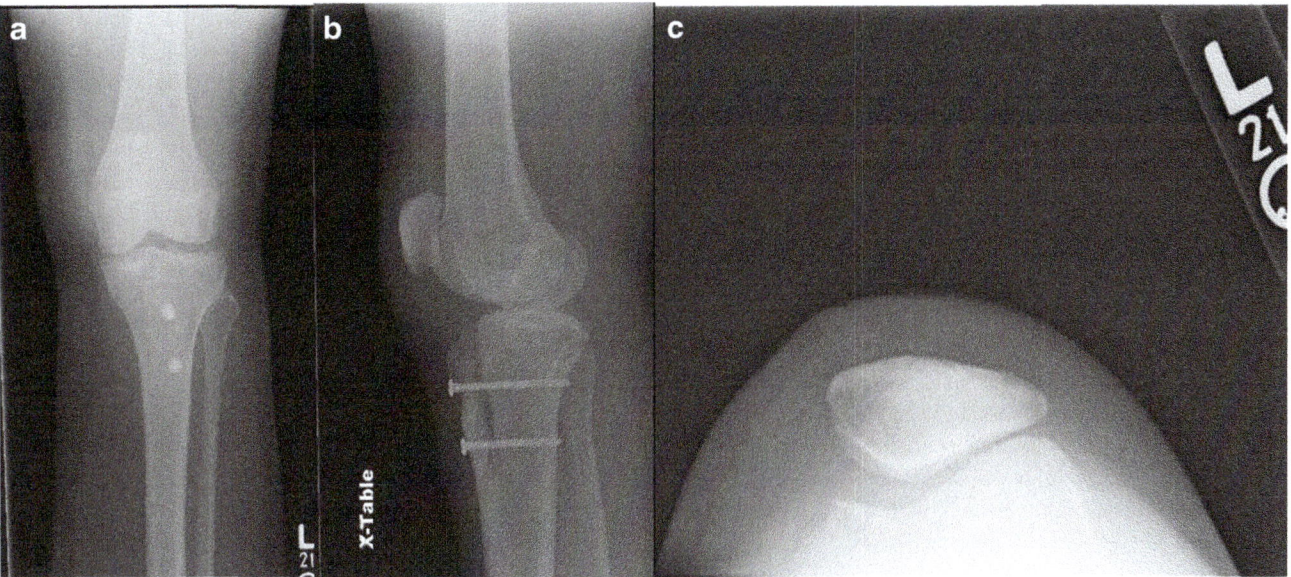

Fig. 9.6 Initial postoperative radiographs, showing fixation of the tibial tubercle (**a**, **b**) osteotomy and correction of excessive patellar tilt (**c**)

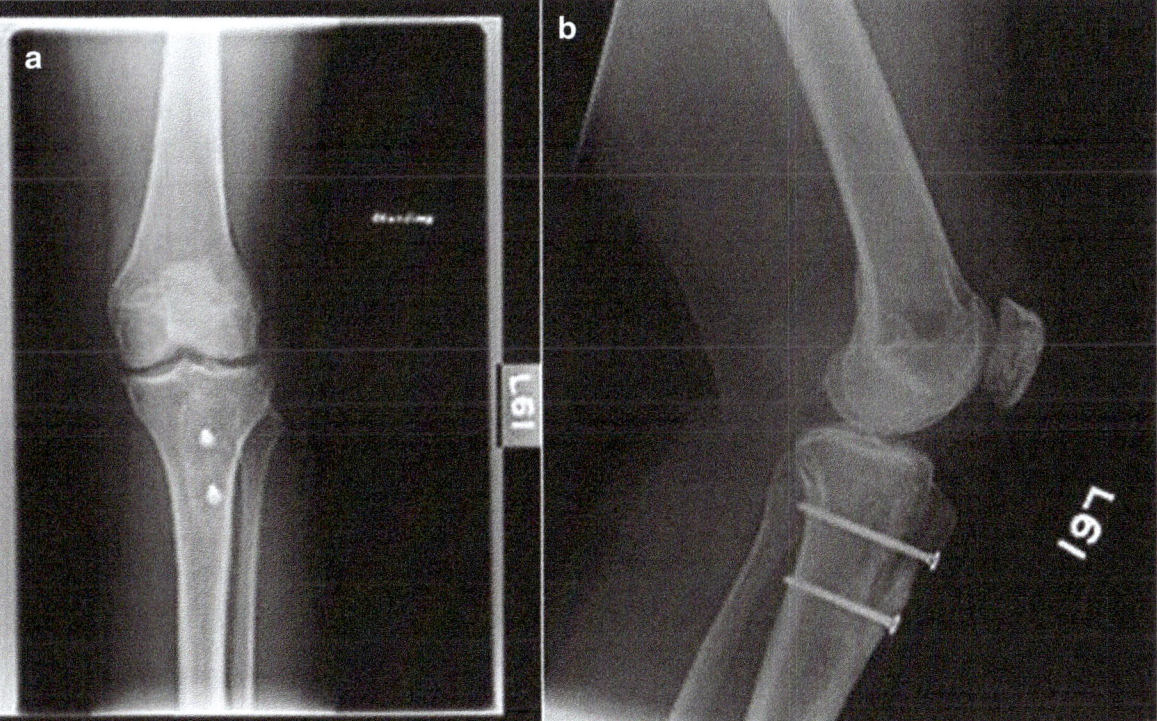

Fig. 9.7 (**a**, **b**) Final PA and lateral radiographs demonstrating a healed tibial tubercle osteotomy

Discussion

- General indications for combined proximal and distal procedures in patellar maltracking
- Essential steps for proper execution of tibial tubercle osteotomy, MPFL reconstruction

Case 2

History/Exam

A 13-year-old female presented to clinic with bilateral knee pain, left greater than right, since early childhood. There was no history of specific injury; however, the patient reportedly had subluxation of both kneecaps with every step, and pain was worsened by any prolonged activities. Prior to her presentation, she had received no operative treatment, but had failed a trial of physical therapy and activity modification. On initial examination, the patient was noted to have external rotation and valgus alignment of both her lower extremities. There was an effusion at the knees bilaterally, with patellar crepitus, tenderness, and apprehension. There was a markedly positive J sign with gross subluxation of the patella requiring manual reduction for the knee to flex. Essentially, her patellas dislocated constantly. The remaining examination findings were unremarkable.

Imaging

On initial imaging, the patient was noted to have a Caton–Deschamps ratio of 1.14 bilaterally, with severe trochlear dysplasia (Dejour type D) with a supratrochlear spur on the left and less severe on the right (Fig. 9.8a–d). There was evidence of MPFL insufficiency bilaterally, with patellar subluxation and excessive lateral tilt. The femoral tibial anatomic axis was 7°, and there was bowing of the femur and tibia resulting in mechanical axis displacement lateral to the joint center. A bilateral lower extremity computed tomography scan was ordered for surgical planning (Fig. 9.9a, b). On the left lower extremity, the femoral neck was retroverted 12° relative to the femoral condylar axis. There was marked trochlear dysplasia, with lateral subluxation and tilt. There was a chronic ossicle of the medial patella, suggestive of chronic avulsion injury from the patella. The TT-TG distance was 23 mm. On the right lower extremity, the femoral neck was retroverted 5°, with trochlear dysplasia and less severe lateral patellar subluxation and tilt. The TT-TG distance was measured at 28 mm. If desired, a 3D reconstruction CT scan can also be obtained for preoperative planning (Fig. 9.9c).

Based on the patients' findings of increased TT-TG distance, excessive patellar tilt, and severe trochlear dyspla-

sia, she was indicated for surgery consisting of anteromedialization osteotomy of the tibial tubercle, lateral retinacular release, MPFL reconstruction with hamstring autograft, and sulcus deepening trochleaplasty. Since the left knee showed more severe symptoms at the time of her presentation, the decision was made for staged reconstruction starting with the left lower extremity. The patient did well clinically following her initial procedure and was indicated for her contralateral knee at 6 months postoperatively. The surgical sequence was similar, and to avoid redundancy, presented findings are based on the patient's second procedure only.

Surgery

On the patient's second procedure date, an examination under anesthesia was performed, confirming gross instability and maltracking of the right patella. Next, a standard medial parapatellar arthrotomy was placed. First, the tibial tubercle osteotomy was prepared, and a cut was made at 45°, leaving a distal periosteal hinge intact. Translation of 13 mm was achieved, based on the preoperative TT-TG distance of 28 mm to achieve a final distance of 15 mm, and the fragment was provisionally fixed with a clamp. Two bicortical 4.5 mm screws were placed after verifying correction of patellar tracking through a full range of motion.

Attention was then turned to the trochlea. After exposing the supratrochlear spur, which showed elevation approximately 1 cm off the anterior femoral cortex, the central trochlea was marked, and two additional markings for the planned osteotomy of the medial and lateral facets were placed (Fig. 9.10a). Alternatively, if a tubercle osteotomy is not performed, the TT-TG can also be improved by marking and creating a new trochlear groove lateral to the native groove, with the distance to the new groove at the proximal extent reflecting the improvement in the TT-TG distance. An osteotome was used to create a subchondral osteotomy around the superior borders of the trochlea, and a small oval burr was used to remove a portion of the bone deep to the subchondral shell to create a cavity (Fig. 9.10b). The bone was removed to the point that the shell would "trampoline" with moderate pressure and to the depth necessary to drop the deepest point of the new trochlear groove to be flushed with the anterior cortex of the femur. Next a #20 blade was used to cut the osteochondral shell along the medial and lateral facets and centrally within the trochlea. Suture anchor fixation was placed at the top of the notch (i.e., the base of the groove) and proximally over the proximal midpoint of each leaflet (Fig. 9.10c, d). A suture bridge with #2 Vicryl allowed the osteotomy to be held in the reduced position.

Next, attention was turned to harvest of the gracilis tendon for MPFL reconstruction. This was then taken to the

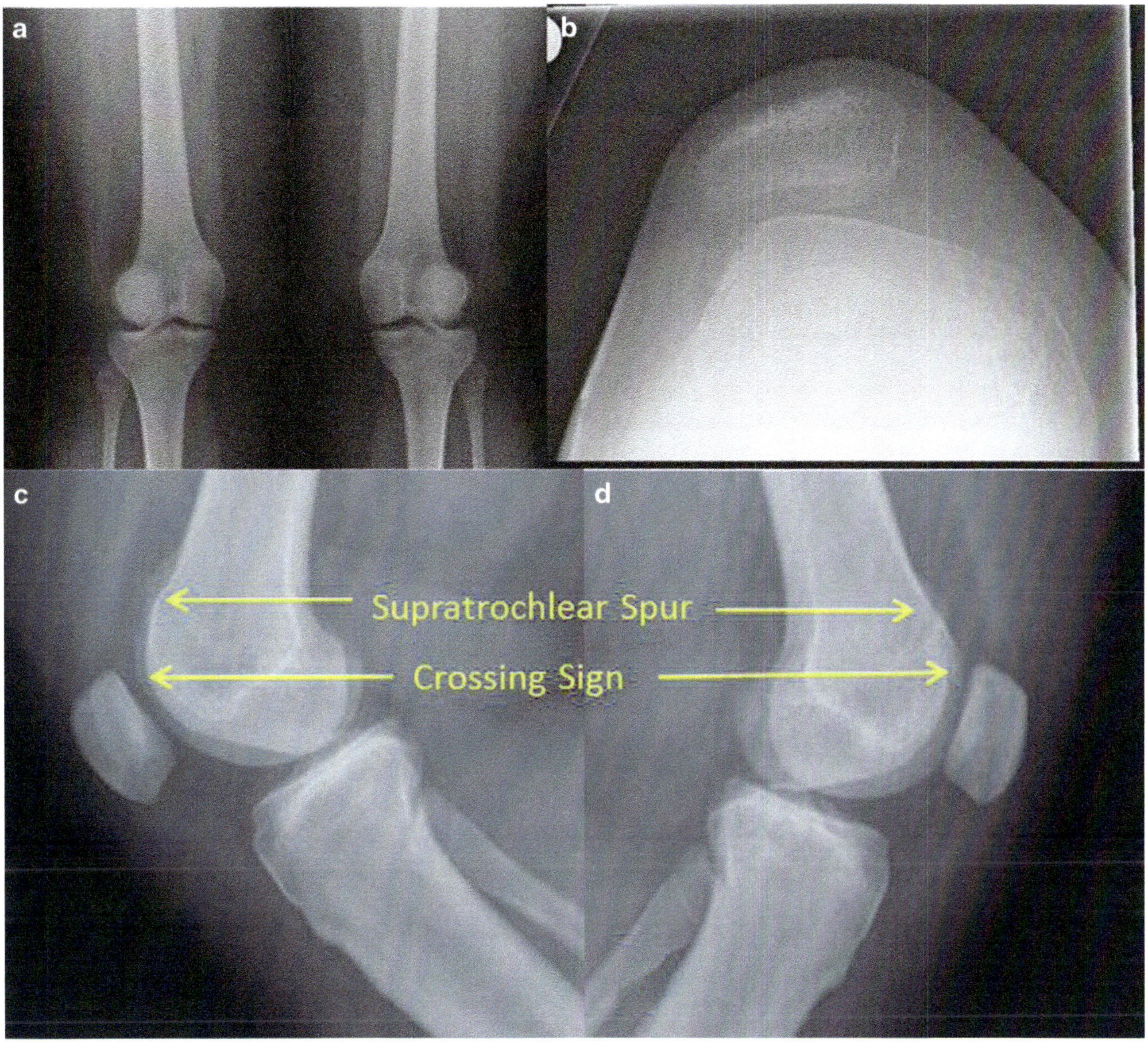

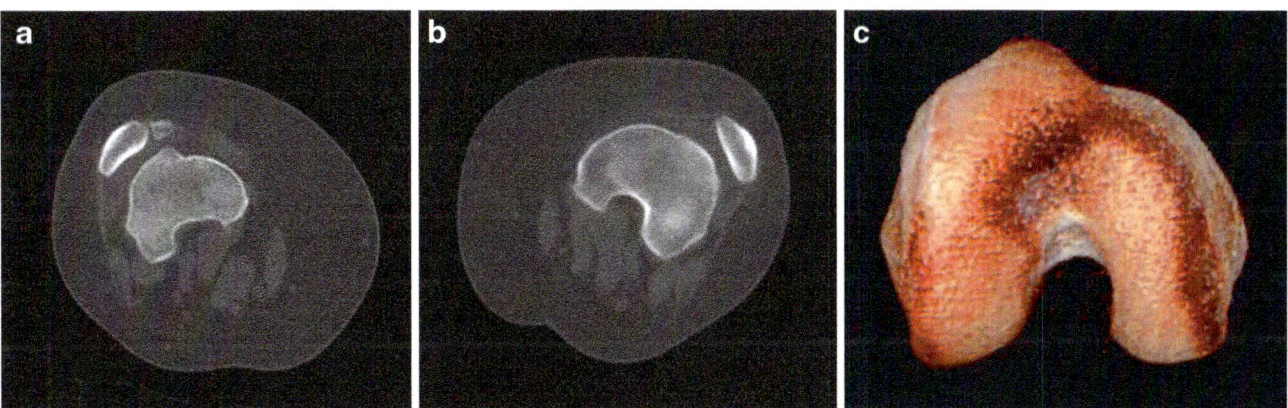

Fig. 9.8 (**a–d**) PA, merchant (R knee), and lateral radiographs, demonstrating Dejour type D trochlear dysplasia bilaterally (*arrows*), more severe on the left. The crossing sign represents the point at which the trochlea is flattened

Fig. 9.9 (**a**) Right lower extremity CT showing a supratrochlear spur, patellar ossicle, and abnormal femoral rotation. (**b**) Left lower extremity CT showing a more severe rotational abnormality of the femur, with chronic patellar subluxation and trochlear dysplasia. (**c**) 3D reconstruction of CT scan for visualization of trochlear dysplasia

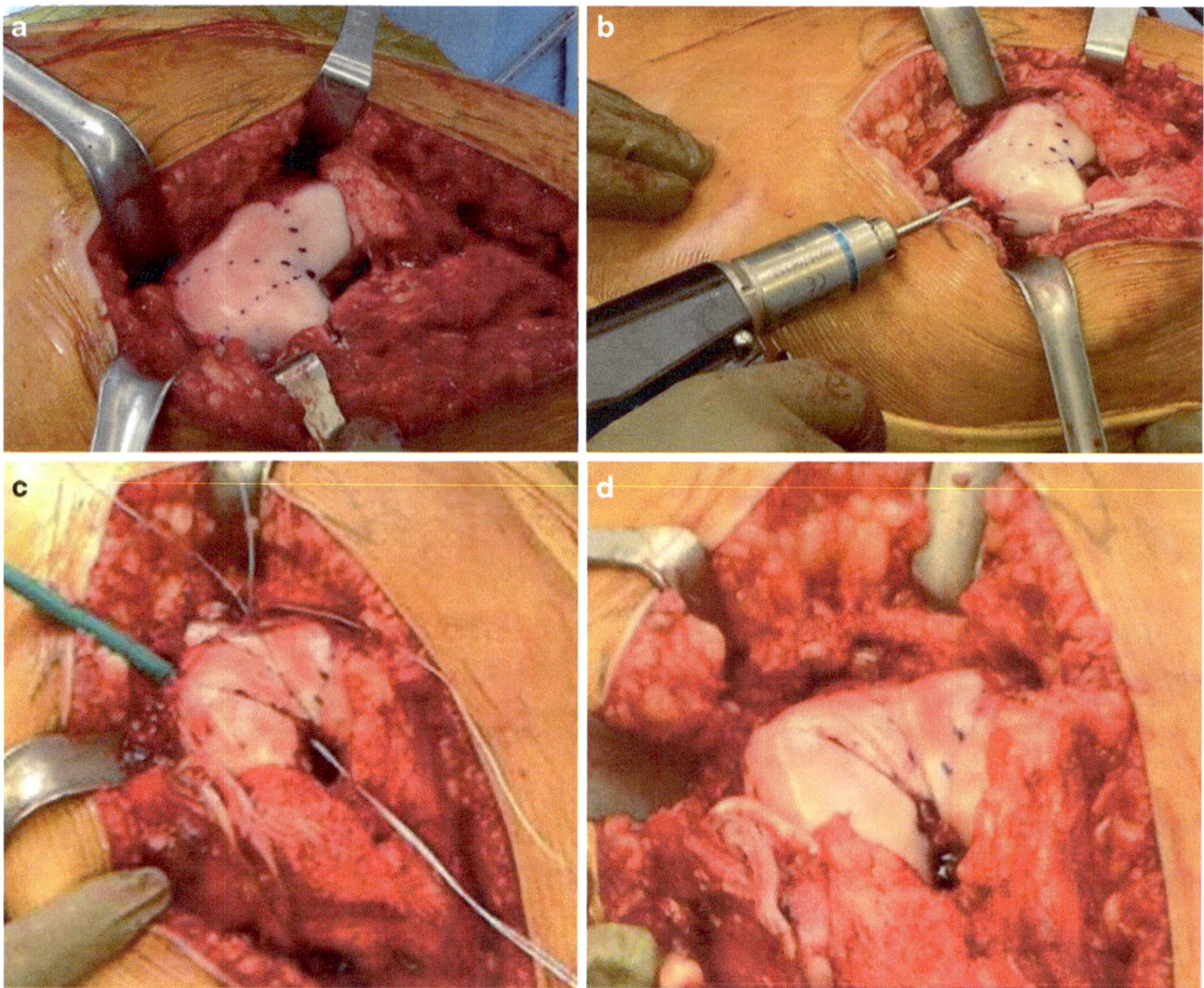

Fig. 9.10 (**a**) *Dotted lines* representing planned osteotomy sites. (**b**) Undermining of the bone deep to osteotomy with oval burr. (**c**) Placement of suture anchors in preparation for fixation of medial and lateral leaflets. (**d**) Final fixation of medial and lateral leaflets with #2 Vicryl sutures. Note improvement in the final depth of groove compared to A

back table for further preparation. After tendon harvesting, an open release of the lateral patellar retinaculum was completed, with care taken to avoid the superior lateral geniculate artery. MPFL reconstruction followed a similar sequence as is outlined in Case 1 (Fig. 9.11a, b). The medial patellar ossicle was excised.

Postoperatively, the patient was initially restricted to 50 % weight bearing until the osteotomy was healed (Fig. 9.12a–c). Flexion began at 0–60° and increased by 30° every 2 weeks in a hinged brace. On the right leg, postoperative range of motion had plateaued at 2 months postoperatively at 90°, and therefore, a manipulation under anesthesia was performed. Otherwise, the patient has progressed to uneventful healing bilaterally, with excellent reduction in pain and improved function.

Discussion

- Indications and technical considerations for performing trochleaplasty
- Surgical sequence for complex combined proximal and distal realignment procedures

Case 3

History/Exam

A 29-year-old female presented to clinic with long-standing right knee pain which was exacerbated following a motor vehicle crash. She previously was treated by another physician

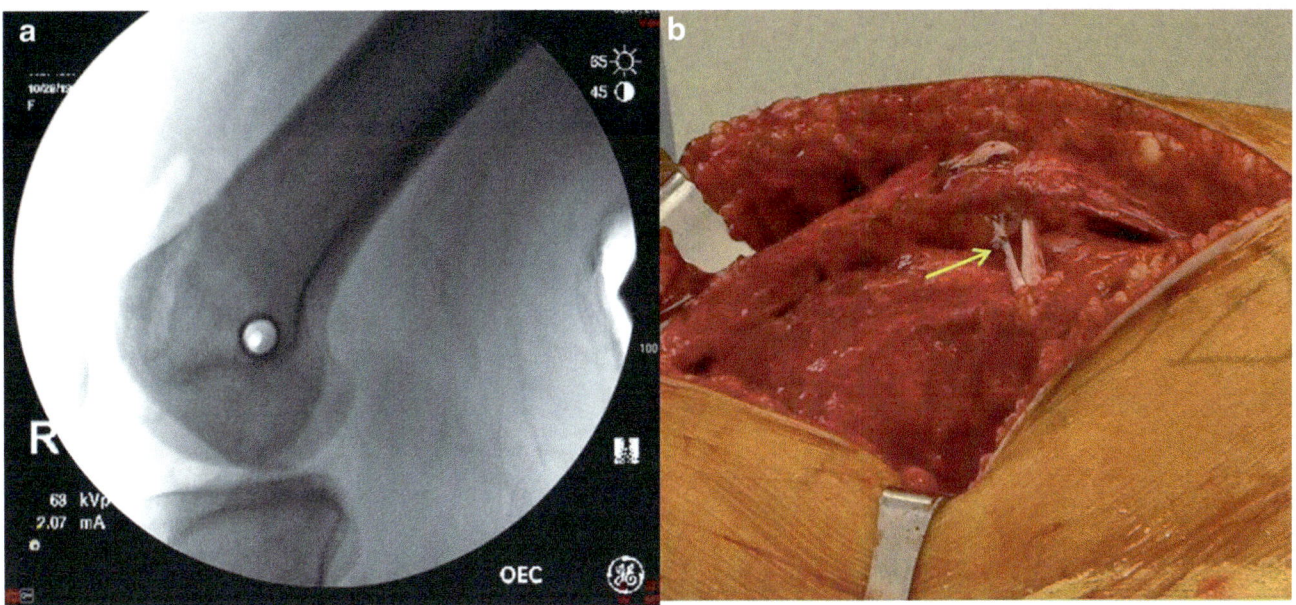

Fig. 9.11 (**a**) Schottle's point, for femoral tunnel entry in MPFL reconstruction. (**b**) Final graft in position for MPFL reconstruction (*arrow*)

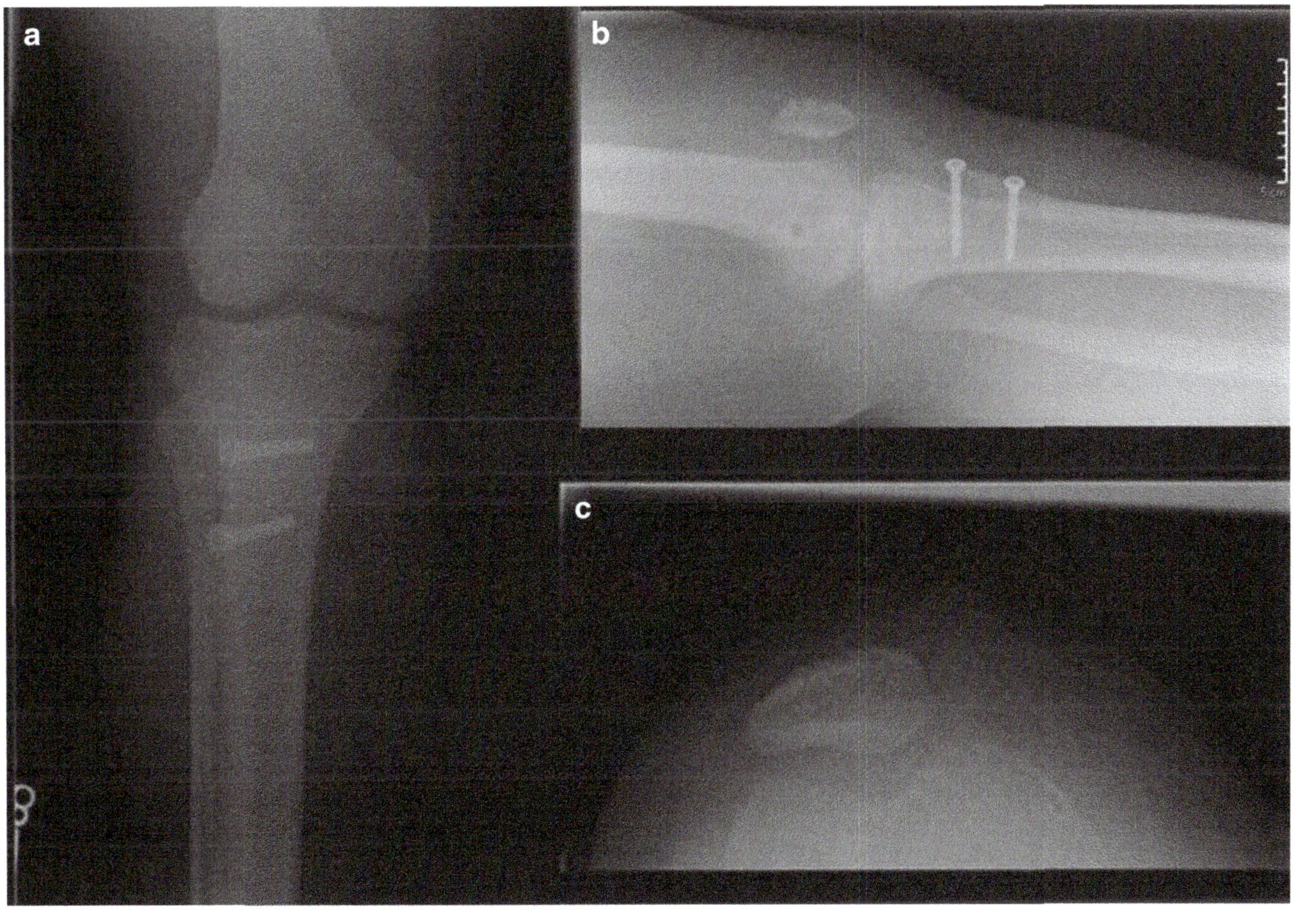

Fig. 9.12 (**a–c**) PA, lateral, and merchant views demonstrating tibial tubercle fixation and improvement in patellar tracking and tilt

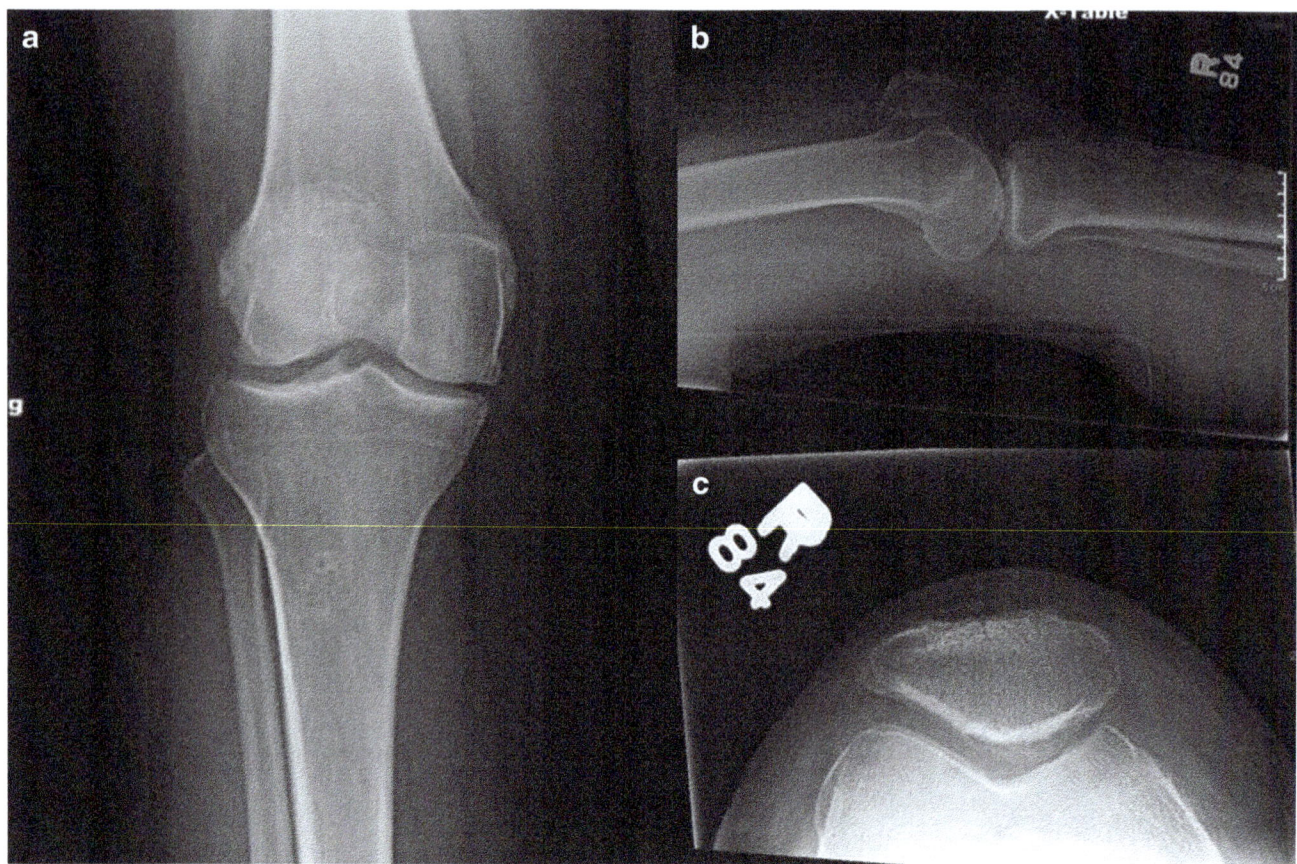

Fig. 9.13 (**a–c**) PA, lateral, and merchant views demonstrating normal patellar tracking, normal trochlear morphology, and healed osteotomy of the tibial tubercle

for multiple surgeries over a 3-year period. Initial surgery involved a plica excision, and subsequently she underwent lateral meniscus repair with proximal and distal extensor mechanism realignment. A third procedure involved the removal of previous hardware and a fourth a shaving chondroplasty of the patellofemoral joint. Her primary complaint upon presentation to our clinic was anterior knee pain, aggravated by stairs and activity. In addition to her multiple surgeries, the patient had failed nonoperative attempts with physical therapy, bracing, anti-inflammatories, steroid injections, and activity modification. On initial physical examination, there was significant patellar tenderness and crepitus, as well as a trace effusion. The patient also endorsed medial joint line tenderness and a positive McMurray. She did not have patellar apprehension, and her patella tracked normally. There was no lateral retinacular tightness, and there was a firm endpoint on MPFL testing. The remainder of her examination was remarkable only for generalized ligamentous laxity.

Imaging

Initial imaging included plain radiographs, which demonstrated mild joint line narrowing medially, with evidence of prior surgery and anteromedialization tibial tubercle osteotomy.

The patellofemoral joint did not show evidence of maltracking or excessive tilt. Trochlear morphology appeared normal (Fig. 9.13a–c). MRI demonstrated evidence of postsurgical changes of the lateral meniscocapsular junction and full-thickness lesions of the proximal mid-patella and trochlea measuring 1.3 cm and 0.8 cm, respectively (Fig. 9.14a, b). The TT-TG distance was measured at 12 mm.

Based on her continued complaints of pain localized to the patellofemoral joint and her documented full-thickness cartilage loss, the patient was indicated for diagnostic arthroscopy with possible allograft cartilage transplantation with the particulated juvenile chondrocyte implantation technique.

Surgery

At the time of surgery, a diagnostic knee arthroscopy demonstrated Outerbridge grade IV cartilage loss over a 22×20 mm area of the patella, with a depth of 3 mm. On the trochlea, a 15×18 mm area was identified with Outerbridge grade IV cartilage loss, also at a 3 mm depth (Fig. 9.15a, b). There was mild degenerative change to the cartilage in the medial compartment, but no evidence of a medial meniscus tear. Next, a medial parapatellar arthrotomy was made, and the patella was partially everted. The patellar lesion and trochlear lesion were sharply

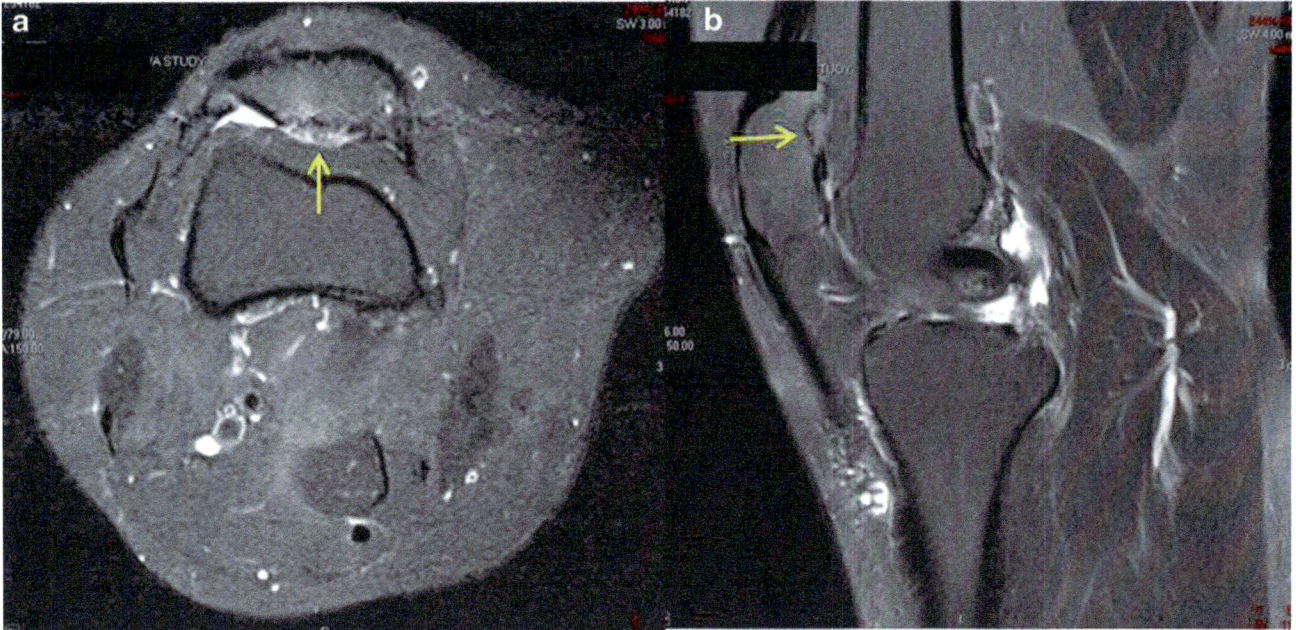

Fig. 9.14 (a, b) T2 imaging sequences demonstrating full-thickness cartilage defects of the proximal mid-patella and trochlea

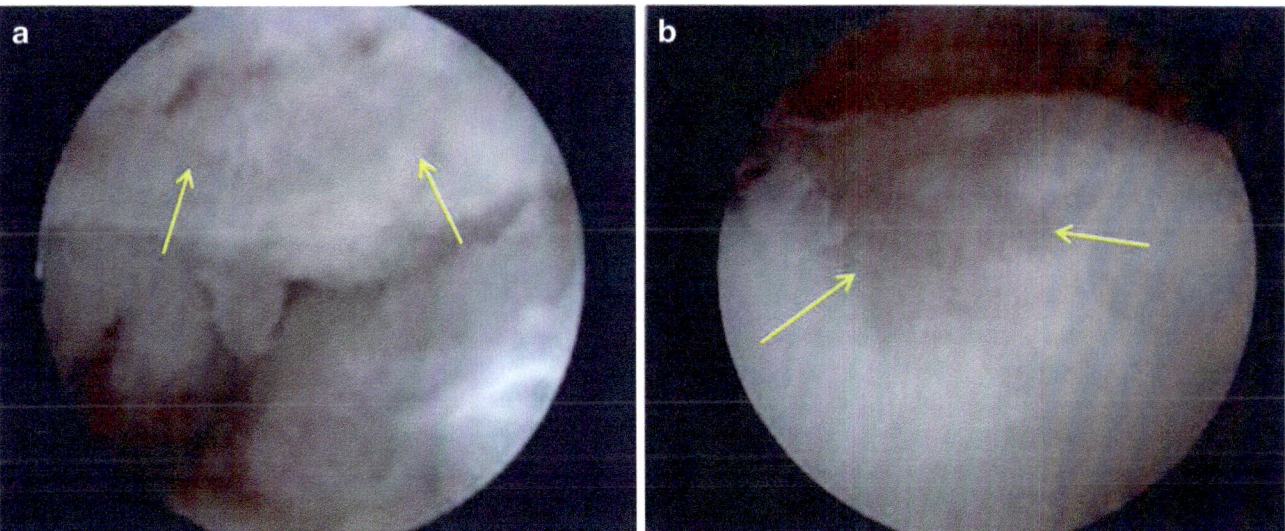

Fig. 9.15 Arthroscopic images confirming full-thickness cartilage loss of the mid-patella (a) and trochlear groove (b)

curetted to a stable rim of cartilage, and the particulated juvenile chondral implant was prepared on the back table (Fig. 9.16a). After placing a layer of fibrin glue at the base of the lesions, the minced chondral allograft was added and a final layer of fibrin glue placed on top (Fig. 9.16b, c). It is important to adhere closely to the manufacturer's recommendations regarding the timing of implantation/preparation of the graft and to monitor the density of the implanted cartilage, to avoid overgrowth.

In the initial postoperative phase, the patient was restricted to 25 % weight bearing and was placed in a hinged knee brace. She was gradually allowed to resume full weight bearing at 6 weeks. Range of motion was advanced as tolerated. At her most recent postoperative visit, she had regained full range of motion and has progressed with strengthening. Her pain level is significantly improved from the preoperative level.

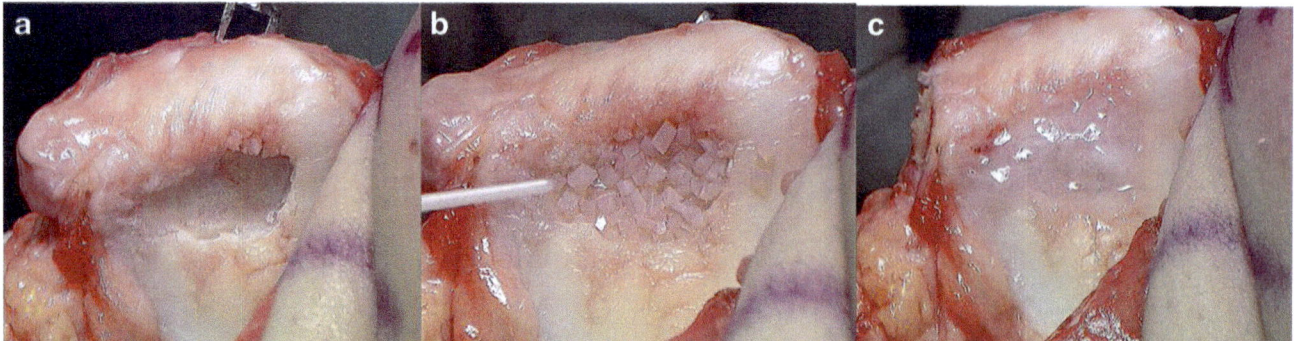

Fig. 9.16 (**a**) Patellar lesion curetted to stable rim. (**b**) Fibrin glue layer added to the base followed by minced chondral allograft. (**c**) The final layer of fibrin glue added over the top of minced chondral allograft

Discussion

- Strategies for management of full-thickness cartilage lesions of the patellofemoral joint
- Technical considerations for the use of allograft particulated juvenile chondrocytes

Conclusion

In the treatment of patellofemoral disorders, as demonstrated by each of the presented cases, it is essential to thoroughly correlate the radiographic findings to the patient's history and physical examination. This comprehensive approach offers the best chance of achieving successful outcomes, but in some cases, despite appropriate management, patients may continue to experience discomfort related to patellofemoral joint disorders. In these isolated cases, consideration of patellofemoral arthroplasty may be reasonable as a final alternative to total knee arthroplasty; however, it is important to set appropriate patient expectations prior to surgery. Patellofemoral arthroplasty may significantly delay additional surgeries, but for most patients is not viable as a definitive strategy, as may often be the case for the various other reconstructive procedures discussed.

References

1. Fithian DC, Paxton EW, Stone ML, Silva P, Davis DK, Elias DA, White LM. Epidemiology and natural history of acute patellar dislocation. Am J Sports Med. 2004;32:1114–21.
2. Hawkins RJ, Bell RH, Anisette G. Acute patellar dislocations. The natural history. Am J Sports Med. 1986;14:117–20.
3. Colvin AC, West RV. Patellar instability. J Bone Joint Surg Am. 2008;90:2751–62.
4. Dejour H, Walch G, Nove-Josserand L, Guier C. Factors of patellar instability: an anatomic radiographic study. Knee Surg Sports Traumatol Arthrosc. 1994;2:19–26.
5. Dejour D, Le Coultre B. Osteotomies in patello-femoral instabilities. Sports Med Arthrosc. 2007;15:40.
6. Berg EE, Mason SL, Lucas MJ. Patellar height ratios. A comparison of four measurement methods. Am J Sports Med. 1996;24: 218–21.
7. Alemparte J, Ekdahl M, Burnier L, Hernández R, Cardemil A, Cielo R, Danilla S. Patellofemoral evaluation with radiographs and computed tomography scans in 60 knees of asymptomatic subjects. Arthroscopy. 2007;23(2):170–7.
8. Sanders TG, Morrison WB, Singleton BA, Miller MD, Cornum KG. Medial patellofemoral ligament injury following acute transient dislocation of the patella: MR findings with surgical correlation in 14 patients. J Comput Assist Tomogr. 2001;25: 957–62.
9. Pihlajamäki HK, Kuikka PI, Leppänen VV, Kiuru MJ, Mattila VM. Reliability of clinical findings and magnetic resonance imaging for the diagnosis of chondromalacia patellae. J Bone Joint Surg Am. 2010;92(4):927–34.
10. Mäenpää H, Lehto MU. Patellar dislocation-the long term results of non-operative management in 100 patients. Am J Sports Med. 1997;25:213–7.
11. Stefancin JJ, Parker RD. First-time traumatic patellar dislocation. A systematic review. Clin Orthop Relat Res. 2007;455:93–101.
12. McConnell J. Rehabilitation and non-operative treatment of patellar instability. Sports Med Arthrosc. 2007;15:95–104.
13. Fulkerson JP. Diagnosis and treatment of patients with patellofemoral pain. Am J Sports Med. 2002;30(3):447–56.
14. Smith TO, Walker J, Russell N. Outcomes of medial patellofemoral ligament reconstruction for patellar instability. A systematic review. Knee Surg Sports Traumatol Arthrosc. 2007;15(11):1301–14.
15. Steiner TM, Torga-Spak R, Teitge RA. Medial patellofemoral ligament reconstruction in patients with lateral patellar instability and trochlear dysplasia. Am J Sports Med. 2006;34(8):1254–61.
16. Schöttle PB, Fucentese SF, Pfirrmann C, Bereiter H, Romero J. Trochleaplasty for patellar instability due to trochlear dysplasia. A minimum 2-year clinical and radiological follow-up of 19 knees. Acta Orthop. 2005;76(5):693–8.
17. Utting MR, Mulford JS, Eldridge JD. A prospective evaluation of trochleaplasty for the treatment of patellofemoral dislocation and instability. J Bone Joint Surg Br. 2008;90(2):180–5.
18. Schottle PB, Schell H, Duda G, Weiler A. Cartilage viability after trochleoplasty. Knee Surg Sports Traumatol Arthrosc. 2004;12: 300–6.
19. Von Knoch F, Bohm T, Burgi ML, et al. Trochleaplasty for recurrent patellar dislocation in association with trochlear dysplasia. A 4 to 14-year follow-up study. J Bone Joint Surg Br. 2006;88:1331–5.

Synovial Disorders of the Knee

10

10

Ryan A. Mlynarek, James R. Ross, David Paul Fessell, and Asheesh Bedi

Introduction

The synovium is a specialized tissue derived from mesenchymal cell lineage that is essential for the proper function of joints. Synovial membranes are comprised of two layers, the synovial intima and subsynovial tissue. The synovial intima is one to four cell layers thick and is composed of synoviocytes, macrophages, and fibroblasts [1]. This overlies the subsynovium, which consists of loosely organized connective tissue, adipocytes, macrophages, lymphatics, and blood vessels [2, 3]. Beneath this connective tissue lies the dense, fibrous joint capsule. The synovium functions as a mechanical shock absorber and filter system to secrete hyaluronic acid and synovial fluid to lubricate and nourish the articular surface [4]. It lines intra-articular structures, including tendons, ligaments, and the bare, intra-capsular periosteal surfaces not covered by cartilage.

The synovium of the knee is the most extensive and complex in the body. Anteriorly, the synovium attaches to the articular borders of the patella. At the upper border of the patella, it extends on each side of the patella posterior to the aponeuroses of the vastus medialis, vastus lateralis, and quadriceps tendon to attach to the anterior femoral shaft, forming the suprapatellar bursa. From the inferior patella, it extends posterior to the infrapatellar fat pad to its insertion on the anterior tibia. Medially and laterally from the patella,

the membrane travels inferiorly, forming redundant alar folds (plicae) of synovium that may project into the joint [5]. The infrapatellar plica (ligamentum mucosum) is the most common plica in the knee and extends from the inferior pole of the patella through the infrapatellar fat pad, anterior to the anterior cruciate ligament (ACL) to insert in the anterior intercondylar notch [6]. The synovial membrane lines the anterior, medial and lateral aspects of the ACL and posterior cruciate ligament (PCL), before reflecting posteriorly to join the posterior fibrous capsule. This functionally divides the knee into medial and lateral compartments [7]. The medial and lateral borders of the joint are defined as the synovial membrane passes inferiorly from the femur to the medial and lateral attachments of the menisci, leaving the peripheral borders of the menisci devoid of synovial membrane [8]. The synovium then extends from the inferior portion of the meniscal attachments to form the medial and lateral perimeniscal recesses. Between the lateral meniscus and the popliteus tendon, the synovial membrane forms the popliteal recess. The synovial membrane extends posteriorly from the femur to the proximal origins of the lateral and medial heads of the gastrocnemius, thus forming the posterior femoral recess [9].

Pathology of the synovium can be part of a systemic process or primary synovial disease affecting a single articulation. Degenerative, traumatic, inflammatory, infectious, or neoplastic processes can affect the synovium. The most common primary synovial disorders are pigmented villonodular synovitis, synovial chondromatosis, synovial hemangioma, and lipoma arborescens [4, 10].

Magnetic resonance (MR) imaging provides excellent soft tissue contrast with multi-planar capabilities by noninvasive means to effectively evaluate the synovium. MR imaging with intravenous (IV) gadolinium-based contrast is most beneficial when characterizing synovial disease, as the synovial membrane is difficult to distinguish from adjacent joint effusion on T1-weighted imaging (both low in signal intensity) and T2-weighted imaging (both high in signal intensity) [4, 11]. The normal synovium avidly enhances on

R.A. Mlynarek, MD • A. Bedi, MD (✉)
Department of Orthopedic Surgery, University of Michigan School of Medicine, Ann Arbor, MI, USA
e-mail: mlynarek@med.umich.edu; abedi@med.umich.edu

J.R. Ross, MD
Department of Orthopedic Surgery, Broward Orthopedic Specialists, Fort Lauderdale, FL, USA
e-mail: orthodocjimross@gmail.com

D.P. Fessell, MD
Department of Radiology, University of Michigan School of Medicine, Ann Arbor, MI, USA
e-mail: fessell@med.umich.edu

post-gadolinium images and this enhancement aids evaluation of synovial disorders.

The primary focus of this chapter is to present the most common synovial disorders affecting the knee, review characteristic MR imaging findings, and discuss surgical treatment options.

Case 1: Pigmented Villonodular Synovitis

A 36-year-old male presents with complaints of progressively worsening right knee pain over the past 2–3 years with no history of antecedent trauma. He describes mechanical symptoms and intermittent effusions without antecedent trauma. The pain is not clearly localized and affects the anterior as well as the posterior aspect of the knee. Nonsteroidal anti-inflammatory medications and physical therapy did not improve the patient's symptoms and advanced imaging was obtained.

Introduction

Pigmented villonodular synovitis (PVNS) is a benign but disabling proliferative disorder of the synovial lining of joints first described by Jaffe et al. in 1941 [12]. It is characterized by the development of villi and nodular thickening of the synovial membrane and deposition of hemosiderin-laden macrophages [13–15]. The etiology of PVNS remains controversial, but recent studies support the theory that a combination of reactive inflammatory disease and chromosomal translocation result in neoplastic proliferation of the synovium [16–18]. It is a rare disease with an incidence of 1.8 per 1,000,000 people, affecting males and females with equal prevalence and most commonly occurs between the ages of 20 and 50 years [19, 20].

Clinical Presentation

PVNS can affect any synovial joint but has a predilection to impact the knee (75 %), hip (15 %), ankle, and shoulder [20]. Monoarticular involvement of the knee occurs in 66–80 % of cases, and involvement of more than one joint is rare [21]. Synovial involvement can be focal; however, diffuse involvement of the affected joint is more common.

Patients with localized PVNS may present with a tender, confined bulging of the synovium. Mechanical symptoms of catching and locking are frequently reported (38 %) and can often lead to a misdiagnosis of meniscal pathology [22]. Diffuse involvement of the synovium typically presents with generalized joint effusion, limited range of motion, and tenderness to palpation. Relevant laboratory studies (ESR, CRP,

WBC) are usually within normal limits. Joint fluid aspiration can aid in the diagnosis, as the aspirate often contains an elevated cholesterol content in the setting of normal blood cholesterol levels, and it is serosanguinous in nature with a prevalence of hemarthrosis in 75 % of PVNS cases [21–25].

Histopathology

The gold standard for diagnosis of PVNS is synovial biopsy. The predominant lesion-defining cells are proliferating, polyhedral, mononuclear synovial cells that contain vesicular nuclei, abundant cytoplasm, and hemosiderin pigment. The cell population within the lesion contains foamy histiocytes, mononuclear cells, and giant cells [20, 26].

Imaging

Conventional radiographs alone are often nondiagnostic when evaluating a patient for PVNS. Joint effusion and dense soft tissue swelling are common but nonspecific. Few exhibit cystic changes or osteophyte formation, and there is usually an absence of periarticular osteopenia, which is helpful to differentiate PVNS from an inflammatory arthritis [15, 17, 27]. Advanced disease may result in joint space narrowing and periarticular erosion of bone particularly in the hip and ankle. Although less common in the knee secondary to the relatively lower intra-articular pressure, bony change may occur in response to the soft tissue proliferation (Fig. 10.1) [24, 28–31].

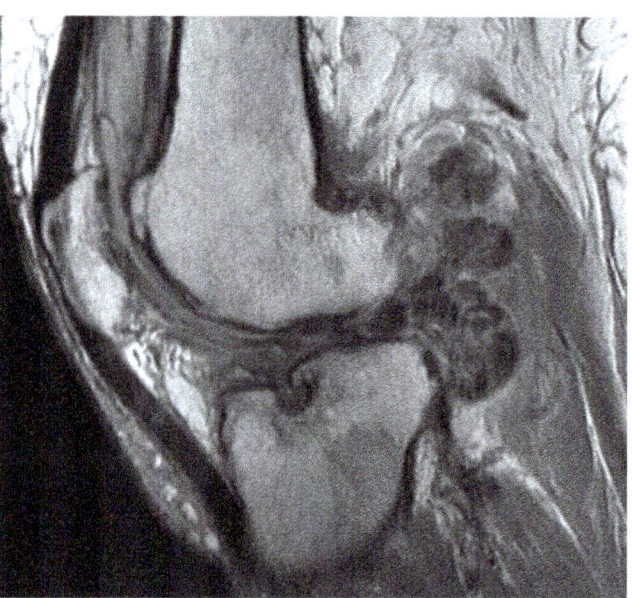

Fig. 10.1 Sagittal proton-density magnetic resonance image without fat saturation illustrating pigmented villonodular synovitis with bony erosion of medial tibial plateau

MR imaging is the method of choice for diagnosis, surgical planning, and evaluation of PVNS [14, 15, 32, 33]. Characteristic MR imaging features of PVNS enable a diagnosis to be made in 83–95 % of cases [24, 32].

In localized or focal PVNS, the classic MR image appearance is a solitary ovoid lesion with low signal intensity on both T1- and T2-weighted imaging. The most common location is the infrapatellar fat pad but areas may also include the suprapatellar pouch, intercondylar notch, and lateral synovial gutter [15, 22, 32].

In diffuse PVNS, MR images of the knee reveal synovial thickening, hypertrophy, and irregularity most commonly in the regions of the suprapatellar bursa and posterior joint recess. The most reliable diagnostic feature is the deposition of hemosiderin-laden macrophages viewed on T1- and T2-weighted images and on echo gradient imaging. As seen in Fig. 10.2, the synovial thickening can produce diffuse low-signal-intensity masses. On gradient echo imaging, these demonstrate a characteristic "blooming" artifact of hemosiderin deposition due to the paramagnetic effects of the iron [15, 32]. Diffuse PVNS exhibits an extensive pattern of hemosiderin deposition within the synovium resulting in frond-like low signal irregularities within the joint capsule. Enhancement is seen on T1-weighted images after IV gadolinium injection. Diffuse disease can extend beyond the joint capsule, and common extra-articular sites of involvement around the knee include the semimembranosus bursa, the popliteus tendon sheath, and previous arthroscopy portals.

Treatment

Localized PVNS

Lesions can be sessile or pedunculated and are often limited to a single location, most commonly intra-articular in location. Nonoperative management may include physical therapy and intra-articular corticosteroid injections; however, these are of limited utility in transiently improving mechanical symptoms and offer no benefit for definitive treatment.

Nodular excision with partial synovectomy (Fig. 10.3) can often be performed arthroscopically with relief of symptoms and 0 % recurrence rate at short- and mid-term follow-up [22, 27, 34–37]. Open local excision may be performed for extra-articular involvement and for inaccessible intra-articular disease such as the posterior knee or fixed synovial disease [17].

Diffuse PVNS

Although considered to be a benign disease, diffuse PVNS can be locally aggressive and cause joint damage. Like local PVNS, nonoperative management may include physical therapy and corticosteroid injections to temporarily improve localized pain and swelling; however, this will not treat the underlying disease pathology. External beam radiation therapy has been described as primary treatment for unresectable lesions or in nonoperative candidates with recurrence rates of 7–67 % [38–40].

Surgical treatment for diffuse PVNS remains controversial and depends on the extent of the disease. Some authors advocate arthroscopic excision with complete synovectomy as the treatment of choice [34, 35, 41]. Arthroscopic treatment

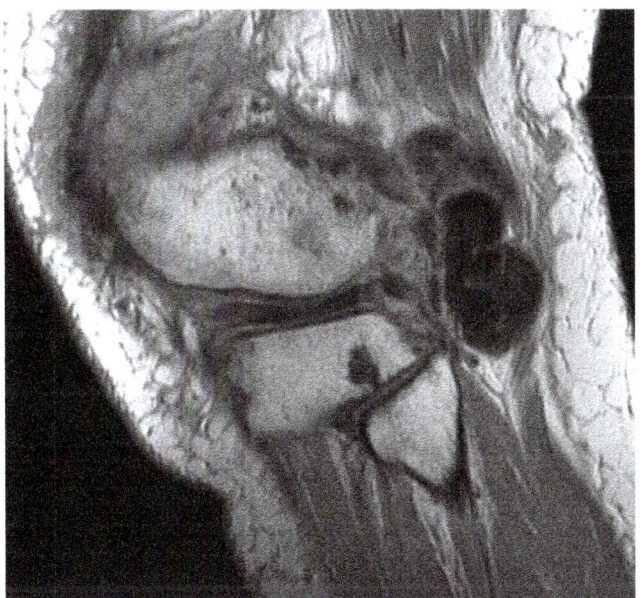

Fig. 10.2 Sagittal proton-density magnetic resonance image without fat saturation reveals low-signal mass extending from the posterior joint space of the knee

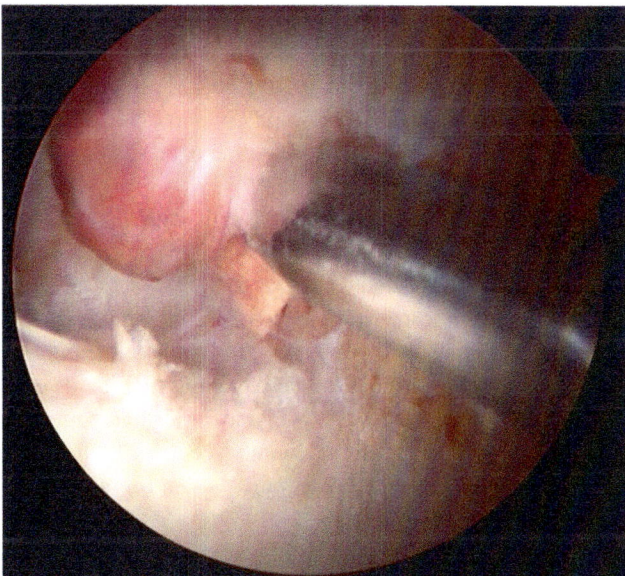

Fig. 10.3 Arthroscopic view of focal, localized pigmented villonodular synovitis lesion

offers the patient a faster postoperative recovery to baseline function and decreased likelihood of stiffness [17, 27]. However, incomplete excision is not uncommon and often leads to recurrence. Recurrence rates approach 25 % for intra-articular involvement and 50 % for extra-articular disease, depending on the extent of the primary excision [20, 42]. For this reason, many surgeons prefer open arthrotomy excision with complete synovectomy, particularly for large-volume diffuse PVNS [17, 26, 42–44]. An open, posterior approach may also be necessary to excise extra-articular extension along tendons within the popliteal fossa. Adjuvant radiosynovectomy with intra-articular injection of yttrium-90 can be used after synovectomy to decrease recurrence rates of intra-articular lesions; however, there is a paucity of evidence and limited case series [45–47].

Case 2: Synovial Chondromatosis

A 46-year-old male presents with insidious-onset pain, swelling, crepitus, and decreased range of motion in his right knee for the past 2 years. He denies any history of trauma. On physical examination, an effusion is present and there is a palpable suprapatellar mass.

Introduction

Primary synovial chondromatosis is a benign disease first described by Leannac in 1813 but not formally named until 1958 by Jaffe [48–51]. It is rare and has an incidence of 1 per 100,000 people [52, 53]. It is two to four times more likely to develop in men and most commonly presents in the third to fifth decades of life [48, 49, 54]. Although clonal abnormalities and rare malignant changes have been reported in synovial chondromatosis, the disease process is generally categorized as a metaplastic rather than neoplastic disease of synovial cells [55–59]. It is characterized by chondroid metaplasia of synovial mesenchymal cells with resultant formation of lobulated, pedunculated intra-articular chondral bodies. These often shed into the joint, which may then ossify (osteochondromatosis). In 1977, Milgram described a clinical progression of this disease process by delineating its course into three phases: (1) active intrasynovial disease only with no loose bodies; (2) transitional lesions with both active, intrasynovial proliferation and free loose bodies; and (3) multiple, free osteochondral bodies with no demonstrable intrasynovial disease [60].

Secondary synovial chondromatosis is associated with mechanical or arthritic joint abnormalities, which result in the formation of loose, intra-articular chondral bodies [61].

Clinical Presentation

Synovial chondromatosis is classically a monoarticular disease, although polyarticular involvement has been described in up to 5 % of cases [53, 62]. The knee is the most commonly involved joint (50–65 %), followed by the hip, elbow, and shoulder [49, 53, 63]. Bilateral knee involvement has been reported in up to 10 % of cases; however, most cases are likely a representation of secondary synovial chondromatosis [54]. Primary synovial chondromatosis is most commonly diffuse, involving the entire synovium of the affected joint; however, localized disease has been described [64, 65].

The most common sites of involvement within the knee are the suprapatellar pouch, infrapatellar fat pad, and the anterior interval between the ACL and the infrapatellar fat pad [66, 67]. Less commonly, the posterior compartment (posterior to the PCL) may be involved [65, 66, 68, 69].

Patients present with a subacute onset of pain (85–100 %), swelling (40–58 %), and limited range of motion (35–55 %). Patients seldom recall an antecedent trauma to the knee and have no apparent systemic signs of infection or illness. On physical exam, patients often have an effusion, tenderness to palpation, articular crepitus (20–33 %), locking (5–10 %), palpable nodules, or a distinct mass (5–20 %) [54, 64, 70–72].

Histopathology

The gross appearance of synovial chondromatosis consists of hyperplastic synovium overlying white, nodular projections of hyaline cartilage diffusely scattered across the entire joint surface [49, 54, 73–75]. This often gives the synovium a "cobblestone" appearance. The nodules may detach from the synovium, thus creating free chondral bodies within the affected joint. The number of nodules can range from a few to thousands, depending on the stage of the disease. They vary in size from a few millimeters to a few centimeters in diameter [49, 54]. As the nodules increase in size, the central zone can undergo calcification and, rarely, endochondral ossification. Multiple detached nodules may coalesce to form a large mass termed giant synovial chondromas, though this is rare [54, 76].

Imaging

As seen in Fig. 10.4, conventional roentgenograms reveal intra-articular ossified bodies in 70–95 % of cases of primary synovial chondromatosis. Characteristically, they are innumerable, similar in size and shape, and evenly dispersed throughout the synovial lining of the affected joint

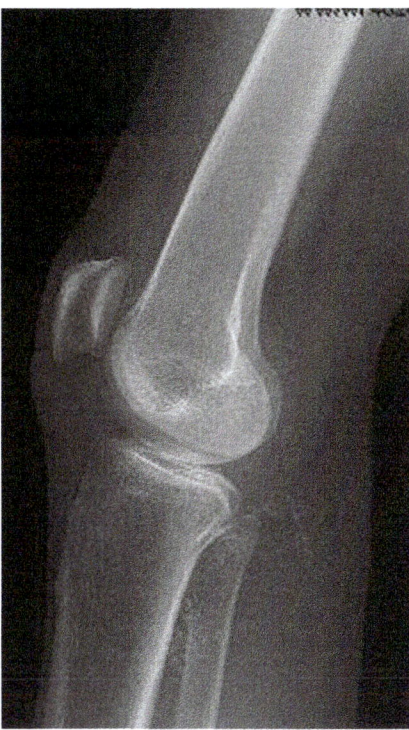

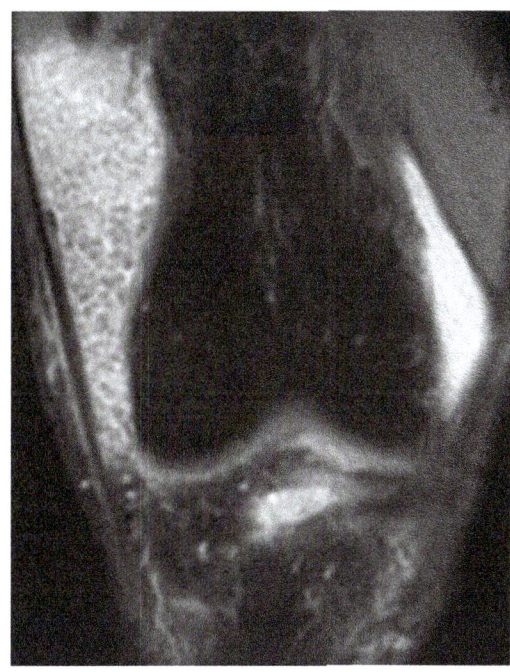

Fig. 10.5 Coronal fat-saturated T2-weighted magnetic resonance image revealing numerous low-signal osteochondral bodies

Fig. 10.4 Lateral radiograph of the knee, revealing multiple ossified bodies in the posterior compartment

[48, 49, 54, 73, 75, 77]. Periarticular bony erosions are common in more constrained joints such as the wrist, elbow, and hip; however, these are less likely in the knee and shoulder [78].

Computed tomography (CT) imaging of the knee can be useful in differentiating primary synovial chondromatosis from other causes of soft tissue lesions, particularly when conventional roentgenograms are equivocal. Hyaline cartilage has a high water content and therefore low attenuation on CT imaging, which can be appreciated in the nonmineralized synovial thickening caused by synovial chondromatosis. Furthermore, the majority of nodules caused by synovial chondromatosis contain central and peripheral ossification which CT imaging delineates as a "ring-and-arc" pattern of mineralization or a target appearance [53, 54]. However, purely chondral lesions are better defined by magnetic resonance imaging.

MR imaging of the knee provides the optimal modality to aid in the diagnosis and treatment plan for primary synovial chondromatosis. Due to the heterogenous makeup of calcification and ossification of the nodules, variable signal characteristics are identified, as illustrated in Figs. 10.5 and 10.6 [54, 76, 79–81]. The most common pattern (77 %) demonstrates low/intermediate signal intensity on T1-weighted sequences and high signal intensity on T2-weighted sequences. This correlates clinically with the Milgram phase 2 lesions, as described above [54, 76].

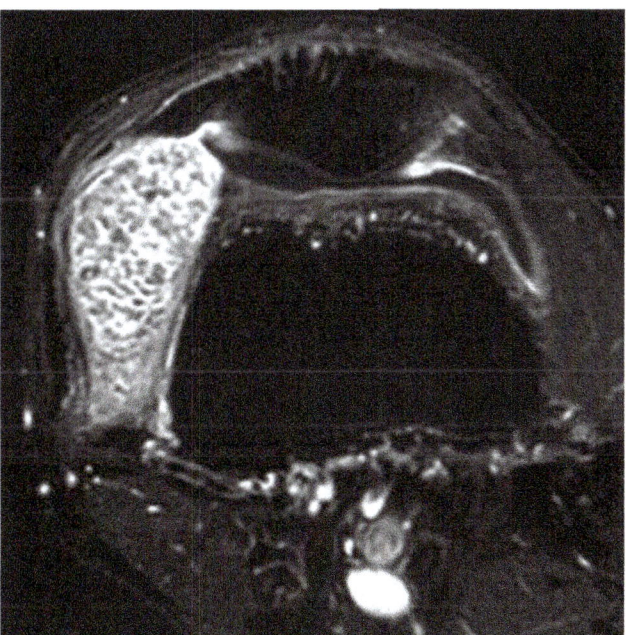

Fig. 10.6 Axial fat-saturated T1-weighted magnetic resonance image post IV gadolinium demonstrates multiple low-signal osteochondral bodies within the enhancing synovium

Treatment

Patients presenting with recurrent pain, swelling, and mechanical symptoms refractory to nonoperative management are candidates for surgical intervention. Primary synovial chondromatosis is generally a benign and self-limiting disease; however, it may be progressive and complicated by osteoarthritis. On rare occasions, synovial chondrosarcoma can arise in the setting of synovial chondromatosis (5 % incidence) [54, 75, 82]. Therefore, the treatment of choice is surgical excision of the osteochondral nodules with or without partial or complete synovectomy, depending on the extent of the disease. Surgical excision can be performed by open or arthroscopic approach, and the technique should be selected based upon ability to safely access and thoroughly remove all the diseased synovium and nodules.

Arthroscopic excision offers the surgeon better visualization of the intra-articular synovium and decreased pain, stiffness, and postoperative rehabilitation course for the patient [65, 69, 83]. The need for partial or complete synovectomy for treatment of primary synovial chondromatosis remains controversial. Milgram recommended treating patients with phase 1 primary synovial chondromatosis (active intrasynovial disease only with no loose bodies) with synovectomy. For phase 2 (transitional form with active intrasynovial disease and chondral bodies), he recommended synovectomy with chondral body retrieval. Lastly, for phase 3 (late inactive intrasynovial disease with chondral bodies but no synovial abnormality), he recommended chondral body retrieval alone [60]. With this treatment regimen, Milgram observed recurrence rates of 12.5 %, 10 %, and 0 % for phases 1, 2, and 3, respectively [54, 60]. The recurrence rate for larger series ranges from 3 to 23 % and recurrence is most likely related to incomplete primary excision [63, 64, 70]. Ogilvie-Harris and Saleh reported nearly a 60 % recurrence rate when treating patients with loose chondral body retrieval alone [84]. Therefore, arthroscopic retrieval of chondral loose bodies and complete synovectomy is the treatment of choice for primary synovial chondromatosis. This was performed in our patient, as seen in Figs. 10.7 and 10.8.

Case 3: Synovial Hemangioma

An otherwise healthy 13-year-old female with no history of trauma presents with recurrent effusions and decreased range of motion in her right knee.

Introduction

Hemangiomas and hemangiohamartomas are types of rare, benign vascular tumors that may affect the musculoskeletal system. Hemangiohamartomas, more commonly known as arteriovenous malformations, are differentiated from hemangiomas in that they contain fat, connective tissue, and peripheral nerve structures [29]. Hemangiomas, however,

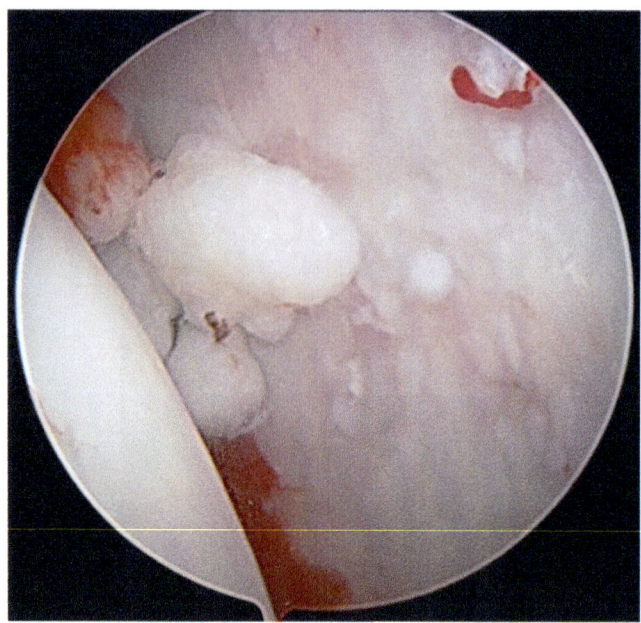

Fig. 10.7 Arthroscopic view of numerous osteochondral bodies embedded within the synovium

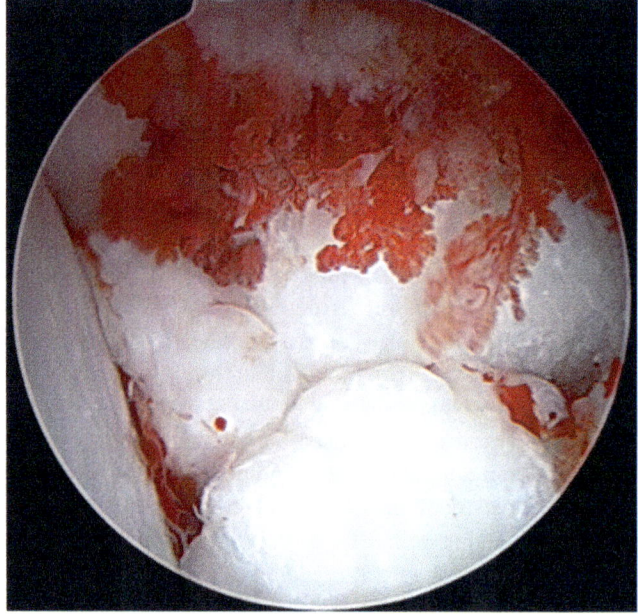

Fig. 10.8 Arthroscopic view of multiple osteochondral bodies and inflamed synovium

are composed primarily of closely packed thin-walled capillaries. Depending on their location in relation to the joint, hemangiomas may be described as juxta-articular (outside the joint capsule but in relation to it), intra-articular, extra-articular, or intermediate (both intra- and extra-articular) [85–87]. Both the intra-articular and intermediate types generally involve the synovial membrane. Synovial hemangiomas were first described by Bouchut in 1856 and further categorized as being either localized or diffuse in character by Bennett and Cobey in 1939 [88, 89]. They are exceedingly rare, with approximately 200 reported cases [90, 91]. Most commonly, they occur in children and adolescents with the average age of onset of 10.9 years in females and 12.5 years in males [92, 93]. Synovial hemangiomas are slightly more common in females (53 %) [91, 94, 95].

Clinical Presentation

Synovial hemangiomas have been reported in the wrist, ankle, and elbow, but they most commonly involve the knee [87, 91, 92, 96, 97]. The tumor may be localized and well circumscribed or diffuse in character. Patients often present with an insidious onset of knee pain and recurrent effusions with associated limitation in range of motion. Atrophy of the quadriceps muscle is common in patients with a synovial hemangioma [87, 95, 98]. Patients with localized and pedunculated synovial hemangiomas may have a palpable soft tissue mass and often experience mechanical symptoms. Diffuse involvement can lead to more pronounced synovial venous congestion and hemorrhagic synovitis. Patients with both localized and diffuse subtypes often have a diagnostic delay, because of the rarity of synovial hemangiomas [99–102]. This delay leads to many patients having a history of spontaneous swelling and recurrent hemarthrosis in the absence of coagulopathy. In up to 40 % of cases, the patient may present with overlying cutaneous hemangiomas and venous congestion of the knee [91, 93, 103, 104].

Histopathology

Synovial hemangiomas can be classified as cavernous, capillary, mixed, or arteriovenous [91, 105]. Most commonly, they exhibit features of cavernous hemangiomas with lobulated proliferation of capillary-sized vascular channels. Inflammatory cells and hemosiderin-laden macrophages are frequently identified, thus resembling pigmented villonodular synovitis. However, the existence of dilated, thin-walled capillaries with cavernous appearance differentiates PVNS from synovial hemangiomas [91, 97].

Imaging

Conventional roentgenograms may reveal the presence of an effusion, soft tissue mass, phleboliths, advanced maturation of the epiphysis, or periosteal reaction [95, 100, 103, 106].

Frequently, however, radiographs show no abnormalities and further imaging is necessary. CT imaging can aid in the diagnosis to rule out bony abnormality; however, the demarcation between soft tissue mass and muscle is limited.

MR imaging does not use ionizing radiation and provides better soft tissue differentiation to demonstrate the extent of involvement of the synovial hemangioma [105, 107–109]. In conventional MR imaging without contrast, the lesions are lobulated with well-defined margins and exhibit homogenous, low-to-iso-signal intensity on T1-weighted imaging and heterogeneous, high signal intensity on T2-weighted imaging, as seen in Figs. 10.9 and 10.10 [90, 100, 103, 106, 110, 111]. The use of gadolinium contrast has been advocated by some authors to differentiate synovial hemangiomas from ganglion cysts, cystic synovial hyperplasia, synovial sarcoma, leiomyoma, and synovial chondromatosis [90]. With Gd-enhancement, synovial hemangiomas exhibit heterogeneous enhancement (Fig. 10.11). This has been useful to differentiate synovial hemangiomas from other intra-articular synovial lesions with the exception of synovial sarcomas which can display similar characteristics. However, these malignant lesions most commonly arise extra-articularly [90, 112]. MR imaging allows for accurate preoperative assessment in the classification of the lesion, thus guiding a definitive treatment strategy.

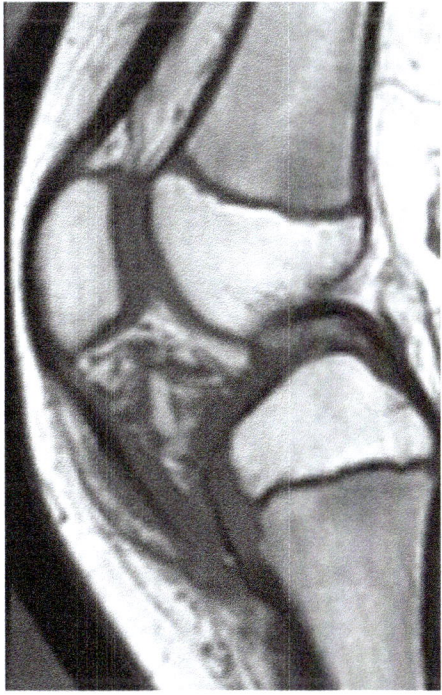

Fig. 10.9 Sagittal T1-weighted magnetic resonance image revealing infrapatellar lesion with internal fat signal

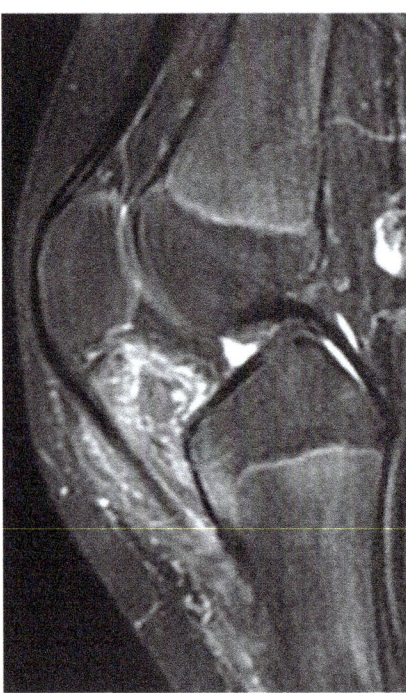

Fig. 10.10 Sagittal T2-weighted magnetic resonance image revealing infrapatellar lesion with internal high T2 signal and suggestion of peripheral vessels

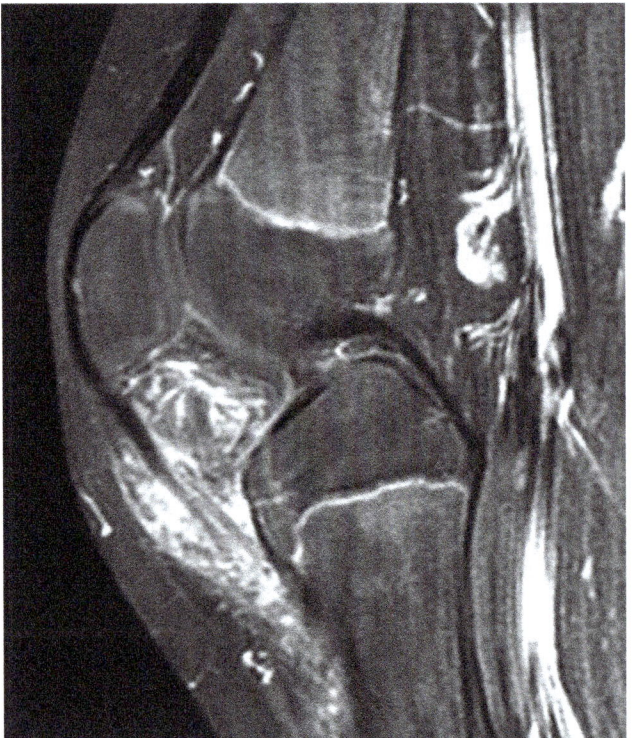

Fig. 10.11 Sagittal fat-saturated T1-weighted magnetic resonance image post IV gadolinium enhancement demonstrates discrete vessels and strong enhancement consistent with synovial hemangioma

Treatment

Aside from pain, mechanical symptoms, and decreased range of motion, synovial hemangiomas frequently cause recurrent hemarthrosis, which can lead to early destruction of the articular surface of the knee. Therefore, several treatment options have been described for synovial hemangiomas including embolization and open or arthroscopic surgical excision with and without partial synovectomy. Like other synovial disorders, the treatment of choice depends on the classification and extent of involvement.

Localized synovial hemangiomas can often be treated successfully with arthroscopic surgical excision, especially when the lesion is pedunculated and well circumscribed [91, 105, 113, 114]. Frequently, localized lesions will have a single vascular supply that can be managed arthroscopically with minimal bleeding.

Diffusely involved synovial hemangiomas in a single compartment of the knee are better treated with open arthrotomy, surgical excision, and partial synovectomy [95, 98, 115, 116]. They often have multiple feeding vessels; therefore, preoperative angiography with embolization may improve surgical results and decrease postoperative bleeding [91, 99, 101]. However, in diffuse synovial hemangiomas that involve multiple compartments of the knee, nonoperative management with repeat imaging to evaluate progression has been encouraged [91, 98].

Case 4: Lipoma Arborescens

A 45-year-old male with diabetes mellitus presents with complaints of mechanical symptoms in his right knee and a palpable, tender mass over the superior aspect of his patella.

Introduction

Lipoma arborescens (diffuse articular lipomatosis) is a rare, benign intra-articular disease affecting the synovial membrane. First described by in 1957 by Arzimanoglu, it is characterized as a diffuse substitution of the joint's subsynovial layer by mature adipocytes, resulting in the formation of villous projections [117–125]. Numerous villous lipomatous synovial proliferations differentiate lipoma arborescens from an intra-articular lipoma [120, 121, 126]. The etiology of lipoma arborescens remains unclear; however, developmental, traumatic, inflammatory, and neoplastic origins have been postulated [118, 123, 124]. Since its first description, there have been approximately 75 case reports presented in the literature [127]. There is a slight male preponderance (56–70 %) and the age range of disease onset is 10–90 years with a mean age of 37 years [127–129]. Associated conditions include osteoarthritis, rheumatoid arthritis, psoriatic arthritis, gout, joint trauma, and diabetes mellitus [118, 128, 130–133].

Clinical Presentation

Lipoma arborescens is a rare disorder that can affect the hip, shoulder, wrist, elbow, and ankle, but it most commonly affects the knee [117, 119, 124, 128, 129, 134]. Most cases are monoarticular; however, bilateral knee involvement has been described in up to 16 % of cases [127, 129]. The suprapatellar pouch is invariably involved. Other common sites include the condylar gutters and the premeniscal regions [117]. Patients with lipoma arborescens typically present with painless swelling of the knee, which leads to progressive restriction of range of motion. They often have intermittent exacerbations with resultant mechanical symptoms, as the villous projections can become trapped within the joint resulting in catching and locking [124]. Laboratory testing (ESR, CRP, WBC, uric acid, rheumatoid factor, HLA-B27) in patients with lipoma arborescens is normal [123, 129, 135]. Joint fluid aspiration reveals a serious appearance, is negative for cells and crystals, and is sterile on culture [124].

Histopathology

Macroscopically, lipoma arborescens is a fatty tissue mass with frond-like appearance. The finger-shaped synovial projections are numerous with broad bases [123, 127, 129, 136, 137]. Histologically, the disease is characterized by diffuse replacement of the subsynovial layer with mature adipocytes. Focal infiltration of perivascular mononuclear inflammatory cells is often appreciated [118, 119, 129].

Imaging

Conventional roentgenogram is of limited utility in the diagnosis of lipoma arborescens but may indicate the presence of a soft tissue mass and help to rule out bony involvement. CT imaging often demonstrates a soft tissue synovial mass and the characteristic synovial fronds may be outlined by an adjacent effusion. Low attenuation measurements are consistent with fat, and there is little or no enhancement after contrast administration [123, 130, 135, 138].

MR imaging is the modality of choice when evaluating a patient for lipoma arborescens. MR imaging reveals villous synovial thickening with fatty frond-like projections, usually

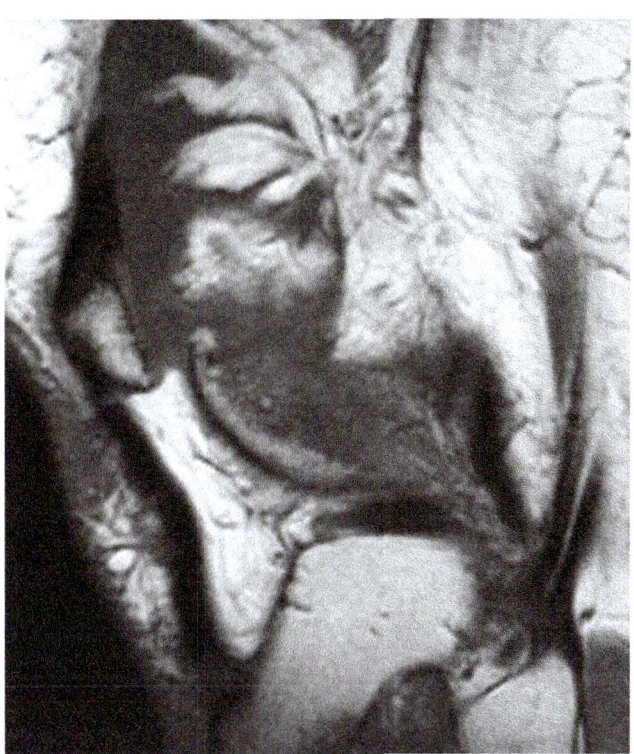

Fig. 10.12 Sagittal T1-weighted magnetic resonance image showing frond-like, villous proliferation of fat within the suprapatellar synovium, consistent with lipoma arborescens

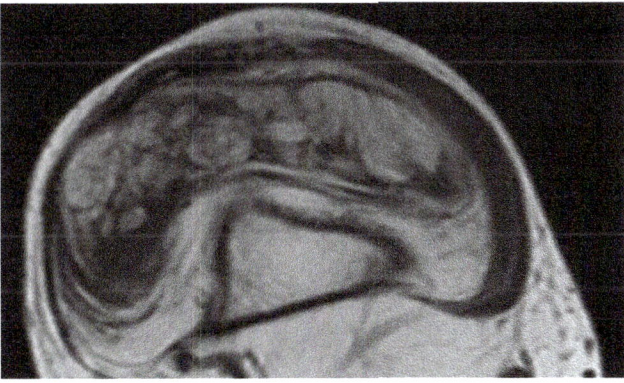

Fig. 10.13 Axial T1-weighted magnetic resonance image reveals frond-like, villous proliferation of fat within suprapatellar synovium, consistent with lipoma arborescens

with an effusion. The uniform fat signal and lack of hemosiderin aid diagnosis and differentiation from other lesions. (Fig. 10.12) [117, 133, 134, 139, 140]. Associated findings on MR imaging include chondral degenerative changes (87 %) and meniscal tears (72 %) [141]. Similar to that of subcutaneous fat, lipoma arborescens has high signal intensity on T1 (Fig. 10.13) and low signal on fat-saturated and STIR sequences (Fig. 10.14) [127, 141].

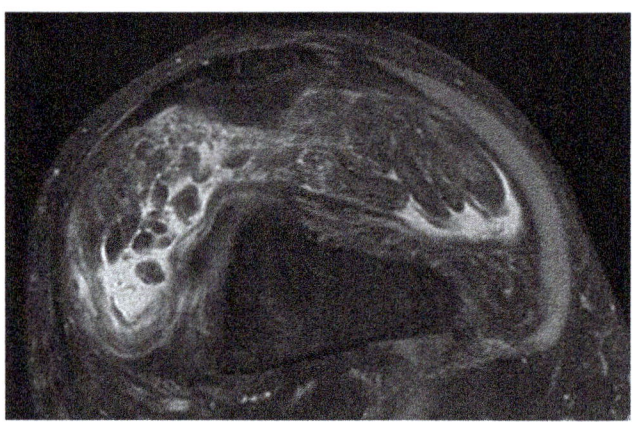

Fig. 10.14 Axial fat-saturated T2-weighted magnetic resonance image shows complete saturation of the signal forming the villous structures, therefore confirming their fatty composition

Treatment

Lipoma arborescens causes recurrent painless swelling of the knee that often leads to mechanical symptoms. Nonoperative management may consist of physical therapy and corticosteroid injections to abate frequent exacerbations. Asymptomatic and incidentally identified lesions do not require a surgical intervention.

Our patient presented with symptoms unresponsive to nonoperative treatment and elected to undergo an excision with partial synovectomy, as is the treatment of choice [123, 124]. Prior to 1998, reported lesions were excised via arthrotomy with partial or total synovectomy leading to low rates of recurrence. Sola and colleagues were the first to report successful arthroscopic excision of a lipoma arborescens lesion without recurrence [123]. Currently, the preferred treatment is arthroscopic excision of the mass with anterior synovectomy [117, 127, 142, 143]. Although some patients may have recurrent effusions postoperatively, likely secondary to arthritic changes, actual recurrence of lipoma arborescens is rare [142, 144].

References

1. Smith MD. The normal synovium. Open Rheumatol J. 2011; 5:100–6.
2. Cohen MJ, Kaplan L. Histology and ultrastructure of the human flexor tendon sheath. J Hand Surg Am. 1987;12(1):25–9.
3. Schmidt D, Mackay B. Ultrastructure of human tendon sheath and synovium: implications for tumor histogenesis. Ultrastruct Pathol. 1982;3(3):269–83.
4. Chung CB, Boucher R, Resnick D. MR imaging of synovial disorders of the knee. Semin Musculoskelet Radiol. 2009;13(4): 303–25.
5. Garcia-Valtuille R, Abascal F, Cerezal L, Garcia-Valtuille A, Pereda T, Canga A, et al. Anatomy and MR imaging appearances of synovial plicae of the knee. Radiographics. 2002;22(4): 775–84.
6. Kosarek FJ, Helms CA. The MR appearance of the infrapatellar plica. AJR Am J Roentgenol. 1999;172(2):481–4.
7. Lee SH, Petersilge CA, Trudell DJ, Haghighi P, Resnick DL. Extrasynovial spaces of the cruciate ligaments: anatomy, MR imaging, and diagnostic implications. AJR Am J Roentgenol. 1996;166(6):1433–7.
8. Fenn S, Datir A, Saifuddin A. Synovial recesses of the knee: MR imaging review of anatomical and pathological features. Skeletal Radiol. 2009;38(4):317–28.
9. De Maeseneer M, Van Roy P, Shahabpour M, Gosselin R, De Ridder F, Osteaux M. Normal anatomy and pathology of the posterior capsular area of the knee: findings in cadaveric specimens and in patients. AJR Am J Roentgenol. 2004;182(4):955–62.
10. O'Connell JX. Pathology of the synovium. Am J Clin Pathol. 2000;114(5):773–84.
11. Boegard T, Johansson A, Rudling O, Petersson I, Forslind K, Jonsson K. Gadolinium-DTPA-enhanced MR imaging in asymptomatic knees. Acta Radiol. 1996;37(6):877–82.
12. Jaffe HL, Lichtenstein L, Sutro CJ. Pigmented villonodular synovitis, bursitis and tenosynovitis. Arch Pathol. 1941;31:731–65.
13. Barile A, Sabatini M, Iannessi F, Di Cesare E, Splendiani A, Calvisi V, et al. Pigmented villonodular synovitis (PVNS) of the knee joint: magnetic resonance imaging (MRI) using standard and dynamic paramagnetic contrast media. Report of 52 cases surgically and histologically controlled. Radiol Med. 2004;107(4):356–66.
14. Hughes TH, Sartoris DJ, Schweitzer ME, Resnick DL. Pigmented villonodular synovitis: MRI characteristics. Skeletal Radiol. 1995;24(1):7–12.
15. Masih S, Antebi A. Imaging of pigmented villonodular synovitis. Semin Musculoskelet Radiol. 2003;7(3):205–16.
16. West RB, Rubin BP, Miller MA, Subramanian S, Kaygusuz G, Montgomery K, et al. A landscape effect in tenosynovial giant-cell tumor from activation of CSF1 expression by a translocation in a minority of tumor cells. Proc Natl Acad Sci U S A. 2006;103(3):690–5.
17. van der Heijden L, Gibbons CL, Dijkstra PD, Kroep JR, van Rijswijk CS, Nout RA, et al. The management of diffuse-type giant cell tumour (pigmented villonodular synovitis) and giant cell tumour of tendon sheath (nodular tenosynovitis). J Bone Joint Surg Br. 2012;94(7):882–8.
18. Nilsson M, Hoglund M, Panagopoulos I, Sciot R, Dal Cin P, Debiec-Rychter M, et al. Molecular cytogenetic mapping of recurrent chromosomal breakpoints in tenosynovial giant cell tumors. Virchows Arch. 2002;441(5):475–80.
19. Beguin J, Locker B, Vielpeau C, Souquieres G. Pigmented villonodular synovitis of the knee: results from 13 cases. Arthroscopy. 1989;5(1):62–4.
20. de St. Aubain Somerhausen N. Diffuse-type giant cell tumour. In: Fletcher C, Unni K, Mertens F, editors. Pathology and genetics of tumours of soft tissue and bone (Series). Lyon: IARC; 2002.
21. Dorwart RH, Genant HK, Johnston WH, Morris JM. Pigmented villonodular synovitis of the shoulder: radiologic-pathologic assessment. AJR Am J Roentgenol. 1984;143(4):886–8.
22. Dines JS, DeBerardino TM, Wells JL, Dodson CC, Shindle M, DiCarlo EF, et al. Long-term follow-up of surgically treated localized pigmented villonodular synovitis of the knee. Arthroscopy. 2007;23(9):930–7.
23. Breimer CW, Freiberger RH. Bone lesions associated with villonodular synovitis. Am J Roentgenol Radium Ther Nucl Med. 1958;79(4):618–29.
24. Ottaviani S, Ayral X, Dougados M, Gossec L. Pigmented villonodular synovitis: a retrospective single-center study of 122 cases and review of the literature. Semin Arthritis Rheum. 2011;40(6): 539–46.

25. Zwass A, Abdelwahab IF, Klein MJ. Case report 463: pigmented villonodular synovitis (PVNS) of knee. Skeletal Radiol. 1988; 17(1):81–4.
26. Sharma H, Rana B, Mahendra A, Jane MJ, Reid R. Outcome of 17 pigmented villonodular synovitis (PVNS) of the knee at 6 years mean follow-up. Knee. 2007;14(5):390–4.
27. Flandry F, McCann SB, Hughston JC, Kurtz DM. Roentgenographic findings in pigmented villonodular synovitis of the knee. Clin Orthop Relat Res. 1989;247:208–19.
28. Merry P, Williams R, Cox N, King JB, Blake DR. Comparative study of intra-articular pressure dynamics in joints with acute traumatic and chronic inflammatory effusions: potential implications for hypoxic-reperfusion injury. Ann Rheum Dis. 1991; 50(12):917–20.
29. Visuri T, Kiviluoto O. Arthroscopic volume of the knee joint in young male adults. Scand J Rheumatol. 1986;15(3):251–4.
30. Draeger RW, Singh B, Parekh SG. Quantifying normal ankle joint volume: an anatomic study. Indian J Orthop. 2009;43(1):72–5.
31. Yen CH, Leung HB, Tse PY. Effects of hip joint position and intra-capsular volume on hip joint intra-capsular pressure: a human cadaveric model. J Orthop Surg Res. 2009;4:8.
32. Cheng XG, You YH, Liu W, Zhao T, Qu H. MRI features of pigmented villonodular synovitis (PVNS). Clin Rheumatol. 2004;23(1):31–4.
33. Steinbach LS, Neumann CH, Stoller DW, Mills CM, Crues 3rd JV, Lipman JK, et al. MRI of the knee in diffuse pigmented villonodular synovitis. Clin Imaging. 1989;13(4):305–16.
34. Ogilvie-Harris DJ, McLean J, Zarnett ME. Pigmented villonodular synovitis of the knee. The results of total arthroscopic synovectomy, partial, arthroscopic synovectomy, and arthroscopic local excision. J Bone Joint Surg Am. 1992;74(1):119–23.
35. De Ponti A, Sansone V, Malchere M. Result of arthroscopic treatment of pigmented villonodular synovitis of the knee. Arthroscopy. 2003;19(6):602–7.
36. Kim SJ, Choi NH, Lee SC. Tenosynovial giant-cell tumor in the knee joint. Arthroscopy. 1995;11(2):213–5.
37. Ozalay M, Tandogan RN, Akpinar S, Cesur N, Hersekli MA, Ozkoc G, et al. Arthroscopic treatment of solitary benign intra-articular lesions of the knee that cause mechanical symptoms. Arthroscopy. 2005;21(1):12–8.
38. Berger B, Ganswindt U, Bamberg M, Hehr T. External beam radiotherapy as postoperative treatment of diffuse pigmented villonodular synovitis. Int J Radiat Oncol Biol Phys. 2007;67(4): 1130–4.
39. Horoschak M, Tran PT, Bachireddy P, West RB, Mohler D, Beaulieu CF, et al. External beam radiation therapy enhances local control in pigmented villonodular synovitis. Int J Radiat Oncol Biol Phys. 2009;75(1):183–7.
40. O'Sullivan B, Cummings B, Catton C, Bell R, Davis A, Fornasier V, et al. Outcome following radiation treatment for high-risk pigmented villonodular synovitis. Int J Radiat Oncol Biol Phys. 1995;32(3):777–86.
41. Blanco CE, Leon HO, Guthrie TB. Combined partial arthroscopic synovectomy and radiation therapy for diffuse pigmented villonodular synovitis of the knee. Arthroscopy. 2001;17(5):527–31.
42. Schwartz HS, Unni KK, Pritchard DJ. Pigmented villonodular synovitis. A retrospective review of affected large joints. Clin Orthop Relat Res. 1989;247:243–55.
43. Akinci O, Akalin Y, Incesu M, Eren A. Long-term results of surgical treatment of pigmented villonodular synovitis of the knee. Acta Orthop Traumatol Turc. 2011;45(3):149–55.
44. Mankin H, Trahan C, Hornicek F. Pigmented villonodular synovitis of joints. J Surg Oncol. 2011;103(5):386–9.
45. Ozturk H, Bulut O, Oztemur Z, Bulut S. Pigmented villonodular synovitis managed by Yttrium 90 after debulking surgery. Saudi Med J. 2008;29(8):1197–200.
46. Shabat S, Kollender Y, Merimsky O, Isakov J, Flusser G, Nyska M, et al. The use of surgery and yttrium 90 in the management of extensive and diffuse pigmented villonodular synovitis of large joints. Rheumatology (Oxford). 2002;41(10):1113–8.
47. Kat S, Kutz R, Elbracht T, Weseloh G, Kuwert T. Radiosynovectomy in pigmented villonodular synovitis. Nuklearmedizin. 2000; 39(7):209–13.
48. Crotty JM, Monu JU, Pope Jr TL. Synovial osteochondromatosis. Radiol Clin North Am. 1996;34(2):327–42, xi.
49. Dorfman HD, Czerniak B. Synovial lesions. In: Dorfman HD, Czerniak B, editors. Bone tumors (Series). St. Louis, MO: Mosby; 1998.
50. Fanburg-Smith JC. Cartilage and bone-forming tumors and tumor-like lesions. In: Miettinen M, editor. Diagnostic soft tissue pathology (Series). Philadelphia, PA: Churchill-Livingstone; 2003.
51. Jaffe HL. Tumours and tumorous conditions of bones and joints. 1st ed. Philadelphia, PA: Lea & Fabiger; 1958.
52. Felbel J, Gresser U, Lohmoller G, Zollner N. Familial synovial chondromatosis combined with dwarfism. Hum Genet. 1992;88(3):351–4.
53. McKenzie G, Raby N, Ritchie D. A pictorial review of primary synovial osteochondromatosis. Eur Radiol. 2008;18(11):2662–9.
54. Murphey MD, Vidal JA, Fanburg-Smith JC, Gajewski DA. Imaging of synovial chondromatosis with radiologic-pathologic correlation. Radiographics. 2007;27(5):1465–88.
55. Nakanishi S, Sakamoto K, Yoshitake H, Kino K, Amagasa T, Yamaguchi A. Bone morphogenetic proteins are involved in the pathobiology of synovial chondromatosis. Biochem Biophys Res Commun. 2009;379(4):914–9.
56. Mertens F, Jonsson K, Willen H, Rydholm A, Kreicbergs A, Eriksson L, et al. Chromosome rearrangements in synovial chondromatous lesions. Br J Cancer. 1996;74(2):251–4.
57. Sciot R, Dal Cin P, Bellemans J, Samson I, Van den Berghe H, Van Damme B. Synovial chondromatosis: clonal chromosome changes provide further evidence for a neoplastic disorder. Virchows Arch. 1998;433(2):189–91.
58. Sperling BL, Angel S, Stoneham G, Chow V, McFadden A, Chibbar R. Synovial chondromatosis and chondrosarcoma: a diagnostic dilemma. Sarcoma. 2003;7(2):69–73.
59. Davis RI, Foster H, Arthur K, Trewin S, Hamilton PW, Biggart DJ. Cell proliferation studies in primary synovial chondromatosis. J Pathol. 1998;184(1):18–23.
60. Milgram JW. Synovial osteochondromatosis: a histopathological study of thirty cases. J Bone Joint Surg Am. 1977;59(6): 792–801.
61. Villacin AB, Brigham LN, Bullough PG. Primary and secondary synovial chondrometaplasia: histopathologic and clinicoradiologic differences. Hum Pathol. 1979;10(4):439–51.
62. Seckley J, Anderson SG, Snow TM, Benjamin M. A rare case of polyarticular synovial osteochondromatosis. J Anat. 2002; 200(5):524.
63. Maurice H, Crone M, Watt I. Synovial chondromatosis. J Bone Joint Surg Br. 1988;70(5):807–11.
64. Murphy FP, Dahlin DC, Sullivan CR. Articular synovial chondromatosis. J Bone Joint Surg. 1962;44(1):77–86.
65. Jesalpura JP, Chung HW, Patnaik S, Choi HW, Kim JI, Nha KW. Arthroscopic treatment of localized synovial chondromatosis of the posterior knee joint. Orthopedics. 2010;33(1):49.
66. Kyung BS, Lee SH, Han SB, Park JH, Kim CH, Lee DH. Arthroscopic treatment of synovial chondromatosis at the knee posterior septum using a trans-septal approach: report of two cases. Knee. 2012;19(5):732–5.
67. Bozkurt M, Ugurlu M, Dogan M, Tosun N. Synovial chondromatosis of four compartments of the knee: medial and lateral tibiofemoral spaces, patellofemoral joint and proximal tibiofibular joint. Knee Surg Sports Traumatol Arthrosc. 2007;15(6):753–5.

68. Church JS, Breidahl WH, Janes GC. Recurrent synovial chondromatosis of the knee after radical synovectomy and arthrodesis. J Bone Joint Surg Br. 2006;88(5):673–5.

69. Pengatteeri YH, Park SE, Lee HK, Lee YS, Gopinathan P, Han CW. Synovial chondromatosis of the posterior cruciate ligament managed by a posterior-posterior triangulation technique. Knee Surg Sports Traumatol Arthrosc. 2007;15(9):1121–4.

70. Roulot E, Le Viet D. Primary synovial osteochondromatosis of the hand and wrist. Report of a series of 21 cases and literature review. Rev Rhum Engl Ed. 1999;66(5):256–66.

71. Trias A, Quintana O. Synovial chondrometaplasia: review of world literature and a study of 18 Canadian cases. Can J Surg. 1976;19(2):151–8.

72. Butt SH, Muthukumar T, Cassar-Pullicino VN, Mangham DC. Primary synovial osteochondromatosis presenting as constrictive capsulitis. Skeletal Radiol. 2005;34(11):707–13.

73. Resnick D. Tumors and tumor-like lesions of soft tissues. In: Resnick D, editor. Diagnosis of bone and joint disorders (Series). 4th ed. Philadelphia, PA: Saunders; 2002.

74. Unni KK, Inwards CY, Bridge JA, Kindblom LG, Wold LE. Synovial tumors. In (Editor) Unni K. Krishnan, published by the American Registry of Pathology, ISBN #9781881041931. Tumors of the bone and joints (Series). 4th ed. Silver Spring, MD: ARP; 2005.

75. Weiss SW, Goldblum JR. Cartilaginous soft tissue tumors. In (Editor) Sharon W. Weiss, published by Mosby, ISBN #0323012000. Enzinger and Weiss's soft tissue tumors (Series). 4th ed. Philadelphia, PA: Mosby; 2001.

76. Garner HW, Bestic JM. Benign synovial tumors and proliferative processes. Semin Musculoskelet Radiol. 2013;17(2):177–8.

77. Dunn EJ, McGavran MH, Nelson P, Greer 3rd RB. Synovial chondrosarcoma. Report of a case. J Bone Joint Surg Am. 1974; 56(4):811–3.

78. Norman A, Steiner GC. Bone erosion in synovial chondromatosis. Radiology. 1986;161(3):749–52.

79. Sheldon PJ, Forrester DM, Learch TJ. Imaging of intraarticular masses. Radiographics. 2005;25(1):105–19.

80. Kramer J, Recht M, Deely DM, Schweitzer M, Pathria MN, Gentili A, et al. MR appearance of idiopathic synovial osteochondromatosis. J Comput Assist Tomogr. 1993;17(5):772–6.

81. Jaganathan S, Goyal A, Gadodia A, Rastogi S, Mittal R, Gamanagatti S. Spectrum of synovial pathologies: a pictorial assay. Curr Probl Diagn Radiol. 2012;41(1):30–42.

82. Kransdorf MJ, Murphey MD. Imaging of soft tissue tumors. 2nd ed. Philadelphia, PA: Lippincott Williams & Wilkins; 2006.

83. Mubashir A, Bickerstaff DR. Synovial osteochondromatosis of the cruciate ligament. Arthroscopy. 1998;14(6):627–9.

84. Ogilvie-Harris DJ, Saleh K. Generalized synovial chondromatosis of the knee: a comparison of removal of the loose bodies alone with arthroscopic synovectomy. Arthroscopy. 1994;10(2):166–70.

85. DePalma AF, Mauler GG. Hemangioma of synovial membrane. Clin Orthop Relat Res. 1964;32:93–9.

86. Mastragostino S, Fares GC. [Synovial hemangioma of the knee]. Riv Anat Patol Oncol. 1959;15:824–36.

87. Halborg A, Hansen H, Sneppen HO. Haemangioma of the knee joint. Acta Orthop Scand. 1968;39(2):209–16.

88. Bouchut ME. Tumeur erectile de l'articulation du genou. Gaz Hop (Paris). 1856;29:379.

89. Bennett GE, Cobey MC. Hemangioma of joints. Arch Surg. 1939;38:487.

90. Sasho T, Nakagawa K, Matsuki K, Hoshi H, Saito M, Ikegawa N, et al. Two cases of synovial haemangioma of the knee joint: Gd-enhanced image features on MRI and arthroscopic excision. Knee. 2011;18(6):509–11.

91. Akgun I, Kesmezacar H, Ogut T, Dervisoglu S. Intra-articular hemangioma of the knee. Arthroscopy. 2003;19(3):E17.

92. Moon NF. Synovial hemangioma of the knee joint. A review of previously reported cases and inclusion of two new cases. Clin Orthop Relat Res. 1973 Jan–Feb;(90):183–90.

93. Ramseier LE, Exner GU. Arthropathy of the knee joint caused by synovial hemangioma. J Pediatr Orthop. 2004;24(1):83–6.

94. Rogalski R, Hensinger R, Loder R. Vascular abnormalities of the extremities: clinical findings and management. J Pediatr Orthop. 1993;13(1):9–14.

95. Suh JT, Cheon SJ, Choi SJ. Synovial hemangioma of the knee. Arthroscopy. 2003;19(7):E27–30.

96. Atkinson TJ, Wolf S, Anavi Y, Wesley R. Synovial hemangioma of the temporomandibular joint: report of a case and review of the literature. J Oral Maxillofac Surg. 1988;46(9):804–8.

97. Winzenberg T, Ma D, Taplin P, Parker A, Jones G. Synovial haemangioma of the knee: a case report. Clin Rheumatol. 2006;25(5):753–5.

98. Yilmaz E, Karakurt L, Ozdemir H, Serin E, Incesu M. [Diffuse synovial hemangioma of the knee: a case report]. Acta Orthop Traumatol Turc. 2004;38(3):224–8.

99. Aalberg JR. Synovial hemangioma of the knee. A case report. Acta Orthop Scand. 1990;61(1):88–9.

100. Cotten A, Flipo RM, Herbaux B, Gougeon F, Lecomte-Houcke M, Chastanet P. Synovial haemangioma of the knee: a frequently misdiagnosed lesion. Skeletal Radiol. 1995;24(4):257–61.

101. Ryd L, Stenstrom A. Hemangioma mimicking meniscal injury. A report on 10 years of knee pain. Acta Orthop Scand. 1989; 60(2):230–1.

102. Devaney K, Vinh TN, Sweet DE. Synovial hemangioma: a report of 20 cases with differential diagnostic considerations. Hum Pathol. 1993;24(7):737–45.

103. Greenspan A, Azouz EM, Matthews 2nd J, Decarie JC. Synovial hemangioma: imaging features in eight histologically proven cases, review of the literature, and differential diagnosis. Skeletal Radiol. 1995;24(8):583–90.

104. Reutter G, Klug S, Rompel O. Synoviales Hämangiom als seltene Ursache eines Hämarthros. Monatsschr Kinderheilkd. 2001; 149(2):150–3.

105. Price NJ, Cundy PJ. Synovial hemangioma of the knee. J Pediatr Orthop. 1997;17(1):74–7.

106. Llauger J, Monill JM, Palmer J, Clotet M. Synovial hemangioma of the knee: MRI findings in two cases. Skeletal Radiol. 1995; 24(8):579–81.

107. Cohen JM, Weinreb JC, Redman HC. Arteriovenous malformations of the extremities: MR imaging. Radiology. 1986;158(2): 475–9.

108. Levine E, Wetzel LH, Neff JR. MR imaging and CT of extrahepatic cavernous hemangiomas. AJR Am J Roentgenol. 1986; 147(6):1299–304.

109. Petasnick JP, Turner DA, Charters JR, Gitelis S, Zacharias CE. Soft-tissue masses of the locomotor system: comparison of MR imaging with CT. Radiology. 1986;160(1):125–33.

110. De Filippo M, Rovani C, Sudberry JJ, Rossi F, Pogliacomi F, Zompatori M. Magnetic resonance imaging comparison of intra-articular cavernous synovial hemangioma and cystic synovial hyperplasia of the knee. Acta Radiol. 2006;47(6):581–4.

111. Okahashi K, Sugimoto K, Iwai M, Tanaka M, Fujisawa Y, Takakura Y. Intra-articular synovial hemangioma; a rare cause of knee pain and swelling. Arch Orthop Trauma Surg. 2004;124(8): 571–3.

112. Tuncbilek N, Karakas HM, Okten OO. Dynamic contrast enhanced MRI in the differential diagnosis of soft tissue tumors. Eur J Radiol. 2005;53(3):500–5.

113. Kroner K, Fruensgaard S. Synovial venous hemangioma of the knee joint. Arch Orthop Trauma Surg. 1989;108(4):253–4.

114. Wirth T, Rauch G, Ruschoff J, Griss P. Synovial haemangioma of the knee joint. Int Orthop. 1992;16(2):130–2.

115. Aynaci O, Ahmetoglu A, Reis A, Turhan AU. Synovial hemangioma in Hoffa's fat pad (case report). Knee Surg Sports Traumatol Arthrosc. 2001;9(6):355–7.

116. Neel MD, Toy PC, Kaste SC, Jenkins JJ, Daw N, Rao BN. Painful limp in a 10-year-old boy. Clin Orthop Relat Res. 2003; 410:326–33.

117. Franco M, Puch JM, Carayon MJ, Bortolotti D, Albano L, Lallemand A. Lipoma arborescens of the knee: report of a case managed by arthroscopic synovectomy. Joint Bone Spine. 2004;71(1):73–5.

118. Arzimanoglu A. Bilateral lateral arborescent lipoma of the knee— a case report. J Bone Joint Surg. 1957;39(4):976–9.

119. Bernstein AD, Jazrawi LM, Rose DJ. Arthroscopic treatment of an intra-articular lipoma of the knee joint. Arthroscopy. 2001; 17(5):539–41.

120. Hill JA, Martin 3rd WR, Milgram JW. Unusual arthroscopic knee lesions: case report of an intra-articular lipoma. J Natl Med Assoc. 1993;85(9):697–9.

121. Gao J, Gillquist J, Messner K. An unusual case of extraarticular lipoma of the knee joint. Knee Surg Sports Traumatol Arthrosc. 1996;4(3):164–6.

122. Margheritini F, Villar RN, Rees D. Intra-articular lipoma of the hip. A case report. Int Orthop. 1998;22(5):328–9.

123. Sola JB, Wright RW. Arthroscopic treatment for lipoma arborescens of the knee—a case report. J Bone Joint Surg. 1998; 80A(1):99–103.

124. Hallel T, Lew S, Bansal M. Villous lipomatous proliferation of the synovial membrane (lipoma arborescens). J Bone Joint Surg. 1988;70A(2):264–70.

125. Blais RE, LaPrade RF, Chaljub G, Adesokan A. The arthroscopic appearance of lipoma arborescens of the knee. Arthroscopy. 1995;11(5):623–7.

126. Pudlowski RM, Gilula LA, Kyriakos M. Intraarticular lipoma with osseous metaplasia: radiographic-pathologic correlation. AJR Am J Roentgenol. 1979;132(3):471–3.

127. Xue J, Alario AJ, Nelson SD, Wu H. Progressive bilateral lipoma arborescens of the knee complicated by juvenile spondyloarthropathy: a case report and review of the literature. Semin Arthritis Rheum. 2013;43(2):259–63.

128. Siva C, Brasington R, Totty W, Sotelo A, Atkinson J. Synovial lipomatosis (Lipoma arborescens) affecting multiple joints in a patient with congenital short bowel syndrome. J Rheumatol. 2002;29(5):1088–92.

129. Davies AP, Blewitt N. Lipoma arborescens of the knee. Knee. 2005;12(5):394–6.

130. Armstrong SJ, Watt I. Lipoma arborescens of the knee. Br J Radiol. 1989;62(734):178–80.

131. Chaljub G, Johnson PR. In vivo MRI characteristics of lipoma arborescens utilizing fat suppression and contrast administration. J Comput Assist Tomogr. 1996;20(1):85–7.

132. Hubscher O, Costanza E, Elsner B. Chronic monoarthritis due to lipoma arborescens. J Rheumatol. 1990;17(6):861–2.

133. Soler R, Rodriguez E, Bargiela A, Da Riba M. Lipoma arborescens of the knee: MR characteristics in 13 joints. J Comput Assist Tomogr. 1998;22(4):605–9.

134. Erol B, Ozyurek S, Guler F, Kose O. Lipoma arborescens of the knee joint. BMJ Case Rep. 2013;2013. pii:bcr2013009271.

135. Grieten M, Buckwalter KA, Cardinal E, Rougraff B. Case report 873. Skeletal Radiol. 1994;23(8):652–5.

136. Kloen P, Keel SB, Chandler HP, Geiger RH, Zarins B, Rosenberg AE. Lipoma arborescens of the knee. J Bone Joint Surg Br. 1998;80(2):298–301.

137. Hirano K, Deguchi M, Kanamono T. Intra-articular synovial lipoma of the knee joint (located in the lateral recess): a case report and review of the literature. Knee. 2007;14(1):63–7.

138. Martinez D, Millner PA, Coral A, Newman RJ, Hardy GJ, Butt WP. Case report 745—synovial lipoma. Skeletal Radiol. 1992;21(6):393–5.

139. Ryu KN, Jaovisidha S, Schweitzer M, Motta AO, Resnick D. MR imaging of lipoma arborescens of the knee joint. AJR Am J Roentgenol. 1996;167(5):1229–32.

140. Kim RS, Song JS, Park SW, Kim L, Park SR, Jung JH, et al. Lipoma arborescens of the knee. Arthroscopy. 2004;20(8): e95–9.

141. Vilanova JC, Barcelo J, Villalon M, Aldoma J, Delgado E, Zapater I. MR imaging of lipoma arborescens and the associated lesions. Skeletal Radiol. 2003;32(9):504–9.

142. Yan CH, Wong JW, Yip DK. Bilateral knee lipoma arborescens: a case report. J Orthop Surg (Hong Kong). 2008;16(1):107–10.

143. Ji JH, Lee YS, Shafi M. Spontaneous recurrent hemarthrosis of the knee joint in elderly patients with osteoarthritis: an infrequent presentation of synovial lipoma arborescens. Knee Surg Sports Traumatol Arthrosc. 2010;18(10):1352–5.

144. Coventry MB, Harrison Jr EG, Martin JF. Benign synovial tumors of the knee: a diagnostic problem. J Bone Joint Surg Am. 1966; 48(7):1350–8.

Part II

The Shoulder

Section Editor: Stephen F. Brockmeier

Diagnostic Shoulder Arthroscopy and Arthroscopic Anatomy

Abdurrahman Kandil and Stephen F. Brockmeier

Overview and Brief History

Shoulder arthroscopy is becoming more popular with advancements in technology and instrumentation. The number of shoulder disorders being treated arthroscopically has increased steadily in recent years.

Shoulder arthroscopy has transformed the way we manage shoulder pathology. Although its popularity has increased in the past two decades, it is not a recent advancement. The first clinical use of shoulder arthroscopy was in 1965 [1]. Over the years, our understanding of shoulder disorders and pathology has improved as a result of this surgical technique. For example, the in situ anatomy of the superior labrum and biceps anchor and the spectrum of pathologic superior labrum anterior and posterior (SLAP) lesions were described by Snyder in 1990 in large part due to shoulder arthroscopy [2]. Shoulder arthroscopy has many uses today, spanning from diagnostic arthroscopy to complex reconstructive procedures. In addition to glenohumeral arthroscopy, subacromial arthroscopy has also expanded in the past two decades. More recently, subdeltoid arthroscopy is being utilized as a newer way to access the anterior shoulder.

Compared to open techniques, shoulder arthroscopy offers many advantages. First, arthroscopy is associated with smaller incisions and less muscle and soft tissue trauma [3]. It provides better visualization of intra-articular structures [3]. Shoulder arthroscopy is associated with decreased pain immediately postoperatively due to smaller incisions and less tissue damage [4]. In addition, many patients prefer

arthroscopic procedures due to improved cosmesis. As with any surgery, a thorough understanding of the normal anatomy and common variations is important, but more so in shoulder arthroscopy as fluid extravasation and swelling may distort anatomic landmarks and potentially lead to increased complications and neurologic injury.

Many decisions need to be made prior to an arthroscopic shoulder procedure. These include selection of anesthesia, patient positioning, and portal placement. This chapter will discuss the various options and considerations for shoulder arthroscopy. In addition, it will aid in portal selection, go over a diagnostic shoulder arthroscopy, and discuss the pertinent applied anatomy of the shoulder.

Anesthesia Options

There are two main anesthesia options for shoulder arthroscopy and both advantages and disadvantages for each.

General anesthesia is the preferred choice for shoulder arthroscopy in many centers for select reasons. It provides for greater control of the surgical field as there is less risk of patient movement. The presence of a secured airway is advantageous in the setting of any unanticipated increase in the duration of a procedure or intraoperative complication. In addition, there is some fear among patients about the nerve injury risks associated with regional anesthesia.

Regional (primarily interscalene block) anesthesia has been shown to be a viable option for the performance of shoulder arthroscopy and is increasing in popularity. There is no difference in surgical and anesthesia time between regional and general anesthesia. In patients in the beach chair position, regional anesthesia has been associated with a decreased rate of desaturations [5]. This supports the notion that regional anesthesia leads to improved cerebral perfusion in patients in the beach chair position. Regional anesthesia provides patients with improved pain control in the early postoperative period and has been shown to decrease narcotic use [6]. Newer techniques such as ultrasonographic

A. Kandil, MD (✉)
Department of Orthopedics, University of Virginia
Medical Center, Charlottesville, VA, USA
e-mail: Ak3ue@hccmail.mcc.virginia.edu

S.F. Brockmeier, MD
Department of Orthopedic Surgery, University of Virginia,
Charlottesville, VA, USA
e-mail: Sfb2e@hcsmail.mcc.virginia.edu

S.F. Brockmeier (ed.), *MRI-Arthroscopy Correlations: A Case-Based Atlas of the Knee, Shoulder, Elbow and Hip*,
DOI 10.1007/978-1-4939-2645-9_11, © Springer Science+Business Media New York 2015

localization and guidance have led to a decrease in the incidence of neurologic complications. Liu et al. looked at a series of 1,169 patients who underwent either ultrasound-guided interscalene or supraclavicular blocks for ambulatory shoulder surgery [7]. They reported a 99.8 % frequency of successful pain relief with a 0 % incidence of vascular puncture or intravascular injection. The incidence of postoperative neurological symptoms (PONS) was very low (0.4 %) and there was a 0 % incidence of permanent nerve injury. They concluded that ultrasound-guided interscalene and supraclavicular blocks are effective and safe for shoulder arthroscopy.

Many arthroscopic shoulder procedures are done with a combination of regional anesthesia and sedation, where sedation is defined as a continuum that ranges from anxiolysis to general anesthesia. The primary aim of sedation is patient comfort. Sedation has been shown to increase patient satisfaction during regional anesthesia [8] and may be considered as a means to increase the patient's acceptance of regional anesthetic techniques.

Indwelling regional catheters are another option for postoperative pain control after shoulder surgery. Bryan et al. looked at outcomes of 144 interscalene catheter placements and found a successful placement rate of 98 % and a complication rate of 0.7 % [9]. Their patients had excellent pain control. This study only looked at inpatients, but outpatient indwelling regional catheters are becoming more popular.

Hypotensive anesthesia is commonly employed in shoulder arthroscopy. It is a safe technique, which can improve visualization in the shoulder joint and diminish bleeding and blood loss during surgery [10]. The goal is to keep the pressure difference between the systolic blood pressure (SBP) and pump pressure (PP) less than 49 mmHg.

After careful evaluation of risks and benefits of each, the choice of anesthesia is ultimately a decision to be made between the patient, surgeon, and anesthesiologist.

Setup and Positioning: Beach Chair vs. Lateral Decubitus

Shoulder arthroscopy is generally performed with the patient in one of two positions: beach chair or lateral decubitus. The decision of which position to use is strongly influenced by the surgeon's preference.

The beach chair position was described by Skyhar et al. in 1988 in an effort to decrease the neuropathies seen with the lateral decubitus position [11]. For the beach chair position, the patient is positioned supine on a bed equipped with a headrest and movable back and leg sections. Care is taken to limit any pressure on nerves and bony prominences. There are a variety of ways to set up the beach chair position, with a number of commercially available tables or torso attachments to a standard OR table. At our institution, the patient is first placed in a reflex position whereby the back and hips are flexed, followed by adjustment of knee flexion with pillows behind the knees, and, finally, placing the back upright. The final position should be a neutrally positioned head, upright back, about 60° of hip flexion, and 30° of knee flexion. The nonsurgical arm is then placed on an armrest and the operative arm is placed on an articulated arm holder which can also provide traction or a static arm stand (Fig. 11.1).

For the lateral decubitus position, the patient is positioned laterally on a padded table with the operative side up. Commonly, a bean bag support is used to aid with positioning and keep the patient stable in the desired position; alter-

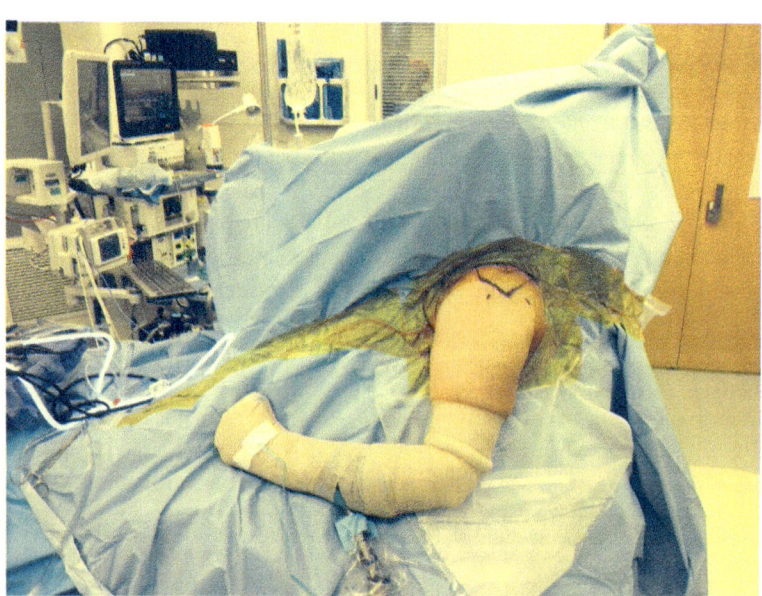

Fig. 11.1 Beach chair position for shoulder arthroscopy

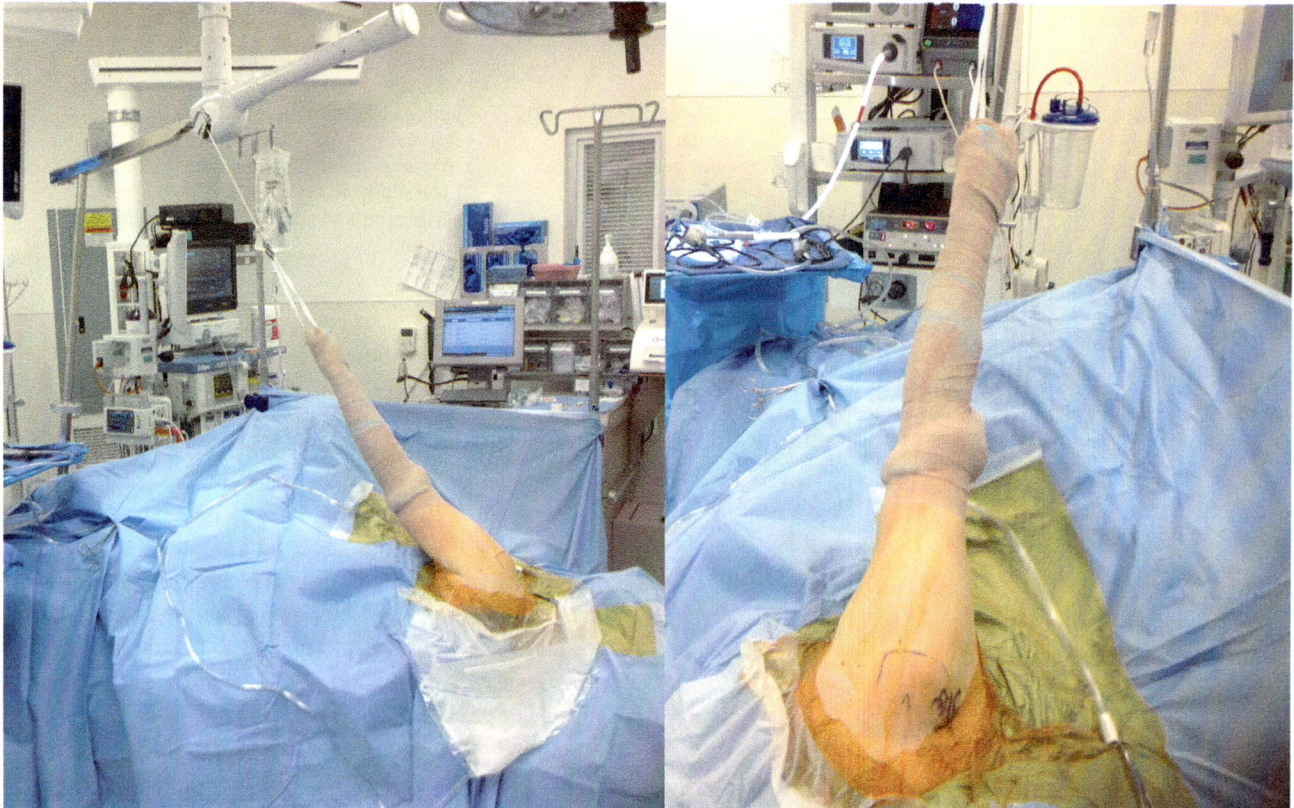

Fig. 11.2 Lateral decubitus position for should arthroscopy

natively, padded anterior and posterior positioner pads that attach directly to the table can be employed to stabilize the patient's torso. Adequate padding is important to prevent skin and neurologic complications. In addition, an axillary roll is placed under the nonoperative arm to limit pressure over the brachial plexus and vascular supply to the limb. The head should be secured in a neutral position and the contralateral elbow and knees in flexion. The surgical arm is then placed in a sling with longitudinal traction. Commonly, a pulley system is used where the surgical arm is suspended in the air by a sling connected by a rope, through a pulley, to a stack of traction weights. The amount of traction weights used is roughly based on the size of the patient (Fig. 11.2). Hennrikus et al. discussed the importance of the ischemic consequences of shoulder traction as it can cause neuropraxia and markedly reduce local and distal tissue perfusion [12]. Regardless of arm position, Peruto et al. suggest traction should be limited to 15–20 lb. [13]. An additional sling attached to the upper arm can be used to assist with lateral traction to the operative extremity. In order to improve orientation and visualization, Gross and Fitzgibbons modified the lateral decubitus position by tilting the table 20–30° posteriorly [14]. This modified position made the glenoid parallel to the floor, thereby improving visualization and making the

relationship of structures more constant. Klein et al. studied the effect of arm position on brachial plexus strain and found that 45° of flexion combined with either 0 or 90° of abduction maximized visibility while minimizing strain [15].

Advantages and disadvantages of the beach chair position and the lateral decubitus position are highlighted in Table 11.1.

Pertinent Shoulder Anatomy and Portal Locations

Following prepping, draping, and setup in either the lateral decubitus or beach chair position, the bony landmarks are palpated and marked. First, mark the posterolateral edge of the acromion. Then, the following landmarks should be marked: scapular spine, acromion, clavicle, coracoid, and AC joint. Accurately identifying and marking these landmarks is important as anatomical correlations and nerve/vascular anatomy is defined with respect to these landmarks. Knowledge of the locations and courses of nerve and vascular structures is important for portal placement and minimizing injuries.

Table 11.1 Beach chair vs. lateral decubitus

	Beach chair	Lateral decubitus
Advantages	– Upright, anatomic position – Decreased incidence of nerve injury – Decreased risk of neurovascular complications during portal placement – Easier conversion to an open procedure utilizing deltopectoral approach – Easier exam under anesthesia – Can mobilize operative arm easier	– Increased visualization of the glenohumeral joint and subacromial space due to joint distraction – No additional traction assistance needed – Lateral distraction of the GH joint allows easier access to the posterior and inferior GH joint
Disadvantages	– Maintenance of cerebral perfusion – Intraoperative hypotension – Airway complications – More difficult to access posterior shoulder pathology – Cost (if using arm holder)	– 10 % incidence of nerve injury with traction – Nonanatomic orientation – Poorer tolerance of regional anesthesia

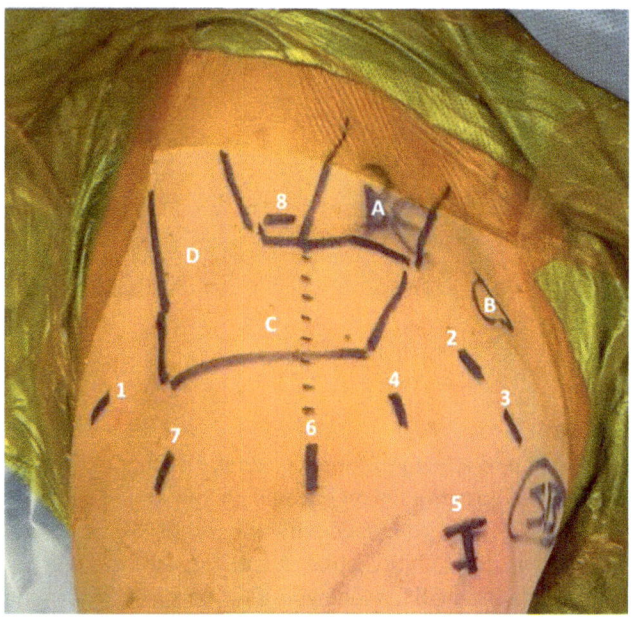

Fig. 11.3 Intraoperative photograph of a prepped and draped shoulder with anatomical landmarks and select portal locations. A, clavicle; B, coracoid; C, acromion; D, scapular spine; 1, posterior portal; 2, anterior portal; 3, low anterior portal for Bankart repair; 4, anterosuperior portal; 5, low anterolateral tenodesis portal; 6, lateral portal; 7, posterolateral portal; 8, Neviaser (supraspinatus) portal

There are three primary portals and many secondary portals that can be used in shoulder arthroscopy cases (Fig. 11.3). These various portals are used for better visualization of certain structures and pathology or for assistance in certain procedures. See Table 11.2 for portal use by common procedures.

Primary Portals

1. **Posterior**: The posterior portal is the primary viewing portal and the first portal established in diagnostic shoulder

arthroscopy. It is located 2 cm inferior and 1–2 cm medial to the posterolateral corner of the acromion. A skin incision is made, followed by a blunted arthroscopic obturator and its sheath directed toward the coracoid tip. This can either pass through the substance of the infraspinatus muscle or pass between the infraspinatus and teres minor. It is usually located in the "soft spot" between the humeral head and the glenoid posteriorly. Proper portal placement is important to decrease injury risk to the axillary and suprascapular nerves. According to a study by Meyer et al., the posterior portal is located an average 49 mm from the axillary nerve and 29 mm from the suprascapular nerve [16].

2. **Anterior**: The anterior portal is an essential working portal in most shoulder arthroscopy procedures. It is located just lateral to the coracoid process and anterior to the AC joint. The portal passes between the pectoralis major and deltoid muscles. The portal is usually placed under direct supervision from the posterior portal with the aid of a spinal needle. The needle is placed within the rotator interval using an outside-in technique. Care must be taken to ensure that all anterior portals are lateral to the coracoid in order to minimize the risk of neurovascular injury to the brachial plexus and axillary vessels. A study by Lo et al. found that, on average, the musculocutaneous nerve lies approximately 33 mm inferior to the tip of the coracoid [17].

3. **Lateral**: The lateral portal, primarily used for procedures in the subacromial space and to address AC pathology, is located 2–3 cm lateral to the lateral edge of the acromion. The portal passes through the deltoid muscle. As with all portals, the location may be adjusted based on pathology. A study by Burkhead et al. found that the axillary nerve can be found as close as 31 mm distal to the anterolateral border of the acromion so care should be taken not to make this portal too inferior [18].

Table 11.2 Portal use by common procedure

Procedure	Posterior	Anterior	Lateral	Posterolateral	Anterosuperior	Anteroinferior (5 o'clock)	Posteroinferior (7 o'clock)	Anterolateral (Port of Wilmington)	Neviaser	Axillary pouch	Inferolateral (pec-portal)
Diagnostic arthroscopy	+	+	−	−	−	−	−	−	−	−	−
Rotator cuff repair	+	+	+	+	−	−	−	−	−	−	−
Subacromial decompression	+	+	+	−	−	−	−	−	−	−	−
Anterior labral repair	+	−	−	−	+/−	+	−	−	−	−	−
Multidirectional instability	+	+	−	−	+/−	+	+	−	−	+	−
SLAP repair	+	+	−	−	+	−	−	+/1	−	−	−
Biceps tenodesis	+	+	−	−	−	−	−	−	−	−	+
Distal clavicle excision	+	+	+	+	−	−	−	−	−	−	−

Secondary Portals

4. **Posterolateral**: The posterolateral portal is primarily utilized for subacromial decompression, rotator cuff, and labral repairs. It is located 2–3 cm lateral to the posterolateral edge of the acromion. Using an outside-in technique, the portal is made and the trocar is aimed medial to the subacromial bursa [16]. Inferior placement places the axillary nerve at risk.

5. **Anterosuperior**: The anterosuperior portal provides good access for procedures involving the anterior capsule. It is created using an outside-in technique at a location halfway between the coracoid and acromion. Placing this portal more laterally can allow access to both the glenohumeral and subacromial spaces. Care should be taken to avoid the cephalic vein and axillary nerve.

6. **Anteroinferior (5 o'clock)**: The anteroinferior portal's main function is to assist in placement of anterior labral repair anchors. It is commonly used together with an anterosuperior portal. It is located slightly inferior to the coracoid and is commonly done through an inside-out technique. The cephalic vein, axillary vein, and axillary artery are all at risk with this portal, especially if placed too inferior. As a result, many surgeons have questioned the safety of this portal.

7. **Posteroinferior (7 o'clock)**: The posteroinferior portal's main function is to assist in placement of posterior labral repair anchors or for loose body removal. This is commonly done through an inside-out technique at the 7 o'clock position of the glenoid. Structures at risk are the suprascapular nerve and artery, axillary nerve, and posterior circumflex humeral artery.

8. **Anterolateral (Port of Wilmington)**: The anterolateral portal is used in the evaluation and repair of posterior SLAP and rotator cuff lesions. It is located 1 cm lateral and 1 cm anterior to the posterolateral corner of the acromion. It pierces the rotator cuff just medial to the musculotendinous junction and is aimed toward the coracoid at an angle 45° to the glenoid surface. Care should be taken to make the portal medial to the musculotendinous junction as rotator cuff tears have been reported with use of cannulas in this portal [19].

9. **Neviaser (supraspinatus)**: The Neviaser portal's main function is to provide the best visualization of the anterior glenoid primarily for SLAP repairs. It is located in the soft spot between the clavicle, acromion, and scapular spine. A needle is placed from this location anteriorly and laterally and goes through the supraspinatus muscle. The suprascapular nerve and artery are at risk with this portal as they are only 3 cm from the supraglenoid tubercle [20].

10. **Axillary pouch**: This is the preferred portal for access to inferior glenohumeral recess and removal of loose bodies.

It is developed by making an incision 2–3 cm inferior to the posterolateral acromion and 2 cm lateral to the posterior viewing portal.

11. **G portal**: Also called the suprascapular nerve (SSN) portal, this portal is used in SSN decompression procedures. This portal is located 7 cm medial to the lateral border of the acromion or 2 cm medial to the Neviaser portal. The obvious structures at risk are the SSN within the suprascapular notch and the suprascapular artery above the transverse scapular ligament.

12. **Pec-portal**: Also called the inferolateral portal, this portal is primarily used in subdeltoid arthroscopy. It is established and is positioned at the inferolateral corner of the subdeltoid space, the junction of the superior margin of the pectoralis major tendon, and the long head of the biceps tendon.

Diagnostic Shoulder Arthroscopy

Diagnostic shoulder arthroscopy should be uniform, comprehensive, and systematic process where all pertinent anatomic structures are visualized and examined. Although the specific order is not important, it is important to make a checklist of the following important structures to ensure completeness. See Fig. 11.4a–i for some intra-articular anatomic structures seen during shoulder arthroscopy.

Glenohumeral Joint

The diagnostic glenohumeral joint arthroscopy can be divided into two portions: The first portion is with the arthroscope in the posterior portal. The second portion is with the arthroscope in the anterior portal. The diagnostic arthroscopy begins with the arthroscope in the posterior portal and a probe in the anterior portal.

The following structures or groups of structures are visualized with the arthroscope in the posterior portal:

1. **Glenoid articular cartilage**: The glenoid is evaluated, noting any chondromalacia or traumatic lesions to the articular surface. A hole in an area of thin articular cartilage in the center of the glenoid may appear to be a defect but is a normal anatomical finding.

2. **Humeral head articular cartilage**: It is important to view the entire humeral head by rotating the shoulder and viewing the entire surface. The bare area is visualized posteroinferiorly on the humeral head. This should be distinguished from a true Hill–Sachs lesion, which has articular cartilage superior and inferior to the area of exposed bone.

3. **Biceps tendon**: Located in the anterosuperior aspect of the joint, the biceps anchor and tendon are evaluated for

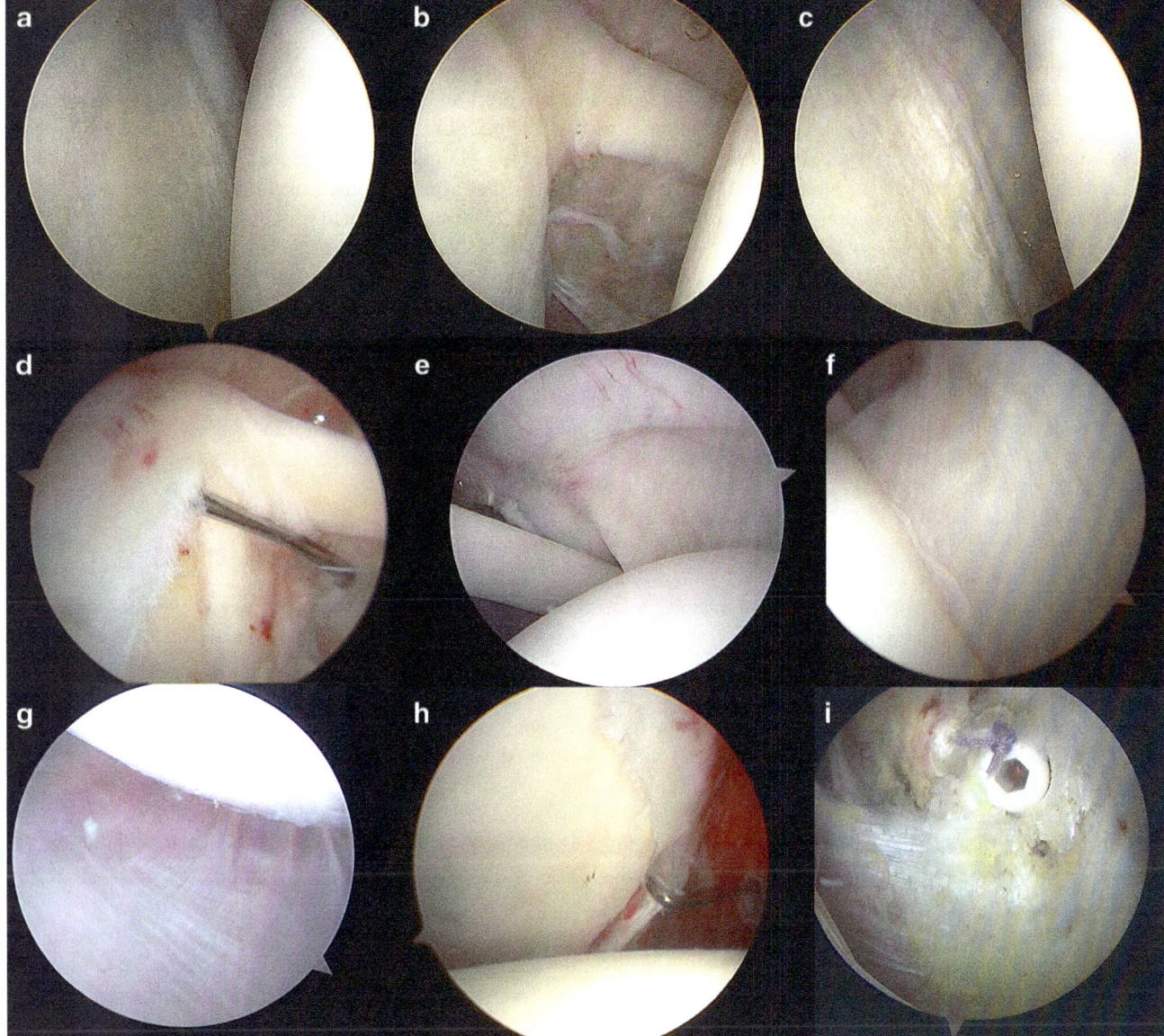

Fig. 11.4 (**a**–**i**) Select intraoperative anatomic structures with patient in beach chair position. (**a**) Glenoid and humeral head articular cartilage. (**b**) Long head of biceps tendon and subscapularis. (**c**) Anterior inferior labrum. (**d**) Superior labrum and long head of biceps tendon origin. (**e**) Biceps sling and anterosuperior rotator cuff insertion. (**f**) Rotator cuff insertion. (**g**) Inferior capsule and recess. (**h**) Posterior labrum tear. (**i**) Arthroscopic biceps tenodesis anchor with pectoralis major insertion

tendinopathy and partial tearing. The biceps tendon can be retracted into the joint to better visualize the extra-articular portion to evaluate any pathology.

4. **Superior labrum**: Should be probed and examined for any tears. A SLAP lesion may be found and should be probed for stability.

5. **Rotator interval with superior and middle glenohumeral ligaments and subscapularis tendon**: These structures can be more clearly visualized by placing the shoulder in various positions to tighten the ligaments or tendons. The superior glenohumeral ligament, which often is a rudimentary structure, may be observed just

inferior to the biceps tendon. A Buford complex, which is a congenital labral variant where the anterosuperior labrum is absent in the 1–3 o'clock position and the MGHL is cord like, is often visualized. The superior tendinous edge ("rolled border") of the subscapularis is examined as is its attachment to the lesser tuberosity of the humerus.

6. **Anterior inferior labrum**: The anterior labrum is examined for fraying or detachment indicating glenohumeral instability. This region is evaluated for detachment, which represents a Bankart tear. Another tool for assessment of shoulder instability is the "drive-through

sign," which is the ability to maneuver the arthroscope in between the humeral head and the glenoid fossa.

7. **Anterior capsule and anterior band of the inferior glenohumeral ligament**: Synovitis or fraying on the anterior capsule indicates repeated trauma or inflammation. The anterior band of the inferior glenohumeral ligament attaches to the glenoid neck between the 2-o'clock and 4-o'clock positions.
8. **Inferior capsule and recess**: This area is assessed for laxity, redundancy, or tearing. In addition, a humeral avulsion (HAGL lesion) may be seen.
9. **Posterior labrum and capsule**: The posterior labrum and capsule are visualized by retracting the arthroscope and pointing it inferiorly.
10. **Rotator cuff supraspinatus attachment**: This is viewed by rotating the arthroscope superiorly. Visualization of this region is aided by positioning the arm in slight abduction and 45° of flexion and applying gentle traction to place the rotator cuff under some tension and open up the viewing space. The rotator cuff insertion into the tuberosity is carefully evaluated for fraying, partial tear, or complete tear of the rotator cuff. Fraying or partial tears of the rotator cuff should be evaluated by examining the thickness with a probe.

The following structures or groups of structures are visualized with the arthroscope in the anterior portal:

1. **Posterior labrum**: This time viewed from the anterior portal, should be smooth with tight attachment to the glenoid. Fraying or subtle clefting in this region can be indicative of a *Kim lesion*, which represents shear injury to the posterior labrum secondary to recurrent posterior subluxations or laxity.
2. **Posterior capsule and rotator cuff**: This should be evaluated for redundancy, synovitis, fraying from instability, or inflammatory processes.
3. **Anterior inferior labrum and the anterior inferior glenohumeral ligament**: Careful observation for the ligamentous insertion to the humerus is indicated to rule out humeral avulsion of the glenohumeral ligament (HAGL).
4. **Middle glenohumeral ligament and medial subscapularis tendon and recess**.
5. **Lateral subscapularis tendon and anterior humeral head and biceps**.

Subacromial Space

The diagnostic shoulder arthroscopy may or may not include evaluation of the subacromial space. The subacromial space is accessed through the posterior portal by redirecting the obturator tip just beneath the posterior acromion and advancing it anteriorly to the region just behind the coracoacromial ligament. After confirming entry into the space, a lateral

portal is established. The subacromial space should be examined thoroughly, which may require partial or subtotal bursectomy to effectively visualize the bursal surface of the rotator cuff and the undersurface of the acromion clearly.

The inferior aspect of the acromion is evaluated. The coracoacromial ligament is then identified. The anterior, lateral, and medial aspects of the acromion are then cleared of the bursal tissue and evaluated for spurring. The acromioclavicular joint is then evaluated and the distal clavicle is brought into view by placing a downward force on the distal clavicle. Afterwards, the arthroscope is pointed downwards and the rotator cuff insertion is carefully evaluated for any tears using a probe. The rotator cuff should be palpated for roughness, fraying, or calcifications. Rotation of the shoulder can aid in visualization of the entire footprint.

Subdeltoid Space

Subdeltoid space arthroscopy is a newer exposure technique for a number of procedures such as biceps tenodesis or transfer, extracompartmental anterior shoulder arthroscopy, and arthroscopic-assisted CC ligament repair or reconstruction. Its popularity has increased in recent years and the technique is best described by O'Brien et al. [21]. The subdeltoid space is extra-articular and defined superiorly by the acromion and coracoacromial ligament, medially by the coracoid and the conjoined tendon, inferiorly by the musculotendinous insertion of the pectoralis major to the humerus, and laterally by the lateral border of the humerus (Fig. 11.5).

First, an inferolateral, or pec-portal, is established and is positioned at the inferolateral corner of the subdeltoid space, the junction of the superior margin of the pectoralis major tendon, and the long head of the biceps tendon. The subdeltoid space is then insufflated with saline and additional portals may be placed to improve visualization and functional access as needed. It is important that incisions only be "skin deep followed by passage of blunt obturator.

It is recommended that this approach only be done in the beach chair position due to inadequate visualization and medial fluid extravasation due to gravity in the lateral decubitus position. First, the operative extremity is positioned in the "90-90-15 position" where the shoulder is flexed 90°, the elbow is flexed 90°, and the arm is abducted 15°. Per O'Brien, this position allows the humeral head to fall posteriorly, which facilitates exposure of the subdeltoid space anteriorly. Second, with the arthroscope in the posterior portal, an anterolateral working portal is established that is 1–2 cm distal to and 1–2 cm posterior to the anterolateral edge of the acromion. This working portal is later converted into a viewing portal. Third, the subdeltoid space is exposed using radiofrequency ablation.

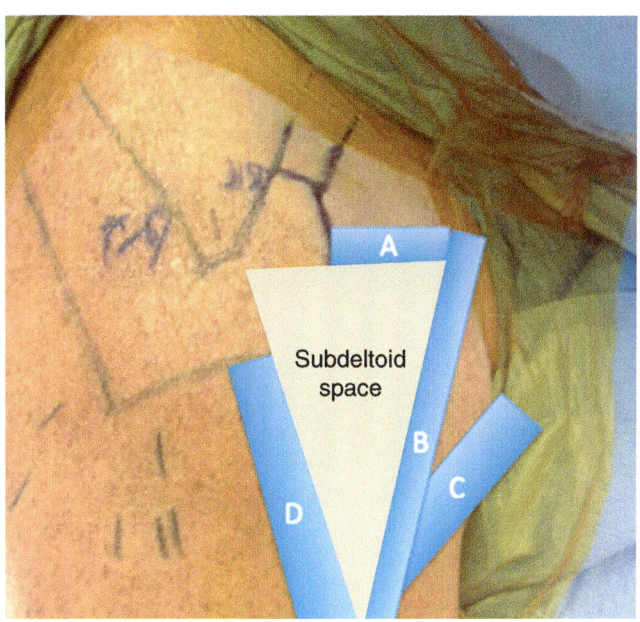

Fig. 11.5 The subdeltoid is defined superiorly by the acromion and coracoacromial ligament (A), medially by the coracoid and the conjoint tendon (B), inferiorly by the musculotendinous insertion of the pectoralis major to the humerus (C), and laterally by the lateral border of the humerus (D)

The following structures are exposed and visualized:

1. Coracoacromial ligament.
2. Coracoid.
3. Conjoint tendon is exposed at its attachment to the coracoid and dissected distally.
4. Pectoralis major tendon is visualized and exposed at its humeral insertion.
5. Long head of the biceps is just medial to the pectoralis major tendon.
6. Humeral shaft is tracked proximally to the anterolateral border of the acromion.

Summary

Shoulder arthroscopy is a common procedure and is becoming more popular with advancements in technology and instrumentation. Glenohumeral, subacromial, and subdeltoid arthroscopy are each tailored to view and treat various shoulder pathologies. Selection of anesthesia, patient positioning, and portal use are important considerations to be made prior to shoulder arthroscopy. The two main anesthesia options are general and regional, and each has its own set of advantages and disadvantages. A combination of both types is often employed where the patient is placed under sedation after a regional block is administered. Patient positioning for shoulder arthroscopy is surgeon dependent and while the beach

chair or lateral decubitus positions can be used for the majority of shoulder arthroscopy procedures, there are some cases where one of the positions can aid in visualization of and access to the desired pathology. Numerous portals have been described for shoulder arthroscopy and the specific shoulder procedure usually guides portal selection. The surgeon should be wary of neurovascular risks when making the portals, thereby emphasizing the importance of a thorough understanding of the normal anatomy and common variations in shoulder arthroscopy. In conclusion, knowledge of the different preoperative and intraoperative options in shoulder arthroscopy can significantly aid in the visualization and treatment of shoulder pathology.

References

1. Andren L, Lundberg BJ. Treatment of rigid shoulders by joint distention during arthroscopy. Acta Orthop Scand. 1965;36:45–53.
2. Snyder SJ, Karzel RP, Del Pizzo W. SLAP lesion of the shoulder. Arthroscopy. 1990;6:274–9.
3. Yamaguchi K, Levine WN, Marra G, Galatz LM, Klepps S, Flatow EL. Transitioning to arthroscopic rotator cuff repair: the pros and cons. Instr Course Lect. 2003;52:81–92.
4. Bishop JY, Sprague M, Gelber J. Interscalene regional anesthesia for shoulder surgery. J Bone Joint Surg Am. 2005;87(5):974–9.
5. Yadeau JT, Liu SS, Bang H. Cerebral oximetry desaturation during shoulder surgery performed in a sitting position under regional anesthesia. Can J Anaesth. 2011;58(11):986–92.
6. Wu CL, Rouse LM, Chen JM, Miller RJ. Comparison of postoperative pain in patients receiving interscalene block or general anesthesia for shoulder surgery. Orthopedics. 2002;25:45–8.
7. Liu SS, Gordon MA, Shaw PM, Wilfred S, Shetty T, Yadeau JT. A prospective clinical registry of ultrasound-guided regional anesthesia for ambulatory shoulder surgery. Anesth Analg. 2010;111(3): 617–23.
8. Wu CL, Naqibuddin M, Fleisher LA. Measurement of patient satisfaction as an outcome of regional anesthesia and analgesia: a systematic review. Reg Anesth Pain Med. 2001;26:196–208.
9. Bryan NA, Swenson JD, Greis PE, Burks RT. Indwelling interscalene catheter use in an outpatient setting for shoulder surgery: technique, efficacy, and complications. JSES. 2007;16(4):388–95.
10. Rains DD, Rooke GA, Wahl CJ. Pathomechanisms and complications related to patient positioning and anesthesia during shoulder arthroscopy. Arthroscopy. 2011;27(4):532–41.
11. Skyhar MJ, Altchek DW, Warren RF, Wickiewicz TL, O'Brien SJ. Shoulder arthroscopy with the patient in the beach-chair position. Arthroscopy. 1988;4(4):256–9.
12. Hennrikus WL, Mapes RC, Bratton MW, Lapoint JM. Lateral traction during shoulder arthroscopy: Its effect on tissue perfusion measured by pulse oximetry. Am J Sports Med. 1995;23(4): 444–6.
13. Peruto CM, Ciccotti MG, Cohen SB. Shoulder arthroscopy positioning: lateral decubitus versus beach chair. Arthroscopy. 2009; 25(8):891–6.
14. Gross RM, Fitzgibbons TC. Shoulder arthroscopy: a modified approach. Arthroscopy. 1985;1(3):156–9.
15. Klein AH, France JC, Mutschler TA, Fu FH. Measurement of brachial plexus strain in arthroscopy of the shoulder. Arthroscopy. 1987;3:35–64.

16. Meyer M, Graveleau N, Hardy P, Landreau P. Anatomic risks of shoulder arthroscopy portals: anatomic cadaveric study of 12 portals. Arthroscopy. 2007;23(5):529–36.
17. Lo IK, Burkhart SS, Parten PM. Surgery about the coracoid: neurovascular structures at risk. Arthroscopy. 2004;20(6): 591–5.
18. Burkhead Jr WZ, Scheinberg RR, Box G. Surgical anatomy of the axillary nerve. J Shoulder Elbow Surg. 1992;1(1):31–6.
19. Stephenson DR, Hurt JH, Mair SD. Rotator cuff injury as a complication of portal placement for superior labrum anterior-posterior repair. J Shoulder Elbow Surg. 2012;21(10):1316–21.
20. Bigliani LU, Dalsey RM, McCann PD, April EW. An anatomical study of the suprascapular nerve. Arthroscopy. 1990;6(4):301–5.
21. O'Brien SJ, Taylor SA, DiPietro JR, Newman AM, Drakos MC, Voos JE. The arthroscopic "subdeltoid approach" to the anterior shoulder. J Shoulder Elbow Surg. 2013;22:e6–10.

Anterior Shoulder Instability

12

Kathryne J. Stabile, E. Michael Chester,
Julie A. Neumann, and Dean C. Taylor

Introduction

Shoulder instability can present as symptomatic and asymptomatic laxity, dislocation, and subluxation. This mixed clinical presentation can be the result of a variety of causes. Specifically, for anterior shoulder instability, there are several mechanisms that contribute to instability. These include soft tissue injuries to the anterior and posterior capsule, glenohumeral ligaments, biceps tendon, and articular cartilage and bony injuries to the humeral head or glenoid. These injuries typically occur with initial shoulder dislocation and can also occur with subsequent dislocation and subluxation events. Diagnosis is paramount to determining treatment algorithm as these associated injuries can increase with time and repeated instability events [1–3].

The focus of treatment is to improve stability of the shoulder and minimize pathologic translation. To accomplish these goals, the surgeon must address both the associated bony and soft tissue structures that are injured. The types of associated injuries have three main categories: labral and cartilage, fractures and bone defects, and combinations of both. Labral and cartilage injuries include Bankart lesions, humeral avulsions of the glenohumeral ligament (HAGL), glenoid labral articular defect (GLAD), and anterior labral periosteal sleeve avulsion (ALPSA). Fractures and bone defects primarily consist of Hill–Sachs lesions, bony Bankarts, as well as greater and lesser tuberosity fractures [4].

K.J. Stabile, MD, MS (✉) • J.A. Neumann, MD
D.C. Taylor, MD
Department of Orthopedic Surgery, Duke University
Medical Center, Durham, NC, USA
e-mail: kastabile@hotmail.com; Julie.neumann.md@gmail.com;
Dean.taylor@duke.edu

E.M. Chester, MD
Department of Radiology, Duke University Medical Center,
Durham, NC, USA
e-mail: Mike.chester@dm.duke.edu

Due to the complexity of cases, not every type of injury can be illustrated in this chapter. There are however some key points that will guide the clinician in diagnosis and management of anterior shoulder instability. The key physical exam, MRI, and surgical findings are highlighted in the following four cases: (1) Bankart with inverted labrum, (2) glenoid labral articular defect (GLAD), (3) Bankart, and (4) Hill–Sachs with bony Bankart.

Case 1: Bankart with Inverted Anterior Labrum

History/Exam

The patient is a 15-year-old right-hand-dominant male who sustained a left shoulder dislocation during football practice requiring a manual reduction. He subsequently had two additional dislocations, but no subluxation events. His physical exam in the clinic revealed a range of motion: 170° of flexion (passive), 90° of abduction, and 50° of external rotation at the side. Provocative maneuvers included the following: anterior apprehension, relocation, and load and shift (anterior).

At the time of surgery (6 weeks after his initial dislocation), his exam under anesthesia revealed a grade 2 anterior load shift and a grade 2 posterior load shift. There was 1 cm of inferior humeral head translation in internal rotation and 1 cm in external rotation.

Imaging

Initial left shoulder radiographs were normal without evidence of shoulder dislocation or fracture. The patient then had an interval shoulder dislocation, which was reduced prior to additional imaging. A complete shoulder MR arthrogram was then obtained with axial, oblique, and oblique coronal fat-suppressed T2-weighted FSE sequences as well

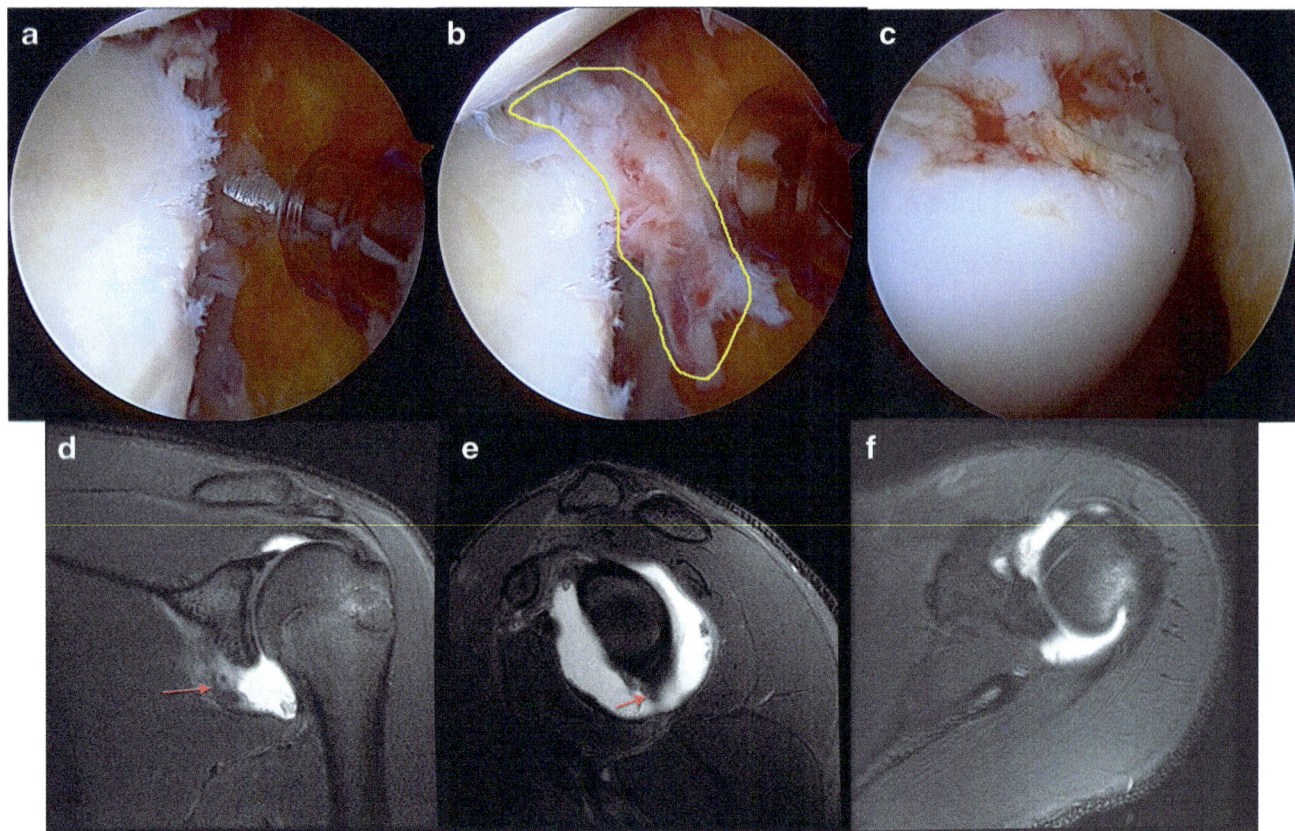

Fig. 12.1 (**a**) The anterior labrum was detached from approximately 6 o'clock to 11 o'clock and was folded and inverted medially and inferiorly. (**b**) The labrum is outlined in *yellow* after being freed from the glenoid rim and scapular neck. (**c**) Arthroscopic view of medium-sized Hill–Sachs lesion. (**d**) T2 fat-suppressed oblique coronal left shoulder MR arthrogram. The anteroinferior labrum (*arrow*) is abnormal in signal and folded, inverted, and flipped medially and inferiorly in respect to the glenoid. (**e**) T2 fat-suppressed oblique sagittal left shoulder MR arthrogram. There is abnormal T2 signal involving the anteroinferior labrum which is folded, inverted, and flipped medially and inferiorly in respect to the glenoid (*arrow*). (**f**) T2 fat-suppressed axial left shoulder MR arthrogram. There is marrow edema surrounding a moderate-sized well-defined impaction fracture of the posterolateral humeral head

as oblique sagittal T1-weighted sequences. The shoulder MR demonstrated evidence of an associated Bankart lesion with detachment of the anteroinferior labrum which was folded, inverted, and displaced medially and inferiorly as seen on the T2 oblique coronal and sagittal series (Fig. 12.1d, e). In addition, there was a recent anterior shoulder dislocation with a moderate-sized Hill–Sachs lesion (Fig. 12.1f).

Arthroscopy

The patient was taken to the operating room and placed in the lateral decubitus position. A standard diagnostic arthroscopy of the right shoulder was completed. Arthroscopic findings demonstrated a medium-sized Hill–Sachs lesion (Fig. 12.1c). The anterior labrum was detached from approx-

imately 6 o'clock to 11 o'clock and was folded and inverted medially and inferiorly (Fig. 12.1a, b). There was a split in the labrum and capsule inferiorly and the labrum was split superiorly. The posterior labrum was normal. The biceps anchor and tendon were normal. The rotator cuff tendons were normal.

To repair this injury, the anterior capsulolabral complex was mobilized from the glenoid rim and scapular neck. The glenoid rim and scapular neck were abraded with an arthroscopic shaver to create a bleeding bony surface. The inferior capsular split was repaired with a #2 high-strength, polyethylene core suture passed with a suture lasso. The labrum was then repaired back to the glenoid rim using three 2.4 mm biocomposite suture anchors. The sutures were passed using a suture lasso and then tied in a simple fashion arthroscopically. Superiorly, the labrum and capsule were repaired utilizing the two suture

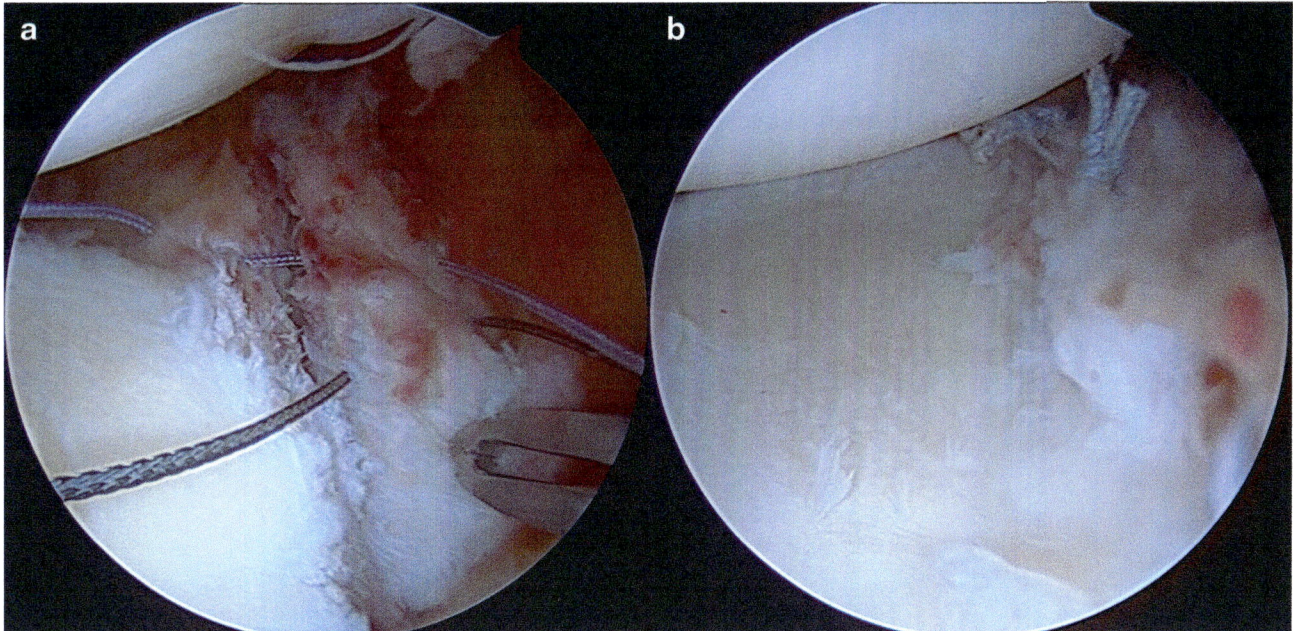

Fig. 12.2 (**a**) Suture passing through the labrum. (**b**) Stable repair construct

limbs from the anchor. This resulted in stable repair of the labrum and restoration of the normal tension within the inferior glenohumeral ligament complex (Fig. 12.2a, b).

Discussion

This case illustrates the importance of careful MRI and arthroscopic evaluation. The inverted labrum was not initially appreciated on MRI. It was not until further evaluation that the labrum was found to be inverted and scarred to the glenoid rim and scapular neck.

There are two variants of the soft tissue Bankart lesion, Perthes and ALPSA. In a Perthes lesion the scapular periosteum remains intact and is stripped medially. In the anterior labroligamentous periosteal sleeve avulsion (ALPSA), the anterior scapular periosteum is not disrupted. This allows the capsulolabral complex to displace medially and rotate inferiorly on the scapular neck. In the case of an ALPSA lesion, the capsulolabral junction scars medially on the scapular neck. In the Perthes and Bankart lesions, the capsulolabral complexes do not displace medially [5]. This distinction is important when determining the anatomy on MRI and arthroscopically. It is also important to distinguish with regard to patient outcomes. Reports for recurrent instability after arthroscopic repair of an ALPSA lesion are twice as high compared with Bankart lesions [4, 6].

Case 2: GLAD

History/Exam

The patient is a 28-year-old right-hand-dominant male who injured his right shoulder when falling forward during a landing while skydiving. He presented to the clinic 5 weeks after this injury due to persistent right shoulder pain. He did not describe a dislocation or subluxation.

Physical exam in the clinic revealed range of motion: forward elevation 145°, external rotation 50°, internal rotation T10, and IGHE 90°. Provocative maneuvers included anterior apprehension, posterior apprehension, and 1+ anterior drawer, with an otherwise normal exam.

At the time of surgery his exam under anesthesia revealed 145° of forward elevation, 80° of external rotation in abduction, 40° of internal rotation, and 75° of external rotation with the arm at the side. There was a 1+ anterior load shift and a 1+ posterior load shift. There was a 0.5 cm sulcus sign in internal rotation, neutral rotation, and external rotation.

Imaging

Initial right shoulder radiographs of the patient were unremarkable. The patient then underwent an MR arthrogram of the right shoulder with axial and oblique coronal fat-saturated

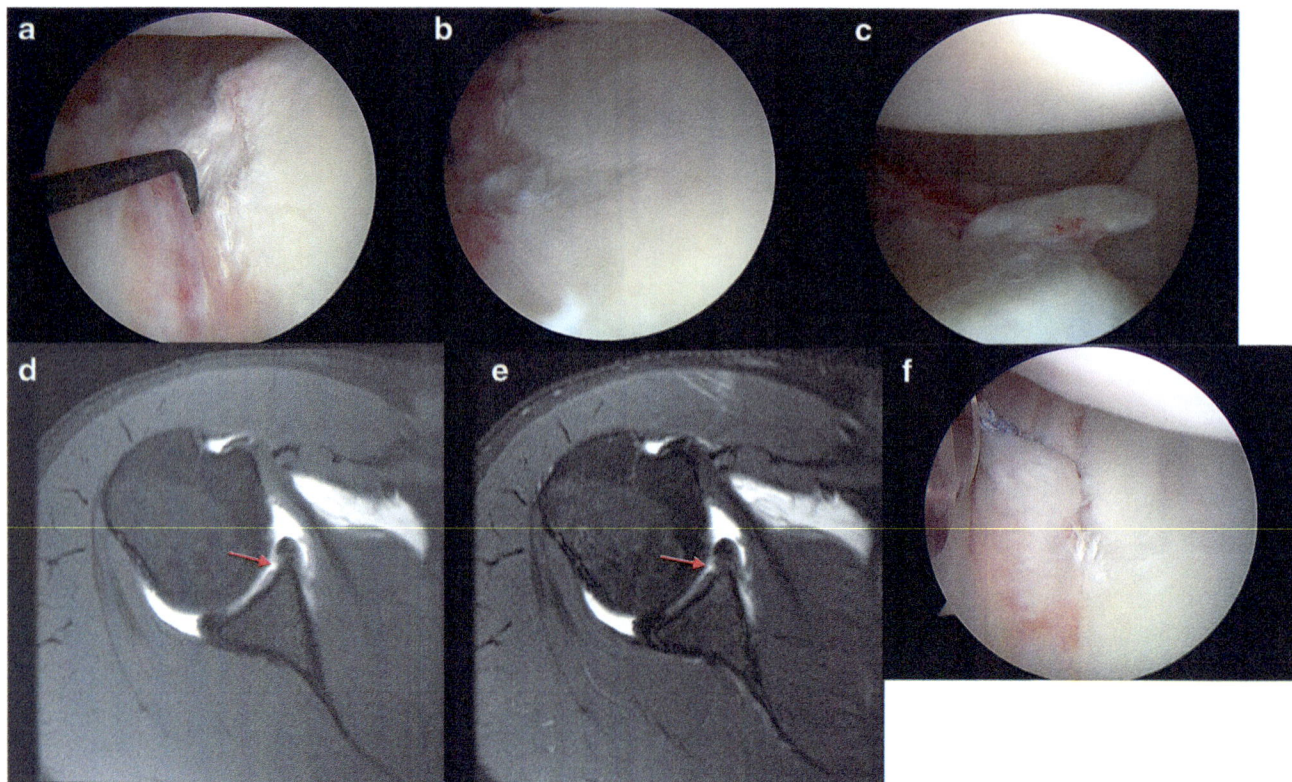

Fig. 12.3 (**a**) Detachment of the anterior labrum associated with the GLAD lesion. (**b**) Articular cartilage defect associated with GLAD lesion. (**c**) Articular cartilage flap flipped into the axillary pouch. (**d**) Axial T1 fat-suppressed right shoulder MR arthrogram. There is a focal chondral defect involving the anteroinferior glenoid. There is faint signal abnormality extending into the anteroinferior labrum consistent with a partial tear. (**e**) Axial T2 fat-suppressed right shoulder MR arthrogram. There is a focal chondral defect involving the anteroinferior glenoid. There is faint signal abnormality extending into the antero-inferior labrum consistent with a partial tear. (**f**) Suture was passed through the labrum and tied reapproximating the labrum into the defect resulting in stable fixation

T1- and T2-weighted imaging and oblique sagittal T1-, fat-saturated T1-, and fat-saturated T2-weighted imaging. MR demonstrated a partial tear of the anteroinferior labrum with a focal chondral defect at the 4–6 o'clock position consistent with a glenolabral articular disruption (GLAD)-type lesion shown in Fig. 12.3d, e. There was also degenerative fraying of the posterosuperior labrum (not shown).

Arthroscopy

The patient was taken to the operating room and placed in the lateral decubitus position. A standard diagnostic arthroscopy of the right shoulder was completed. This demonstrated normal glenoid and humeral articular cartilage in the areas away from the lesion. The biceps tendon and rotator cuff tendons were normal. The posterior labrum had some fraying but was intact in a meniscoid configuration. The anterior–inferior labrum had an articular cartilage and labral flap that was flipped into the axillary pouch (Fig. 12.3b, c). There was a partial detachment of the anterior labrum associated with this GLAD lesion (Fig. 12.3a). There was no sublabral hole.

With an arthroscopic shaver, the flap of the articular cartilage and anterior–inferior labrum was resected. The remaining defect in the anterior–inferior articular cartilage of the glenoid as well as detachment of the labrum was further explored. We elected to repair the anterior–inferior labrum into the glenoid defect. A single 3.0 mm PEEK suture anchor was placed into the defect. Suture was passed through the labrum which was then tied reapproximating the labrum into the defect resulting in stable fixation (Fig. 12.3f).

Discussion

With GLAD lesions the articular cartilage defect can be subtle and often missed on imaging. A high index of suspicion is needed to appreciate the articular cartilage defect. Additionally, the piece of cartilage from the defect can occasionally be seen as in Fig. 12.3b, c. It is important to identify the articular cartilage lesion to prepare for possible microfracture or other treatment that may be necessary at the time of arthroscopy.

Case 3: Bankart

History/Exam

The patient is a 34-year-old left-hand-dominant male who sustained a traumatic right shoulder dislocation approximately 1 year prior to presentation during a paint ball match. He subsequently had four dislocations. His most recent dislocation was from sneezing, but he was able to relocate his shoulder within a few minutes.

Physical exam in the clinic revealed a normal range of motion with no generalized laxity. Provocative maneuvers included anterior apprehension and anterior relocation, 1+ load and shift (anterior), and 1+ load and shift (posterior) with a 1+ sulcus (neutral).

At the time of surgery his exam under anesthesia revealed 150° of forward elevation, 90° of external rotation in abduction, 30° of internal rotation, and 30° of external rotation

with the arm at the side. There was a grade 2 anterior load shift and a grade 2 posterior load shift. There was 0 cm of inferior humeral head translation in internal rotation and 0 cm in external rotation.

Imaging

Initial shoulder radiographs were unremarkable for fracture or dislocation. A complete MRI arthrogram of the shoulder with axial, oblique, sagittal, and oblique coronal fat-suppressed T2 FSE sequences as well as oblique sagittal T1-weighted sequence was obtained. The MRI arthrogram demonstrated irregularity/partial detachment of the antero-inferior labrum with possible scarring consistent with a labral Bankart lesion (Fig. 12.4e). In addition, there was increased marrow signal in the posterolateral humeral head consistent with a small Hill–Sachs impaction fracture (Fig. 12.4d).

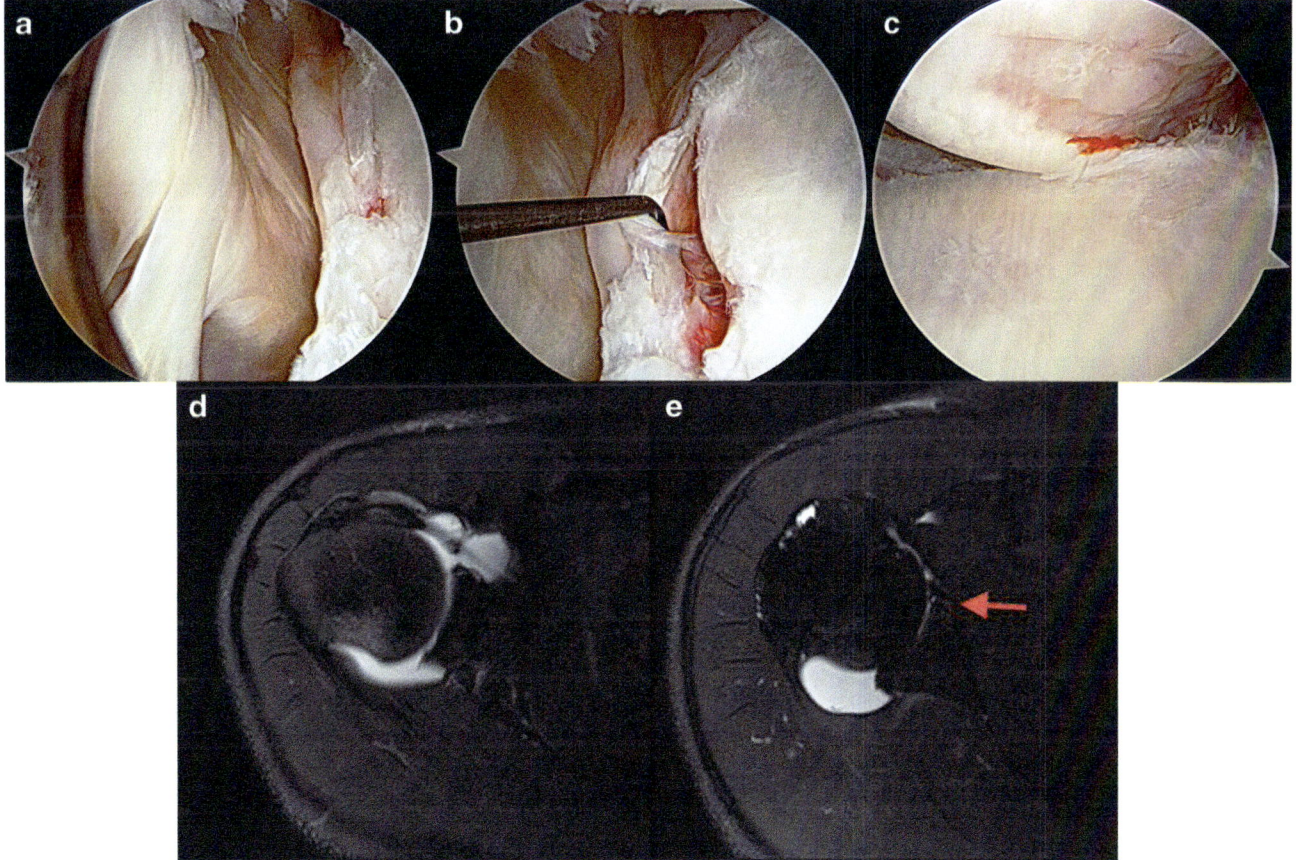

Fig. 12.4 (**a, b**) The anterior labrum was detached from approximately 1 o'clock to 5 o'clock. (**c**) Medium-sized Hill–Sachs. (**d**) Axial T2 fat-suppressed right shoulder MR arthrogram. There is abnormal flattening of the posterolateral humeral head with associated increased marrow signal consistent with a Hill–Sachs impaction fracture. (**e**) Axial T2 fat-suppressed right shoulder MR arthrogram. There is abnormal T2 signal between the glenoid and the anteroinferior labrum consistent with a labral Bankart lesion (*arrow*)

Arthroscopy

The patient was taken to the operating room and placed in the lateral decubitus position. Arthroscopic findings demonstrated a medium-sized Hill–Sachs lesion (Fig. 12.4c). The anterior labrum was detached from approximately 1 o'clock to 5 o'clock (Fig. 12.4a, b). The posterior labrum was normal. The biceps anchor and tendon were normal. The subscapularis tendon was normal. There was a partial (20 %) articular sided tear of the supraspinatus. The remainder of the rotator cuff tendons was normal.

With an arthroscopic elevator, the anterior capsule labral complex was mobilized from the glenoid rim and scapular neck. The glenoid rim and scapular neck were abraded with an arthroscopic shaver to create a bleeding bony surface. The labrum was then repaired back to the glenoid rim using five 2.4 mm biocomposite suture anchors. The sutures were passed using a suture lasso and then tied in a simple fashion arthroscopically. This resulted in stable repair of the labrum and restoration of the normal tension within the inferior glenohumeral ligament complex shown in Fig. 12.5a, b.

Discussion

This case is exemplary of a soft tissue Bankart injury and repair. The Hill–Sachs lesion should routinely be graded by size. Evaluating stability and how the Hill–Sachs lesion engages with the glenoid can help guide the surgeon on whether to address it surgically [7]. The surgical options for large Hill–Sachs can be bony or soft tissue. Preoperative physical exam and imaging can help guide the surgeon which treatment is best suited for the patient.

Case 4: Bony Bankart with a Large Hill–Sachs

History/Exam

The patient is a 20-year-old male with epilepsy initially presented with recurrent anterior shoulder instability associated with a bony Bankart lesion and a very large Hill–Sachs lesion (Fig. 12.6a–f). The patient underwent an open Bankart repair with humeral head allograft transplantation to the large Hill–Sachs defect for instability (Fig. 12.7a–d). Patient did well until 4 months postoperatively when he dislocated his right shoulder after slipping on ice. He then went on to fracture through the Bankart repair (Fig. 12.8) and required a Latarjet procedure as described below.

After his fall on ice his physical exam in the clinic revealed tenderness to palpation along the anterior glenohumeral joint. Provocative maneuvers included apprehension with any abduction and with only 10° of external rotation and a positive belly press with associated pain.

At the time of surgery his exam under anesthesia revealed marked instability of the glenohumeral joint. There was a 3+ anterior load shift and 1+ posterior load shift. There was 1 cm of inferior translation with internal rotation, neutral rotation,

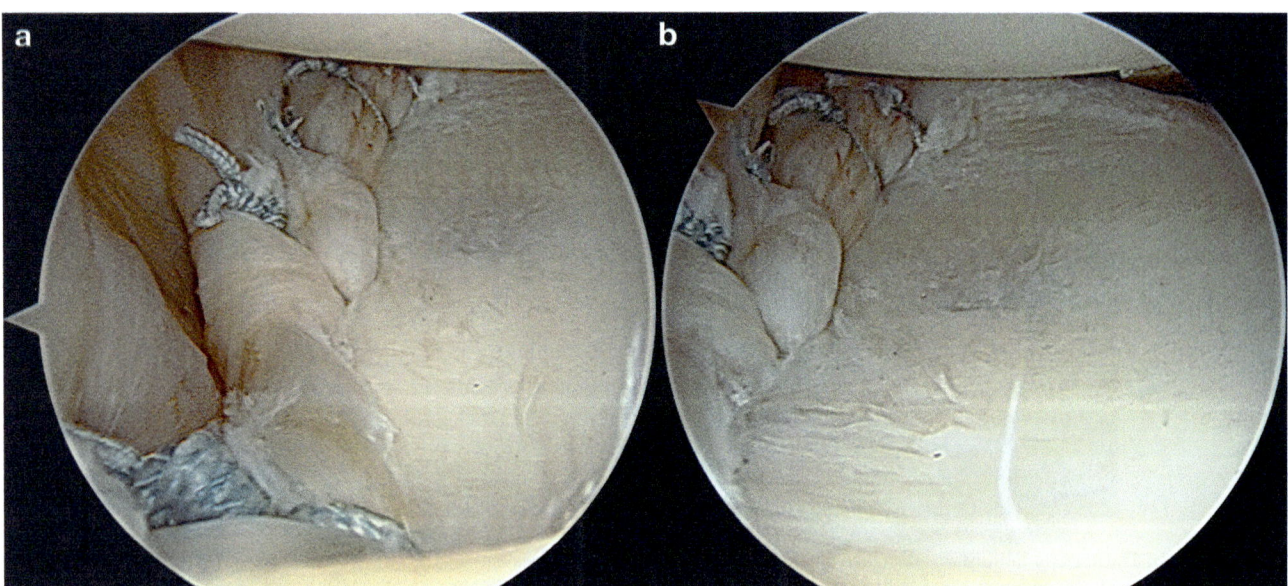

Fig. 12.5 (**a, b**) Multiple views of the final Bankart repair construct with five total anchors

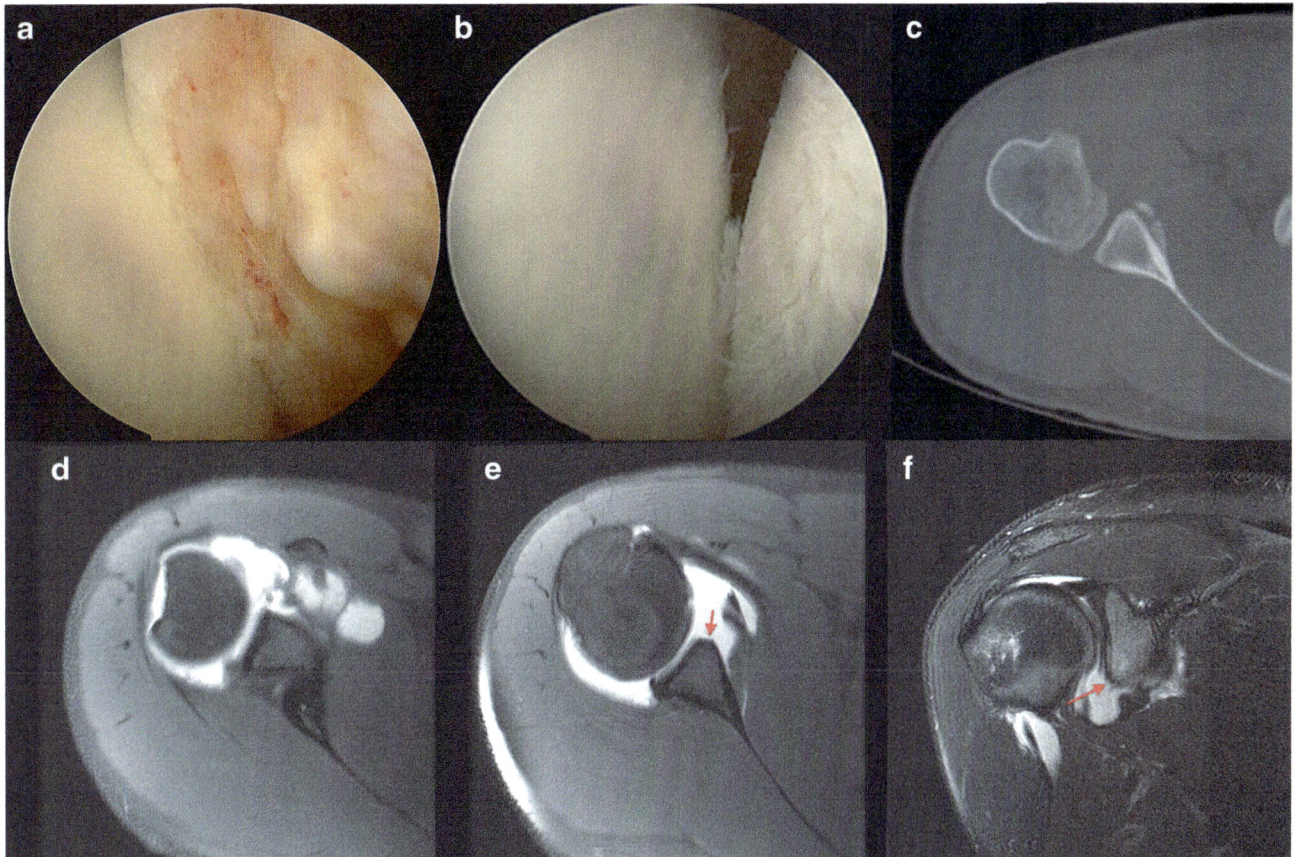

Fig. 12.6 (**a**–**f**) Initial injury images. (**a**) Arthroscopic view of large engaging Hill–Sachs with bony Bankart. (**b**) Arthroscopic view of remaining glenoid. (**c**) CT scan illustrating amount of bone loss from Bankart injury. (**d**) Axial T1 fat-suppressed right shoulder MR arthrogram. There is a large area of flattening involving the posterolateral humeral head consistent with a Hill–Sachs impaction fracture. (**e**) Axial T1 fat-suppressed right shoulder MR arthrogram. There is blunting of the anteroinferior glenoid (*arrow*) with associated detachment of the anteroinferior labrum consistent with a small bony Bankart lesion. (**f**) Coronal T2 fat-suppressed right shoulder MR arthrogram. There is blunting of the anteroinferior labrum (*arrow*) with associated abnormal marrow signal consistent with a small bony Bankart lesion

and external rotation. There was 135° of forward elevation, 80° of external rotation in abduction, 30° of internal rotation, and 50° of external rotation with the arm at the side.

Imaging

Initial injury shoulder radiographs showed a large Hill–Sachs impaction fracture of the posterolateral humeral head. CT scan of the right shoulder demonstrated a large Hill–Sachs impaction fracture and blunting of the anteroinferior glenoid with a small adjacent ossific fragment consistent with a bony Bankart (Fig. 12.6c). MR shoulder arthrogram with oblique coronal, sagittal, and axial T2 fat-suppressed sequences, axial PD sequences, and sagittal and axial T1 fat-suppressed sequences was obtained. The MR demonstrated a large Hill–Sachs impaction fracture of the posterolateral humeral head (Fig. 12.6d). In addition, there was blunting of the anteroinferior glenoid consistent with a Bankart fracture with associated detachment of the labrum (Fig. 12.6e, f).

Arthroscopy

The patient was taken to the operating room and placed in the lateral decubitus position. Arthroscopic findings demonstrated diffuse synovitis as well as multiple small cartilaginous loose bodies throughout the glenohumeral joint. There were cartilage flaps as well as wear of the articular cartilage on the superior aspect of the humeral head. The anterior 1/3 of the glenoid was eroded (Fig. 12.7a–c). Previously placed sutures could be seen exiting the scapular neck and glenoid rim (Fig. 12.7b). The anterior labrum was completely detached. The rotator cuff tendons were intact.

Open findings demonstrated an intact subscapularis tendon; however it was encased in scar. The anterior capsule appeared to be scarred to the subscapularis tendon. The remainder of the open findings was consistent with the arthroscopic findings.

The shoulder was approached through a deltopectoral approach. With sharp and blunt dissection, the deltopectoral interval was developed. The coracoid process was exposed.

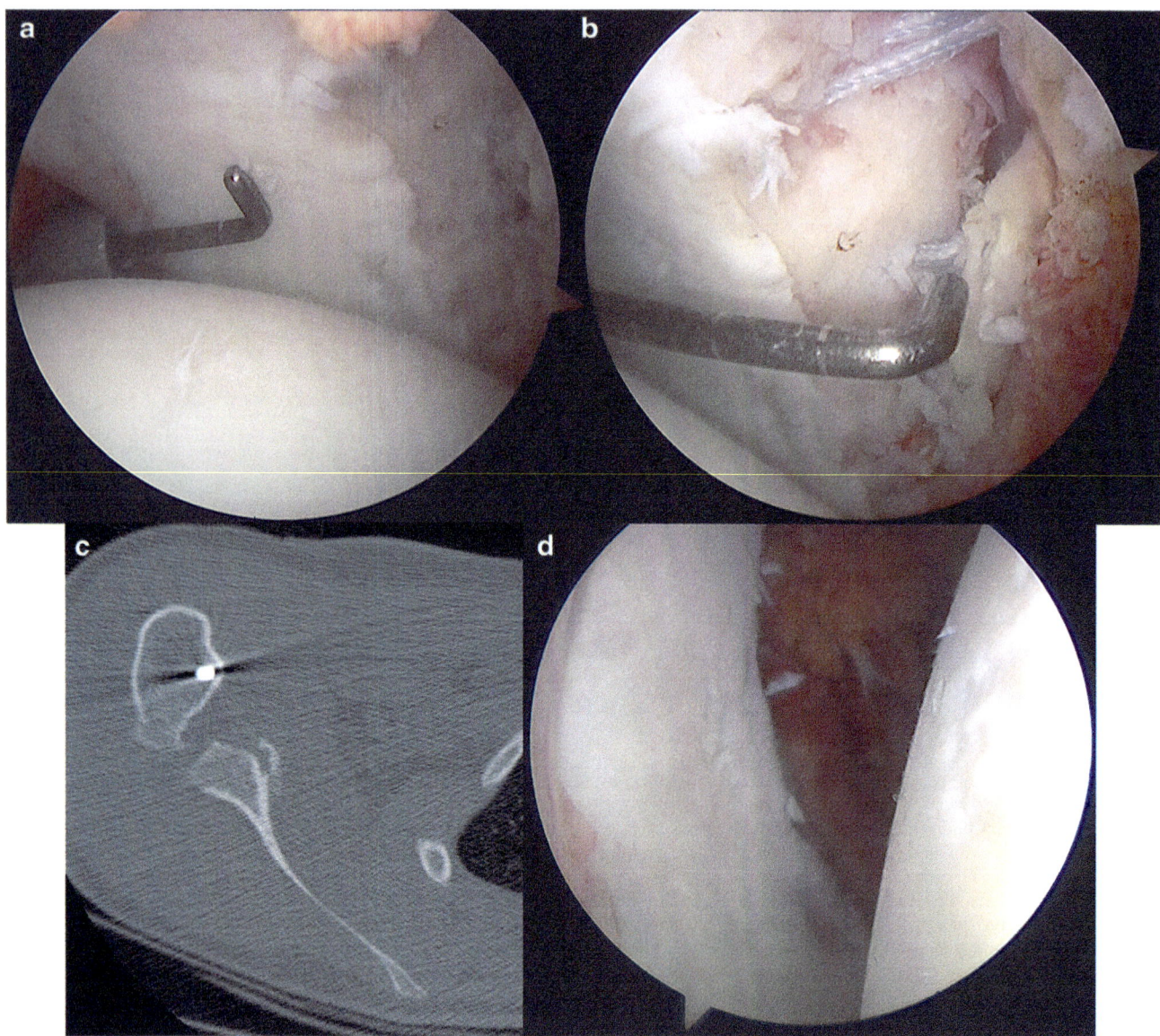

Fig. 12.7 (**a**) The anterior 1/3 of the glenoid was eroded as shown. (**b**) Arthroscopic view of previously placed anchors and sutures. (**c**) CT scan illustrating degree of glenoid bone deficiency from subsequent fall. (**d**) Arthroscopic view of remaining glenoid

The coracoacromial ligament was transected approximately 1 cm lateral to the coracoid process. The pectoralis minor was released from the coracoid process. A coracoid osteotomy was made at the base of the coracoid. The musculocutaneous and axillary nerves were identified and protected throughout the case. A rongeur and a high-speed bur were used to create a flat cancellous surface on the underside of the coracoid to encourage healing to the scapular neck. Adhesions to the conjoined tendon were carefully lysed.

The subscapularis tendon and anterior capsule were split transversely to expose the glenohumeral joint. The labrum was transected and then elevated off the glenoid rim and scapular neck to expose the area of bony deficiency. The glenoid rim and scapular neck were abraded to a flat surface

using a high-speed bur. Suture and hardware from the previous operation were removed (Fig. 12.8).

The coracoid process was drilled with a 2.5 drill bit. Two drill holes were made. The glenoid rim was then drilled using a 2.5 drill bit. The depth was measured. A 4.0 screw was placed through the inferior coracoid drill hole and then into the drill hole in the glenoid and scapular neck. This resulted in good positioning of the coracoid fragment onto the glenoid rim and scapular neck. There was a slight offset of approximately 1–2 mm medial to the glenoid. A second drill hole was made into the scapular neck through the previously placed drill hole in the coracoid. The fragment was fixed with a second 4.0 screw. The screws were tightened and provided excellent fixation for the coracoid (Fig. 12.9).

The anterior labrum was repaired back to the glenoid using two 2.4 mm biocomposite suture anchors. Sutures were placed through the inferior labrum and the superior labrum to restore the soft tissue buttress. The labrum and anterior capsule were also sewn to the coracoacromial ligament stump that remained on the lateral aspect of the coracoid process. The split in the anterior capsule and subscapularis was repaired with imbricating #2 high-strength, polyethylene core sutures. The shoulder was manipulated and could not be dislocated anteriorly or posteriorly. There were 90° of abduction and 75° of external rotation without undue stress on the repair.

Discussion

This case shows the challenge that can be associated with shoulder instability in the setting of bone loss. This patient's initial injury required a humeral head allograft to address the large Hill–Sachs and also an open procedure to address the bony Bankart. Unfortunately the patient reinjured himself. In the revision case his glenoid defect was so significant that he required a Latarjet to provide stability.

Revision cases possess a unique set of challenges for the surgeon. There is often hardware to remove. Bony injuries can be worse and there is less bone stock to hold anchors. It is imperative that the surgeon use all imaging studies necessary to understand the extent of injury. In the case of bony defects, this often means a CT scan. Preoperative planning and imaging are a crucial factor to determining how to best address these injuries.

Conclusions

As illustrated in each of these cases, there is a myriad of injuries that can be associated with anterior shoulder instability. The key to treatment lies in close scrutiny of preoperative images and clinical exam. Observation of occult signs of

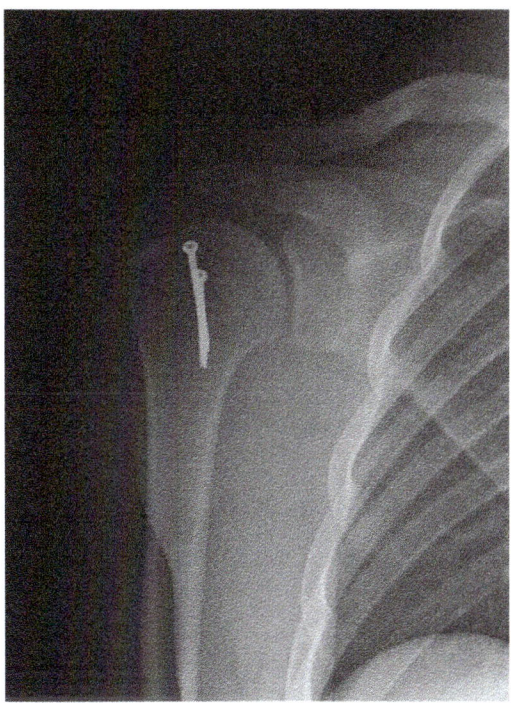

Fig. 12.8 Grashey radiographic view of shoulder illustrating screw placement for humeral head allograft to fill large Hill–Sachs lesion

Fig. 12.9 Postoperative radiographic AP and axillary views of shoulder after Latarjet procedure. Screws are well placed into the glenoid without hardware complications

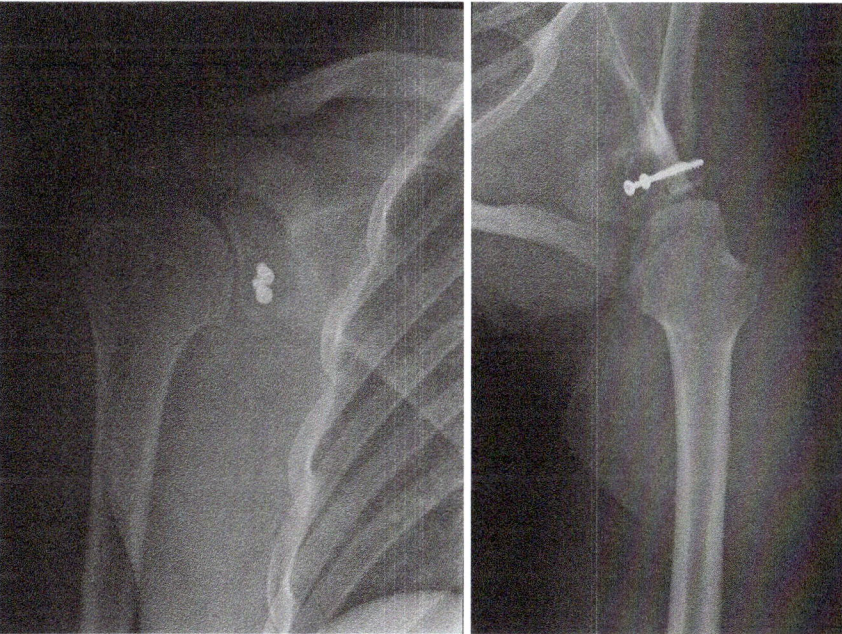

injury such as paralabral cysts, bony edema, and bone loss helps to clue the surgeon into the specific etiology of injury. There are also pitfalls that can mislead the surgeon. These include variants in anterior anatomy such as sublabral foramen versus labral avulsion. Additionally, a cord-like middle glenohumeral ligament with a sublabral foramen (Buford complex) can often be mistaken for a labral injury [8, 9]. Contrary to this, a non-displaced Perthes lesion can masquerade as a functional intact labrum since the labrum is still attached to the periosteum when in reality it provides no stability [10, 11].

Having a thorough understanding of how the MRI translates to what is seen clinically and arthroscopically can be challenging [12–14]. Even though the majority of radiographs were not shown, they remain the first line of imaging that is obtained. Quality radiographs can often tip off the surgeon to bony injury. However, they often cannot fully illustrate the extent of bony injury. It is in these cases where CT scan may be necessary. MRI continues to be the imaging modality of choice for evaluating soft tissue pathology. With ever-increasing magnets and resolution, the ability to correlate what is seen on the MRI and arthroscopically continues to improve.

References

1. Kim YK, Cho SH, Son WS, Moon SH. Arthroscopic repair of small and medium-sized bony Bankart lesions. Am J Sports Med. 2014;42(1):86–94.

2. Owens BD, Dickens JF, Kilcoyne KG, Rue JP. Management of mid-season traumatic anterior shoulder instability in athletes. J Am Acad Orthop Surg. 2012;20(8):518–26.

3. Piasecki DP, Verma NN, Romeo AA, Levine WN, Bach Jr BR, Provencher MT. Glenoid bone deficiency in recurrent anterior shoulder instability: diagnosis and management. J Am Acad Orthop Surg. 2009;17(8):482–93.

4. Kim DS, Yoon YS, Kwon SM. The spectrum of lesions and clinical results of arthroscopic stabilization of acute anterior shoulder instability. Yonsei Med J. 2010;51(3):421–6.

5. Lee BG, Cho NS, Rhee YG. Anterior labroligamentous periosteal sleeve avulsion lesion in arthroscopic capsulolabral repair for anterior shoulder instability. Knee Surg Sports Traumatol Arthrosc. 2011;19(9):1563–9.

6. Ozbaydar M, Elhassan B, Diller D, Massimini D, Higgins LD, Warner JJ. Results of arthroscopic capsulolabral repair: Bankart lesion versus anterior labroligamentous periosteal sleeve avulsion lesion. Arthroscopy. 2008;24(11):1277–83.

7. Wolf EM, Arianjam A. Hill-Sachs remplissage, an arthroscopic solution for the engaging Hill-Sachs lesion: 2- to 10-year follow-up and incidence of recurrence. J Shoulder Elbow Surg. 2014;23(6): 814–20.

8. Tirman PF, Feller JF, Palmer WE, Carroll KW, Steinbach LS, Cox I. The Buford complex—a variation of normal shoulder anatomy: MR arthrographic imaging features. AJR Am J Roentgenol. 1996;166(4):869–73.

9. Williams MM, Snyder SJ, Buford Jr D. The Buford complex—the "cord-like" middle glenohumeral ligament and absent anterosuperior labrum complex: a normal anatomic capsulolabral variant. Arthroscopy. 1994;10(3):241–7.

10. Wischer TK, Bredella MA, Genant HK, Stoller DW, Bost FW, Tirman PF. Perthes lesion (a variant of the Bankart lesion): MR imaging and MR arthrographic findings with surgical correlation. AJR Am J Roentgenol. 2002;178(1):233–7.

11. Neviaser TJ. The anterior labroligamentous periosteal sleeve avulsion lesion: a cause of anterior instability of the shoulder. Arthroscopy. 1993;9(1):17–21.

12. Mutlu S, Mahirogullari M, Guler O, Ucar BY, Mutlu H, Sonmez G, et al. Anterior glenohumeral instability: classification of pathologies of anteroinferior labroligamentous structures using MR arthrography. Adv Orthop. 2013;2013:473194.

13. Waldt S, Burkart A, Imhoff AB, Bruegel M, Rummeny EJ, Woertler K. Anterior shoulder instability: accuracy of MR arthrography in the classification of anteroinferior labroligamentous injuries. Radiology. 2005;237(2):578–83.

14. Yeh L, Kwak S, Kim YS, Pedowitz R, Trudell D, Muhle C, et al. Anterior labroligamentous structures of the glenohumeral joint: correlation of MR arthrography and anatomic dissection in cadavers. AJR Am J Roentgenol. 1998;171(5):1229–36.

Posterior Instability and Labral Pathology

Bastian Uribe-Echevarria Marbach and Brian R. Wolf

Introduction

Posterior labral lesions are associated with posterior and, occasionally, multidirectional instability [1, 2]. Posterior–superior labral tears may also occur as part of a posterior SLAP 2 or posterior peel-back lesions, in which pathologies are further discussed in Chaps. 15 and 16 in this book.

Compared with anterior instability, posterior shoulder instability is relatively uncommon, accounting for somewhere between 2 and 11 % of all shoulder instability cases [1, 3–5]. Less than half of the posterior instability cases is thought to occur secondary to trauma [4]. Recurrent posterior subluxations are more common compared with recurrent posterior dislocations [4–6].

Traumatic posterior dislocations typically result from a direct blow to the anterior shoulder or a fall on a forward flexed arm (94 %). Less frequent (6 %) are indirect forces such as seizures and electric shock, producing flexion, internal rotation, and adduction [1, 5, 6].

Posterior subluxations are common in overhead throwers, tennis players, butterfly and freestyle swimmers, weightlifters, and football linemen, resulting from repetitive microtrauma to the posterior capsule producing attenuation of the posterior capsular tissue [5, 6].

Less frequently, posterior labral tears can be present in the setting of multidirectional instability, being part of a more global pathology including labrum, capsule (inferior glenohumeral ligament complex), and the rotator interval.

B.U.-E. Marbach, MD (✉)
Institute for Orthopedic Sports Medicine and Rehabilitation, University of Iowa Hospitals and Clinics, Iowa City, IA, USA
e-mail: Bastian-uribe@uiowa.edu

B.R. Wolf, MD, MS
Department of Orthopedics and Rehabilitation, University of Iowa, Iowa City, IA, USA
e-mail: Brian-wolf@uiowa.edu

Clinical Presentation

Posterior shoulder instability, especially recurrent posterior subluxation, often presents with poorly localized shoulder pain associated with laxity of the posterior capsule and/or fatigue of the static and dynamic stabilizers [5–7].

Pain and discomfort when doing activities such as a push-up or bench-press, when the arm is flexed and internally rotated, suggest posterior instability. Pain, numbness, and tingling when carrying heavy objects occurring secondary to traction of the brachial plexus suggest inferior instability.

The presence of hyperlaxity in the contralateral shoulder and elbows and the patient's ability to bring the thumb to the forearm may signify a syndrome of generalized ligamentous laxity [8].

Provocative maneuvers such as the jerk test (painful posterior translation of the glenohumeral joint in internal rotation) and the posterior apprehension test (apprehension or involuntary guarding with flexion, adduction, and internal rotation) have a high correlation with posterior instability [8–10]. Posterior drawer tests and anterior and posterior load-and-shift tests evaluate for laxity in this direction [9], the latter being more reliable [2, 11].

Imaging Technique

The historically low accuracy of MRIs in assessing the glenoid labrum has improved significantly with greater understanding of the anatomic and pathologic variants that may occur. In addition, specific pulse sequences (fat-suppressed gradient-recalled echoes) [4, 12] and the availability of direct magnetic resonance arthrography produce sensitivities between 86 and 91 % and specificities of 86–98 % [13–16].

The posterior labrum and capsule are best visualized on axial images. An intact labrum has a low intensity signal on all pulse sequences. Labral tears are best detected on T2 and proton-density sequences as increased signal intensity that extends to the surface [1].

There is a lower diagnostic accuracy of the posterior compared to anterior labral lesions, showing sensitivity of 0.50 and a specificity of 0.92 [17]. Contrary to the ABER position, flexion, adduction, and internal rotation positioning appear to be a useful adjunct in evaluating patients with equivocal or subtle posteroinferior labral abnormalities on conventional MRI arthrography sequences [7, 18].

Imaging

Similar to anterior labral tears, posterior tears present themselves with an absence of the labrum, morphologic distortion or contrast, or fluid extending into the substance of the labrum [19]. Posterior labral and capsular tears have a lower and more variable prevalence in patients with posterior instability than the anteroinferior labrocapsular lesions in patients with anterior instability [4, 6, 20].

Reverse Bankart lesions and posterior labrocapsular sleeve avulsion lesions are present in 52–58 % of patients with posterior instability [3, 21]. Kim's lesion is a superficial tearing between the posteroinferior labrum and the glenoid articular cartilage without complete detachment of the labrum (marginal crack) [15, 22, 23]. The posteroinferior labrum had lost its normal height and flattened, with subsequent retroversion of the chondrolabral glenoid. It may be concealed at arthroscopy.

Posterior labral tears may be classified into three types using MR arthrograms and into four types arthroscopically, according to Kim et al. [15, 22]. The MR type I lesion is a separation without displacement, type II is an incomplete avulsion (cystic lesion), and type III is a loss of contour. The arthroscopic type I lesion is an incomplete detachment (36 %), type II is a marginal crack or incomplete and concealed avulsion of posterior–inferior labrum (39 %), type III is a chondrolabral erosion (19 %), and type IV is a flap tear (6 %).

The posterior labrocapsular periosteal sleeve avulsion (POLPSA) is a detachment of the posterior labrum and the intact posterior scapular periosteum from the glenoid, producing a redundant recess that communicates with the joint space [20].

The reverse osseous Bankart lesion, defined as an avulsion of a fragment of the posterior osseous glenoid, can be seen in one third of traumatic posterior dislocations [3].

Findings that can accompany posterior instability include a redundant posterior capsule (43–67 %) [2, 21], reverse Hills–Sachs or McLaughlin fractures (an impact fracture of the anteromedial humeral head after posterior humeral dislocation [24], seen in up to 86 % of traumatic cases), and rota-

tor cuff lesions, present in up to 42 % of traumatic posterior shoulder dislocations [3].

The reverse HAGL represents an avulsion of the posterior joint capsule from the humerus superior to the posterior band of the inferior GHL [4]. The posterior band of the inferior GHL is variable in size and often not visualized.

Glenoid hypoplasia, posterior glenoid rim deficiency, and glenoid dysplasia represent a range of developmental anomalies associated with multidirectional and posterior instability [2, 3, 20, 25].

Indications for surgery after a posterior dislocation include a displaced tuberosity or glenoid fracture requiring reduction or inability to maintain reduction due to a humeral or glenoid defect. For recurrent posterior instability, consideration for surgical intervention follows 3–6 months of conservative treatment, though more aggressive management may be warranted in severe cases and elite athletes [9].

In this chapter, clinical cases will be used to demonstrate the correlation between MRI and arthroscopy for posterior labral tears, reviewing the diagnosis and management of each patient.

Four cases will be presented, including:
- Posterior shoulder instability with posterior labral tear and associated posterior capsular tear
- Reverse bony Bankart
- Concealed posterior labral tear (Kim lesion)
- Traumatic posterior labral re-tear

Case 1: Posterior Labral Tear

History/Exam

A 17-year-old young man came to the clinic with persistent pain in both shoulders for over a year. His pain was greater on his dominant right side. It began during the last football season, with pain posteriorly and superiorly in both shoulders during physical activity. He continued to play football but transitioned from linebacker to safety for the last year, which was less painful for his shoulders. Occasionally, he had a slipping and cracking sensation while playing football or lifting weights.

On physical examination, he was noted to have mild pain over the posterior joint line on the right shoulder, a positive O'Brien maneuver bilaterally less painful with the arm supinated, and no anterior apprehension on either side. Jerk test was positive for pain on both shoulders, more so on the right than the left, but no subluxation was felt or provoked. No tenderness over the AC joint or anteriorly over the biceps was noted. Rotator cuff strength was 5/5.

Imaging

Plain shoulder films were unremarkable. His acromion had a normal shape and contour. There was no evidence of arthritic changes, glenoid rim, or humeral head bony insufficiency that could lead to instability.

Given his lasting pain and the findings during the physical examination, bilateral shoulder MRI arthrograms were obtained.

T1 sequences with fat saturation were obtained in coronal, axial, and sagittal planes, plus a T2 with fat saturation in the coronal plane. Additionally, T1 with fat saturation imaging sequence was performed in the abduction external rotation (ABER) position. Images were obtained after the instillation of 12 cc of a dilute gadolinium solution into the shoulder joint.

Axial T1-weighted images on the right shoulder (Fig. 13.1a–d) show a moderate-sized tear of the posterior labrum without changes on the posterior capsule.

The ABER position sequence also shows the posterior labrum detachment (Fig. 13.1e).

The same axial images on the left shoulder (Fig. 13.1f–i) show a similar posterior labral tear, this time accompanied with a more patulous posterior capsule, without an obvious capsule tear. This redundancy of the posterior capsule can also be observed on sagittal images (Fig. 13.1f–m), and the extension of the posterior labral detachment can be evaluated in a more medial sagittal image (Fig. 13.1n) showing the glenoid rim without bone loss.

Because of his worsening symptoms over the last year, a concordant physical exam, and a bilateral MRI with evidence of a posterior labrum tear and instability, he was indicated for arthroscopy with posterior labrum tear repair and capsulorrhaphy at the end of the season.

Arthroscopy

The operations were staged 6 weeks apart, starting with the right shoulder.

The procedure was performed in beach chair position under combined anesthesia. The right shoulder was examined under anesthesia prior to prepping and draping. It was stable anteriorly and inferiorly, but grade III posterior instability was found on jerk testing.

A posterior arthroscopy portal was established slightly lateral to the standard position, adjacent to the humeral head in anticipation of posterior repair. Anterior and high lateral rotator interval portals were created under needle localization.

Diagnostic arthroscopy revealed an intact anterior, superior, and inferior labrum to 6 o'clock. His posterior labrum was detached and frayed (Fig. 13.1o, p), and he had a capacious posterior capsule.

The posterior labrum was debrided to stable tissue and was found to be detached from approximately the 6:30 position to the 11 o'clock position. The posterior glenoid was debrided with a shaver down to bleeding bone. A total of five single loaded 3.0 mm absorbable anchors were placed posteriorly, using a suture lasso to shuttle sutures throughout the posterior capsule and then around the detached labrum using a two-bite technique, shifting the capsule superiorly and medially on the glenoid (Fig. 13.1q, r).

The posterior cannula was removed, and the resulting capsule defect was closed with a single #0 PDS suture.

The same setting was used for performing the surgery on his left shoulder 6 weeks later.

During examination under anesthesia, his left shoulder was stable anteriorly and inferiorly and had a grade II posterior clunk.

The posterior labrum was detached and frayed, and the posterior capsule was patulous with a posterior capsule tear (Fig. 13.1s–u). This was an oblique capsule split that went toward the humeral anatomic neck with cuff muscle evident through the tear posterior inferiorly.

The posterior capsule tear was repaired with a total of 3 #0 PDS sutures placed side to side with the joint using a suture lasso across the tear (Fig. 13.1v).

The posterior labrum tear was localized between 2 and 6 o'clock, and a total of four anchors were placed, repairing the posterior labrum anatomically into its appropriate position with generous bites of capsule also taken (Fig. 13.1w). The posterior cannula was withdrawn, and a final PDS suture was placed across the capsular defect from where the cannula was inserted.

Discussion

This case demonstrates several things common with posterior shoulder instability. Posterior shoulder instability is often seen in football [26] due to the repetitive blocking and engagement of other players with the arms outstretched in flexion. This places a lot of repetitive load on the posterior joint and can result in damage. Posterior capsule tears and reverse humeral avulsion of the glenoid ligaments (rHAGL) lesions can present in addition to posterior labrum tears or in isolation. In an acute setting, rHAGL and posterior capsule tears result in intra-articular contrast leaking into the posterior cuff musculature on the axial views or seen tracking down along the proximal humerus on the sagittal oblique cuts. These lesions can be a challenge to see on the MRI, in a chronic setting. Once scarring has occurred, imaging findings are limited, making the interpretation of the MRI more

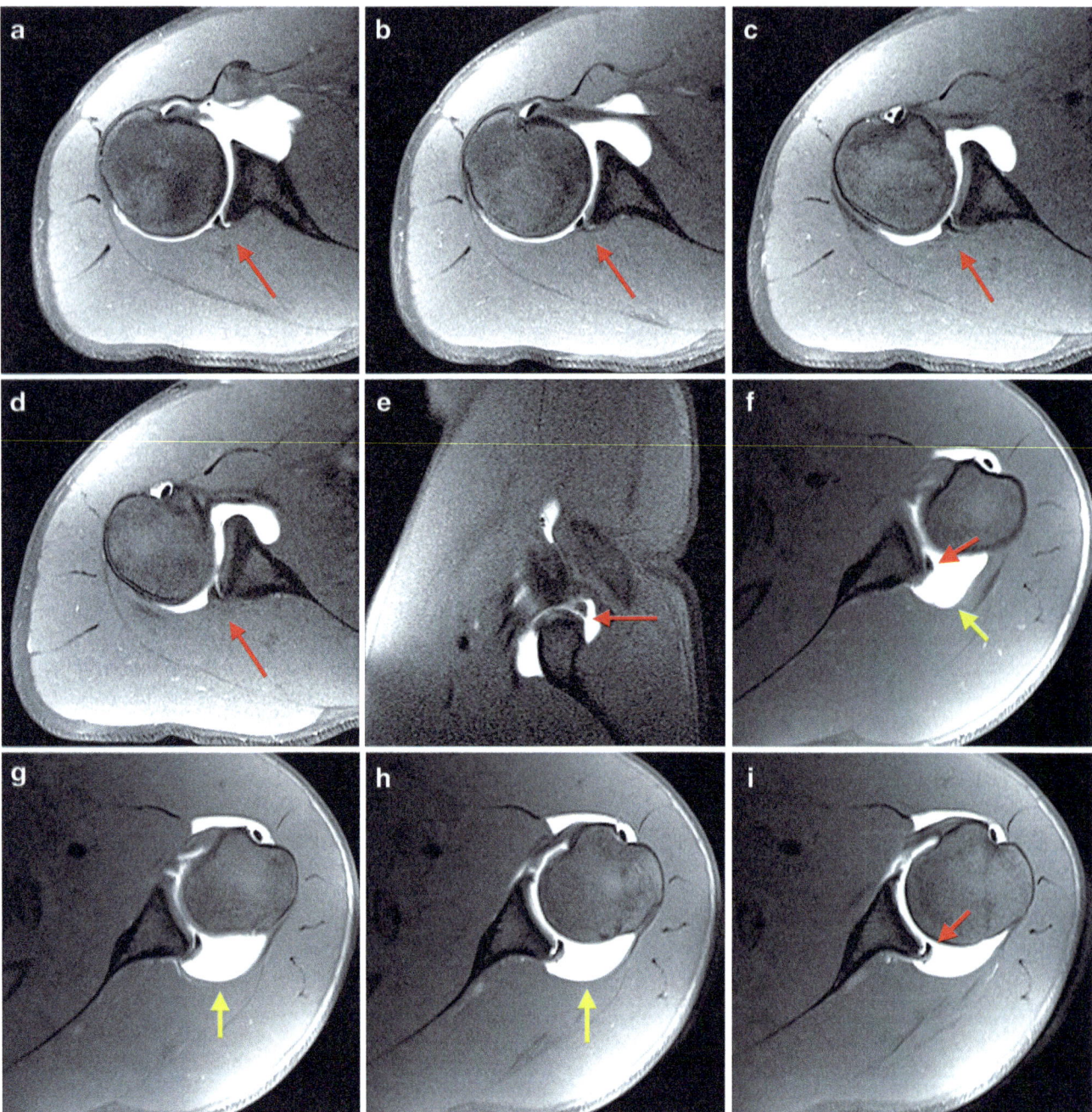

Fig. 13.1 (**a–d**) Right shoulder T1-weighted images showing a moderate-sized tear of the posterior labrum (*red arrow*) without changes on the posterior capsule. These findings are consistent with a Type I posteroinferior labral tear. (**e**) ABER position sequence showing the posterior labrum detachment. (**f–i, f–n**) Axial and sagittal T1-weighted images of a left shoulder showing a posterior labral tear (*red arrow*) accompanied with a patulous posterior capsule (*yellow arrow*), without an obvious capsule tear. (**j, n**) Medial sagittal images of the right and left shoulders, respectively, showing the extension of the posterior labral detachment and the intact osseous glenoid rim (*red arrow*), with the associated more patulous posterior capsule on the *left side* (*yellow arrow*). (**o, p**) Detached and frayed posterior labrum on a right shoulder (*red arrows*). (**q, r**) Right shoulder. Debrided posterior labrum and posterior capsule secured with anchors (*green arrows*). Shifting the capsule superiorly and medially on the glenoid can be noted. Suture of the defect of the posterior cannula with PDS (*blue arrow*). (**s–u**) Left shoulder. Detached and frayed labrum (*red arrow*) and patulous posterior capsule with a posterior capsule tear (*yellow arrows*) with muscle evident through the tear. (**v**) Repaired posterior capsule tear with PDS sutures placed side to side (*blue arrows*). (**w**) Repaired posterior labral tear on a left shoulder (*green arrow*). PDS sutures of the side-to-side repair of the posterior capsule tear are visible (*blue arrows*)

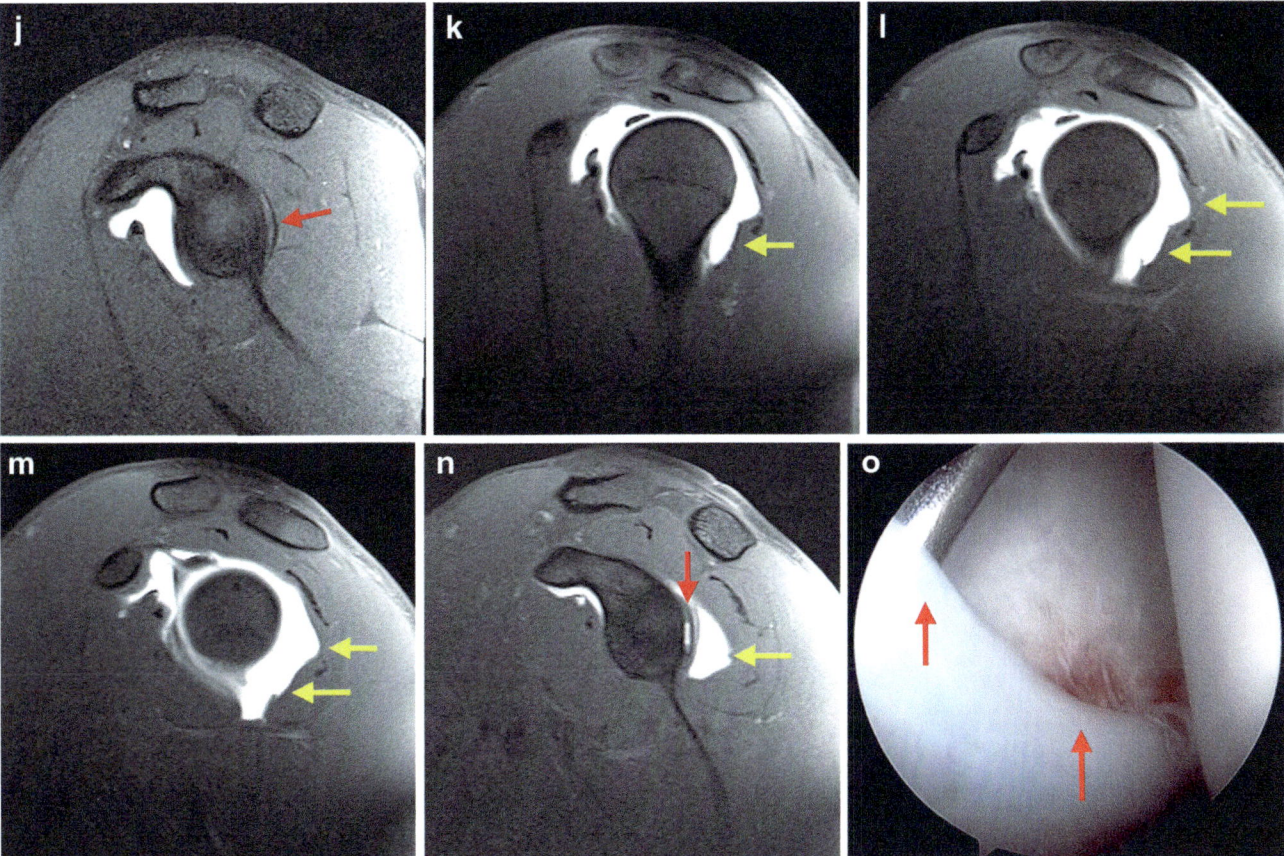

Fig. 13.1 (continued)

challenging. The torn stump cannot be distinguished from remodeled scar, and there is no edema or hemorrhage. A redundancy of the posterior capsule can be present (Fig. 13.1f–i), and a pseudo-pouch may form distally along the humeral neck (Fig. 13.1f–m). In addition, close inspection of the posterior and inferior capsule should be done at the time of arthroscopy to look for the lesions since they can often be missed on imaging.

There are several technical tips for repairing the posterior labrum and tears of the posterior capsule. First, the senior author prefers to use a posterior portal that is approximately 2 cm more lateral than a standard portal, which brings the cannula just along the posterior humeral head. This provides a much better angle for placing anchors in the posterior glenoid. If a standard posterior portal is used, then an additional lateralized posterior portal or percutaneous suture anchor portal will be needed to place anchors. It is recommended to repair the labrum from inferior to superior while visualizing from a superior rotator interval portal. Posterior capsule tears and rHAGL lesions can be repaired arthroscopically as well.

Pearls for these repairs include using a suture passer and/or bird-beak penetrator to shuttle sutures across the capsule tears side to side. Often an additional anchor in the anatomic neck of the humerus will be needed for rHAGL lesions to restore the capsule attachment to the humerus. These sutures can be placed from the posterior portal or using a suture passer from an anterior portal, depending on the location. Sutures should be placed from inferior to superior. Suture knots may be tied on the internal or external surface of the capsule depending on how the sutures are passed and shuttled. A 70° arthroscope may be helpful to visualize rHAGL lesions or very low posterior capsule tears. Lastly, the authors prefer to always close the defect of the posterior created by the posterior cannula for cases of posterior shoulder instability. This defect often becomes large due to the thin nature of the posterior capsule and the frequent manipulation and stress on the posterior cannula. This capsule cannula defect is done at the very end of the procedure by withdrawing the cannula just outside the capsule and shuttling an absorbable (0-PDS) suture or two across the defect.

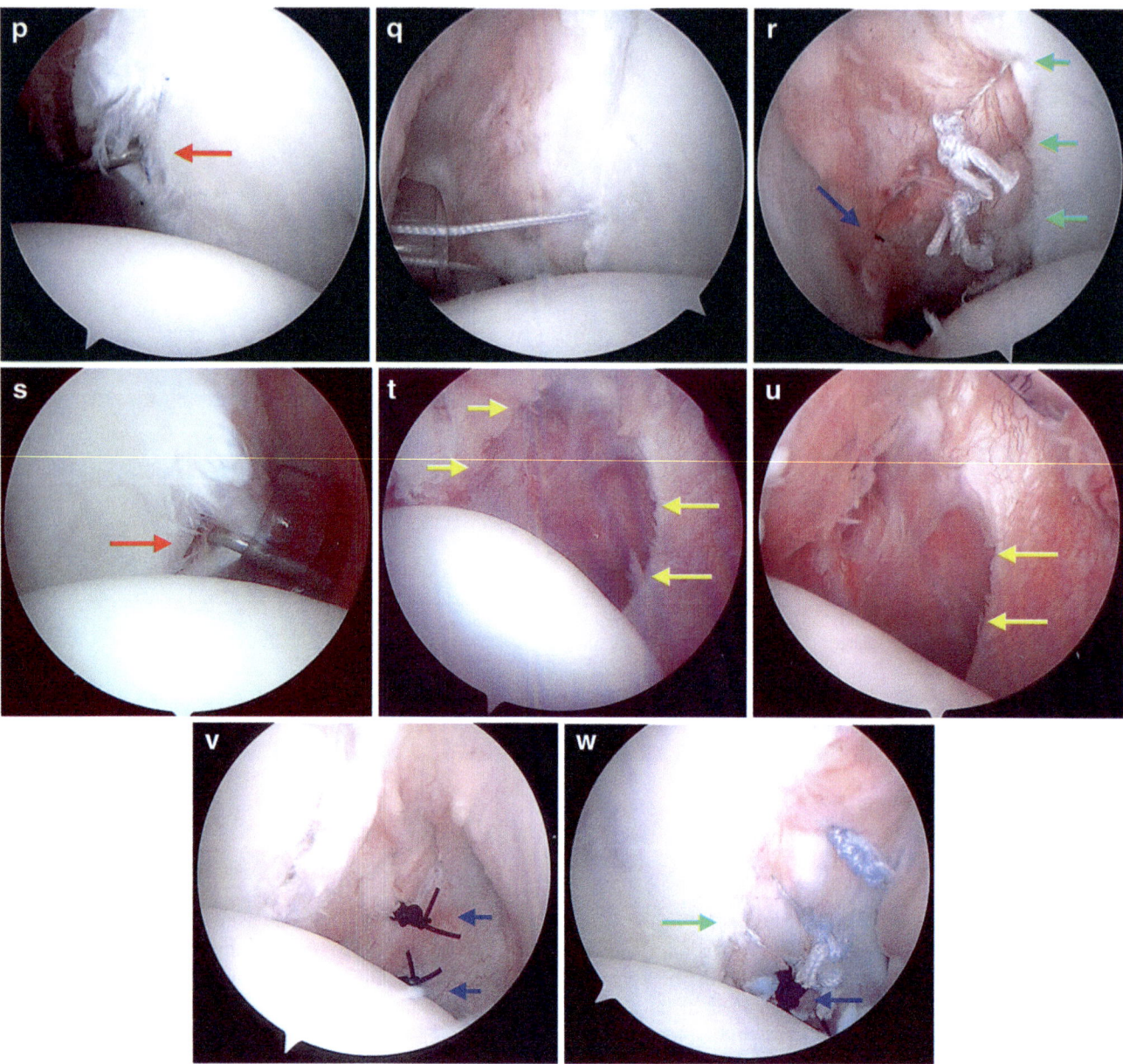

Fig. 13.1 (continued)

Case 2: Reverse Bony Bankart

History/Exam

A 19-year-old member of a college football team presented to the clinic complaining of left shoulder difficulties the entire prior season. He had an injury end of the prior season which had worsened, with several injuries during the recent season despite use of a shoulder stabilizing brace. He noted no pain with regular daily activities but occasionally crepitus and popping sensations.

On physical examination, the left shoulder demonstrated full range of motion and excellent strength. He had some pain on posterior loading but presents with a no subluxation on jerk test. He had pain with O'Brien testing and has no anterior apprehension.

Imaging

Plain X-rays show a reverse bony Bankart lesion (Fig. 13.2a, b) of considerable size, displaced 2 mm. An MRI arthrogram of the left shoulder was performed.

Axial T2 images with fat saturation (Fig. 13.2c–f) show a posterior glenoid fracture with articular cartilage defect and a chronic appearing tear of the posterior and posteroinferior labrum with avulsion of the posterior scapular periosteum.

The ABER position T1 fat saturation sequence shows the reverse Bankart and the bony fragment in the most distal cuts (Fig. 13.2g). Sagittal T2 images with fat saturation (Fig. 13.2h–j) show the bony fragment and the area of the glenoid articular surface affected by the fracture.

There is no apparent femoral head lesion on the MRI. The bone marrow signal intensity is within normal limits. Other structures, like the biceps tendon, acromioclavicular joint, rotator cuff, and subacromial space, appear normal.

Having repeated posterior injuries on his left shoulder and imaging studies showing a posterior bony Bankart lesion, the patient was indicated for arthroscopy with posterior Bankart repair. An open repair was also considered, but because of the size of the bony lesion, it was anticipated that it could be addressed arthroscopically.

Arthroscopy

The procedure was performed in beach chair position under combined anesthesia. The left shoulder was examined under anesthesia showing a grade 1 posterior translation. The patient had full range of motion and was stable anteriorly.

A posterior arthroscopy portal was created slightly lateral to the standard position, and anterior and high rotator interval portals were made under needle localization.

Diagnostic arthroscopy revealed an intact rotator cuff and long head of the biceps. The patient's subscapularis, anterior labrum, and superior labrum were normal. There were two small cartilage loose bodies in the axillary recess that were approximately 5–6 mm in diameter that were removed.

There was a reverse bony Bankart injury involving the entire posterior glenoid (Fig. 13.2k), approximately 5–7 mm from an anterior to posterior dimension, and the posterior labrocapsular complex was associated with this. The reverse Bankart lesion had partially healed medially on the glenoid neck.

The reverse bony Bankart lesion was mobilized using a liberator as well as a shaver. When reduced, it sat flush with the posterior aspect of the glenoid.

The glenoid was prepared down to bleeding bone, as was the bony surface of the bony Bankart fragment. A two-row suture bridge repair of the bony fragment and the labrum was performed with two 3.0 mm absorbable anchors placed medially on the glenoid neck. The sutures from these anchors were shuttled around the fragment and associated labrocapsular

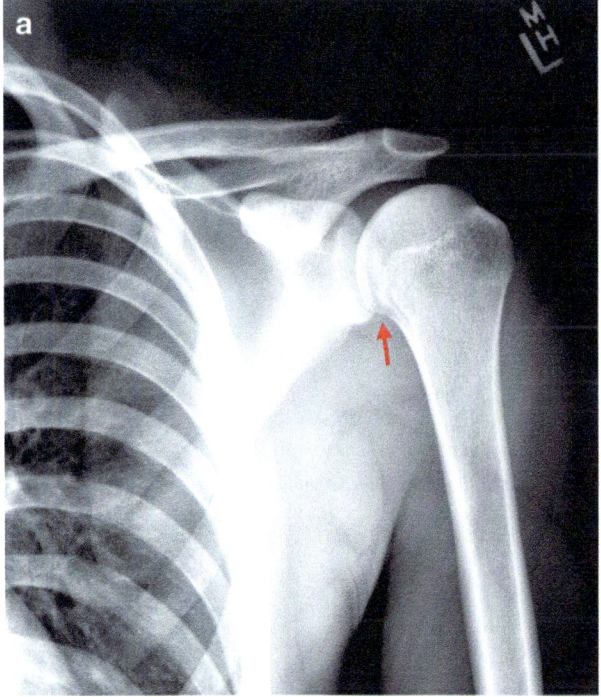
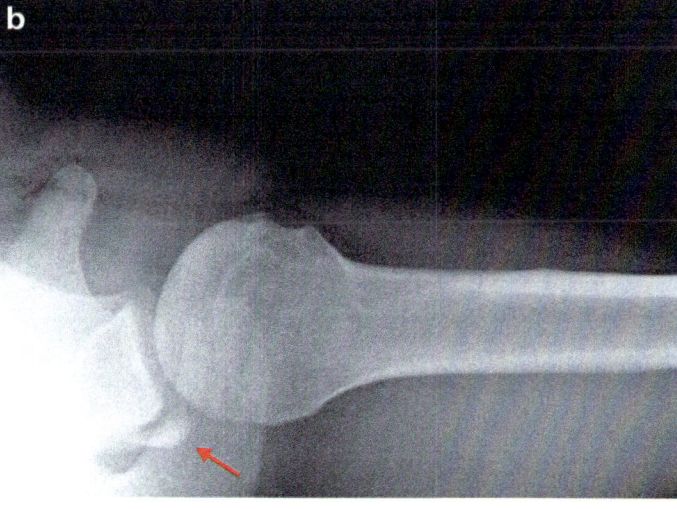

Fig. 13.2 (**a, b**) AP and axial views X-rays of a left shoulder showing a reverse bony Bankart lesion with 2 mm of displacement (*red arrows*). (**c–f**) Axial T2 images with fat saturation showing a posterior glenoid fracture (*red arrow*) with an articular cartilage defect (*pink arrow*) and a chronic appearing tear of the posterior and posteroinferior labrum with avulsion of the posterior scapular periosteum (*orange arrow*) and a patulous posterior capsule (*yellow arrow*). (**g**) ABER position T1 fat saturation sequence showing a reverse bony Bankart (*red arrow*). (**h–j**)

Sagittal T2 images with fat saturation showing a bony Bankart (*red arrow*). The area of the affected glenoid articular surface can be visualized. (**k**) Left shoulder with a reverse bony Bankart injury involving the entire posterior glenoid and associated posterior labrocapsular complex (*red arrow*). (**l**) Two-row construct repair around the reverse bony Bankart and associated labrocapsular complex (*green arrow*). Additional anchors were used to repair the labrum above and below this two-row construct around the bony fragment (*yellow arrows*)

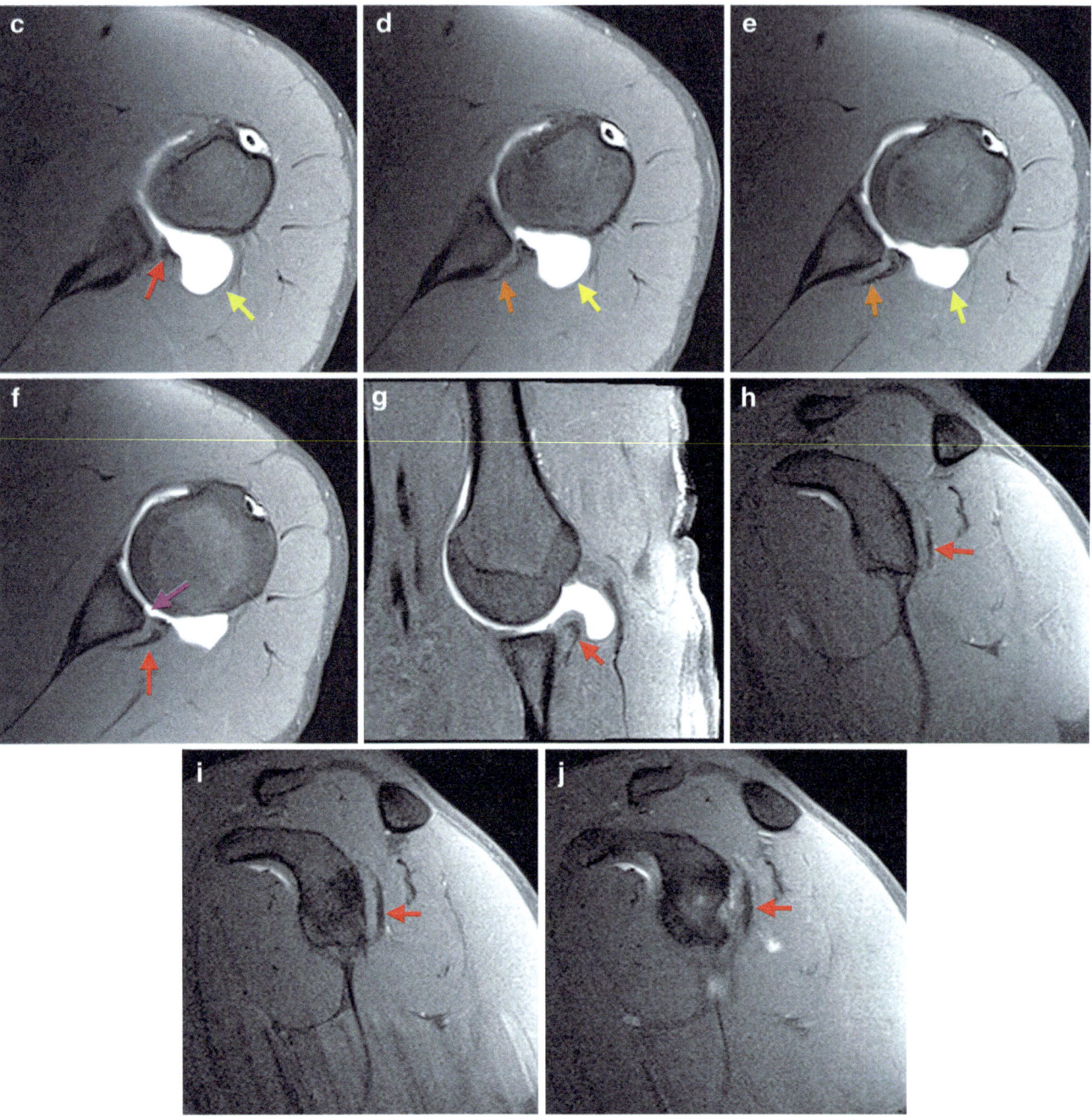

Fig. 13.2 (continued)

complex using a suture lasso. The sutures were brought around the bony Bankart lesion and secured to the edge of the glenoid using knotless anchors. Additional anchors were used to repair the labrum above and below this two-row construct around the bony fragment (Fig. 13.2l).

A single #0 PDS suture was used to close the posterior portal site.

Discussion

The case also demonstrates the association of football with posterior shoulder instability, as also seen in case 1. Reverse bony Bankart lesions are technically more challenging to repair than pure labrum injuries. Options for repair include open fixation with suture anchors or screws. The authors

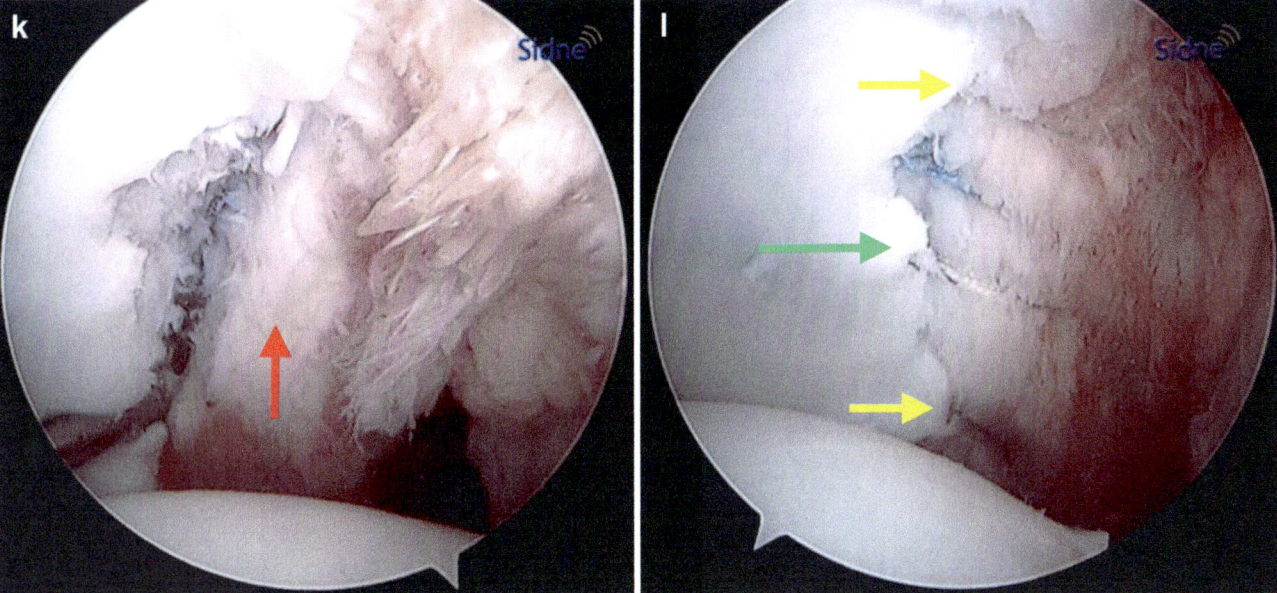

Fig. 13.2 (continued)

prefer to do arthroscopic repair using a suture compression technique when feasible. Reverse bony Bankart injuries will often have some bony healing on the medial neck but not bony union at the level of the joint. It is important to mobilize the bony fragment and associated labrum. This is done with an arthroscopic liberator. It can be used like an osteotome if medial bony bridging needs to be taken down to reduce the fragment appropriately and to prepare the bony edges of the fragment and the native glenoid. The two-row repair technique for bony Bankart lesions has been described by Millett et al. [27]. Anchor placement along the medial neck of the glenoid can be technically challenging but does allow for a suture compression fixation of osseous Bankart lesions anteriorly and posteriorly.

Case 3: Kim Lesion

History/Exam

A 16-year-old right-hand-dominant young man with right shoulder pain for 6 months came to the clinic after 3 months of physical therapy with a shoulder therapist without any relief of his symptoms. He was referred to the clinic for posterior shoulder instability involving the right shoulder. He wrestled the previous semester but denied any traumatic injuries. He located his pain posteriorly and felt his shoulder dislocated posteriorly whenever he raised it above his head.

On physical exam, his right shoulder demonstrated subluxation posteriorly with forward flexion to 90°. He had a grossly positive jerk test that produced pain, as did the posterior loading. He had posterior apprehension with flexion, adduction, and internal rotation. He fired his rotator cuff well but had posterior pain with resistance. External rotation with the arm abducted was 90°. Sulcus was slightly positive compared to the left side and improved with external rotation.

Imaging

Plain films were unremarkable. There was no evidence of arthritic changes, glenoid rim, or humeral head bony insufficiency.

An external MRI arthrogram showed on axial images (T2 fat suppression) a possible small split in the posterior inferior labrum (Fig. 13.3a–d). Most of the posterior labrum appeared intact except for one cut that showed slight leaking of the contrast. Posterior capsule was slightly more patulous posteroinferiorly, as was the anterior capsule. Glenohumeral ligaments appeared to be intact.

After several months of physical therapy without improvement and persisting posterior subluxation, the patient was indicated for arthroscopy and stabilization.

Arthroscopy

The procedure was performed in beach chair position under combined anesthesia. The right shoulder was examined under anesthesia prior to prepping and draping. It was found

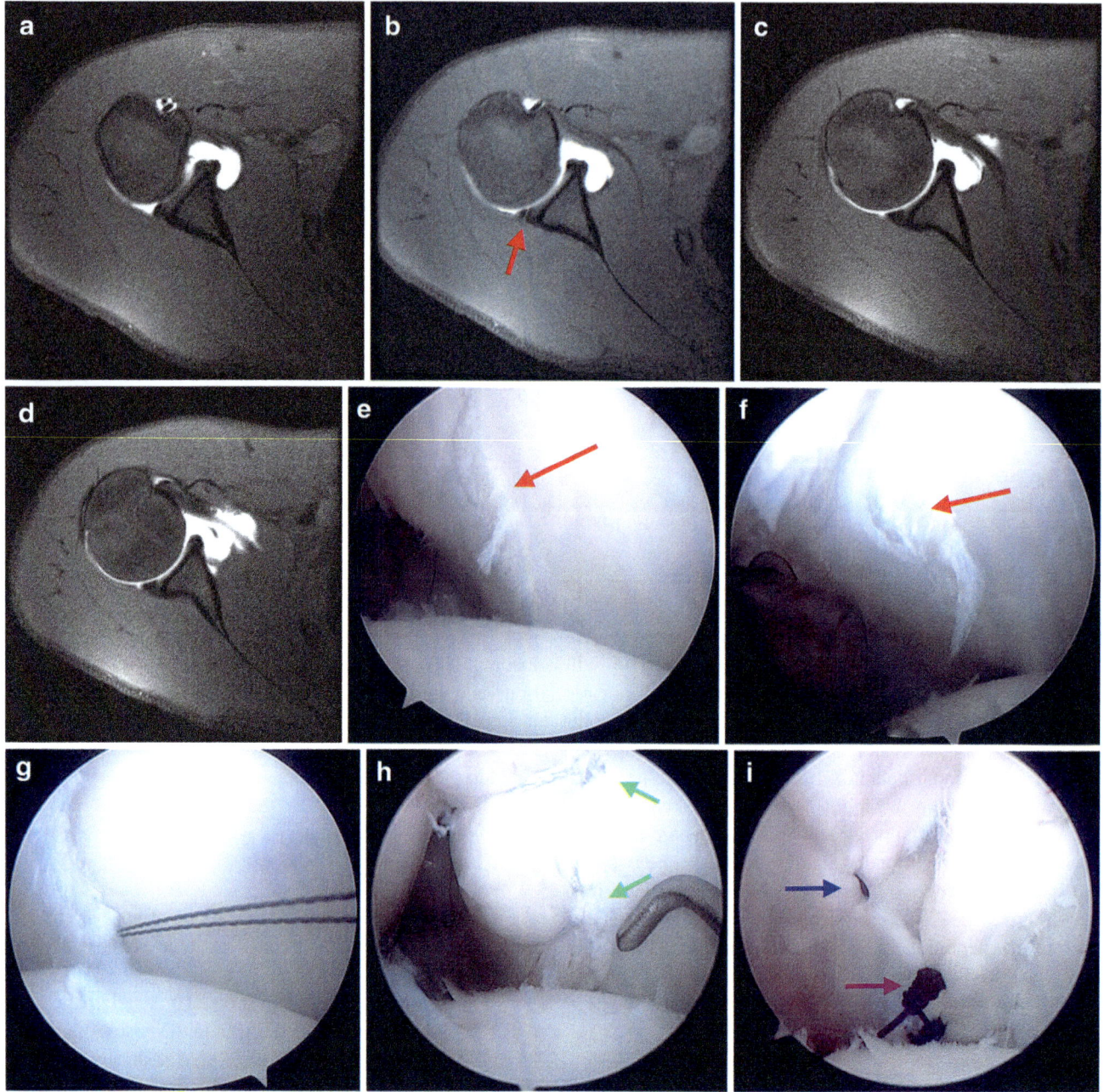

Fig. 13.3 (**a–d**) MRI arthrogram, axial T2 fat suppression images showing a small split (**b**) in the posterior inferior labrum (*red arrow*). (**e, f**) Right shoulder arthroscopy showing slightly frayed posterior labrum without frank detachment. Once probed, it revealed a bigger defect con-sistent with a Kim lesion (*red arrow*). (**g–i**) Posterior capsulorrhaphy (*purple arrows*) and repair of the posterior labrum with anchors (*green arrows*), including repair of the defect left by the posterior cannula (*blue arrow*)

to have a grade 2 posterior subluxation. He was stable anteriorly and had full range of motion.

Portals were placed as described in previous cases in anticipation of a posterior repair. Superior, anterior, and inferior labrum were outwardly normal, and the humeral head had no lesions. The rotator cuff and biceps tendon were normal.

The posterior labrum was slightly frayed and showed evidence of posterior subluxation (Fig. 13.3e, f). It was not frankly detached, but once probed, it revealed a bigger defect consistent with a Kim lesion (concealed lesion of the posterior labrum). He had a patulous posterior capsule.

The posterior labrum was liberated using a soft tissue and labrum liberator, showing an abnormal attachment. Surfaces were prepared with a rasp.

A double-bite technique was used to perform a posterior capsulorrhaphy as well as repair the posterior labrum for each anchor. A suture lasso was then used to shuttle #2 FiberWire sutures around the posterior abnormal labrum and a second bite of posterior inferior capsule. The labrum and capsule were repaired using a total of four absorbable anchors (Fig. 13.3g, h).

In addition, a #0 PDS suture was placed to perform additional capsulorrhaphy tightening of the posterior capsule after labrum repair was complete. The posterior capsule was repaired where the cannula had come through (Fig. 13.3i).

Discussion

This case highlights the classic Kim lesion that can be seen with posterior instability. The posterior labrum often shows signal abnormalities on MRI arthrograms imaging but is not grossly abnormal on initial inspection during arthroscopy. However, probing often demonstrates the labrum to be abnormal with cracking and scuffing consistent with posterior subluxation. If the labrum is at all abnormal on imaging and arthroscopy in the setting of posterior instability, then the authors prefer to take down the suspicious area of labrum and repair it while tightening the posterior capsule, as described by Kim et al. [23].

Case 4: Posterior Dislocation Recurrence

History/Exam

A 16-year-old male, 8 months post-op right shoulder arthroscopy from a combined posterior labrum and SLAP repair, presented to the clinic. Figure 13.4a, b shows the posterior labral tear he suffered after falling on an outstretched arm in football camp last summer. At that time, he did feel his shoulder slide, but it did not come all the way out of joint.

He underwent a posterior labral repair (Fig. 13.4c, d).

He recovered well and returned to play football as a lineman. Ten days before presenting in clinic, he tackled someone and heard a pop, resulting in recurrent pain, mostly over the anterior aspect of his shoulder. He did not perceive the shoulder dislocating but continued to have discomfort.

Examination demonstrated no swelling, but did show tenderness over the anterior joint line and biceps. He had a positive O'Brien test and pain with Jobe's maneuver. Relocation maneuver was positive but had a negative jerk test and no posterior joint line tenderness.

Imaging

Plain radiographs were unremarkable.

An MRI arthrogram was obtained, showing a linear signal evident within the superior labrum extending in the anterior–posterior direction and consistent with underlying SLAP tear (Fig. 13.4e) and showing also the anchor sites from the prior surgery.

On axial T2 fat suppression images (Fig. 13.4f–i), an abnormal linear signal was also seen extending in the superior to inferior direction within the posterior labrum, involving the 2:30–4:30 region. On these cuts, previous anchors were also visible in glenoid bone. When correlating with the previous study, findings indicated potential for re-tear of the posterior labrum.

He was indicated for revision posterior stabilization after failing to improve with conservative measures.

Arthroscopy

The procedure was performed in beach chair position under combined anesthesia.

The right shoulder was examined under anesthesia, showing a grade 2 posterior instability and stable anteriorly. Portals were placed as described in previous cases in anticipation of a posterior repair.

Diagnostic arthroscopy showed that the anterior labrum and superior labrum were intact. His rotator cuff was intact as was his biceps tendon.

His posterior labrum demonstrated partial re-tearing from approximately the 3 o'clock position to the 6 o'clock position, and sutures were still in place (Fig. 13.4j, k).

Prior sutures were removed. The posterior glenoid was prepared using a rasp as well as a shaver and then repaired with a total of five anchors in a double-bite technique to generously plicate the posterior capsule and also capture the posterior labrum (Fig. 13.4l).

The anterior and posterior cannulas were withdrawn, and the capsule defects were closed with 0 PDS sutures without performing an interval closure (Fig. 13.4m).

Discussion

As with all shoulder instability cases treated with surgery, there exists a risk for recurrent injury. This is especially true when the patient returns to high-risk sport activities such as football. MRI imaging of the labrum and capsule becomes more difficult to interpret after prior surgical repair. The labrum often does not look normal even in cases where it has healed appropriately. Hence, the physical examination findings

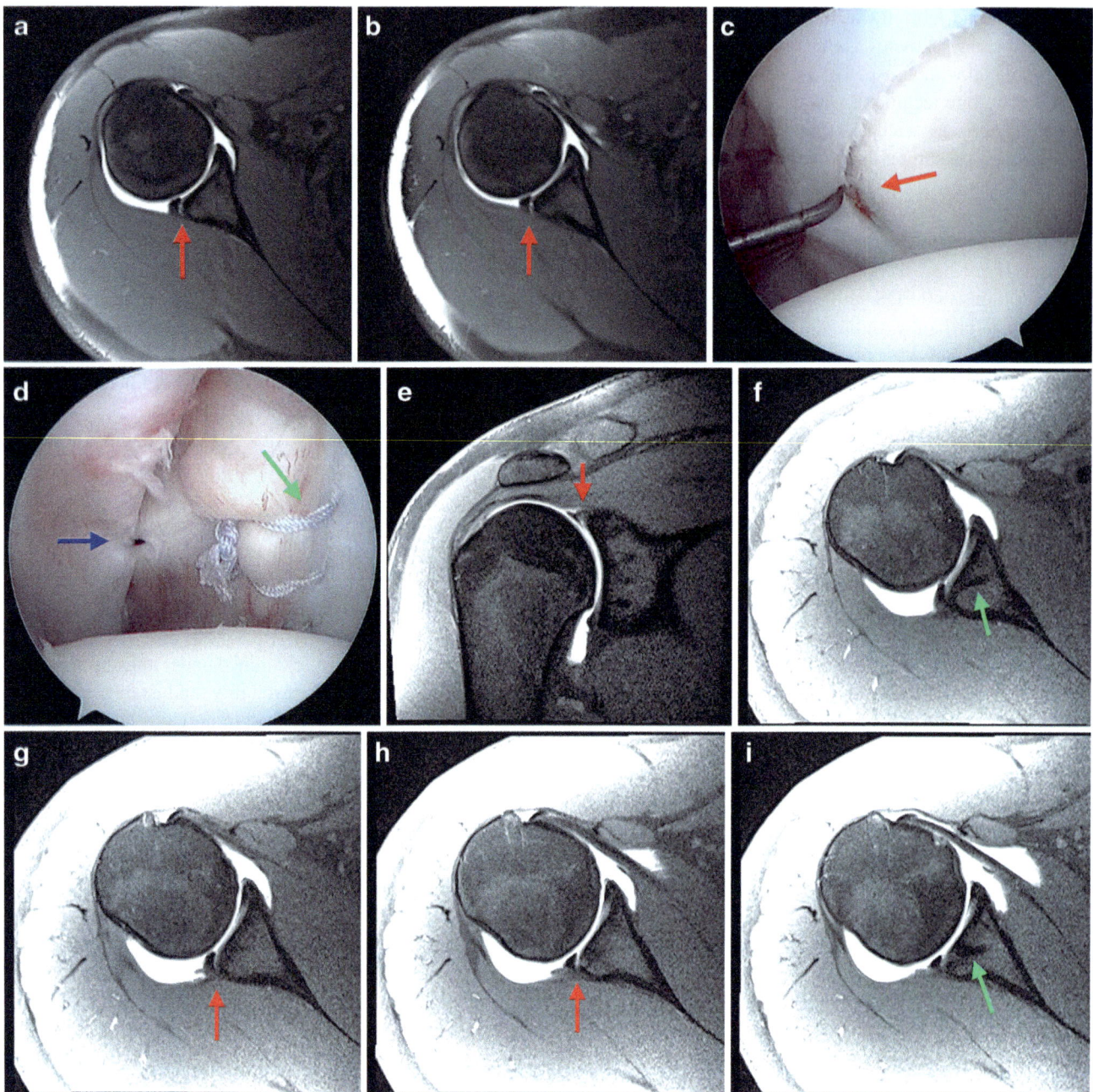

Fig. 13.4 (**a**, **b**) T2 fat suppression axial images showing a posterior labral tear (*red arrow*). (**c**, **d**) Posterior labral repair with anchors (*green arrow*) and repair of the defect left by the posterior cannula (*blue arrow*). (**e**) MRI arthrogram showing concomitant SLAP tear in a patient with posterior instability. A linear signal is evident within the superior labrum (*red arrow*). (**f–i**) Axial T2 fat suppression images showing a linear signal consistent with a posterior labral re-tear (*red arrow*). Anchors from a previous surgery are visible in glenoid (*green arrow*). (**j**, **k**) Arthroscopy of a right shoulder demonstrating partial re-tearing of the posteroinferior labrum (*red arrow*). Sutures of the previous surgery are still in place (*green arrow*). (**l**) After removing prior sutures, the posterior labrum was repaired with a double-bite technique, plicating the posterior capsule (*green arrow*). (**m**) Closure of portal capsule defects with PDS sutures

are even more crucial for diagnosis and treatment decisions than usual. Options for treating a failed arthroscopic posterior labrum repair and stabilization include repeat arthroscopic stabilization versus open repair and capsulorrhaphy. When revision arthroscopic stabilization is done, the authors prefer to include more capsular plication and increased suture anchor fixation points to increase posterior stability as much as possible. The authors also use a slower rehabilitation program and slower return to sport program after revision instability cases.

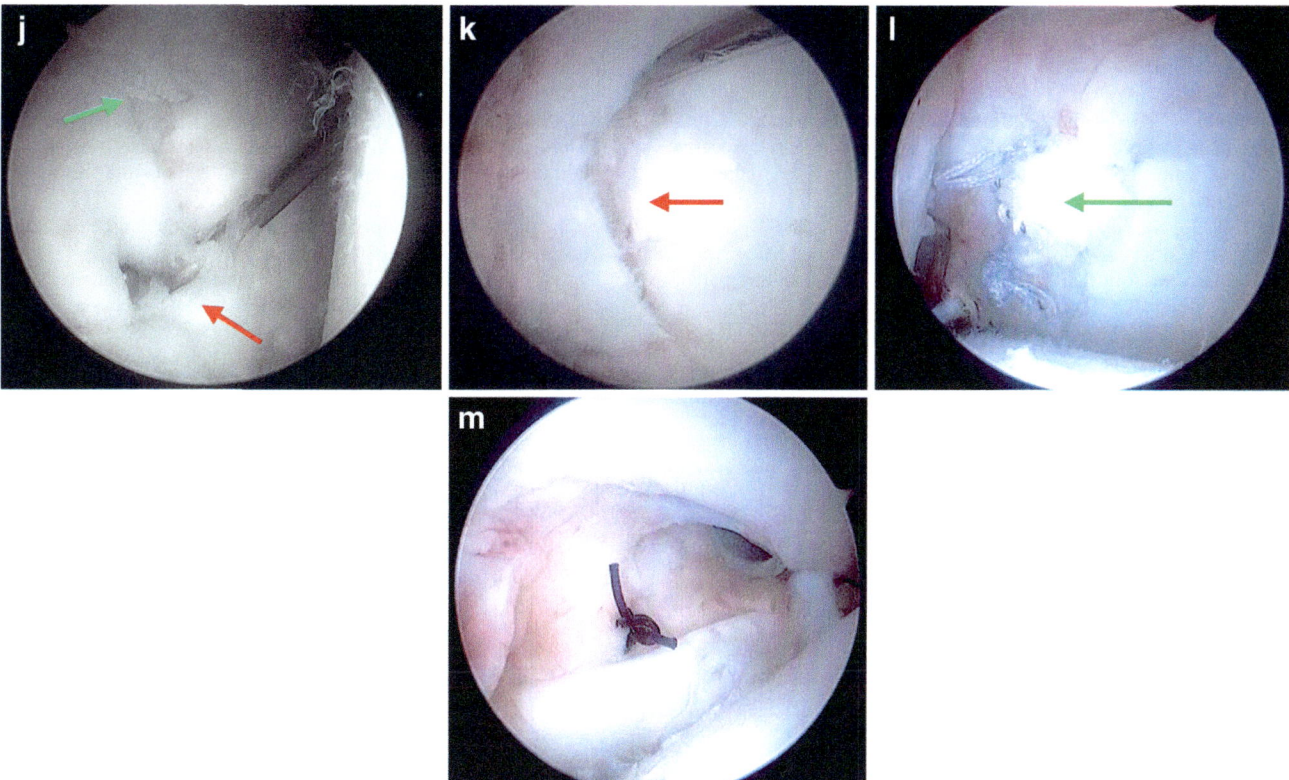

Fig. 13.4 (continued)

Summary

Posterior shoulder instability and labrum pathology is common after trauma and with American football. There are standard physical examination tests that can help elucidate posterior shoulder instability such as the jerk test and posterior joint line tenderness. MRI arthrograms imaging is extremely helpful to accurately define structural pathology that may be present. Arthroscopic techniques are available to restore anatomy and stability for patients suffering from posterior shoulder instability.

References

1. Stoller DW. Magnetic resonance imaging in orthopaedics and sports medicine. 3rd ed. Philadelphia, PA: Lippincott Williams and Wilkins; 2007.
2. Tischer T, Vogt S, Kreuz PC, Imhoff AB. Arthroscopic anatomy, variants, and pathologic findings in shoulder instability. Arthroscopy. 2011;27(10):1434–43.
3. Saupe N, White LM, Bleakney R, Schweitzer ME, Recht MP, Jost B, Zanetti M. Acute traumatic posterior shoulder dislocation: MR findings. Radiology. 2008;248(1):185–93.
4. Macmahon PJ, Palmer WE. Magnetic resonance imaging in glenohumeral instability. Magn Reson Imaging Clin N Am. 2012;20(2): 295–312.
5. Diane Bergin MD. Imaging shoulder instability in the athlete. Magn Reson Imaging Clin N Am. 2009;17(4):595–615.
6. Tung GA, Hou DD. MR arthrography of the posterior labrocapsular complex: relationship with glenohumeral joint alignment and clinical posterior instability. AJR Am J Roentgenol. 2003;180(2): 369–75.
7. Chiavaras MM, Harish S, Burr J. MR arthrographic assessment of suspected posteroinferior labral lesions using flexion, adduction, and internal rotation positioning of the arm: preliminary experience. Skeletal Radiol. 2010;39(5):481–8.
8. Millett PJ, Clavert P, Warner JJ. Arthroscopic management of anterior, posterior, and multidirectional shoulder instability: pearls and pitfalls. Arthroscopy. 2003;19 Suppl 1:86–93.
9. Forsythe B, Ghodadra N, Romeo AA, Provencher MT. Management of the failed posterior/multidirectional instability patient. Sports Med Arthrosc. 2010;18(3):149–61.
10. Cuellar R, Gonzalez J, de la Herran G, et al. Exploration of glenohumeral instability under anesthesia: the shoulder jerk test. Arthroscopy. 2005;21:672–9.
11. Kim SH, Kim HK, Sun JI, Park JS, Oh I. Arthroscopic capsulolabroplasty for posteroinferior multidirectional instability of the shoulder. Am J Sports Med. 2004;32:594–607.
12. Murray PJ, Shaffer BS. Clinical update: MR imaging of the shoulder. Sports Med Arthrosc. 2009;17(1):40–8.
13. De Maeseneer M, Jaovisidha S, Jacobson JA, Tam W, Schils JP, Sartoris DJ, Fronek J, Resnick D. The Bennett lesion of the shoulder. J Comput Assist Tomogr. 1998;22(1):31–4.
14. Weishaupt D, Zanetti M, Nyffeler RW, Gerber C, Hodler J. Posterior glenoid rim deficiency in recurrent (atraumatic) posterior shoulder instability. Skeletal Radiol. 2000;29(4):204–10.
15. Kim SH. Arthroscopic treatment of posterior and multidirectional instability. Oper Tech Sports Med. 2004;12(2):111–21.

16. Major NM, Browne J, Domzalski T, Cothran RL, Helms CA. Evaluation of the glenoid labrum with 3-T MRI: is intraarticular contrast necessary? AJR Am J Roentgenol. 2011;196(5): 1139–44.

17. Kalson NS, Geoghegan JM, Funk L. Magnetic resonance arthrogram and arthroscopy of the shoulder: a comparative retrospective study with emphasis on posterior labral lesions and radiologist locality. Shoulder Elbow. 2011;3:210–4.

18. Modi CS, Karthikeyan S, Marks A, Saithna A, Smith CD, Rai SB, Drew SJ. Accuracy of abduction-external rotation MRA versus standard MRA in the diagnosis of intra-articular shoulder pathology. Orthopedics. 2013;36(3):e337–42.

19. Steinbach LS. MRI of shoulder instability. Eur J Radiol. 2008;68(1):57–71.

20. Shah N, Tung GA. Imaging signs of posterior glenohumeral instability. AJR Am J Roentgenol. 2009;192(3):730–5.

21. Savoie III FH, Holt MS, Field LD, et al. Arthroscopic management of posterior instability: evolution of technique and results. Arthroscopy. 2008;24(4):389–96.

22. Kim SH, Ha KI, Park JH, et al. Arthroscopic posterior labral repair and capsular shift for traumatic unidirectional recurrent posterior subluxation of the shoulder. J Bone Joint Surg Am. 2003;85(8): 1479–87.

23. Kim SH, Ha KI, Yoo JC, et al. Kim's lesion: an incomplete and concealed avulsion of the posteroinferior labrum in posterior or multidirectional posteroinferior instability of the shoulder. Arthroscopy. 2004;20(7):712–20.

24. McLaughlin HL. Posterior dislocation of the shoulder. J Bone Joint Surg Am. 1952;24-A-3:584–90.

25. Kim SH, Noh KC, Park JS, Ryu BD, Oh I. Loss of chondrolabral containment of the glenohumeral joint in atraumatic posteroinferior multidirectional instability. J Bone Joint Surg Am. 2005;87(1):92–8.

26. Wolf BR, Strickland S, Williams RJ, Allen AA, Altchek DW, Warren RF. Open posterior stabilization for recurrent posterior glenohumeral instability. J Shoulder Elbow Surg. 2005;14(2):157–64.

27. Millett PJ, Braun S. The "bony Bankart bridge" procedure: a new arthroscopic technique for reduction and internal fixation of a bony Bankart lesion. Arthroscopy. 2009;25(1):102–5.

Rotator Cuff Disease

14

Robert Z. Tashjian

Introduction

Rotator cuff disorders are the most commonly treated cause of shoulder pain and dysfunction by orthopedic surgeons [1]. Similarly, rotator cuff repair surgery has dramatically increased over the past two decades with increased usage of arthroscopic repairs and outpatient surgery [2]. Despite this dramatic increase in the operative treatment of rotator cuff tears, surgical indications still remain controversial and lack standardization [3]. This lack of consensus is partly attributable to a lack of information regarding the natural history of nonoperatively treated rotator cuff tears. Recently, several authors have published on the natural history of nonoperatively treated rotator cuff tears allowing an improved understanding of the risks involved [4–7]. Utilizing this information along with the wealth of data on the healing rates after surgical treatment of rotator cuff tears, reasonable indications and timing of surgical and nonsurgical treatment of rotator cuff tears can be outlined [8–14].

We have previously published a data-driven algorithm for the treatment of rotator cuff disease [15]. Patients can be grouped into three different categories based upon the risk of tear progression and development of irreversible changes with nonoperative treatment versus the likelihood of healing after rotator cuff repair: group I, low risk for development of irreversible rotator cuff changes with nonoperative management; group II, high risk for development of irreversible rotator cuff changes with nonoperative management as well as a high likelihood for rotator cuff healing if repaired; and group III, irreversible changes have already occurred to the rotator cuff and/or a low likelihood for healing after rotator cuff repair (Table 14.1). Groups I and III can be initially

treated with nonoperative measures, whereas group II should be considered for early initial surgical repair [15].

The purpose of this chapter will utilize a case-based approach to highlight each group of patients. In groups I and III, nonoperative management was utilized initially in each of the cases. Cases were chosen in these groups that failed initial conservative treatment to review arthroscopic aspects of each case. Group II patients underwent initial early surgical repair. Cases were chosen not only to highlight the indications for surgical versus nonsurgical treatment but also to review specific aspects of surgical management that can be recognized on preoperative MRI and then translated to the arthroscopic repair. Topics reviewed will include tear pattern recognition (L-shaped tear, reverse L-shaped tear, U-shaped tear) requiring margin convergence, recognition of rotator cuff muscle and tendon quality, and improved identification of subscapularis tears.

Case 1: Group I—Partial Thickness Undersurface Subscapularis Rotator Cuff Tear

History and Exam

This is a 42-year-old right-hand-dominant miner with two years of anterior shoulder pain. He reports over a 20-year history of overhead work use as a miner. He has had prior intra-articular corticosteroid injections as well as multiple rounds of physical therapy. The injections temporarily improved his symptoms. He currently has difficulty with work relegating him to work out of the mine.

On physical examination, he has symmetric range of motion of the effected shoulder compared with the opposite shoulder. He has tenderness over his biceps tendon anteriorly and pain with Speeds maneuver and the active compression test. He has no tenderness over his acromioclavicular joint and no pain with cross shoulder adduction. He has pain with a bear-hug test, lift-off test, and abdominal compression

R.Z. Tashjian (✉)
Department of Orthopedic Surgery, University of Utah,
Salt Lake City, UT, USA
e-mail: Robert.tashjian@hsc.utah.edu

S.F. Brockmeier (ed.), *MRI-Arthroscopy Correlations: A Case-Based Atlas of the Knee, Shoulder, Elbow and Hip*,
DOI 10.1007/978-1-4939-2645-9_14, © Springer Science+Business Media New York 2015

181

Table 14.1 Treatment algorithm for rotator cuff disease

Group I—initial nonoperative treatment

- Tendonitis
- Partial-thickness tears (except maybe larger bursal-sided tears)
- Maybe small (<1 cm) full-thickness tears

Group II—consider early surgical repair

- All acute tears full-thickness (except maybe small [<1 cm] tears)
- All chronic full-thickness tears in a young (<65) age group (except maybe small [<1 cm] tears)

Group III—initial nonoperative treatment

- All chronic full-thickness tears in an older (>65 or 70) age group
- Irreparable tears (based on tear size, retraction, muscle quality, and migration)

Used with permission from Tashjian RZ. Epidemiology, natural history, and indications for treatment of rotator cuff tears. Clin Sports Med 2012;31:589–604

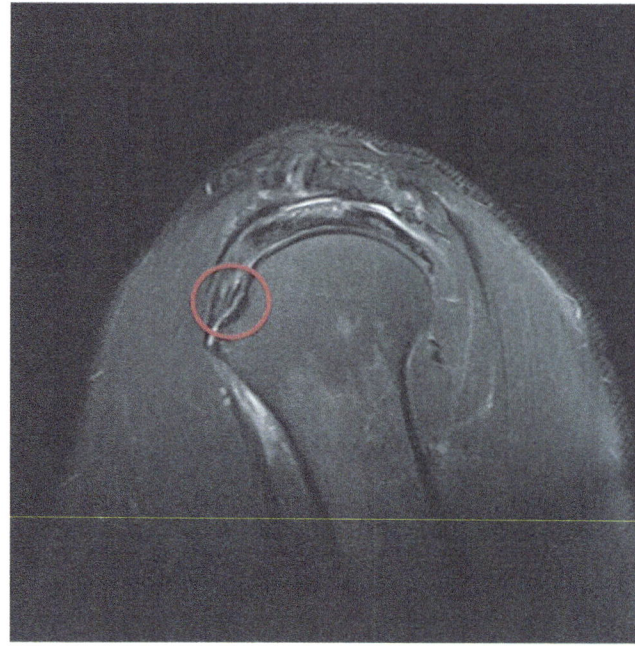

Fig. 14.2 Sagittal T2 MRI image showing exposed lesser tuberosity footprint of undersurface partial-thickness subscapularis tear (*circle*)

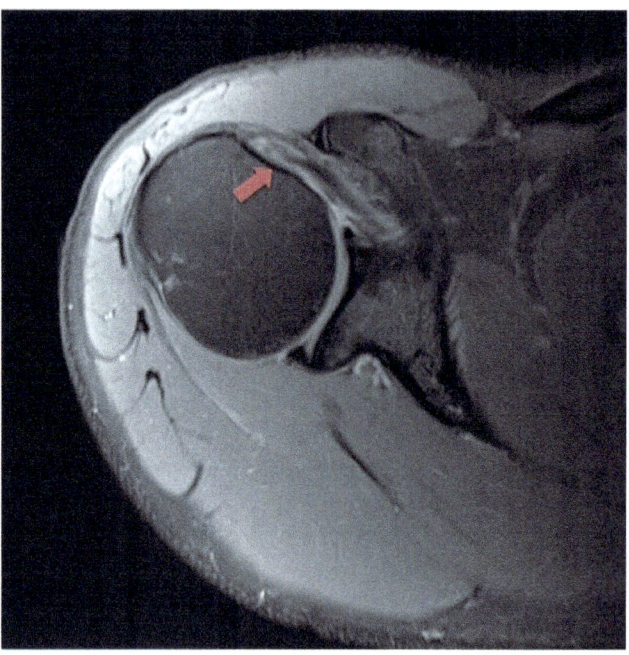

Fig. 14.1 Axial T2 MRI image with a partial-thickness undersurface upper third subscapularis tear (*arrow*)

testing although he has no weakness with these maneuvers. He has no pain and full strength with thumbs-down scapular plane elevation at 90° of elevation and external rotation at the side.

Imaging

Axial T2 MRI images reveal partial undersurface detachment (red arrow) of the subscapularis tendon (Fig. 14.1). Waviness in the subscapularis tendon is a marker for probable tearing at the insertion. Sagittal T2 MRI images reveal the same partial undersurface tear of the upper third of the subscapularis tendon (red circle) (Fig. 14.2). While biceps tendon deep

subluxation was not noted in this patient (not shown), in the presence of subscapularis tearing, either partial or full thickness, biceps instability/subluxation should be presumed to be present and should be specifically looked for during review of axial images. Anterior humeral head subluxation should also be investigated on both plain radiographs and MRI since this is typically prognostic for a very large, chronic subscapularis injury that may not be completely reparable.

Arthroscopy

The patient was considered a group I patient and was initially treated conservatively. Due to failure of conservative treatment, the patient was indicated for arthroscopic subscapularis repair and open subpectoral biceps tenodesis.

At the time of arthroscopic subscapularis repair, the biceps tendon was noted to have significant fraying and partial-thickness tearing; therefore, it was cut for later tenodesis (Fig. 14.3). The upper third of the subscapularis was noted to have undersurface tearing although the footprint was not obviously visible using a 30° arthroscope (Fig. 14.4). After application of a "posterior level push" and the switching to a 70° scope, the lesser tuberosity footprint was well visualized [16] (Fig. 14.5). A single triple-loaded 5.5 mm metal anchor was placed into the bed of the lesser tuberosity, and three stitches were passed (inferior two as simple stitches and superior stitch as a lasso loop) and tied completing the all intra-articular repair [17] (Fig. 14.6).

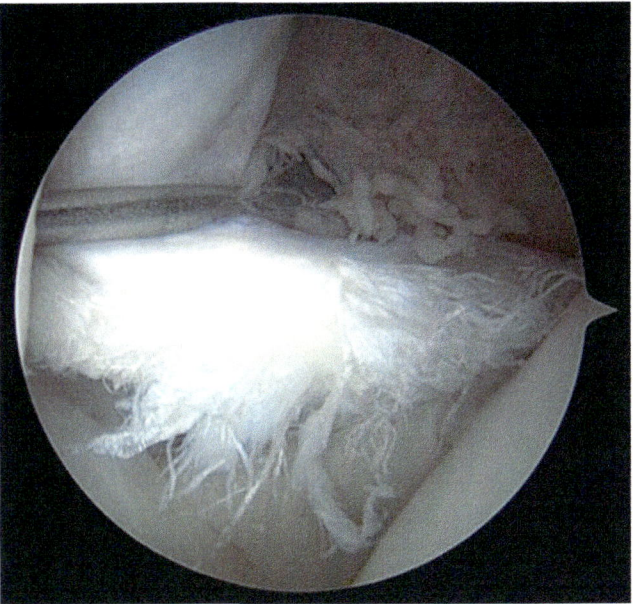

Fig. 14.3 High-grade partial-thickness tear of the intra-articular portion of the biceps tendon long head

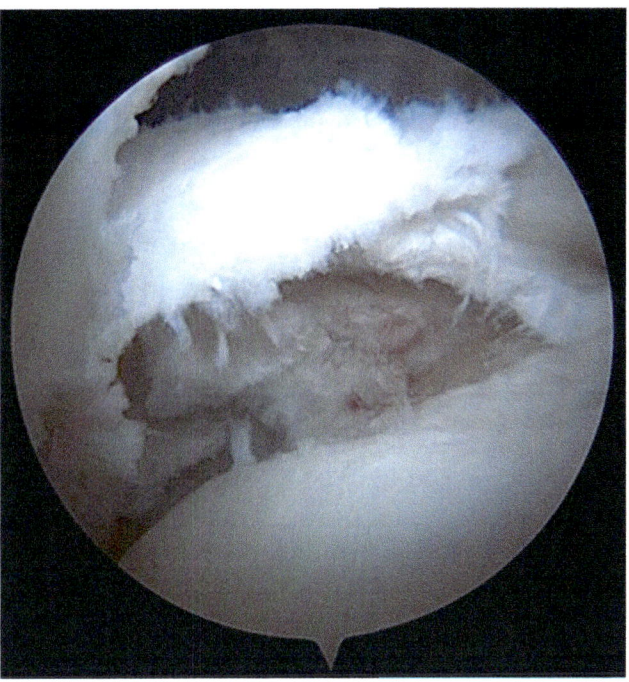

Fig. 14.5 Improved arthroscopic visualization of the lesser tuberosity footprint of the partial undersurface subscapularis tear using a 70-degree arthroscope and a "posterior lever push"

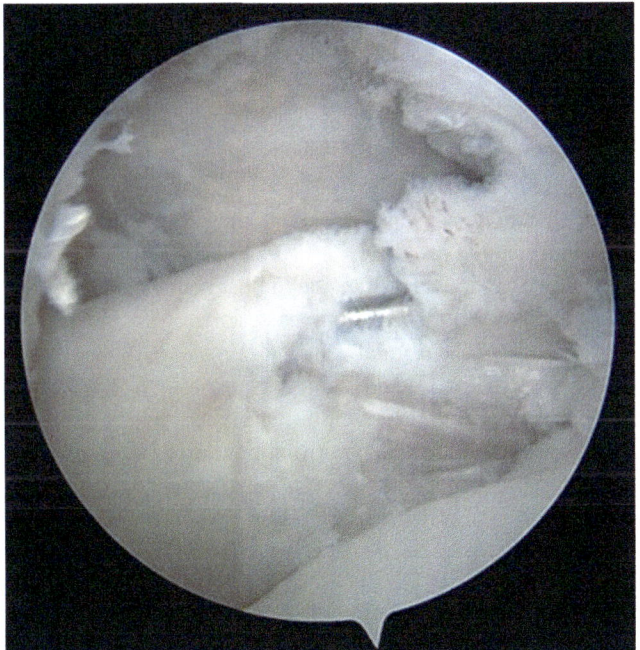

Fig. 14.4 Arthroscopic view of the partial undersurface subscapularis tear utilizing a 30-degree arthroscope

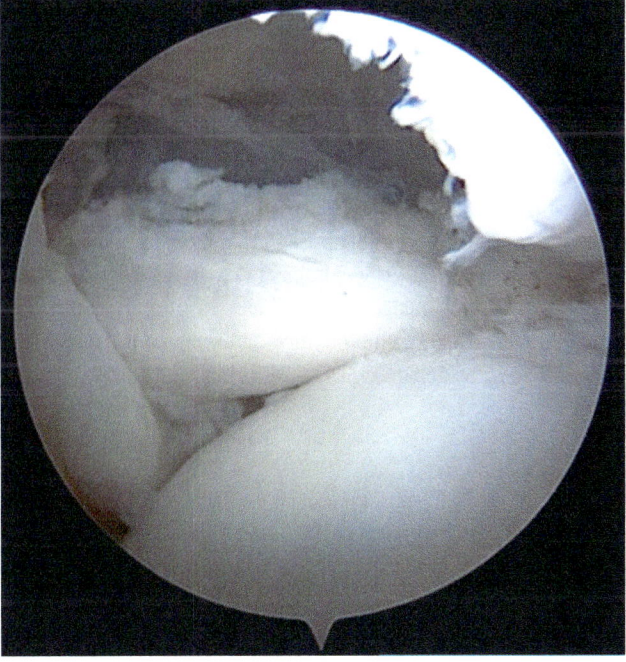

Fig. 14.6 Arthroscopic view of the final subscapularis tendon repair

Discussion

All partial-thickness rotator cuff tears can be initially treated conservatively and are therefore considered group I patients. In general, partial-thickness tears have shown good response to conservative treatment and have also shown a very slow, low risk for tear enlargement or progression making nonop-erative treatment safe and effective [4]. Maman et al. evaluated 26 symptomatic partial-thickness rotator cuff tears and determined that 8 % of tears had increased in tear size over 5 mm at an average of 1.5 years with 92 % having no change [4]. Consequently, it is reasonable to consider nonoperative treatment for partial thickness tears and proceed with surgical repair only if there is a failure of conservative management.

Arthroscopic repair of subscapularis tears has shown excellent outcomes in improving pain and function with very high healing rates [18, 19]. MRI can sometimes be difficult to clearly define injuries, especially partial thickness under-surface tears. A tip on identifying these injuries is to be aware of waviness in the subscapularis tendon and deep sublux-ation of the biceps tendon on axial views as well as evaluat-ing the lesser tuberosity footprint on the sagittal MRI views which can often more clearly show the detachment as in this case. Tips to improve visualization and access to the lesser tuberosity during the procedure include a "posterior lever push" and use of the 70-degree scope.

Case 2: Group II—Chronic Full-Thickness Rotator Cuff Tear in a Young (<65 Years Old) Patient and Failed Arthroscopic Rotator Cuff Repair: Lateral Failure

History and Exam

This is a 54-year-old right-hand-dominant female with six months of chronic shoulder pain. She reports no recent trauma to her shoulder. Her pain is in the anterolateral loca-tion worsened by overhead activities. She cannot sleep due to shoulder pain. She has only tried anti-inflammatory medica-tions without improvement.

On physical examination, she has symmetric scapular plane elevation to 160° and external rotation to 50°. She has pain with resisted rotator cuff testing in thumbs-down for-ward elevation at 90° of scapular plane elevation as well as weakness. She has mild weakness in external rotation at the side as well. She has a positive Neer impingement test as well as Hawkins test. She has no tenderness over either her biceps tendon or acromioclavicular joint.

Imaging

Plain radiographs of the shoulder show no signs of glenohu-meral or acromioclavicular joint arthritis with a well-centered humeral head. Coronal T2 MRI images of the shoulder show a 2.5 cm full-thickness, mildly retracted rotator cuff tear of the supraspinatus tendon with grade I Goutallier changes of the supraspinatus muscle (Fig. 14.7). She has limited signal heterogeneity of the tendon on MRI. The tendon length is over 25 mm, and the musculotendinous junction of the supra-spinatus is laterally positioned to the glenoid face.

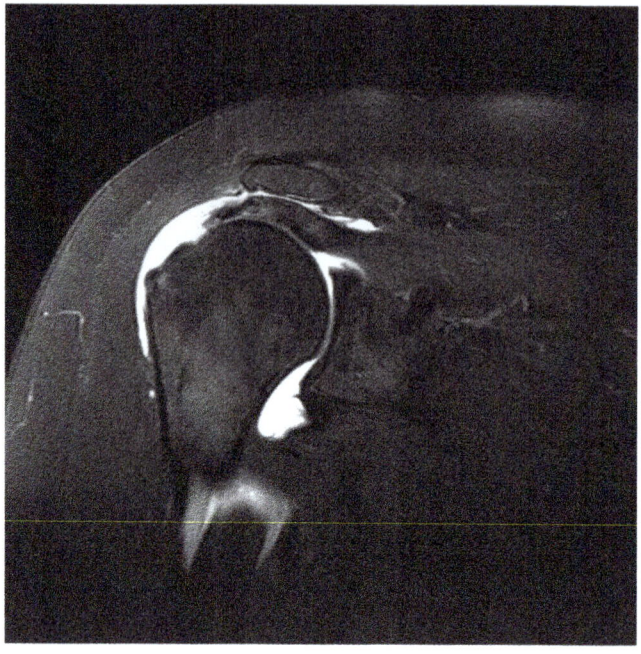

Fig. 14.7 Coronal T2 MRI image of a full-thickness supraspinatus tear with mild retraction

Arthroscopy

Because this is a full-thickness symptomatic rotator cuff tear of substantial size in a young (<65 years old) patient, this was considered a group II patient therefore indicated for early surgical repair.

The patient had an arthroscopy in the beach chair position and was viewed through both posterior and lateral portals while in the subacromial space during the repair. Intra-articular exam revealed no significant pathology, and the sub-scapularis was normal. A mobile crescent-shaped tear was found of the supraspinatus with mild tendinopathic changes (Fig. 14.8). A double-row transosseous-equivalent repair was performed with limited tension (Fig. 14.9).

Postoperative Course

The patient underwent conservative postoperative care including sling wear for 6 weeks as well as passive motion starting at 2 weeks. Active and active-assisted motion started at 6 weeks, and strengthening commenced at three months postoperative. At 6 months postoperative, the patient still had lateral-based pain and pain with resisted cuff testing. Her motion had returned to normal and had reasonable strength with rotator cuff testing.

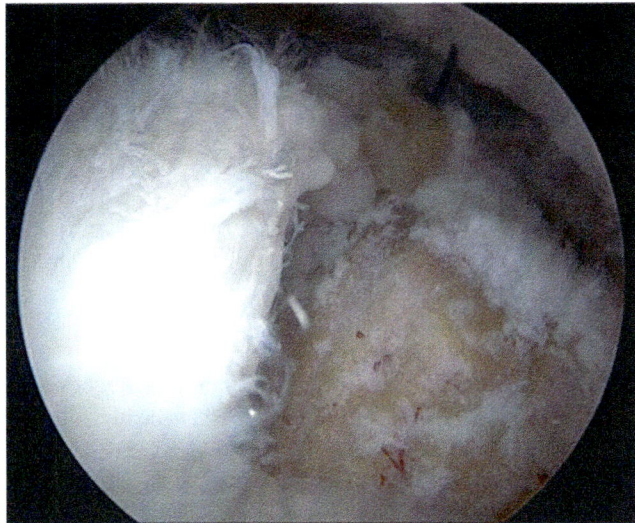

Fig. 14.8 Arthroscopic view from the posterior portal of a crescentic full-thickness supraspinatus tear. There are obvious tendinopathic changes of the rotator cuff tissue

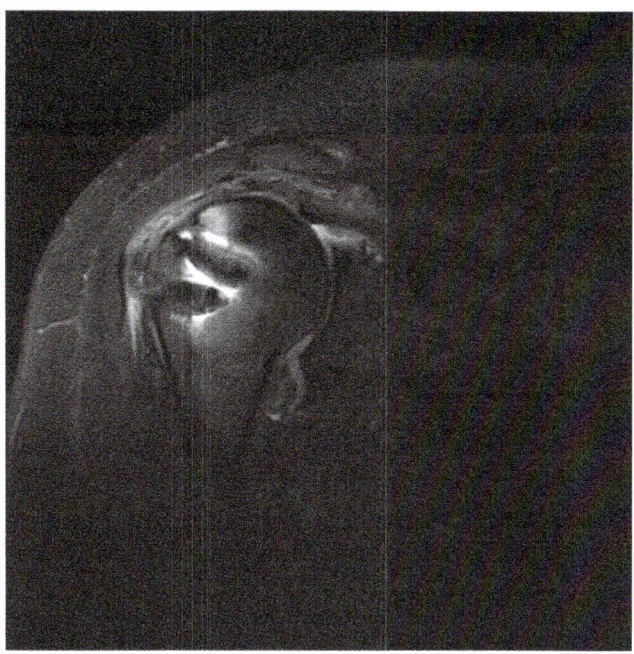

Fig. 14.10 Coronal T2 MRI image of a full-thickness retear of the supraspinatus repair with increased retraction compared to preoperative imaging but preserved tendon length

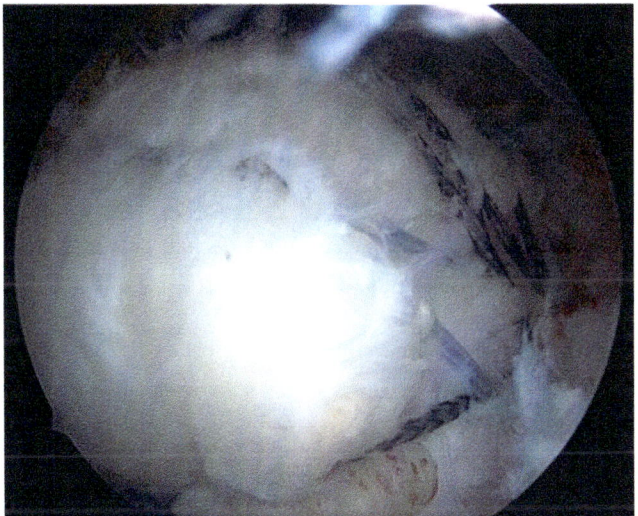

Fig. 14.9 Arthroscopic view from the posterior portal of the complete transosseous equivalent double-row rotator cuff repair

Imaging

Repeat MRI was performed which showed evidence of repair failure with scar tissue interposed between the tendon edge and the tuberosity (Fig. 14.10). The supraspinatus had waviness of the tendon also suggesting the tissue at the footprint was only scar and not healed tendon. Sagittal T1 MRI image of the shoulder shows Goutallier grade II changes to the supraspinatus and infraspinatus muscles (Fig. 14.11). The residual

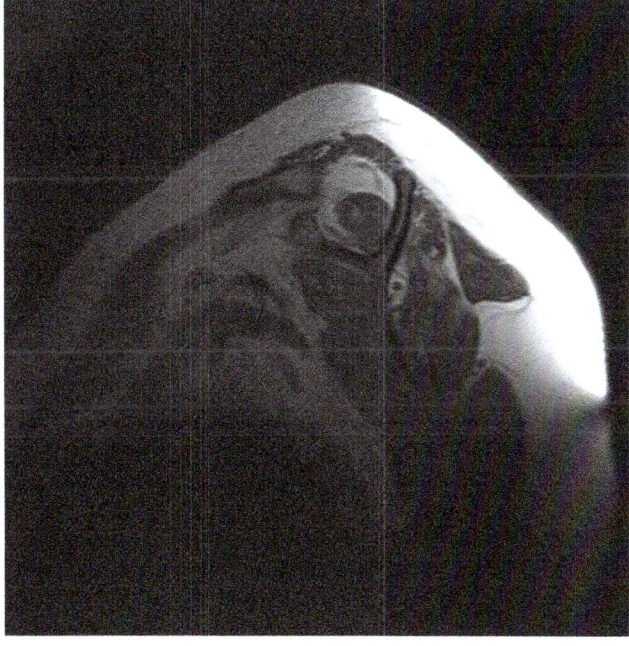

Fig. 14.11 Sagittal T1 MRI image showing Goutallier grade II changes to the supraspinatus and infraspinatus muscles

tendon length was still 25 mm although the musculotendinous junction of the supraspinatus was now approximately at the level of the glenoid face.

Arthroscopy

The patient returned for revision rotator cuff repair and was found to have only fibrous tissue overlaying the greater tuberosity (Fig. 14.12). The tissue was debrided, and anchors were removed leaving moderate amounts of tuberosity cavitation at the site of the prior anchors (Fig. 14.13). A single-row repair was performed with limited tension with three

triple-loaded anchors placed at the anatomic neck using nine simple stitches (Fig. 14.14). Microfracture of the greater tuberosity was also performed to stimulate repair healing.

Discussion

Rotator cuff repair was indicated in both instances because each time the patient had a reparable chronic rotator cuff tear in a young (<65-year-old) patient (group II). Substantially sized (>1 cm) chronic reparable full-thickness rotator cuff tears in young patients are indicated for early surgical repair due to the risk for tear progression as well as the high chance for healing if repair is performed [5, 9, 14]. Safran et al. followed 51 patients under the age of 60 with symptomatic full-thickness rotator cuff tears treated conservatively and found that 49 % of tears increased in size at an average of 29 months [5]. Pain at the time of follow-up correlated with significant tear progression. They recommended that young patients with conservatively treated full-thickness tears be monitored with an ultrasound for increases in tear size especially if they remain symptomatic. Tashjian et al. and Boileau et al. determined that younger age correlated with significantly improved healing rates after arthroscopic double-row and single-row repairs, respectively [9, 14]. Given the increased risk for tear progression and the improved chance for healing in a young aged population, early surgical repair was indicated in this patient.

Failure of rotator cuff healing can occur despite healing rates after transosseous equivalent arthroscopic rotator

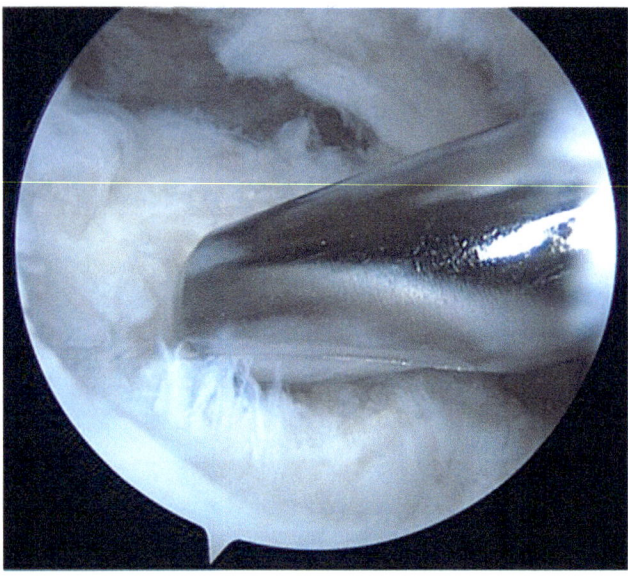

Fig. 14.12 Fibrous scar tissue being debrided from the greater tuberosity footprint in the location of the prior repair

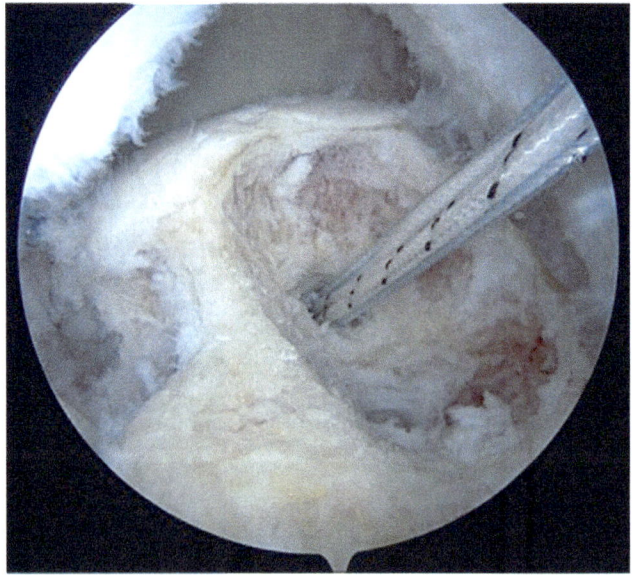

Fig. 14.13 Arthroscopic view from the lateral portal after preparation of the footprint and tendon for re-repair. The cavitary defect left from the prior anchor is obvious, and a new anchor was placed near the articular margin for the re-repair

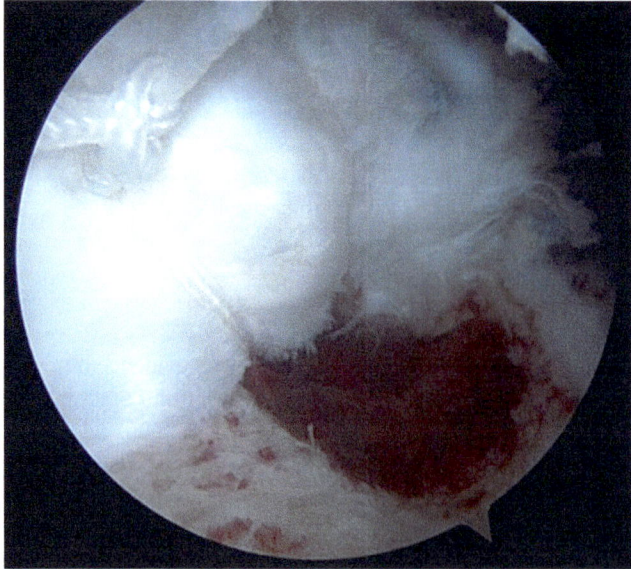

Fig. 14.14 Arthroscopic view from the posterior portal of the final revision repair construct using a single-row technique and triple-loaded suture anchors

cuff repairs being reported to be very high (<3 cm—92 % healing; >3 cm—83 %) [20, 21]. Not all patients with failure of rotator cuff healing have significant disability. Maintenance of clinical improvement has been documented even after repair failure at long term with 95 % satisfaction [22]. Despite these promising results, there are likely subgroups of patients that do poorly including younger patients, patients with a worker's compensation claim, patients with lower education levels, and patients with labor-intensive jobs [23, 24]. This patient was younger than the average rotator cuff repair patient although otherwise she didn't have any other risk factors for a clinical failure.

In the setting of full-thickness recurrent tears in young patients, the major factor that might influence the indication of revision repair is the residual quality of the rotator cuff—both muscle and tendon. In this case, the patient had Goutallier stage II changes to the supraspinatus and infraspinatus muscles and a preoperative tendon length of 25 mm with minimal retraction (Fig. 14.11). Goutallier originally described the quality of the rotator cuff muscles on CT scan, and Fuch's et al. translated the grading to MRI [25, 26]. The Goutallier grades are as follows: 0, normal muscle; I, streaks of fat; II, less fat than muscle; III, equal fat and muscle; and IV, more fat than muscle. Liem et al. have previously shown a correlation of healing after rotator cuff repair with quality of the rotator cuff muscle with worse healing rates with Goutallier stage II and above [13]. Despite having slightly worsened fatty degeneration, re-repair was still indicated in this young patient.

Other MRI findings that should be scrutinized prior to surgical re-repair include the preoperative tendon length, tendon retraction, and position of the musculotendinous junction. Meyer et al. have shown the importance of preoperative tendon length on the likelihood for healing after rotator cuff repair [27]. They reported that if the supraspinatus had Goutallier grade II or III changes and a tendon length of less than 15 mm, then the failure rate was 92 %, but if the tendon length was greater than 15 mm, then the failure rate was only 33 %. With Goutallier grade 0 or I changes, then failure rates were 57 % and 25 % for tears with preoperative tendon lengths less than 15 mm and greater than 15 mm, respectively. Tashjian et al. reported on the importance of the musculotendinous junction position relative to the face of the glenoid on preoperative MRIs [28]. Healing rates after arthroscopic rotator cuff repair were 93 % compared to 55 % if the musculotendinous junction of the supraspinatus was either lateral or medial to the glenoid face, respectively. In the current case, the musculotendinous junction was approaching the glenoid face but still stayed lateral and there was preserved tendon length; therefore, re-repair was indicated with a reasonable chance for healing.

Few series have reported the results of revision arthroscopic rotator cuff repair. In general, repair will allow improved function and reduced pain and reasonable patient satisfaction although healing rates are often inferior to those of primary repairs [29, 30]. Female sex, lower preoperative forward elevation, higher preoperative pain scores, and greater than one prior shoulder surgery are poor prognostic risk factors for obtaining a satisfactory result [31, 32]. Keener et al. evaluated 21 patients after arthroscopic revision rotator cuff repair and found an overall healing rate of 48 % with improved healing in smaller tears (70 % healing rate in single tendon tears, 27 % healing rate in multiple tendon tears) and a younger age group [29]. Nevertheless, complication rates after revision cuff repair have been reported to be about double the rate of primary arthroscopic repairs [33]. In general, patients need to be counseled prior to revision repair of the potential for worse tendon healing and higher complication rates compared to their primary surgery.

Case 3: Group II—Revision Arthroscopic Rotator Cuff Repair After Medial Failure Using Margin Convergence Stitches

History and Exam

The patient is a 58-year-old male that underwent an arthroscopic rotator cuff repair using a single-row technique approximately nine months prior. Despite therapy, the patient still felt pain with overhead activities and reported symptoms of weakness. On exam, he could elevate to 150° in forward elevation but with weakness. External rotation strength was preserved.

Imaging

A postoperative MRI revealed a Cho type II rotator cuff repair failure with healing of a lateral stump of tissue to the greater tuberosity and minimal residual tendon lateral to the supraspinatus muscle [10]. Muscle quality of the supraspinatus was still preserved with Goutallier grade I changes (Fig. 14.15).

Arthroscopy

The patient was considered a group II patient because of his young age (<65 years), reasonable muscle quality (Goutallier grade I) and the full-thickness nature of the tear. The tear was not considered irreparable based upon the MRI images.

At the time of revision surgery, the patient had a large U-shaped retracted tear (Fig. 14.16). We were not able to mobilize the tendon edge directly to the anatomic neck of the greater

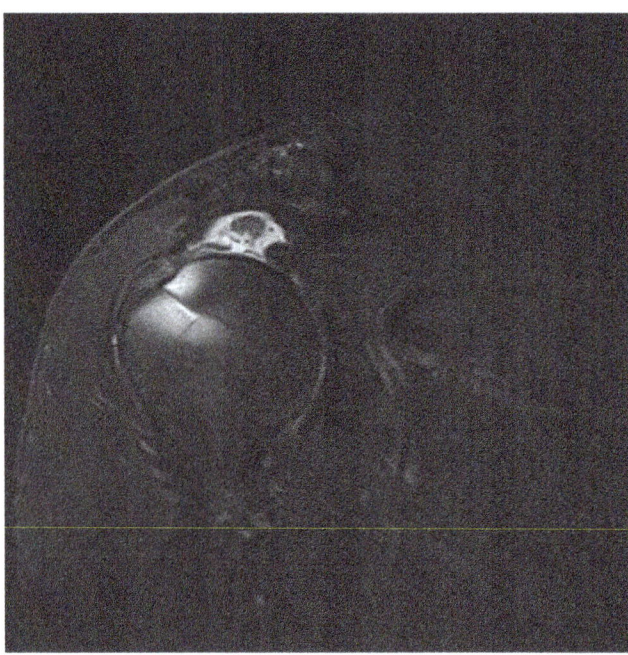

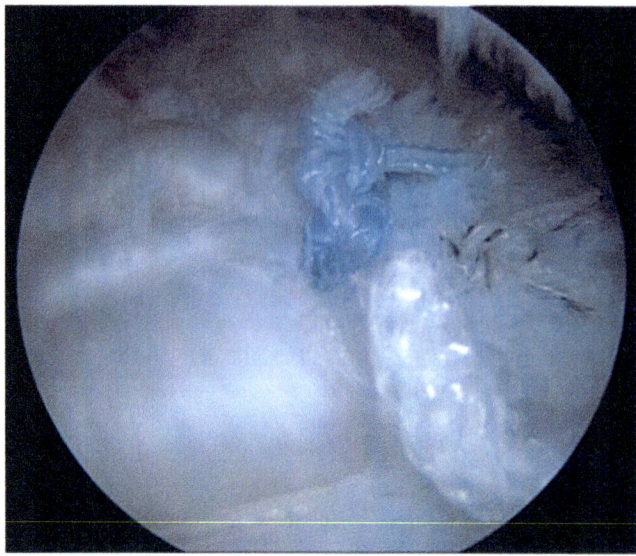

Fig. 14.17 Arthroscopic view of the final revision repair using multiple margin convergence stitches

Fig. 14.15 Coronal T2 MRI image of a recurrent full-thickness tear with a remnant of rotator cuff attached laterally to the greater tuberosity (Cho type II)

Discussion

Margin convergence repair was originally described by Burkart et al. to fix large, chronically retracted rotator cuff tears (U-shaped pattern) [34]. MRI images will often reveal a very small stump of tendon lateral to the muscle of the rotator cuff. These images should alert the surgeon that the tear pattern is likely to be either a U-shaped, L-shaped, or reverse L-shaped pattern instead of a simple crescent pattern [35] (Figs. 14.18a–c and 14.19a–c). Crescent-shaped tears often have a medial-to-lateral length less than the total width of the tear with a length less than 2 cm. L-shaped, reverse L-shaped, or U-shaped will typically have an anteroposterior width less than the length of the tear with the width less than 2 cm. Massive contracted tears are considered those where the length and width are both greater than 2 cm and can often only be partially repaired and not directly repaired to the bone. Identifying these tear patterns (crescent vs. L-shaped, reverse L-shaped, U-shaped vs. massive contracted) prior to surgery will alert the surgeon that during arthroscopy, margin convergence will likely be required in order to improve the ability to perform a tension-free repair.

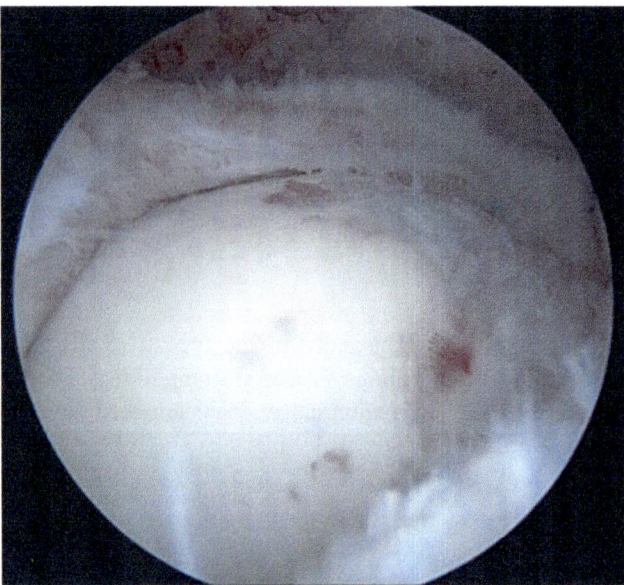

Fig. 14.16 Arthroscopic view from the posterior portal showing a large U-shaped recurrent tear

tuberosity. Several side-to-side margin convergence stitches were utilized to close the rent and allow re-approximation of the cuff back to the anatomic neck of the greater tuberosity (Fig. 14.17).

Medial-based retears are much more common after double-row repairs as opposed to single-row repairs although both failure mechanisms can occur with both types of repairs [10]. Medial failures are often more difficult to repair and often a direct tendon-to-bone re-repair is not achievable and will often require margin convergence stitches as in this case. Awareness should be made of significant tendon heterogeneity or delamination on MRI as this will likely be associated with

Fig. 14.18 (**a–c**) U-shaped tear and repair configuration (Used with permission from Davidson J, Burkhart SS. The geometric classification of rotator cuff tears: a system linking tear pattern to treatment and prognosis. Arthroscopy 2010;26(3):41–24.)

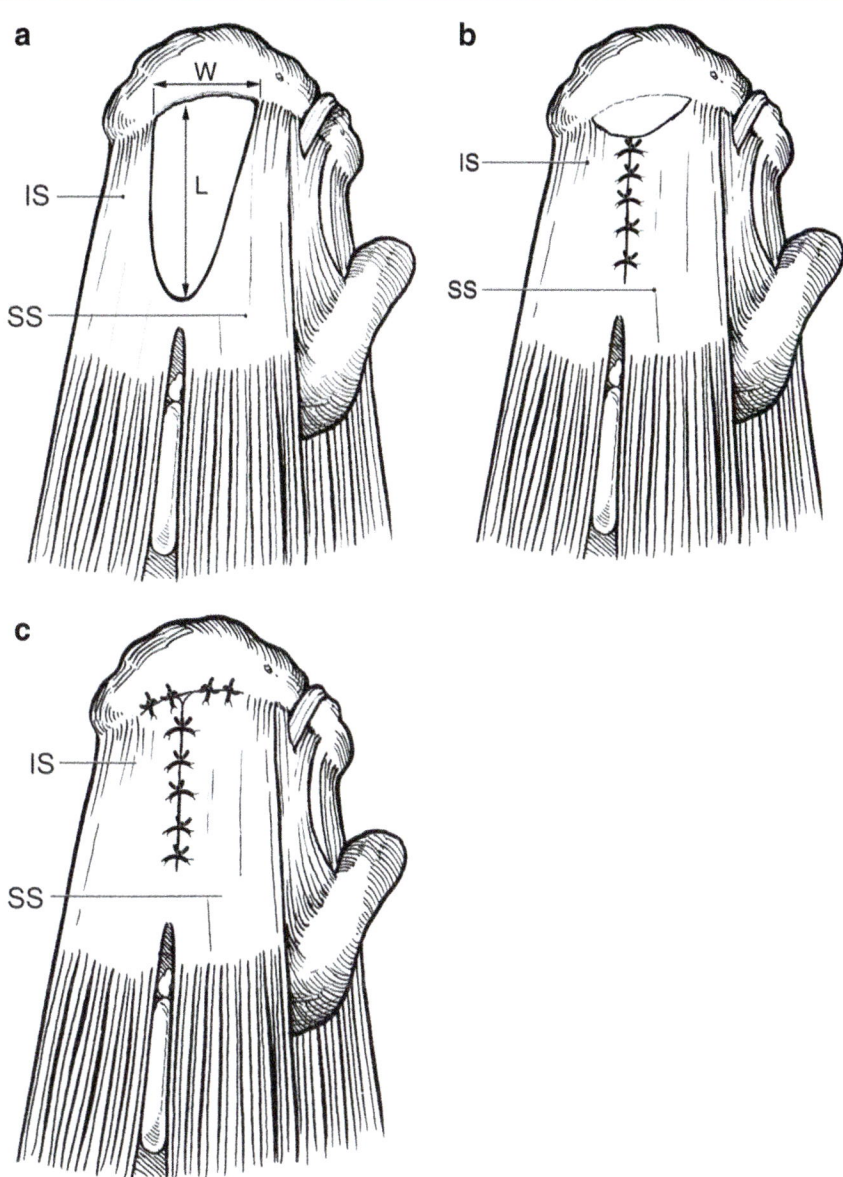

poor tissue quality at the time of repair. Augmentation with an acellular dermal matrix graft as an augmentation patch may be considered to strengthen the repair in the setting of poor tissue quality [36].

Case 4: Group III—Massive Irreparable Full-Thickness Rotator Cuff Tear With a Reverse L-Shaped Pattern

History and Exam

The patient is a 57-year-old right-hand-dominant female with chronic right shoulder pain for 10 months. She had an insidious onset of lateral shoulder pain and progressive weakness. She has difficulty sleeping, working overhead, and performing her part-time job working as a clerk in a store. She has attempted both physical therapy and subacromial injection without significant improvement.

On physical examination, she can elevate her arm to 160 of forward elevation although she has both weakness and pain with forward elevation and external rotation at the side. She has obvious atrophy of her supraspinatus and infraspinatus fossa. She has a negative belly press and negative Hornblower's sign.

Imaging

MRI of her shoulder is consistent and shows a large retracted rotator cuff tear involving the supraspinatus and infraspinatus (4 cm anteroposterior width and 4 cm of retraction).

Fig. 14.19 (**a–c**) L-shaped tear and repair configuration (Used with permission rom Davidson J, Burkhart SS. The geometric classification of rotator cuff tears: a system linking tear pattern to treatment and prognosis. Arthroscopy 2010;26(3):41–24.)

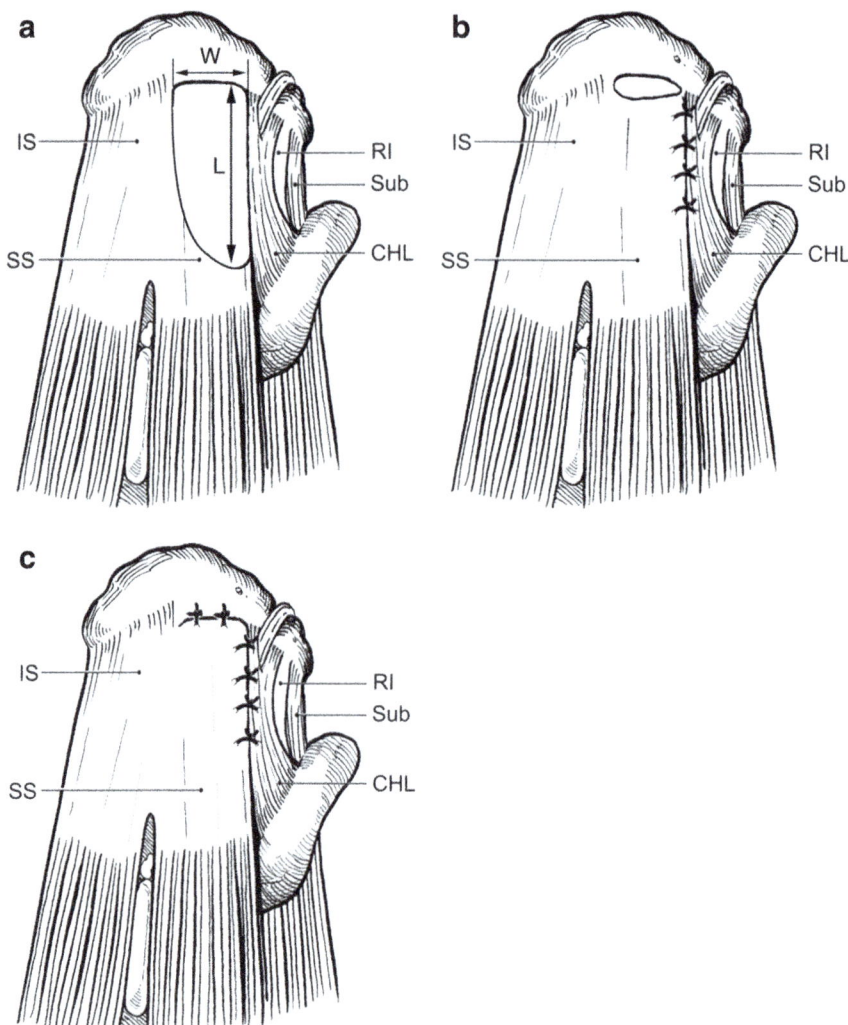

Coronal MRI T2 sections show retraction of the tendon to the glenoid with minimal tendon length at the posterior portion of the supraspinatus (Fig. 14.20). Sagittal MRI T1 sections show Goutallier grade III changes to the supraspinatus and grade IV changes to the infraspinatus (Fig. 14.21).

Arthroscopy

The patient was considered a group III patient because the tear size (massive), tendon retraction (to the glenoid), and cuff fatty degeneration (grade III and IV) were severe enough to consider the tear irreparable despite the young age of the patient. The initial surgical plan was to perform an arthroscopic debridement for pain as well as a biceps tenotomy.

At the time of arthroscopy, a reverse L-shape tear pattern was recognized (Fig. 14.22). Despite what appeared to be a completely irreparable tear preoperatively, there was a very large anterior rotator cuff leaf of the supraspinatus tendon that could be easily reduced back to the infraspinatus by placing several side-to-side stitches (Fig. 14.23).

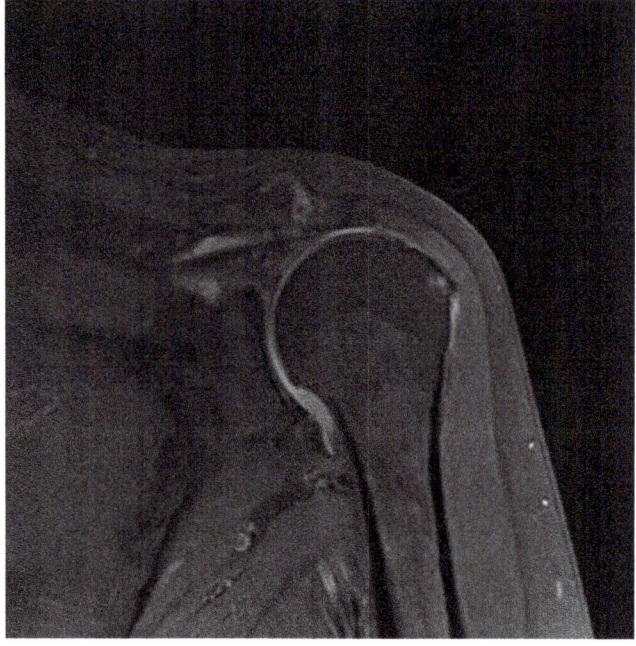

Fig. 14.20 Coronal T2 MRI image of a massive retracted rotator cuff tear with limited residual lateral tendon length

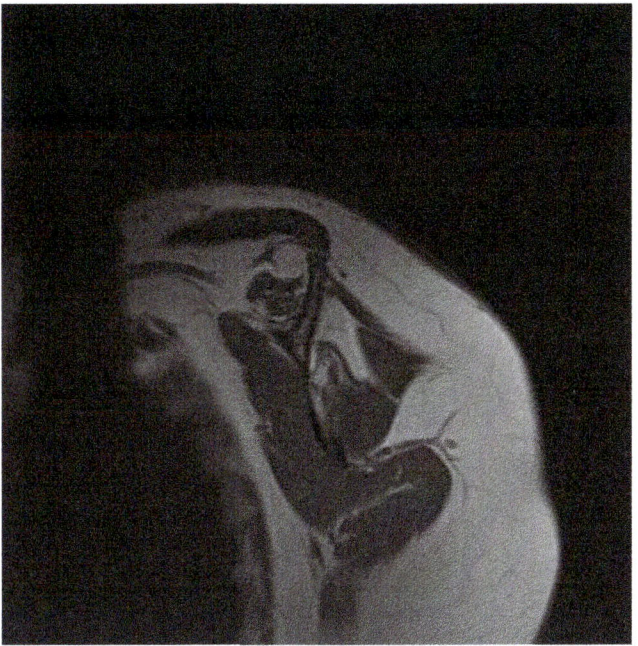

Fig. 14.21 Sagittal T1 MRI image showing Goutallier grade III changes to the supraspinatus and grade IV changes to the infraspinatus

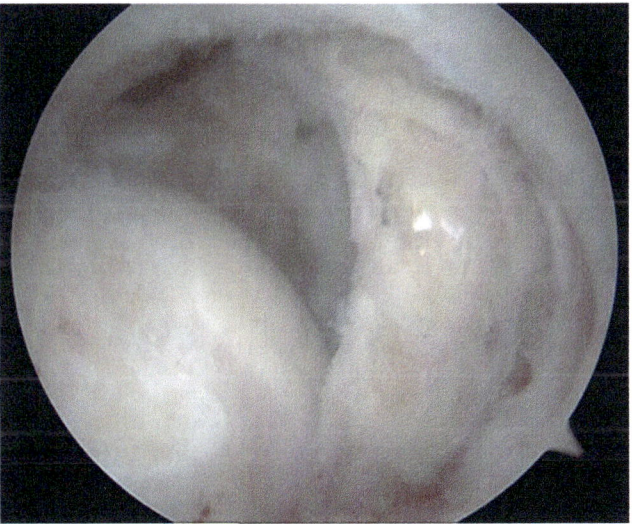

Fig. 14.22 Arthroscopic view from the posterior portal showing a large reverse L-shaped tear pattern

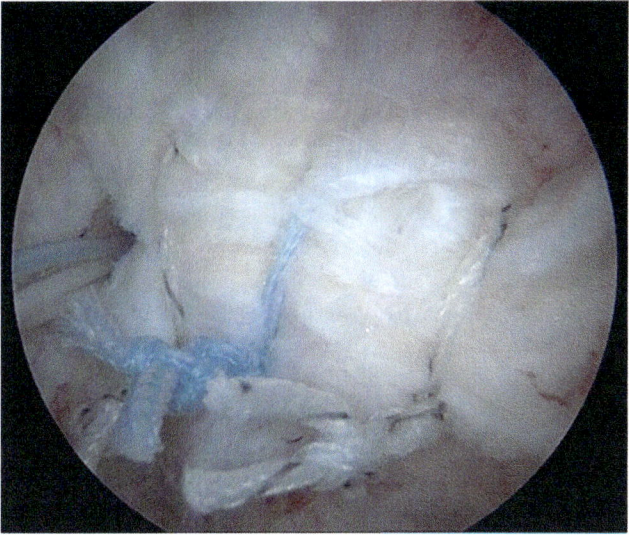

Fig. 14.23 Arthroscopic view from the posterior portal showing closure of the posterior interval re-approximating the entire supraspinatus back to the greater tuberosity with minimal tension

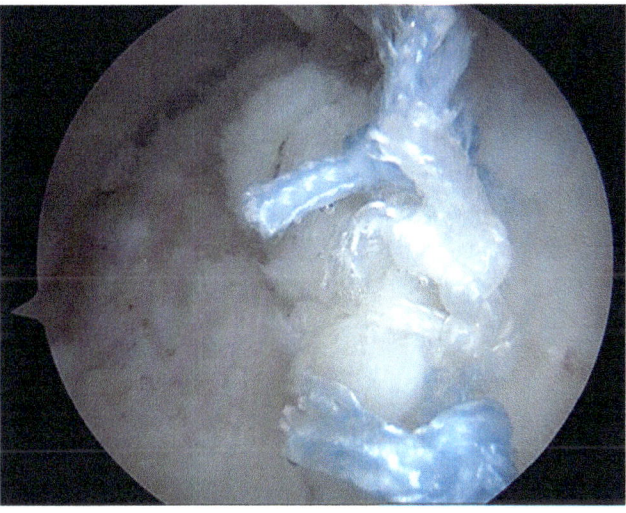

Fig. 14.24 Arthroscopic view from the posterior portal showing the final single-row repair construct with multiple triple-loaded suture anchors and simple stitches

After re-approximation of this leaf, the tear was reduced back to the midportion of the greater tuberosity, and a single-row low-tension repair was performed using three triple-loaded suture anchors and nine simple stitches (Fig. 14.24).

Discussion

Very limited data exists on the outcomes of L-shaped and reverse L-shaped tears requiring repair. Typically, most rotator cuff repair healing and outcome studies lump tears by anteroposterior tear size instead of by pattern. Crescent tears are often lumped with other tear patterns despite these more complex patterns likely having an effect on outcomes and healing. Davidson et al. were the first to geometrically classify tears based upon preoperative MRI measurements [37]. Van der Zwaai et al. have confirmed that the Davidson classification of rotator cuff tears using magnetic resonance arthrography has good-to-excellent intraobserver agreement and moderate-to-good interobserver agreement among experienced observers [38]. The only clinical study evaluating the effect of tear pattern on final rotator cuff outcomes or healing was by Park et al. [39]. These authors grouped a series of large rotator cuff tears into either crescent/L-shaped/reverse

L-shaped tears or U-shaped tears and evaluated healing rates and outcomes. At 24 months postoperative, initial rotator cuff tear pattern had no effect on final healing rates or Constant scores [39]. Consequently, the key with tear patterns is that if correctly recognized and anatomically repaired, there is likely little consequence with regard to outcomes. If unrecognized, these more complex tear patterns are most likely to fail due to excessively high tension levels placed upon the repairs due to a nonanatomic reduction.

Based upon the MRI criteria of Davidson et al., the tear would be considered irreparable, and bone-to-tendon repair would not be able to be performed [37]. Intraoperatively, the tear was determined to not be a massive contracted tear (Davidson group III) but rather a reverse L-shaped tear (Davidson group II) [35]. Consequently, re-approximation of the supraspinatus posteriorly pulled the tendon back to the greater tuberosity like a curtain, and almost no tension was placed on the repair. Davidson et al. reported only a 76.5 % positive predictive value using the L>2 cm and W>2 cm criteria to predict irreparability [37]. The current case represents a failure of the criteria to predict the repair pattern. Nevertheless, the Davidson criteria can be very useful and should still be considered to assist preoperatively in determining intraoperative tear patterns identified at the time of arthroscopy.

Conclusions

With improvements in the understanding of structural outcomes after rotator cuff surgery as well as the risk of developing irreversible changes with nonoperative management of rotator cuff tears, reasonable guidelines can be created to aid in the appropriate management of patients with rotator cuff tears. Groups I and III should be treated nonoperatively initially due to a low risk for the development of irreversible changes (group I) or that irreversible changes have already occurred (group III), or the likelihood for healing after repair is relatively low (group III). Group II patients should be considered for early surgical repair due to a high risk for tear progression and a high likelihood for healing. The previous cases highlight several scenarios from each treatment group.

Preoperative MRI evaluation can significantly assist in the planning for arthroscopic rotator cuff surgery. At a base level, understanding tear size and muscle quality can aid in indicating patients for repair as well as predicting reparability at the time of surgery. More sophisticated analysis of the imaging can further improve the preoperative planning process by including assessments of tendon length, musculotendinous junction position and tear pattern recognition as part of the MRI measurements. Many of these additional findings on MRI will often translate into improved arthroscopic injury recognition and repair techniques that will ultimately lead to improved clinical outcomes.

References

1. Chakravarty K, Webley M. Shoulder joint movement and its relationship to disability in the elderly. J Rheumatol. 1993;20:1359–61.
2. Colvin AC, Egorova N, Harrison AK, Moskowitz A, Flatow EL. National trends in rotator cuff repair. J Bone Joint Surg Am. 2012;94(3):227–33.
3. Dunn WR, Schackman BR, Walsh C, et al. Variation in orthopaedic surgeons' perceptions about the indications for rotator cuff surgery. J Bone Joint Surg Am. 2005;87:1978–84.
4. Maman E, Harris C, White L, Tomlinson G, Shashank M, Boynton E. Outcome of nonoperative treatment of symptomatic rotator cuff tears monitored by magnetic resonance imaging. J Bone Joint Surg Am. 2009;91(8):1898–906.
5. Safran O, Schroeder J, Bloom R, Weil Y, Milgrom C. Natural history of nonoperatively treated symptomatic rotator cuff tears in patients 60 years old or younger. Am J Sports Med. 2011;39(4):710–4.
6. Fucentese SF, von Roll AL, Pfirrmann CW, Gerber C, Jost B. Evolution of nonoperatively treated symptomatic isolated full-thickness supraspinatus tears. J Bone Joint Surg Am. 2012;94(9):801–8.
7. Mall NA, Kim HM, Keener JD, Steger-May K, Teefey SA, Middleton WD, Stobbs G, Yamaguchi K. Symptomatic progression of asymptomatic rotator cuff tears: a prospective study of clinical and sonographic variables. J Bone Joint Surg Am. 2010;92(16):2623–33.
8. Bjornsson HC, Norlin R, Johansson K, et al. The influence of age, delay of repair, and tendon involvement in acute rotator cuff tears: structural and clinical outcomes after repair of 42 shoulders. Acta Orthop. 2011;82(2):187–92.
9. Boileau P, Brassart N, Watkinson DJ, et al. Arthroscopic repair of full-thickness tears of the supraspinatus: does the tendon really heal? J Bone Joint Surg Am. 2005;87:1229–40.
10. Cho NS, Lee BG, Rhee YG. Arthroscopic rotator cuff repair using a suture bridge technique. Is the repair integrity actually maintained? Am J Sports Med. 2011;39:2108–16.
11. Gulotta LV, Nho SJ, Dodson CC, et al. Prospective evaluation of arthroscopic rotator cuff repairs at 5 years: part II – prognostic factors for clinical and radio- graphic outcomes. J Shoulder Elbow Surg. 2011;20:941–6.
12. Harryman DT, Mack LA, Wang KY, et al. Repairs of the rotator cuff. Correlation of functional results with integrity of the cuff. J Bone Joint Surg Am. 1991;73:982–9.
13. Liem D, Lichtenberg S, Magosch P, et al. Magnetic resonance imaging of arthroscopic supraspinatus tendon repair. J Bone Joint Surg Am. 2007;89:1770–6.
14. Tashjian RZ, Hollins AM, Kim HM, et al. Factors affecting healing rates after arthroscopic double-row rotator cuff repair. Am J Sports Med. 2010;38:2435–42.
15. Tashjian RZ. Epidemiology, natural history, and indications for treatment of rotator cuff tears. Clin Sports Med. 2012;31:589–604.
16. Burkhart SS, Brady PC. Arthroscopic subscapularis repair: surgical tips and pearls A to Z. Arthroscopy. 2006;22(9):1014–27.
17. Lafosse L, Van Raebroeckx A, Brzoska R. A new technique to improve tissue grip: "the lasso-loop stitch". J Arthroscopy. 2006;22(11):1246.e1-3.
18. Lafosse L, Jost B, Reiland Y, Audebert S, Toussaint B, Gobezie R. Structural integrity and clinical outcomes after arthroscopic repair of isolated subscapularis tears. J Bone Joint Surg Am. 2007;89(6):1184–93.
19. Nove-Josserand L, Hardy MB, Leandro Nunes Ogassawara R, Carrillon Y, Godeneche A. Clinical and structural results of arthroscopic repair of isolated subscapularis tear. J Bone Joint Surg Am. 2012;94(17):e125.

20. Keener JD, Galatz LM, Stobbs-Cucchi G, Patton R, Yamaguchi K. Rehabilitation following arthroscopic rotator cuff repair: a prospective randomized trial of immobilization compared with early motion. J Bone Joint Surg Am. 2014;96(1):11–9.

21. Sethi PM, Noonan BC, Cunningham J, Shreck E, Miller S. Repair results of 2-tendon rotator cuff tears utilizing the transosseous equivalent technique. J Shoulder Elbow Surg. 2010;19(8):1210–7.

22. Jost B, Zumstein M, Pfirrmann CW, Gerber C. Long-term outcome after structural failure of rotator cuff repairs. J Bone Joint Surg Am. 2006;88(3):472–9.

23. Kim HM, Caldwell JM, Buza JA, Fink LA, Ahmad CS, Bigliani LU, Levine WN. Factors affecting satisfaction and shoulder function in patients with a recurrent rotator cuff tear. J Bone Joint Surg Am. 2014;96(2):106–12.

24. Namdari S, Donegan RP, Chamberlain AM, Galatz LM, Yamaguchi K, Keener JD. Factors affecting outcome after structural failure of repaired rotator cuff tears. J Bone Joint Surg Am. 2014;96(2):99–105.

25. Fuchs B, Weishaupt D, Zanetti M, Hodler J, Gerber C. Fatty degeneration of the muscles of the rotator cuff: assessment by computed tonography versus magnetic resonance imaging. J Shoulder Elbow Surg. 1999;8(6):599–605.

26. Goutallier D, Postel JM, Bernageau J, Lavau L, Voisin MC. Fatty muscle degeneration in cuff ruptures. Pre- and postoperative evaluation by CT scan. Clin Orthop Relat Res. 1994;304:78–83.

27. Meyer DC, Wieser K, Farshad M, Gerber C. Retraction of supraspinatus muscle and tendon as predictors of success of rotator cuff repair. Am J Sports Med. 2012;40(10):2242–7.

28. Tashjian RZ, Hung M, Burks RT, Greis PE. Influence of preoperative musculotendinous junction position on rotator cuff healing using single-row technique. Arthroscopy. 2013;29(11):1748–54.

29. Keener JD, Wei AS, Kim HM, Paxton ES, Teefey SA, Galatz LM, Yamaguchi K. Revision arthroscopic rotator cuff repair: repair integrity and clinical outcome. J Bone Joint Surg Am. 2010;92(3):590–8.

30. Ladermann A, Denard PJ, Burkhart SS. Midterm outcome of arthroscopic revision repair of massive and nonmassive rotator cuff tears. Arthroscopy. 2011;27(12):1620–7.

31. Ladermann A, Denard PJ, Burkhart SS. Revision arthroscopic rotator cuff repair: systematic review and authors' preferred surgical technique. Arthroscopy. 2012;28(8):1160–9.

32. Piasecki DP, Verma NN, Nho SJ, Bhatia S, Boniquit N, Cole BJ, Nicholson GP, Romeo AA. Outcomes after arthroscopic revision rotator cuff repair. Am J Sports Med. 2010;38(1):40–6.

33. Parnes N, DeFranco M, Wells JH, Higgins LD, Warner JJ. Complications after arthroscopic revision rotator cuff repair. Arthroscopy. 2013;29(9):1479–86.

34. Burkhart SS, Athanasiou KA, Wirth MA. Margin convergence: a method of reducing strain in massive rotator cuff tears. Arthroscopy. 1996;12(3):335–8.

35. Davidson J, Burkhart SS. The geometric classification of rotator cuff tears: a system linking tear pattern to treatment and prognosis. Arthroscopy. 2010;26(3):417–24.

36. Barber FA, Burns JP. Deutsch A, Labbe MR, Litchfield RB. A prospective, randomized evaluation of acellular human dermal matrix augmentation for arthroscopic rotator cuff repair. Arthroscopy. 2012;28(1):8–15.

37. Davidson JF, Burkhart SS, Richards DP, Campbell SE. Use of preoperative magnetic resonance imaging to predict rotator cuff tear pattern and method of repair. Arthroscopy. 2005;21(12):1428.

38. Van der Zwaai P, Thomassen BJ, Urlings TA, de Rooy TP, Swen JW, van Arkel ER. Preoperative agreement on the geometric classification and 2-dimensional measurement of rotator cuff tears based upon magnetic resonance arthrography. Arthroscopy. 2012;28(10):1329–36.

39. Park JY, Jung SW, Jeon SH, Cho HW, Choi JH, Oh KS. Arthroscopic repair of large U-shaped rotator cuff tears without margin convergence versus repair of crescent- or L-shaped tears. Am J Sports Med. 2014;42(1):103–11.

SLAP Lesions and Biceps Tendon Pathology

Brian C. Werner and Stephen F. Brockmeier

Introduction

Pathology of the superior glenoid labrum, biceps anchor, and long head biceps tendon is a well-established etiology of shoulder pain [1]. Tears of the superior labrum from anterior to posterior (SLAP) were first described by Andrews et al. in 1985 [2]. Snyder et al. later classified these injuries into types I–IV in 1990 based on location and stability of the tear [3]. Later, types V–VII to the classification scheme [4]. Morgan and Burkhart later subclassified type II lesions into three groups based on location (anterior, posterior, or anterior and posterior) [5]. The biceps anchor and long head biceps tendon are often involved in a pathologic continuum with superior labrum lesions, involving a range of disorders including tendinopathy, tenosynovitis, subluxation, and degenerative tendinosis [6].

SLAP tears are typically a result of traction injury, compression injury, or repetitive overhead activity. Although discussed frequently in the literature, the incidence of SLAP tears is low, reported only in 6 % of operative cases [7]. Neither the incidence or prevalence of biceps tendon pathology is reported; however, long head biceps tendinitis commonly is found in combination with other shoulder conditions, including SLAP tears, impingement, and rotator cuff disease [8–10].

The clinical diagnosis of SLAP or long head biceps pathology is challenging, as coexistent pathology is frequently present, and symptoms of pathology at each site are often indistinguishable. A careful history, physical examination including provocative maneuvers, and imaging as dictated from the exam are key in establishing an appropriate diagnosis. Magnetic resonance imaging (MRI) remains the imaging technique of choice for patients with suspected SLAP tears or long head biceps pathology. MRI is also useful in identifying concomitant shoulder pathology. Unfortunately, even with a contrast arthrogram, MRI lacks the sensitivity and specificity to consistently diagnose all biceps pathology that is found at arthroscopy [6, 11].

A standard management protocol for SLAP and long head biceps pathology begins with nonsurgical treatment. Conservative options focus on improving flexibility, strengthening the rotator cuff and scapular stabilizers, and normalizing scapular mechanics. Intra-articular glenohumeral injections may be utilized in both a diagnostic and therapeutic fashion early in the treatment course of patients with suspected SLAP or biceps pathology.

Surgical intervention can be pursued when nonsurgical measures have failed a 3-month course, and clinical suspicion is high for SLAP or long biceps pathology that can be improved with surgery. After the pathology is characterized by diagnostic arthroscopy, treatment options are numerous, including arthroscopic SLAP repair, arthroscopic or open biceps tenodesis, or arthroscopic biceps tenotomy. Concomitant pathology, including labral tears causing instability, rotator cuff tears, or bony impingement, can be addressed in the same setting.

This chapter will utilize a case-based format to demonstrate the correlation between MRI and arthroscopy for SLAP and long head biceps pathology and review the diagnosis and management of each patient. Four cases will be presented, including:

1. A Type II SLAP tear requiring arthroscopic repair
2. A high-grade partial long head biceps tendon tear requiring biceps tenodesis
3. A failed prior SLAP repair treated with arthroscopic suprapectoral biceps tenodesis
4. A degenerative SLAP tear with biceps tendon degeneration treated with biceps tenotomy

B.C. Werner, MD (✉) • S.F. Brockmeier, MD
Department of Orthopedic Surgery, University of Virginia,
Charlottesville, VA, USA
e-mail: Bcw4x@hscmail.mcc.virginia.edu;
Sfb2e@hcsmail.mcc.virginia.edu

S.F. Brockmeier (ed.), *MRI-Arthroscopy Correlations: A Case-Based Atlas of the Knee, Shoulder, Elbow and Hip*,
DOI 10.1007/978-1-4939-2645-9_15, © Springer Science+Business Media New York 2015

Case 1: SLAP Tear

History/Exam

An 18-year-old collegiate baseball pitcher presented to the orthopedic clinic reporting 8 months of shoulder pain in his dominant arm. He denied any symptoms previously in his career, including high school. He had sought advice from his trainer and team physical therapist, but his symptoms persisted despite conservative measures. He eventually moved from pitcher to shortstop due to difficulty with repetitive overhead motion. Finally, he was moved to designated hitter due to significant pain with any attempt at throwing.

On physical examination, the patient was found to have a grossly positive O'Brien's active compression test, with notable discomfort with his thumb down that was alleviated with changing to thumb up. His Speed's test was negative, as was Yergason's. He did not have any pain with palpation of his bicipital groove and he had a negative Thrower's test. He denied symptoms over his acromioclavicular joint. The patient was otherwise neurovascularly intact and without symptoms in his contralateral shoulder. Given that the patient had already failed extensive nonsurgical options and was regressing in his chosen sport, a decision was made to proceed with imaging studies.

Imaging

Plain radiography did not demonstrate any significant pathology. His acromion had a normal shape and contour. There was no evidence of arthritic changes or glenoid rim or humeral head bony abnormality. Magnetic resonance imaging with contrast arthrography was obtained to further evaluate the patient's labrum, biceps tendon, and rotator cuff, given his persistent symptoms. A complete sequence of images was obtained, including oblique coronal fat-saturated T1 and T2 sequences, oblique sagittal T1 and fat-saturated T2, axial T1 and fat-saturated T2, and oblique axial T1 sequences. Coronal T2-weighted images are demonstrated in Fig. 15.1a–d and axial T1-weighted images are demonstrated in Fig. 15.2a–c.

A labral tear extending from the posterior labrum at the level of the equator, through the superior labrum and into the anterosuperior labrum to the near level of the equator is demonstrated in both Figs. 15.1a–d and 15.2a–c. Mild signal heterogeneity and globular morphology of the anteroinferior labrum were noted, particularly in the axial images, without a discrete tear noted. A multilobulated paralabral cyst measuring 4×13 mm along the posterosuperior labrum was also demonstrated. The biceps tendon, visualized best in Fig. 15.2a–c, was intact without subluxation or increased signal. No rotator cuff or articular cartilage pathology was noted. Incidental note was made of moderate AC joint degeneration with intraosseous edema within the distal clavicle and acromion without significant mass effect upon the underlying supraspinatus.

Given the identified SLAP tear on MRI consistent with the patient's clinical examination, risks and benefits of operative intervention were discussed with the patient, as he had failed extensive nonsurgical management. He elected to proceed with diagnostic arthroscopy and likely SLAP repair, given his age and activity level and desire to return to collegiate baseball.

Arthroscopy

The patient was taken to the operating room and placed in the beach chair position. A standard diagnostic arthroscopy of the right shoulder was completed. A type II SLAP tear was noted as demonstrated in Fig. 15.3a, b, both by probing and by an arthroscopic "peel-back" maneuver. The biceps tendon was intact. The anteroinferior labrum was also found to be intact. This correlated well with the findings on MRI: an isolated SLAP tear.

Given the absence of biceps pathology or subluxation or significant degeneration of the superior labrum, the decision was made to proceed with arthroscopic SLAP repair in this young, athletic patient. The joint was insufflated, and a high rotator interval portal was established anteriorly for working purposes. Inside the joint, the detached tear of the superior labrum that involved a segment from approximately the 1 o'clock position anteriorly to approximately the 9 o'clock position posteriorly was easily mobilized with a probe. Additionally, with an arthroscopic peel-back maneuver, the patient was found to have mobility of the labrum off the glenoid surface superiorly in an abnormal fashion.

The superior and posterior aspects of the glenoid neck were debrided with a 4.2 mm shaver to bleeding subchondral bone. Two anchors were placed, one just posterior to the biceps anchor and one down at the 3 o'clock position. Sutures were then shuttled in a simple configuration and tied utilizing an arthroscopic knot tying technique (Fig. 15.4a–d). After repair, the superior labrum was probed and found to be stable with normalization of labral position with arthroscopic "peel-back" testing.

The patient was placed in a shoulder immobilizer sling for 4 weeks postoperatively. Passive and active assisted shoulder range of motion was emphasized during the first phase of postoperative rehab (weeks 0–6), followed by active range of motion, terminal capsular mobilization, and strengthening beginning at week 6 and terminating at around 3.5 months

Fig. 15.1 (**a–d**) Coronal T2-weighted images of an 18-year-old baseball pitcher with 8 months of shoulder pain. A superior labral tear was identified, which is also clarified in the axial images of Fig. 15.2a–c. No rotator cuff or articular cartilage pathology was noted

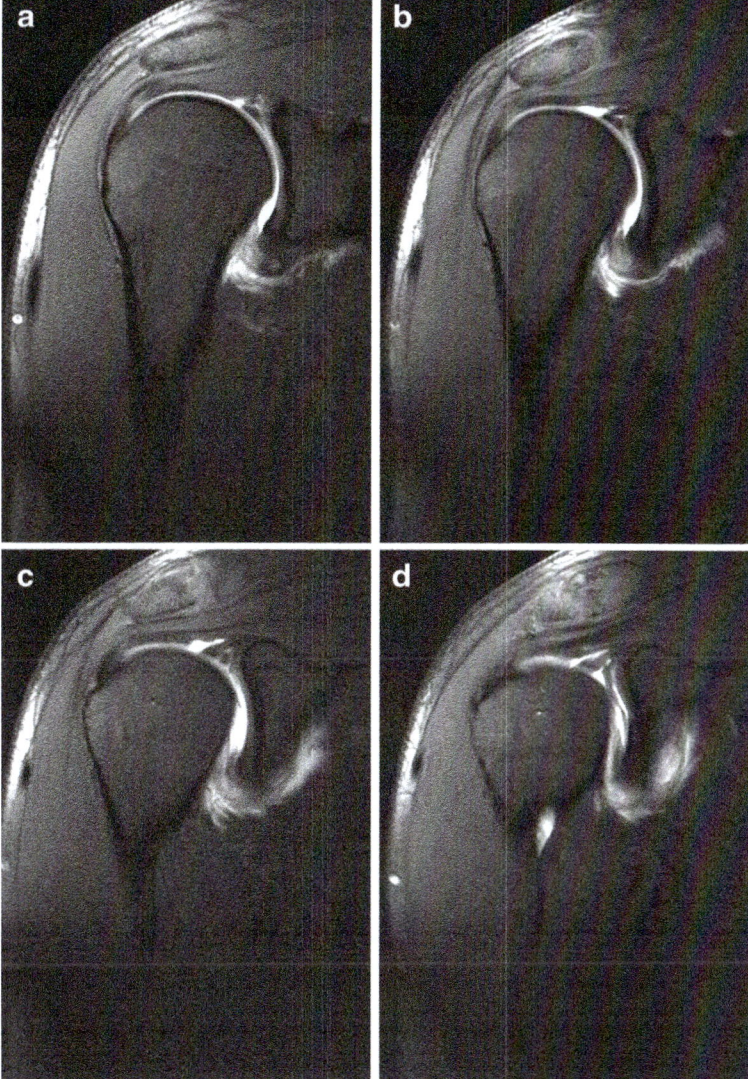

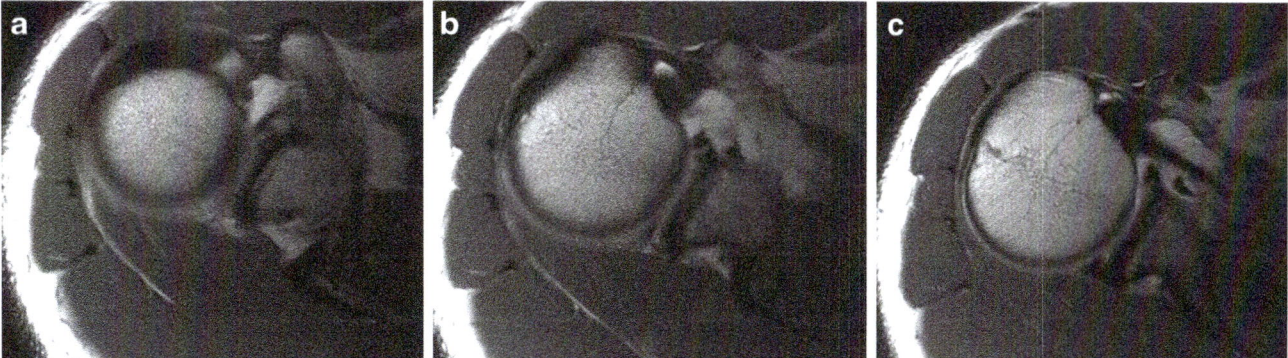

Fig. 15.2 (**a–c**) Axial T1-weighted images of the 18-year-old baseball pitcher discussed in Fig. 15.1a–d. The superior labral tear extends from the posterior labrum at the level of the equator to near the level of the equator in the anterosuperior labrum. A paralabral cyst was noted along the posterosuperior labrum. The biceps tendon is intact without subluxation or change in signal

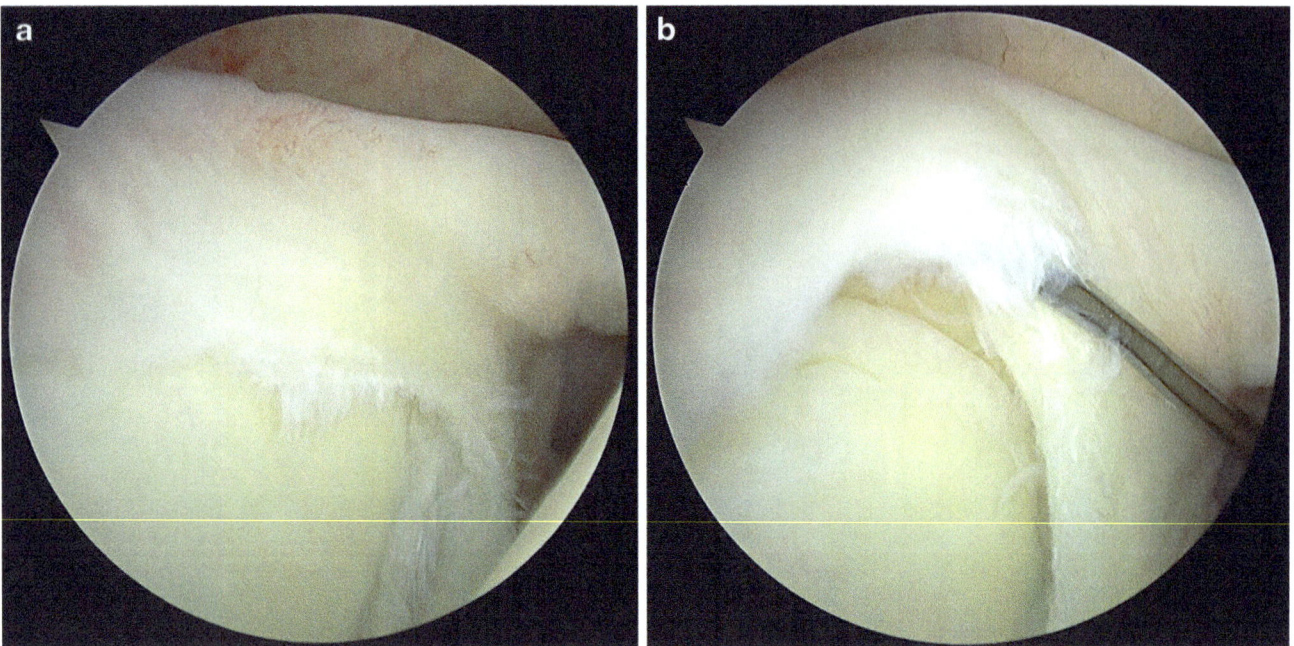

Fig. 15.3 (**a, b**) Arthroscopic images in the beach chair position demonstrating a type II SLAP tear, confirmed with an arthroscopic "peel" back maneuver. The biceps tendon was intact

postoperatively. The patient initiated a phased throwing program at 14 weeks postoperatively and was allowed to return to athletics and overhead sports at approximately 6 months postoperatively.

Discussion

The clinical presentation of a SLAP tear in an overhead athlete can be nonspecific, with the most common presenting complaints being pain with throwing and loss of velocity or accuracy as was noted in this patient. Exam findings including anterior or posterior joint line tenderness, the O'Brien's active compression test, and biceps-specific tests such as Speed's and Yergason's tests can cumulatively be suggestive of a superior labral lesion. Imaging, consisting of an MRI with intra-articular gadolinium, can help with confirming a type II SLAP lesion. Arthroscopic SLAP repair most commonly yields successful outcomes, especially in the setting of a young patient, a traumatic onset of symptoms, and absent concomitant pathology. Outcomes in patients over the age of 35 or in throwing athletes can be less predictable, and thus patients in these groups should be counseled.

Case 2: Long Head Biceps Tendon Tear

History/Exam

A 39-year-old male presented to sports medicine clinic with a chief complaint of right shoulder pain, which was chronic in nature but worsening over the past 2 years prior to presentation. He reported the onset of symptoms when he was in college. He endorsed a distant history of two shoulder subluxations during sporting events but denied ever having a full dislocation. He noted significant exacerbation of his symptoms with overhead movements. He was able to play golf without symptoms, but his shoulder pain prohibited any overhead sports, such as tennis. He denied any recent subluxation events or feelings of instability.

On physical examination, he was found to have a positive O'Brien's sign. His Speed's test was positive as was his Yergason's. He had mild tenderness over his bicipital groove. He had some very subtle apprehension. His strength and range of motion were normal, and he was otherwise neurovascularly intact and without symptoms in his contralateral shoulder. His long-standing symptoms and recent progressive deterioration warranted additional investigation with imaging.

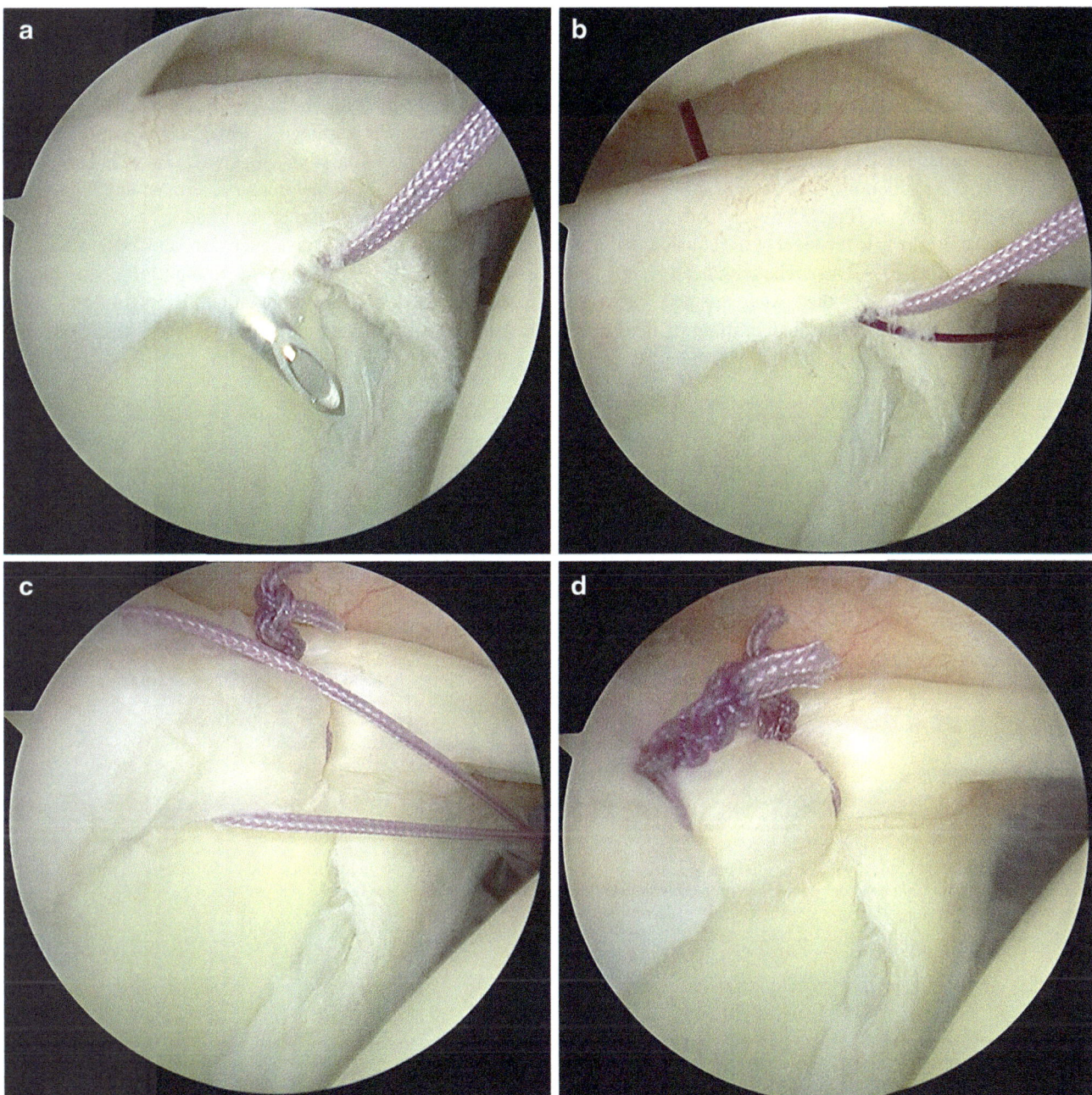

Fig. 15.4 (**a–d**) Arthroscopic images in the beach chair position demonstrating arthroscopic SLAP repair. The superior and posterior aspects of the glenoid neck were debrided with a 4.2 mm shaver to bleeding subchondral bone. Two anchors were placed, one just posterior to the biceps anchor and one down at the 3 o'clock position. Sutures were then shuttled in a simple configuration and tied utilizing an arthroscopic knot tying technique

Imaging

Initially, plain radiographs were obtained, which were unremarkable. There was no evidence of arthritic changes or glenoid or humeral head bony changes indicative of bony insufficiency leading to instability. Magnetic resonance imaging with contrast arthrography was obtained to further evaluate the patient's labrum, biceps tendon, and rotator cuff, due to his worsening symptoms. A complete sequence of images was obtained, including oblique coronal fat-saturated T1 and T2 sequences, oblique sagittal T1 and fat-saturated T2, axial T1 and fat-saturated T2, and oblique axial T1 sequences. Coronal fat-saturated T1-weighted images are demonstrated in Fig. 15.5a–c, and axial T2-weighted images are demonstrated in Fig. 15.6a–c.

The coronal images (Fig. 15.5a–c) demonstrate tearing of the superior labrum with contrast undermining the labrum. The inferior labrum as demonstrated on coronal imaging appears intact. This superior labral tear is further characterized on the axial images (Fig. 15.6a–c). The tear extends anteriorly and posteriorly to the level of the equator, confirming the diagnosis of a SLAP tear. The long head biceps tendon is best evaluated on the axial imaging provided (Fig. 15.6a–c). There is longitudinal splitting of the biceps

tendon within the bicipital groove. Furthermore, there is subluxation of the biceps tendon, as the groove appears empty as the axial images move cephalad (Fig. 15.6b, c). Incidental note was made of mild narrowing of the anterior aspect of the glenoid articular cartilage. A low-grade undersurface and bursal irregularity of the supraspinatus tendon were also noted, most obvious in the coronal imaging, without any high-grade partial or full-thickness tearing identified.

The patient's history, physical exam, and MRI were consistent with a SLAP tear and concomitant long head biceps tendon partial tear with subluxation. His symptoms were present and worsening over a several year period and were

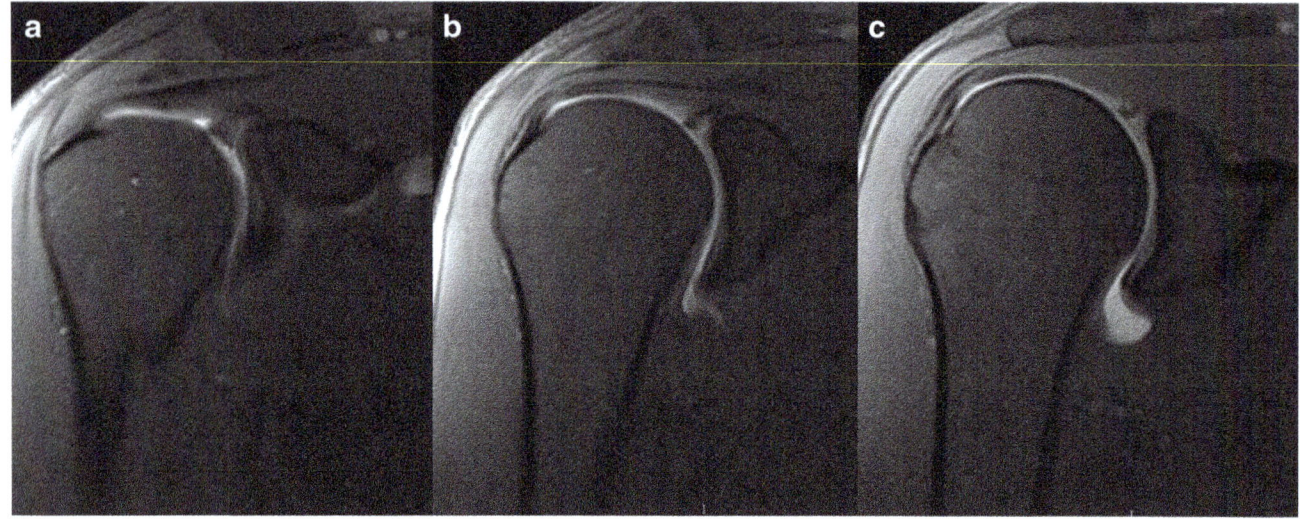

Fig. 15.5 (**a–c**) Coronal fat-saturated T1-weighted MRI of a 39-year-old male with chronic right shoulder pain. The coronal images demonstrate tearing of the superior labrum with contrast undermining the labrum. A low-grade undersurface and bursal irregularity of the supraspinatus tendon is also noted

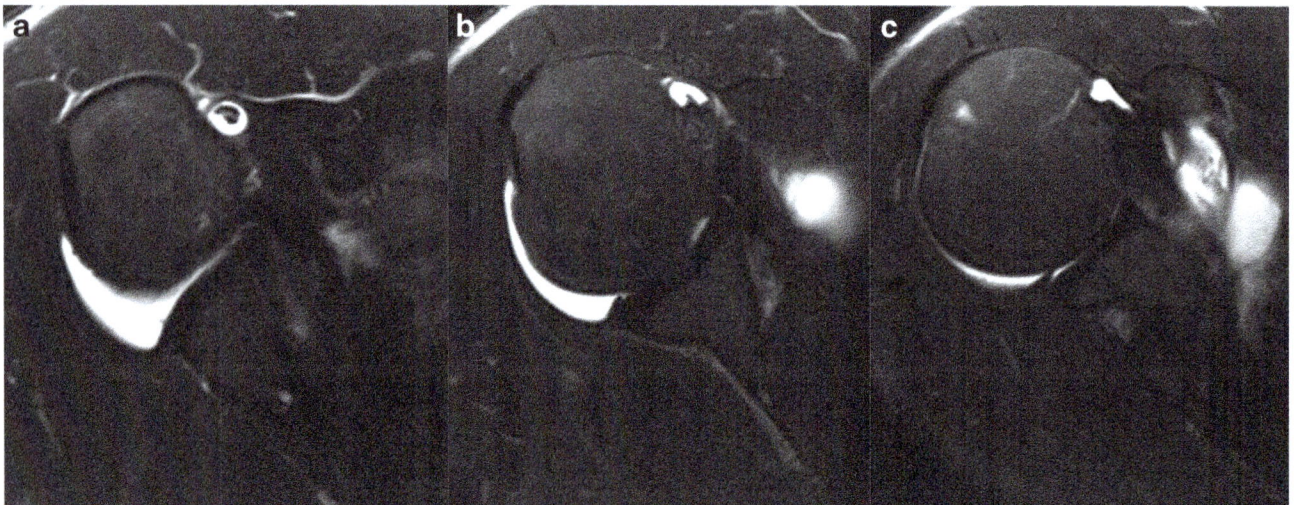

Fig. 15.6 (**a–c**) Axial T2-weighted images of the same patient allow further characterization of the superior labral tear. The tear extends anteriorly and posteriorly to the level of the equator. There is subluxation of the biceps tendon, as the groove appears empty on the more cephalad images. There is also longitudinal splitting of the biceps tendon

recalcitrant to conservative measures. Surgical intervention was offered, with a plan to address his biceps pathology with biceps tenodesis and to evaluate the superior labrum following this for potential concomitant repair. His low-grade rotator cuff irregularities noted on MRI were not suspected to be of consequence, given his lack of related symptoms on exam.

Arthroscopy

The patient was taken to the operating room and placed in the beach chair position. Given his questionable history of instability, an examination under anesthesia was carried out prior to skin incision. The patient was noted to have a low-grade anterior and posterior load and shift with a grade one sulcus sign. Diagnostic arthroscopy was then carried out. Through a standard posterior portal, the glenohumeral joint was entered. An anterior portal was then immediately established. Intra-articularly, the joint was inspected thoroughly. The chondral surfaces were intact. The patient was found to have a labral tear extending from approximately the anterior aspect of the biceps anchor into the posterior aspect of the labrum down to approximately the 9 o'clock position, confirming the diagnosis from MRI (Fig. 15.7a–d). There was fraying of the labrum itself. There was damage to the biceps anchor encompassing at least 25 % of the thickness of the biceps tendon itself. A second but substantially higher-grade injury to a long head biceps tendon was encountered at the groove entrance (Fig. 15.7a, b). This was at least 80 % if not 90 % of the caliber of the biceps itself with only a few small fibers remaining intact. The biceps was probed and the extent of this damage was confirmed down into the intertubercular groove region, confirming the findings noted on MRI. The biceps was substantially damaged. The rotator cuff was visualized. The patient has a low-grade articular sided rotator cuff tear involving only the far anterior aspect supraspinatus, as was noted on the MRI. This was debrided and contoured to a stable edge. The remainder of the labrum was intact. The subscapularis was also intact.

A decision was made at this point to proceed with labral repair and biceps tenodesis to address his areas of pathology. The labrum was debrided back to a stable edge at the glenoid neck superiorly and into the posterior superior glenoid region. Two anchors were used to repair the labrum, the first one placed at approximately the 11:30 position and the second placed at approximately the 10 o'clock position (Fig. 15.8a, b).

Following labral repair, a biceps tenotomy was performed after tagging the biceps with a #0 PDS suture. At this point, the arthroscope was repositioned into the subacromial space. The patient was found to have a normal bursal space with no evidence of bursitis. The bursal surface of the rotator cuff was visualized and found to be intact and without abnormality.

Given this patient's biceps pathology and extension down into the intertubercular segment, as well as his age and activity level, a decision was made to proceed with an open subpectoral tenodesis.

A skin incision was created at the region of the inferior border of the pectoralis major tendon just lateral to the axillary crease. Soft tissue dissection was carried down to the anterior fascia and flaps were raised. The inferior border of the pectoralis major was identified and was mobilized superiorly. Deep retractors were placed in order to well visualize the biceps tendon as it exited the pectoralis major region (Fig. 15.8c, d). The tendon was then externalized with digital traction and prepared for a tenodesis with a whipstitch. A 6.5-mm blind-ended hole in the region of the inferior aspect of the bicipital groove was created, deep to the pectoralis major tendon which was retracted superiorly. The tendon was then docked into a place and fixed with a 6.25 × 15-mm bioabsorbable tenodesis screw (Fig. 15.8c, d). This was then augmented with suture fixation for the tendon itself and tied to secure the repair.

Discussion

Concomitant superior labral and long head biceps pathology is not uncommon. This case serves as a good example of a patient with a high-grade partial long head biceps tendon tear in the region of the bicipital groove entrance with a coexisting type 2 SLAP lesion. Options for surgical management in this patient include biceps tenodesis with possible concurrent SLAP repair. Given his age and activity level, biceps tenotomy is less ideal. Tenodesis can be performed arthroscopically in the region of the bicipital groove or in the suprapectoral region or using a mini-open subpectoral technique as described by Mazzocca. Our preference in the young, highly active male patient is open subpectoral tenodesis.

Case 3: Failed SLAP Repair

History/Exam

A 43-year-old female presented to orthopedic clinic with pain in her nondominant shoulder that returned 6 months following an arthroscopic SLAP repair. She initially did well after her SLAP repair, but unfortunately, now noted 4 weeks of substantial pain similar to her initial symptoms. She did not recall any new injury. She had tried nonsteroidal anti-inflammatories, muscle relaxants, physical therapy, and stretching prior to presentation without relief.

On physical examination, she was noted to have pain over her bicipital groove, with a negative O'Brien's, negative Speed's, and negative Yergason's tests. She was somewhat

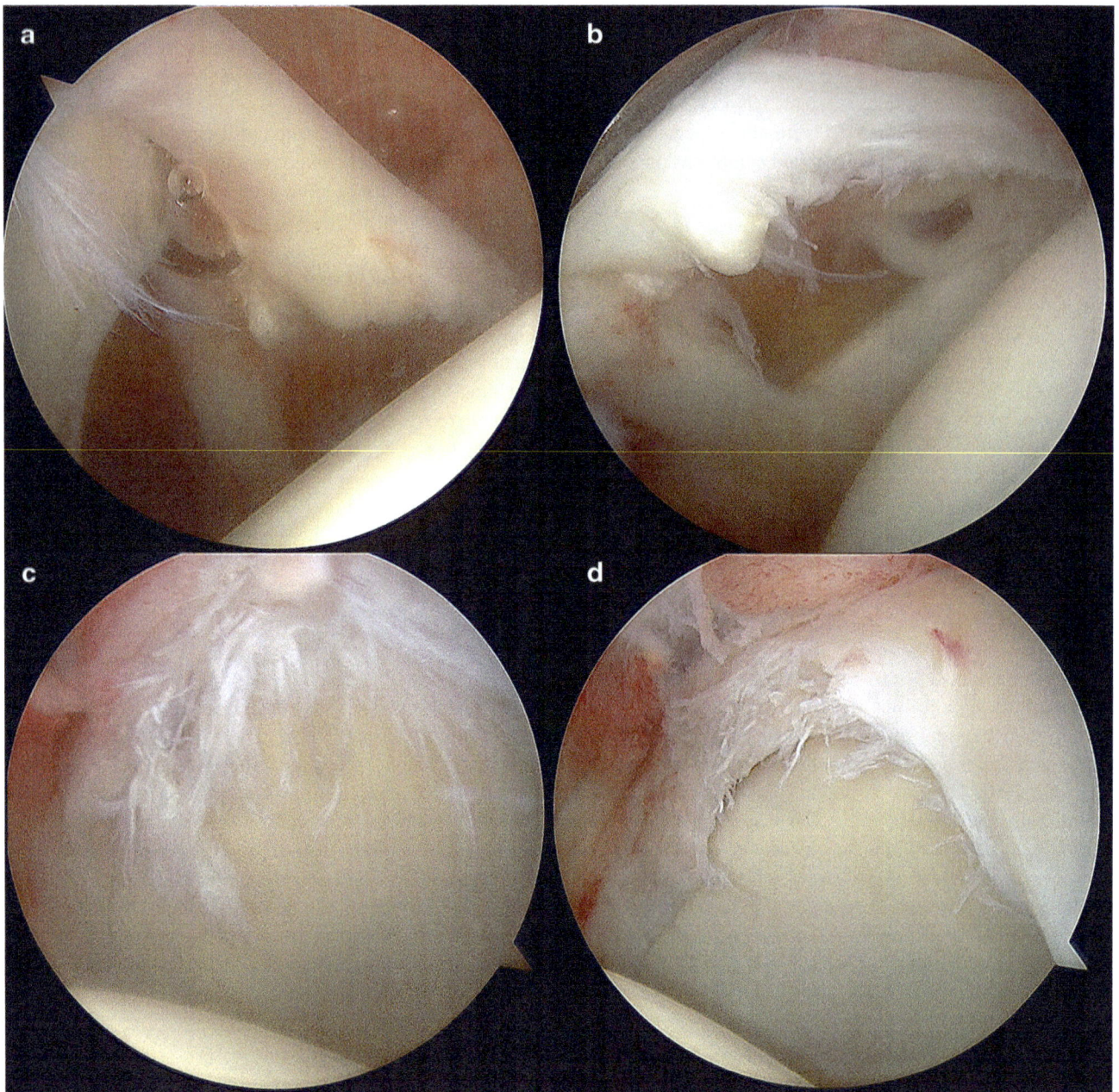

Fig. 15.7 (**a–d**) Arthroscopic images in the beach chair position demonstrate a labral tear extending from approximately the anterior aspect of the biceps anchor into the posterior aspect of the labrum down to approximately the 9 o'clock position, confirming the diagnosis from MRI. There was fraying of the labrum itself. There was damage to the biceps anchor encompassing at least 25 % of the thickness of the biceps tendon itself. A second but substantially higher-grade injury to a long head biceps tendon was encountered at the groove entrance

weak in her rotator cuff, with 4/5 strength in the supraspinatus and infraspinatus that was somewhat limited by pain.

Given her initial improvement and subsequent decline after arthroscopic SLAP repair and failure of repeat nonsurgical treatments, a decision was made to proceed with advanced imaging. Bioabsorbable anchors had been used during her SLAP repair, making MRI the diagnostic modality of choice.

Imaging

Standard MRI sequences of the affected shoulder were obtained as described in the previous case examples, including an arthrogram. Coronal T2-weighted images are demonstrated in Fig. 15.9a–c with corresponding axial T2-weighted images in Fig. 15.10a–c. The MRI demonstrates postsurgical changes of SLAP tear repair with three suture anchors noted

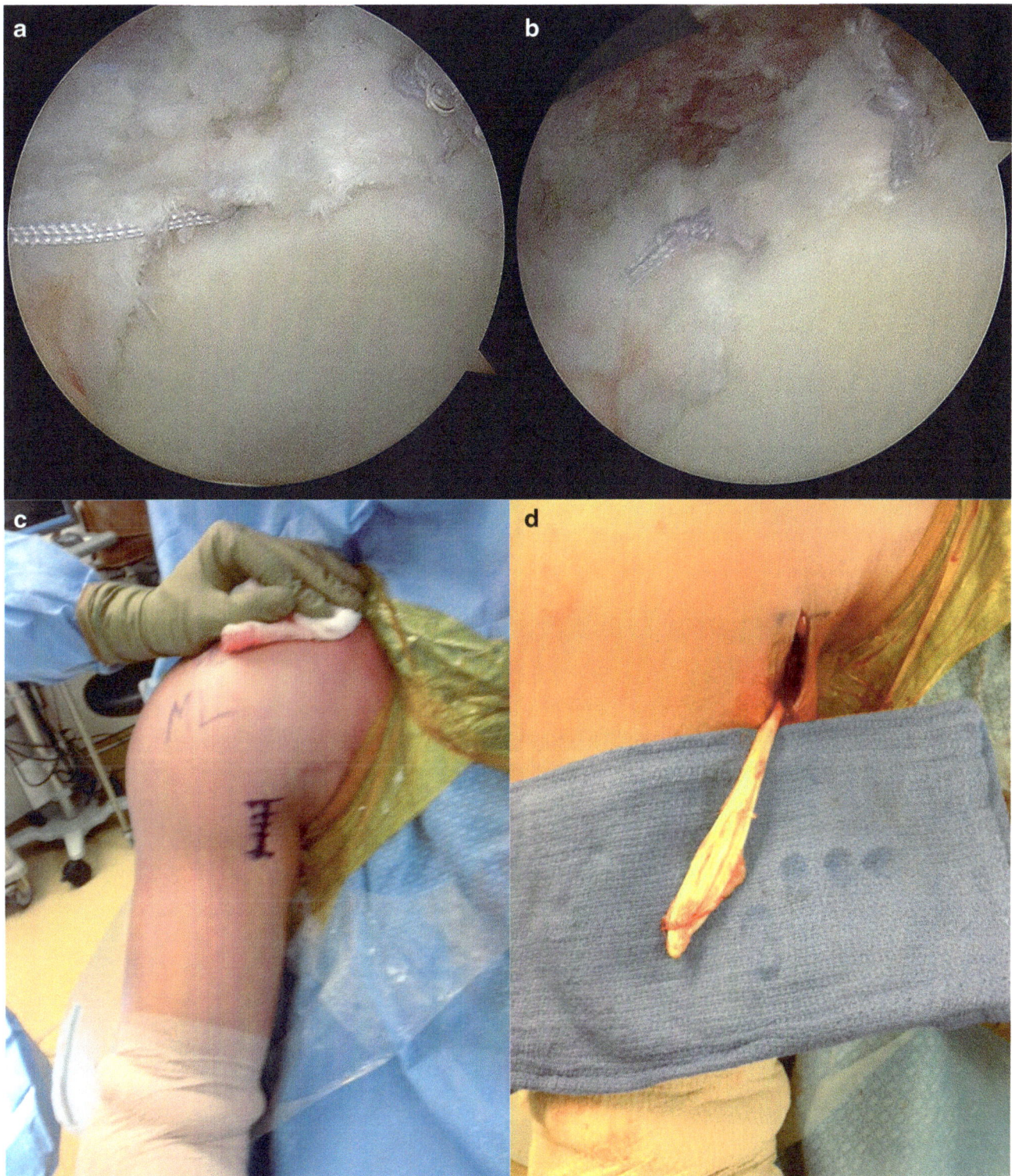

Fig. 15.8 (**a–d**) The decision was made to proceed with arthroscopic SLAP repair and open subpectoral biceps tenodesis. Two anchors were used to repair the labrum, one placed at approximately the 11:30 position and the second placed at approximately the 10 o'clock position (**a, b**). An open subpectoral biceps tenodesis with an interference screw was performed through an incision just lateral to the axillary crease (**c, d**)

within the glenoid. The SLAP tear had worsened with extension into the biceps tendon superficial to the head of the superior most anchor (Fig. 15.9a–c). The SLAP tear extended superiorly from the anterior 2 o'clock position to the posterior 10 o'clock position, seen best on the axial imaging (Fig. 15.10a–c).

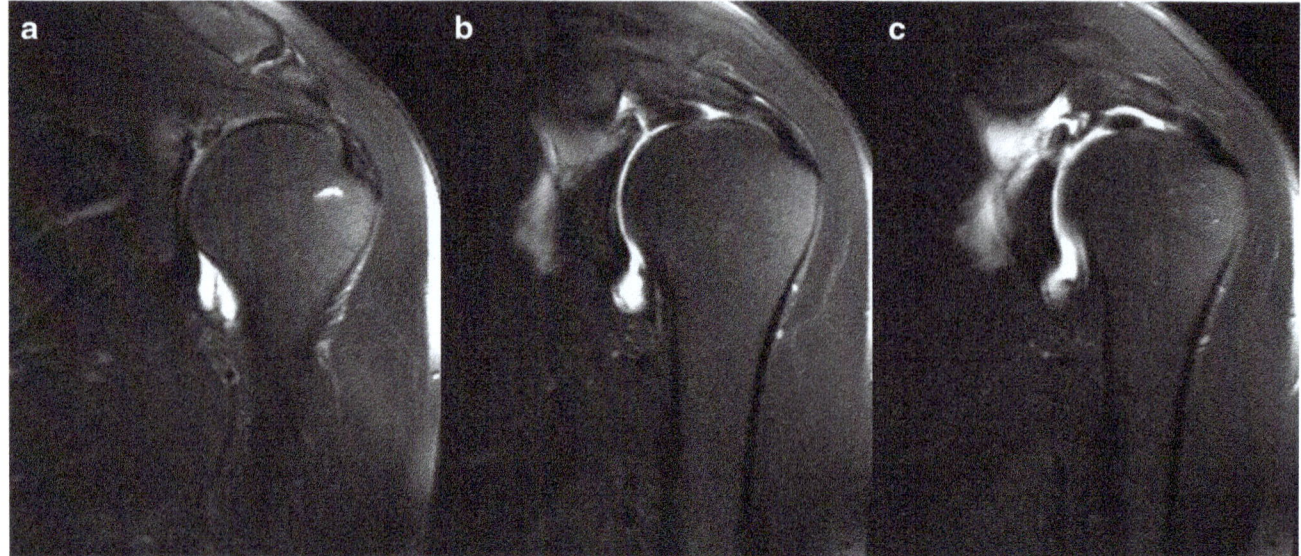

Fig. 15.9 (**a–c**) Coronal T2-weighted MR images of a 43-year-old female with pain in her nondominant shoulder that returned 6 months following an arthroscopic SLAP repair. Her current symptoms were similar to her symptoms prior to her SLAP repair. Postsurgical changes were noted on her coronal images, but the SLAP tear had worsened with extension into the biceps tendon superficial to the most superior anchor

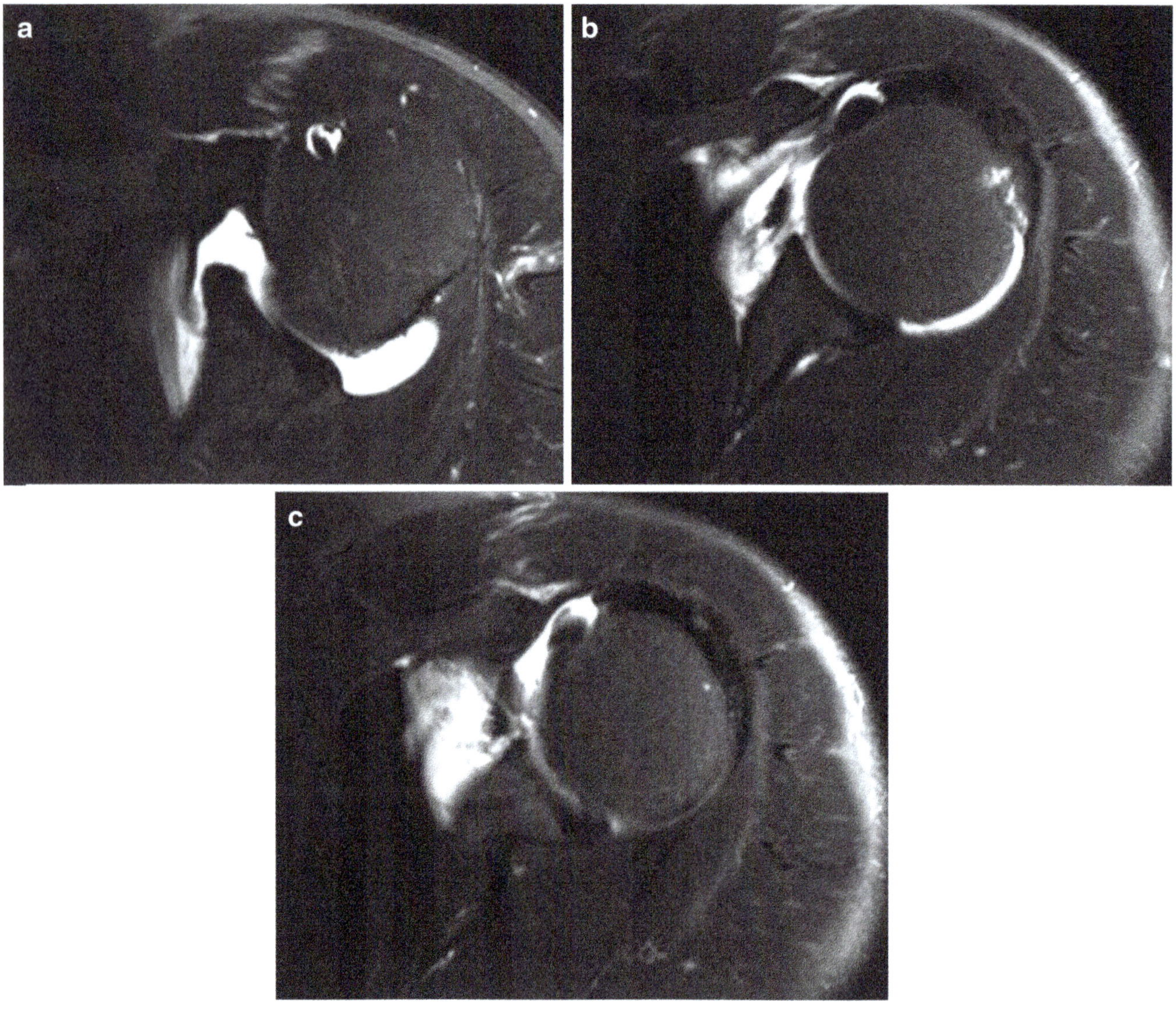

Fig. 15.10 (**a–c**) Axial T2-weighted images of the same patient demonstrate that the SLAP tear extended superiorly from the anterior 2 o'clock position to the posterior 10 o'clock position

Conservative measures were exhausted, including physical therapy, subacromial injections, and glenohumeral injections, all of which provided mild but unsustained relief. At 9 months postoperatively from her SLAP repair, she elected to proceed with revision surgery.

Arthroscopy

The patient was placed in the beach chair position and diagnostic arthroscopy of the shoulder was performed. Her articular surfaces were inspected and found to be intact. The anterior and inferior labrum were inspected next and found to be intact. The glenohumeral ligaments were also visualized and no significant damage was noted. Then the superior labrum and biceps tendon anchor were inspected. The previously placed sutures were identified and found to be frayed (Fig. 15.11a–c). The superior labrum was noted to be poorly healed to the glenoid rim and was quite unstable and degenerative when probed (Fig. 15.11a–c). The SLAP tear had now extended into the biceps anchor as had been predicted from MRI.

A decision was made to proceed with biceps tenodesis, given the involvement of the biceps anchor and her lack of a healing response in her previous SLAP repair. The biceps tendon was tenotomized from the superior labrum, and the residual labrum debrided with an arthroscopic shaver (Fig. 15.11d). The arthroscopic instruments were moved to the subacromial space. Moving anteriorly along the bicipital groove, the biceps tendon was identified just proximal to the pectoralis major insertion. A suprapectoral location for tenodesis was identified and cleared using electrocautery. A guide pin was reamed to 7.5 mm. A 7 mm tenodesis screw was placed, and sutures were subsequently sewn overtop to reinforce the fixation (Fig. 15.11e, f).

Discussion

Management of patients after a failed prior SLAP repair can be challenging. While revision SLAP repair is an option, we generally favor biceps tenodesis in this setting, especially in patients over the age of 30 and those with clearly delineated long head biceps tendon degeneration or partial tearing. This patient was managed with a revision arthroscopic suprapectoral biceps tenodesis with successful mitigation of her symptoms.

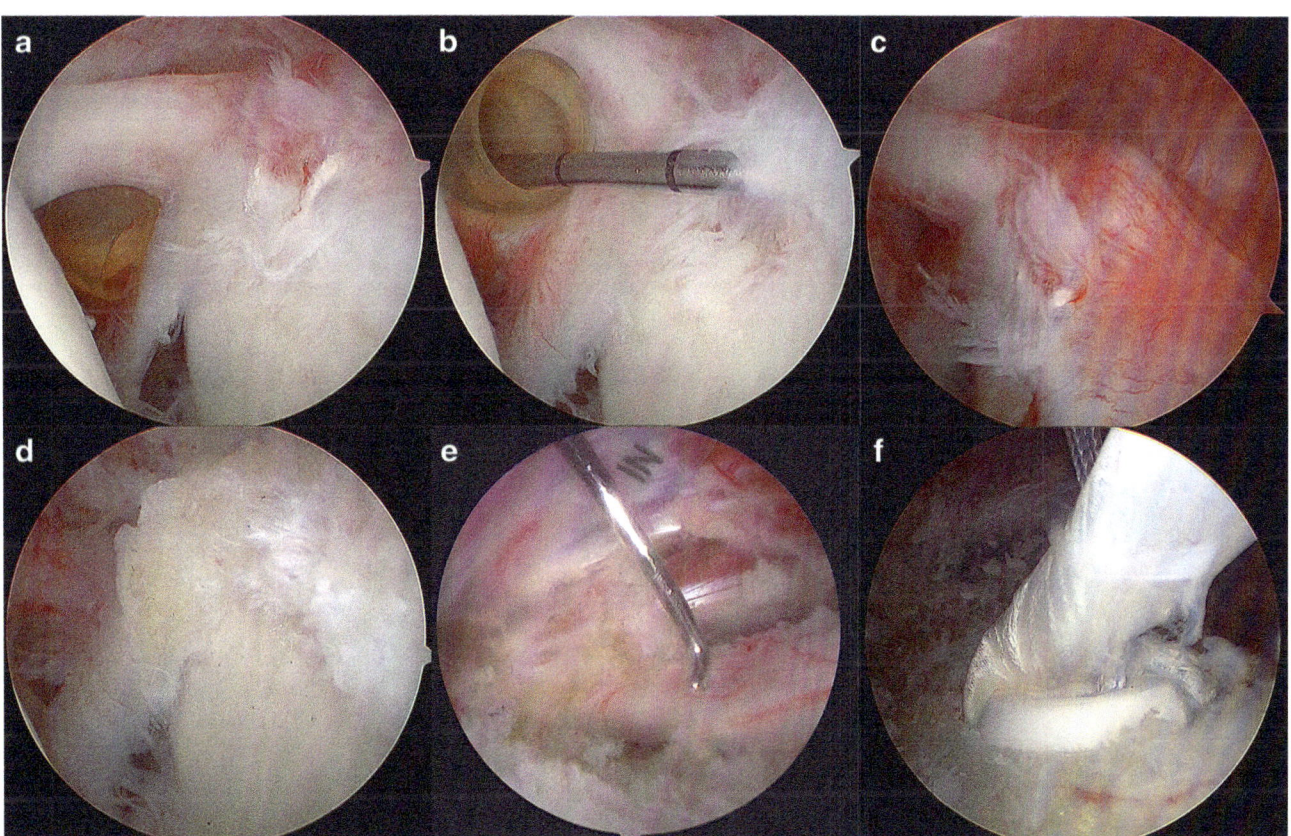

Fig. 15.11 (**a–f**) Arthroscopic images in the beach chair position. The previously placed sutures were identified and found to be frayed. The superior labrum had not healed and was quite unstable upon probing (**a–c**). The biceps was tenotomized and the residual labrum debrided (**d**). An arthroscopic biceps tenodesis using an interference screw was performed (**e, f**)

Case 4: Degenerative SLAP and Biceps Tear

History/Exam

A 68-year-old otherwise healthy right-hand dominant male presented to orthopedic clinic for initial evaluation of his left shoulder. He had been noting gradually worsening left antero-lateral shoulder pain over 6–8 months prior to presentation. He denied any inciting event or previous injury to the shoulder. He noted mild baseline pain but significant worsening with activities. Prior to presentation, he tried oral anti-inflammatories and physical therapy without significant relief.

On physical examination, he was found to have normal range of motion. Positive impingement signs were noted.

Rotator cuff strength testing demonstrated mild-to-moderate weakness to supraspinatus testing with normal infraspinatus strength. His Speed's test was normal. He had a positive O'Brien's. Due to his failure of nonoperative management and physical examination demonstrating possible rotator cuff or labral etiology for his symptoms, advanced imaging was pursued.

Imaging

Standard MRI sequences of the affected shoulder were obtained as described in the previous case examples, including an arthrogram. Coronal T2-weighted images are demonstrated in Fig. 15.12a–f with corresponding axial T2

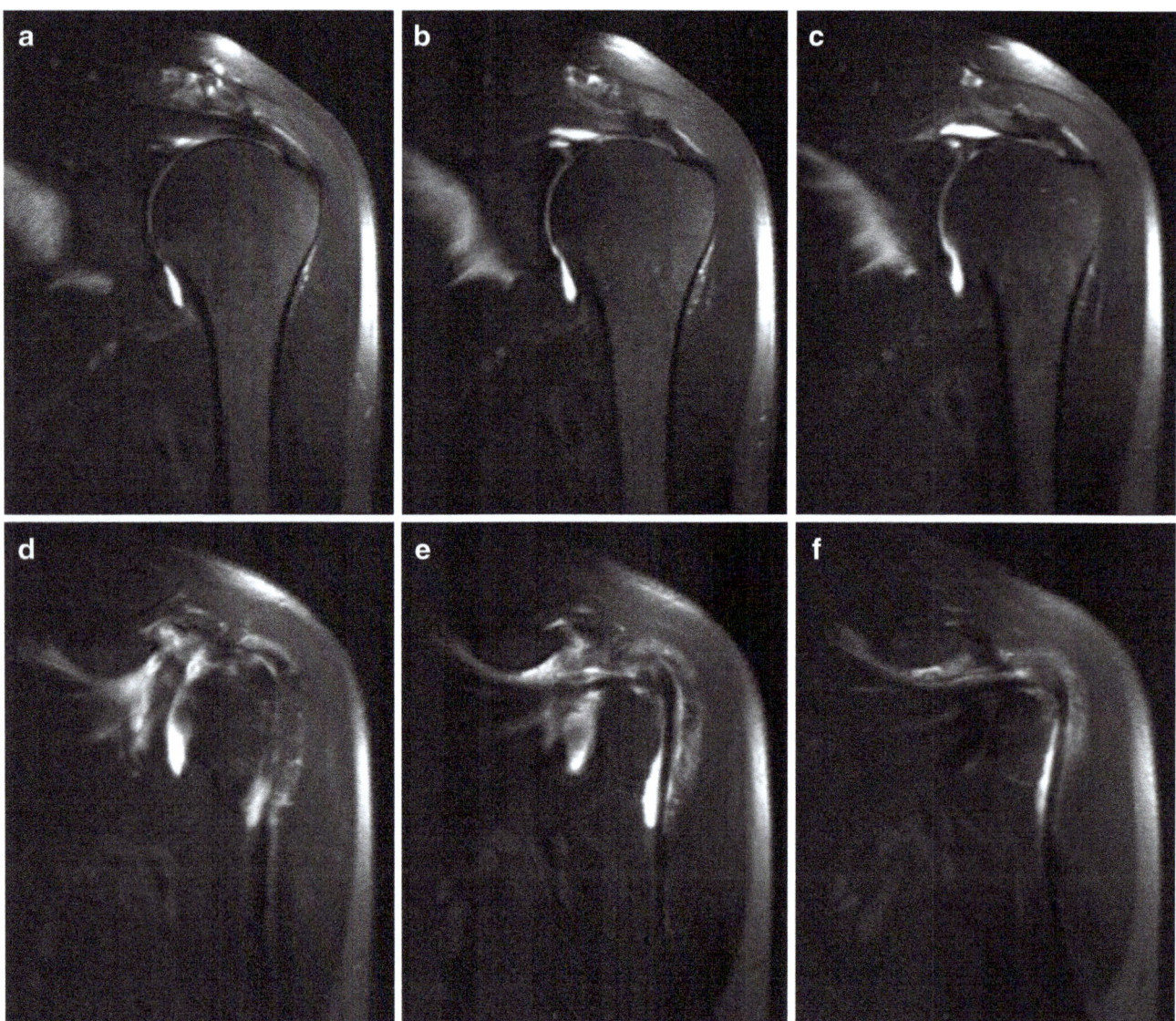

Fig. 15.12 (**a–f**) Coronal T2-weighted MR images of a 68-year-old male with left shoulder pain. Moderate degenerative changes of the acromioclavicular joint were noted (**a**). Mild edema was noted in the subacromial and subdeltoid bursa

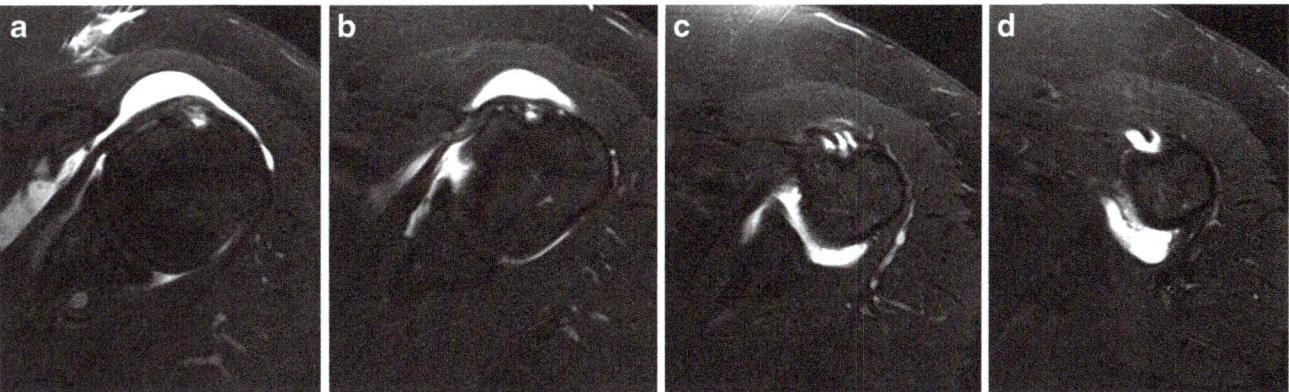

Fig. 15.13 (**a–d**) Axial T2 fat-saturated MR images of the same patient demonstrate thinning and medial subluxation of the biceps tendon with partial tearing. Signal abnormality in the superior and posterior labrum was consistent with a degenerative SLAP tear

fat-saturated images in Fig. 15.13a–d. The MRI demonstrated moderate degenerative changes of the acromioclavicular joint (Fig. 15.12a). Mild edema within the subacromial and subdeltoid bursa was also seen, suggestive of bursitis. Tendinosis of the mid to distal supraspinatus tendon was noted without evidence of focal tear (Fig. 15.12a–f). There was mild atrophy and thinning of the subscapularis tendon. The infraspinatus and teres minor tendons were all intact. The long head of the biceps tendon was thinned and subluxed medially with partial tearing, best demonstrated on axial imaging (Fig. 15.13a–d). Linear signal is seen extending along the intra-articular portion of the long head biceps tendon suggestive of a split tear, which can be seen on both the axial and coronal imaging (Figs. 15.12a–f and 15.13a–d). Signal abnormality within the superior labrum that extended into the superior aspect of the posterior labrum was also found, consistent with a degenerative SLAP tear. Despite his age, he had intact articular cartilage. The patient's symptoms persisted despite exhaustive conservative management; he elected to proceed with surgical intervention.

Arthroscopy

At arthroscopy, the findings on MRI were confirmed; there was significant fraying at the biceps root and an obvious SLAP tear, as well as significant partial tearing of the biceps tendon (Fig. 15.14a–d). The overall glenoid and humeral articular surfaces were noted to have minimal degenerative changes, as was suspected from MRI. The undersurface of the rotator cuff was thoroughly probed and found to be somewhat irregular with fraying on the anterior edge but no obvious full-thickness tear. This was debrided with an arthroscopic shaver. The anterior labrum had some mild fraying which was also debrided using a shaver. Given his age and the condition of the superior labrum and biceps

tendon itself, a biceps tenotomy was performed with a straight punch. The tendon stump was then debrided with an arthroscopic shaver (Fig. 15.15a–d).

Discussion

Biceps tenotomy is a fast, technically simple, and predictable treatment option in patients over the age of 60, low demand patients, and patients with high-grade longitudinal tearing of the long head biceps tendon. Patients should be counseled regarding the likelihood of a popeye deformity as well as the potential for fatigue discomfort and/or spasm of the biceps with heavy labor or athletics.

Conclusions

Pathology of the superior glenoid labrum, biceps anchor, and long head biceps tendon is a well-established etiology of shoulder pain. The clinical diagnosis of SLAP or long head biceps pathology is challenging, as coexistent pathology is frequently present, and symptoms of pathology at each site are often indistinguishable. A careful history, physical examination including provocative maneuvers, and imaging as dictated from the exam are key in establishing an appropriate diagnosis. Magnetic resonance imaging (MRI) remains the imaging technique of choice for patients with suspected SLAP tears or long head biceps pathology. MRI is also useful in identifying concomitant shoulder pathology. Surgical intervention can be pursued when nonsurgical measures have failed. Treatment options are numerous and should be individualized to the patient based on age, functional status, and injury characteristics and include arthroscopic SLAP repair, arthroscopic or open biceps tenodesis, or arthroscopic biceps tenotomy.

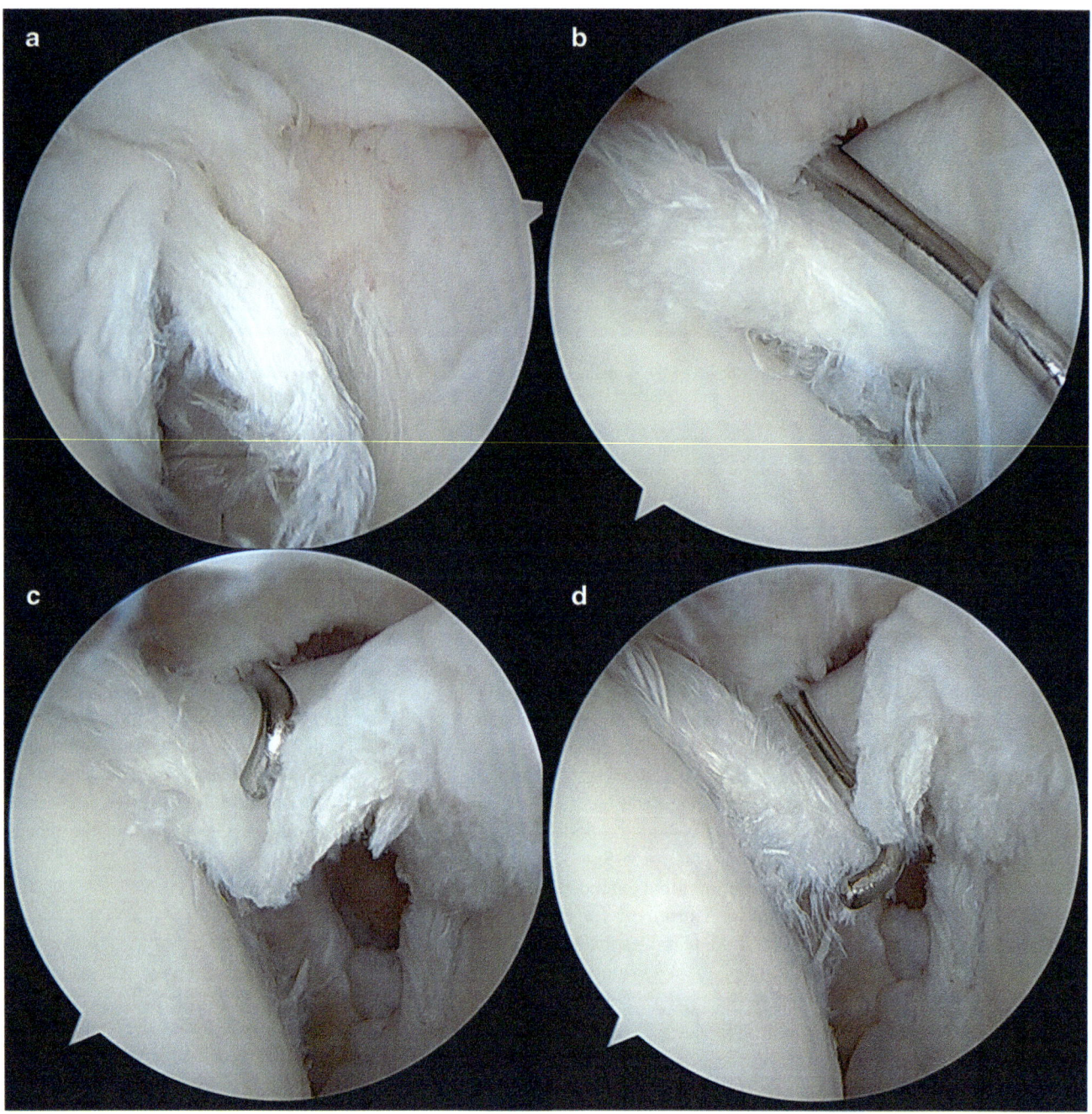

Fig. 15.14 (**a–d**) Arthroscopic images in the beach chair position. There was significant fraying at the biceps root and an obvious SLAP tear, as well as significant tearing of the biceps tendon

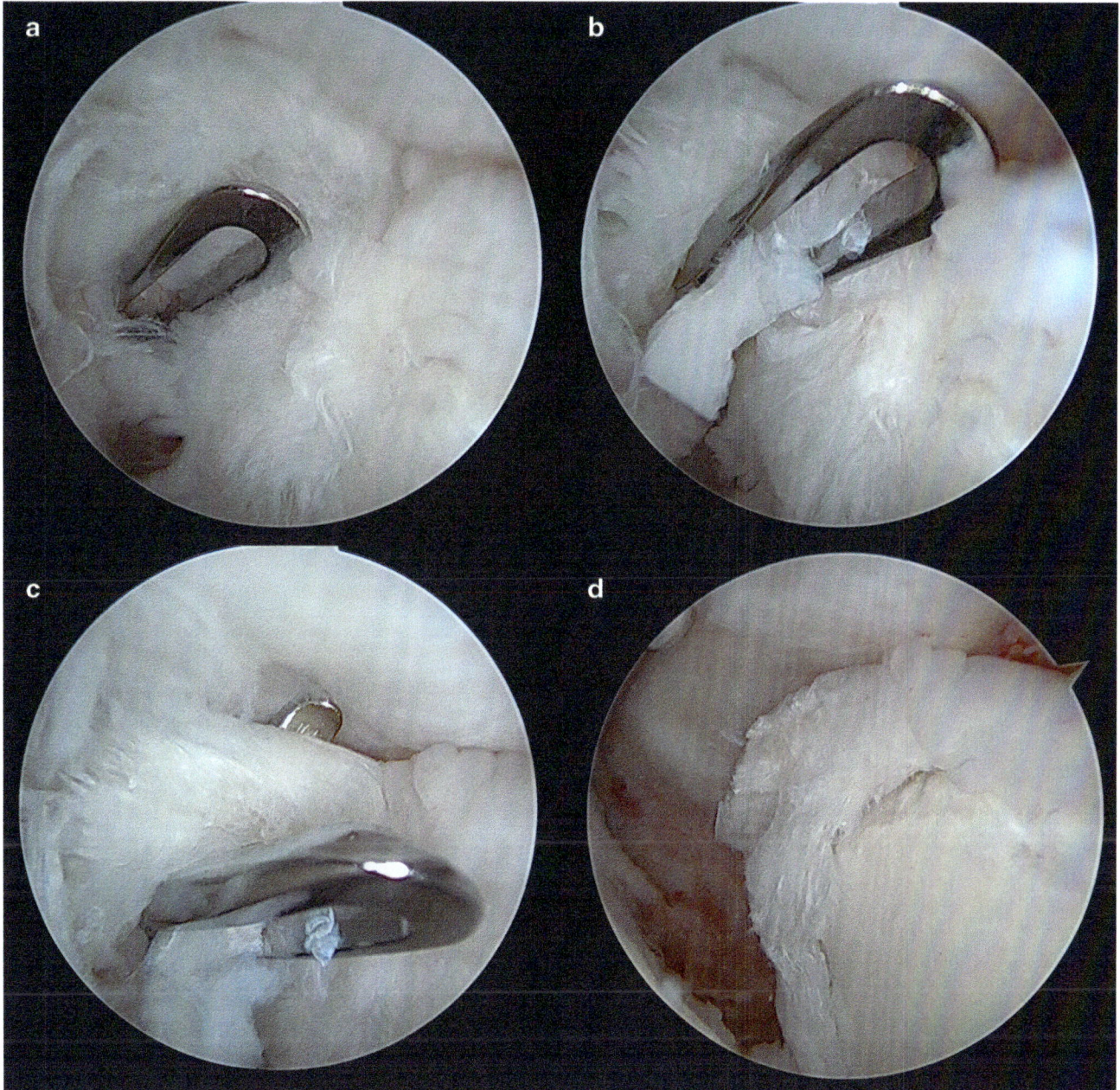

Fig. 15.15 (**a–d**) Given the patient's age and the condition of the superior labrum and biceps tendon, a biceps tenotomy was performed with a straight punch. The remaining stump was then debrided with an arthroscopic shaver

References

1. Keener JD, Brophy RH. Superior labral tears of the shoulder: pathogenesis, evaluation, and treatment. J Am Acad Orthop Surg. 2009;17:627–37.
2. Andrews JR, Carson Jr WG, McLeod WD. Glenoid labrum tears related to the long head of the biceps. Am J Sports Med. 1985; 13:337–41.
3. Snyder SJ, Karzel RP, Del Pizzo W, Ferkel RD, Friedman MJ. SLAP lesions of the shoulder. Arthroscopy. 1990;6:274–9.
4. Maffet MW, Gartsman GM, Moseley B. Superior labrum-biceps tendon complex lesions of the shoulder. Am J Sports Med. 1995;23:93–8.
5. Morgan CD, Burkhart SS, Palmeri M, Gillespie M. Type II SLAP lesions: three subtypes and their relationships to superior instability and rotator cuff tears. Arthroscopy. 1998;14: 553–65.

6. Nho SJ, Strauss EJ, Lenart BA, et al. Long head of the biceps tendinopathy: diagnosis and management. J Am Acad Orthop Surg. 2010;18:645–56.

7. Snyder SJ, Banas MP, Karzel RP. An analysis of 140 injuries to the superior glenoid labrum. J Shoulder Elbow Surg. 1995;4:243–8.

8. Mazzocca AD, McCarthy MB, Ledgard FA, et al. Histomorphologic changes of the long head of the biceps tendon in common shoulder pathologies. Arthroscopy. 2013;29:972–81.

9. Chen CH, Hsu KY, Chen WJ, Shih CH. Incidence and severity of biceps long head tendon lesion in patients with complete rotator cuff tears. J Trauma. 2005;58:1189–93.

10. Sethi N, Wright R, Yamaguchi K. Disorders of the long head of the biceps tendon. J Shoulder Elbow Surg. 1999;8:644–54.

11. Ahrens PM, Boileau P. The long head of biceps and associated tendinopathy. J Bone Joint Surg Br. 2007;89:1001–9.

Seth C. Gamradt

Introduction

This chapter will provide a brief introduction to the patho-physiology of shoulder pain in the throwing athlete. In addition, a concise discussion of important physical exam findings is presented. Lastly, cases illustrating MRI findings correlated with arthroscopic findings will be presented.

Injury to the throwing shoulder is common due to the high forces placed on the joint during overhead athletic activity [1]. The shoulder is subjected to high rotational, distraction, and compressive forces that can damage the structures of the shoulder acutely or as a buildup of repetitive microtrauma [2, 3].

There has been extensive clinical and biomechanical research interest in the normal and disabled throwing shoulder. This research has led to numerous theories explaining the pathologic mechanism (or mechanisms) by which shoulder injuries result in the overhead athlete. While a complete discussion of the pathophysiology of the throwing shoulder is beyond the scope and goals of this book, these overlapping theories should each be introduced. Historically, the cause of shoulder pain in the thrower included theories proposed by some of the giants of shoulder surgery:

1. In 1959, Bennett noted a posterior glenoid exostosis in throwing shoulders on radiographs and postulated that it was caused by posterior capsule traction [4].
2. In 1972, Neer described subacromial impingement of the rotator cuff on the anterior acromion [5]. This condition is thought to also affect throwers. Acromioplasty in throwing athletes has been used with moderate success [6].
3. Jobe and colleagues described anterior instability in the throwing athlete as a cause of shoulder pain. Anterior

capsulolabral reconstruction has also been used with moderate success in the throwing athlete [7, 8].

More recently, several newer concepts have been introduced that attempt to explain injuries to the throwing shoulder in the athlete:

1. *Glenohumeral internal rotation deficit (GIRD)*: This concept describes the phenomenon of an overhead athlete gaining external rotation at the expense of internal rotation. This gain of external rotation is a common physiologic adaptation in thrower's shoulder but is often considered pathologic when the total arc of motion (abducted internal rotation plus abducted external rotation) differs from the contralateral non-throwing shoulder. This pathologic internal rotation deficit is then thought to lead to internal impingement [9–11].
2. *Internal impingement*: is described as abnormal contact between the posterosuperior glenoid and rotator cuff. It can be seen both in biomechanical studies and at the time of arthroscopy. Repetitive contact between the cuff and labrum in internal impingement is thought to place the throwing shoulder at risk for SLAP tears and partial thickness articular sided rotator cuff tears [10, 12–14].
3. *Scapular dyskinesis*: overhead athletes can develop abnormal scapular position and periscapular weakness which can not only decrease velocity but place the shoulder at further risk for injury [15].
4. *Kinetic chain*: Pitching mechanics have been studied extensively in motion analysis laboratories. These studies evaluate how the athlete delivers power from the trunk and legs to the shoulder. These studies underscore the fact that the throwing motion is the end result of converting power from the legs and trunk to a rotational force in the shoulder and eventually into velocity on the ball. Problems anywhere along the kinetic chain can lead to poor mechanics and can contribute to injury risk and shoulder dysfunction [15, 16].

These theories are generally applied to the young throwing or pitching athlete who has overused the shoulder in competition or practice. Acute trauma to the previously

S.C. Gamradt, MD (✉)
Keck Medical Center of USC, University of Southern California, Los Angeles, CA, USA
e-mail: gamradt@usc.edu

well-functioning throwing shoulder considerably widens the differential diagnosis, and the aforementioned discussion is less applicable. Lastly, the aging athlete presents with more garden-variety shoulder conditions as a result of overhead athletics such as subacromial impingement syndrome, rotator cuff tears, and coracoid impingement.

Physical Exam Evaluation of the Throwing Shoulder

The physical examination of the thrower's shoulder is an indispensable part of the evaluation of these athletes. Mcfarland et al. have published an excellent review of the pertinent exam findings that can be found in the throwing athlete [17]. Because MRI is extremely sensitive and because overhead athletes commonly have incidental findings [18–20], MRI should be interpreted in the context of the history and physical exam of the patient. When the symptoms, history, and physical exam all match the MRI findings, it is likely that a correct diagnosis has been made. When the MRI findings do not match the physical exam findings, it is critical to interpret the results with caution. An old adage in treating the overhead athlete's shoulder is to "operate on the patient, not the MRI." Put another way, when obtaining advanced imaging such as MRI of a throwing athlete, damage and/or adaptations of the shoulder are to be expected; surgery should only be indicated after failure of a carefully crafted rehabilitation program.

Table 16.1 shows a non-exhaustive differential diagnosis of various conditions that can be present in the throwing shoulder with the corresponding physical exam findings that can indicate the presence of the condition. As mentioned, these physical exam maneuvers should be correlated with the history, physical exam, and imaging findings to accurately diagnose the painful shoulder in the overhead athlete. It is important to note that many of these tests are not specific, meaning that no one physical exam test definitively diagnoses a shoulder condition.

MRI Findings in the Throwing Shoulder

MRI is commonly ordered in the injured or dysfunctional throwing shoulder to evaluate the presence or absence of structural damage as well as the extent of the damage. Conventional MRI and MR arthrography can be used to evaluate the disabled throwing shoulder. There is some evidence that MRI arthrography is more sensitive in the diagnosis of both labral tear and partial thickness rotator cuff tears [21, 22]. MRI is taken in standard coronal/sagittal/axial views; in addition, MR arthrography in the abducted external rotated position has been advocated in the overhead athlete as an effective adjunct to identify partial thickness rotator cuff tears [23, 24].

A systematic approach to evaluate the MRI in the throwing athlete is critical. It is common for multiple areas of pathology to be present (e.g., SLAP tear and partial thickness rotator cuff tear). Interpretation of the rotator cuff images should include an evaluation of not only the tendon and tendon insertion but also the muscle belly to document the presence or absence of atrophy. Evaluation of the labrum is obviously centered on evaluating the superior labrum, biceps anchor, and long head biceps tendon. However, the labrum should be inspected on MRI circumferentially as superior labral tears can extend both anteriorly and posteriorly. MRI should also be used to evaluate acromial morphology, the AC joint, glenohumeral articular cartilage, and surrounding structures to ensure proper diagnosis of concomitant pathology.

Case 1: Superior Labral Tear with Posterosuperior Paralabral Cyst

A 19-year-old collegiate water polo player with 12 months of low-grade shoulder pain presented with an acute exacerbation of pain in his dominant right shoulder after a game. He reported an inability to throw hard and a feeling of a dead-arm.

Table 16.1 Non-exhaustive differential diagnosis of conditions present in the throwing shoulder with the corresponding physical exam findings

Condition	Physical exam signs
Cervical radiculopathy and/or neuroforaminal stenosis	Cervical range of motion and Spurling's maneuver
AC joint osteoarthritis or distal clavicle osteolysis	Cross body adduction and acromioclavicular (AC) tenderness
Abnormal scapular position or motion	Scapular dyskinesia or scapular winging
SLAP tear	Active compression (O'Brien's) test
Anterior instability	Apprehension/relocation/load and shift
Subacromial impingement	Hawkins'/Neer's signs
Multidirectional instability	Sulcus sign, load and shift
Biceps tenosynovitis	Speed and Yergason's test, palpation of long head biceps tendon
Glenohumeral internal rotation deficit	Decreased abducted internal rotation with decreased total arc of motion
Thoracic outlet syndrome	Adson's test (diminished pulse with forward elevation and neck rotation)
Rotator cuff tendonitis/rotator cuff tear/suprascapular neuropathy (partial or full)	Direct rotator cuff strength testing

The patient had normal cervical spine exam and a negative Spurling's maneuver. He had no tenderness to palpation over the AC joint but mild tenderness to palpation over the biceps tendon. Inspection revealed no muscle atrophy or scapular winging. Strength was 5/5 throughout except for slight (5–/5) weakness with external rotation in the dominant shoulder. Range of motion was full, and there was no glenohumeral internal rotation deficit. Provocative testing revealed negative apprehension/relocation testing, 2+ load and shift anteriorly/1+ load and shift posteriorly (symmetric to left shoulder), and

positive active compression (O'Brien's test) with relief of symptoms with supination of the hand. Speed's and Yergason's tests were negative, as were Neer and Hawkins' tests.

Due to the duration and severity of the symptoms, plain radiographs and MRI arthrography were performed. Plain radiographs were unremarkable. MRI arthrography revealed a type 2 superior labral tear with multiloculated posterosuperior labral cyst just superior to the spinoglenoid notch (Fig. 16.1a–d). Anterior labrum, posterior labrum, and rotator cuff were intact.

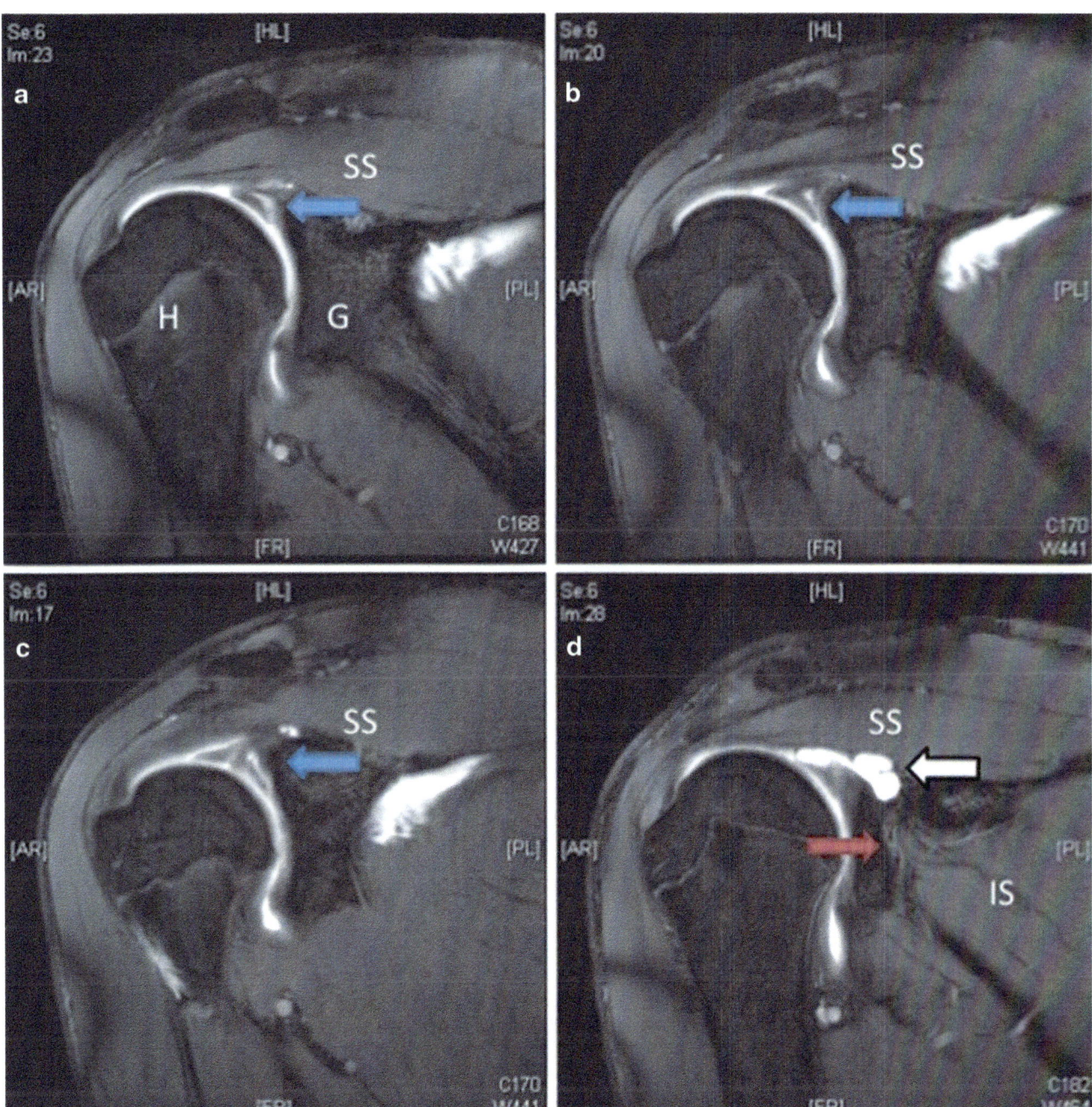

Fig. 16.1 Coronal T1-fat suppressed MR arthrography images reveal intact rotator cuff and significant superior labral tearing (**a–c**) with contrast extending under and within the superior labrum (*blue arrows*). In addition, a spinoglenoid notch cyst (**d**) was present at the posterior aspect of the superior glenoid (*white arrow*). This cyst effaced the suprascapular neurovascular bundle (*red arrow*) as it exits the spinoglenoid notch toward the infraspinatus. *H* humerus, *G* glenoid, *SS* supraspinatus, *IS* infraspinatus

The patient failed 6 weeks of conservative treatment that included rest, physical therapy, and NSAIDs and was still unable to throw or swim comfortably after an attempted return to play.

Arthroscopic surgery was recommended (Fig. 16.2a–f). At the time of surgery, diagnostic arthroscopy revealed intact biceps tendon, type 2 superior labral tear (10:00–12:00) with a small, displaced flap of labrum, intact posterior and anterior labrum, intact glenohumeral cartilage, and normal supraspinatus/infraspinatus/subscapularis.

Two working portals were established. The paralabral cyst was entered and debrided with a 3.5 mm shaver through

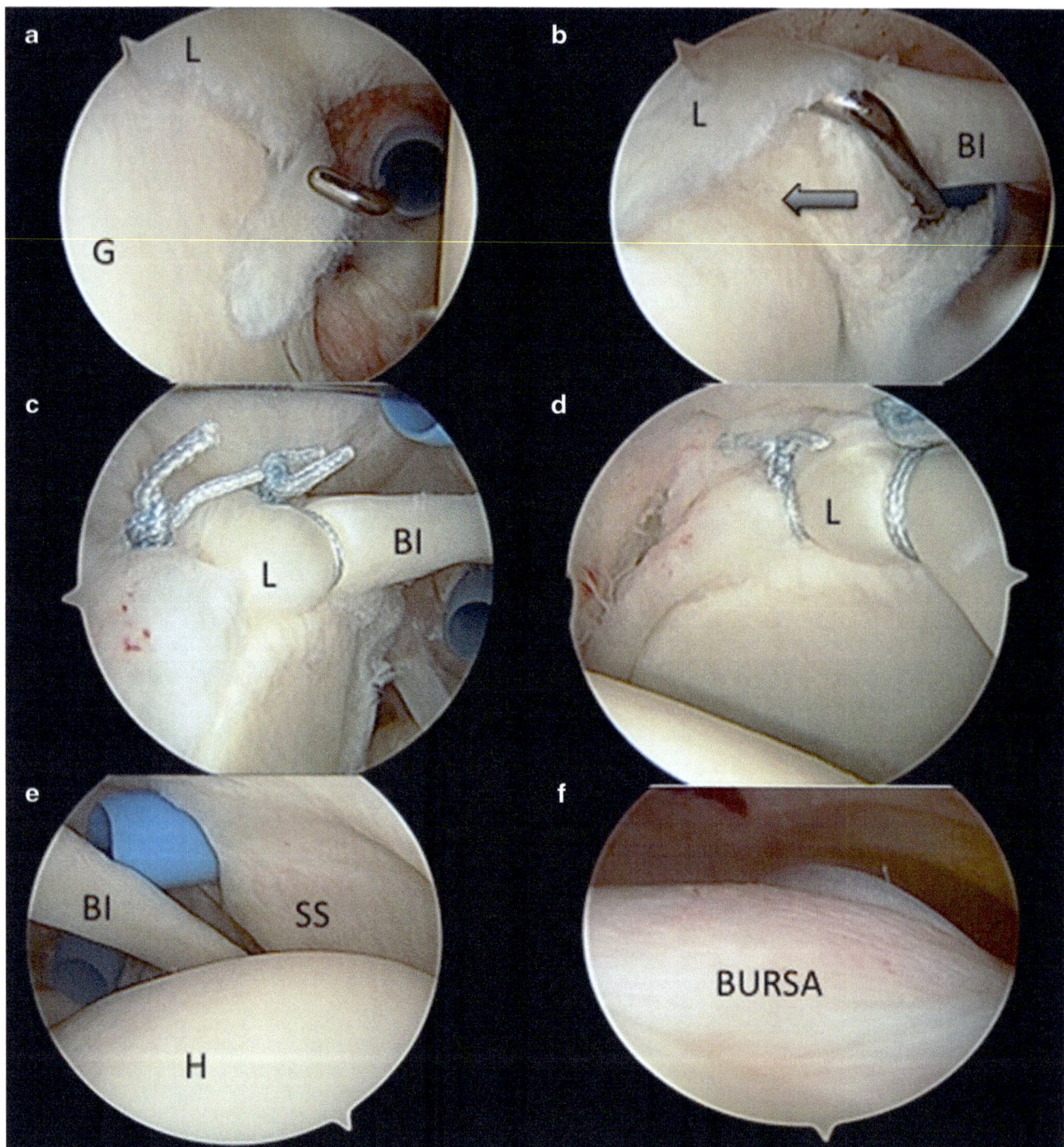

Fig. 16.2 (**a–f**) Arthroscopic images. (**a**) Probe demonstrates small interposed labral flap. (**b**) Probe demonstrates type 2 SLAP tear from 10:00 to 12:00 (*black arrow*). (**c**) Superior labral repair with two suture anchors viewed from the posterior portal. (**d**) Repair viewed from the anterosuperior portal. (**e**) Pristine articular supraspinatus. Note the low rotator interval portal (working) and the high lateral rotator interval just anterior to the supraspinatus above the biceps tendon (used for anchor placement). (**f**) Normal subacromial space and subacromial bursa. *L* labrum, *G* glenoid, *H* humerus, *BI* biceps, *SS* Supraspinatus

the posterior extent of the tear. The superior labral repair was accomplished using two 2.4 mm bioabsorbable suture anchors with sutures tied in a simple fashion. The subacromial space was pristine.

Postoperatively, immobilization was 3 weeks. Passive range of motion was permitted. Full range of motion was restored at 10 weeks. Strengthening was permitted at 12 weeks. Throwing program was initiated at 18 weeks. Successful return to competition was accomplished at 6 months. The patient subsequently competed for 2 years in collegiate water polo.

Discussion

While early results in the throwing athlete were very promising after the arthroscopic repair of SLAP lesions [25, 26], more recent literature reporting outcome scores more sensitive for overhead activity have tempered the enthusiasm for labral repair in the throwing athlete; return to previous level of activity may not be as high as once thought [27–29]. Brockmeier et al. showed that acute traumatic SLAP tears may be better candidates for surgery with better short-term results [30]. A study by Provencher et al. revealed a high rate of continued pain after SLAP repair in the military population sometimes leading to reoperation [27]. In addition, there is evidence that older athletes with SLAP tears may be better served with biceps tenodesis [31] and that SLAP tears can possibly be ignored in the setting of rotator cuff repair [32, 33]. Certainly good to excellent outcomes can be obtained with SLAP repair in the overhead athlete, but recent literature suggests following a conservative course and ensuring the athlete have realistic expectations following surgery.

Case 2: Internal Impingement with SLAP Tear and Partial Thickness Rotator Cuff Tear

A 27-year-old former junior college baseball player who now plays recreational softball complains of years of right shoulder pain. He has found it difficult over the last 12 months to throw. He complains of posterior shoulder pain in the cocking phase of his throwing motion. He reports no trauma in the shoulder but does report a history of successful cortisone injections to his shoulder years ago.

The patient had normal cervical spine exam and a negative Spurling's maneuver. He had no tenderness to palpation over the AC joint but mild tenderness to palpation over the biceps tendon. Inspection revealed no muscle atrophy or scapular winging. Strength was 5/5 throughout. Range of motion was full in forward elevation bilaterally, but there was a glenohumeral internal rotation deficit of 20°. Abducted

external rotation in the right shoulder was 105°; abducted internal rotation in the right shoulder was 35°. Abducted external rotation in the left shoulder was 95°; abducted internal rotation in the left shoulder was 65°. Provocative testing revealed negative apprehension/relocation testing, 1+ load and shift anteriorly/1+ load and shift posteriorly (symmetric to left shoulder), and positive active compression (O'Brien's test) with relief of symptoms with supination of the hand. Speed's and Yergason's tests were negative. Neer and Hawkins' tests were slightly positive.

Plain radiographs revealed a type 2 acromion and early AC joint osteoarthritis but were otherwise negative.

Because he had success with a corticosteroid injection in the past, a subacromial injection was prescribed; this partially relieved his baseline shoulder pain over the next several weeks. A course of physical therapy was prescribed to include restoration of right shoulder internal rotation using sleeper stretches. The patient returned to softball but still had pain while throwing. Due to the duration and severity of the symptoms, MRI arthrography was performed. MRI arthrography revealed a small posterosuperior labral tear. In addition, contrast was observed in a delaminated partial thickness articular sided rotator cuff tear in the posterior supraspinatus (Fig. 16.3a–d). Anterior labrum and posterior labrum were intact, but there was MRI evidence of subacromial impingement.

The patient elected to undergo arthroscopic surgery (Fig. 16.4a–f). At the time of surgery, diagnostic arthroscopy revealed intact biceps tendon and a peel-back type 2 superior labral tear (9:30–10:30) with an Ellman grade 1A partial thickness articular sided rotator cuff tear in the posterior aspect of the supraspinatus. There was intact posterior and anterior labrum, intact glenohumeral cartilage, and normal infraspinatus/subscapularis. Contact between the rotator cuff tear and posterosuperior labrum was observed in the abducted-externally rotated position at the time of arthroscopy.

Two working portals were established. The superior labral repair was accomplished using one double loaded 2.4 mm bioabsorbable suture anchor with sutures tied in a simple fashion. The rotator cuff was debrided back to stable tissue. The subacromial space was entered. A subacromial bursectomy and conservative acromioplasty were performed.

Postoperatively, immobilization was 3 weeks. Passive range of motion was permitted. Full range of motion was restored at 10 weeks. Strengthening was permitted at 12 weeks. Throwing program was initiated at 18 weeks. Successful return to competition was accomplished at 6 months. The patient improved and competed in recreational softball postoperatively with improvement but still with some mild, occasional pain during throwing.

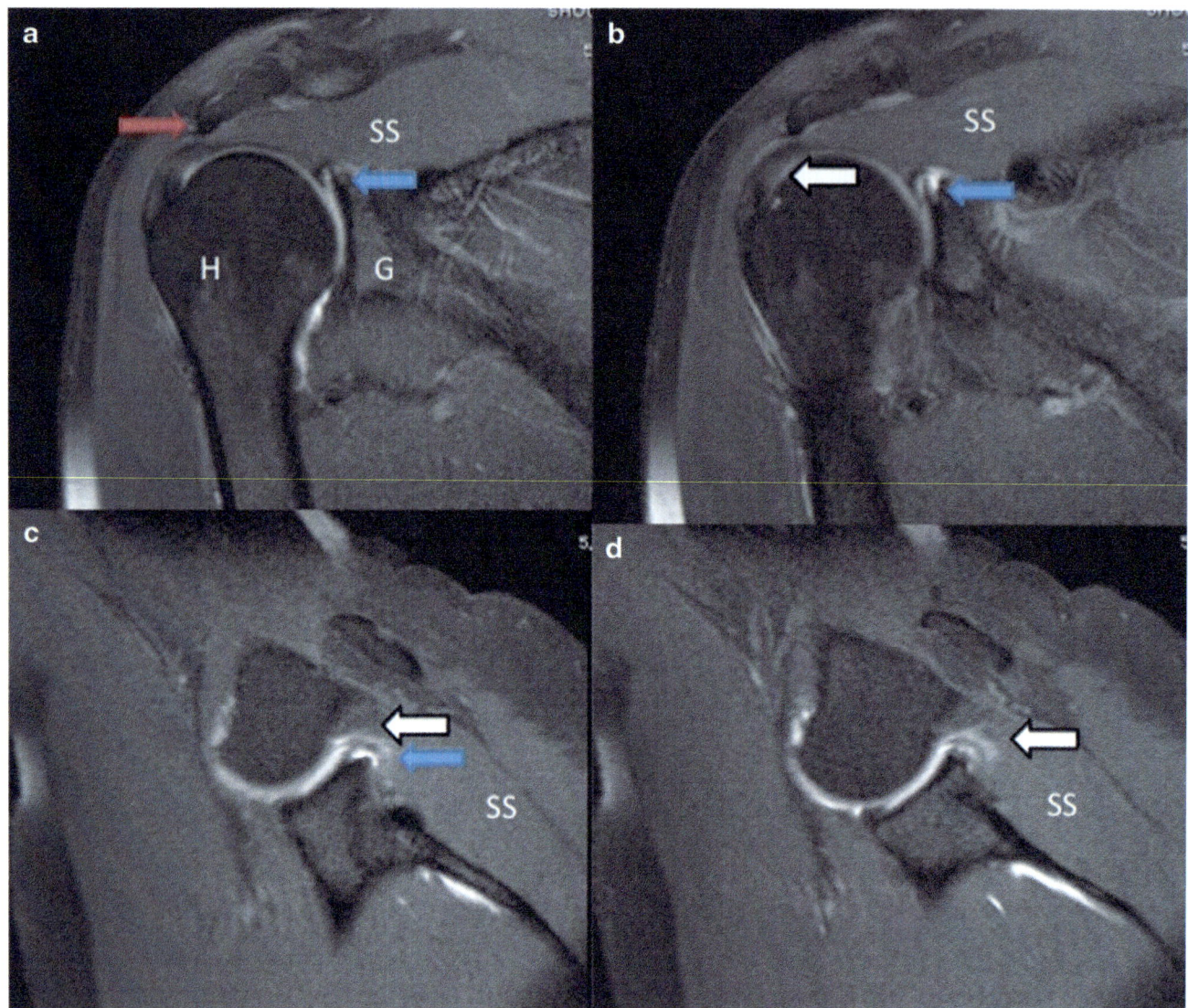

Fig. 16.3 (**a–d**) Coronal T1-fat suppressed MR arthrography images reveal downsloping acromion (*red arrow*). The rotator cuff was largely intact but with some high signal in the articular surface of the posterior supraspinatus (*white arrow* in **b**). There was superior labral tearing (*blue arrows* in **a–c**) with contrast extending under and within the supe-rior labrum. The ABER views (**c, d**) revealed contact of the rotator cuff with the superior glenoid. In addition, contrast was observed in a delaminated partial thickness articular sided rotator cuff tear in the posterior supraspinatus (*white arrows* **c, d**). *H* humerus, *G* glenoid, *SS* supraspinatus

Case 3: Repair of Partial Thickness Rotator Cuff Tear

A 22-year-old shot-putter acutely injured his right shoulder throwing shot. He complained of acute weakness and inability to participate in practice. He did not feel the shoulder dislocate or subluxate. Plain radiographs were negative. He reported no history of shoulder trouble in the past.

The patient had normal cervical spine exam and a negative Spurling's maneuver. He had no tenderness to palpation over the AC joint or biceps tendon. Inspection revealed no

muscle atrophy or scapular winging. Strength was 5/5 throughout except for the supraspinatus in his right shoulder, which was 4/5 with significant pain. Range of motion was full in forward elevation bilaterally but painful on the right. There was no glenohumeral internal rotation deficit. Provocative testing revealed pain in the apprehension position which did not resolve with relocation testing, 1+ load and shift anteriorly/1+ load and shift posteriorly (symmetric to left shoulder), and positive active compression (O'Brien's test) with no relief of symptoms with supination of the hand. Speed's and Yergason's tests were negative. Neer and Hawkins' tests were slightly positive.

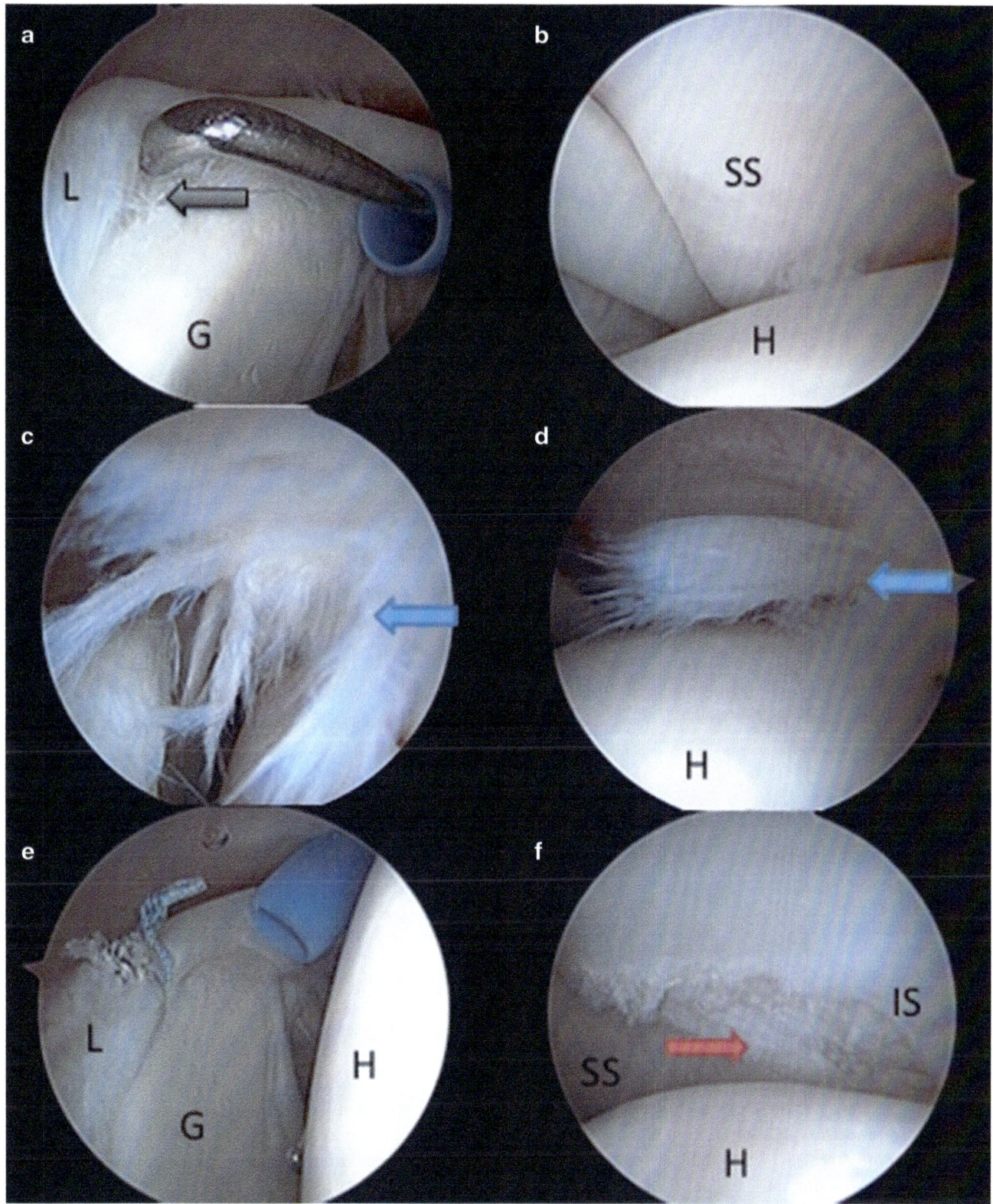

Fig. 16.4 (**a**–**f**) Arthroscopic images. (**a**) Probe demonstrates a small peel-back type 2 superior labral tear (9:30–10:30) (*black arrow*). (**b**) Intact supraspinatus. (**c**) ABER position arthroscopically reveals contact between torn articular side of supraspinatus and posterosuperior glenoid. (**d**) Partial articular sided rotator cuff tear viewed with the arm in the neutral, adducted position. (**e**) Superior labral repair with a single anchor, double loaded suture. (**f**) After debridement of the rotator cuff to stable tissue, no repair of the rotator cuff was performed. *L* labrum, *G* glenoid, *H* humerus, *BI* biceps, *SS* supraspinatus

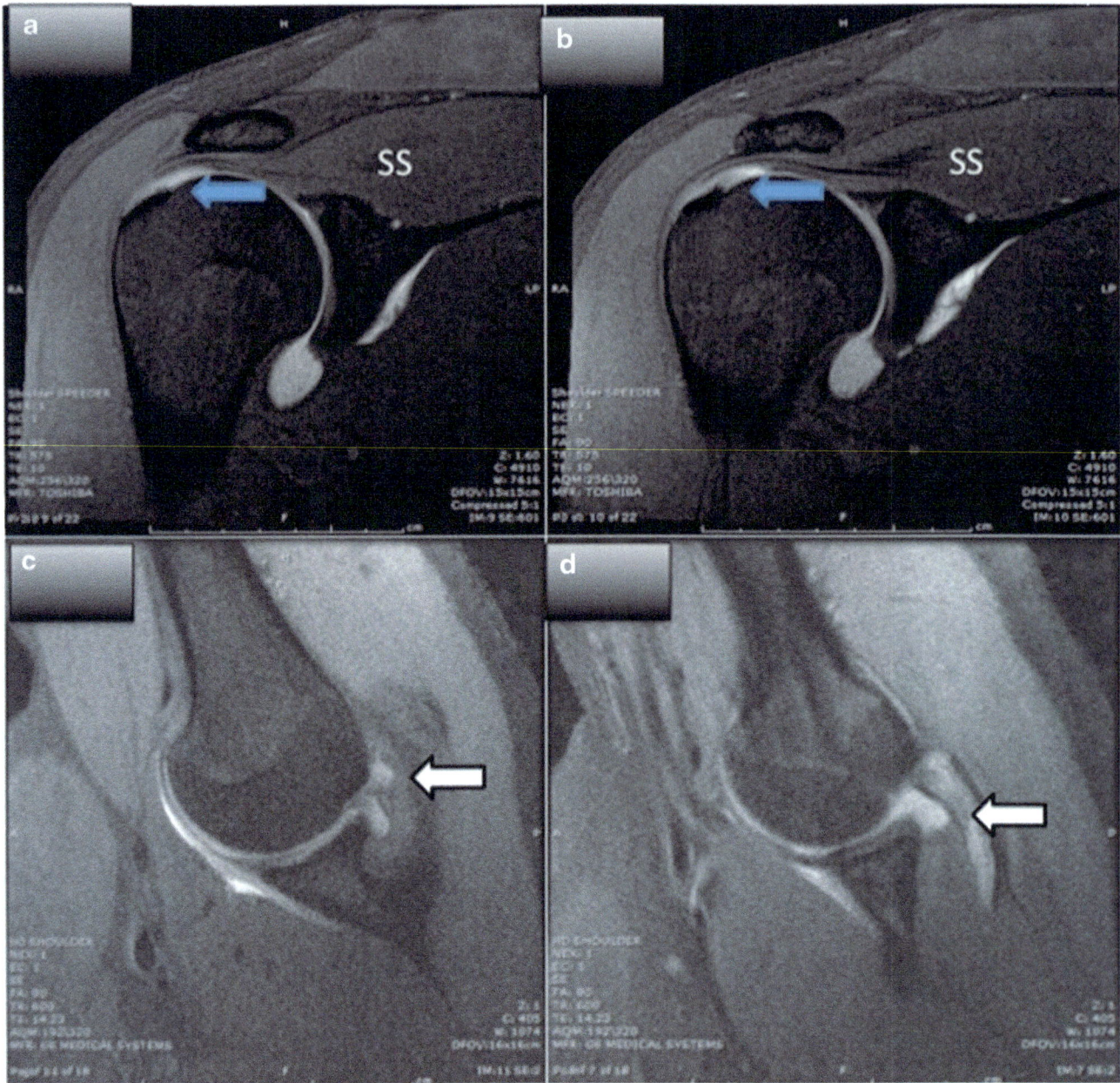

Fig. 16.5 (**a–d**) Coronal T1-fat suppressed MR arthrography images reveal a type 1 acromion. In **a**, **b**, the rotator cuff had high signal on the articular surface (*blue arrows*). There was superior labrum intact. The ABER views (**c**, **d**) revealed that the tear was more extensive and that there was delamination of the cuff, allowing contrast within the tear (*white arrows*). *SS* supraspinatus

Due to the acute weakness in the shoulder, the decision was made to proceed with MRI arthrogram (Fig. 16.5a–d). MR arthrogram revealed partial thickness articular sided supraspinatus tear with intralaminar tracking of the dye along the cuff tear in the ABER position. The labrum and glenohumeral cartilage were normal. There was no bone bruising to suggest instability. Acromion was type 1.

The patient was prescribed NSAIDs for pain and immobilized for 1 week as the shoulder had discomfort with daily activities. He then started rehabilitation. Despite restoring normal range of motion at 8 weeks, his strength remained 4+/5 and he could not compete. The decision was made at that point to proceed with arthroscopic rotator cuff repair versus debridement.

The patient elected to undergo arthroscopic surgery (Fig. 16.6a–f). At the time of surgery, diagnostic arthroscopy revealed intact biceps tendon and superior labrum. There was an Ellman grade 3A partial thickness articular sided

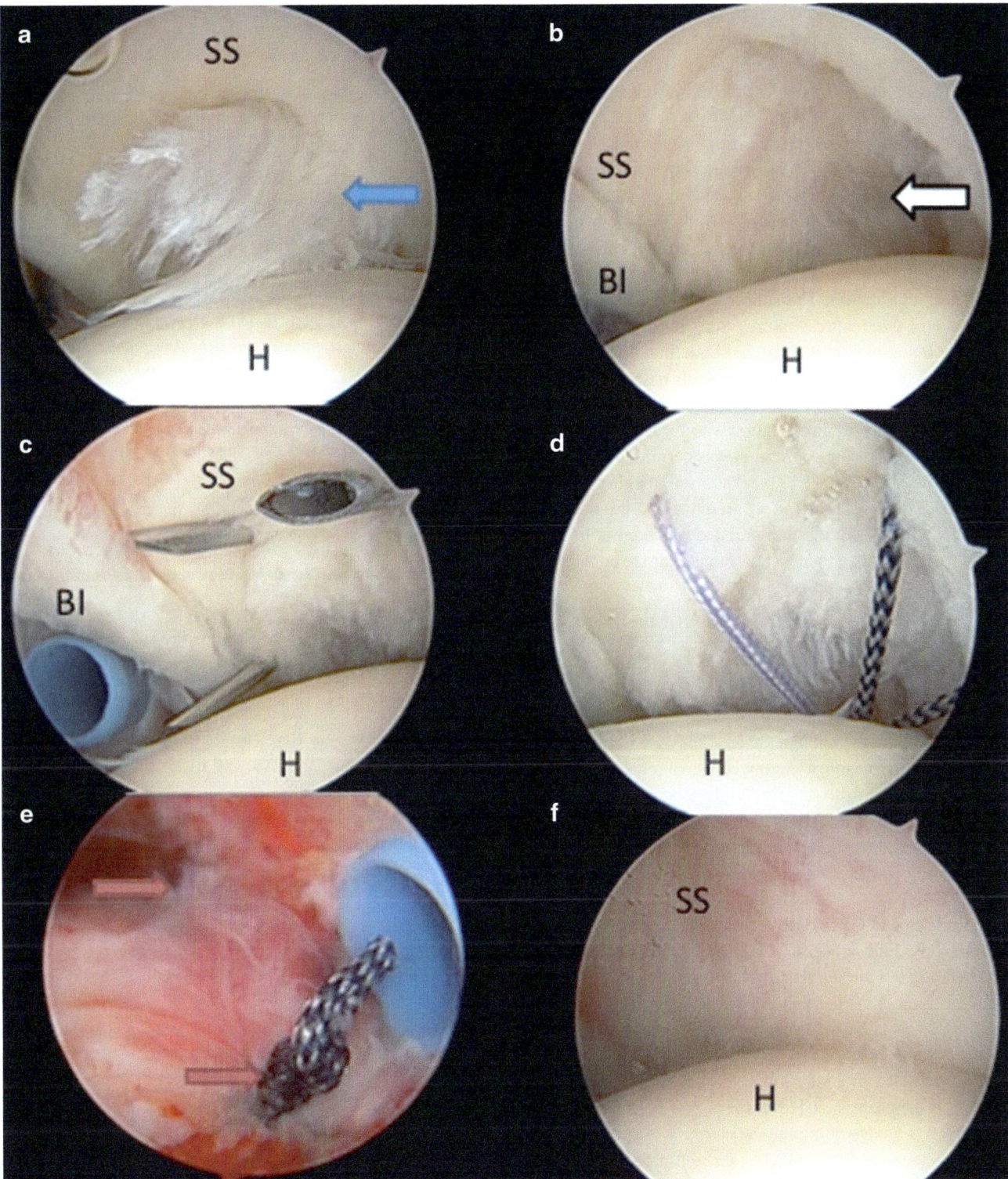

Fig. 16.6 (**a–f**) Arthroscopic images. (**a**) *Blue arrow* demonstrates partial thickness articular sided rotator cuff tear. (**b**) Debridement reveals deep Ellman grade 3A supraspinatus tear (*white arrow*). (**c**) Multiple spinal needles passed percutaneously to be used as suture passers to shuttle sutures through cuff. (**d**) After anchor placement and suture passage. (**e**) Tying of knots in the subacromial space (*red arrows*) (**f**) Final view in the glenohumeral joint reveals excellent restoration of supraspinatus footprint after repair. *H* humerus, *BI* biceps, *SS* supraspinatus

rotator cuff tear in the supraspinatus. There was intact posterior and anterior labrum, intact glenohumeral cartilage, and normal infraspinatus/subscapularis.

The rotator cuff was debrided, and the exposed rotator cuff footprint on the greater tuberosity was debrided. Next, a subacromial bursectomy was performed in standard fashion to aid in suture tying in the subacromial space. A bioabsorbable rotator cuff anchor was inserted in a transtendinous fashion into the greater tuberosity. Multiple spinal needles were used as suture passers. Prolene sutures were used to shuttle four limbs of suture from the anchor through the edges of the torn cuff tissue. The subacromial space was entered again and the two mattress sutures were tied arthroscopically. The glenohumeral joint was entered for a final time to inspect the repair. Excellent coaptation of the cuff tissue to bone was observed.

Postoperatively, immobilization was 4 weeks in an abduction sling. Passive range of motion was permitted. Full range of motion was restored at 10 weeks. Strengthening was permitted at 12 weeks. Throwing program was not initiated until 6 months. Successful return to practice was accomplished at 9 months albeit with a lighter shot. Final return to competition has not yet been accomplished.

Discussion

Rotator cuff tears and labral pathology can be normal findings in the overhead athletes' shoulder even if they are throwing well [20, 34]. For this reason, a lengthy course of rehab is appropriate before proceeding to surgery. While good results have been reported for overhead athletes undergoing arthroscopic repair of partial thickness rotator cuff tears [35, 36], the trend is toward erring on the side of debridement in the high-level athlete [37]. Repair of partial thickness rotator cuff tears are rarely indicated in GIRD/internal impingement unless the tear is extremely high-grade or the athlete has already failed debridement and an attempted return to play [3]. The hypermobility of the shoulder that allows generation of high rotational forces can be lost after rotator cuff repair. Repair of full thickness rotator cuff tearing in the throwing athlete carries a poor prognosis with a very low rate of return to competitive pitching at the professional level [38].

Disclosure The senior author (SCG) is a consultant for Biomet.

References

1. Dillman CJ, Fleisig GS, Andrews JR. Biomechanics of pitching with emphasis upon shoulder kinematics. J Orthop Sports Phys Ther. 1993;18(2):402–8.
2. Cohn RM, Jazrawi LM. The throwing shoulder: the orthopedist perspective. Magn Reson Imaging Clin N Am. 2012;20(2):261–75, x.
3. Economopoulos KJ, Brockmeier SF. Rotator cuff tears in overhead athletes. Clin Sports Med. 2012;31(4):675–92.
4. Bennett GE. Elbow and shoulder lesions of baseball players. Am J Surg. 1959;98:484–92.
5. Neer 2nd CS. Anterior acromioplasty for the chronic impingement syndrome in the shoulder: a preliminary report. J Bone Joint Surg Am. 1972;54(1):41–50.
6. Tibone JE, Jobe FW, Kerlan RK, Carter VS, Shields CL, Lombardo SJ, et al. Shoulder impingement syndrome in athletes treated by an anterior acromioplasty. Clin Orthop Relat Res. 1985;198:134–40.
7. Jobe FW, Giangarra CE, Kvitne RS, Glousman RE. Anterior capsulolabral reconstruction of the shoulder in athletes in overhand sports. Am J Sports Med. 1991;19(5):428–34.
8. Kvitne RS, Jobe FW. The diagnosis and treatment of anterior instability in the throwing athlete. Clin Orthop Relat Res. 1993;291:107–23.
9. Lintner D, Mayol M, Uzodinma O, Jones R, Labossiere D. Glenohumeral internal rotation deficits in professional pitchers enrolled in an internal rotation stretching program. Am J Sports Med. 2007;35(4):617–21.
10. Myers JB, Laudner KG, Pasquale MR, Bradley JP, Lephart SM. Glenohumeral range of motion deficits and posterior shoulder tightness in throwers with pathologic internal impingement. Am J Sports Med. 2006;34(3):385–91.
11. Tokish JM, Curtin MS, Kim YK, Hawkins RJ, Torry MR. Glenohumeral internal rotation deficit in the asymptomatic professional pitcher and its relationship to humeral retroversion. J Sports Sci Med. 2008;7(1):78–83.
12. Burkhart SS. Internal impingement of the shoulder. Instr Course Lect. 2006;55:29–34.
13. Drakos MC, Rudzki JR, Allen AA, Potter HG, Altchek DW. Internal impingement of the shoulder in the overhead athlete. J Bone Joint Surg Am. 2009;91(11):2719–28.
14. Burkhart SS, Morgan CD, Kibler WB. The disabled throwing shoulder: spectrum of pathology part I: pathoanatomy and biomechanics. Arthroscopy. 2003;19(4):404–20.
15. Burkhart SS, Morgan CD, Kibler WB. The disabled throwing shoulder: spectrum of pathology part III: the SICK scapula, scapular dyskinesis, the kinetic chain, and rehabilitation. Arthroscopy. 2003;19(6):641–61.
16. Braun S, Kokmeyer D, Millett PJ. Shoulder injuries in the throwing athlete. J Bone Joint Surg Am. 2009;91(4):966–78.
17. McFarland EG, Tanaka MJ, Papp DF. Examination of the shoulder in the overhead and throwing athlete. Clin Sports Med. 2008; 27(4):553–78.
18. Lesniak BP, Baraga MG, Jose J, Smith MK, Cunningham S, Kaplan LD. Glenohumeral findings on magnetic resonance imaging correlate with innings pitched in asymptomatic pitchers. Am J Sports Med. 2013;41(9):2022–7.
19. Connor PM, Banks DM, Tyson AB, Coumas JS, D'Alessandro DF. Magnetic resonance imaging of the asymptomatic shoulder of overhead athletes: a 5-year follow-up study. Am J Sports Med. 2003;31(5):724–7.
20. Miniaci A, Mascia AT, Salonen DC, Becker EJ. Magnetic resonance imaging of the shoulder in asymptomatic professional baseball pitchers. Am J Sports Med. 2002;30(1):66–73.
21. Meister K, Thesing J, Montgomery WJ, Indelicato PA, Walczak S, Fontenot W. MR arthrography of partial thickness tears of the undersurface of the rotator cuff: an arthroscopic correlation. Skeletal Radiol. 2004;33(3):136–41.
22. Chandnani VP, Yeager TD, DeBerardino T, Christensen K, Gagliardi JA, Heitz DR, et al. Glenoid labral tears: prospective evaluation with MRI imaging, MR arthrography, and CT arthrography. AJR Am J Roentgenol. 1993;161(6):1229–35.
23. Iyengar JJ, Burnett KR, Nottage WM, Harwin SF. The abduction external rotation (ABER) view for MRI of the shoulder. Orthopedics. 2010;33(8):562–5.

24. Jung JY, Jee WH, Chun HJ, Ahn MI, Kim YS. Magnetic resonance arthrography including ABER view in diagnosing partial-thickness tears of the rotator cuff: accuracy, and inter- and intra-observer agreements. Acta Radiol. 2010;51(2):194–201.

25. Burkhart SS, Morgan CD, Kibler WB. Shoulder injuries in overhead athletes. The "dead arm" revisited. Clin Sports Med. 2000;19(1):125–58.

26. Burkhart SS, Morgan C. SLAP lesions in the overhead athlete. Orthop Clin North Am. 2001;32(3):431–41, viii.

27. Provencher MT, McCormick F, Dewing C, McIntire S, Solomon D. A prospective analysis of 179 type 2 superior labrum anterior and posterior repairs: outcomes and factors associated with success and failure. Am J Sports Med. 2013;41(4):880–6.

28. Gorantla K, Gill C, Wright RW. The outcome of type II SLAP repair: a systematic review. Arthroscopy. 2010;26(4):537–45.

29. Knesek M, Skendzel JG, Dines JS, Altchek DW, Allen AA, Bedi A. Diagnosis and management of superior labral anterior posterior tears in throwing athletes. Am J Sports Med. 2013;41(2): 444–60.

30. Brockmeier SF, Voos JE, Williams 3rd RJ, Altchek DW, Cordasco FA, Allen AA. Outcomes after arthroscopic repair of type-II SLAP lesions. J Bone Joint Surg Am. 2009;91(7):1595–603.

31. McCormick F, Bhatia S, Chalmers P, Gupta A, Verma N, Romeo AA. The management of type II superior labral anterior to posterior injuries. Orthop Clin North Am. 2014;45(1):121–8.

32. Abbot AE, Li X, Busconi BD. Arthroscopic treatment of concomitant superior labral anterior posterior (SLAP) lesions and rotator cuff tears in patients over the age of 45 years. Am J Sports Med. 2009;37(7):1358–62.

33. Franceschi F, Longo UG, Ruzzini L, Rizzello G, Maffulli N, Denaro V. No advantages in repairing a type II superior labrum anterior and posterior (SLAP) lesion when associated with rotator cuff repair in patients over age 50: a randomized controlled trial. Am J Sports Med. 2008;36(2):247–53.

34. Miniaci A, Dowdy PA, Willits KR, Vellet AD. Magnetic resonance imaging evaluation of the rotator cuff tendons in the asymptomatic shoulder. Am J Sports Med. 1995;23(2):142–5.

35. Brockmeier SF, Dodson CC, Gamradt SC, Coleman SH, Altchek DW. Arthroscopic intratendinous repair of the delaminated partial-thickness rotator cuff tear in overhead athletes. Arthroscopy. 2008;24(8):961–5.

36. Conway JE. Arthroscopic repair of partial-thickness rotator cuff tears and SLAP lesions in professional baseball players. Orthop Clin North Am. 2001;32(3):443–56.

37. Reynolds SB, Dugas JR, Cain EL, McMichael CS, Andrews JR. Debridement of small partial-thickness rotator cuff tears in elite overhead throwers. Clin Orthop Relat Res. 2008;466(3):614–21.

38. Mazoue CG, Andrews JR. Repair of full-thickness rotator cuff tears in professional baseball players. Am J Sports Med. 2006; 34(2):182–9.

Frozen Shoulder

Stephen R. Thompson

Introduction

Frozen shoulder, or adhesive capsulitis, is a disabling condition that severely restricts shoulder range of motion. The condition was originally recognized by Duplay in 1872, and he coined the disease as "peri-arthritis." In 1934, Codman more fully elaborated on the condition and termed it frozen shoulder [1]. Then, in 1945, Neviaser introduced the phrase adhesive capsulitis, based on his findings at surgery of adhesions of the capsule along the humerus [2]. All of these authors described the condition as a painful shoulder of insidious onset with associated loss of motion in forward elevation and external rotation.

Frozen shoulder is a common condition. It is estimated to affect approximately 2 % of the population [3]. Frozen shoulder typically occurs in the sixth decade of life, with women slightly more frequently affected than men. The peak age of onset is 56 years old, and it is rarely seen in patients under 40 or over 70 years old. The non-dominant shoulder is more commonly affected than the dominant side. Recurrence in the same shoulder is extremely rare, but approximately 20 % of individuals will develop frozen shoulder in the contralateral side.

The phrase "frozen shoulder" is useful when describing the clinical presentation and natural history. There is a "freezing" phase which is characterized by painful range of motion secondary to inflammation of the synovial lining of the joint, a "frozen" phase with little pain but significant stiffness, and a "thawing" phase with some pain and gradual resolution of stiffness. Symptoms in the freezing phase begin insidiously with a history of worsening pain, particularly at night. Occasionally, there may be a history of minor trauma, such as a fall onto the shoulder. This phase typically occurs

for 1–3 months. The frozen phase is characterized by a gradual decrease in pain. Patients will have often developed compensatory mechanisms to avoid shoulder motion during the freezing phase and may not immediately recognize the significant loss of glenohumeral range of motion. The characteristic physical examination is that of active range of motion equaling that of passive range of motion. Loss of passive external rotation is the most frequently reported directional loss. This phase often lasts for 4–18 months. Finally, in the thawing phase, range of motion is gradually restored. This is often accompanied by some pain, but is less intense than that encountered during the freezing phase. This phase may last for 3–12 months.

Diagnosis of frozen shoulder is clinical. Although formal diagnostic criteria are currently lacking in the literature, loss of active and passive external rotation of the shoulder along with the classic pain pattern should lead to the correct diagnosis. The two most frequently encountered conditions that can also demonstrate a loss of selective external rotation are glenohumeral osteoarthritis and a locked posterior glenohumeral dislocation. Both of the conditions are readily diagnosed on routine radiographs. Magnetic resonance imaging (MRI) is not routinely necessary to confirm a diagnosis of frozen shoulder but may occasionally be used to rule out associated pathologies, such as rotator cuff tears.

Despite being recognized over a hundred years ago, the true natural history of frozen shoulder remains uncertain. It is a protracted disease that can take up to 2 years to resolve. As such, it has necessitated a "patient" patient to endure the condition [4]. This 2-year rule, while useful when discussing the condition with patients, may underestimate the long-term disability of frozen shoulder. In the longest reported follow-up of frozen shoulder, approximately 60 % had some degree of stiffness, and approximately half had mild persistent pain [5].

The cause of frozen shoulder is unknown [6]. A variety of mechanisms have been postulated, including immunologic, inflammatory, and fibrosing. Given the history of pain followed by stiffness, the most apparent mechanism would be

S.R. Thompson, MD, MEd, FRCSC (✉)
Department of Orthopedics, Eastern Maine Medical Center, Bangor, ME, USA
e-mail: theskip@gmail.com

S.F. Brockmeier (ed.), *MRI-Arthroscopy Correlations: A Case-Based Atlas of the Knee, Shoulder, Elbow and Hip*, DOI 10.1007/978-1-4939-2645-9_17, © Springer Science+Business Media New York 2015

of inflammation followed by fibrosis. Biopsy samples demonstrate both inflammatory cells and evidence of fibrosis on histologic analysis. Further, there is a dense matrix of type-III collagen containing fibroblasts and myofibroblasts that appears very similar to that seen in Dupuytren's disease. However, frozen shoulder also disproportionally affects individuals who have diabetes mellitus or thyroid disease. As such, there is suggestion that immunologic or microvascular contributions could also play a causative role.

The goals of treatment are to alleviate pain and to restore range of motion. Overwhelmingly, the majority of patients can be treated nonoperatively. Many modes of nonoperative management exist, including physical therapy, corticosteroid injection, nonsteroidal anti-inflammatory medication, and distension arthrography. Typically, approximately 90 % of patients do not require surgical intervention. Those patients who do fail nonoperative management are offered arthroscopic capsular release.

This chapter will use a case-based format to demonstrate many of the correlations between MRI and arthroscopy for frozen shoulder. Given that most patients neither require MRI or arthroscopy, specific illustrative cases will be used to illustrate examples of how the diagnosis could have been made or treatment altered.

Case 1

A 59-year-old right-hand dominant man presented to the orthopedic clinic with the chief complaint of left shoulder pain. The pain began insidiously approximately 3 months ago. He specifically denies a history of trauma. He describes the pain as being dull in nature and moderate in intensity. It is worse when he reaches to the side or with overhead activities. He has found sleeping very difficult secondary to his pain. Treatment to date has included use of an over-the-counter anti-inflammatory medication. He is otherwise well and takes no regular medications.

On physical examination, he appears well and is in no distress. His cervical spine examination is normal. General inspection demonstrates a trace amount of deltoid atrophy. Palpation reveals tenderness over the coracoid process and over the anterior aspect of the deltoid. Range of motion analysis demonstrates 100° of passive and active forward elevation, 5° of passive and active external rotation, and 40° of pure passive abduction. Manual muscle strength testing is limited secondary to pain, but is grossly intact.

Imaging

A standard series of plain radiographs were obtained, including AP shoulder in internal rotation, AP shoulder in external rotation, Grashey (Fig. 17.1), Scapular Y, and axillary (Fig. 17.2). These demonstrated preservation of the glenohumeral joint space without evidence of arthrosis. The axillary radiograph confirmed that the joint was located.

An MRI was also available for review, having been ordered by the patient's primary care physician. MRI of the left shoulder was performed in the axial plane and in the long and short axes of the supraspinatus muscle and tendon with spin density technique without and with fat suppression as well as T1-weighted and T2-weighted techniques. Sequential

Fig. 17.1 True anteroposterior (AP) (Grashey) X-ray demonstrating preservation of the glenohumeral joint space without evidence of arthrosis

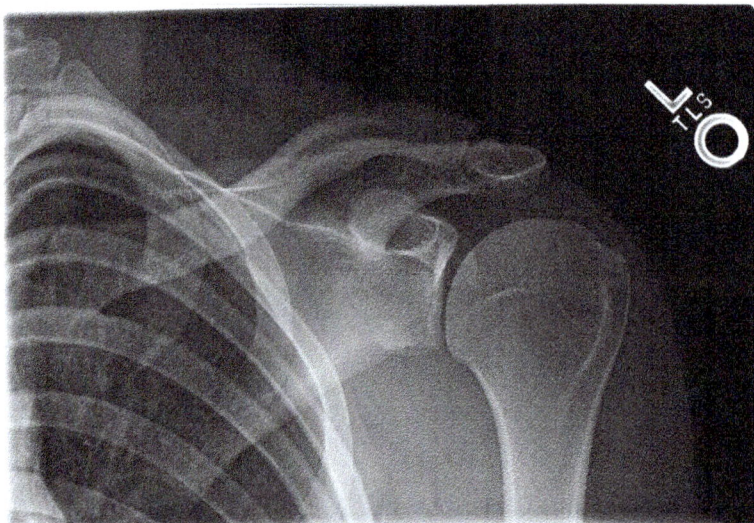

Fig. 17.2 Axillary radiograph demonstrating the glenohumeral joint is located

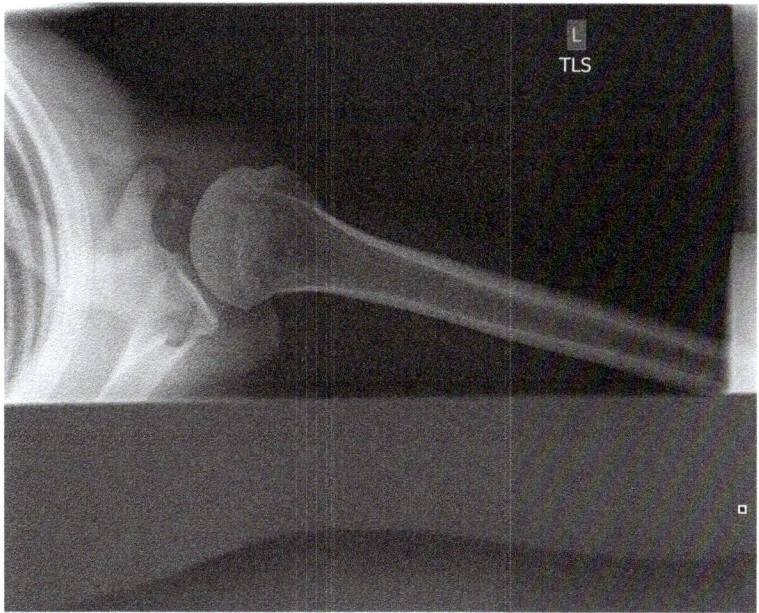

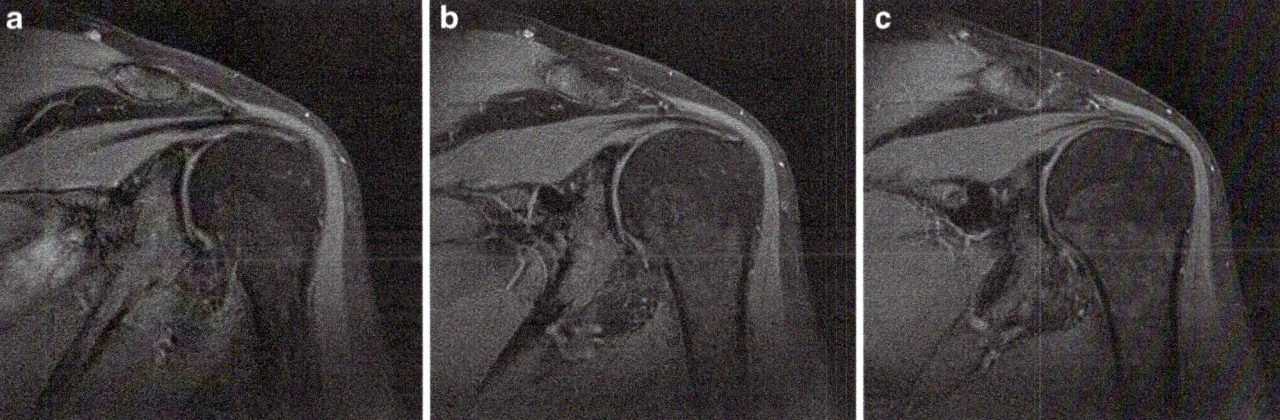

Fig. 17.3 (**a–c**) Sequential T2 fat-saturated BLADE coronal oblique images demonstrating significant thickening and loss of definition of the inferior capsule

T2 fat-saturated BLADE coronal oblique images are shown in Fig. 17.3a–c.

MRI findings are subtle in frozen shoulder. To be certain, frozen shoulder is a clinical diagnosis, and there are no specific direct signs that are pathognomonic for frozen shoulder. Described direct signs suggestive of frozen shoulder include:

- Thickening of the glenohumeral joint capsule along the axillary pouch
- Thickening of the coracohumeral ligament
- Obliteration of the subcoracoid fat triangle
- Rotator interval synovitis

In the present patient, Fig. 17.3a–c demonstrates significant thickening and loss of definition of the inferior capsule.

The supraspinatus tendon has mild thinning and increased signal consistent with tendinosis.

Management

Given the patient's symptoms of insidious onset of pain and a physical examination where active and passive range of motion were equal, a clinical diagnosis of frozen shoulder was established. Radiographs failed to demonstrate arthritic change to account for the loss of motion, and there was no evidence of posterior shoulder dislocation. As such, the diagnosis was confirmed. Findings at MRI failed to demonstrate

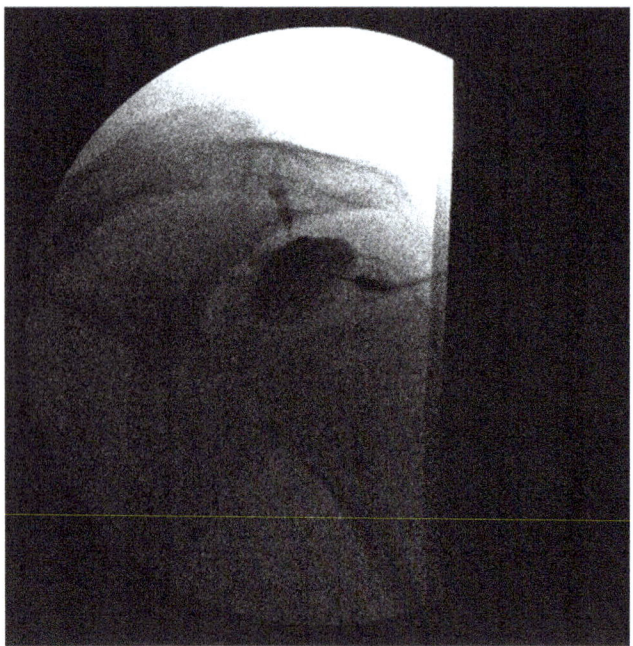

Fig. 17.4 Fluoroscopic image from image-guided glenohumeral corticosteroid injection. There is a complete lack of capsular filling, particularly in the inferior axillary recess

a secondary cause for frozen shoulder, such as concomitant rotator cuff tear. The decision was made to proceed with nonoperative management.

The patient was sent for supervised physical therapy with a structured home exercise program. An evidence-based program of pendulum circumduction, combined with passive shoulder stretching exercises in forward elevation, external rotation, horizontal adduction, and internal rotation, was initiated. An overhead pulley was supplied, and the home exercise program performed five times daily.

The patient returned 6 weeks later with little improvement. Range of motion had increased by only 5–10° in each plane of motion. The pain was slightly diminished. At that juncture, the decision was made to proceed with intraarticular glenohumeral corticosteroid injection. Given the significant capsular contraction and thickening, we prefer not to inject patients in the office. Rather, intra-articular injection achieved via arthrographic confirmation is our recommended technique. As demonstrated in Fig. 17.4, there is a complete lack of capsular filling, particularly in the inferior axillary recess.

The patient returned to the orthopedic clinic approximately 5 weeks later and had near complete resolution of his pain. His forward elevation was now 140°, and passive external rotation was 45°. At 3 months post-injection, he had complete resolution of his symptoms with full range of motion.

Discussion

- Nonspecific findings of MRI for frozen shoulder
- Nonoperative management of frozen shoulder

Case 2

A 54-year-old right-hand dominant woman presented to the orthopedic clinic with a 3-month history of right shoulder pain. Her pain began suddenly after a ground level mechanical fall onto her right side. Since that time, she has had progressively worsening shoulder pain that has particularly bothered her at night. However, over the last 3 weeks, she states that her pain has somewhat abated. She has taken an over-the-counter anti-inflammatory with some relief. She has not done any physical therapy. Her previous medical history is notable for hypothyroidism for which she takes levothyroxine. She has seen a different orthopedic surgeon who referred her after obtaining an MRI.

On physical examination, she is well and in no obvious distress. Examination of the cervical spine does not reveal any pathologic findings. General inspection is normal. Palpation reveals tenderness over the greater tuberosity. Evaluation of range of motion demonstrates 80° of forward elevation both actively and passively, 0° of active and passive external rotation, and 35° of pure passive abduction. Manual muscle strength testing reveals 4+/5 supraspinatus strength and 5/5 internal and external rotation strength. Neer and Hawkins signs are unable to be elicited secondary to lack of motion.

Imaging

A standard radiographic series was obtained, and this demonstrated a preserved glenohumeral joint space without evidence of arthrosis. There was no evidence of posterior glenohumeral dislocation.

Standard MRI sequences without contrast arthrography were obtained. Proton density (PD) (intermediate-weighted) fat-suppressed coronal oblique images are shown in Fig. 17.5a–c. Proton density (intermediate-weighted) sagittal oblique images are shown in Fig. 17.6a–c. Figure 17.5a–c demonstrates the anterior aspect of the supraspinatus tendinous insertion into the greater tuberosity. There is severe tendinopathy at the insertion with suggestion of a full-thickness tear of approximately 13 mm anterior-to-posterior and 10 mm medial-to-lateral. There was no evidence of fatty atrophy of the supraspinatus muscle belly. On sagittal oblique imaging shown in Fig. 17.6a–c, there is partial obliteration of the subcoracoid fat triangle. The subcoracoid fat triangle is a

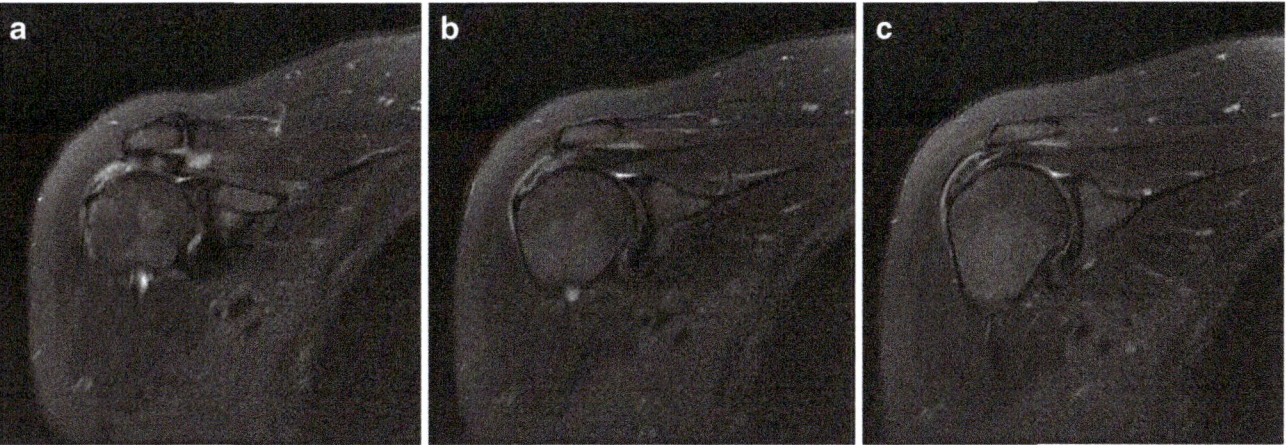

Fig. 17.5 (**a–c**) Sequential proton density (PD) (intermediate-weighted) fat-suppressed coronal oblique images demonstrating severe tendinopathy suggestive of a full-thickness rotator cuff tear

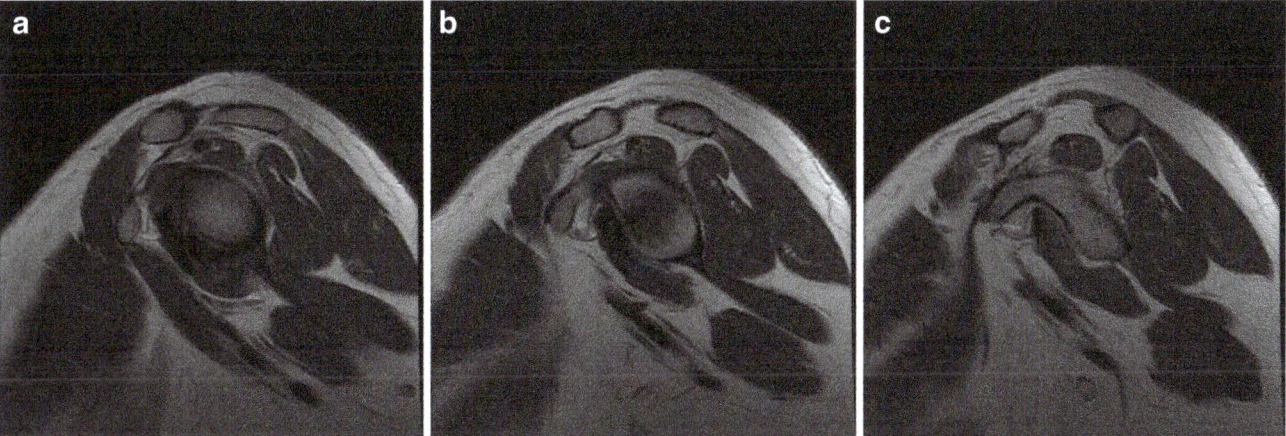

Fig. 17.6 (**a–c**) Sequential proton density (intermediate-weighted) sagittal oblique demonstrating partial obliteration of the subcoracoid fat triangle

radiologic space defined anterosuperiorly by the coracoid process, superiorly by the coracohumeral ligament, and posteroinferiorly by the joint capsule. Partial or complete obliteration of this fat triangle is highly suggestive of adhesive capsulitis.

In this case, the radiologists' report failed to mention any findings suggestive of frozen shoulder. This is not uncommon [7]. It has been suggested that this is due to the relative hypointensity of the tissue on all pulse sequences and is often unrecognized on fat-suppressed imaging. When fat suppression is employed, it can be particularly difficult to detect margins of the axillary recess. This results in decreased sensitivity in detecting one of the most common findings of frozen shoulder on MRI, thickening of the glenohumeral joint capsule along the axillary pouch. The detection of fro-

zen shoulder on MRI can be improved [7] by evaluating three features with different pulse sequences: (1) the rotator interval on sagittal T1 without fat suppression; (2) capsular thickness on coronal imaging with either T1 or T2 non-fat-suppressed sequences; and (3) capsular edema on T2-weighted, fat-suppressed images.

Management

Given the clinical examination, management proceeded with regard to the frozen shoulder. Consideration of management regarding the rotator cuff tear would be delayed until the stiffness had passed. After 6 weeks of guided physical therapy, significant gains in motion were observed, and her pain had decreased. At 12 weeks of follow-up, there was almost complete resolution of stiffness and pain, with normal strength on manual muscle strength testing.

Case 3

A 59-year-old left-hand dominant man presented to the orthopedic clinic with a 5-month history of right shoulder pain and associated shoulder dysfunction. His pain began insidiously without history of trauma. It initially worsened in severity but then decreased, prompting him not to seek earlier medical treatment. However, over the last 6 weeks, he has noticed a decrease in his ability to reach overhead and reach outward with his right arm. His pain is primarily at night, and he rates it as 2/10. He has not done any physical therapy to date and has taken naproxen irregularly for the pain. His previous medical history is notable for type 2 diabetes, diagnosed at the age of 41. He takes metformin and controls his sugar with diet. His last hemoglobin A1C, evaluated 4 weeks ago, was 7.1.

On examination, he has full range of motion of his cervical spine, without evidence of neurologic involvement. Active forward elevation of his left shoulder is to 160°, and active external rotation is to 60°. On the right side, active forward elevation is to 45°, and external rotation is to 0°. Passive range of motion evaluation reveals the same values. He is quite tender over the coracoid. He has 5/5 internal and external rotation strength, while the supraspinatus cannot be adequately isolated secondary to stiffness.

Imaging

Standard radiographs were obtained and failed to demonstrate abnormality. An MRI had been obtained by the patient's referring physician. Standard spin echo sequences, fast low angle shot (FLASH) gradient echo sequences, and short tau inversion recovery (STIR) inversion recovery sequences were obtained. STIR coronal images are shown in Fig. 17.7a–c. Axial plane FLASH sequences are shown in Fig. 17.8a–c. STIR sagittal images are shown in Fig. 17.9a–c. Figure 17.7a–c illustrates substantial thickening of the capsule within the axillary pouch. Figure 17.8a–c demonstrates fairly extensive soft tissue within the rotator interval. Figure 17.9a–c demonstrates almost complete obliteration of the subcoracoid fat triangle. The coracohumeral ligament is also thickened.

Arthroscopy

The patient was sent for physical therapy for 8 weeks. When he returned, he had made virtually no gains in his range of motion and his mild pain persisted. At that juncture, given his history of diabetes, the decision was made to proceed with arthroscopy and capsular release.

Surgery was performed under the control of general anesthesia and a supplementary interscalene block. Prior to positioning, an examination under anesthesia was performed so as to confirm the diagnosis of adhesive capsulitis. Next, using the T-MAX shoulder positioner (Smith and Nephew, Andover, MA), the patient was placed in the beach-chair position with the acromion parallel to the floor. Although some authors advocate for performing a manipulation under anesthesia prior to arthroscopy, we do not believe this is beneficial, as it creates intra-articular bleeding and significantly impairs visualization during surgery. Further, it carries an unnecessarily high risk for fracture. Bony landmarks were carefully marked prior to initiation of surgery.

A standard posterior viewing portal was employed. Given the significant capsular contracture and capsular thickening,

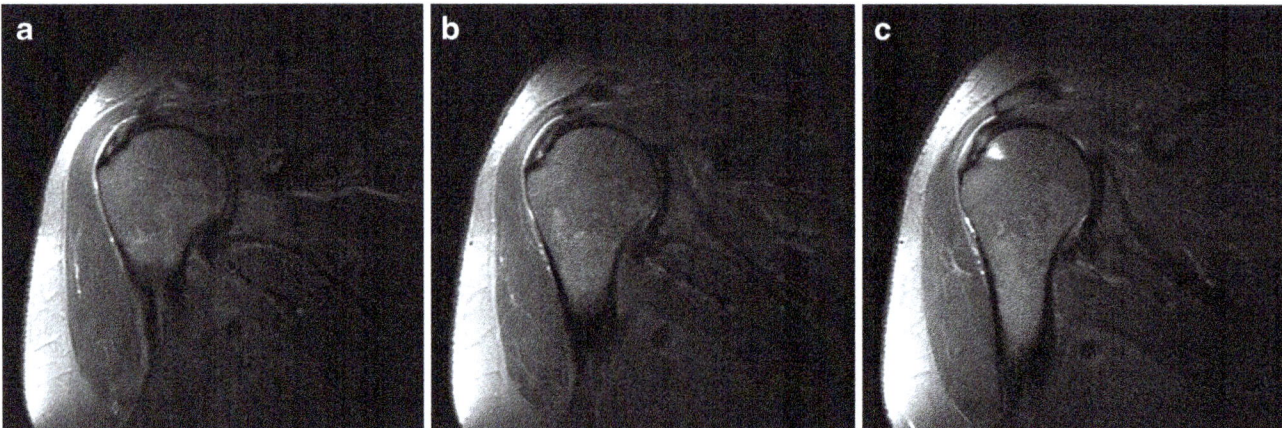

Fig. 17.7 (**a–c**) Sequential STIR coronal images demonstrating substantial thickening of the capsule within the axillary pouch

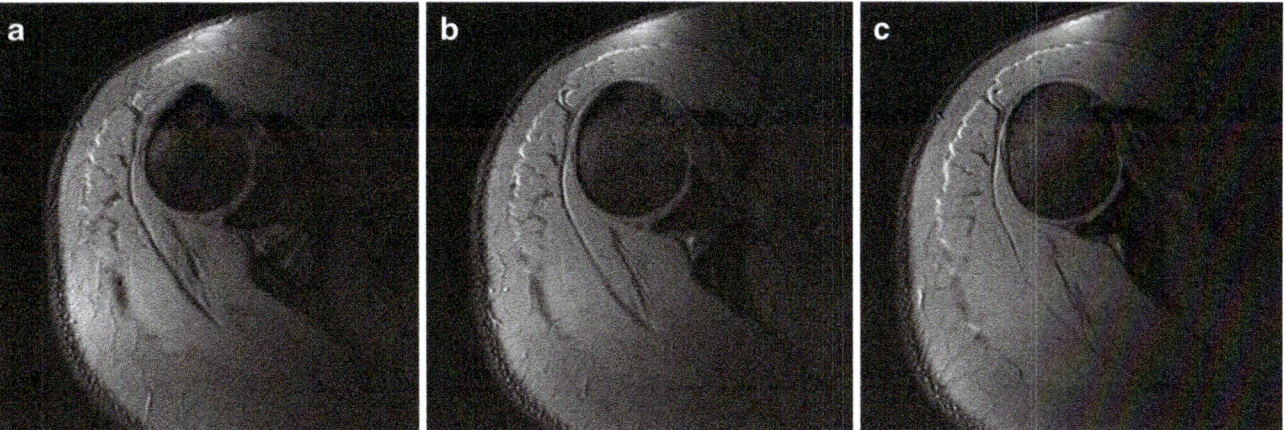

Fig. 17.8 (**a–c**) Sequential axial FLASH images demonstrating fairly extensive soft tissue within the rotator interval

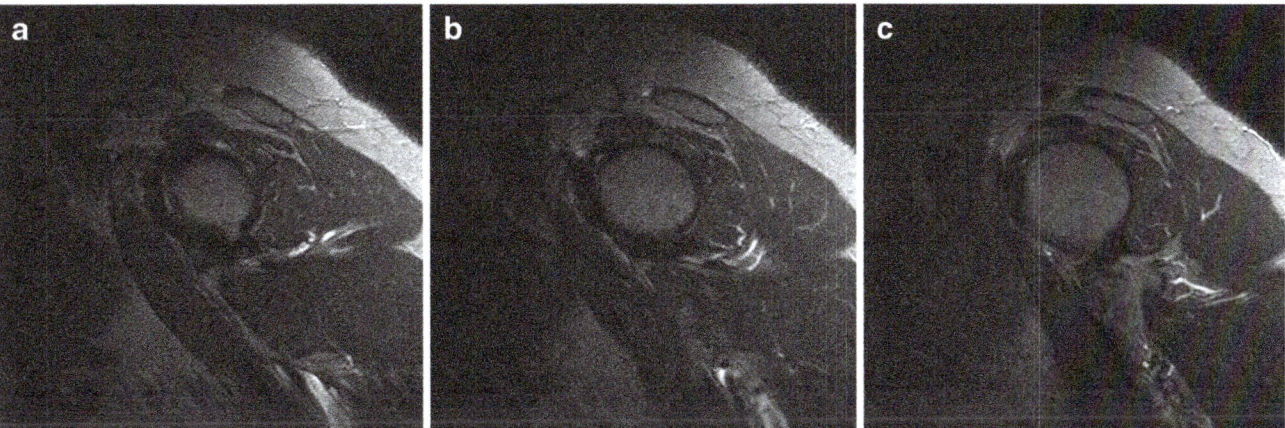

Fig. 17.9 (**a–c**) Sequential STIR sagittal images demonstrating near complete obliteration of the subcoracoid fat triangle

it can be extremely difficult to enter the joint with the arthroscope in patients with frozen shoulder. To reduce the risk of iatrogenic damage, the proper trajectory is gleaned from insertion of a spinal needle into the glenohumeral joint. Using approximately 20 ml of saline, the joint was distended and intra-articular placement was confirmed by removing the syringe and observing return of saline. The spinal needle is left in place as a guide for the obturator of the arthroscopic sheath.

Once the arthroscope was introduced into the joint, a spinal needle was inserted into the joint through the rotator interval, and the obturator is removed (Fig. 17.10). This permits for immediate outflow and visualization. Next, an anterior–superior portal is created in the rotator interval using an outside-in technique. A standard diagnostic arthroscopy was undertaken. The rotator interval was extremely thickened (Fig. 17.10). The biceps tendon was intact without evidence of erythema, as is typical in adhesive capsulitis (Fig. 17.11). The rotator cuff was intact (Fig. 17.12). The space of the

inferior axillary recess was almost completely obliterated (Fig. 17.13).

A standard 90° radiofrequency (RF) ablation wand was inserted through the anterior interval portal. The very thick tissue in the rotator interval was then carefully ablated (Fig. 17.14) to reveal the tip of the coracoid and coracoacromial ligament. The middle glenohumeral ligament was released simultaneously. Careful attention was given to the subscapularis to ensure it was preserved.

Attention was next turned to antero-inferior capsular release. A threaded cannula was inserted through the anterior interval portal. Rather than employing an arthroscopic punch or continue using a standard 90° RF wand that would require switching portals, we prefer to use a flexible RF wand that is typically used in hip arthroscopy [8]. The flexible RF ablator probe (EFLEX Ablator ElectroThermal Probe, Smith and Nephew, Andover, MA) was inserted through the anterior interval portal, and the remainder of the anterior–inferior capsular release was performed with the device fully extended (Fig. 17.15).

Fig. 17.10 Arthroscopic image demonstrating a spinal needle in the very thickened rotator interval

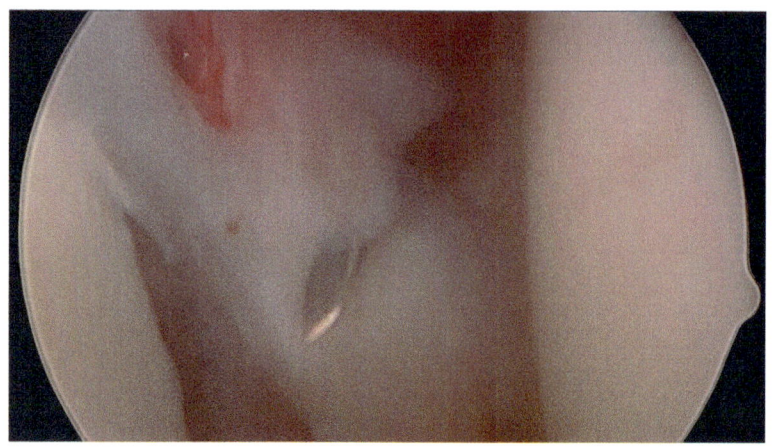

Fig. 17.11 Arthroscopic image demonstrating a normal biceps tendon

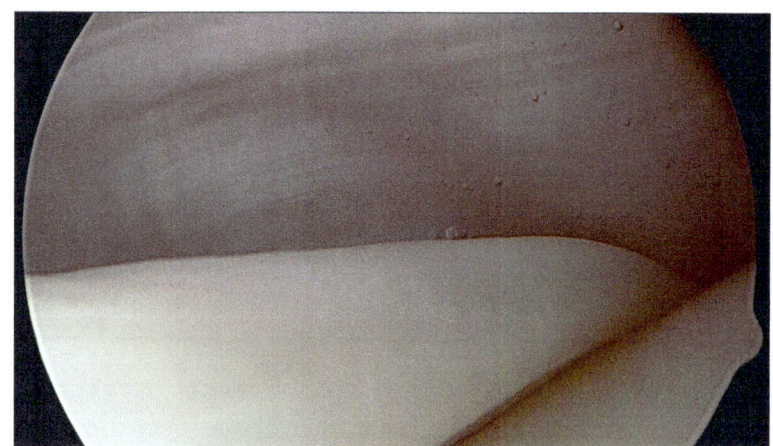

Fig. 17.12 Arthroscopic image demonstrating an intact rotator cuff

Fig. 17.13 Arthroscopic image demonstrating near complete obliteration of the inferior axillary recess

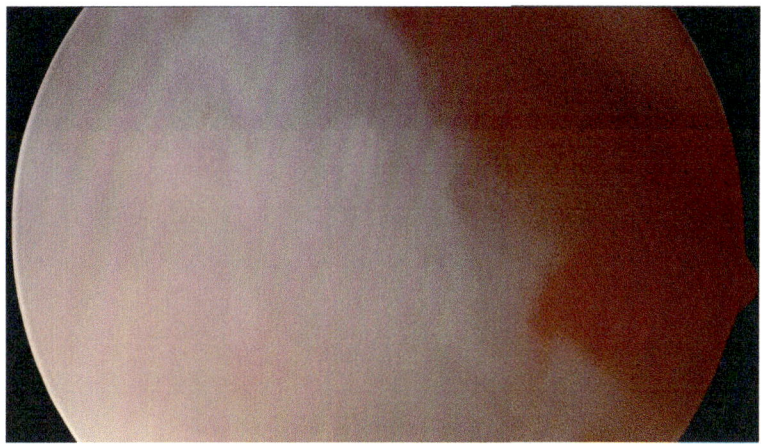

Fig. 17.14 Arthroscopic image demonstrating the radiofrequency ablation wand through the anterior interval portal and a thickened rotator interval being ablated

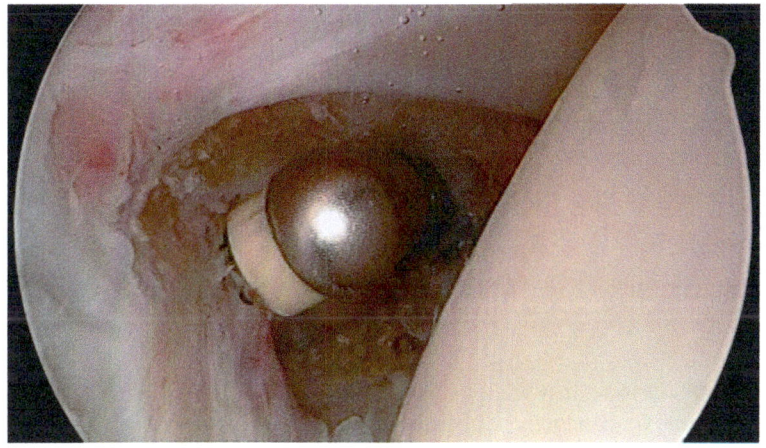

Fig. 17.15 Arthroscopic image demonstrating the flexible radiofrequency ablator probe through the anterior interval portal, ablating the anterior–inferior capsule

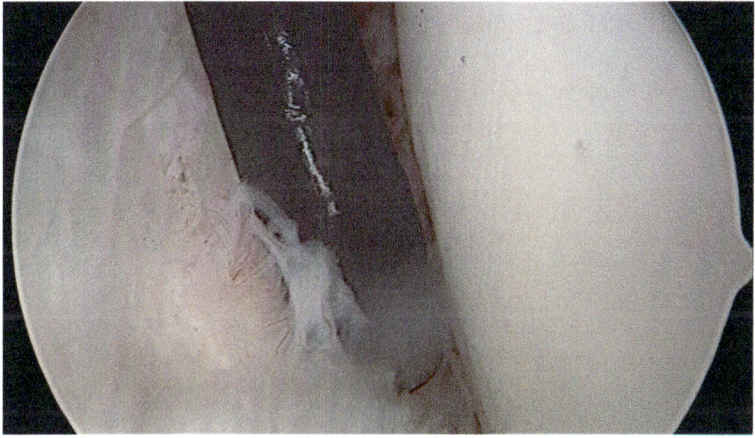

Fig. 17.16 Arthroscopic image demonstrating the flexible radiofrequency ablator probe through the anterior interval portal, ablating the inferior capsule

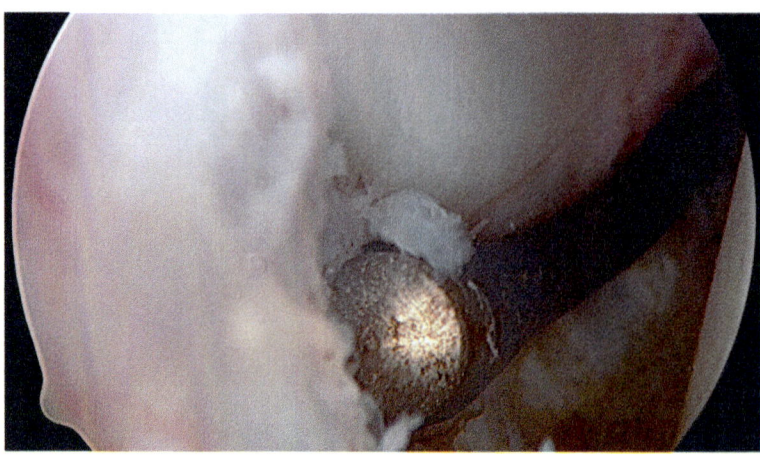

Once the 4:30 o'clock position of the glenoid face was reached, the flexible RF ablator probe was progressively flexed to match the curvature of the glenoid and adjacent labrum (Fig. 17.16). This allowed the capsule to be released while maximizing the distance away from the axillary nerve. Lastly, the need for posterior release was assessed. Internal rotation was assessed and found to be acceptable. As such, posterior release was not performed. The procedure was completed by performing subacromial bursectomy.

Discussion

- Indications for surgical release of frozen shoulder, particularly in diabetics
- Operative management of frozen shoulder

Conclusion

The frozen shoulder is a commonly encountered condition that is often mistaken for other, potentially concomitant, pathologies. The diagnosis can be made clinically with a loss of external rotation that is present both actively and passively. Radiographs are essential to rule out the other two major causes of rotation loss: glenohumeral osteoarthritis and locked posterior dislocation. Magnetic resonance imaging (MRI) is unnecessary for the diagnosis. However, many patients present to the orthopedic clinic with an MRI already having been obtained. Regrettably, there are few specific findings on MRI. The four most commonly observed direct signs that suggest the diagnosis of frozen shoulder on MRI include thickening of the glenohumeral joint capsule in the axillary pouch, thickening of the coracohumeral ligament, obliteration of the subcoracoid fat triangle, and synovitis of the rotator interval. Management is overwhelmingly nonoperative, with 90 % of patients reporting resolution of symptoms. In those patients who fail to improve, arthroscopic capsular release may be indicated.

References

1. Codman EA. The shoulder; rupture of the supraspinatus tendon and other lesions in or about the subacromial bursa. Boston, MA: T. Todd; 1934.
2. Neviaser JS. Adhesive capsulitis of the shoulder. A study of the pathological findings in periarthritis of the shoulder. J Bone Joint Surg. 1945;27(2):211.
3. van der Windt DA, Koes BW, de Jong BA, Bouter LM. Shoulder disorders in general practice: incidence, patient characteristics, and management. Ann Rheum Dis. 1995;54(12):959.
4. Miller MD, Wirth MA, Rockwood Jr CA. Thawing the frozen shoulder: the "patient" patient. Orthopedics. 1996;19(10):849.
5. Shaffer B, Tibone JE, Kerlan RK. Frozen shoulder. A long-term follow-up. J Bone Joint Surg Am. 1992;74(5):738.
6. Robinson CM, Seah KT, Chee YH, Hindle P, Murray IR. Frozen shoulder. J Bone Joint Surg Br. 2012;94(1):1.
7. Polster JM, Schickendantz MS. Shoulder MRI: what do we miss? AJR Am J Roentgenol. 2010;195(3):577.
8. Thompson SR, Lebel ME. Use of a hip arthroscopy flexible radiofrequency device for capsular release in frozen shoulder. Arthrosc Tech. 2012;1(1):e75.

Disorders of the AC Joint and Suprascapular Nerve Compression Syndrome

18

Elaine J. Ahillen, Jonathan P. Braman and Marc Tompkins

Introduction

The acromioclavicular (AC) joint is a diarthrodial joint comprised of the distal clavicle, the medial facet of the acromion, the joint capsule, and the acromioclavicular ligament. A fibrocartilaginous disk is interposed in the joint and helps with force distribution [1]. The coracoclavicular ligaments also play a role in maintaining the position of the distal clavicle relative to the acromion.

A common AC joint pathology is degenerative osteoarthritis. This is not acutely traumatic but can be the chronic sequela of trauma to the AC joint, or it may just develop over time due to overuse or repetitive stress to the joint. It is not uncommon in weight lifters or other individuals commonly doing heavy lifting, especially overhead lifting. Like arthritis in other joints, symptoms do not inherently correlate with severity of arthritis on imaging. On X-ray, the AC joint space is narrowed or obliterated, with bone spurs, sclerosis, subchondral cysts, and other common radiographic signs of osteoarthritis. An MRI is not routinely used for diagnosis, but in cases where one is obtained, increased severity of degenerative joint changes is noted in symptomatic patients when compared with MRI scans of asymptomatic individuals. Additionally, reactive bone edema is more likely to indicate symptomatic pathology than degenerative changes [2].

Traumatic AC joint injury usually occurs from a direct force onto the lateral shoulder—either a fall onto the point of the shoulder or a direct blow—but may also result from a fall onto the elbow [3]. When the force is from a direct lateral impact, the acromion is forced into distal clavicle, impacting at the articular surfaces (type 1 injury). When the injuring force is delivered from a superior-lateral direction, the scapula is externally rotated. This rotation first disrupts the acromioclavicular ligaments (type 2 injury) and, as the force continues, the coracoclavicular ligaments are disrupted (type 3 injury) [4]. As the capsule-ligamentous joint complex is injured, the acromion also moves inferiorly due to the weight of the extremity, while the clavicle is pulled superiorly by the trapezius [5].

Traumatic injuries to the AC joint have been classified based on which anatomic structures are injured and the direction that the distal clavicle dislocates relative to the acromion. Type 1–3 AC sprains were described by Allman in 1967, based on increasing extent of ligamentous injury [3]. Type 1 sprains involve only a portion of the fibers of the acromioclavicular ligament and joint capsule, with no laxity of the AC joint. The relative positions of the acromion and clavicle are maintained, and plain X-rays do not show any change in the acute period. Type 2 sprains are injuries where the capsule and acromioclavicular ligaments are torn, but the coracoclavicular ligaments are intact. On plain X-rays, the distal clavicle is superior to the acromion, but not by more than the width of the clavicle, and this relationship is maintained even when stressed by downward force on the arm. Type 3 sprains involve disruption of the joint capsule, the acromioclavicular ligament, and the coracoclavicular ligaments. Plain X-rays will show the acromion translated inferior to the distal clavicle, and there is also increased distance between the coracoid and clavicle [3]. Physical examination will demonstrate focal tenderness over the AC joint, with visibly greater degrees of deformity of the AC joint depending on grade of injury.

Later on, Rockwood added types 4–6 to this classification. In each of these grades, the AC and CC ligaments are torn, and the grade is determined by the location of the lateral end of the clavicle relative to its normal relationship with the acromion. In a type 4 injury, the acromion has displaced anteriorly, which makes it appear that the distal clavicle has displaced posteriorly. This is radiographically

E.J. Ahillen, MD (✉)
Department of Orthopedic Surgery, TRIA Orthopedic Center, Bloomington, MN, USA
e-mail: Elaine.ahillen@tria.com

J.P. Braman, MD • M. Tompkins, MD
Department of Orthopedic Surgery, University of Minnesota Medical School, Minneapolis, MN, USA
e-mail: Brama011@umn.edu; tompkinsm@hotmail.com

best seen on an axillary X-ray but can also be identified on three-dimensional imaging, such as a CT or MRI. In a type 5 injury, the acromion has displaced inferiorly, with rupture of the deltotrapezial fascia. Type 6 injuries are those where the distal clavicle becomes displaced inferior to or under the coracoid. This is a rare injury, with three cases described in 1987 by Gerber and Rockwood [6].

Injuries to AC joint are more common in the first three decades of life, with lower-grade injuries more common than complete separations. Type 1 and 2 injuries are frequently treated with sling immobilization, early motion, and physical therapy. Optimal treatment of type 3 injuries is debated, and treatment should be individualized as some patients who are overhead athletes or otherwise place high demands on their shoulders may benefit from consideration of operative reduction and coracoclavicular ligament reconstruction. For those patients with type 4–6 injuries, operative management is indicated with reduction, coracoclavicular ligament reconstruction, and deltotrapezial fascial repair [7].

In addition to ligamentous injury, discussions of traumatic injury in the region of the AC joint also frequently include mention of distal clavicle fractures. These fractures are described based on their location relative to the CC ligaments and based on the integrity or injury of these ligaments. Some of these injuries are most appropriately treated with coracoclavicular ligament reconstruction, similar to high-grade AC joint sprains.

The suprascapular nerve bears mentioning here both because it innervates the AC joint and similar arthroscopic techniques that can be used to address AC joint pathology may also be employed to address suprascapular nerve compression. The suprascapular nerve is a peripheral nerve that arises from the superior trunk of the brachial plexus and provides sensory innervations about the shoulder and motor innervation to supraspinatus and then the infraspinatus muscles. Prior to innervating either muscle, this nerve passes deep to the trapezius and omohyoid muscle and then travels with the suprascapular artery to enter the suprascapular notch, where the artery travels superficial and the nerve travels deep to the transverse scapular ligament [8, 9]. Within 1 cm of passing under this ligament, the nerve gives off two branches that innervate the supraspinatus muscle. The main nerve then continues inferiorly through the spinoglenoid notch before innervating the infraspinatus muscle. Throughout its course, the nerve also gives off sensory branches to the coracoclavicular and coracohumeral ligaments, the AC joint, the subacromial bursa, and the posterior glenohumeral joint capsule [8]. There is a variable sensory role in the overlying skin and soft tissues of the shoulder [10].

Suprascapular nerve dysfunction has an unclear prevalence. It has been estimated to account for approximately 1–4.3 % of shoulder complaints, although the true prevalence may be higher [8, 10]. It is more common in patients less than 35 years old, and 3–4 times more common in males [9]. The most common site of compression of this nerve is at the suprascapular notch [11]. The nerve makes a sharp turn at the suprascapular notch and may be compressed against the undersurface of the bony notch or the ligament at this point, which is referred to as the sling effect and was described in 1979 by Rangrery et al. [11] Nerve irritation in this manner may be exaggerated by shoulder depression, retraction, or hyperabduction, and this mechanism of nerve compression is frequently associated with athletic or overuse injury [8]. It has also been suggested that compression of the nerve may be associated with calcification of the transverse scapular ligament, as well as ligament variants that are bifid, trifid, or hypertrophied [8]. Traction injury on the suprascapular nerve can be seen at the suprascapular notch, as well, in patients with a massive rotator cuff tear. It is unclear if a nerve decompression should accompany rotator cuff repair in these patients or if rotator cuff repair alone will relieve the compression [12].

Patients with suprascapular nerve pathology will frequently complain of vague aching shoulder pain and weakness. On exam, they may have gross atrophy of the supraspinatus and/or the infraspinatus muscles [10]. Nonoperative treatment of suprascapular nerve compression involves 4–6 weeks of oral anti-inflammatories, avoidance of exacerbating overhead activities, and physical therapy. The therapy is focused on strengthening of the rotator cuff and scapular stabilizers [8]. Corticosteroid injections may also be employed [9]. Operative treatment is indicated in those patients that have electrodiagnostically proven nerve compression or those patients who fail 3–6 the nonoperative treatment stated above [9]. Electrodiagnostic findings in abnormal studies are prolonged motor latency, denervation potentials, and delayed conduction time [10]. A 2011 study by Boykin et al. evaluated 40 patients with an electrodiagnostic study positive for suprascapular nerve pathology and found that 88 % had abnormal motor unit action potentials and 33 % had EMG abnormalities [10]. Operative treatment is decompression of the suprascapular nerve at the suprascapular notch by release of the transverse scapular ligament.

Case 1: AC Joint Arthritis

History/Exam

A 42-year-old man presented to the orthopedic clinic reporting 18 months of right shoulder pain. He first noticed the pain after doing push-ups and had off and on pain with increasing frequency since, mostly after strenuous activity (re-aggravated cleaning up after a flood) or attempted throwing. He had previously been seen at an orthopedic clinic closer to his home, where he had undergone multiple injections. A subacromial injection did not seem to help, but two separate injections into the AC joint both relieved his symptoms almost completely for 1 week's duration.

On physical examination, the patient had full and painless shoulder range of motion, symmetric to his contralateral shoulder. He had a positive O'Brien's active compression test, with pain localized to his AC joint. He had focal tenderness to palpation over his AC joint. His Speed's and Yergason's tests were negative. He did not have any pain with palpation of his bicipital groove. He was neurovascularly intact in this extremity and without symptoms in his contralateral shoulder.

Imaging

In this case, the patient had a recent prior MRI that he brought with him on a disk to clinic, and plain radiography was obtained that day. These are presented below in Figs. 18.1a, b and 18.2a–d.

The findings of AC joint arthritis on plain radiographs and MRI were consistent with the patient's clinical presentation, with symptoms suggesting AC joint pathology and pain relived with AC joint injection. No other structures had pathology identified on the MRI. Specifically, the rotator cuff, biceps tendon, labrum, and articular cartilage of the glenohumeral joint were all intact. At this point, conservative management had not adequately controlled his symptoms, and the risks and benefits of operative intervention were discussed with the patient. He elected to proceed with arthroscopic distal clavicle excision.

Arthroscopy

Anesthesia was interscalene block plus local infiltration.

The patient was placed into the beach chair position. Arthroscopy was limited to only the AC joint, as no other shoulder pathology was suspected.

The plane of the AC joint was identified using a 1.5 inch 22-guage needle. A posterior viewing portal was then made directly posterior to the AC joint and a size 2.7 mm arthroscope was inserted into the AC joint. An anterior portal was then made and a 4.0 mm shaver was introduced into the AC joint.

There was a significant amount of degenerated intraarticular meniscus, which was debrided with a shaver and an ablator. A burr was then used to remove bone from the lateral end of the clavicle until there was a 1 cm gap between the remaining clavicle and the acromion. In this case, approximately 8 mm of bone from the distal clavicle was resected to achieve a 1 cm gap between the remaining bone ends.

Arthroscopic findings correlated well with the findings on X-ray and MRI: AC joint arthritis.

Discussion

Radiographic changes of AC joint arthritis are a common finding and frequently deemed incidental when the patient does not have clinical evidence of symptoms attributable to the AC joint. When AC joint arthritis is symptomatic, this is frequently confirmed with plain radiographs, and an MRI may not be needed.

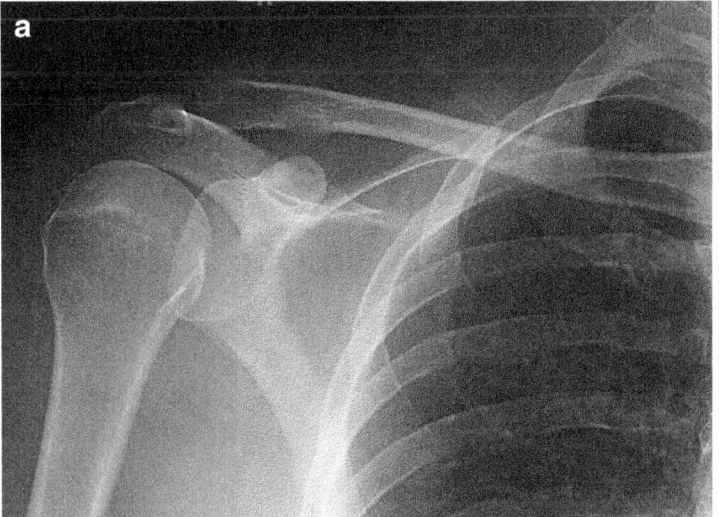 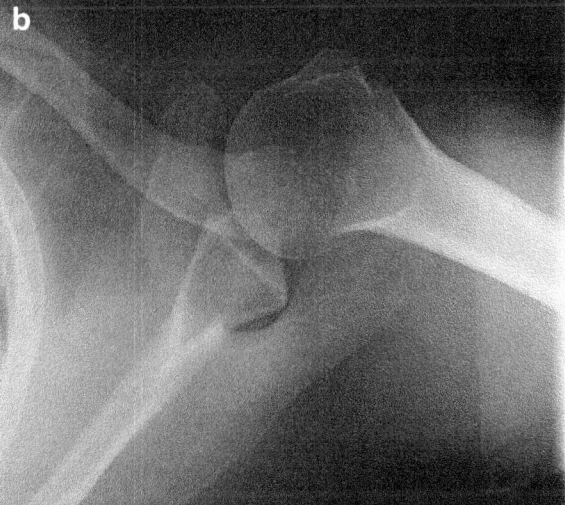

Fig. 18.1 (**a, b**) PA and axillary plain radiographs demonstrate arthritis of the acromioclavicular joint with narrowing of the joint space, osteophyte formation on both the acromion and distal clavicle, sclerosis and subchondral cystic change

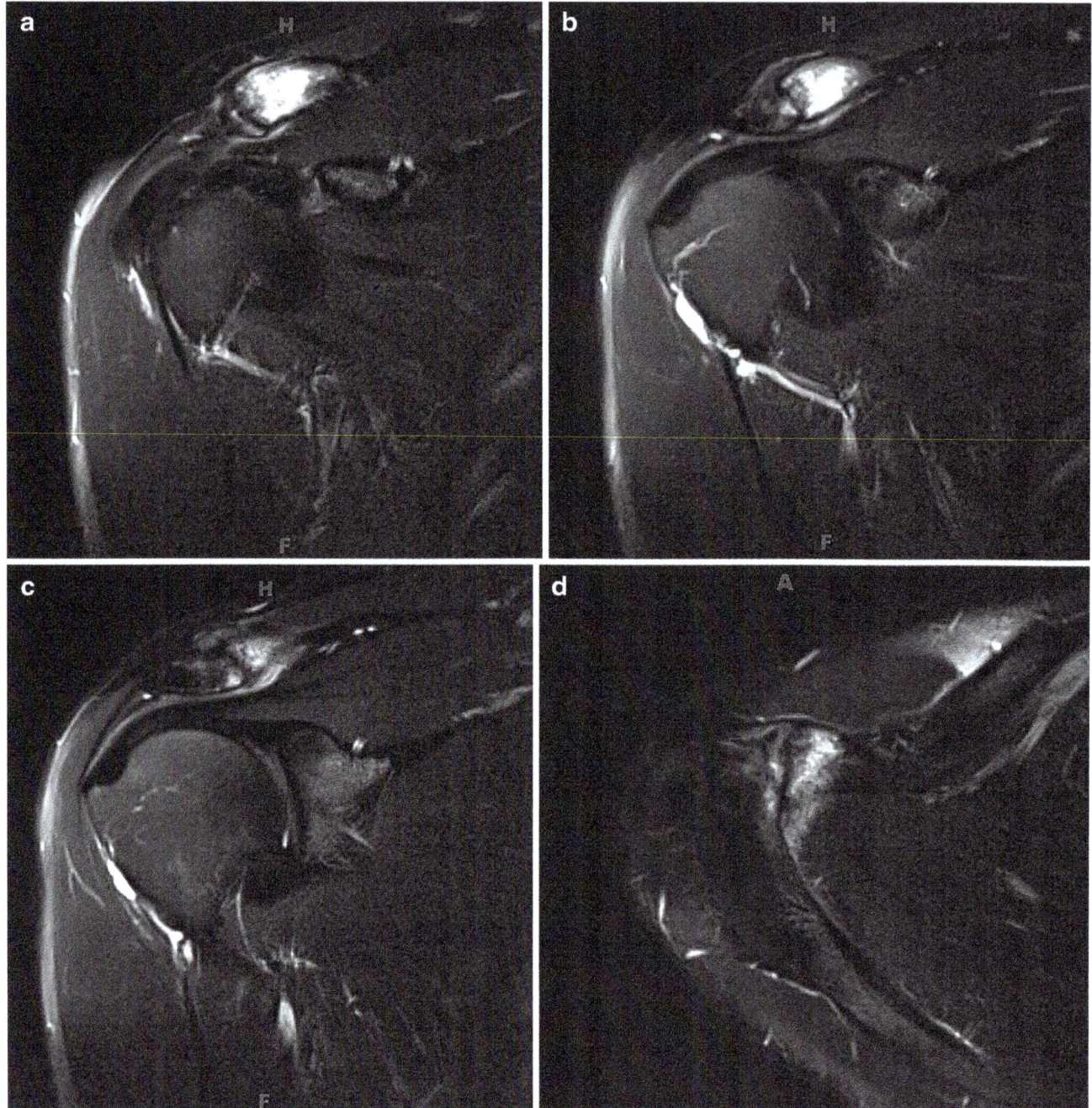

Fig. 18.2 **a–c** show a series of coronal MRI images, and **d** shows an axillary MRI image. These T2 MRI slices show edema in the distal clavicle and acromion as well as confirm degenerative changes seen on plain radiographs

AC joint arthritis may be addressed with arthroscopic distal clavicle excision. This may be done through an isolated arthroscopy of the AC joint, as in the case above, or as a component of a subacromial arthroscopy. postoperative PA and axillary plain radiographs are shown in Fig. 18.3a, b, and the arthroscopy images are shown in Fig. 18.4a–e.

Case 2: AC Joint Separation

History/Exam

A 25-year-old man presented to the orthopedic clinic 2 months after a fall directly onto his right shoulder. He had gone to an urgent care on the day of his injury and was

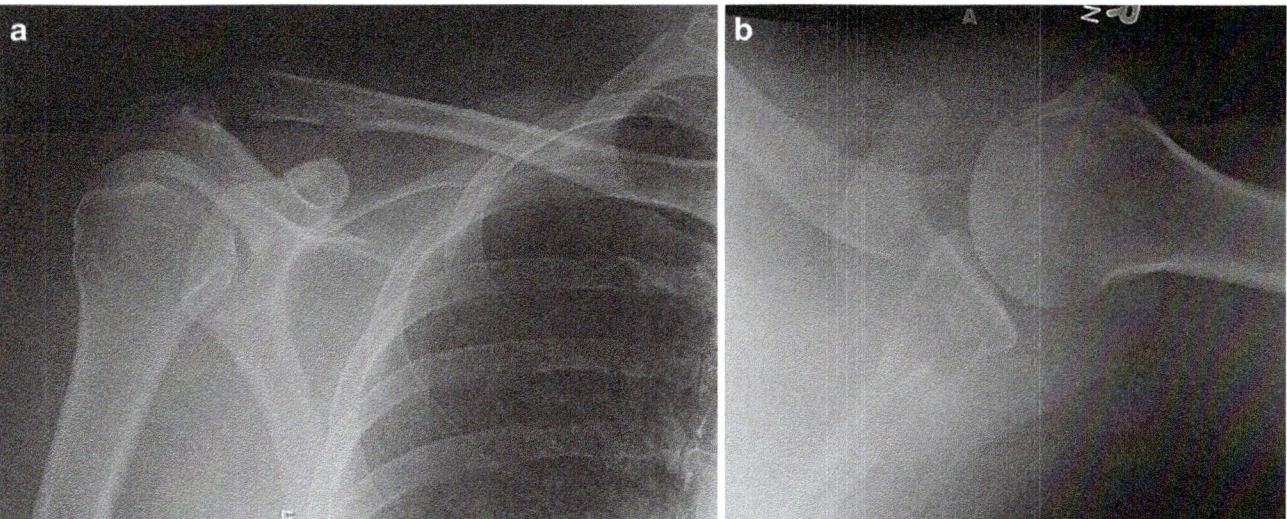

Fig. 18.3 (**a, b**) Postoperative PA and axillary radiographs demonstrate increased distance between the acromion and distal clavicle

diagnosed with a type III AC separation. Subsequently, he wore a sling intermittently and was seen by an orthopedist and a physical therapist. Two months later, he presented to our clinic with continued pain localized to his right AC joint. Symptoms were exacerbated by certain arm motions, such as elevating his arm above his head, lifting items with this arm, and rolling onto this shoulder while sleeping.

On physical examination, the patient had a prominence over the AC joint consistent with type V AC separation. Additionally, he was tender to palpation over the AC joint. His shoulder range of motion was full and equal to the contralateral side. He was neurovascularly intact in the extremity and without symptoms in his contralateral shoulder. The remainder of his exam was unremarkable.

Imaging

Three views of the right shoulder were taken at the urgent care facility including a PA, a scapular Y, and an axillary X-ray (Fig. 18.5a–c). They demonstrate inferior displacement of the acromion relative to the distal clavicle; the coracoclavicular distance has increased greater than 100 %. The glenohumeral joint is located. The radiographic impression is a type V AC separation.

The findings of AC joint separation on plain radiographs were consistent with the patient's clinical presentation. At this point, continued conservative management was recommended. It was discussed with the patient that many people with this injury do not require surgery. We discussed the high success rate of nonoperative treatment and that delayed reconstruction was no less successful than acute repair.

One month later, he returned to the clinic, noting no improvement in his symptoms. At this time, the risks and benefits of operative intervention were discussed with the patient. He elected to proceed with arthroscopically assisted coracoclavicular ligament reconstruction.

Arthroscopy

Anesthesia was an interscalene nerve block. The patient was placed into a well-padded beach chair position. Standard anterior and posterior arthroscopy portals were made, and a diagnostic arthroscopy of the glenohumeral joint was completed.

The arthroscope was then moved into the subacromial space and a lateral portal was created. The subacromial space was debrided using a radiofrequency device exposing the coracoacromial ligament. An anterolateral portal was then created and the arthroscope moved into the lateral portal. The radiofrequency device was then used through the anterolateral portal to clear bursal tissue from around the coracoid exposing the superior, lateral, and inferior portions of the coracoid. Care was taken to maintain the working surface of the device against the coracoid and to avoid proceeding medial or distal on the coracoid, in order to avoid neurovascular injury.

A 3 cm incision was made over the distal clavicle 2–3 cm medial to the distal end of the clavicle. A suture shuttling device was introduced anterior to the clavicle through the clavicular incision. It was visualized through the arthroscope on the medial side of the coracoid and passed inferior to the coracoid. The loop was retrieved with a looped suture grasper, and No. 5 nonabsorbable suture was shuttled around

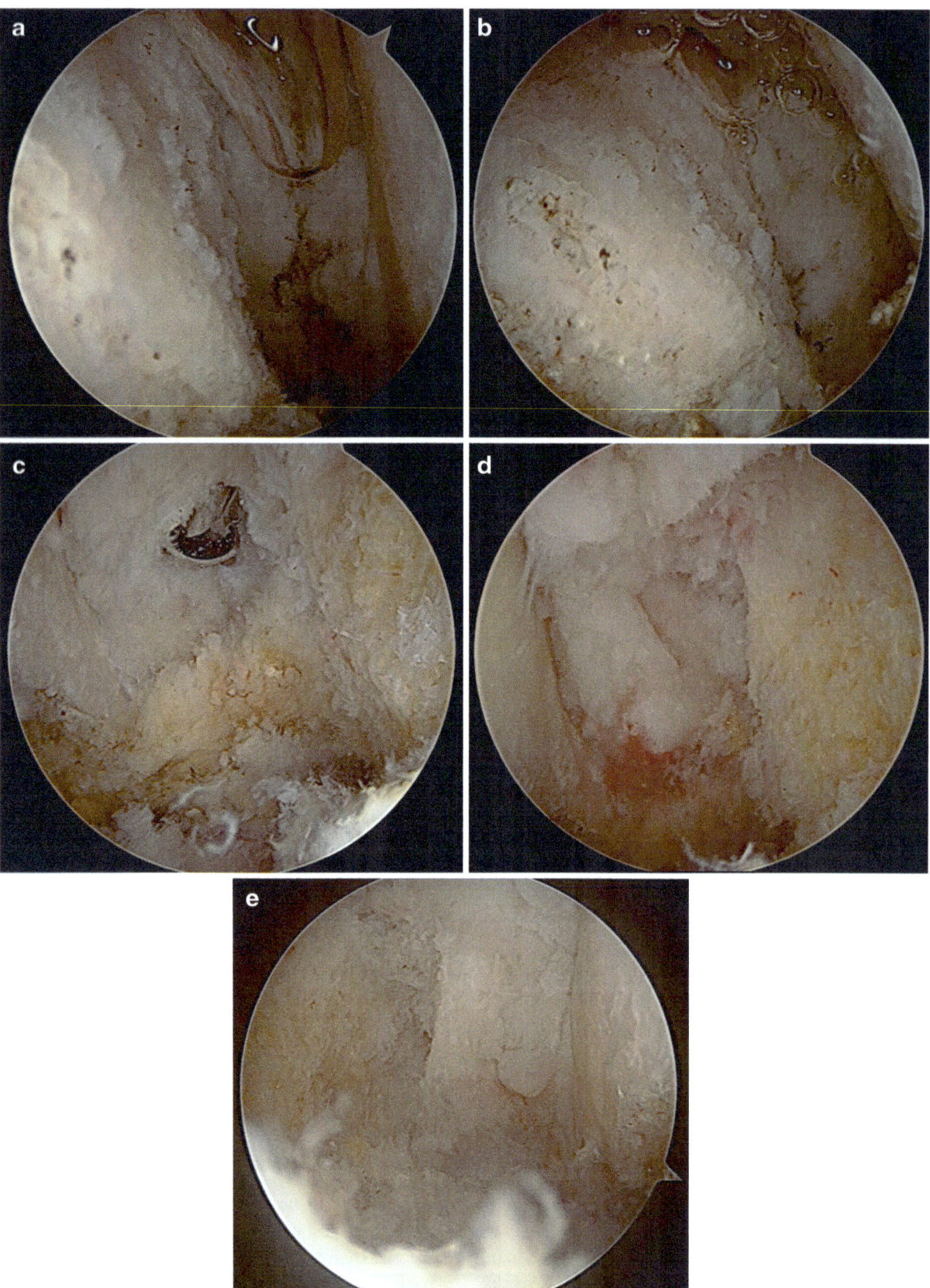

Fig. 18.4 (**a–e**) Images from the arthroscopy. **a** and **b** show the arthritic acromioclavicular joint from the posterior portal prior to any resection. **c** is viewed from the anterior portal, and a shaver is seen entering the AC joint from the posterior portal. **d** and **e** show the space created in the AC joint after the distal clavicle is resected; **d** is viewed from the anterior portal and **e** from the posterior portal

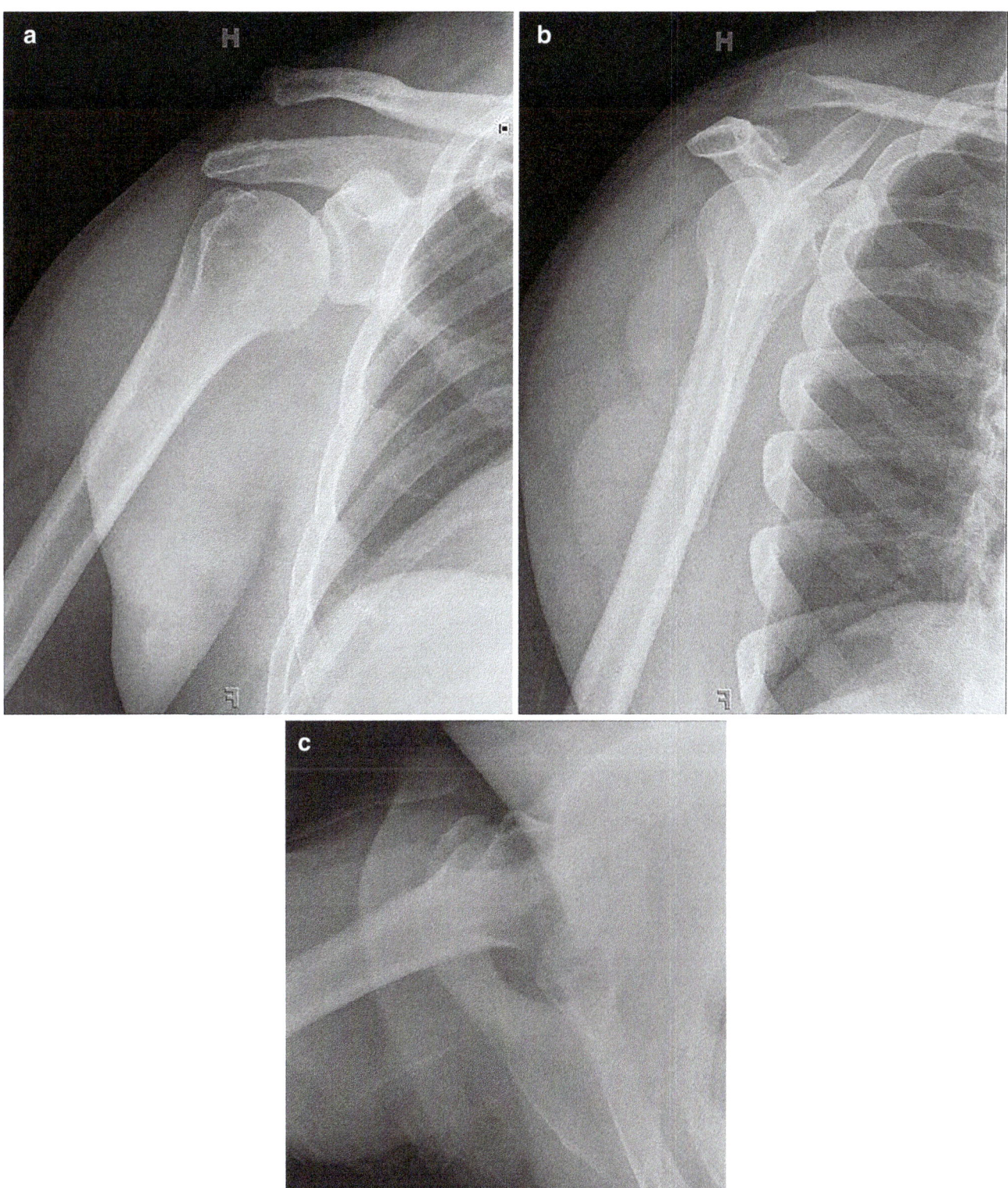

Fig. 18.5 **a–c** demonstrate PA, scapular Y, and axillary plain radiographs of a right shoulder with a type V AC separation

the coracoid. On the clavicle, a 6 mm hole was drilled approximately 1.5 cm medial to the AC joint, followed by a second hole drilled 2 cm medial to the first. The suture shuttling device was passed through each clavicular tunnel

and used to shuttle one end of the No. 5 nonabsorbable suture through each clavicular tunnel.

One end of the No. 5 nonabsorbable suture was tied to the suture placed through a semitendinosus allograft as well as

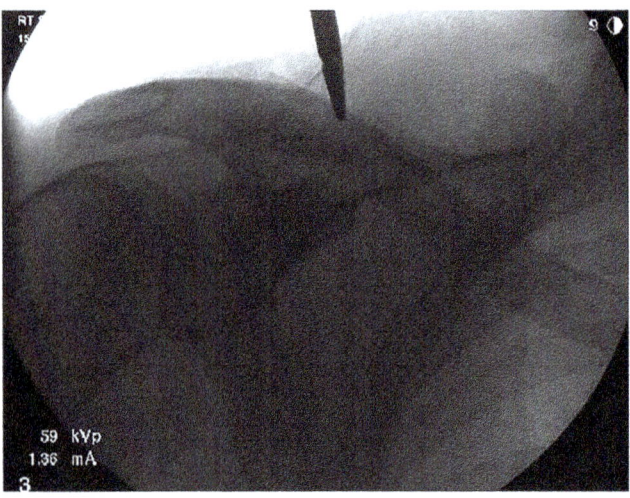

Fig. 18.6 Intraoperative PA fluoroscopy showing provisional reduction of an AC joint separation. The clamp in this image is maintaining this reduction by holding appropriate tension on the two ends of the cores suture placed around the coracoid and through clavicular tunnels

to one end of a core suture with a braided exterior. Both the core suture and the suture attached to the graft were then passed through one tunnel, around the coracoid, and through the second tunnel. Tension on the suture attached to the graft then allowed the graft to be advanced around the coracoid and into position. The AC joint was manually reduced, and the core suture was clamped over the bony bridge between the clavicle tunnels for provisional fixation. Fluoroscopy was used to verify that acceptable reduction was obtained and then maintained with longitudinal traction on the arm and the core suture was tied. This intraoperative image is seen in Fig. 18.6. Tension was then applied to both limbs of the graft and interference screws were advanced, while manual reduction was again used to keep the AC joint reduced during final fixation. Repeat fluoroscopic exam was similar to the previous images, and the wounds were closed.

Operative findings correlated well with the findings on X-ray: type V AC joint separation.

Figure 18.7a–d shows arthroscopic images taken in a cadaver to allow for more extensive removal of bursal tissue in order to enhance visualization of the anatomic structures.

Discussion

AC separation is a diagnosis frequently made clinically and confirmed by plain radiograph, with no MRI obtained. In those cases of type III AC separation or higher where an MRI is obtained, the MRI will show disruption of the coracoclavicular ligaments and associated edema in addition to findings seen on plain radiographs such as displacement of the lateral clavicle relative to the acromion. Figure 18.8a–d

shows representative coronal images from an MRI in a patient with an AC separation.

A trial of conservative treatment for this patient was reasonable. Traditionally, patients with type V AC separation, where there is a coracoclavicular distance that has increased greater than 100 % and often have rupture of the deltotrapezial fascia, are recommended to have surgery. Some patients, however, can have improvements in symptoms and tolerate the new position of the distal clavicle well, especially if it is not directly subcutaneous. In those patients who do need surgery, the coracoclavicular ligament reconstruction may be done acutely or in a delayed fashion.

Case 3: Suprascapular Nerve Compression

History/Exam

A 38-year-old woman presented to the orthopedic clinic with over a year of increasing pain and weakness in her right shoulder. Sixteen months prior, she had a fall down a flight of stairs. She had shoulder pain and an MRI was done immediately after the fall. She reports that she had an aching pain in her shoulder at the end of the day but was able to tolerate her symptoms and sought no further intervention at that time. Months later, she increased her activity level to include daily workouts. This caused her shoulder pain, and she noticed that her right shoulder was weaker and fatigued more quickly than the contralateral side. After 4 weeks, she was unable to tolerate her symptoms, so she stopped her workouts and presented to her physician. An MR arthrogram and EMG were ordered, and she was referred to the orthopedic clinic. She denies having numbness and tingling at any point.

The patient had weakness (four out of five) with resisted external rotation at the side. Her strength testing was otherwise symmetric to the contralateral extremity. She had a normal belly press and lift-off test bilaterally. Her shoulder active and passive range of motion was full and equal to the contralateral side. She was neurovascularly intact in this extremity and without symptoms in her contralateral shoulder. The remainder of her exam was unremarkable.

The EMG was abnormal with evidence of both acute and chronic denervation of the right infraspinatus and supraspinatus muscles. In addition, there were no signs of more diffuse pathology.

Imaging

At presentation, the patient had both the MRI from immediately after the injury and the recent MR arthrogram. Additionally, plain radiographs of the shoulder were obtained on the day of clinic evaluation.

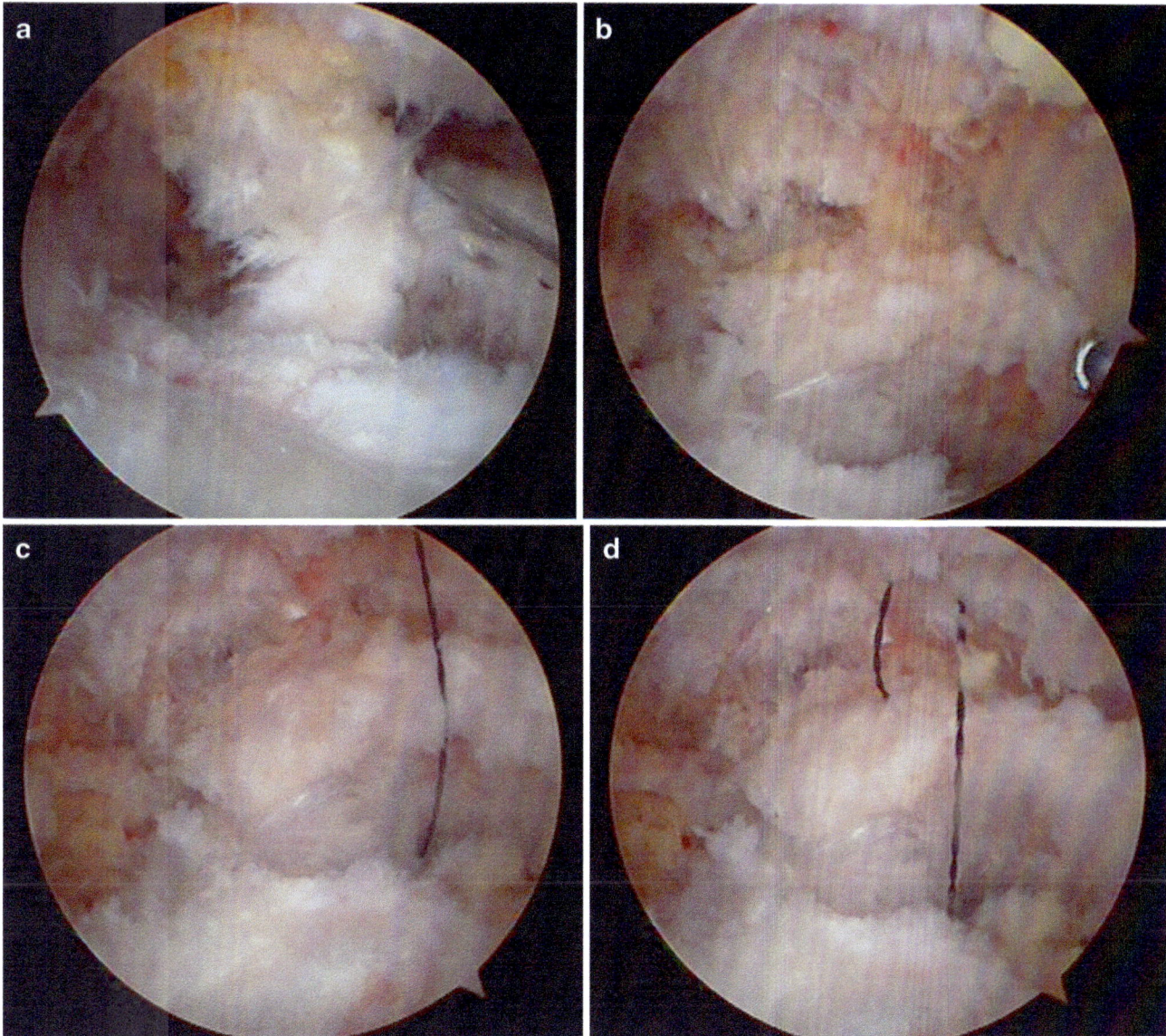

Fig. 18.7 (**a–d**) Series of arthroscopic images taken in a cadaver to allow for more extensive removal of bursal tissue in order to enhance visualization of the anatomic structures. (**a**) Intact coracoclavicular ligaments. (**b**) Coracoclavicular ligaments are torn, and the coracoid is visible. (**c, d**) A suture lasso being passed around the coracoid

These radiographs of the right shoulder were normal (Fig. 18.9a–c).

The MRI immediately following the injury is displayed in Fig. 18.10.

The MR arthrogram showed progressive perimuscular edema of supraspinatus and infraspinatus muscles from the initial MRI, with no discreet mass or cyst identified in the suprascapular notch, spinoglenoid notch, or quadrilateral space. The tendons of the rotator cuff were intact without tear. A comparison between the initial MRI and the MR arthrogram is displayed in Fig. 18.11a–d.

The findings of atrophy or reactive edema of the supraspinatus and infraspinatus muscles without tendon tear are consistent with the EMG findings of denervation injury to these muscles and the clinical presentation. At this point, arthroscopic suprascapular nerve decompression at the suprascapular notch was discussed. Despite no discreet mass identified in this region on the MR imaging, decompression of the nerve was suggested with the goal of stopping progressive damage to the nerve from continued compression. It was discussed with the patient that it was unclear if the weakness she already had would improve.

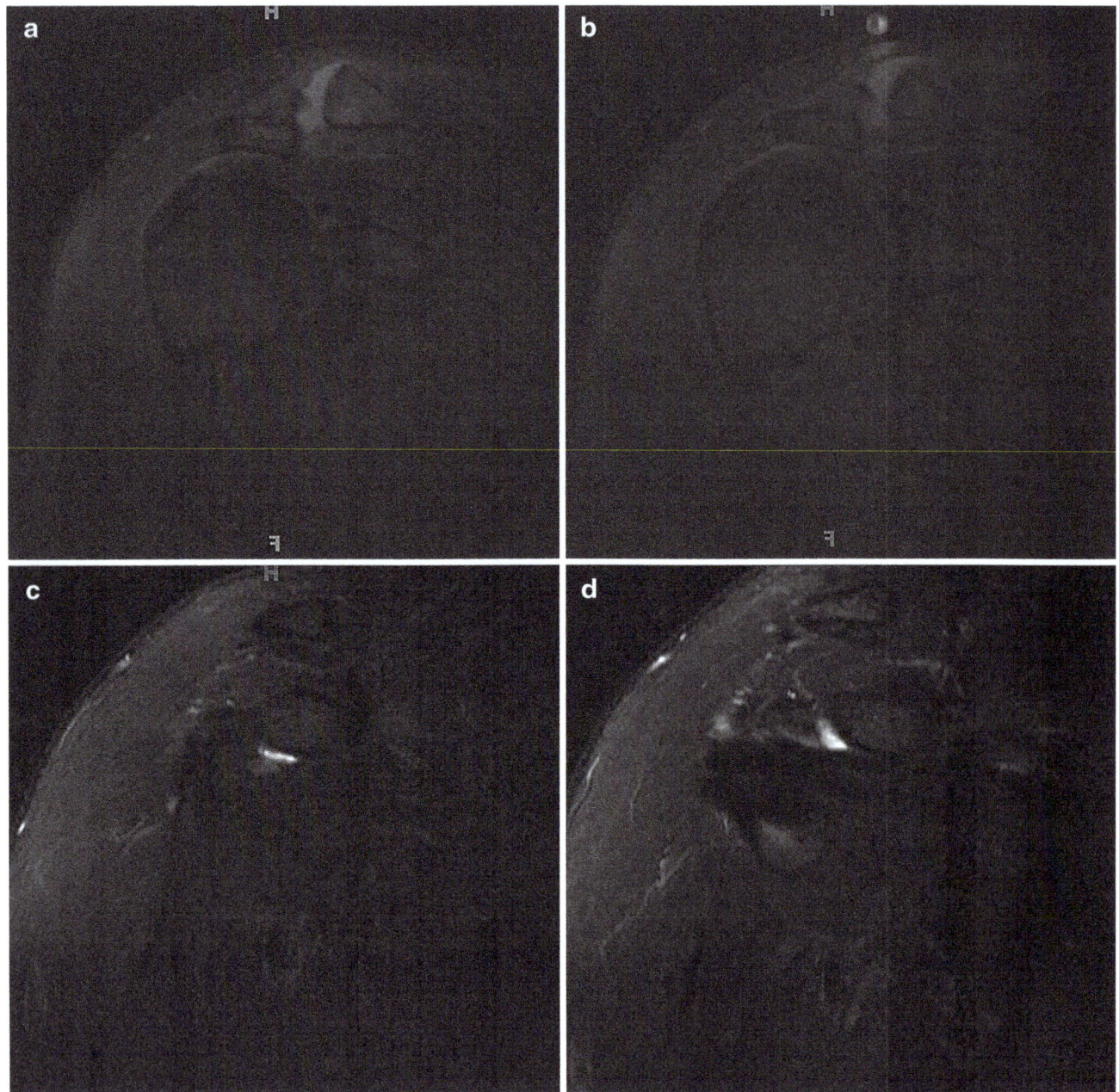

Fig. 18.8 **a** and **b** show tearing of the AC ligaments and elevation of the clavicle relative to the acromion. **c** and **d** demonstrate tearing of the CC ligaments

Arthroscopy

Anesthesia was an interscalene nerve block. The patient was placed into a well-padded beach chair position.

Two portals were marked 3 cm distal to the anterolateral raphe, with one 1 cm anterior to the raphe and one 1 cm posterior to the raphe. The posterior of these portals was made and the scope inserted. The more anterior anterolateral portal was then made under direct visualization. A significant amount of bursitis and an intact rotator cuff were identified.

The coracoacromial ligament was identified and followed to its attachment at the base of the coracoid. At the level of

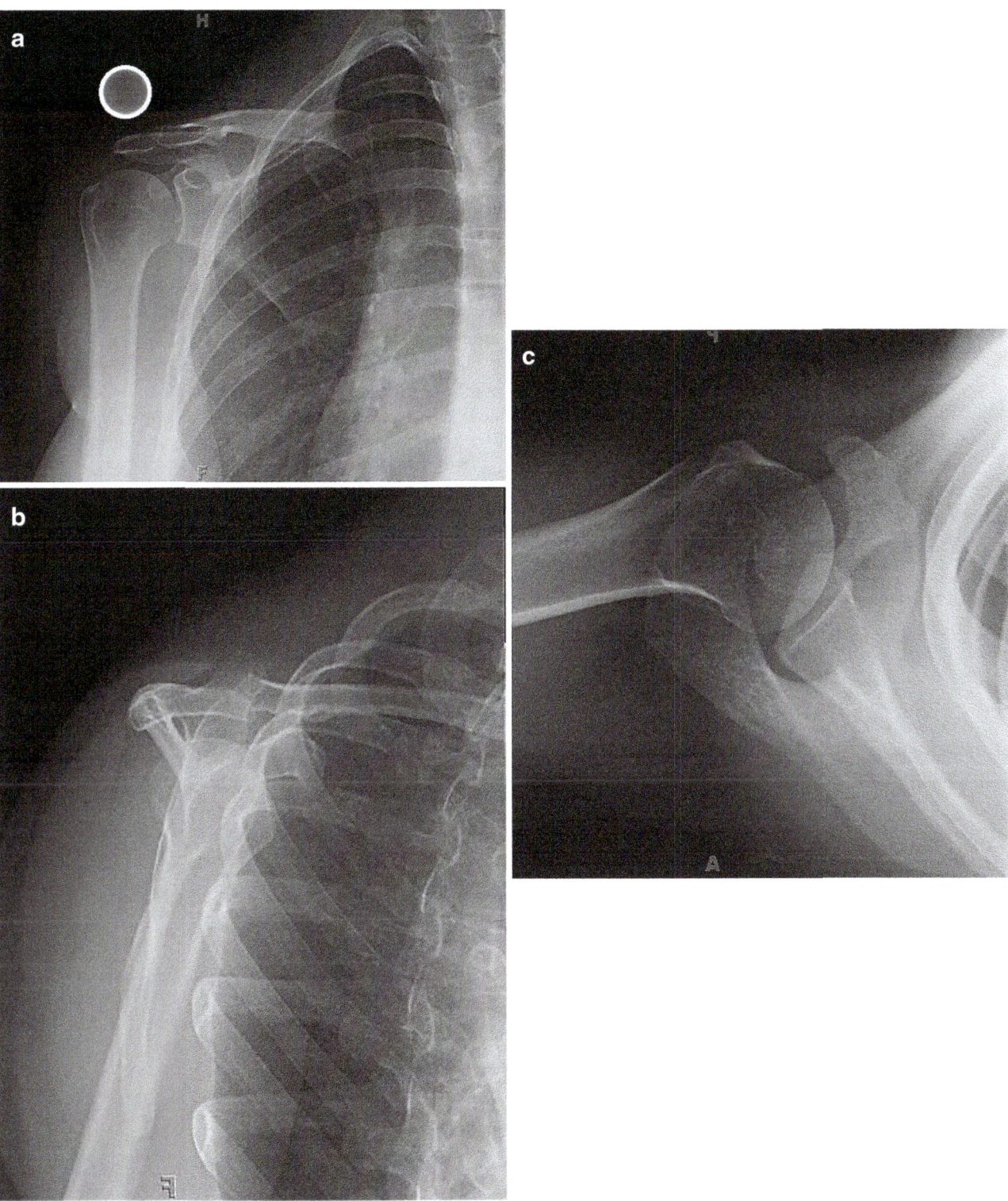

Fig. 18.9 (**a–c**) The plain radiographs demonstrate no abnormal findings

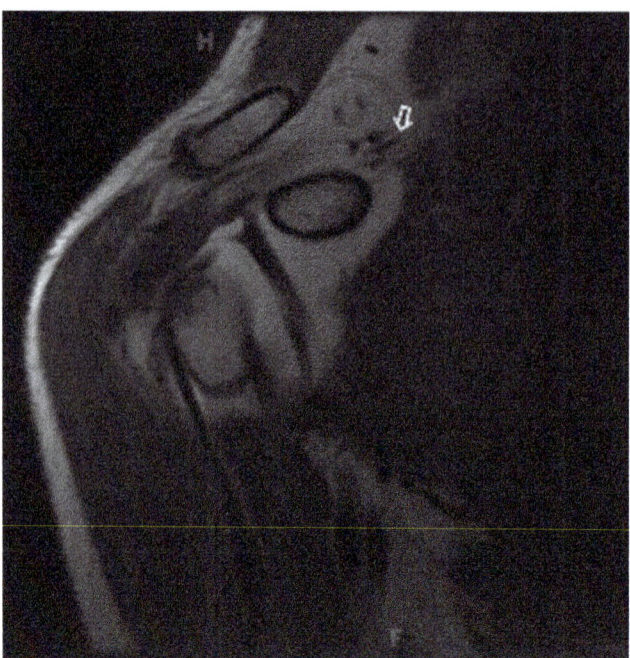

Fig. 18.10 This is a coronal image demonstrating the transverse scapular ligament (*white arrow*) with the suprascapular artery above and the suprascapular nerve below the ligament

the coracoid, the anterior aspect of the supraspinatus and the trapezoid ligament's origin were identified.

A third portal was then made posterior to the clavicle and dilated with a blunt trocar. Using a blunt switching stick through this portal, the supraspinatus tendon was swept medially and posteriorly. Tissue was then bluntly swept out

of the way following the base of the coracoid medially until the transverse scapular ligament was identified. The artery was identified and found running above the ligament. There was a significant amount of adipose tissue in this region, with some globular fat underneath the transverse scapular ligament, which was removed to reveal the suprascapular nerve deep to the ligament.

With care taken to remain between the artery and nerve, the ligament was cut with a 1.5 mm up-biter. The suprascapular nerve was mobilized using a probe and the blunt switching stick. A stenotic region was seen in the nerve, located where it had run beneath the ligament. Operative findings, therefore, correlated well with the clinical diagnosis: suprascapular nerve compression at the suprascapular notch.

Images from the arthroscopy are shown in Fig. 18.12a–d.

Figure 18.13a–c shows arthroscopic images from a cadaver, where tissue was more aggressively resected to provide improved visualization of the anatomy.

Discussion

The goal of suprascapular nerve decompression is to relieve ongoing nerve compression and diminish the potential for permanent nerve injury. While pain relief is frequently achieved postoperatively, the recovery of muscle that had already atrophied is less predictable [8]. Active range of motion should start within 2 weeks postoperatively. Despite physical therapy, patients should be warned that improvement of muscular atrophy and weakness can be less predictable [9].

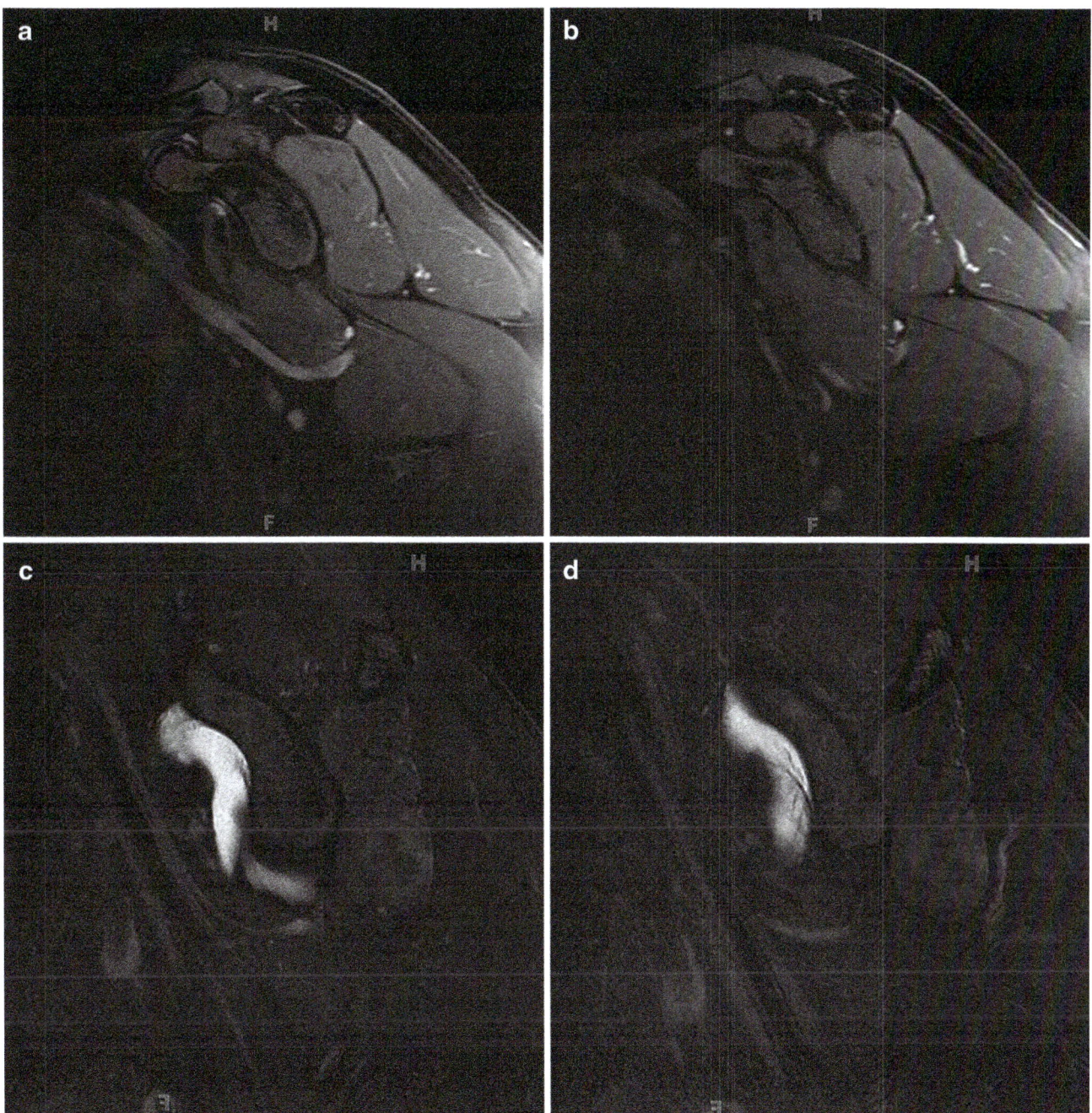

Fig. 18.11 (**a–d**) Adjacent MRI cuts taken two and three slices medial to the glenoid. **a** and **b** demonstrate images from the initial MRI, and **c** and **d** show similar images from the MR arthrogram done 16 months later. There has been interval progressive perimuscular edema of the supraspinatus and infraspinatus muscles, as well as the teres minor

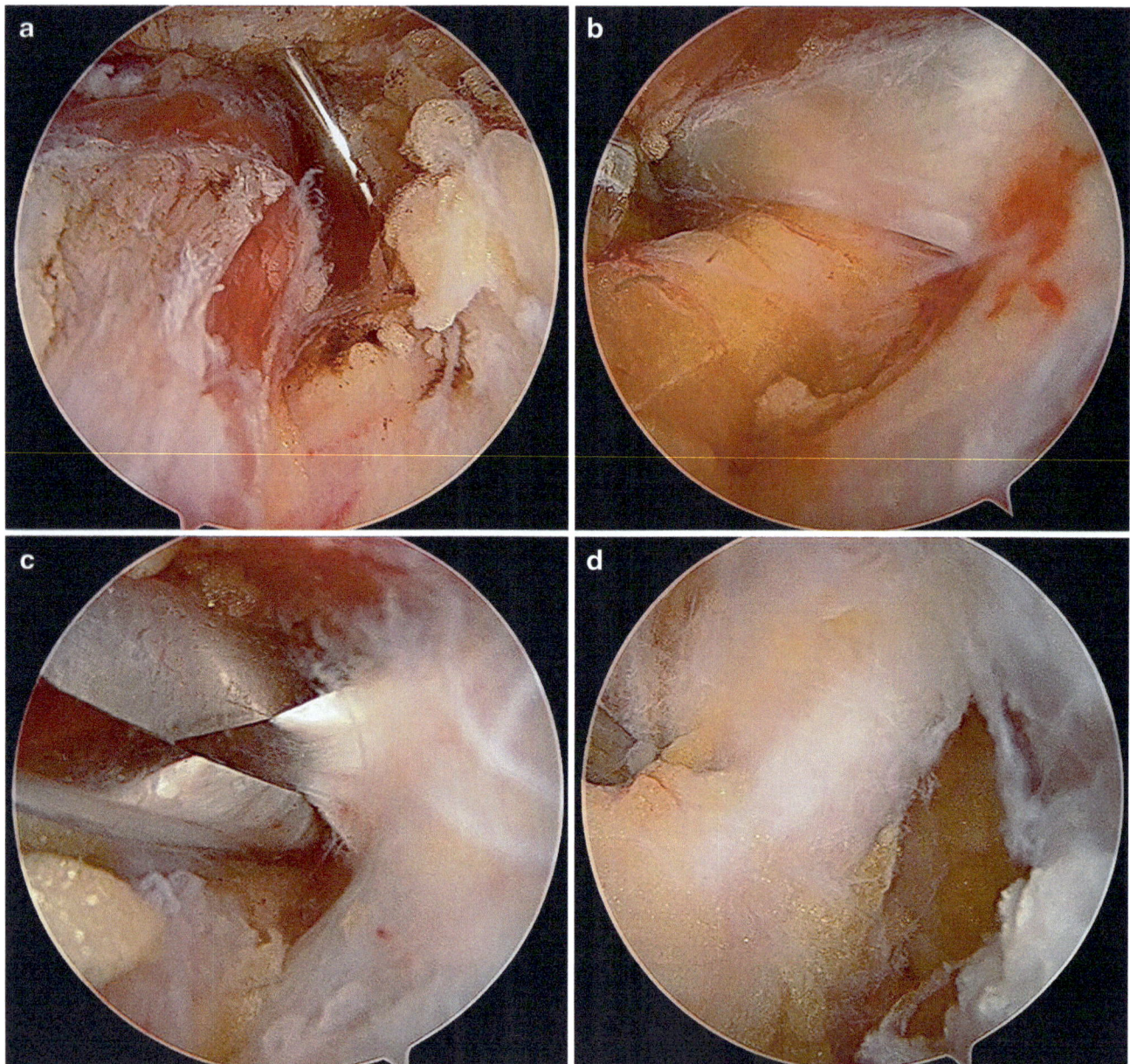

Fig. 18.12 (**a**) Anterior edge of the supraspinatus and a blunt retractor sweeping tissue away for visualization. (**b**) Transverse scapular ligament. (**c**) Ligament being cut. (**d**) Suprascapular nerve that is freed after the ligament has been severed

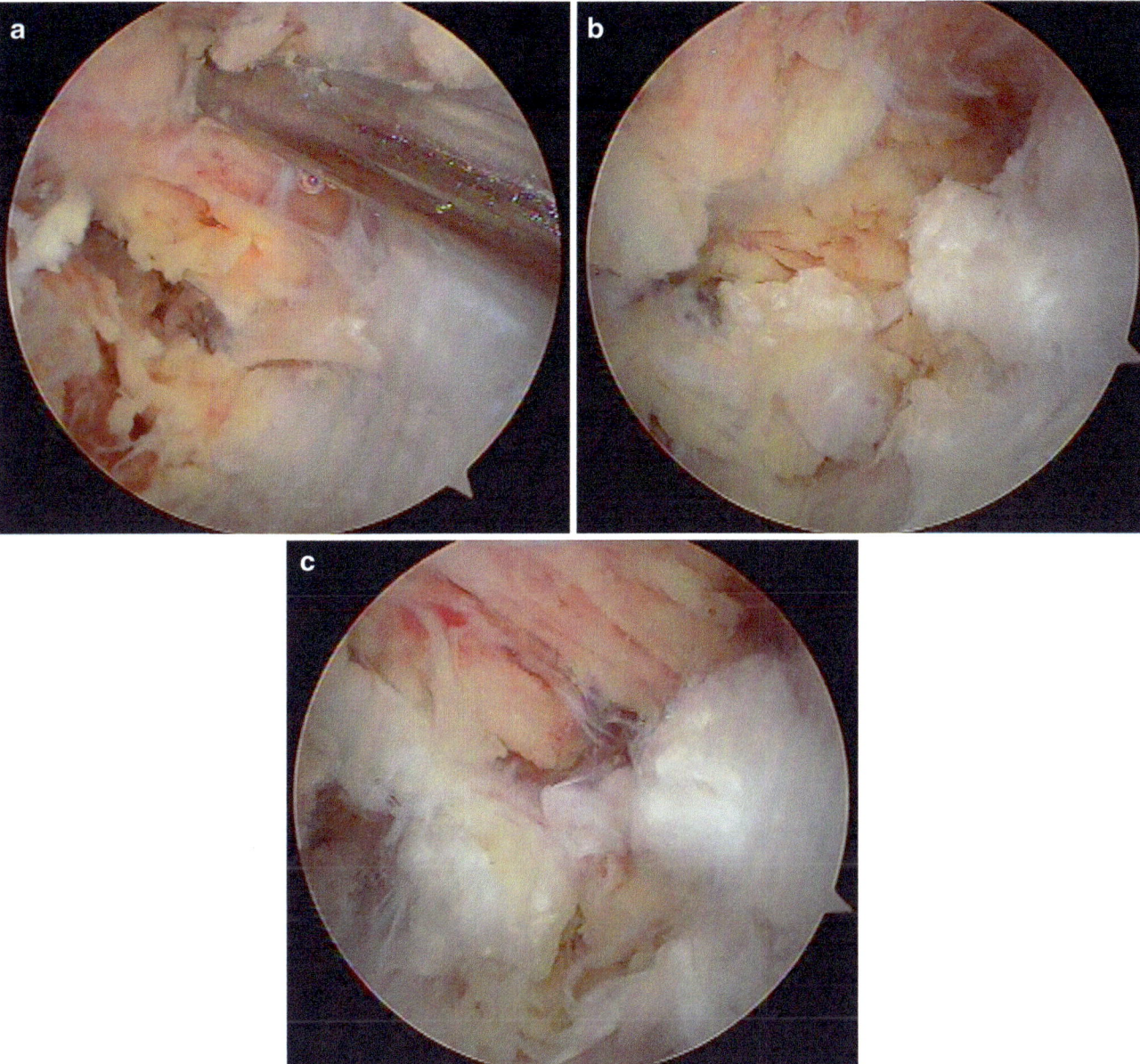

Fig. 18.13 (**a–c**) Arthroscopic images from a cadaver, where tissue was more aggressively resected to provide improved visualization of the anatomy. (**a**) Probe identifying the suprascapular artery superior to the transverse scapular ligament. (**b**) Transverse scapular ligament after it has been transected. (**c**) Relationship of the artery and transected ligament

References

1. Lemos MJ. The evaluation and treatment of the injured acromioclavicular joint in athletes. Am J Sports Med. 1998;26(1):137–44.
2. Moen TC, Babatunde OM, Hsu SH, Ahmad CA, Levine WN. Suprascapular neuropathy: what does the literature show? J Shoulder Elbow Surg. 2012;21(6):835–46.
3. Allman Jr FL. Fractures and ligamentous injuries of the clavicle and its articulation. J Bone Joint Surg Am. 1967;49(4):774–84.
4. Weaver JK, Dunn H. Treatment of acromioclavicular injuries, especially complete acromioclavicular separation. J Bone Joint Surg. 1972;54-A(6):1187–94.
5. Fialka C, Stampfl P, Oberleitner G, Vecsei V. Traumatic acromioclavicular joint separation—current concepts. Eur Surg. 2004; 36(1):20–4.
6. Gerber C, Rockwood Jr CA. Subcoracoid dislocation of the lateral end of the clavicle. A report of three cases. J Bone Joint Surg Am. 1987;69(6):924–7.
7. Li X, Ma R, Bedi A, Dines DM, Altchek DW, Dines JS. Current concepts review: management of acromioclavicular joint injuries. J Bone Joint Surg Am. 2014;96-A(1):73–84.
8. Amendola NA, Richmond J, Sgaglione NA. Chapter 27, Arthroscopic suprascapular nerve release. In: Barber FA, Bynum JA, editors. Operative arthroscopy [internet]. Philadelphia, PA: Lippincott Williams & Wilkins; 2012. p. 318–26.

9. Lubahn JD, Cermak MB. Uncommon nerve compression syndromes of the upper extremity. J Am Acad Orthop Surg. 1998;6(6):378–86.

10. Boykin RE, Friedman DJ, Zimmer ZR, Oaklander AL, Higgins LD, Warner JP. Suprascapular neuropathy in a shoulder referral practice. J Shoulder Elbow Surg. 2011;20(6):983–8.

11. Polguj M, Sibiński M, Grzegorzewski A, Grzelak P, Majos A, Topol M. Variation in morphology of suprascapular notch as a factor of suprascapular nerve entrapment. Int Orthop. 2013;37(11): 2185–92.

12. Shubin Stein BE, Ahmad CS, Pfaff CH, Bigliani LU, Levine WN. A comparison of magnetic resonance imaging findings of the acromioclavicular joint in symptomatic versus asymptomatic patients. J Shoulder Elbow Surg. 2006;15(1):56–9.

Imaging Evaluation of the Painful or Failed Shoulder Arthroplasty

Phillip Williams, Gabrielle Konin, and Lawrence V. Gulotta

Background

Shoulder arthroplasty has led to successful results in over 90 % of cases with an estimated complication rate of about 15 % [1–5]. Not all complications, however, lead to undesirable outcomes for the patient. Conversely, the absence of complications does not ensure a good clinical result, such as with stiffness or unexplained pain [6]. For this reason, shoulder arthroplasty failure is a broader term that also encompasses patient dissatisfaction with the result of the procedure, regardless of the severity of symptoms or physical findings [7]. Using this definition, Hasan and colleagues studied 144 shoulder arthroplasties and observed the following characteristics of failure in descending order: stiffness, instability, rotator cuff tear, nonunion of the tuberosities or surgical neck, glenoid component loosening, glenoid erosion, glenoid polyethylene wear, component malposition, humeral component loosening, periprosthetic fracture, infection, nerve injury, and heterotopic bone [6].

Similar to the findings by Hasan et al. [6], other investigators have identified common trends in complications after shoulder arthroplasty, although the complication rate varies depending on the study. Matsen et al. [5] analyzed the results of 18 reports on TSA with a minimum 2-year follow-up and observed a mean overall complication rate of 16 % (range, 0–62 %). They listed the following factors in descending frequency: component loosening, instability, rotator cuff tear, periprosthetic fracture, infection, implant failure including dissociation of a modular prosthesis, and deltoid dysfunction. In another study, Cofield [4] reported a 14 % complication rate and identified eight major causes in decreasing frequency: instability, rotator cuff tear, heterotopic ossification, glenoid component loosening, intraoperative fracture, nerve injury, infection, and humeral component loosening. More recently Bohsali and colleagues [8] performed a large retrospective review of 39 studies involving 2810 TSA and reported a 14.7 % complication rate. The most common complications, in order of frequency, were component loosening, instability, periprosthetic fracture, rotator cuff tears, neural injury, infection, and deltoid muscle dysfunction. Kalandiak et al. [9] categorized complications with failure into three broad categories: those involving soft tissue (instability, stiffness, tuberosity malunion or nonunion, and rotator cuff tears), those involving the glenoid component, and those involving the humeral component.

The imaging evaluation of the painful or failed shoulder arthroplasty should be used in conjunction with a careful history and physical examination and directed laboratory testing, if indicated. Plain radiographs provide substantial information about bone and soft tissue pathology and thus comprise the initial imaging modality to evaluate a shoulder arthroplasty. At least two mutually orthogonal images should be obtained. The glenohumeral anteroposterior (AP) and axillary lateral projections fulfill this requirement [10]. The true AP view of the glenohumeral joint is a 40° posterior oblique projection taken in the plane of the scapula (i.e., Grashey view). Rotational AP views of the shoulder in the coronal plane are oblique to the joint line and do not adequately image the glenohumeral articulation [11]. The acromioclavicular joint can often be viewed on the coronal AP projection, but it is best imaged with a 10° cephalad tilt view [12]. The axillary lateral projection allows assessment of glenoid anatomy, including version and bone deficiency, the position of the humeral head, and posterior displacement of the greater tuberosity [13, 14].

P. Williams, MD (✉)
Department of Orthopedic Surgery, Hospital for Special Surgery, New York, NY, USA
e-mail: williamsp@hss.edu

G. Konin, MD
Department of Radiology and Imaging, Hospital for Special Surgery, New York, NY, USA
e-mail: koning@hss.edu

L.V. Gulotta, MD
Department of Sports Medicine and Shoulder Service, Hospital for Special Surgery, New York, NY, USA
e-mail: gulottal@hss.edu

Immediate postoperative plain radiography is helpful in evaluating the placement and positioning of prosthetic implants, to assess cement interfaces and to rule out significant bony complications such as tuberosity displacement of humeral fracture. Additionally, the initial postoperative radiographs establish baseline images of the bone/cement, cement/implant, and implant/bone interfaces that can be used in subsequent follow-up for comparison [15]. It is important to note that a true AP image of the glenohumeral joint requires the shoulder to be externally rotated 20°, which is a position that most early postoperative patients cannot tolerate or should avoid.

Unlike hip and knee arthroplasty, there is no established comprehensive protocol for evaluating the optimal position of a shoulder implant [16]. Authors have made general recommendations based on observations. Iannotti et al. [17] suggest the humeral component should sit above the level of the tuberosity by less than 1 cm to avoid impingement and rotator cuff tears. Figgie et al. [18] found that functional outcome correlated with the position of the glenoid and humeral components. When the height of the humeral head above the tuberosity and the glenoid and humeral offsets were restored, there was an improved range of motion and reduced incidence of lucent lines compared with patients without restoration of correct alignment. Long-term vigilance is required when caring for shoulder arthroplasty patients because complications often present in a delayed fashion. Deshmukh et al. [18–20] analyzed complications with respect to the time of occurrence and found that, on the average, component loosening was found at 7.7±4.8 years; infections, at 12.1±2.9 years; dislocations, at 2.1±3.6 years; and periprosthetic fractures, at 5.8±4.7 years. No matter when a patient presents with complaints, a thorough knowledge of the pathological appearance on imaging is essential for quality care.

In this chapter, we will discuss some of the more common causes of TSA failure and the utility of MRI in the diagnosis and management of them. When possible, case vignettes are used to demonstrate the correlation between MRI results and the findings during revision surgery.

Component Loosening

Case 1

A 67-year-old right-hand-dominant man who underwent a left total shoulder replacement approximately 5 years prior to presentation. He now complains of pain with range of motion. His physical exam shows forward flexion to 160°, external rotation of 45°, and internal rotation to the lumbar spine. He demonstrates excellent strength with rotator cuff testing including a negative belly press. Radiographs show some radiolucency around the glenoid component but without

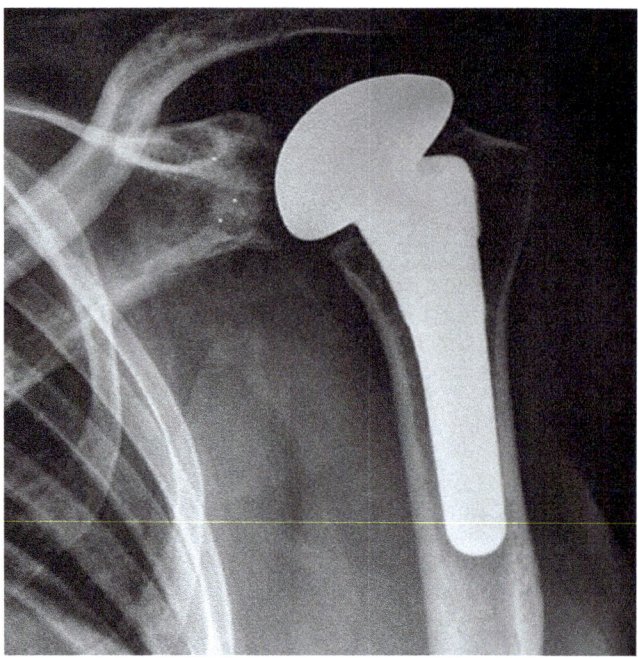

Fig. 19.1 Glenoid component loosening with radiolucent lines

frank loosening (Fig. 19.1). MRI shows evidence of loosening around glenoid component (Fig. 19.2a, b).

Patient then underwent arthroscopic removal of a loose glenoid component (Fig. 19.3a–c). The component was removed through the rotator interval. At the time of arthroscopy, biopsies were taken for culture and were held for 14 days in order to rule out an indolent infection with *P. acnes*. These were negative. The patient went on to pain-free range of motion and elected not to undergo another procedure for glenoid reimplantation.

In the analysis by Bohsali et al., loosening of the glenoid and humeral components occurred frequently, accounting for 39 % of complications [8, 18–20]. Moreover, 83 % of the cases of loosening involved failure of the glenoid component fixation. Loosening of an arthroplasty component is recognized on radiographs as the appearance of a radiolucent line at the implant/cement/bone interface. Line thickness is measured starting with 0.5 mm. The sites of appearance have been divided into eight zones for the humeral component and six zones for the glenoid component [21–24]. Franklin et al. [25] devised criteria to classify radiolucency around the glenoid component for keeled implants (Table 19.1). Similarly, Lazarus et al. [26] developed a classification for pegged implants. For glenoid components, the overall prevalence of radiolucent lines is reported to range from 22 to 95 % [2, 7, 27–29]. However, relying solely on plain radiographs to determine security of fixation may be problematic because obtaining reproducible X-rays of the glenoid can be difficult [30]. Nagels et al. [31] performed a study of loosening of the glenoid component

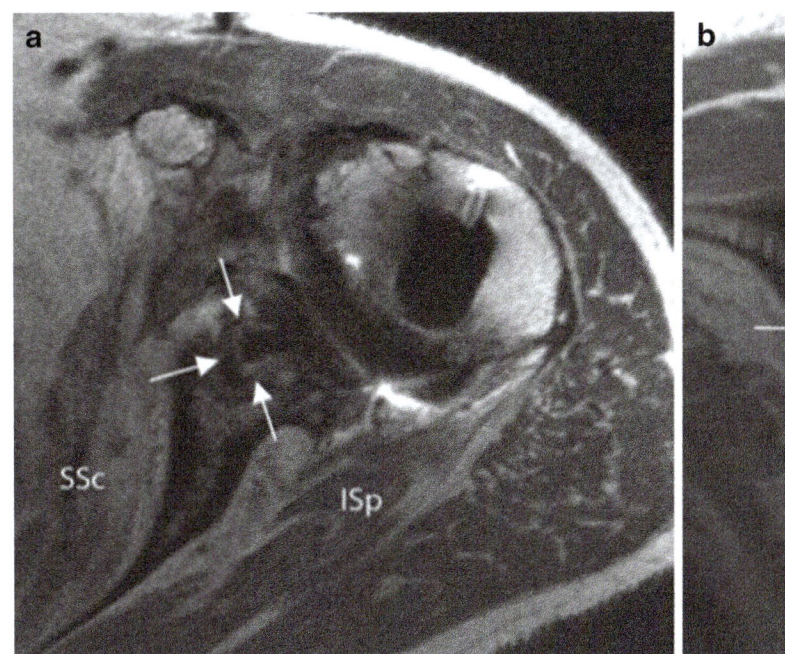
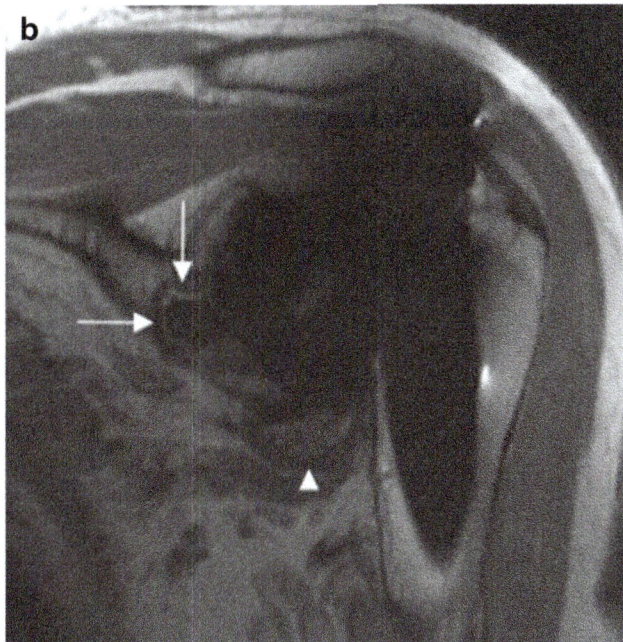

Fig. 19.2 Axial (**a**) and coronal oblique (**b**) FSE PD images demonstrate circumferential hyperintense signal with adjacent thin low-signal rim about the glenoid baseplate and keel indicative of loosening *(arrows)* in two different patients. Wear-induced synovitis is detected on the coronal oblique image at the axillary recess *(arrowhead)*

using digital roentgen stereophotogrammetric analysis and found that it was more accurate in detecting early loosening. Its use in practice, however, is limited to the lack of experience and familiarity with the technique.

In reverse total shoulder arthroplasty, scapular notching is another glenoid complication that can lead to implant failure. This term describes a common complication involving the erosion of the inferior scapular neck related to impingement by the medial rim of the humeral cup during adduction [32–38]. A large multicenter trial found an incidence of 68 % at a mean follow-up of 51 months. It was also shown that notching was accompanied by decreases in strength and anterior elevation as well as an increased incidence in humeral and glenoid radiolucent lines [39]. Nyffeler et al. [40] concluded inferior placement of the baseplate on the glenoid plate to prevent the occurrence of notching and also improve range of motion. Glenospheres with a lateral center of rotation have been shown to produce lower rates of scapular notching [41–43].

With regard to the prosthetic humeral head, analyzing its position relative to the greater tuberosity and the shift of the stem in the frontal plane can identify a humeral component at risk or not at risk of loosening [44]. For additional precision in measuring shift of the stem, authors have devised various terminologies. Subsidence (S) describes the change in the vertical distance between the most superior aspects of the humeral component and the greater tuberosity [22]. The tilt is the medial or lateral change in the components' posi-

tion measured by calculating the distance of the external surface of the humeral component from the external surface of cortical bone in four areas: superolateral (at the border between radiographic zones 1 and 2), inferolateral (zones 2 and 3), superomedial (zones 6 and 7), and inferomedial (zones 5 and 6) [22, 45]. Clinically relevant threshold amounts for subsidence and tilt in humeral component position are ≥5 mm and ≥10 mm, respectively [44].

Instability

Shoulder arthroplasty can disturb the complex interplay of bony and soft tissue restraints of the glenohumeral joint. Instability following shoulder arthroplasty is a common complication with a reported prevalence of 4 % and accounts for 30 % of all complications across multiple studies [8, 18, 19, 46, 47]. Specifically, anterior and superior instability accounted for 80 % of the cases of instability [8, 18, 19, 46, 47]. Superior instability is associated with a deficient rotator cuff or coracoacromial arch [4, 28, 48, 49]. Attributable causes to anterior stability include humeral component malrotation, anterior glenoid deficiency, anterior deltoid muscle dysfunction, and failure of the subscapularis tendon and anterior aspect of the capsule [5, 46, 50].

Plain radiographs can be used to assess prosthesis instability. The axillary radiograph is the gold standard to assess subluxation of the prosthetic head in the sagittal plane.

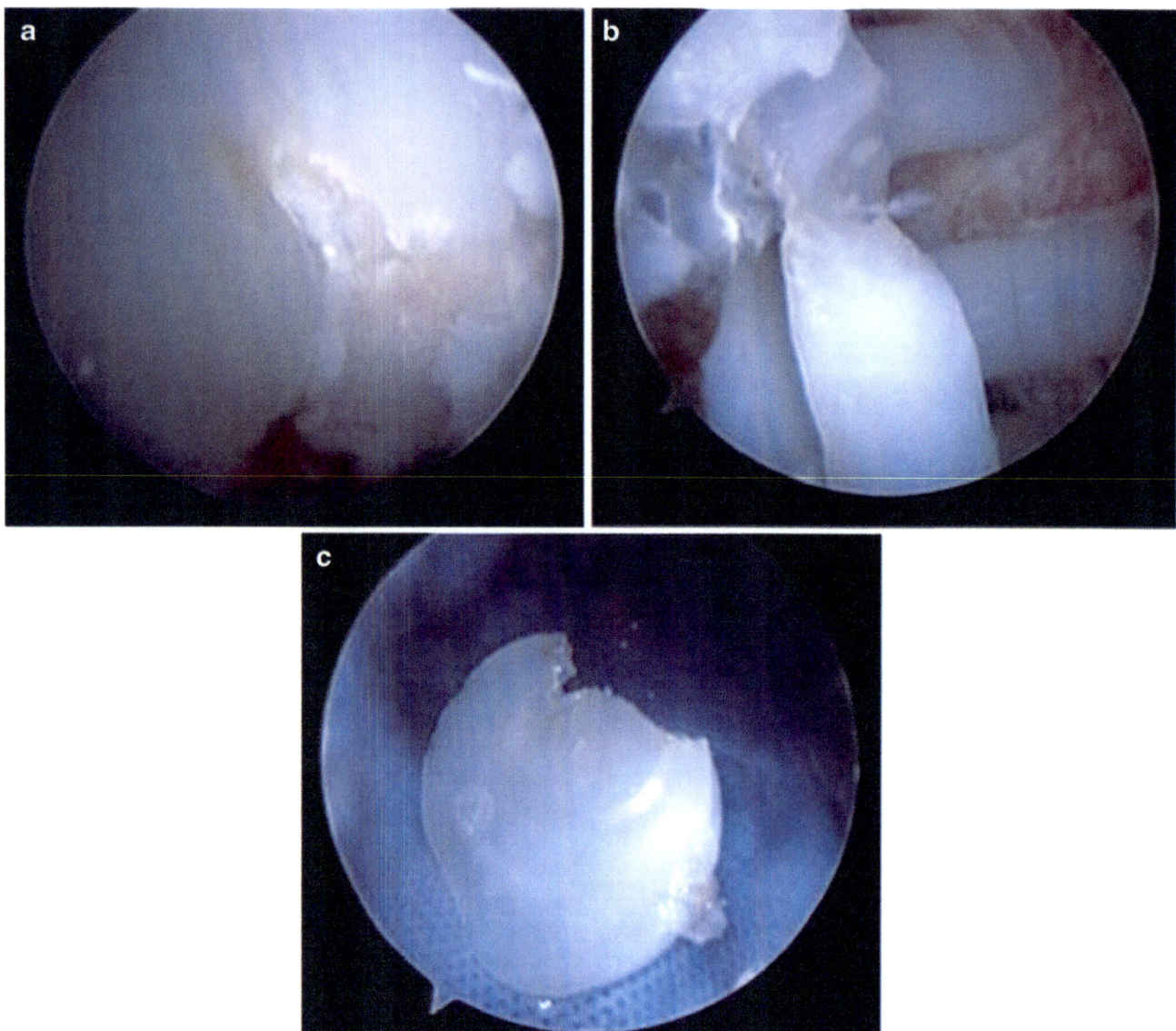

Fig. 19.3 (**a**) Arthroscopic images while viewing from a posterior portal of a cracked and loose glenoid. (**b**) Glenoid was easily removed arthroscopically through an incision made in the rotator interval. (**c**) View of the glenoid on the back table after removal

Table 19.1 Classification of radiolucency around keeled glenoid components

Grade 0	No radiolucency
Grade 1	Radiolucency at superior and/or inferior flange
Grade 2	Incomplete radiolucency at keel
Grade 3	Complete radiolucency (≤2 mm wide) around keel
Grade 4	Complete radiolucency (>2 mm wide) around keel
Grade 5	Gross loosening

Used with permission from Franklin JL, Barrett WP, Jackins SE, Matsen FA. Glenoid loosening in total shoulder arthroplasty. Association with rotator cuff deficiency. J Arthroplasty. 1988;3(1):39–46

Table 19.2 Classification of prosthetic head subluxation

Absent	The humeral head is centered in the glenoid cavity
Slight	<25 % translation of the center of the head component with respect to the glenoid center
Moderate	25–50 % translation of the center of the prosthetic head with respect to the glenoid center
Severe	>50 % translation of the center of the head component with respect to the glenoid center

Used with permission from Sperling JW, Cofield RH, Rowland CM. Minimum fifteen-year follow-up of Neer hemiarthroplasty and total shoulder arthroplasty in patients aged fifty years or younger. J Shoulder Elbow Surg. 2004;13(6):604–13

Furthermore, the degree of subluxation can be classified as either absent, slight, moderate, or severe based on the direction and severity (Table 19.2) [20]. Joint widening on the true AP

views may also indicate instability, possibly due to an undersized humeral component, an excessive osteotomy, or a deficient rotator cuff [44].

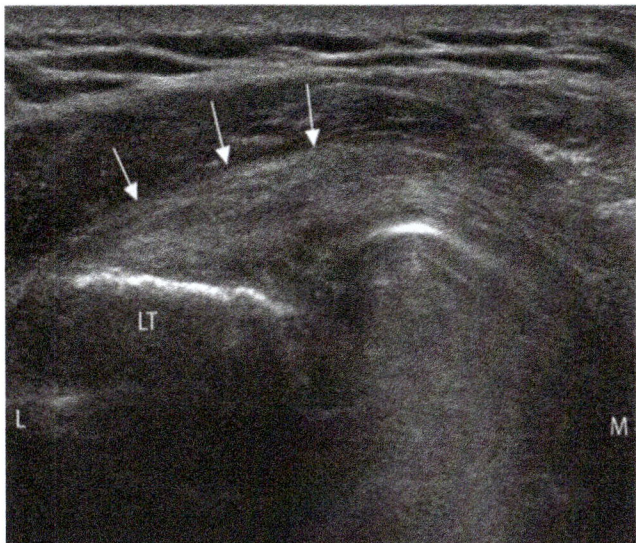

Fig. 19.4 Ultrasound image depicts an intact subscapularis tendon (*arrows*) in the long axis. *LT* lesser tuberosity, *L* lateral, *M* medial

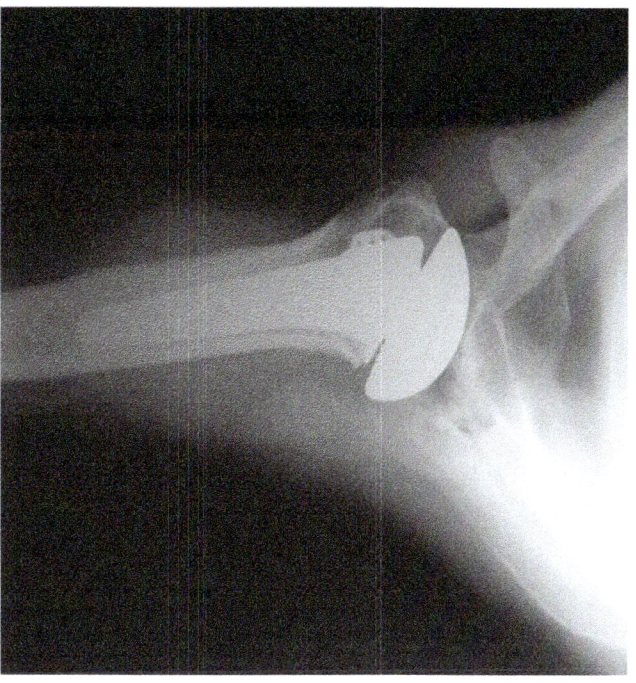

Fig. 19.5 Axillary radiograph showing posterior subluxation of the humeral head component secondary to eccentric posterior glenoid wear

Failure of the subscapularis tendon is implicated in many cases of anterior instability following TSA [51–53], but clear visualization is difficult due to metal artifact. Ultrasound can be extremely accurate in the detection of rotator cuff tears in the postoperative shoulder (Fig. 19.4) [54, 55]. In a study documenting the subscapularis healing rate by the use of postoperative ultrasound after TSA in 30 patients, ultrasound identified four torn tendons, whereas there were no radiographic findings definitively associated with the absence of intact subscapularis tendons [56]. A study by Sofka et al. of 11 shoulder arthroplasty revealed six subscapularis tears [57].

Posterior instability is normally a result of excessive component retroversion [8, 50, 58, 59]. Consequently, posterior glenoid erosion and soft tissue imbalance lead to instability [8]. Posterior subluxation can be seen on the axillary radiograph (Fig. 19.5). A CT can also be used to determine glenoid version accurately [54].

Periprosthetic Fracture

The reported prevalence of periprosthetic humeral fractures has been estimated to be between 1.5 and 3 % [5, 46, 60]. Initial evaluation of a suspected fracture in a patient should include anteroposterior and axillary radiographs. Cofield and Wright developed a classification system for humeral periprosthetic fractures [61]. Type A fractures occur at the tip of the prosthesis and extend proximally. Type B fractures occur at the tip of the prosthesis without extension. Type C fractures occur at the prosthetic tip and have distal extension [62].

Rotator Cuff Tear

Case 2

A 73 year-old right-hand-dominate male who originally underwent a right total shoulder replacement at an outside hospital approximately 18 months prior to presentation with pain and limited function. Physical exam revealed pseuodo-paralysis with attempted elevation and anterosuperior escape. Radiographs show superior and anterior subluxation (Fig. 19.6a, b), and MRI showed subscapularis dehiscence with retraction to the coracoid (Fig. 19.7) and fatty infiltration of the muscle belly.

Patient underwent conversion of his total shoulder replacement to a reverse shoulder arthroplasty (Fig. 19.8). Four years later the patient now has 150° of forward flexion, 15° of external rotation, and internal rotation to the back pocket all with minimal pain.

Rotator cuff tears can be assessed radiographically by observing superior migration of the humeral head and measuring a reduction of the acromio-humeral distance. However, this measurement can be imprecise because it varies according to the projection, size, and sex of the patient. Instead, Skirving [30] advocated the importance of the continuity of the scapulohumeral line (analogous to Shenton's line in the hip) on a true AP of the shoulder taken with the arm in neutral or external rotation. When there is a break in this line,

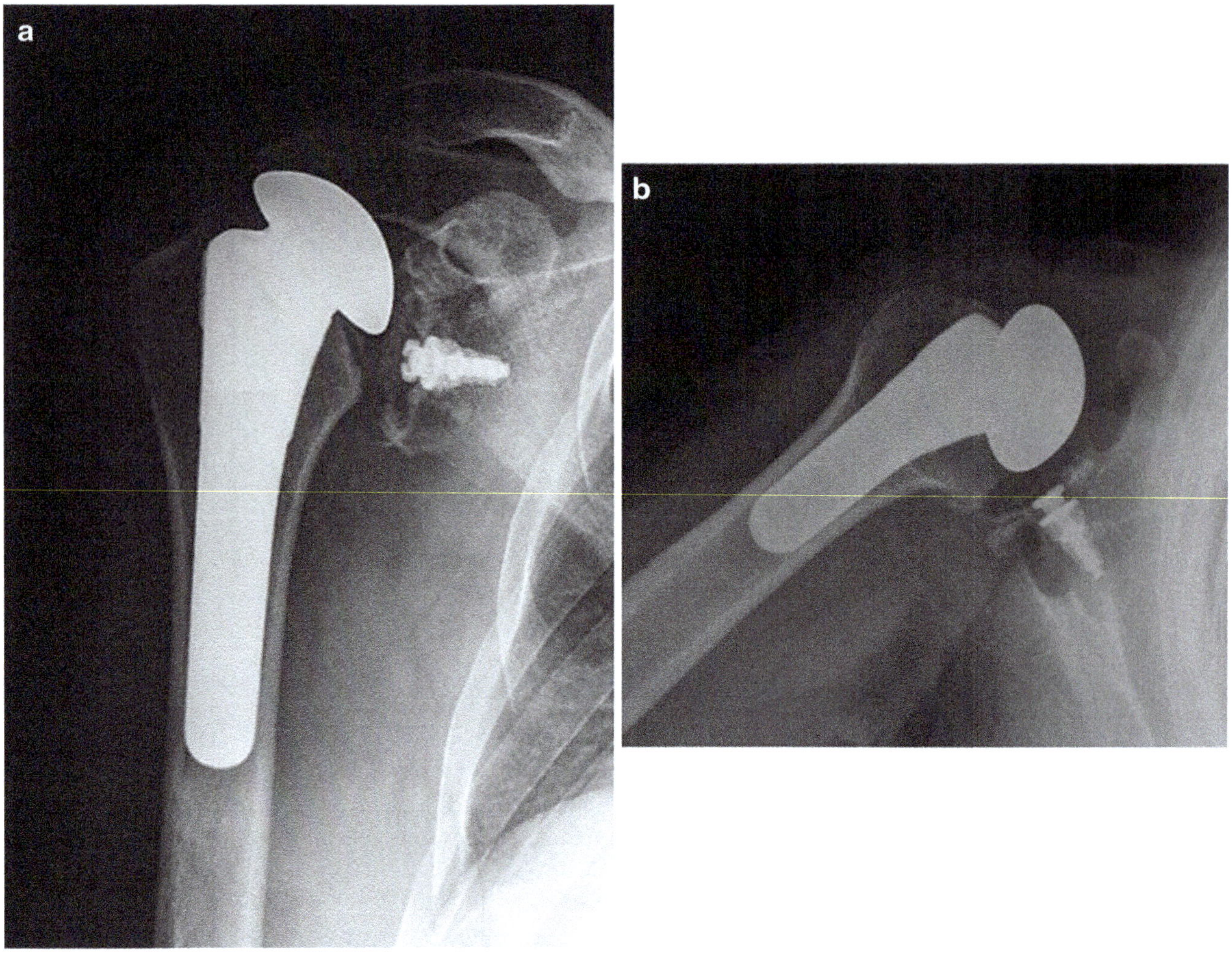

Fig. 19.6 Anteroposterior (**a**) radiograph shows superior migration of the humeral head, and the axillary (**b**) shows anterior subluxation. Both indicative of a rotator cuff tear

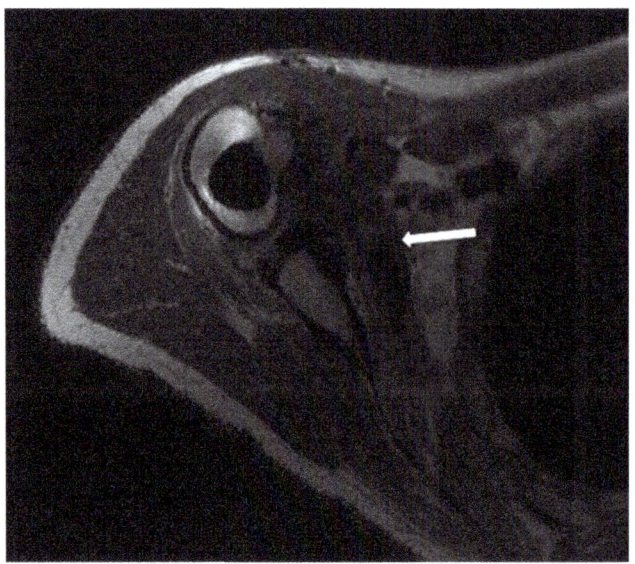

Fig. 19.7 MRI showing dehiscence of the subscapularis with retraction of the main tendon stump past the coracoid (*arrow*)

it is a more sensitive indicator of superior migration of the humeral head and, therefore, of rotator cuff tears. Despite these findings, plain radiographs have limited ability to assess the integrity of the cuff, the quality of the muscle, and the degree of retraction of a torn tendon.

Consequently, MRI has been relied upon to provide a more accurate diagnosis in the face of clinical and conventional imaging limitations [63]. MRI, however, presents its own particular set of imaging challenges in shoulder arthroplasty due to the magnetic susceptibility generated by the implant resulting in local field distortions that obscure the regional structures. The intensity of the susceptibility artifact is a function of the relative ferromagnetism of the components, with titanium being less ferromagnetic (and thus causing less artifact) than cobalt-chrome alloy components, as well as the orientation of the components relative to the external magnetic field. Additionally, the eccentric location of the shoulder relative to the isocenter of the imaging bore and the large spherical component increase the susceptibility artifact of shoulder arthroplasty when compared to knee or hip arthroplasty [63, 64].

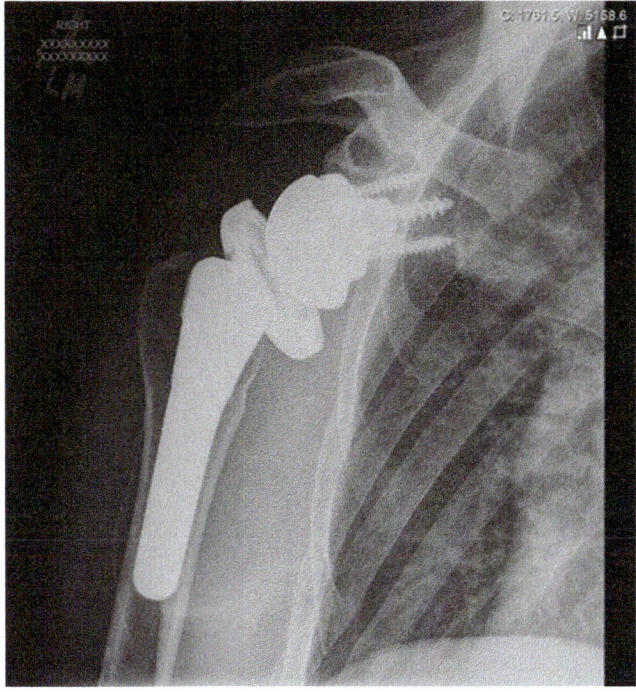

Fig. 19.8 Anteroposterior radiograph after conversion of the total shoulder replacement to a reverse shoulder arthroplasty

Modifications in conventional fast spin echo techniques have improved visualization of the soft tissues around implants. In an MRI study of 42 painful shoulder arthroplasties, Sperling et al. [63] suggested that MR imaging is a useful tool to determine the integrity of the rotator cuff; however, they found that the lesser tuberosity and glenoid component were obscured by artifact created by the proximal spherical humeral component. Relatively new commercially available pulse sequences, multiacquisition variable-resonance image combination (MAVRIC) and slice-encoding metal artifact correction (SEMAC), can further reduce susceptibility artifact near implants [65–67]. These new pulse sequences rely on conventional imaging techniques and can be used with standard clinical 1.5-T and 3-T MRI hardware.

Early studies have shown that MAVRIC images can detect pathology not visible with standard metal artifact-reduction FSE sequences. Hayter et al. [65] evaluated the quality of MAVRIC images compared with that of metal artifact-reduction FSE images of 27 patients who underwent shoulder arthroplasty. Their findings included significantly improved visualization of the synovium, periprosthetic bone, glenoid osteolysis, and supraspinatus tendon. Importantly, detection of supraspinatus tears was significantly increased with MAVRIC compared with FSE imaging alone (Fig. 19.9a, b). Although the lesser tuberosity and subscapularis footprint often remain obscured, the muscle

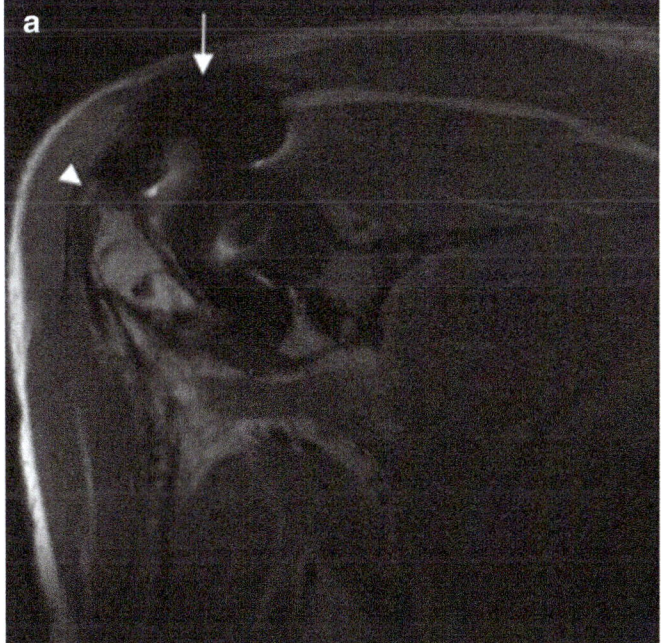
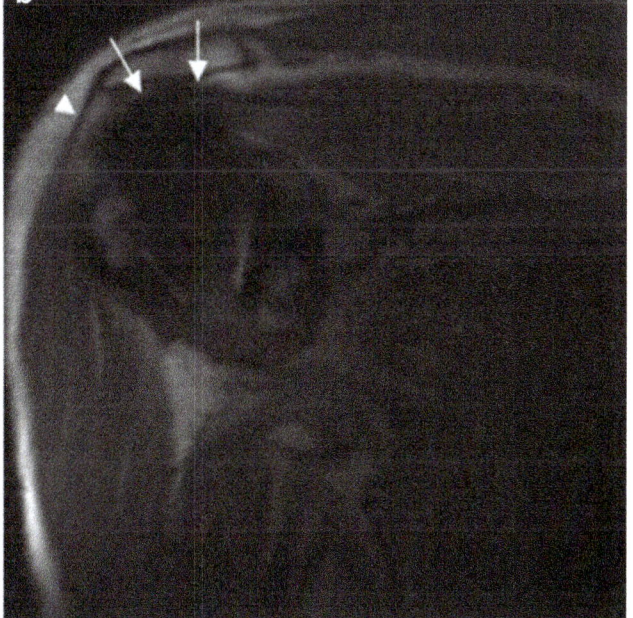

Fig. 19.9 (**a**) Coronal oblique FSE proton density image demonstrates bulky dephasing artifact superiorly obstructing the supraspinatus muscle tendon junction (*arrow*). Note that the supraspinatus footprint (*arrowhead*) remains visualized, which is hyperintense in this case indicating tendinosis but no tear. (**b**) Coronal oblique MAVRIC FSE proton density image allows visualization of the supraspinatus muscle tendon junction (*arrows*), thereby increasing the ability to detect supraspinatus tendon tears and retraction. Note the ability to see the origin of the deltoid (*arrowhead*)

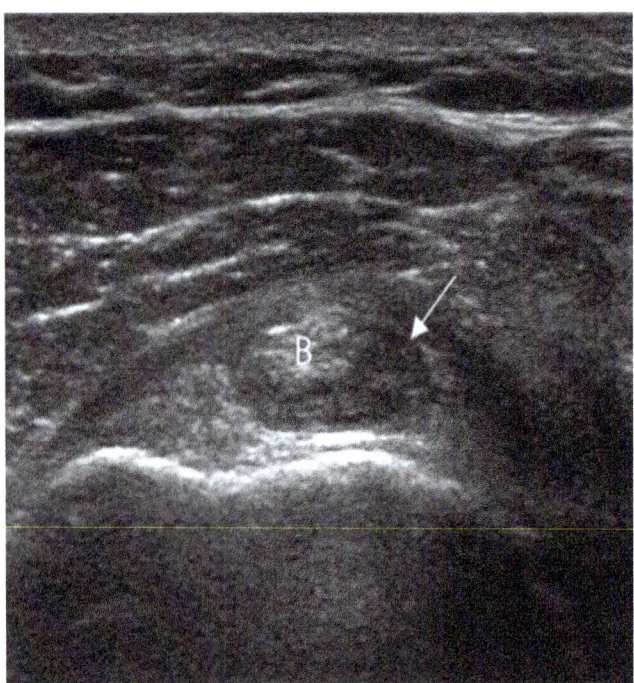

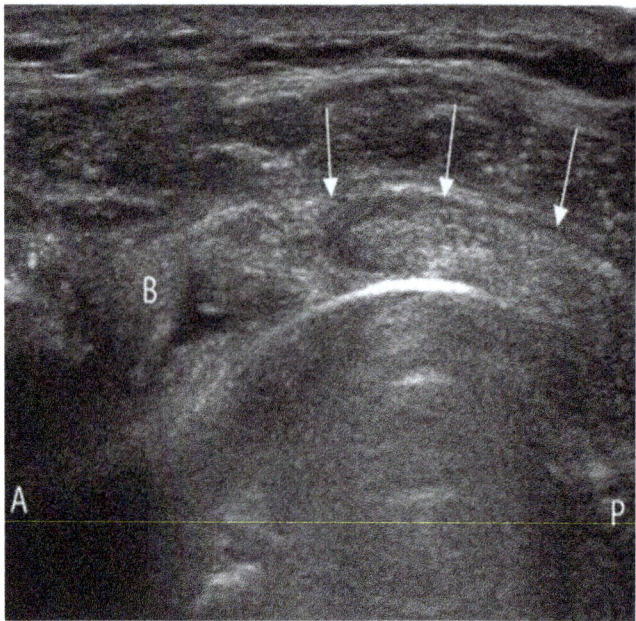

Fig. 19.10 Ultrasound image demonstrates the long head of the biceps tendon (B) in short axis with a hypoechoic rim of synovial fluid and debris (*arrow*) — "halo" sign

Fig. 19.11 Short axis ultrasound image shows an intact supraspinatus tendon (*arrows*). The hyperechoic curvilinear line deep to the supraspinatus is the humeral component. *B* biceps long head tendon

tendon junction and its muscle belly are typically visualized and should be carefully evaluated for failure, as this is a common cause of anterior instability. Application of MAVRIC or SEMAC to axial images could potentially better elucidate subscapularis tears at the footprint (Fig. 19.7).

By decreasing image distortion and improving visualization of the bone-prosthesis interface, these new metal reduction techniques (MAVRIC/SEMAC) serve to complement conventional FSE images, which ultimately offer higher spatial resolution than MAVRIC images, thus providing greater detail of the visualized soft tissues [65].

Similar to MRI, ultrasound is able to assess periarticular soft tissues without radiation; however, sonography has the added benefits of eliminating interference from the implant and allowing dynamic examinations. Westhoff et al. [68] performed static and dynamic ultrasound examinations on 22 patients, and results were correlated with clinical outcome. Pathologic changes within the supraspinatus and infraspinatus tendons were found in several shoulders. A halo sign around the biceps tendon was detected in seven shoulders (Fig. 19.10). This low-echogenic halo around the biceps tendon correlated well with fluid in the synovial sheath and indicated effusion within the glenohumeral joint according to a study by Rupp et al. [69] Increased intra-articular volume was detected in five patients, two of whom also had a halo sign around the biceps tendon. Subdeltoid bursitis was found in only one shoulder. Loosening of the glenoid during dynamic examination was detected in one shoulder. Pathological findings also correlated

well with poorer outcomes, while lack of findings correlated with better outcomes.

Sofka and Adler [57] performed ultrasound examinations on 11 shoulder arthroplasty patients who had clinical suspicion of rotator cuff tear, pain, and decreased range of motion. Sonographic findings included six supraspinatus tendon tears and three infraspinatus tendon tears. Nine patients had biceps tendinosis. The prosthesis did not hinder examination of the rotator cuff in any patient (Fig. 19.11). The authors concluded that sonography is a rapid and reliable method to use for evaluating the periprosthetic soft tissues, including the rotator cuff, in patients who have undergone shoulder replacement. Disadvantages of ultrasound are that it does not give a global picture of the joint and it provides limited evaluation of component loosening [70].

Despite the relatively common use of MRI and ultrasound for evaluation of most soft tissue shoulder abnormalities, CT arthrography can also provide an accurate assessment of the rotator cuff, the capsular-labral-ligamentous structures, and the articular cartilage of the glenohumeral joint [71, 72]. Multi-detector CT (MDCT) is a development that has provided excellent spatial resolution and multiplanar capability, thus markedly improving the diagnostic power of CT arthrography of the shoulder [73]. Some authors [74, 75] prefer MDCT arthrography for imaging patients with shoulder prostheses because the images have minimal artifacts while allowing sufficient assessment of prosthetic and periprosthetic bony and soft tissue abnormalities. Post-processing of volume-rendered 3D CT can also substantially reduce beam-hardening artifacts and can be used to assess hardware integrity [76]. Additionally, joint fluid can be aspirated during the intra-articular administration of contrast medium and sent for culture and sensitivity testing if clinical suspicion of infection warrants [77]. General indications for MDCT arthrography pertain to the inability to perform MRI or failure of MRI to adequately evaluate the shoulder. For example, indications include the presence of metal hardware close to the joint, the presence of MRI-incompatible implanted medical devices, and a history of claustrophobia. In patients who have undergone shoulder surgery, MDCT arthrography has been found to be more accurate than nonarthrographic MRI [78]. However, to date there has not been a direct comparison of MDCT arthrography and MR arthrography.

Infection

Although infection is a rare complication of primary shoulder arthroplasty, it can have devastating consequences. Bohsali [8] found an overall prevalence of 0.7 % across several studies. Susceptible host-related factors for infection include diabetes, rheumatoid arthritis, systemic lupus erythematosus, previous surgery, and remote sources of infection. Extrinsic causes of infection include chemotherapy, systemic corticosteroid therapy, and repeated intra-articular steroid injections [5, 46].

Clinically, pain is usually the most common symptom. Laboratory tests such as measurements of the C-reactive protein level, erythrocyte sedimentation rate, and white blood cell count are important indicators of infection [5, 46, 79, 80]. The two most common organisms responsible for infections after shoulder surgery are *Propionibacterium acnes and Staphylococci*, which are mainly coagulase negative [81]. A well-fixed humeral component that later becomes loose is considered to be infected until proven otherwise [62].

On plain radiographs, there are some nonspecific findings that are suggestive of infection. These include periosteal reaction, scattered foci of osteolysis, or generalized bone resorption in the absence of implant wear [82]. In fact, in the early stages of infection, plain radiographs may be normal in appearance. Radiographs, however, can be extremely helpful in ruling out other conditions such as dislocation and periprosthetic fractures [83].

The current imaging modality of choice for evaluation of suspected joint replacement infection is radionuclide imaging because it is generally not affected by metallic hardware [84]. Advantages of bone scintigraphy are that it is widely available, relatively inexpensive, and easily performed [85]. In a study of 72 total joint replacements, Levitsky and colleagues [86] showed that bone scintigraphy had a sensitivity of 33 %, a specificity of 86 %, a positive predictive value of 30 %, and a negative predictive value of 88 %. A standard protocol of combined radionuclide imaging has been established to improve specificity. The technetium scan is performed first to reveal all areas of high metabolic activity. Next, indium-111, which targets leukocytes, accumulates in regions of inflammation. Superimposing these results can help distinguish true infection from uninflamed areas of high metabolic activity such as fracture or remodeling [82]. F-fluorodeoxyglucose positron emission tomography (FDG PET) appears to have numerous advantages over conventional radionuclide imaging such as improved spatial resolution within a short time [87]. Unfortunately, data on FDG PET suggest there is no additional benefit over conventional nuclear medicine modalities in diagnosing prosthetic joint infections [88–90]. Therefore, radionuclide imaging should be used as an adjunct to support a diagnosis of infection when serologic findings are abnormal or equivocal [82].

Conclusion

While shoulder arthroplasty is extremely successful in the majority of patients, its estimated 15 % complication rate should raise the examining clinician's suspicion when pain is the chief complaint. Common complications include component loosening, instability, periprosthetic fracture, rotator cuff tear, and infection. Correct diagnosis and ultimately improved patient care depend on a careful history and physical combined with the selection of the imaging modality that will best highlight the pathological change suspected.

References

1. Barrett WP, Thornhill TS, Thomas WH, Gebhart EM, Sledge CB. Nonconstrained total shoulder arthroplasty in patients with polyarticular rheumatoid arthritis. J Arthroplasty. 1989;4(1): 91–6.
2. Barrett WP, Franklin JL, Jackins SE, Wyss CR, Matsen FA. Total shoulder arthroplasty. J Bone Joint Surg Am. 1987;69(6):865–72.
3. Cofield RH. Total shoulder arthroplasty with the Neer prosthesis. J Bone Joint Surg Am. 1984;66(6):899–906.
4. Cofield RH, Edgerton BC. Total shoulder arthroplasty: complications and revision surgery. Instr Course Lect. 1990;39:449–62.
5. Matsen III FA, Rockwood CA, Wirth MA, Lippitt SB. Glenohumeral arthritis and its management. In: Rockwood Jr CA, Matsen 3rd FA, editors. The shoulder, vol. 2. Philadelphia, PA: Elsevier Health Sciences; 2009. p. 840–964.
6. Hasan SS, Leith JM, Campbell B, Kapil R, Smith KL, Matsen FA. Characteristics of unsatisfactory shoulder arthroplasties. J Shoulder Elbow Surg. 2002;11(5):431–41.
7. Brenner BC, Ferlic DC, Clayton ML, Dennis DA. Survivorship of unconstrained total shoulder arthroplasty. J Bone Joint Surg Am. 1989;71(9):1289–96.
8. Bohsali KI, Wirth MA, Rockwood CA. Complications of total shoulder arthroplasty. J Bone Joint Surg Am. 2006;88(10): 2279–92.
9. Kalandiak SP, Wirth MA, Rockwood CA. Complications of shoulder arthroplasty. In: Williams GR, editor. Shoulder and elbow

arthroplasty. Philadelphia, PA: Lippincott Williams & Wilkins; 2005. p. 229–49.

10. Norris TR. Fracture and fracture dislocations of the glenohumeral complex. In: Chapman MW, Madison M, editors. Operative Orthopaedics. Philadelphia, PA: Lippincott Williams & Wilkins; 1993. p. 405–24.

11. Liberson F. The value and limitation of the oblique view as compared with the ordinary anteroposterior exposure of the shoulder: a report of the use of the oblique view in 1800 cases. AJR Am J Roentgenol. 1937;37(4):498–509.

12. Zanca P. Shoulder pain: involvement of the acromioclavicular joint. (Analysis of 1,000 cases). Am J Roentgenol Radium Ther Nucl Med. 1971;112(3):493–506.

13. Castagno AA, Shuman WP, Kilcoyne RF, Haynor DR, Morris ME, Matsen FA. Complex fractures of the proximal humerus: role of CT in treatment. Radiology. 1987;165(3):759–62.

14. Friedman RJ, Hawthorne KB, Genez BM. The use of computerized tomography in the measurement of glenoid version. J Bone Joint Surg Am. 1992;74(7):1032–7.

15. Green A, Green A, Norris TR, Norris TR. Imaging techniques for glenohumeral arthritis and glenohumeral arthroplasty. Clin Orthop Relat Res. 1994;307:7–17.

16. Iannotti JP, Gabriel JP, Schneck SL, Evans BG, Misra S. The normal glenohumeral relationships. An anatomical study of one hundred and forty shoulders. J Bone Joint Surg Am. 1992;74(4):491–500.

17. Figgie HE, Inglis AE, Goldberg VM, Ranawat CS, Figgie MP, Wile JM. An analysis of factors affecting the long-term results of total shoulder arthroplasty in inflammatory arthritis. J Arthroplasty. 1988;3(2):123–30.

18. Deshmukh AV, Koris M, Zurakowski D, Thornhill TS. Total shoulder arthroplasty: long-term survivorship, functional outcome, and quality of life. J Shoulder Elbow Surg. 2005;14(5):471–9.

19. Stewart MP, Kelly IG. Total shoulder replacement in rheumatoid disease: 7- to 13-year follow-up of 37 joints. J Bone Joint Surg Br. 1997;79(1):68–72.

20. Sperling JW, Cofield RH, Rowland CM. Minimum fifteen-year follow-up of Neer hemiarthroplasty and total shoulder arthroplasty in patients aged fifty years or younger. J Shoulder Elbow Surg. 2004;13(6):604–13.

21. Orfaly RM, Rockwood CA, Esenyel CZ, Wirth MA. A prospective functional outcome study of shoulder arthroplasty for osteoarthritis with an intact rotator cuff. J Shoulder Elbow Surg. 2003;12(3): 214–21.

22. Sanchez-Sotelo J, Wright TW, O'Driscoll SW, Cofield RH, Rowland CM. Radiographic assessment of uncemented humeral components in total shoulder arthroplasty. J Arthroplasty. 2001; 16(2):180–7.

23. Mileti J, Boardman ND, Sperling JW, et al. Radiographic analysis of polyethylene glenoid components using modern cementing techniques. J Shoulder Elbow Surg. 2004;13(5):492–8.

24. Klepps S, Chiang AS, Miller S, Jiang CY, Hazrati Y, Flatow EL. Incidence of early radiolucent glenoid lines in patients having total shoulder replacements. Clin Orthop Relat Res. 2005;435:118–25.

25. Franklin JL, Barrett WP, Jackins SE, Matsen FA. Glenoid loosening in total shoulder arthroplasty. Association with rotator cuff deficiency. J Arthroplasty. 1988;3(1):39–46.

26. Lazarus MD, Jensen KL, Southworth C, Matsen FA. The radiographic evaluation of keeled and pegged glenoid component insertion. J Bone Joint Surg Am. 2002;84-A(7):1174–82.

27. Amstutz HC, Thomas BJ, Kabo JM, Jinnah RH, Dorey FJ. The Dana total shoulder arthroplasty. J Bone Joint Surg Am. 1988; 70(8):1174–82.

28. Boyd AD, Thomas WH, Scott RD, Sledge CB, Thornhill TS. Total shoulder arthroplasty versus hemiarthroplasty. Indications for glenoid resurfacing. J Arthroplasty. 1990;5(4):329–36.

29. Torchia ME, Cofield RH, Settergren CR. Total shoulder arthroplasty with the Neer prosthesis: long-term results. J Shoulder Elbow Surg. 1997;6(6):495–505.

30. Skirving AP. Total shoulder arthroplasty—current problems and possible solutions. J Orthop Sci. 1999;4(1):42–53.

31. Nagels J, Valstar ER, Stokdijk M, Rozing PM. Patterns of loosening of the glenoid component. J Bone Joint Surg Br. 2002;84(1): 83–7.

32. Boileau P, Watkinson DJ, Hatzidakis AM, Balg F. Grammont reverse prosthesis: design, rationale, and biomechanics. J Shoulder Elbow Surg. 2005;14(1 Suppl S):147S–61.

33. Werner CML, Steinmann PA, Gilbart M, Gerber C. Treatment of painful pseudoparesis due to irreparable rotator cuff dysfunction with the Delta III reverse-ball-and-socket total shoulder prosthesis. J Bone Joint Surg Am. 2005;87(7):1476–86.

34. Sirveaux F, Favard L, Oudet D. Grammont inverted total shoulder arthroplasty in the treatment of glenohumeral osteoarthritis with massive rupture of the cuff. Results of a multicentre study of 80 Shoulders. J Bone Joint Surg Am. 2004;86(3):388–95.

35. Grassi FA, Murena L, Valli F, Alberio R. Six-year experience with the Delta III reverse shoulder prosthesis. J Orthop Surg (Hong Kong). 2009;17(2):151–6.

36. John M, Pap G, Angst F, et al. Short-term results after reversed shoulder arthroplasty (Delta III) in patients with rheumatoid arthritis and irreparable rotator cuff tear. Int Orthop. 2010;34(1):71–7.

37. Farshad M, Gerber C. Reverse total shoulder arthroplasty-from the most to the least common complication. Int Orthop. 2010;34(8): 1075–82.

38. Vanhove B, Beugnies A. Grammont's reverse shoulder prosthesis for rotator cuff arthropathy. A retrospective study of 32 cases. Acta Orthop Belg. 2004;70(3):219–25.

39. Levigne C, Garret J, Boileau P, Alami G, Favard L, Walch G. Scapular notching in reverse shoulder arthroplasty: is it important to avoid it and how? Clin Orthop Relat Res. 2011;469(9):2512–20.

40. Nyffeler RW, Werner C, Gerber C. Biomechanical relevance of glenoid component positioning in the reverse Delta III total shoulder prosthesis. J Shoulder Elbow Surg. 2005;14(5):524–8.

41. Levy JC, Virani N, Pupello D, Frankle M. Use of the reverse shoulder prosthesis for the treatment of failed hemiarthroplasty in patients with glenohumeral arthritis and rotator cuff deficiency. J Bone Joint Surg Br. 2007;89(2):189–95.

42. Cuff D, Pupello D, Virani N, Levy J, Frankle M. Reverse shoulder arthroplasty for the treatment of rotator cuff deficiency. J Bone Joint Surg Am. 2008;90(6):1244–51.

43. Kalouche I, Sevivas N, Wahegaonker A, Sauzieres P, Katz D, Valenti P. Reverse shoulder arthroplasty: does reduced medialisation improve radiological and clinical results? Acta Orthop Belg. 2009;75(2):158–66.

44. Merolla G, Di Pietto F, Romano S, Paladini P, Campi F, Porcellini G. Radiographic analysis of shoulder anatomical arthroplasty. Eur J Radiol. 2008;68(1):159–69.

45. Sperling JW, Cofield RH, O'Driscoll SW, Torchia ME, Rowland CM. Radiographic assessment of ingrowth total shoulder arthroplasty. J Shoulder Elbow Surg. 2000;9(6):507–13.

46. Wirth MA, Rockwood CA. Complications of total shoulder-replacement arthroplasty. J Bone Joint Surg Am. 1996;78(4):603–16.

47. Sperling JW, Cofield RH, Rowland CM. Neer hemiarthroplasty and Neer total shoulder arthroplasty in patients fifty years old or less. Long-term results. J Bone Joint Surg Am. 1998;80(4):464–73.

48. Neer CS. Replacement arthroplasty for glenohumeral osteoarthritis. J Bone Joint Surg Am. 1974;56(1):1–13.

49. Jahnke AH, Hawkins RJ. Instability after shoulder arthroplasty: causative factors and treatment options. Semin Arthroplasty. 1995;6(4):289–96.

50. Brems JJ. Complications of shoulder arthroplasty: infections, instability, and loosening. Instr Course Lect. 2002;51:29–39.

51. Gartsman GM, Russell JA, Gaenslen E. Modular shoulder arthroplasty. J Shoulder Elbow Surg. 1997;6(4):333–9.
52. Hawkins RJ, Bell RH, Jallay B. Total shoulder arthroplasty. Clin Orthop Relat Res. 1989;242:188–94.
53. Middleton WD, Reinus WR, Totty WG, Melson CL, Murphy WA. Ultrasonographic evaluation of the rotator cuff and biceps tendon. J Bone Joint Surg Am. 1986;68(3):440–50.
54. Hennigan SP, Iannotti JP. Instability after prosthetic arthroplasty of the shoulder. Orthop Clin North Am. 2001;32(4):649–59, ix.
55. Stefko JM, Jobe FW, VanderWilde RS, Carden E, Pink M. Electromyographic and nerve block analysis of the subscapularis liftoff test. J Shoulder Elbow Surg. 1997;6(4):347–55.
56. Armstrong A, Lashgari C, Teefey S, Menendez J, Yamaguchi K, Galatz LM. Ultrasound evaluation and clinical correlation of subscapularis repair after total shoulder arthroplasty. J Shoulder Elbow Surg. 2006;15(5):541–8.
57. Sofka CM, Adler RS. Original report. Sonographic evaluation of shoulder arthroplasty. AJR Am J Roentgenol. 2003;180(4):1117–20.
58. Warren RF, Coleman SH, Dines JS. Instability after arthroplasty: the shoulder. J Arthroplasty. 2002;17(4 Suppl 1):28–31.
59. Moeckel BH, Altchek DW, Warren RF, Wickiewicz TL, Dines DM. Instability of the shoulder after arthroplasty. J Bone Joint Surg Am. 1993;75(4):492–7.
60. Kumar S, Sperling JW, Haidukewych GH, Cofield RH. Periprosthetic humeral fractures after shoulder arthroplasty. J Bone Joint Surg Am. 2004;86-A(4):680–9.
61. Wright TW, Cofield RH. Humeral fractures after shoulder arthroplasty. J Bone Joint Surg Am. 1995;77(9):1340–6.
62. Sperling JW, Hawkins RJ, Walch G, Mahoney AP, Zuckerman JD. Complications in total shoulder arthroplasty. Instr Course Lect. 2013;62:135–41.
63. Sperling JW, Potter HG, Craig EV, Flatow E, Warren RF. Magnetic resonance imaging of painful shoulder arthroplasty. J Shoulder Elbow Surg. 2002;11(4):315–21.
64. Potter HG, Foo LF. Magnetic resonance imaging of joint arthroplasty. Orthop Clin North Am. 2006;37(3):361–73, vi–vii.
65. Hayter CL, Koff MF, Shah P, Koch KM, Miller TT, Potter HG. MRI after arthroplasty: comparison of MAVRIC and conventional fast spin-echo techniques. AJR Am J Roentgenol. 2011;197(3):W405–11.
66. Koch KM, Lorbiecki JE, Hinks RS, King KF. A multispectral three-dimensional acquisition technique for imaging near metal implants. Magn Reson Med. 2009;61(2):381–90.
67. Koch KM, Brau AC, Chen W, et al. Imaging near metal with a MAVRIC-SEMAC hybrid. Magn Reson Med. 2011;65(1):71–82.
68. Westhoff B, Wild A, Werner A, Schneider T, Kahl V, Krauspe R. The value of ultrasound after shoulder arthroplasty. Skeletal Radiol. 2002;31(12):695–701.
69. Rupp S, Seil R, Kohn D. [Significance of the hypoechoic area around the long biceps tendon in shoulder sonography—underlying pathology]. Z Orthop Ihre Grenzgeb. 1999;137(1):7–9.
70. McMenamin D, Koulouris G, Morrison WB. Imaging of the shoulder after surgery. Eur J Radiol. 2008;68(1):106–19.
71. Buckwalter KA. CT Arthrography. Clin Sports Med. 2006;25(4):899–915.
72. de Jesus JO, Parker L, Frangos AJ, Nazarian LN. Accuracy of MRI, MR arthrography, and ultrasound in the diagnosis of rotator cuff

73. Cody DD. AAPM/RSNA physics tutorial for residents: topics in CT. Image processing in CT. Radiographics. 2002;22(5):1255–68.
74. Woertler K. Multimodality imaging of the postoperative shoulder. Eur Radiol. 2007;17(12):3038–55.
75. Lee M-J, Kim S, Lee S-A, et al. Overcoming artifacts from metallic orthopedic implants at high-field-strength MR imaging and multidetector CT1. Radiographics. 2007;27(3):791–803.
76. Fayad LM, Johnson P, Fishman EK. Multidetector CT of musculoskeletal disease in the pediatric patient: principles, techniques, and clinical applications. Radiographics. 2005;25(3):603–18.
77. Fritz J, Fishman EK, Small KM, et al. MDCT arthrography of the shoulder with datasets of isotropic resolution: indications, technique, and applications. AJR Am J Roentgenol. 2012;198(3):635–46.
78. De Filippo M, Bertellini A, Sverzellati N, et al. Multidetector computed tomography arthrography of the shoulder: diagnostic accuracy and indications. Acta Radiol. 2008;49(5):540–9.
79. Wolfe SW, Figgie MP, Inglis AE, Bohn WW, Ranawat CS. Management of infection about total elbow prostheses. J Bone Joint Surg Am. 1990;72(2):198–212.
80. Yamaguchi K, Adams RA, Morrey BF. Infection after total elbow arthroplasty. J Bone Joint Surg Am. 1998;80(4):481–91.
81. Dodson CC, Thomas A, Dines JS, Nho SJ, Williams RJ, Altchek DW. Medial ulnar collateral ligament reconstruction of the elbow in throwing athletes. Am J Sports Med. 2006;34(12):1926–32.
82. Bauer TW. Diagnosis of periprosthetic infection. J Bone Joint Surg Am. 2006;88(4):869.
83. Palestro CJ, Love C, Miller TT. Infection and musculoskeletal conditions: imaging of musculoskeletal infections. Best Pract Res Clin Rheumatol. 2006;20(6):1197–218.
84. Love C, Marwin SE, Palestro CJ. Nuclear medicine and the infected joint replacement. Semin Nucl Med. 2009;39(1):66–78.
85. Gemmel F, Wyngaert H, Love C, Welling MM, Gemmel P, Palestro CJ. Prosthetic joint infections: radionuclide state-of-the-art imaging. Eur J Nucl Med Mol Imaging. 2012;39(5):892–909.
86. Levitsky KA, Hozack WJ, Balderston RA, et al. Evaluation of the painful prosthetic joint. Relative value of bone scan, sedimentation rate, and joint aspiration. J Arthroplasty. 1991;6(3):237–44.
87. de Winter F, van de Wiele C, Vogelaers D, de Smet K, Verdonk R, Dierckx RA. Fluorine-18 fluorodeoxyglucose-position emission tomography: a highly accurate imaging modality for the diagnosis of chronic musculoskeletal infections. J Bone Joint Surg Am. 2001;83-A(5):651–60.
88. Love C, Marwin SE, Tomas MB, et al. Diagnosing infection in the failed joint replacement: a comparison of coincidence detection 18F-FDG and 111In-labeled leukocyte/99mTc-sulfur colloid marrow imaging. J Nucl Med. 2004;45(11):1864–71.
89. Zhuang H, Duarte PS, Pourdehnad M, et al. The promising role of 18F-FDG PET in detecting infected lower limb prosthesis implants. J Nucl Med. 2001;42(1):44–8.
90. Kwee TC, Kwee RM, Alavi A. FDG-PET for diagnosing prosthetic joint infection: systematic review and metaanalysis. Eur J Nucl Med Mol Imaging. 2008;35(11):2122–32.

tears: a meta-analysis. AJR Am J Roentgenol. 2009;192(6):1701–7.

Part III

The Elbow

Section Editors: Larry D. Field, Michael J. O'Brien, and Felix H. Savoie III

Diagnostic Elbow Arthroscopy and Arthroscopic Anatomy

20

Benjamin S. Miller and E. Rhett Hobgood

Introduction

The arthroscope has proven itself to be the ideal tool for evaluation and treatment of intra-articular pathology about the elbow. Elbow arthroscopy has become useful for the removal of loose bodies [1–7], synovectomy [8, 9], lysis of adhesions [10, 11], excision of osteophytes [12, 13], debridement of osteochondritis dissecans lesions [5, 14–16], radial head resection [17], plica excision [18, 19], instability [20], septic arthritis [21], and diagnostic arthroscopy for complex elbow pain [5].

Advances in elbow arthroscopy have enabled surgeons to treat a broad spectrum of disorders that were once thought to be unsafe through arthroscopic techniques. Although technically demanding, recent advances in surgical technique, arthroscopic equipment, and an improved understanding of neurovascular and joint anatomy have made this procedure safer and more effective. More recently, indications have been expanded to include autograft replacement for osteochondritis dissecans, treatment of lateral epicondylitis, and reduction and fixation of fractures of the radial head, capitellum, and distal humerus. Elbow arthroscopy can also be useful in the treatment of posterolateral instability [22].

The potential advantages of treating elbow pathology arthroscopically include reducing iatrogenic insult by decreasing incision size, a more thorough evaluation of the intra-articular compartments of the elbow, and possibly reducing scarring and potential stiffness due to limited disruption of the capsule. The disadvantages center squarely on the technical requirements needed to safely and effectively perform the procedure due to the close proximity of neurovascular structures. Understanding of the anatomy of the

elbow as well as the principles and techniques of elbow arthroscopy allows a surgeon to perform these procedures safely and effectively.

Anatomy

Prior to performing arthroscopic surgery of the elbow, a thorough understanding of the relevant anatomy must be obtained. Superficial landmarks can be palpated and marked for reference during surgery [23]. Starting posteriorly, the triceps tendon and olecranon can be palpated. Moving medially, the ulnar nerve should be palpated in the groove along the posterior aspect of the medial epicondyle. Flexing and extending the arm while palpating the ulnar groove is important to recognize whether the nerve subluxes out of the groove. A subluxable ulnar nerve is present in 16 % of the population [24]. Marking the course of the ulnar nerve is imperative to be reminded of the location of the nerve during arthroscopy. Laterally, the lateral epicondyle, radial head, and tip of the olecranon form a triangle marking the boundaries of the "soft spot" of the elbow.

Superficial nervous structures include the medial and lateral antebrachial cutaneous nerves. The lateral antebrachial cutaneous nerve, the termination of the musculocutaneous nerve, emerges from the distal portion of the biceps and travels laterally across the brachioradialis muscle proximal to the antecubital fossa. As it turns laterally, it branches and provides sensation for the lateral aspect of the forearm. The medial antebrachial cutaneous nerve travels along the medial arm with the basilic vein. It branches well proximal to the elbow joint and provides sensation to the medial aspect of the forearm. Damage to superficial nerves can be avoided by incising skin only and using blunt trocars [25].

The deeper neurovascular structures include the median, radial, and ulnar nerves and the brachial artery. The brachial artery emerges between the brachialis and biceps muscles lateral to the median nerve. It travels just medial to the biceps tendon and deep to the biceps aponeurosis. It bifurcates just

B.S. Miller, MD (✉) • E.R. Hobgood, MD
Mississippi Sports Medicine and Orthopedic Center, Jackson, MS, USA
e-mail: Benjimiller7@gmail.com; rhetthobgood@msmoc.com

S.F. Brockmeier (ed.), *MRI-Arthroscopy Correlations: A Case-Based Atlas of the Knee, Shoulder, Elbow and Hip*,
DOI 10.1007/978-1-4939-2645-9_20, © Springer Science+Business Media New York 2015

distal to the joint at the level of the radial head. The median nerve travels along with the brachial artery along the anterior surface of the brachialis muscle. As it crosses the elbow joint, it is just medial to the brachial artery. As it enters the forearm, it courses just deep to the pronator teres but superficial to the deep head of the pronator. The ulnar nerve travels posterior to the medial intermuscular septum. At the level of the elbow, it courses posterior to the medial epicondyle and can often be palpated in this area. As it enters the forearm, the ulnar nerve travels between the flexor digitorum superficialis and the flexor digitorum profundus. The radial nerve curves posteriorly around the humerus and penetrates the lateral intermuscular septum well proximal to the elbow joint. It then travels between the brachialis and brachioradialis muscles. It branches into the superficial radial nerve and posterior interosseous nerve just proximal to the elbow joint. The superficial radial nerve passes into the forearm just deep to the brachioradialis. The posterior interosseous nerve continues distally and courses into the supinator muscle while curving around the lateral aspect of the radial head.

Arthroscopy Basics

Patient Positioning

Supine

Once the patient is positioned supine on the operating table, the operative extremity is lateralized on the operating table so that the shoulder is placed at the edge of the bed. The operative extremity is placed in 90° of shoulder abduction, 90° of elbow flexion, and neutral forearm rotation, and a non-sterile arm tourniquet is applied. The arm is suspended as illustrated in Fig. 20.1. The supine position offers the advantage of conversion to an open procedure if necessary and provides quick access to the patient's airway. Disadvantages of the supine position include the necessity of a suspension setup and the inability to easily visualize and work in the posterior compartment. Another disadvantage is that the arm is not rigidly stabilized in this suspended manner and requires an assistant to provide stability during the procedure (Fig. 20.1).

Prone

The prone position is an additional method of positioning. The greatest benefit of the prone positioning is the excellent access to the posterior compartment of the elbow. Direct visualization of the ulnohumeral joint from posterior is helpful for debridement of excess bone in cases of posterior impingement. The face and chest are padded and supported by a foam airway/head positioner and padded chest rolls. The nonoperative extremity is positioned in 90° of shoulder abduction and external rotation with the elbow in 90° of flexion.

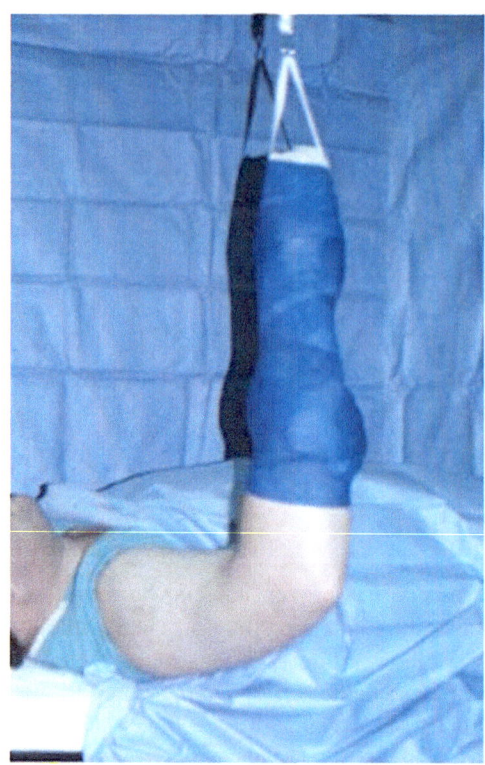

Fig. 20.1 Clinical photo of supine positioning of the arm in suspension for elbow arthroscopy

Often a special arm holder is used to optimize positioning of the operative arm. A non-sterile arm tourniquet is applied, and the arm is place in 90° of shoulder abduction and neutral rotation. The arm is supported at the mid-humeral level by a padded arm holder attached to the operating table allowing for flexion and extension of the arm during arthroscopy (Fig. 20.2a, b).

In the prone position, several advantages are realized. The elbow is easily manipulated from flexion to full extension. The posterior compartment of the elbow is easily accessible for numerous procedures directed by posterior pathology. Open procedures are easily performed if necessary. If the surgeon chooses to perform an open procedure, no change in positioning is needed for posterior procedures. Medial or lateral procedures can be carried out in the prone position by internally or externally rotating the shoulder and supporting the arm on a padded arm board (Figs. 20.3 and 20.4). Drawbacks of the prone position primarily relate to patient positioning, ventilation, and anesthetic options. It is imperative to support the head and face with foam padding to secure the airway, and chest rolls are needed to facilitate ventilation. Regional anesthesia is poorly tolerated and may not provide adequate anesthesia thus necessitating conversion to general anesthesia. In such cases, repositioning is necessary to establish an airway.

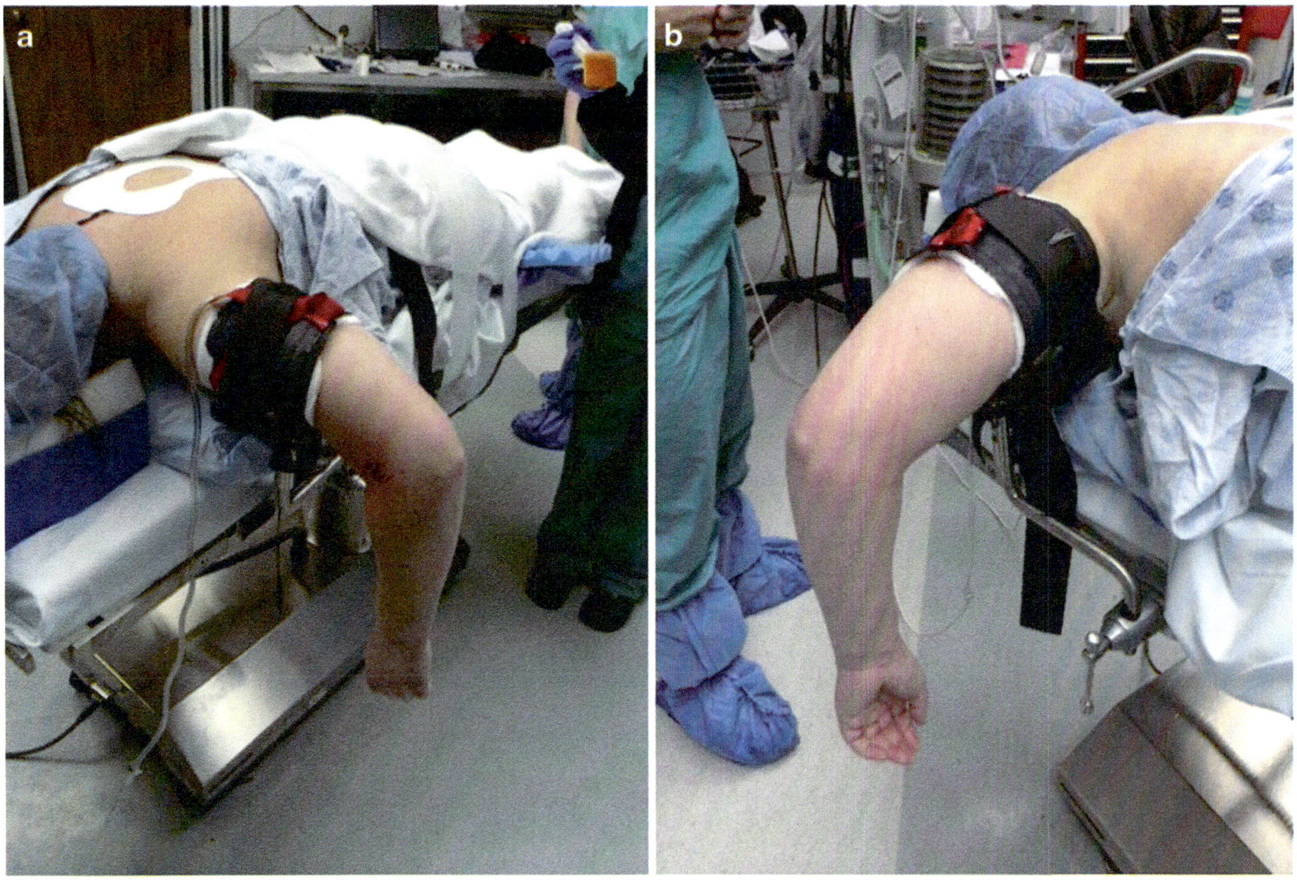

Fig. 20.2 (**a, b**) Author's preferred setup for elbow arthroscopy in prone position with arm holder under mid-humerus giving plenty of room for range of motion during procedure

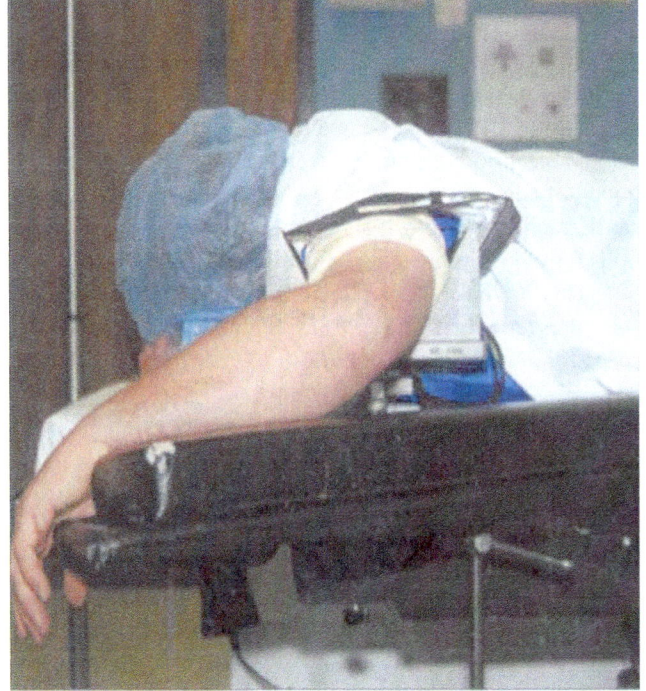

Fig. 20.3 Clinical photo shown demonstrating the ability to externally rotate the shoulder and support the forearm on the arm board in prone position for an open lateral approach to the elbow

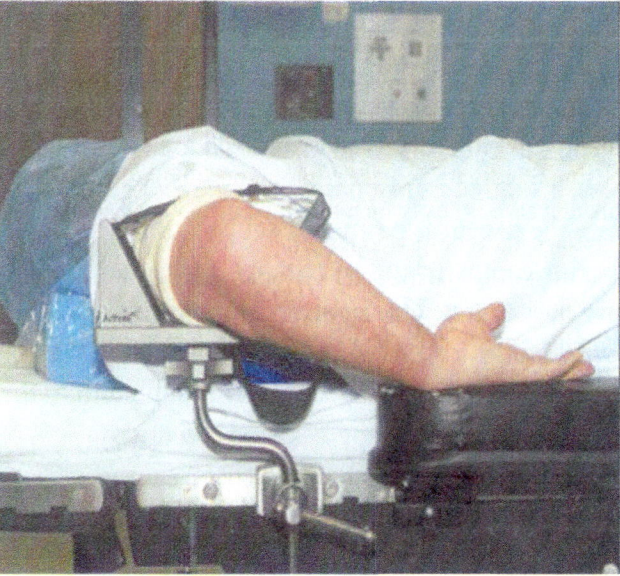

Fig. 20.4 Clinical photo demonstrating the ability to internally rotate the shoulder and rest the forearm on an arm board to gain access to the medial elbow for an open procedure

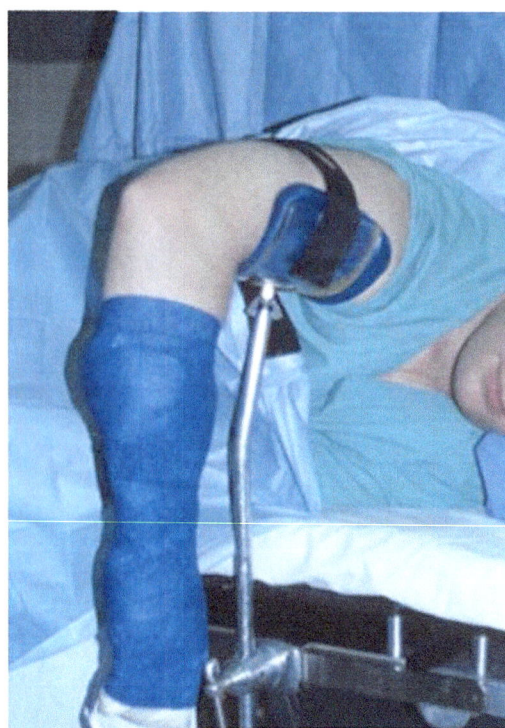

Fig. 20.5 Lateral positioning of the arm in elbow arthroscopy (used with permission from Baker CL, Grant LJ. Arthroscopy of the elbow. Am J Sports Med. 1999;27:251–64)

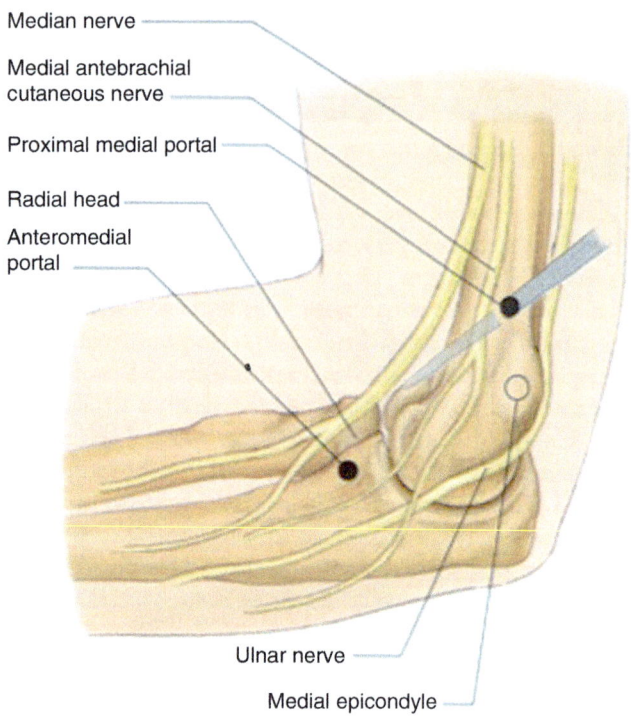

Median nerve

Medial antebrachial cutaneous nerve

Proximal medial portal

Radial head

Anteromedial portal

Ulnar nerve

Medial epicondyle

Medial view

Fig. 20.6 The medial elbow with anteromedial and proximal antero-medial portals shown. The ulnar, median, and medial antebrachial nerves are all in close proximity to these portals as described above. Note that the proximal anteromedial portal is at increased distance from the median nerve as compared to the anteromedial portal (used with permission from Cole BJ, Sekiya JK. Surgical techniques of the shoulder, elbow, and knee in sports medicine. Philadelphia: Elsevier Saunders; 2008)

Lateral Decubitus

The aim of this position is to take advantage of the benefits of both the supine and prone position while avoiding the major pitfalls inherent to each setup. A beanbag is used to place the patient in the lateral decubitus position. An axillary roll is appropriately placed. The operative extremity is positioned over an arm holder or over a padded bolster with the shoulder internally rotated and flexed to 90°. The elbow is maintained in 90° of flexion (Fig. 20.5).

The elbow is maintained in the prone position thus affording the advantages of the prone position. Patient positioning is simplified with respect to prone positioning, and airway maintenance is easily monitored with adequate exposure for the anesthesiologist. Disadvantages include the need for a padded bolster and the potential inconvenience of repositioning should a need for an open procedure arise.

Portal Placement

A thorough understanding of the bony and neurovascular anatomy around the elbow is necessary prior to proceeding with elbow arthroscopy. After adequate positioning, prepping, and draping, the landmarks about the elbow should be palpated and marked with a sterile marker. The medial and lateral epicondyles, the olecranon, and radial head should be marked. Care should also be taken to palpate the ulnar nerve in its groove. It should be noted if the nerve is subluxed or subluxable prior to portal placement as this could lead to injury of the nerve. Its course should be marked with the sterile marker as well. It should also be noted that all positions for elbow arthroscopy allow for flexion of the elbow at 90°. This is vital because flexion moves the neurovascular structures anteriorly further from the joint and provides more space for portal placement [26].

Proximal Anteromedial Portal (Figs. 20.6 and 20.7)

The proximal anteromedial portal is made 2 cm proximal to the medial epicondyle and 1–2 cm anterior to the intermuscular septum. A nick in the skin is made, and the blunt tip trocar is advanced to the anterior surface of the humerus. The trocar is kept in contact with the anterior cortex and then slid distally to the elbow joint. This technique keeps the trocar posterior to the brachialis muscle therefore protecting the median nerve and brachial artery. Blunt dissection stays anterior to the medial intermuscular septum and thus anterior to the ulnar

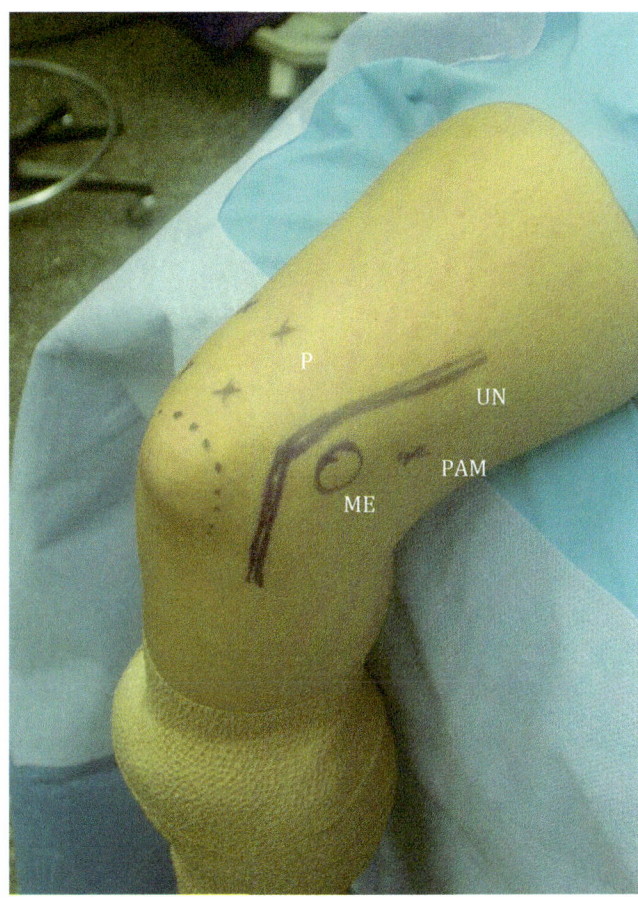

Fig. 20.7 Operative view of the medial elbow. *P* posterior portal, *PAM* proximal anteromedial portal, *UN* ulnar nerve, *ME* medial epicondyle (used with permission from Baker CL, Grant LJ. Arthroscopy of the elbow. Am J Sports Med. 1999;27:251–64)

nerve. Structures at risk during creation of this portal are the medial antebrachial cutaneous, median, and ulnar nerves. The medial antebrachial cutaneous nerve is at risk as it courses approximately 2.3 mm from the portal site. The median nerve is at risk as the trocar is advanced distally between the humerus and brachialis muscle. The average distance from the median nerve to the trocar tip is 12.4–22 mm [22, 27].

Relative contraindications to the creation of this portal include ulnar nerve subluxation or previous ulnar nerve transposition [22, 27, 28]. In the case of prior ulnar nerve transposition, this portal can be utilized if care is taken to identify the course of the nerve with dissection prior to trocar placement. In the absence of ulnar nerve subluxation or history of transposition, the ulnar nerve is located between 12 and 23.7 mm from the portal site and is hence not at risk so long as the trocar entry site is placed anterior to the intermuscular septum [22, 27].

This portal is easily reproducible and provides visualization of the entire anterior compartment from the medial to the lateral gutter. As such, it serves well as the initial portal in elbow arthroscopy.

Anteromedial Portal (Figs. 20.6 and 20.7)

This portal is placed 1–2 cm anterior and 2 cm distal to the medial epicondyle [29]. A nick in the skin is made, and the blunt tip trocar is advanced through the flexor mass aiming for the radial head taking care to stay between the humerus and the brachialis. With the trocar anterior to the medial epicondyle and the ulnar nerve in its normal anatomic position, the ulnar nerve should not be at risk. The greatest risk is to the medial antebrachial cutaneous which passes 1–2 mm from the portal site [22]. Risk of injury can be minimized by incising skin only and using the blunt trocar for the subcutaneous dissection [25, 27]. The median nerve travels approximately 7–14 mm away from the portal site and is at less risk of injury if the surgeon maintains dissection posterior to brachialis [22, 30]. The standard anteromedial portal is therefore almost twice as close to the median nerve as the proximal anteromedial portal determined by the difference between the anatomical measurements mentioned above, 7–14 mm away from the portal in standard anteromedial portal versus 12–23.7 mm away from the portal in the proximal anteromedial portal. The proximal anteromedial portal presents a safer alternative to standard anteromedial portal therefore minimizing the risk of a devastating median nerve injury.

Proximal Anterolateral Portal (Fig. 20.8)

The proximal anterolateral portal in addition to the proximal anteromedial portal can also be used as a starting portal [9, 31, 32]. It is established 2 cm proximal and 2 cm anterior to the lateral epicondyle. This portal was developed as an alternative to the standard anterolateral portal, due to the portal providing greater safe distance from the radial nerve [22, 31]. Anatomic studies with the elbow in 90° of flexion and distended with fluid at the time of proximal anterolateral portal creation reveal a safe distance between 9.9 and 14.2 mm between the trocar and radial nerve [22, 31]. This distance is markedly decreased to 4.9–9.1 mm when the standard anterolateral portal is created [22, 31]. The lateral antebrachial cutaneous nerve passes 6 mm from this portal site [22].

As the trocar is advanced distally, toward the elbow joint, the brachioradialis and brachialis muscle are pierced prior to entering the lateral joint capsule. With the arthroscope placed into the cannula, the anterior capsule, lateral gutter, radial head, capitellum, coronoid, and anterolateral aspect of the ulnohumeral articulation can be visualized. It is believed by some authors that the proximal anterolateral portal provides improved visualization of the lateral aspect of the joint [31].

Anterolateral Portal (Fig. 20.8)

The anterolateral portal was originally described as being made 1 cm anterior and 3 cm distal to the lateral epicondyle [18]. As the blunt trocar is introduced, it passes through the extensor carpi radialis brevis muscle before traversing the lateral joint capsule. This portal position is limited in its

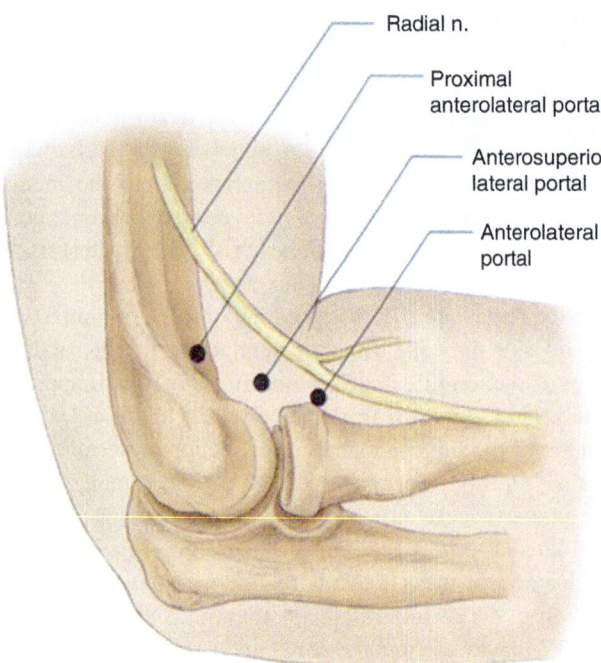

Fig. 20.8 Lateral view of the elbow with anterolateral and proximal anterolateral portals shown. Note that the proximal anterolateral portal is at increased distance from the radial nerve as compared to the anterolateral portal (used with permission from Cole BJ, Sekiya JK. Surgical techniques of the shoulder, elbow, and knee in sports medicine. Philadelphia: Elsevier Saunders; 2008)

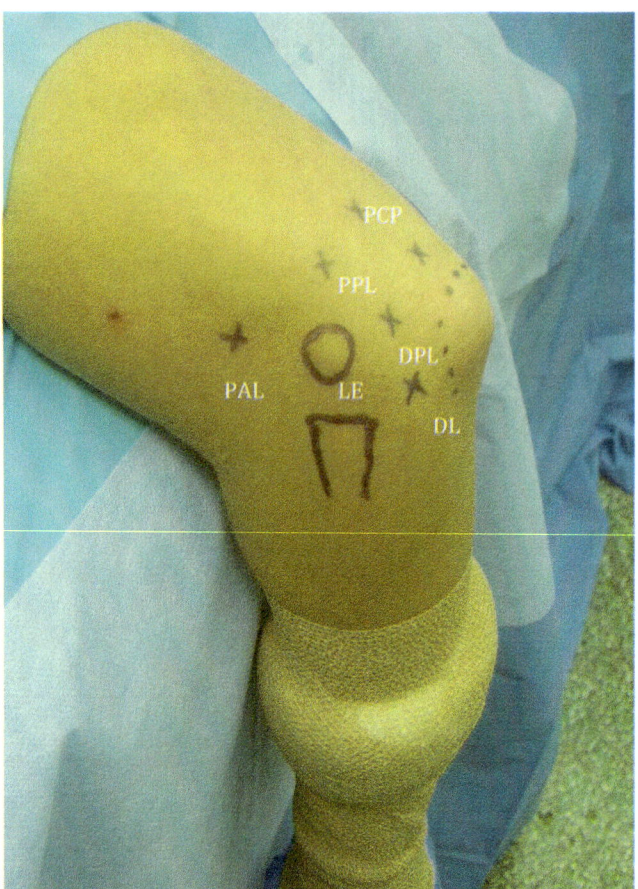

Fig. 20.9 Operative view of the lateral elbow. *PCP* proximal central posterior portal, *PPL* proximal posterolateral portal, *DPL* distal posterolateral portal, *DL* direct lateral portal, *PAL* proximal anterolateral portal, *LE* lateral epicondyle

capabilities with respect to the lateral joint. However, it permits visualization of the anteromedial aspect of the joint including the trochlea, coronoid fossa, coronoid process, and medial aspect of the radial head [31]. Care must be taken not to place the portal distal to the radial head, as the posterior interosseous nerve courses 1–1.5 cm from the radial head around the radial neck. Furthermore, care should be taken not to make the portal distal to the radial head as this can endanger the radial nerve. The radial nerve passes 5–9 mm from this portal site [22, 27, 28].

An inside-out technique allows the arthroscope in the anteromedial or proximal anteromedial portal to be advanced over the radial head and pressed firmly against the joint capsule lateral to the radial head. The camera is exchanged in the cannula for a switching stick which is advanced through the extensor carpi radialis brevis until it tents the skin. Incision is made over the switching stick, and cannula is inserted over the switching stick. This portal provides good access to the radial head and allows visualization of the annular ligament.

Direct Lateral Portal (Figs. 20.9, 20.10, and 20.11)

Also known as the soft spot portal, this portal is often used for the initial insufflation of the joint with an 18-gauge needle. It is found in the soft spot in the triangle marked by the lateral epicondyle, radial head, and tip of the olecranon.

This portal is fairly safe with regard to neurologic structures with the sole risk being injury to the posterior antebrachial cutaneous nerve which courses approximately 7 mm away [33]. The biggest risks of this portal are the risk of fluid extravasation into the soft tissues and postoperative portal drainage [22, 23, 28].

When establishing this portal, the trocar is advanced through the anconeus muscle, and entry to the lateral elbow joint is attained through the posterior elbow capsule. Visualization of the radioulnar joint and inferior aspect of the radial head and capitellum can be achieved through this portal site. In addition, this portal provides a safe entry site for instrumentation of the radiocapitellar joint and lateral gutter. Due to the risk of soft tissue extravasation, it is advisable to delay making this portal until near the end of the operation.

Posterior Portals (Figs. 20.12 and 20.13)

Multiple posterior portals can be established based on the pathology. These include the proximal and distal central posterior portals as well as the proximal and distal posterolateral portals. The distal central posterior portal is made in

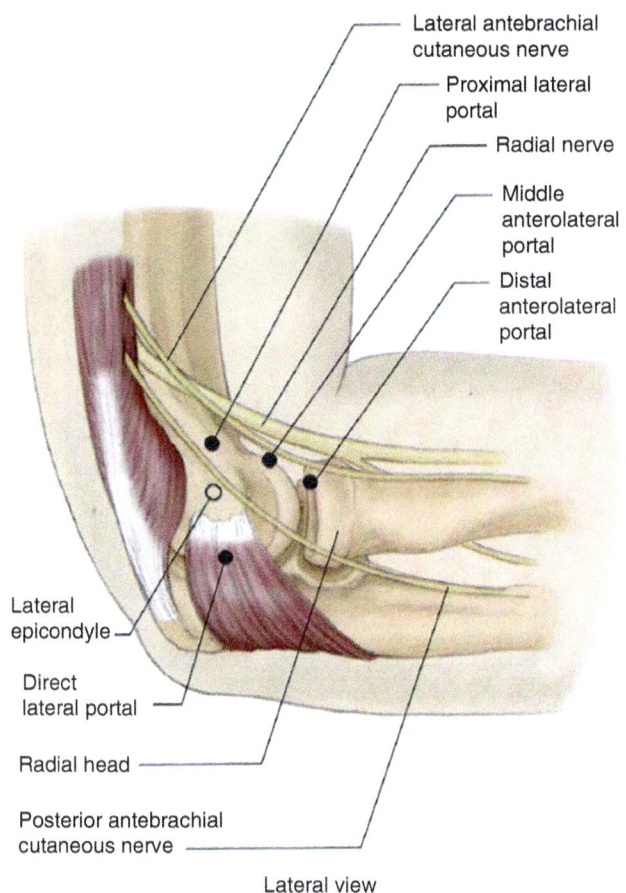

Lateral view

Fig. 20.10 Schematic of lateral view of the elbow with the direct lateral portal shown which is located in the soft spot marked by the lateral epicondyle, radial head, and tip of the olecranon (used with permission from Cole BJ, Sekiya JK. Surgical techniques of the shoulder, elbow, and knee in sports medicine. Philadelphia: Elsevier Saunders; 2008)

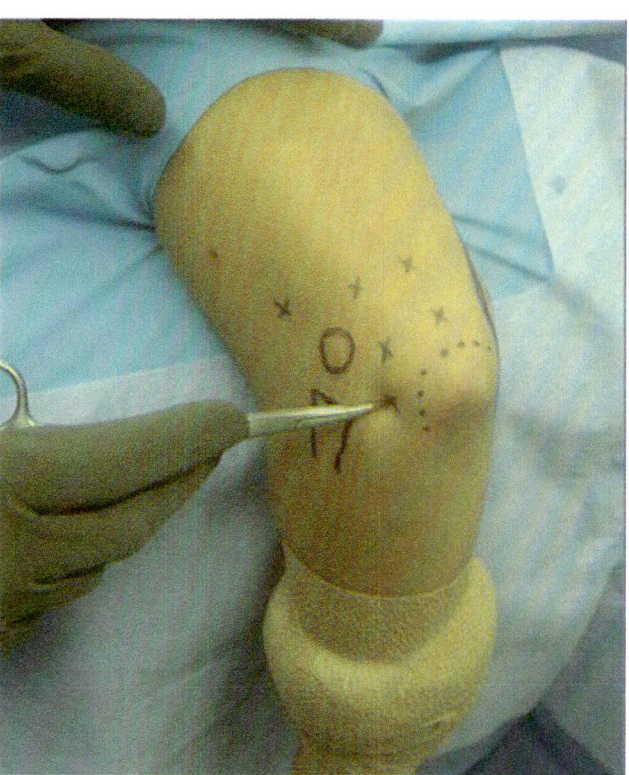

Fig. 20.11 Operative view of the lateral elbow. Instrument pointing to the lateral soft spot and location of the direct lateral portal (used with permission from Baker CL, Grant LJ. Arthroscopy of the elbow. Am J Sports Med. 1999;27:251–64)

the midline, 3 cm proximal to the olecranon tip, through the triceps tendon [23, 34]. Additionally a more proximal central posterior portal can be made 1–2 cm proximal to the distal central posterior portal (4–5 cm proximal to the olecranon tip). The skin is incised, and a blunt trocar is then inserted into the olecranon fossa. The joint capsule is very close to the joint in this position with the elbow flexed. Therefore, it is helpful to have an inflow cannula already placed in one of the anterior portals to allow for maximal joint distension. Furthermore, after the trocar is inserted, the edge of the cannula needs to be advanced down to the bone. It often helps to turn the cannula while advancing, using the tip like a cutting tool to help penetrate the capsule in this region. If the trocar is removed without cannula advancement, the tip of the cannula will still be outside the joint capsule due to the length of the trocar tip. Adequate placement can be confirmed by the return of fluid out of the cannula with removal of the trocar. Care should be taken when visualizing or working in the medial gutter as the ulnar nerve lies just superficial to the joint capsule in this region. These portals provide visualization of

the posterior aspect of the ulnohumeral joint, the olecranon fossa, and the medial and lateral gutters [35]. Several common procedures can be performed through the portal sites including the removal of olecranon spurs and loose bodies and contouring or humeral fenestration of the olecranon fossa for ulnohumeral arthroplasty [28, 35].

The proximal and distal posterolateral portals are very similar to and are often used interchangeably with the central posterior portals. The distal posterolateral portal is made 3 cm proximal to the tip of the olecranon, just lateral to the triceps tendon. The proximal posterolateral portal is made 4–5 cm from the tip of the olecranon, just lateral to the triceps tendon. The trocar is advanced toward the olecranon fossa, and advancement of the cannula through the capsule must be carried out as previously described. However, when making this portal, it is sometimes helpful to bring the elbow to 45° of flexion in order to relax the triceps and posterior capsule [22]. These portals also offer visualization of the ulnohumeral joint as well as the medial and lateral gutters. From this position, the arthroscope can often be advanced into the lateral gutter in order to visualize the radiocapitellar joint and posterior aspect of the radial head. Again, care must be taken to avoid injury to the ulnar nerve when instrumenting the medial gutter as it transverses

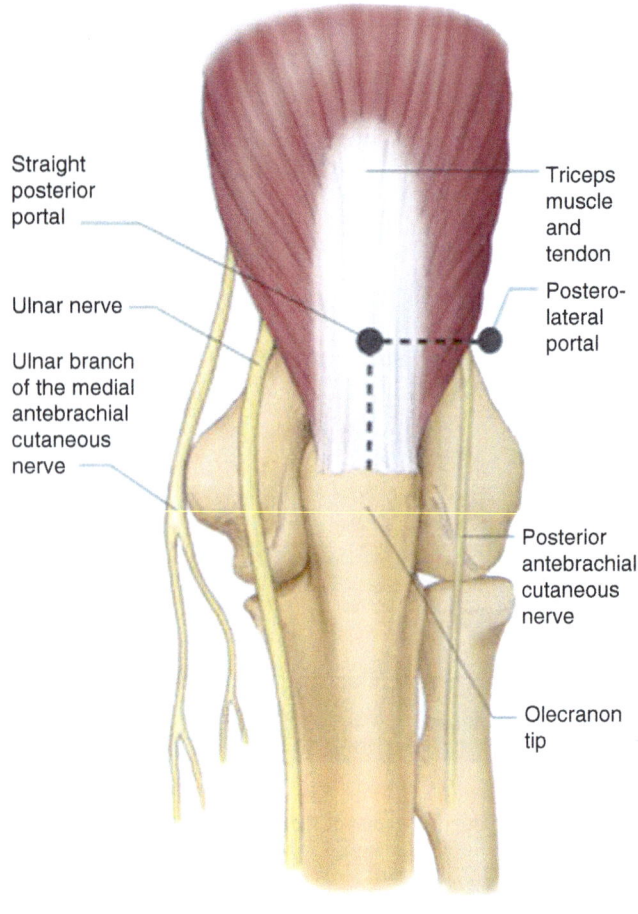

Posterior view

Fig. 20.12 Schematic of the posterior elbow with the distal central posterior portal (named in this figure as straight posterior) and distal posterolateral portal shown (used with permission from Cole BJ, Sekiya JK. Surgical techniques of the shoulder, elbow, and knee in sports medicine. Philadelphia: Elsevier Saunders; 2008)

obliquely just superficial to the medial capsule of the elbow [35] (Fig. 20.13).

The purpose of this chapter is to emphasize the arthroscopic anatomy to allow for safe portal placement to enable the surgeon to safely and effectively perform elbow arthroscopy. The following two case examples illustrate a proper portal placement and diagnostic arthroscopy of the elbow.

Case 1

A 53-year-old female complains of pain in her left elbow. She is left-hand dominant. In the past, she was an intercollegiate softball player. Her main complaint is pain at terminal flexion and extension. The pain interferes with her daily activities now and prevents her from being active in her recreational softball league. She takes anti-inflammatories daily and now gets no pain relief from medications.

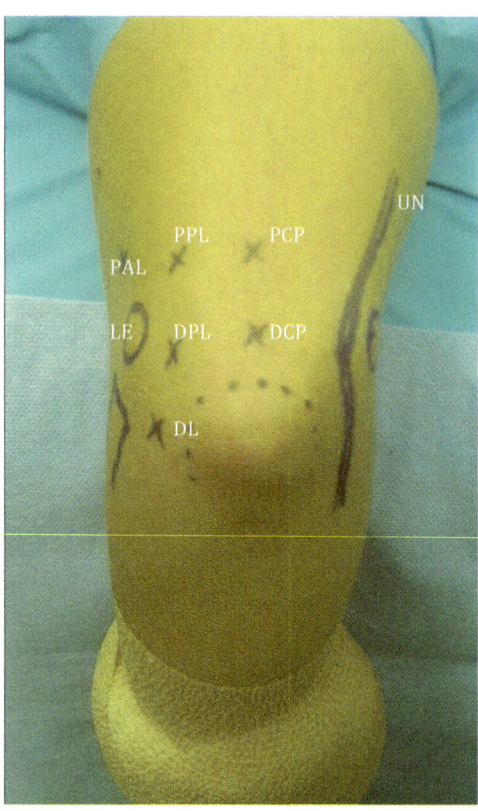

Fig. 20.13 Operative image of the posterior of the elbow showing portals including proximal and distal straight posterior portals and the proximal and distal posterolateral portals. *PCP* proximal central posterior portal, *DCP* distal central posterior portal, *PPL* proximal posterolateral portal, *DPL* distal posterolateral portal, *DL* direct lateral portal, *PAL* proximal anterolateral portal, *LE* lateral epicondyle, *UN* ulnar nerve

Physical Exam

Left upper extremity: The left elbow active and passive range of motion is −30° of extension to 130° of flexion. She has pain at the end point of extension and flexion of her elbow. She has full forearm supination and pronation equal to the right upper extremity. The left elbow is stable to varus and valgus stress. She has crepitus throughout the elbow range of motion. Neurovascular exam in the left upper extremity is unremarkable.

Imaging

Radiographs (Figs. 20.14 and 20.15): Views of the left elbow include AP and lateral views, which reveal osteophyte formation of the olecranon tip and anterior process of coronoid.

MRI (Figs. 20.16, 20.17, and 20.18): Images demonstrate pathology in the elbow of the patient. Figure 20.16 demonstrates a sagittal view of the elbow with osteophytes seen posterior along the olecranon and olecranon fossa as well as

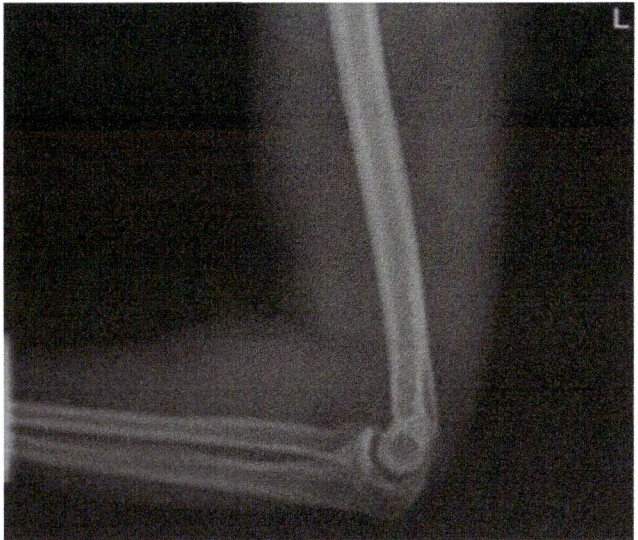

Fig. 20.14 Lateral radiograph of the left elbow

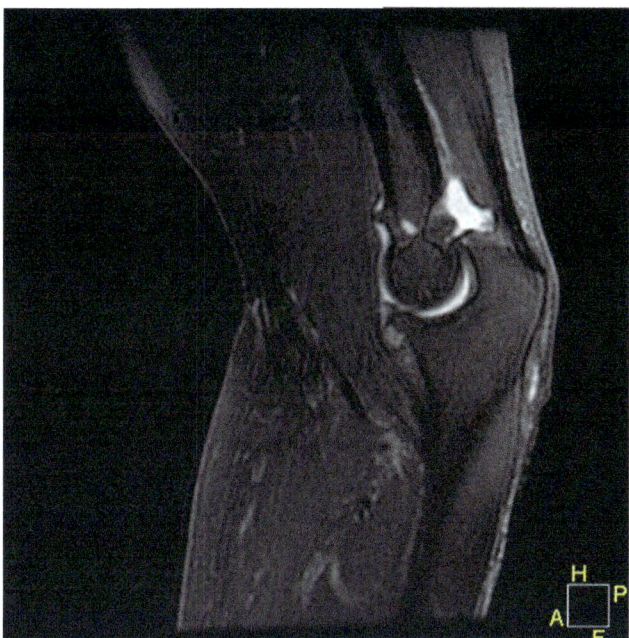

Fig. 20.16 Sagittal T2 MRI image demonstrating osteophyte formation posteriorly around the olecranon fossa, on the tip of the olecranon, and anteriorly around the coronoid tip and coronoid fossa

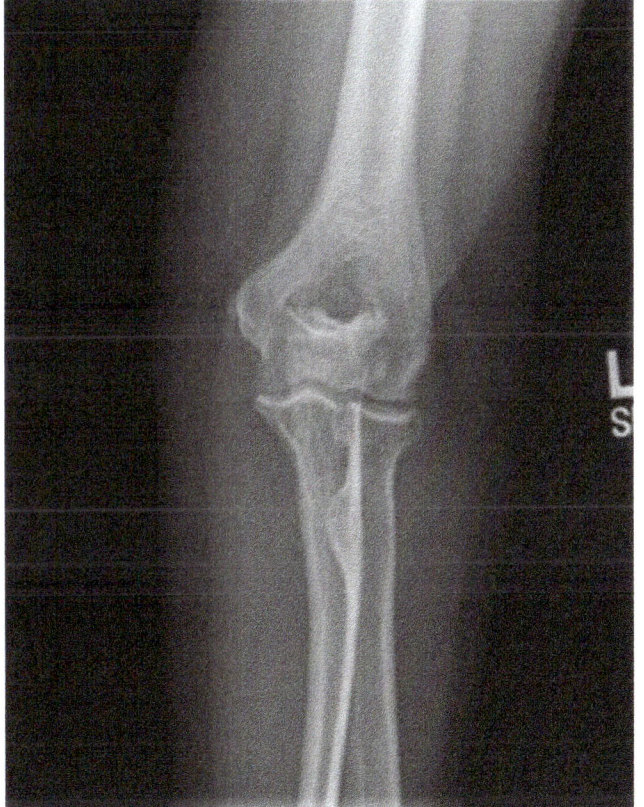

Fig. 20.15 AP radiograph of the left elbow

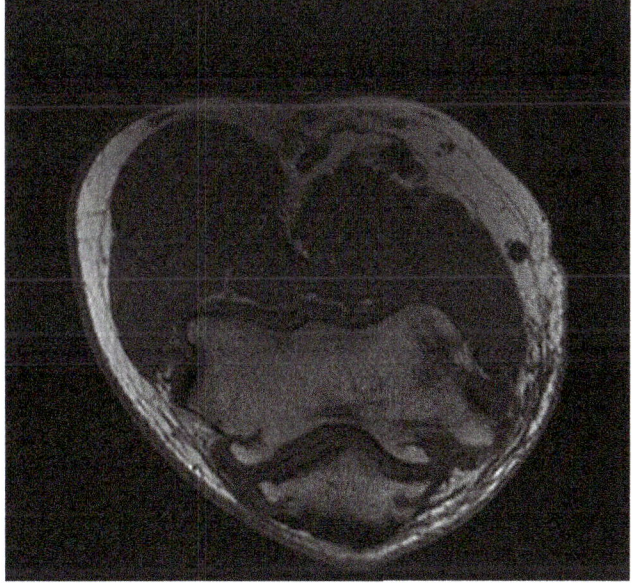

Fig. 20.17 Axial T1 MRI image demonstrating osteophytes along the articulation of the olecranon posteriorly and the olecranon fossa more anterior

anteriorly in the coronoid fossa which causes decreased range of motion in our physical exam. Figures 20.17 and 20.18 are both axial MRI image T1 sequence and T2 sequence, respectively. The images both demonstrate osteophytes seen along the olecranon fossa in addition to osteophytes lining the olecranon.

After the patient had failed conservative treatment, risks and benefits of the procedure of elbow arthroscopy with extensive debridement was discussed with the patient. She elected to proceed with elbow arthroscopy.

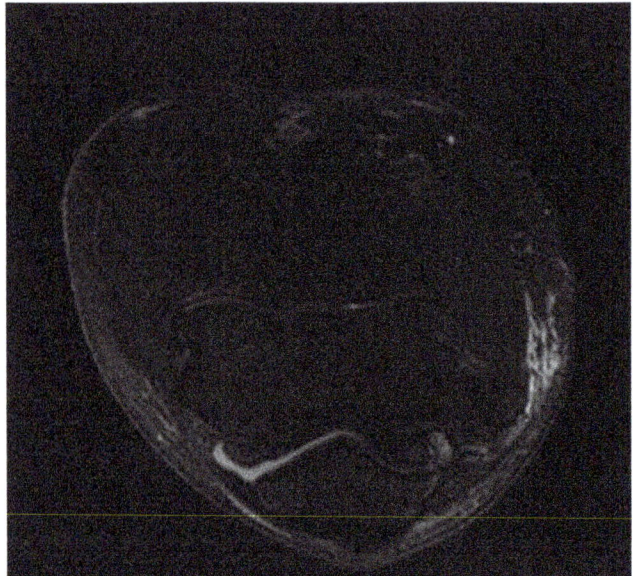

Fig. 20.18 Axial T2 MRI again demonstrating osteophytes lining the olecranon fossa with corresponding osteophytes along the periphery of the olecranon

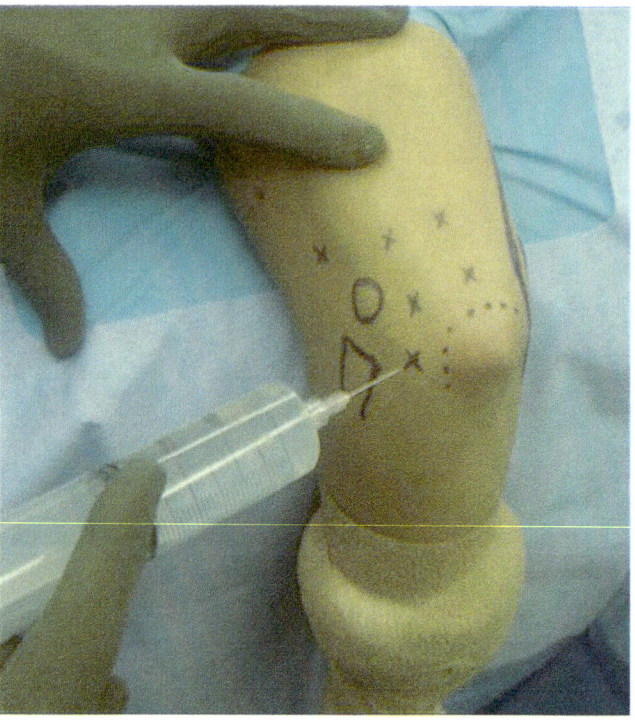

Fig. 20.19 Operative image shown with syringe injecting saline into the straight lateral portal in the soft spot

Surgical Technique

After prone positioning, a tourniquet is placed on the upper arm taking care to place tourniquet proximal enough to ensure exposure for portal placement after draping. A non-sterile upper arm tourniquet is applied. An arm holder is attached to the operating table, which supports the arm at mid-humerus (Figs. 20.2a, b and 20.5). A Chloraprep™ (CareFusion, San Diego, CA) solution is used to prep the arm and forearm. An impervious, sterile stockinet is applied to the hand and covered with self-adherent Coban™ (3M, St. Paul, MN) to seal the hand and forearm contents from the operative field. Standard sterile draping is conducted followed by exsanguination of the limb with an esmarch bandage. The tourniquet is inflated. After prepping and draping, bony landmarks are marked with a sterile marker. Also, the ulnar nerve is palpated and marked in the ulnar groove. The ulnar nerve is evaluated for subluxation. An 18-guage spinal needle is introduced into the straight lateral portal site, and the joint is insufflated with 20–30 cm^3 of sterile saline until resistance is felt (Fig. 20.19).

The proximal anteromedial portal (Figs. 20.4 and 20.6) site is established; the portal is placed 2 cm proximal to the medial epicondyle and 1–2 cm anterior to the intermuscular septum [18]. A blunt trocar with 4.5 mm metal cannula is introduced through a nick made in the skin with a No. 11 blade knife and advanced distally toward the radiocapitellar joint. The trocar is advanced palpating the intermuscular septum to ensure the surgeon is anterior to this structure. Next, the trocar is advanced to make contact with the anterior

aspect of the humerus. Palpation of the anterior humerus while advancing ensures protection of the anterior neurovascular structures, by the brachialis muscle. An egress of fluid with trocar removal confirms intra-articular placement. The 30° 4.0 mm arthroscope is introduced, and a diagnostic arthroscopy of the anterior compartment ensues.

The proximal anteromedial portal, if appropriately placed, permits a systematic evaluation of the medial gutter, trochlea, coronoid process, anterior capsule, capitellum, radial head, and lateral gutter. The radiocapitellar joint is assessed for instability and articular cartilage damage with pronation and supination aiding the evaluation. Next, the 30° arthroscope lens is rotated to facilitate evaluation of the anterior capsule and extensor carpi radialis brevis tendon insertion. The coronoid and trochlea are then evaluated by withdrawing the scope and repositioning the lens of the arthroscope.

Next, the surgeon establishes a proximal anterolateral portal. An "outside-in" technique is used for starting this portal which includes advancing a spinal needle bat the site described for this portal: 2 cm proximal to the lateral epicondyle and 2 cm anteriorly. The spinal needle is removed, and a No. 11 blade knife is used to incise the skin only. A blunt trocar and cannula are inserted into the elbow while maintaining constant contact with the anterior humeral cortex as the trocar is advanced. An alternative method of starting the anterolateral portal is by placing a switching stick within the anteromedial cannula and advancing through the joint and

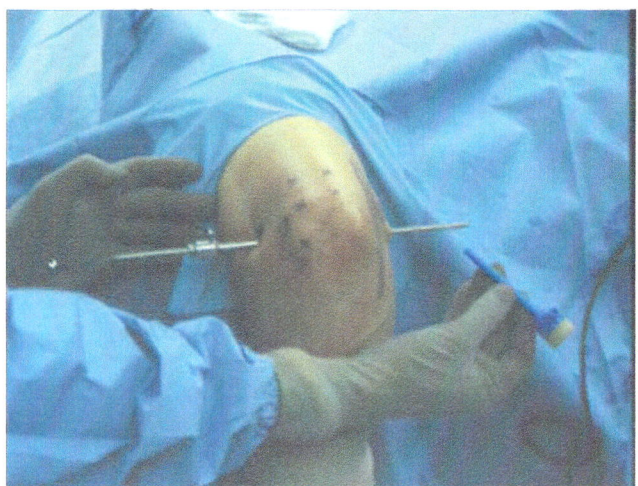

Fig. 20.20 Operative image showing the technique of placing switching stick within the cannula and advancing through the joint and piercing musculature until it is tenting the skin. When it can be palpated subcutaneously, make a small incision over the top of the switching stick. Advance switching stick out the newly made portal and place a cannula over the switching stick. The switching stick can now be removed while the arthroscope is placed in the new cannula

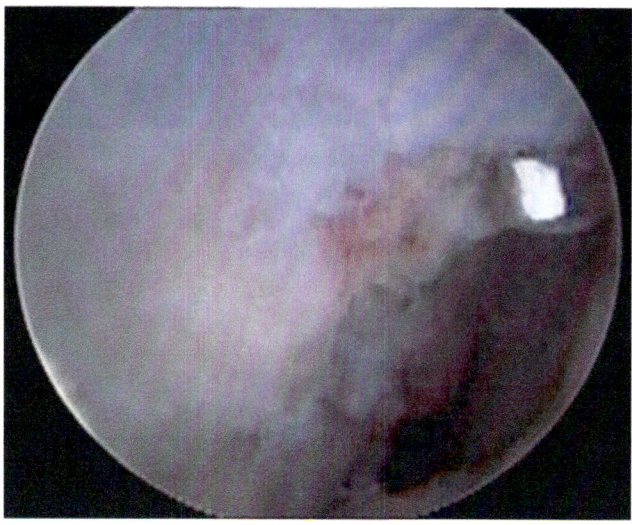

Fig. 20.21 Arthroscopic photo viewing in the anterior compartment demonstrating the removal of the anterior humeral osteophyte in the center of the screen with burr

piercing musculature until it is tenting the skin on the lateral side and placing a cannula over the switching stick (Fig. 20.20). The switching stick can now be removed while being replaced by the arthroscope. The diagnostic arthroscopy ensues with the camera in the proximal anterolateral portal including a systematic evaluation of the lateral gutter, radial head, capitellum, anterior capsule, trochlea, coronoid process, and medial gutter as discussed above.

Arthroscopy of the anterior compartment can also begin from the proximal anterolateral portal. Starting in the proximal anterolateral portal requires starting the portal with an "outside-in" technique as directed in the above discussion of the proximal anterolateral portal. Diagnostic arthroscopy can be pursued from the lateral side of the elbow progressing medially. The proximal anteromedial portal is most safely made by inserting a switching stick into the proximal anterolateral portal and advancing across the joint penetrating capsule and tinting skin in the appropriate area for the proximal anteromedial portal as discussed above. Use a knife to make a small incision over the switching stick advancing the switching stick forward. Insert a cannula over the switching stick to begin working from the portal.

Once the proximal anterior portals are established, diagnostic arthroscopy confirmed the patient to have a large osteophyte on the coronoid tip as well as a corresponding osteophyte on the distal humerus. A burr was then inserted through the anterolateral portal and was used to remove the osteophytes from the anterior humerus and the coronoid tip (Fig. 20.21). This completed the work in the anterior compartment.

Leaving the inflow in the proximal anteromedial portal for insufflation, the distal posterolateral portal was established. When the arthroscope is introduced, the olecranon fossa will come into view. Turning the angle of the scope to look inferiorly will bring the tip of the olecranon into view. The fossa and olecranon were both found to have large osteophytes. The elbow was extended to bring the olecranon tip into contact with the fossa which demonstrated impingement resulting in the decreased range of motion the patient was experiencing clinically. The ulnohumeral articulation can be followed medial into the medial gutter. Care should be taken when instrumenting the medial gutter, as the ulnar nerve lies immediately superficial to the joint capsule in this area. The arthroscope can be retracted back to the olecranon fossa, and then, once again following the ulnohumeral articulation, the lateral gutter can be inspected. The arthroscope can be advanced into the lateral gutter, and the angle of the scope can be rotated to look laterally. In doing so, this will bring the radiocapitellar joint into view showing the posterior aspect of the radial head. The patient demonstrated pathology related to the osteophytes causing impingement posteriorly.

After diagnostic arthroscopy of the posterior compartment, a proximal central posterior portal was established under spinal needle localization. This portal allowed excellent visualization of the olecranon osteophyte. Likewise, an inspection of the olecranon fossa is important to remove any potential osteophytes in the fossa, which may be impeding motion. Due the large size of the osteophyte, the decision was made to perform the excision with a small osteotome. A distal posterolateral portal was established by an "outside-in" technique to aide in excising the osteophyte. The osteotome was introduced through the distal posterolateral portal and viewed from the proximal central posterior portal. After excision of the osteophyte with the osteotome back to the native olecranon, the pieces of bone were removed with an arthroscopic grasper. Last, the burr was used to delicately complete the excision of the osteophyte and to remove a shallow layer of osteophytes from the olecranon fossa. Viewing from the proximal central posterior portal, medial and lateral gutters were again viewed to confirm there were no remaining bony fragments. By extending the elbow under direct visualization from either the distal posterolateral or proximal central posterior portals, the surgeon can confirm full extension has been gained.

Intraoperative fluoroscopy was used at the end of the arthroscopy in flexion and extension to confirm excision of the anterior and posterior osteophytes.

Case 2

A 34-year-old gentleman presented to the clinic for evaluation of his left elbow. He is left-hand dominant. He had a previous history of an elbow dislocation when he was 17. He does not complain of instability, but he does complain of catching and locking while he is performing jujitsu.

Physical Exam

The elbow active and passive range of motion is −10° of extension to 130° flexion. With repeated range of motion, a mechanical block is experienced intermittently, and the patient experiences a loss of extension at −45°. The patient has full supination and pronation, which is equal to the right extremity. The left elbow was stable to varus and valgus stress. Stability tests including a lateral pivot shift test and moving valgus stress test were negative. He has crepitus throughout the range of motion. Neurovascular exam of the left upper extremity is unremarkable.

Imaging

Radiographs (Figs. 20.22 and 20.23): AP/lateral radiographs of the left elbow demonstrate multiple loose bodies and osteophytes lining the olecranon as well as the coronoid and anterior humerus.

CT scan (Figs. 20.24 and 20.25): A CT scan was obtained to outline the specific bony anatomy and visualize extent of osteophytes for arthroscopic planning. Selected images from the CT scan show multiple large intra-articular loose osteochondral fragments with osteophytes and arthrosis along bony surfaces. Figure 20.24 is a sagittal reconstruction of left elbow CT scan demonstrating significant bony impingement

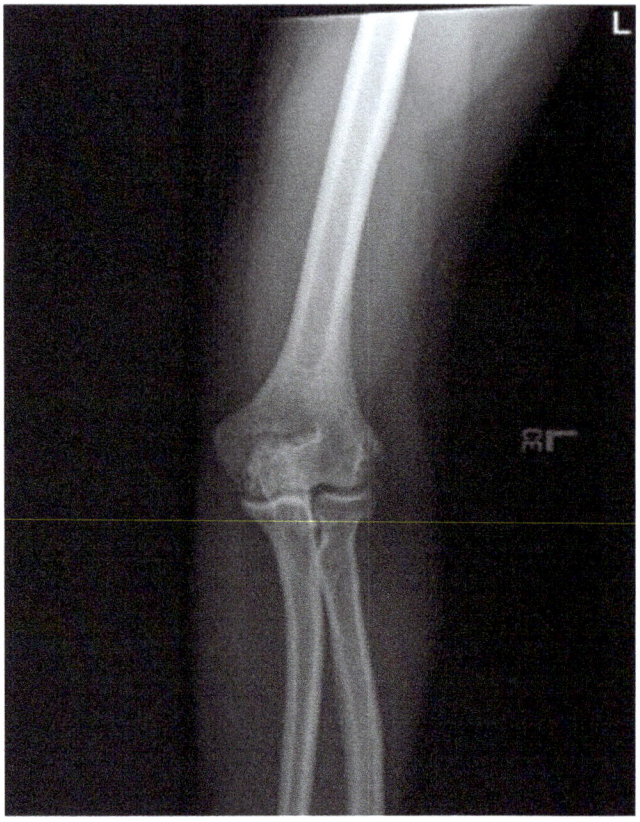

Fig. 20.22 AP radiograph of the left elbow

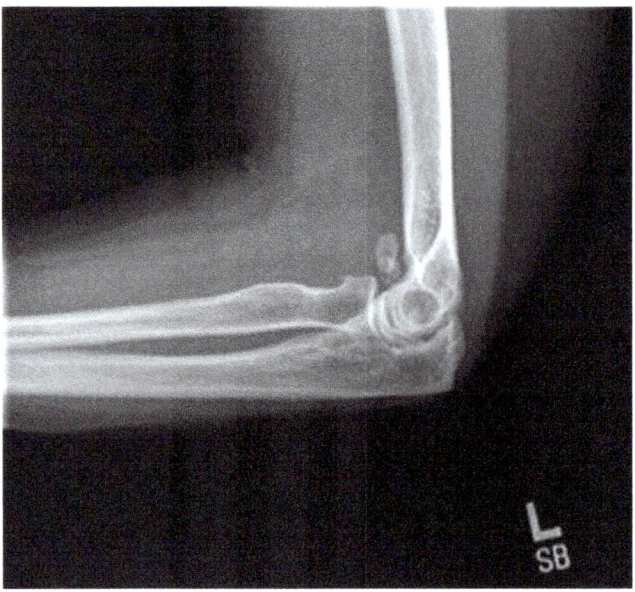

Fig. 20.23 Lateral radiograph of the left elbow

from olecranon osteophyte as well as a loose body visualized posterior to the olecranon tip. Figure 20.25 is a 3-D reconstruction image, which shows many loose bodies and osteophytes along the articular margin of the olecranon as well as the proximal ulna, radial head, and humerus.

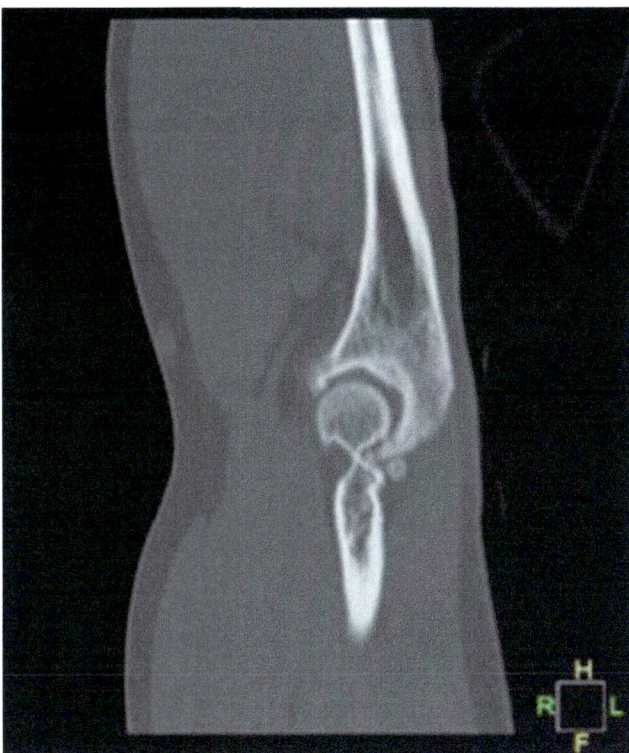

Fig. 20.24 Representative image selected from CT scan

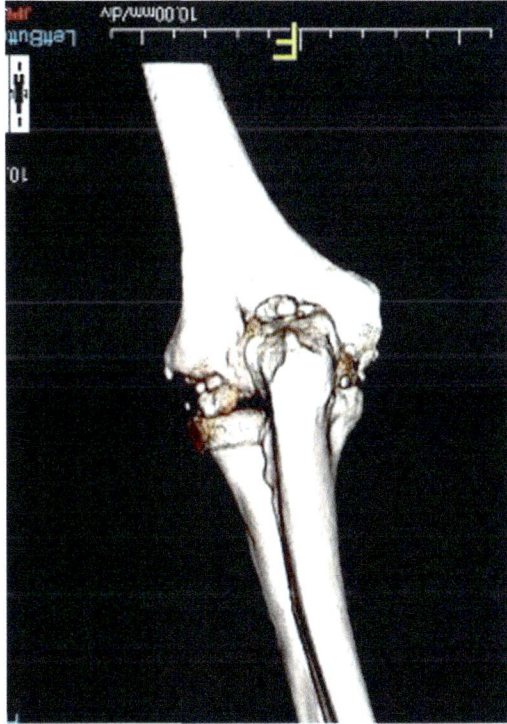

Fig. 20.25 3-D reconstruction from left elbow CT scan

The patient failed all conservative treatment and requested arthroscopic surgery to remove loose bodies and also removal of osteophytes.

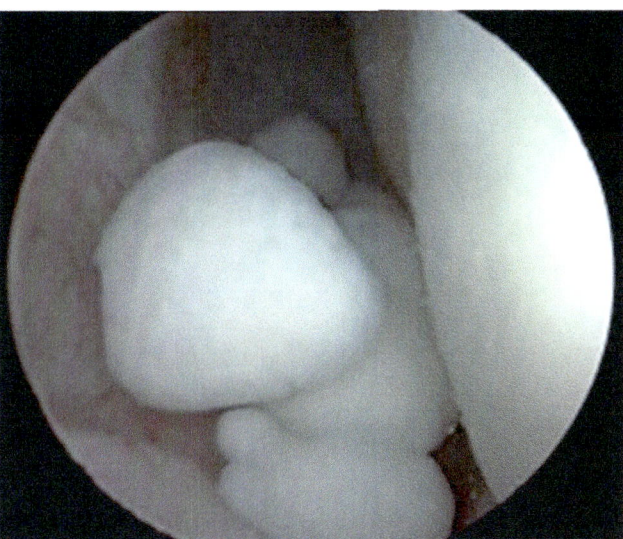

Fig. 20.26 Multiple large loose osteochondral loose bodies are visualized in the anterior compartment of the elbow

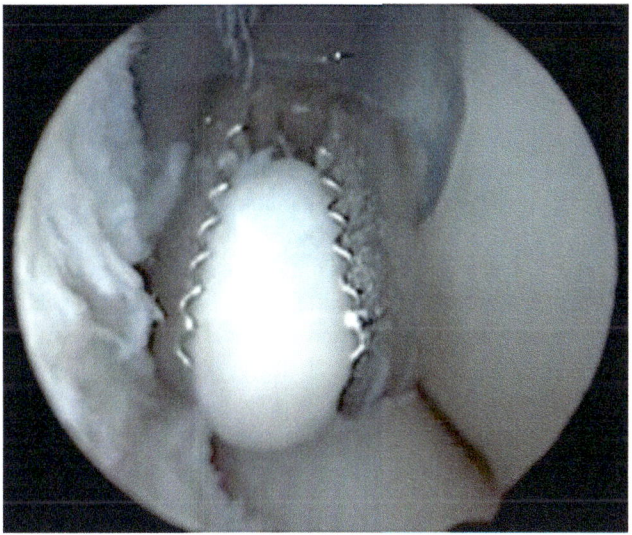

Fig. 20.27 A grasper is utilized for the removal of a large loose body from the anterior compartment of the elbow

Surgical Technique

The patient was prepared for surgery and in the prone position and setup for arthroscopy as described above. Arthroscopy began by making the proximal anteromedial portal as described above with an "outside-in" approach. Once the proximal anteromedial portal was established, a diagnostic arthroscopy ensued as described above viewing from medial to lateral. Large loose bodies were visualized in the anterior compartment as shown in the clinical photo in Fig. 20.26. Next, a proximal anterolateral portal was established by an "outside-in" approach with a spinal needle. A grasper is introduced through the proximal anterolateral portal and used to remove loose bodies as shown in Fig. 20.27.

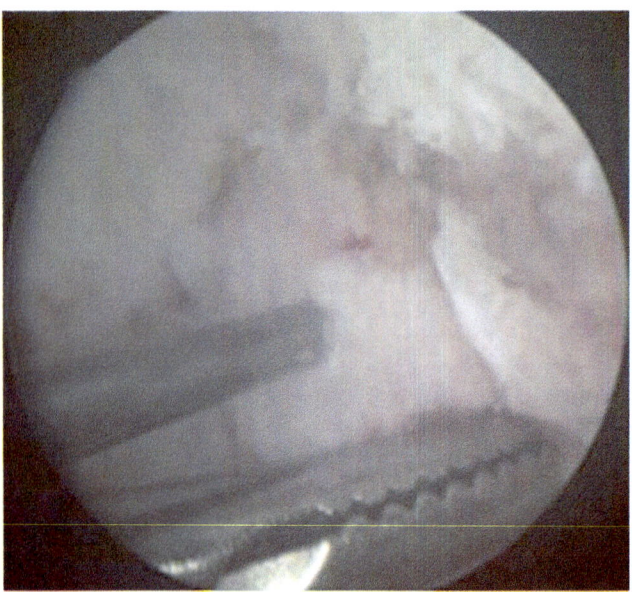

Fig. 20.28 A spinal needle can be used to skewer a large loose body in the posterior compartment of the elbow to facilitate retrieval with a grasper

Should the size of the osteochondral fragment or loose body exceed that of the cannula, it may necessitate piecemeal removal or the use of a motorized shaver. In certain cases, the grasper can be used to pull the cannula and fragment through the soft tissue. This can be accomplished by rotating the grasper as it is removed from the soft tissues while maintaining firm grasp on the fragment. Alternatively, a spinal needle may be needed to skewer and stabilize the loose body for retrieval with a grasper (Fig. 20.28).

After removal of loose bodies, osteophytes were removed from the anterior humerus and coronoid tip with high-speed burr. The elbow was then flexed until the coronoid made contact with the anterior humerus to confirm appropriate removal of osteophytes. With completion of the anterior compartment arthroscopy, the inflow was maintained in the proximal anteromedial portal, and posterior compartment arthroscopy began by making a distal posterolateral portal. With the arthroscope in the distal posterolateral portal, a diagnostic arthroscopy was performed. A large osteophyte on the olecranon process impeded extension. The osteophyte was excised with the combination of high-speed burr and small osteotome. Osteophyte formation in the olecranon fossa was also excised with the use of high-speed burr. Extension of the elbow was confirmed to be restored.

Conclusion

Elbow arthroscopy has an expanding role in elbow surgery, and the indications are increasing. A thorough knowledge of elbow anatomy is vital to prevent complications. Perhaps one the most common indications for elbow arthroscopy as demonstrated in the cases above is arthrosis and loose body removal. The success rates of arthroscopic loose body removal from the elbow approach 90 % when performed safely and methodically [3].

References

1. McKenzie PJ. Supine position. In: Savoie FH, Field LD, editors. Arthroscopy of the elbow. New York: Churchill Livingstone; 1996. p. 35–9.
2. Morrey BF. Arthroscopy of the elbow. In: Anderson LD, editor. Instructional course lectures, vol. 35. Rosemont, IL: American Academy of Orthopaedic Surgeons; 1986. p. 102–7.
3. O'Driscoll SW. Elbow arthroscopy for loose bodies. Orthopaedics. 1992;15:855–9.
4. O'Driscoll SW. Elbow arthroscopy: loose bodies. In: Morrey BF, editor. The elbow and its disorders. 3rd ed. Philadelphia, PA: Saunders; 2000. p. 510–4.
5. O'Driscoll SW, Morrey BF. Arthroscopy of the elbow: diagnostic and therapeutic benefits and hazards. J Bone Joint Surg Am. 1992;74:84–94.
6. Savoie FH. Arthroscopic management of loose bodies of the elbow. Oper Tech Sports Med. 2001;9(4):241–4.
7. Savoie FH. Guidelines to becoming an expert elbow arthroscopist. J Arthroscopic Relat Surg. 2007;23(11):1237–40.
8. Andrews JR, Baumgarten TE. Arthroscopic anatomy of the elbow. Orthop Clin North Am. 1995;26:671.
9. Wiesler ER, Poehling GG. Elbow arthroscopy: introduction, indications, complications, and results. In: McGinty JB, Burkhart SS, Jackson RW, et al., editors. Operative arthroscopy. 3rd ed. Philadelphia, PA: Lippincott-Raven; 2003. p. 661–4.
10. Byrd JW. Elbow arthroscopy for arthrofibrosis after type I radial head fractures. Arthroscopy. 1994;10:162–5.
11. Jones GS, Savoie FH. Arthroscopic capsular release of flexion contractures (arthrofibrosis) of the elbow. Arthroscopy. 1993; 9:277–83.
12. O'Driscoll SW. Arthroscopic treatment for osteoarthritis of the elbow. Orthop Clin North Am. 1995;26:691–706.
13. Ogilvie-Harris DJ, Gordon R, MacKay M. Arthroscopic treatment for posterior impingement in degenerative arthritis of the elbow. Arthroscopy. 1995;11:437–43.
14. Baumgarten TE, Andrew JR, Satterwhite YE. The arthroscopic evaluation and treatment of osteochondritis dissecans of the capitellum. Am J Sports Med. 1998;26:520–3.
15. Ruch DS, Cory JW, Poehling GG. The arthroscopic management of osteochondritis dissecans of the adolescent elbow. Arthroscopy. 1998;14(8):797–803.
16. Savoie FH, Field LD. Basics of elbow arthroscopy. Tech Orthop. 2000;15(2):138–46.
17. Menth-Chiari WA, Ruch DS, Poehling GG. Arthroscopic excision of the radial head: clinical outcome in 12 patients with posttraumatic arthritis after fracture of the radial head or rheumatoid arthritis. Arthroscopy. 2001;17(9):918–23.
18. Andrews JR, Carson WG. Arthroscopy of the elbow. Arthroscopy. 1985;1:97–107.
19. Clarke R. Symptomatic lateral synovial fringe of the elbow joint. Arthroscopy. 1988;4:112–6.
20. Smith 3rd JP, Savoie FH, Field LD. Posterolateral rotatory instability of the elbow. Clin Sports Med. 2001;20(1):47–58.
21. Thomas MA, Fast A, Shapiro DL. Radial nerve damage as a complication of elbow arthroscopy. Clin Orthop Relat Res. 1987;215: 130–1.

22. Savoie 3rd FH, O'Brien MJ, Field LD, Gurley DJ. Arthroscopic and open radial ulnohumeral ligament reconstruction for posterolateral rotatory instability of the elbow. Clin Sports Med. 2010;29(4):611–8.

23. Poehling GG, Ekman EF, Ruch DS. Elbow arthroscopy: introduction and overview. In: McGinty J, Caspari R, Jackson R, et al., editors. Operative arthroscopy. 2nd ed. Philadelphia, PA: Lippincott; 1996. p. 821–8.

24. Poehling GG, Ekman EF. Arthroscopy of the elbow. In: Jackson D, editor. Instructional course lectures, vol. 44. Chicago, IL: AAOS; 1994. p. 214–23.

25. Childress HM. Recurrent ulnar nerve dislocation at the elbow. Clin Orthop. 1986;108:168.

26. Baker CL, Grant LJ. Arthroscopy of the elbow. Am J Sports Med. 1999;27:251–64.

27. Lindenfeld TN. Medial approach in elbow arthroscopy. Am J Sports Med. 1990;18:413.

28. Adolfsson L. Arthroscopy of the elbow joint: a cadaveric study of portal placement. J Shoulder Elbow Surg. 1994;3:53–61.

29. Plancher KD, Peterson RK, Breezenoff L. Diagnostic arthroscopy of the elbow: set-up, portals, and technique. Oper Tech Sports Med. 1998;6:2–10.

30. Stothers K, Day B, Reagan WR. Arthroscopy of the elbow: anatomy, portal sites, and a description of the proximal lateral portal. Arthroscopy. 1995;11:449–57.

31. Field LD, Altchek DW, Warren RF, et al. Arthroscopic anatomy of the lateral elbow: a comparison of three portals. Arthroscopy. 1994;10:602–7.

32. Savoie FH, Field LD. Anatomy. In: Savoie FH, Field LD, editors. Arthroscopy of the elbow. New York: Churchill Livingstone; 1996. p. 3–24.

33. Aboud JA, Ricchetti ET, Tjoumakaris F, Ramsey ML. Elbow arthroscopy: basic setup and portal placement. J Am Acad Orthop Surg. 2006;14:312–8.

34. Poehling G, Whipple T, Sisco L, Goldman B. Elbow arthroscopy: a new technique. Arthroscopy. 1989;5:222.

35. Lyons TR, Field LD, Savoie FH. Basics of elbow arthroscopy. In: Price CT, editor. Instructional course lectures, vol. 49. Rosemont, IL: American Academy of Orthopaedic Surgeons; 2000. p. 239–46.

Lateral and Medial Epicondylitis

21

Patrick M. O'Brien and Felix H. Savoie III

Introduction

Epicondylitis of the elbow involves pathologic alteration in the musculotendinous origins at the lateral and/or medial epicondyle [1]. Runge first described lateral epicondylitis in the German literature in 1873 [2]. Ten years later, in 1883, Morris first noted an association between lateral epicondylitis and lawn tennis [3]. This has led to the commonly used term "tennis elbow" for lateral epicondylitis. Furthermore, medial epicondylitis is often referred to as "golfer's elbow." Both conditions result in pain and discomfort about their respective aspects of the elbow. Lateral epicondylitis, however, is encountered far more often, affecting 1–3 % of the general population and up to 7 % of manual workers [4, 5]. This is 7–20 times more prevalent than medial epicondylitis [6].

Several studies have investigated the etiology and pathogenesis of lateral epicondylitis, including those by Cyriax [7], Goldie [8], as well as Coonrad and Hooper [9]. More recently, Nirschl and associates [10, 11] localized the underlying lesion to involve the origin of the extensor carpi radialis brevis (ECRB). Repetitive overuse, either from recreational or occupational activities, leads to microtears within the ECRB tendon origin. Attempted healing of these tears, however, is unsuccessful, leading to replacement with immature reparative tissue. Histologically, this tissue demonstrates a noninflammatory degenerative tendinosis, with fibroblasts, disorganized collagen, and neovascularization. This has been termed "angiofibroblastic tendinosis" [11]. Similar findings are seen in medial epicondylitis, though the pathologic fibrotic tissue is noted within the origin of the

P.M. O'Brien, MD (✉)
Mississippi Sports Medicine and Orthopedic Center,
Jackson, MS, USA
e-mail: patrick.m.obrien2@gmail.com

F.H. Savoie III, MD
Department of Orthopedic Surgery, Tulane University School of Medicine, Tulane Medical Center, New Orleans, LA, USA
e-mail: fsavoie@tulane.edu

flexor-pronator mass, most commonly involving the humeral head of the pronator teres (PT) and the flexor carpi radialis (FCR) [12].

Lateral and medial epicondylitis are both encountered most often in the fourth and fifth decades, with an equal distribution between males and females, most often in the dominant arm [1, 10]. While lateral epicondylitis can be encountered in tennis players, medial epicondylitis is rarely seen in golfers. More often, it is observed in baseball pitchers and individuals whose recreational or occupational activities involve repetitive valgus forces about the elbow [6]. Both conditions have an insidious onset of symptoms.

Clinical Presentation

Clinically, patients with lateral epicondylitis will complain of a sharp pain localized about the lateral aspect of the elbow which is exacerbated with activities involving active wrist extension or passive wrist flexion with the elbow extended [13]. On physical examination, pain is maximally elicited at a point slightly distal and anterior to the midpoint of the lateral epicondyle, within the tendinous portion of the ECRB. Pain is worsened with resisted wrist and finger extension with the elbow in extension. Other conditions included in the differential diagnosis of lateral elbow pain that should also be assessed to include cervical radiculopathy, radial tunnel syndrome, osteochondral lesion of the radiocapitellar joint, a synovial elbow plica, and/or posterolateral rotatory instability [13]. Medial epicondylitis will present with two different scenarios: one with burning type pain over the bony tip of the epicondyle and the second type similar to lateral epicondylitis localized more to the muscle of the flexor-pronator origin just distal to the tip of the epicondyle. Pain is sometimes exacerbated with resisted wrist flexion and forearm pronation. Additional conditions that should be assessed to include concomitant valgus elbow instability and ulnar neuritis [12]. Some of the differential diagnoses for lateral and medial elbow pain are summarized in Table 21.1.

S.F. Brockmeier (ed.), *MRI-Arthroscopy Correlations: A Case-Based Atlas of the Knee, Shoulder, Elbow and Hip*,
DOI 10.1007/978-1-4939-2645-9_21, © Springer Science+Business Media New York 2015

Table 21.1 Lateral versus medial elbow pain

Lateral elbow pain	Medial elbow pain
Lateral epicondylitis	Medial epicondylitis
Cervical radiculopathy	Cervical radiculopathy
Radial tunnel syndrome	Flexor-pronator muscle strain/tear
OCD lesion of the radiocapitellar joint	Ulnar collateral ligament injury
	Ulnar neuritis
Synovial elbow plica	Valgus extension overload
Posterolateral rotatory instability	

Summary of the differential diagnoses to be considered when evaluating a patient with either lateral- or medial-sided elbow pain
Published with kind permission. Copyright © Felix H. Savoie, III, MD

Radiographic Evaluation

Though lateral and medial epicondylitis both remain clinical diagnoses, imaging is oftentimes included in the diagnostic workup of patients with either lateral or medial elbow pain. Plain radiographs, including anteroposterior, lateral, and oblique views of the elbow, are frequently obtained and usually are normal. However, calcifications within the soft tissues about the lateral epicondyle may be noted in 22–25 % of patients with lateral epicondylitis, though this has not been found to have a prognostic implication [10].

Magnetic resonance imaging (MRI), while not an essential part of the diagnostic workup, can be a useful adjunct in assessing both conditions. In particular, MRI allows for evaluation of both the surrounding tissue structures and the intra-articular surface, which helps determine if any other potential causes of elbow pain may be present. This is especially useful in patients with medial elbow pain, as the integrity of the UCL can be determined. The typical appearance on MRI shows abnormally high signal intensity on T2-weighted and short TI inversion recovery (STIR) sequences within a thickened common extensor or flexor-pronator tendon origin for lateral and medial epicondylitis, respectively [14]. Overall, MRI has a 90–100 % sensitivity and a 83–100 % specificity for detecting epicondylitis [15]. It may be performed either with or without intra-articular gadolinium contrast injection.

Treatment Options and Outcomes

The majority of cases of both lateral and medial epicondylitis respond well to conservative management. While no consensus treatment algorithm currently exists for either condition, multiple options have been utilized previously. This includes an initial phase of rest, ice, and nonsteroidal anti-inflammatory (NSAIDs) medications. This is often followed by a course of physical therapy, the use of counterforce bracing, and/or corticosteroid injection [13]. Other modalities that have been

investigated include extracorporeal shock wave (ECSW) therapy [16–18], platelet-rich plasma injection [19], and use of low-dose thermal ablation devices [20]. While most patients respond well to nonoperative management, historically noted at up to a 90 % recovery rate within 1–2 years [9, 10], surgical treatment of recalcitrant disease is sometimes required. Bot et al., however, recently found that, while most patients (90 %) obtained at least some improvement with conservative treatment for lateral epicondylitis at 1 year follow-up, only 13 % reported a full recovery at 3 months and 34 % at 1 year [21]. This may indicate an expanded surgical role in the treatment of both lateral and medial epicondylitis.

Regardless of these prior findings, a minimum of 3–6 months of nonoperative treatment is recommended prior to pursuing surgical treatment for either lateral or medial epicondylitis. Traditionally, surgical options involved open debridement of the involved tissue, such as those previously described by Bosworth in 1955 [22], as well as Nirschl and Pettrone in 1979 [10] in treating lateral epicondylitis. Percutaneous approaches for ECRB release have also been described [23, 24]. However, with the advances made in arthroscopic surgery of the elbow, there has been an increased focus on arthroscopic management of epicondylitis. Baker et al. initially reported on 40 patients (42 elbows) with recalcitrant lateral epicondylitis who underwent arthroscopic debridement of the diseased tissue, often combined with decortication of the lateral epicondyle [25]. These arthroscopic techniques have continued to evolve beyond simple debridement, with ECRB repair and plication utilizing both simple suture and suture anchor devices being described [20].

Given its increased prevalence, surgical outcomes regarding the arthroscopic management of lateral epicondylitis have been investigated more extensively than has medial epicondylitis. Several studies comparing open and arthroscopic debridement techniques for the treatment of lateral epicondylitis have been performed. While overall equivalent clinical results have been oftentimes noted, those treated arthroscopically were noted to return to work earlier without restrictions [25–28]. More recently, however, Solheim et al. noted that patients undergoing arthroscopic release had a better QuickDASH score than those that underwent an open surgical debridement [29]. An additional advantage of arthroscopic treatment is that a full intra-articular assessment of the elbow joint can be performed and any concomitant pathology addressed during the same surgical setting, as concurrent intra-articular pathology has been found in up to 44 % of cases [30].

While arthroscopic treatment of lateral epicondylitis has become more prevalent and accepted, concerns exist over the arthroscopic treatment of medial epicondylitis. This is due to the proximity of both the ulnar nerve and the medial ulnar collateral ligament to the flexor-pronator origin at the medial epicondyle. On the other hand, cadaveric models have indicated that these structures lie at a far enough distance away from the debridement site and that arthroscopic debridement for medial epicondylitis can be performed at a low risk of injury to these structures [31]. Relative contraindications to elbow arthroscopy do exist, however, including prior medial elbow surgery with ulnar nerve transposition or the presence of ulnar nerve subluxation. Absolute contraindication includes active infection.

Case Presentation: Concurrent Lateral and Medial Epicondylitis

A 38-year-old, right-hand dominant female presented with a long-standing history of elbow pain. Her pain was localized over both the lateral and medial aspects of her elbow. This had been present over the past several years, and she had been treated by her primary care physician with anti-inflammatory medications, counterforce bracing, and intermittent cortico-steroid injections. Orthopedic consultation had been obtained, and a sequence of injections had been given with some temporary relief, but each time, the pain returned and thought to be more severe with each recurrence. Her pain symptoms had become constant, with worsening both at night and with lifting activities. She denied any traumatic etiology of her symptoms and had not had any previous surgical procedures to her right elbow.

Upon her initial presentation to our orthopedic clinic, her physical examination showed tenderness to palpation about both the medial and lateral epicondyle. She had full active and passive range of motion to elbow flexion and extension, as well as forearm pronation and supination. She had increased pain with active resisted wrist extension over her lateral elbow and with active resisted wrist flexion over her medial elbow. No elbow instability was present clinically, with negative varus/valgus stress testing and a negative lateral elbow pivot shift. She had full motor strength in all key groups and had no sensory deficits or complaints of numbness. She had a negative Tinel's test over the cubital tunnel.

Radiographic assessment was obtained including two view X-rays of the right elbow. These were found to be normal. An MRI obtained by her orthopedic surgeon was reviewed. This revealed the presence of increased signal both within the tendinous portion of the flexor-pronator mass medially and within the common extensor mass laterally, consistent with both medial and lateral epicondylitis, as seen in Fig. 21.1a–d. Further conservative recommendations were made at her initial appointment, including a course of physical therapy, topical and oral anti-inflammatory medications, a wrist brace, and repeat corticosteroid injections to both the medial and lateral epicondyle. This course of treatment provided good initial relief, but her symptoms returned fully within 3 months. Surgical intervention in the form of elbow arthroscopy was then offered, and the patient elected to pursue.

The patient was taken to the operating room, and general anesthesia was induced. She was then placed in the prone position, and her right upper extremity prepped and draped in the normal sterile manner. Following initial joint insufflation with 30 mL of sterile saline, an initial proximal antero-medial portal was created, and the 30° arthroscope inserted into the joint. Inspection was begun on the lateral aspect of the elbow, focusing on the radiocapitellar joint (Fig. 21.2a). Spinal needle localization was then utilized to establish a lateral working portal just anterior to the lateral epicondyle (Fig. 21.2b). An arthroscopic shaver was used to debride the capsule underlying the ECRB tendon insertion. This allowed for visualization of the degenerative "tendinosis" seen within the ECRB, which appears grayish in color (Fig. 21.3a). Debridement of this degenerative tissue reveals the remaining healthy ECRB tendon, which is more shiny and white in color (Fig. 21.3b). Following completion of the tendon release, the muscle fibers of the extensor carpi radialis longus (ECRL) are seen (Fig. 21.3c). A small amount of bony debridement was also performed on the lateral epicondyle.

Attention was then turned medially, with the arthroscope placed through the previous lateral portal. Muscle fibers from the flexor-pronator mass are initially noted (Fig. 21.4a). Debridement of the medial epicondyle is then performed, moving from anterior to posterior, until the tendon fibers of the flexor-pronator mass insertion are encountered. Again, the grayish, degenerative "tendinosis" tissue (Fig. 21.4b) is noted and subsequently debrided until the white, shiny appearing healthy tendon tissue is found (Fig. 21.4c, d). The lateral portal sites were closed to prevent continued drainage and fistula formation. The arm was placed in a posterior splint with the elbow at 90° for her immediate postoperative period.

Conclusions

Epicondylitis of the elbow is a commonly encountered condition in people with elbow pain, with lateral epicondylitis involved more often than medial epicondylitis. Clinically, patients present with an insidious onset of pain about either the lateral or medial epicondyle, worsened with resisted wrist

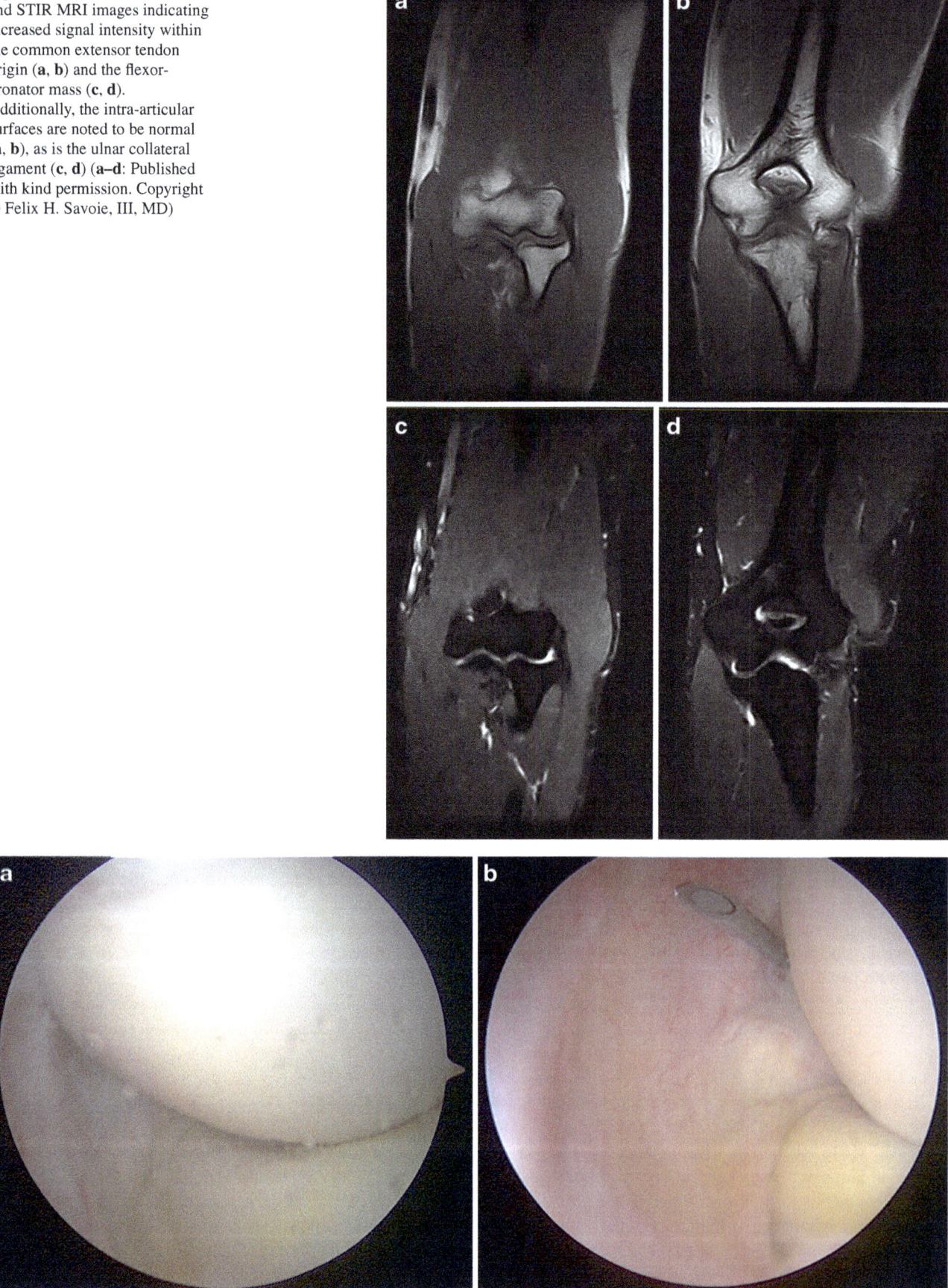

Fig. 21.1 Coronal T1-weighted and STIR MRI images indicating increased signal intensity within the common extensor tendon origin (**a, b**) and the flexor-pronator mass (**c, d**). Additionally, the intra-articular surfaces are noted to be normal (**a, b**), as is the ulnar collateral ligament (**c, d**) (**a–d**: Published with kind permission. Copyright © Felix H. Savoie, III, MD)

Fig. 21.2 (**a**) Arthroscopic visualization of the radiocapitellar joint when viewing from the proximal anteromedial portal. (**b**) Spinal needle being used to create lateral working portal just anterior to the lateral epicondyle. (**a, b**: Published with kind permission. Copyright© Felix H. Savoie, III, MD)

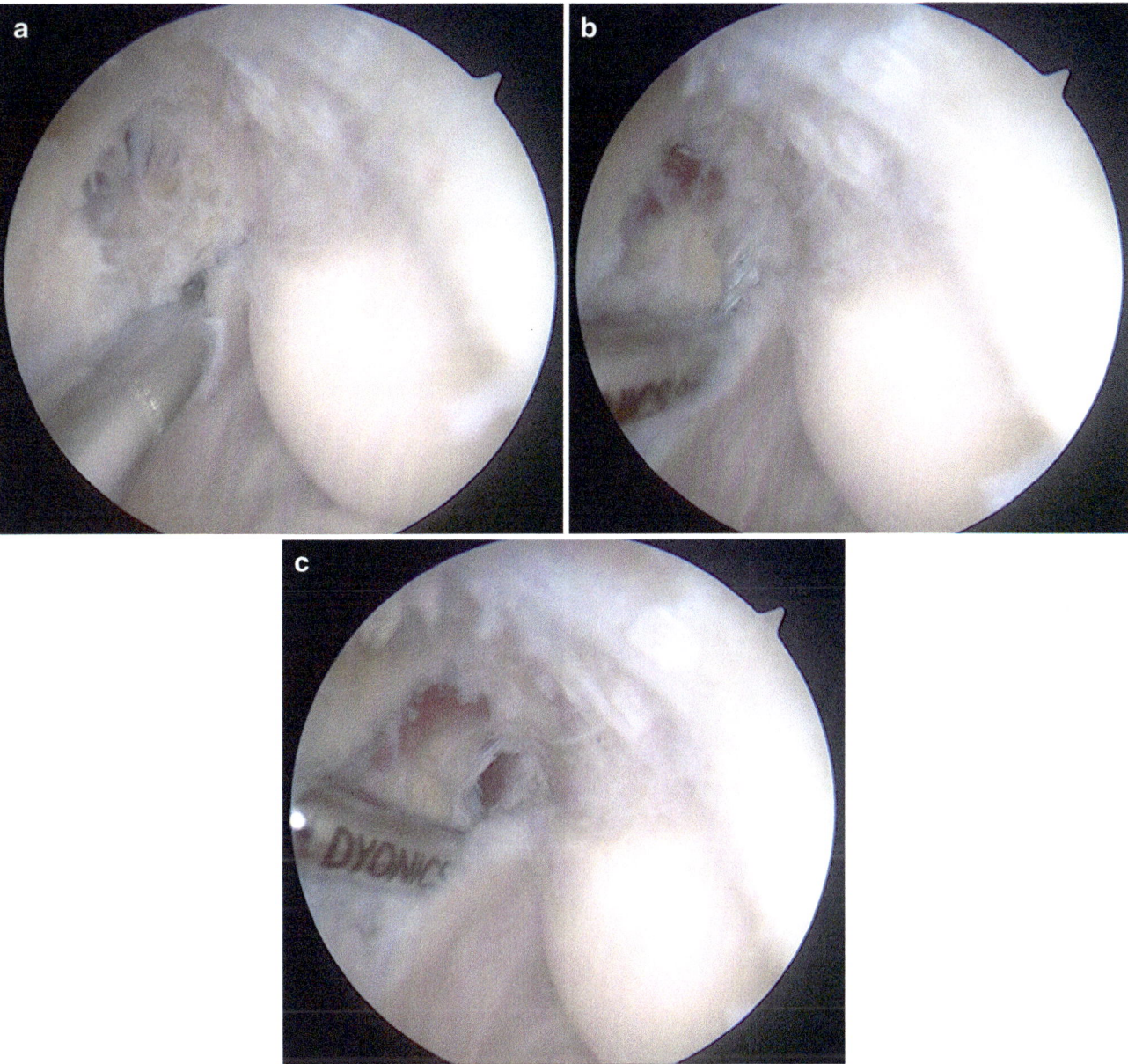

Fig. 21.3 (**a**) Following debridement of the underlying capsule the degenerative, *grayish* "tendinosis" tissue of the ECRB is identified. (**b**) Further debridement of the diseased tissue reveals the *white, shiny* normal ECRB tendon. (**c**) Following complete release of the ECRB ten- don, the muscle fibers of the ECRL are visible. A small bony debridement of the lateral epicondyle has also been performed (**a–c**: Published with kind permission. Copyright © Felix H. Savoie, III, MD)

extension in the former and resisted wrist flexion in the latter. Concurrent conditions, however, may be present and must be evaluated, especially when investigating medial elbow pain. While both conditions remain clinical diagnoses, MRI can provide valuable information, particularly in assessing the adjacent tissue for any concomitant pathology. Numerous conservative treatment options have been described and are usually effective. However, in recalcitrant cases, surgical intervention may be required. While traditionally performed with open surgical debridement of the diseased tissue, arthroscopic treatment of epicondylitis has been shown to provide equivalent, if not superior, clinical improvement with the potential for a quicker return to work and sporting activities.

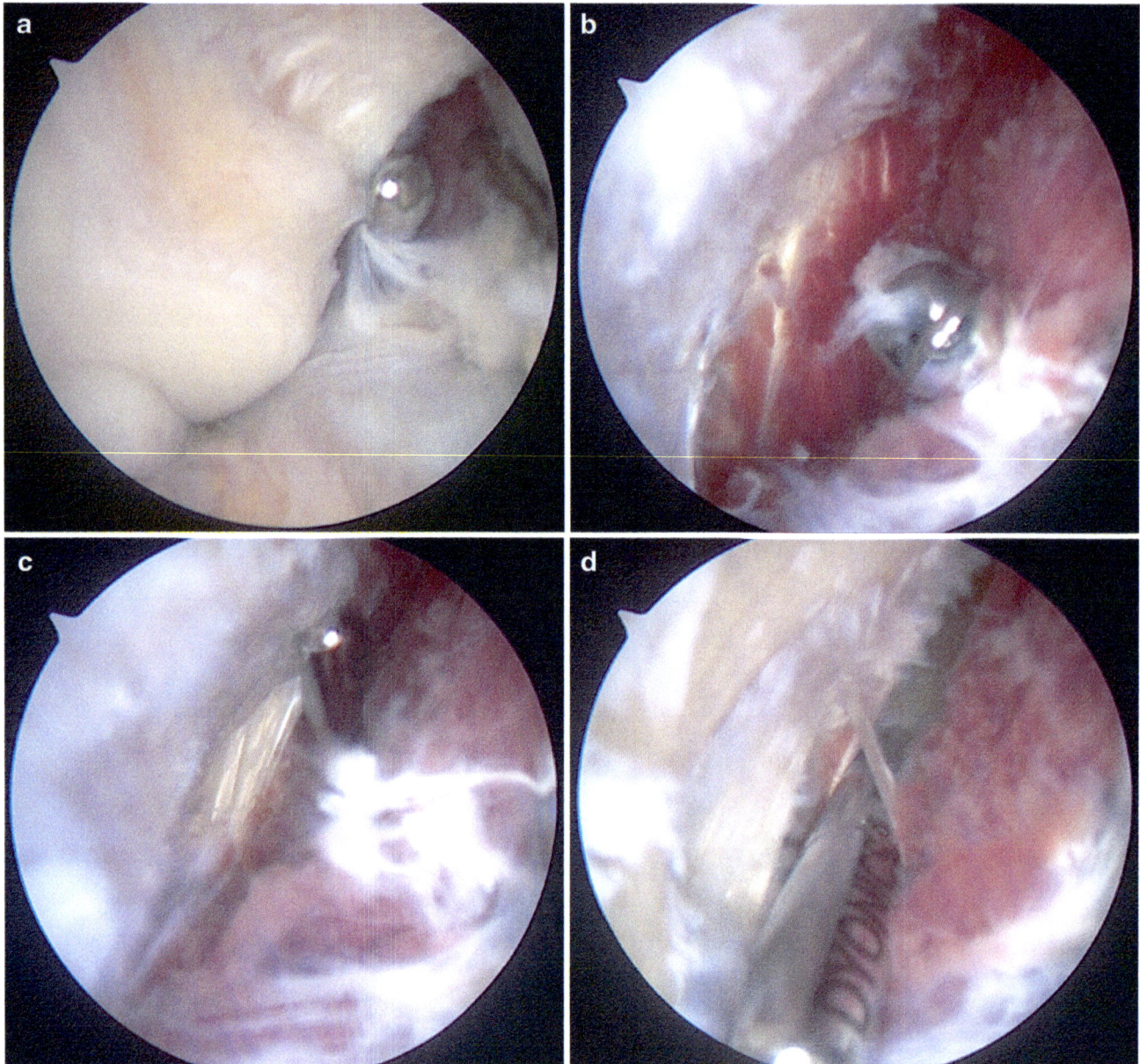

Fig. 21.4 (**a**) The medial side of the elbow is visualized, with the trochlea seen superiorly and the coronoid inferiorly. An arthroscopic shaver has begun debriding back on the medial epicondyle. (**b**) Continued debridement posteriorly reveals the degenerative "tendino- sis" tissue of the flexor-pronator mass, *grayish* in appearance. (**c**, **d**) Following debridement of the diseased tissue, the *white*, *shiny* fibers representing healthy tendon tissue are seen (**a–d**: Published with kind permission. Copyright © Felix H. Savoie, III, MD)

References

1. Jobe FW, Ciccotti MG. Lateral and medial epicondylitis of the elbow. J Am Acad Orthop Surg. 1994;2:1–8.
2. Runge F. Zur genese und behandlung des schreibekramfes. Berl Klin Wochenschr. 1873;10:245.
3. Morris HP. Lawn-tennis elbow. BMJ. 1883;2:557.
4. Shiri R, Vukari-Juntura E, Varonen H, Heliovaara M. Prevalence and determinants of lateral and medial epicondylitis: a population study. Am J Epidemiol. 2006;164:1065–74.
5. De Smedt T, de Jong A, Van Leemput W, Lieven D, Van Glabbeek F. Lateral epicondylitis in tennis: update on aetiology, biomechan- ics and treatment. Br J Sports Med. 2007;41:816–9.
6. Leach RE, Miller JK. Lateral and medial epicondylitis of the elbow. Clin Sports Med. 1987;6:259–72.
7. Cyriax JH. The pathology and treatment of tennis elbow. J Bone Joint Surg Am. 1936;18:921–40.
8. Goldie I. Epicondylitis lateralis humeri (epicondylalgia or tennis elbow): a pathogenetical study. Acta Chir Scand Suppl. 1964;57:339.
9. Coonrad RW, Hooper WR. Tennis elbow: its course, natural history, conservative, and surgical management. J Bone Joint Surg Am. 1973;55:1183–7.

10. Nirschl RP, Pettrone FA. Tennis elbow: the surgical treatment of lateral epicondylitis. J Bone Joint Surg Am. 1979;61:832–9.
11. Kraushaar BS, Nirschl RP. Tendinosis of the elbow (tennis elbow): clinical features and findings of histological, immunohistochemical, and electron microscopy studies. J Bone Joint Surg Am. 1999; 81:259–78.
12. Chen FS, Rokito AS, Jobe FW. Medial elbow problems in the overhead-throwing athlete. J Am Acad Orthop Surg. 2001; 9:99–113.
13. Calfee RP, Patel A, DaSilva MF, Akelman E. Management of lateral epicondylitis: current concepts. J Am Acad Orthop Surg. 2008; 16:19–29.
14. Dewan AK, Chhabra AB, Khanna AJ, Anderson MW, Brunton LM. MRI of the elbow: techniques and spectrum of disease: AAOS exhibit selection. J Bone Joint Surg Am. 2013;95(14):e99 1–13.
15. Miller TT, Shapiro MA, Schultz E, Kalish PE. Comparison of sonography and MRI for diagnosing epicondylitis. J Clin Ultrasound. 2002;30(4):193–202.
16. Haake M, Konig IR, Decker T, Riedel C, Buch M, Muller HH. Extracorporeal shock wave therapy in the treatment of lateral epicondylitis: a randomized multicenter trial. J Bone Joint Surg Am. 2002;84:1982–91.
17. Pettrone FA, McCall BR. Extracorporeal shock wave therapy without local anesthesia for chronic lateral epicondylitis. J Bone Joint Surg Am. 2005;87:1297–304.
18. Buchbinder R, Green SE, Youd JM, Assendelft WJ, Barnsley L, Smidt N. Shock wave therapy for lateral elbow pain. Cochrane Database Syst Rev. 2005;(1):CD003524.
19. Edwards SG, Calandruccio JH. Autologous blood injections for refractory lateral epicondylitis. J Hand Surg Am. 2003;28:272–8.
20. Savoie III FH, VanSice W, O'Brien MJ. Arthroscopic tennis elbow release. J Shoulder Elbow Surg. 2010;19:31–6.
21. Bot SDM, van der Waal JM, Terwee CB, van der Windt DAWM, Bouter LM, Dekker J. Course and prognosis of elbow complaints: a cohort study in general practice. Ann Rheum Dis. 2005;64: 1331–6.
22. Bosworth DM. The role of the orbicular ligament in tennis elbow. J Bone Joint Surg Am. 1955;37:527–34.
23. Baumgard SH, Schwartz DR. Percutaneous release of the epicondylar muscles for humeral epicondylitis. Am J Sports Med. 1982; 10:233–6.
24. Yerger B, Turner T. Percutaneous extensor tenotomy for chronic tennis elbow: an office procedure. Orthopedics. 1995;8:1261–3.
25. Baker Jr CL, Murphy KP, Gottlob CA, Curd DT. Arthroscopic classification and treatment of lateral epicondylitis: two-year clinical results. J Shoulder Elbow Surg. 2000;9:475–82.
26. Owens BD, Murphy KP, Kuklo TR. Arthroscopic release for lateral epicondylitis. Arthroscopy. 2001;17:582–7.
27. Peart RE, Strickler SS, Schweitzer Jr KM. Lateral epicondylitis: a comparative study of open and arthroscopic lateral release. Am J Orthop. 2004;33:565–7.
28. Mullett H, Sprague M, Brown G, Hausman M. Arthroscopic treatment of lateral epicondylitis: clinical and cadaveric studies. Clin Orthop Relat Res. 2005;439:123–8.
29. Solheim E, Hegna J, Oyen J. Arthroscopic versus open tennis elbow release: 3- to 6-year results of a case-control series of 305 elbows. Arthroscopy. 2013;29:854–9.
30. Szabo SJ, Savoie III FH, Field LD, Ramsey JR, Hosemann CD. Tendinosis of the extensor carpi radialis brevis: an evaluation of three methods of operative treatment. J Shoulder Elbow Surg. 2006;15:721–7.
31. Zonno A, Manuel J, Merrell G, Ramos P, Akelman E, DaSilva MF. Arthroscopic technique for medial epicondylitis: technique and safety analysis. Arthroscopy. 2010;26:610–6.

Elbow Injuries in the Overhead Athlete: MUCL Avulsion and Tears

22

Jonathan Capelle, Felix H. Savoie III,
and Michael J. O'Brien

Introduction

The throwing motion of overhead athletes, especially pitchers, creates a large valgus force across the elbow. This repetitive strain can cause microtrauma to the main valgus stabilizer, the medial ulnar collateral ligament (MUCL), which may eventually lead to failure in function.

The anterior bundle of the MUCL is the primary restraint to the valgus force, predominantly from 20 to 120°. The act of pitching nears the max resistive capabilities of this ligament of up to 290N and angular velocities around 3,100°/s [1].

A thorough history is important in evaluating these patients. MUCL injuries typically present with chronic medial-sided elbow pain that is worse with activity, though occasionally may present in an acute fashion after a specific event. Pitchers may note decrease in their velocity or control as well as decreased arm endurance. It is also important to note any evidence of ulnar nerve irritation as this may impact the treatment plan.

Physical examination includes the valgus stress test, moving valgus stress test, and milking maneuver noting any pain or instability elicited. The ulnar nerve should be evaluated for any subluxation and presence or absence of a Tinel's sign. If surgery is a consideration, palpation for presence of the palmaris longus should be performed for possible use as autograft.

Plain radiographs of the elbow with a MUCL injury are often normal, though in an avulsion or a small fleck of bone, most commonly from the humeral aspect, may be seen. In radiographs of the chronic setting, one would more commonly see calcifications in the area of the ligament. Magnetic resonance imaging (MRI) is the primary imaging modality to confirm the diagnosis of a MUCL injury. MRI findings include edema, partial versus full thickness MUCL tear, avulsion injuries, as well as other associated injuries such as loose bodies, flexor-pronator tears, and cartilage injury.

Indications for surgical treatment include athletes who are unable to return to play due to pain or instability associated with a compromised MUCL. Recreational athletes that do not intend to pursue further athletic careers can often forgo surgery, as the function of normal day activities does not stress the elbow to the point of pain or instability even in the presence of MUCL insufficiency.

Before the techniques for surgical reconstruction were developed, tears or avulsions of the MUCL would typically signal the end to a player's career. Nonoperative treatment of these injuries, according to one study, resulted in only 42 % of players returning to their previous level of play [2]. Jobe in 1986 published the first description of a technique for MUCL reconstruction. This technique consisted of an ulnar nerve transposition and figure-of-8 graft construct through bone tunnels in the ulna and medial epicondyle [3]. Since then, multiple technique variations have been developed including interference screws, docking, and hybrid techniques. Due to these advances, return to play at the previous level of competition has been reported between 80 and 90 % [4–7]. Though reconstruction of the MUCL has become the mainstay treatment option for competitive athletes, it should be noted that repair of the ligament, especially in the younger population with isolated proximal or distal injuries to the ligament, can result in successful outcomes [8].

J. Capelle, MD (✉)
Department of Orthopedics, Mississippi Sports Medicine
and Orthopedic Center, Jackson, MS, USA
e-mail: Jcapelle11@gmail.com

F.H. SavoieIII, MD • M.J. O'Brien, MD
Department of Orthopedic Surgery, Division of Sports Medicine,
Tulane University School of Medicine, Tulane Medical Center,
New Orleans, LA, USA
e-mail: fsavoie@tulane.edu; mobrien@tulane.edu

Case 1: MUCL Avulsion

History/Exam

A 17-year-old, right-hand-dominant pitcher injured his elbow throwing during the previous season. He underwent a period of nonoperative treatment including bracing and

Fig. 22.1 (a, b) Plain radiographs (anteroposterior (AP) and lateral) of the elbow do not show any evidence of injury (a, b: Published with kind permission. Copyright © Felix H. Savoie, III, MD)

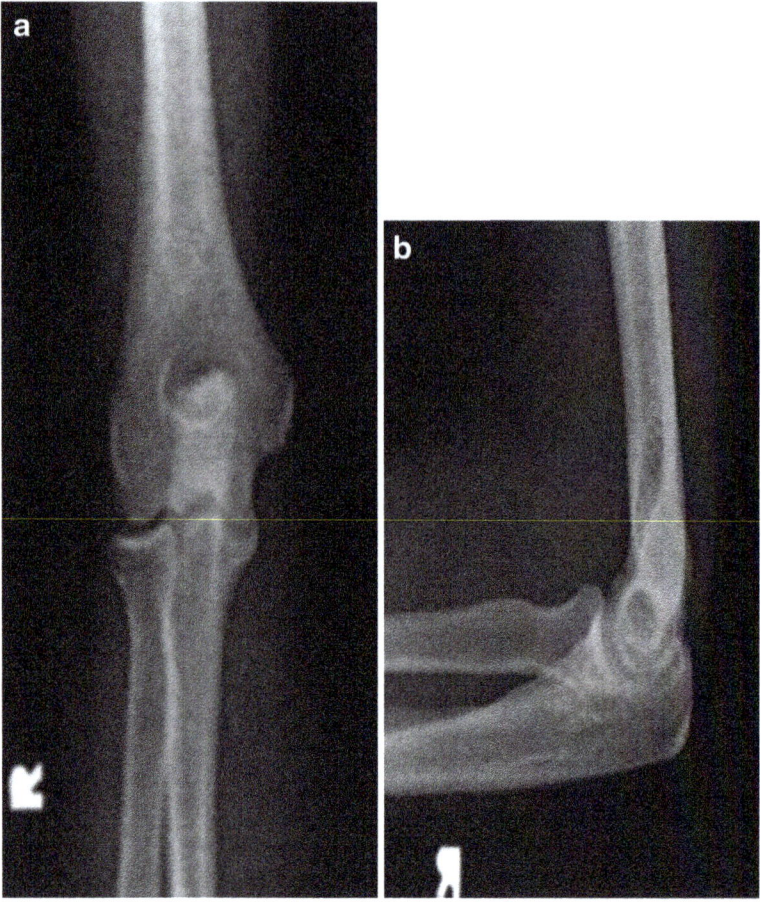

physical therapy, but was unable to achieve pain-free throwing ability; thus he was referred for surgical evaluation.

During physical examination, the patient was found to have a positive moving valgus stress test. He had noted 3+ instability with valgus stress at 30° and palpable tenderness to palpation along the medial aspect of the elbow. Milking maneuver was also positive. Range of motion was full with no loss of extension or flexion. Patient did not have any evidence of lateral-sided pathology.

Imaging

Plain radiographs as seen in Fig. 22.1a, b did not demonstrate any significant pathology. No bony avulsions were observed. No degenerative changes were noted in the olecranon fossa or ulnohumeral and radiocapitellar joints. Magnetic resonance imaging was obtained to further evaluate the medial ulnar collateral ligament. Complete sequences were obtained including coronal T1 and fat-saturated T1 and T2 sequences, sagittal T1 and fat-saturated T2 sequences, and axial T1 and fat-saturated T2 sequences. Coronal fat-saturated T2 sequences are shown in Fig. 22.2a–d and coronal T1 sequence images are shown in Fig. 22.3a–d.

An ulnar-sided avulsion of the MUCL from the sublime tubercle of the ulna is seen in both Figs. 22.1a, b and 22.2a–d. The fragment from the sublime tubercle measures 7×4 mm and has sclerotic margins indicating pathology is likely subacute. Some marrow edema can also be noted on the T2 images. The ulnar collateral ligament can still be seen inserting onto the fragment, and the remainder of the ligament demonstrates no evidence of tearing. Evaluation of the lateral collateral ligament shows no evidence of pathology. Likewise, no chondromalacia or chondral defects are seen on imaging.

Given the clinical and radiographic correlation and failure of nonoperative treatment, the risks and benefits of operative intervention were discussed with the patient and his family. The patient desired to return to his previous level of play; thus, the decision was made to proceed with elbow arthroscopy and open repair of the ulnar collateral ligament.

Operative Treatment

The patient was taken to the operating room and placed in the prone position. A standard diagnostic elbow arthroscopy was performed as seen in Fig. 22.4a–c. The radiocapitellar

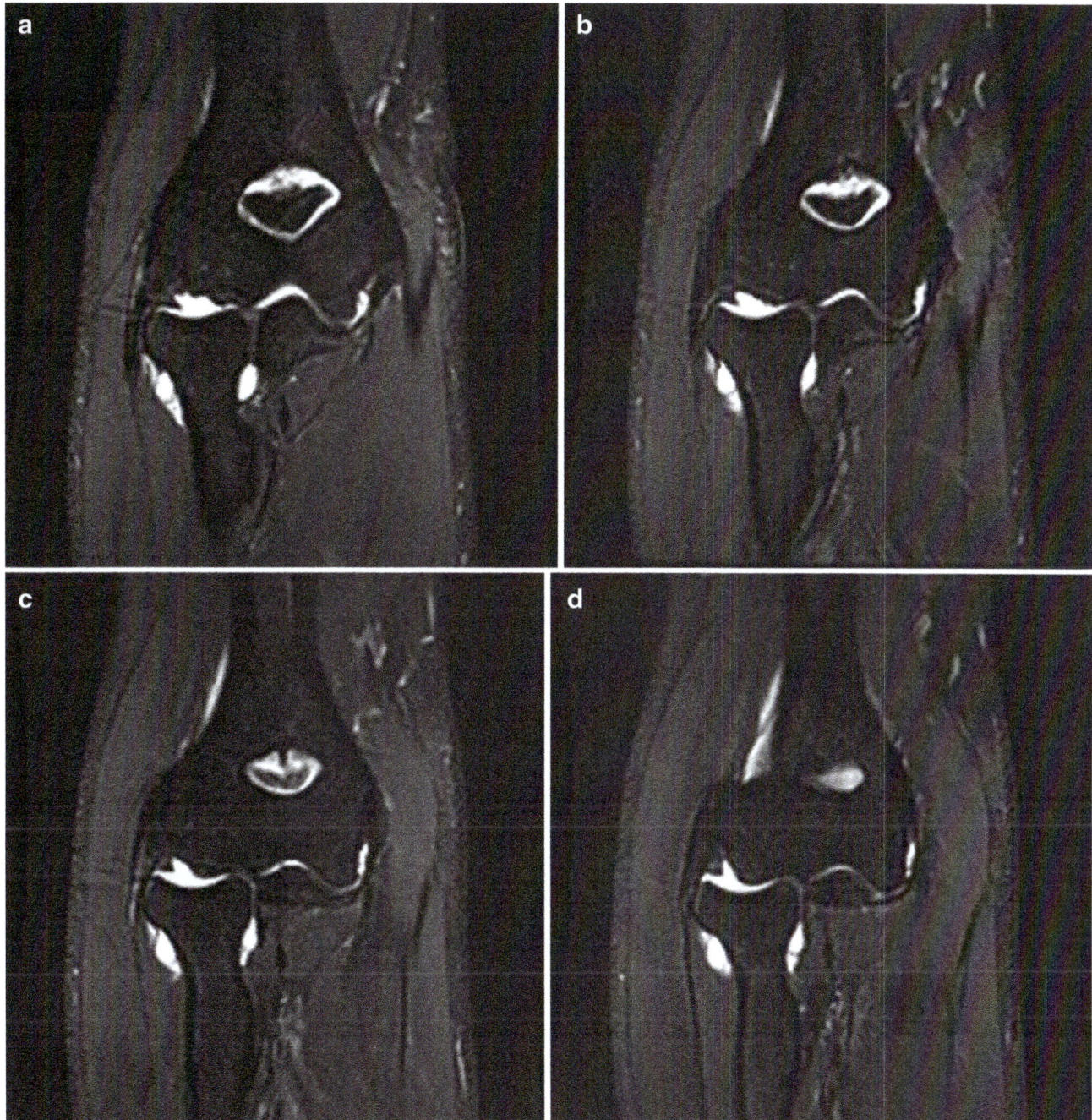

Fig. 22.2 (**a–d**) Coronal T2 fat-saturated images showing signal change and a small bony avulsion of the UCL from the sublime tubercle (**a–d**: Published with kind permission. Copyright © Felix H. Savoie, III, MD)

joint and capsule were found to be normal. The medial aspect showed evidence of instability but no signs of capsular damage. The medial gutter was found to be normal. A thickened plica was noted within the lateral gutter and was excised. The arthroscopic portion was completed.

The arm was then rotated to expose the medial aspect of the elbow and the open portion of the case was completed as seen in Fig. 22.5a–d. A direct approach to the medial ulnar collateral ligament was used. A split in the flexor-pronator

fascia was made posterior to the medial conjoined tendon while keeping a blunt retractor in position to protect the ulnar nerve. Upon inspection of the MUCL, the ligament itself appeared in good condition. The humeral insertion was intact; however, a small ossicle and disruption of the ulnar attachment were noted. The ligament was carefully dissected to visualize the attachment site on the sublime tubercle. The small ossicle was excised, and the bony footprint was roughened to improve healing of the ligament. A double-loaded

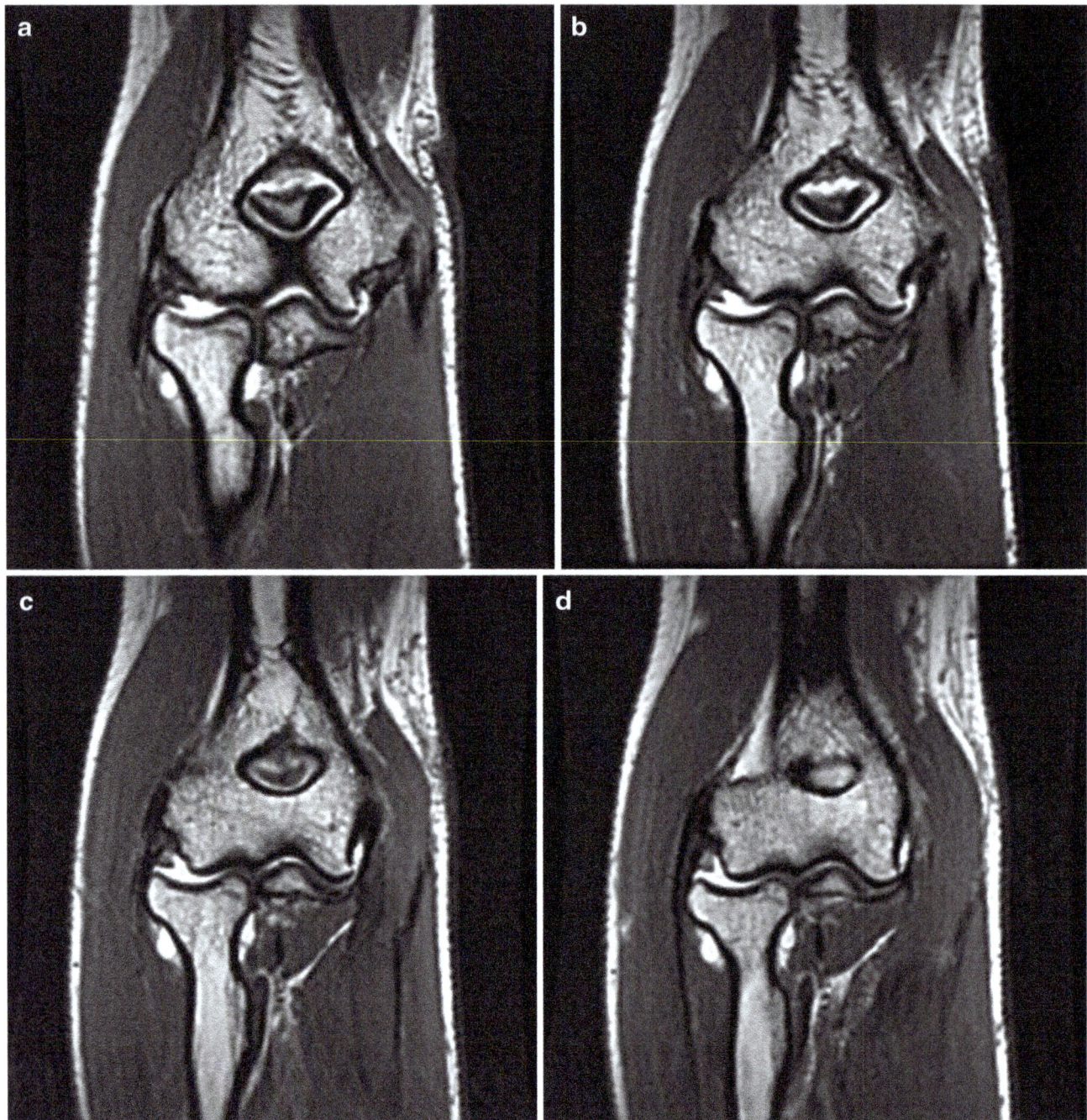

Fig. 22.3 (**a–d**) Coronal T1 images showing the small avulsion from the sublime tubercle of the ulnar insertion of the UCL (**a–d**: Published with kind permission. Copyright © Felix H. Savoie, III, MD)

suture anchor was placed at the footprint. Two limbs of the anchor were placed through the more posterior aspect of the ligament, while the remaining two limbs were placed through the anterior aspect. The two strands were then tied, securing the MUCL to its footprint. A #1 Vicryl was then used to plicate the midportion of the tendon. The elbow was tested and found to be stable. The incision was then irrigated and closed in standard fashion.

MRI Case 2: MUCL Tear

History/Exam

A 19-year-old, right-hand-dominant pitcher injured his elbow while pitching. Despite initial activity modification and therapy, he was unable to return to play due to pain and dysfunction.

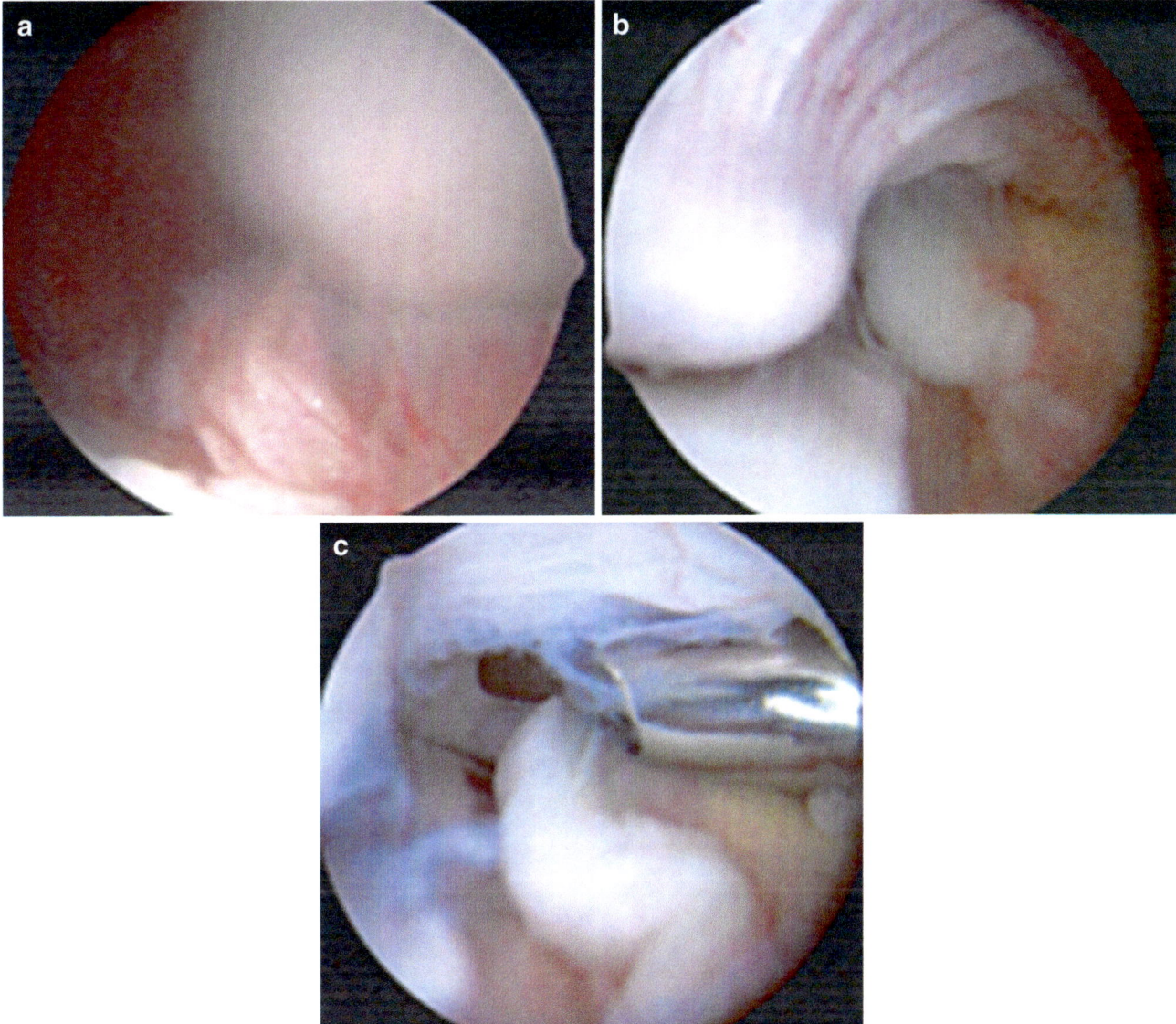

Fig. 22.4 Arthroscopic images showing the lateral gutter and synovitis (**a**, **b**), the medial gutter, and debridement of tissue in the lateral gutter (**c**) (**a–c**: Published with kind permission. Copyright © Felix H. Savoie, III, MD)

A physical examination concluded the patient had no specific tenderness to palpation. He had 3+ instability to valgus stress testing at 30°. Range of motion did not show any flexion or extension deficits. Strength testing was 5/5 in all muscle groups. Patient did not have any evidence of lateral-sided pathology.

Imaging

Plain radiographs in Fig. 22.6a, b show a small bony avulsion from the medial epicondyle. No degenerative changes were noted. Magnetic resonance imaging was obtained to further evaluate the medial ulnar collateral ligament.

Complete sequences were obtained, including coronal fat-saturated T1 and T2 sequences, sagittal fat-saturated T2 sequences, and axial fat-saturated T1 and T2 sequences. Coronal T2-weighted images are shown in Fig. 22.7a–f and coronal T1-weighted images are shown in Fig. 22.8a–e.

A mid-substance tear can be seen in both Figs. 22.7a–f and 22.8a–e close to the medial epicondyle. Signal change and the small bony avulsion from the medial epicondyle are better appreciated on the T2-weighted images in Fig. 22.7a–f. The lateral collateral ligament is shown to be intact. The cartilage of the ulnohumeral and radiocapitellar joints shows no significant cartilage pathology on any of the sequences.

Due to the clinical and radiographic correlation and failure of nonoperative treatment, the risks and benefits of operative

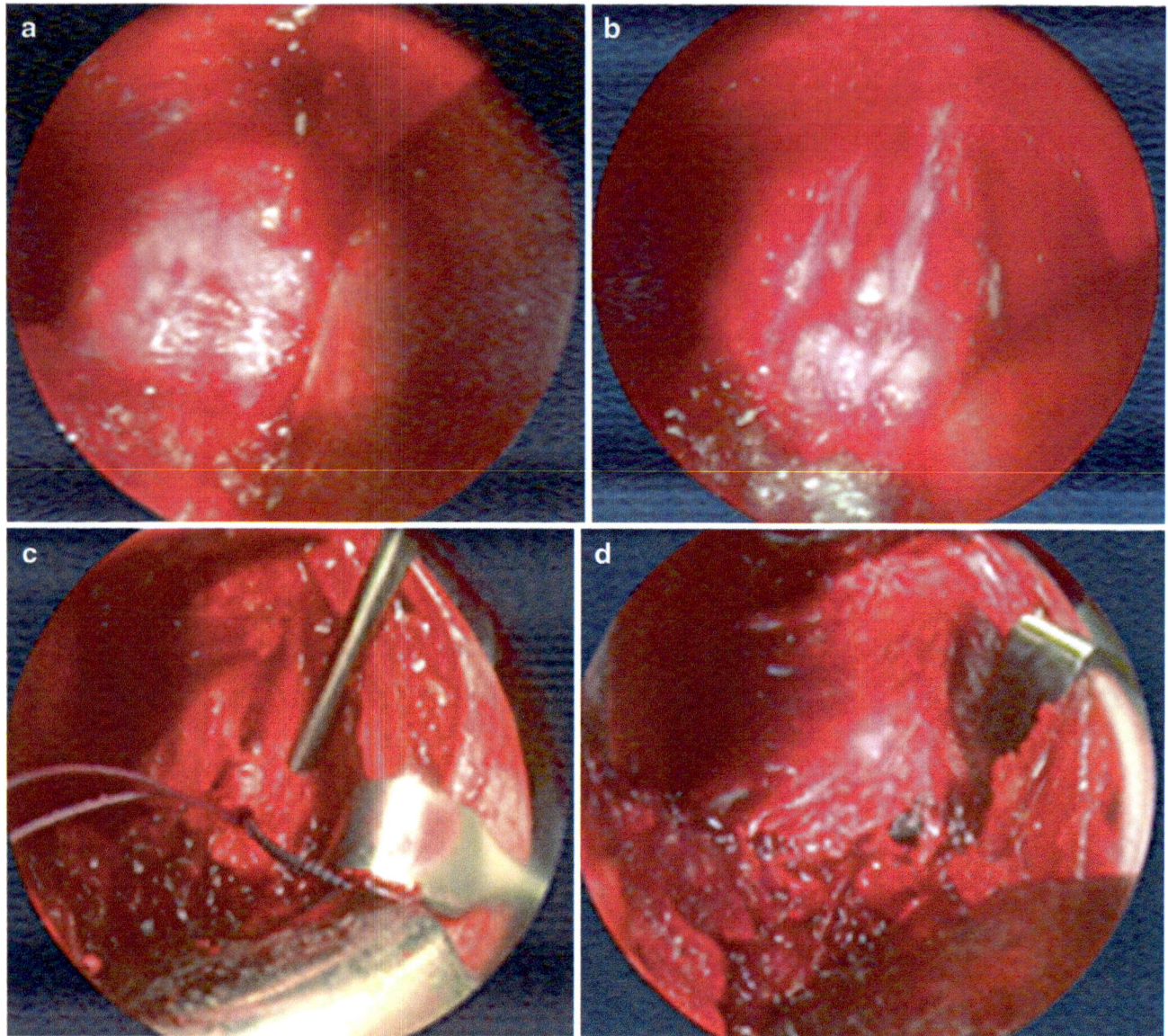

Fig. 22.5 Images of the open portion of the procedure showing (**a**) the intact mid-substance of the MUCL. (**b**) Again a preserved mid-substance of the ligament with avulsion of the ulnar aspect. (**c**) Suture anchor placement into the sublime tubercle. (**d**) Completed repair of the distal MUCL to the sublime tubercle (**a–d**: Published with kind permission. Copyright © Felix H. Savoie, III, MD)

intervention were discussed with the patient and his family. The patient desired to return to play and elected to proceed with elbow arthroscopy and open ulnar collateral ligament reconstruction with palmaris tendon autograft.

Operative Treatment

The patient was taken to the operating room, and an exam under anesthesia was performed. Again, gross instability was noted in the elbow. The patient was placed in the prone position and prepped and draped in standard fashion. The arm was rotated to provide access to the palmaris which was harvested from the proximal wrist crease and transected from the palmar fascia. A second incision, further proximal, was used to dissect out the tendon followed by the use of a tendon stripper to complete the harvest. The tendon was then prepped on the back table.

A standard diagnostic elbow arthroscopy was performed as demonstrated in Fig. 22.9a–d. The lateral aspect of the elbow showed some mild synovitis but no evidence of chondromalacia or an osteochondritis dissecans (OCD) lesion. Gross medial opening was visualized from the medial and lateral portals with no end point. The lateral gutter was

Fig. 22.6 (**a, b**) AP and lateral of the right elbow showing a small bony avulsion from the medial epicondyle (**a, b**: Published with kind permission. Copyright © Felix H. Savoie, III, MD)

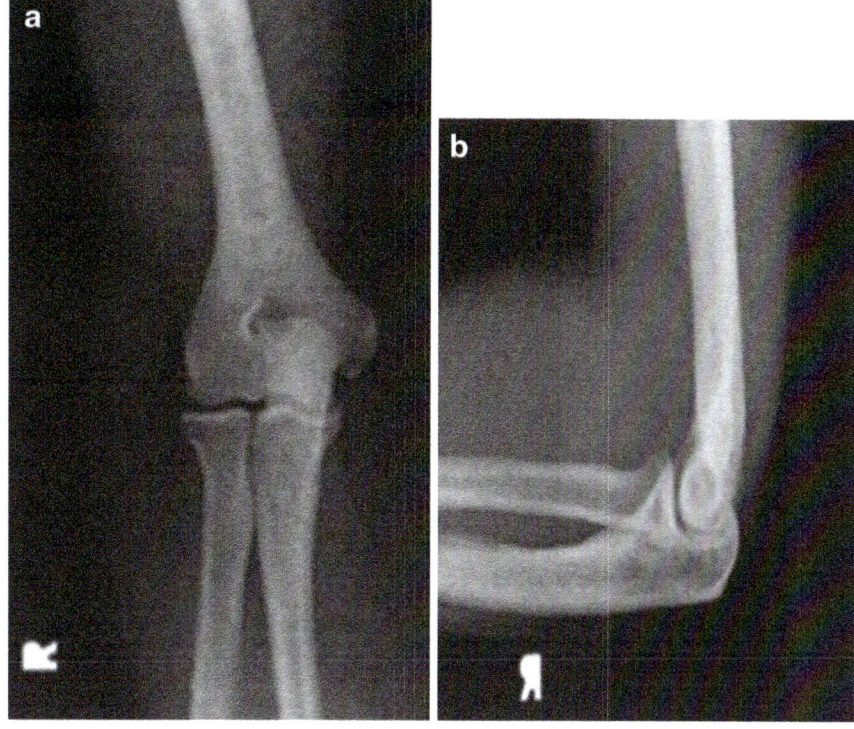

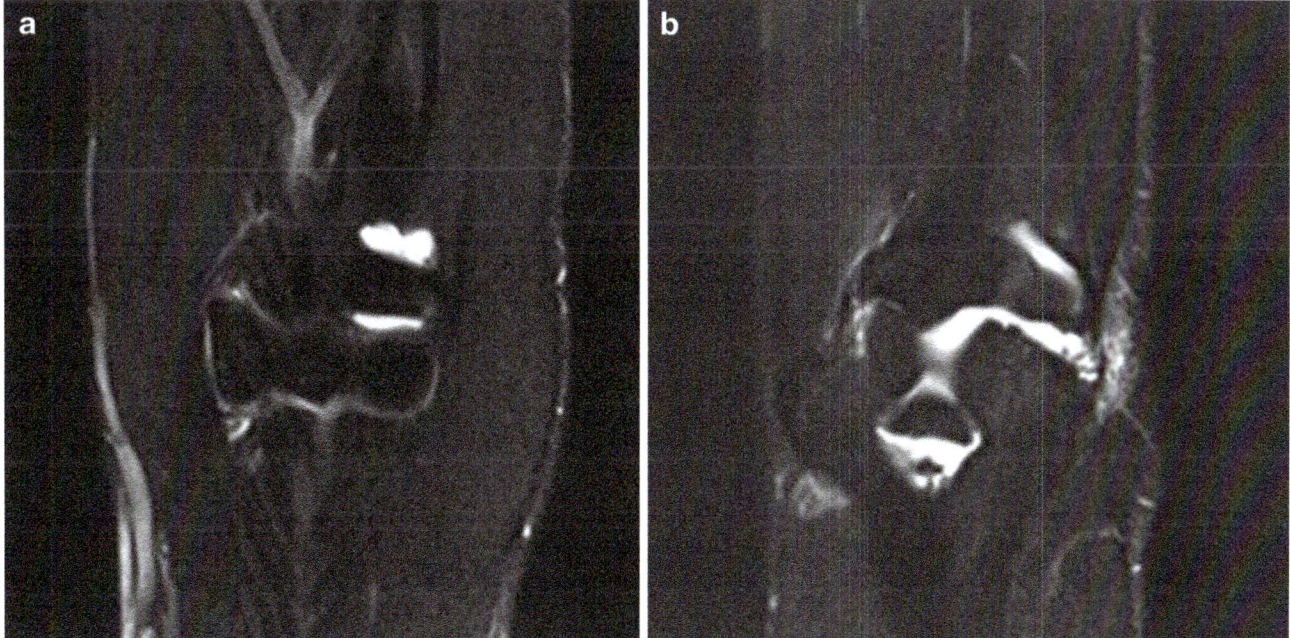

Fig. 22.7 (**a–f**) Coronal T2 fat-saturated images show the avulsed fragment from the medial epicondyle as well as signal change within the ligament indicative of a tear (**a–f**: Published with kind permission. Copyright © Felix H. Savoie, III, MD)

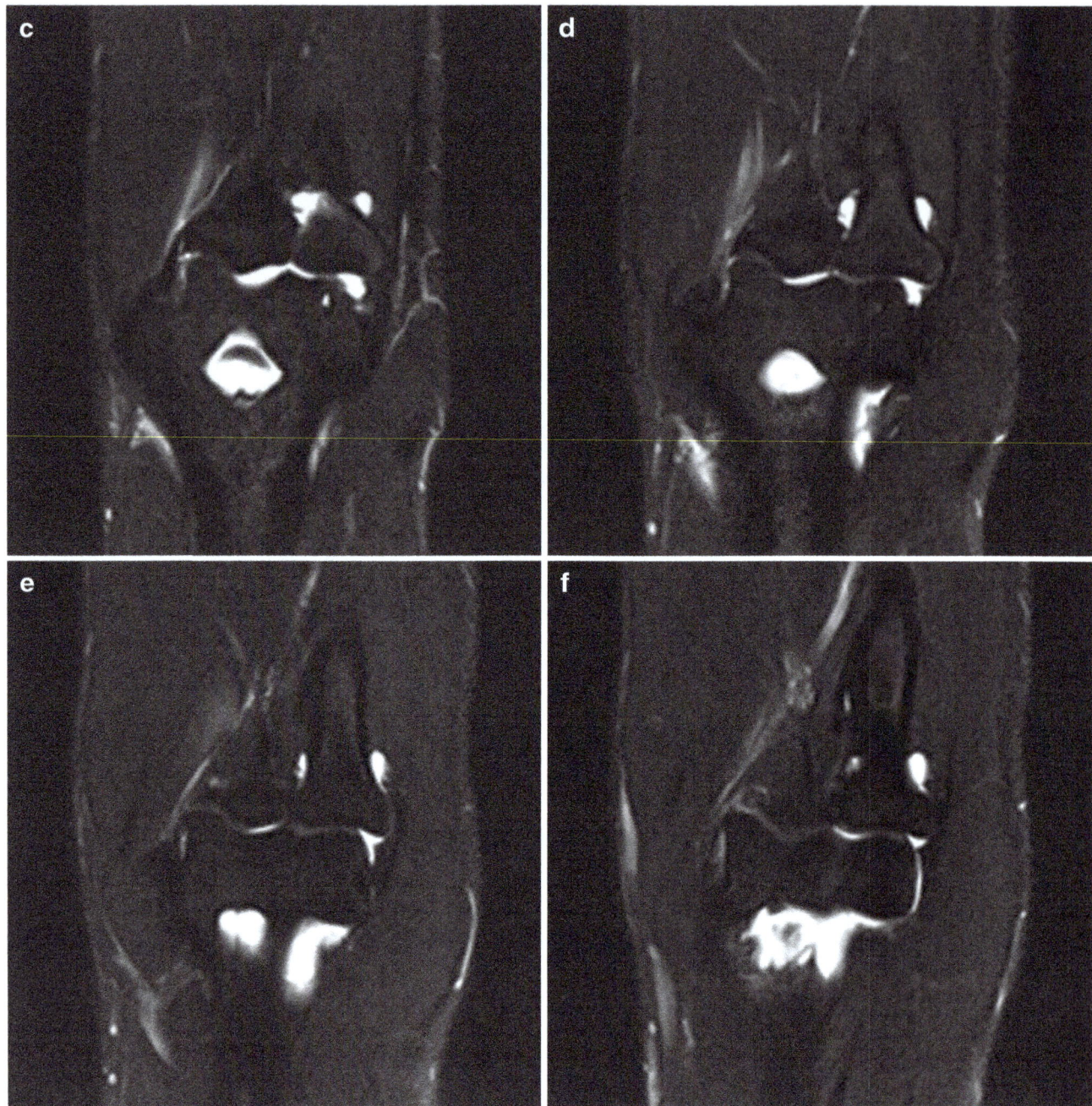

Fig. 22.7 (continued)

visualized and a "drive-through sign" of the elbow was noted again indicative of medial instability. The arthroscopic portion of the procedure was then terminated.

The arm was rotated to gain access to the medial aspect of the elbow; the UCL reconstruction was started as seen in Fig. 22.10a–d. A medial approach to the elbow was made and the ulnar nerve was protected. The flexor-pronator group was incised and split. Upon inspection of the ligament, it was noted that there was a bony avulsion from the medial epicondyle that likely represented an older injury given the ligament was not actually detached from the epicondyle. There was also tearing of the mid-substance of the ligament as well as evidence of avulsing of the ligament from the sublime tubercle. The ligament was dissected posteriorly to obtain

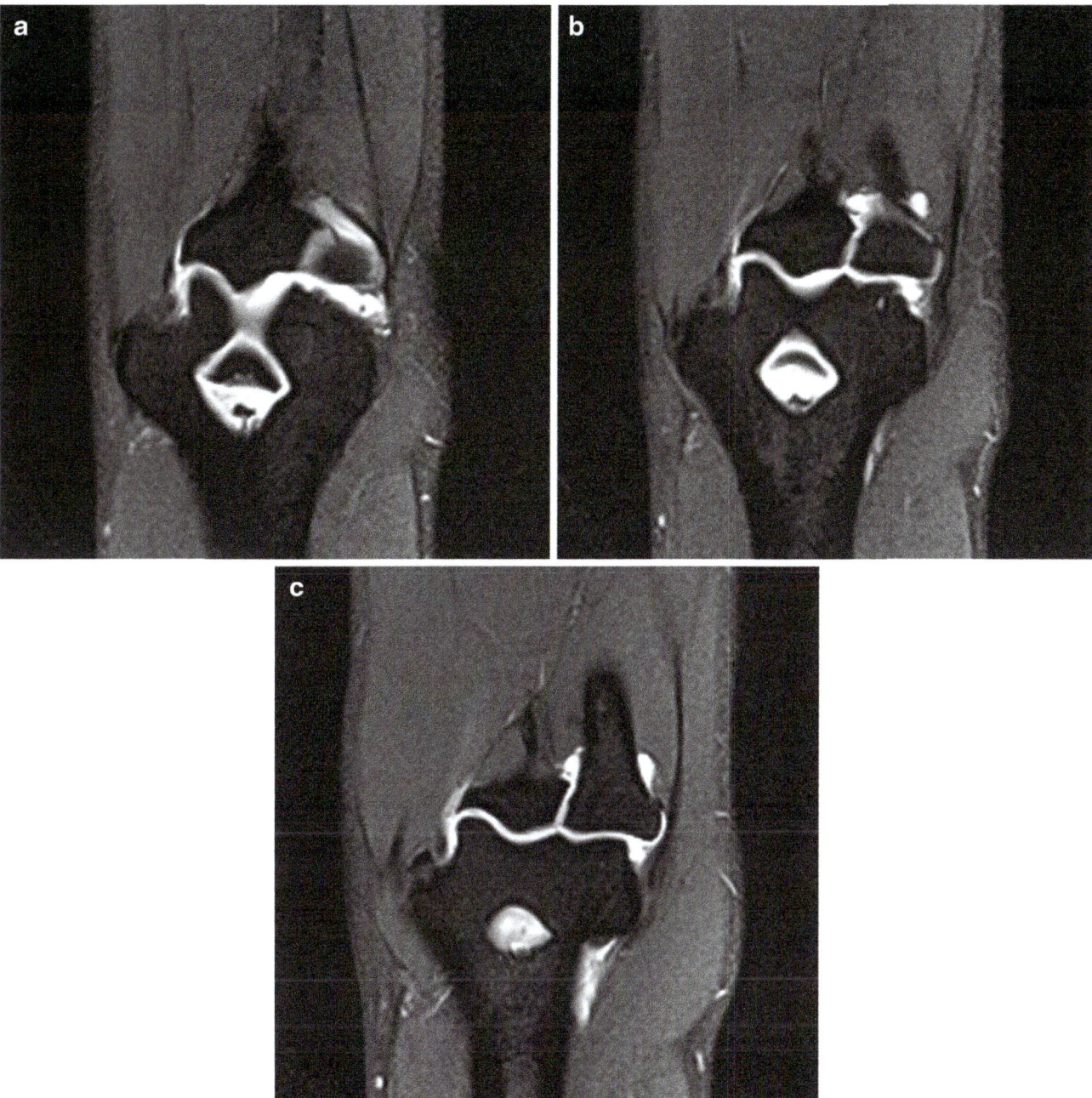

Fig. 22.8 (**a–e**) Coronal T1 fat-saturated images again show the avulsed fragment from the medial epicondyle as well as signal change in the mid-substance of the ligament indicating a tear (**a–e**: Published with kind permission. Copyright © Felix H. Savoie, III, MD)

access to the insertion site. A pilot hole was drilled through the sublime tubercle and reamed with a 5 mm reamer. The prepared palmaris graft was then pulled into the hole and transfixed with an interference screw. A pilot hole was drilled into the origin of the medial epicondyle. A Y-tunnel configuration was made with a 4.5 mm tunnel at the origin and two intersecting 3.5 mm tunnels out posteriorly. The palmaris graft was docked into these tunnels followed by reinforcing of the graft by sewing the remaining MUCL to the graft. The elbow was tested and found to have no gapping medially with a solid end point. The capsule was repaired and the wound closed in standard fashion.

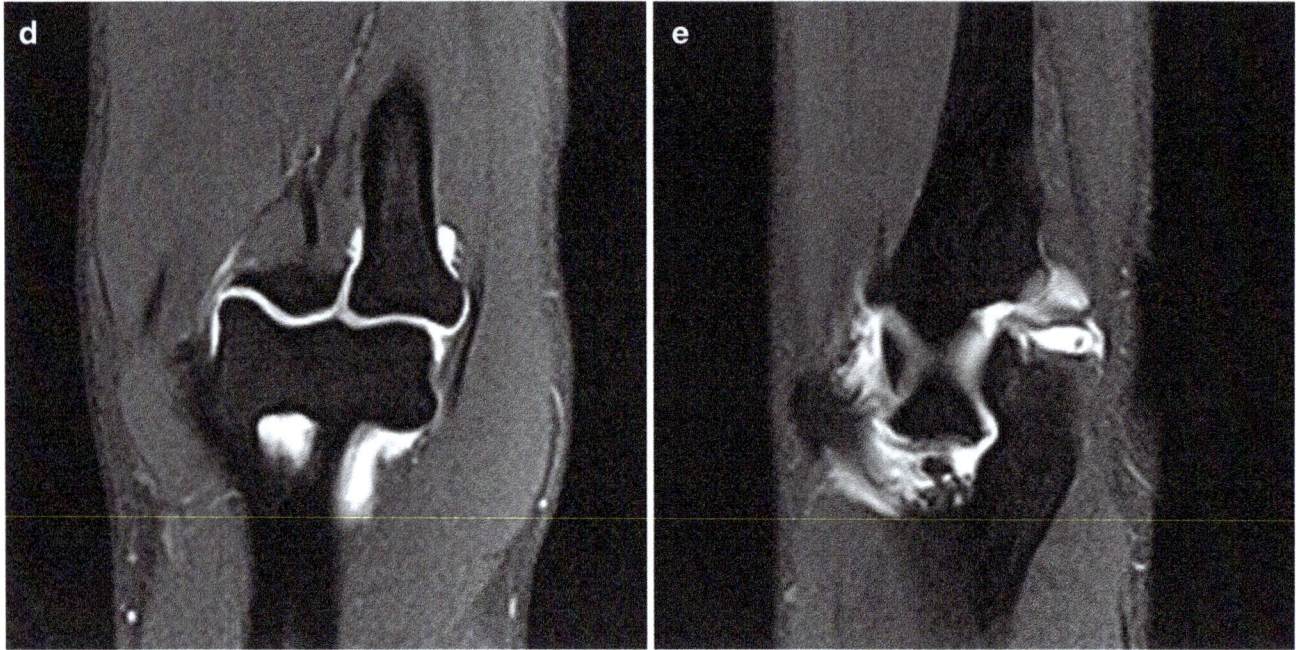

Fig. 22.8 (continued)

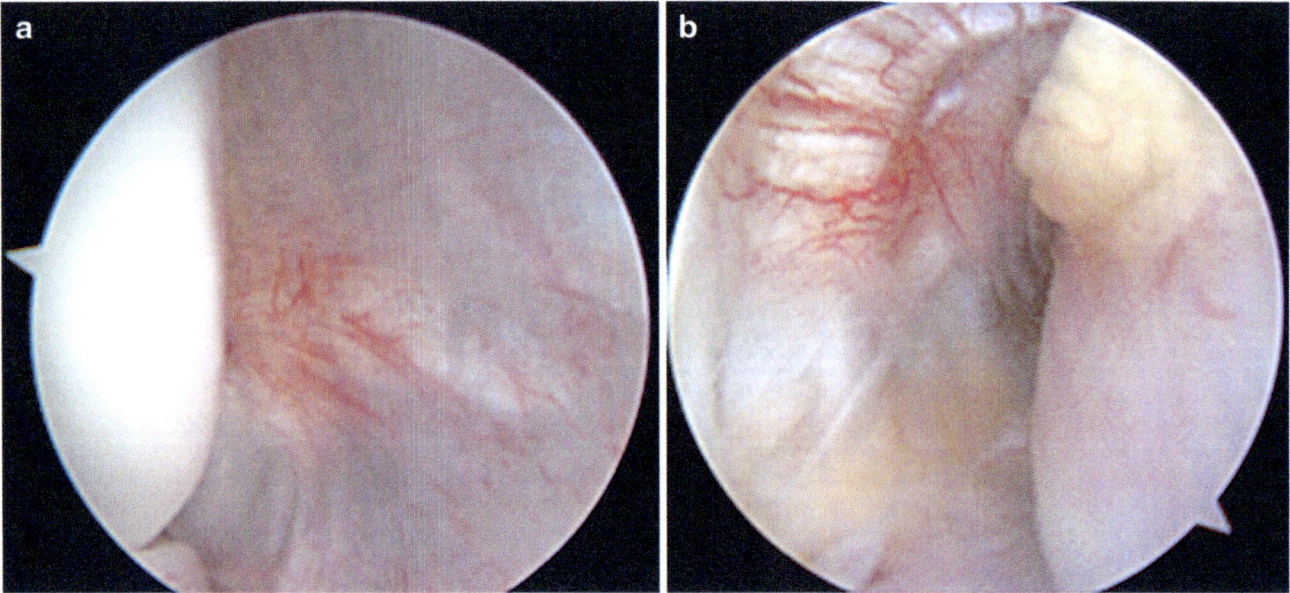

Fig. 22.9 (**a–d**) Arthroscopic images showing lateral synovitis, medial synovitis, and evidence of instability with a "drive-through sign" and medial gapping (**a–d**: Published with kind permission. Copyright © Felix H. Savoie, III, MD)

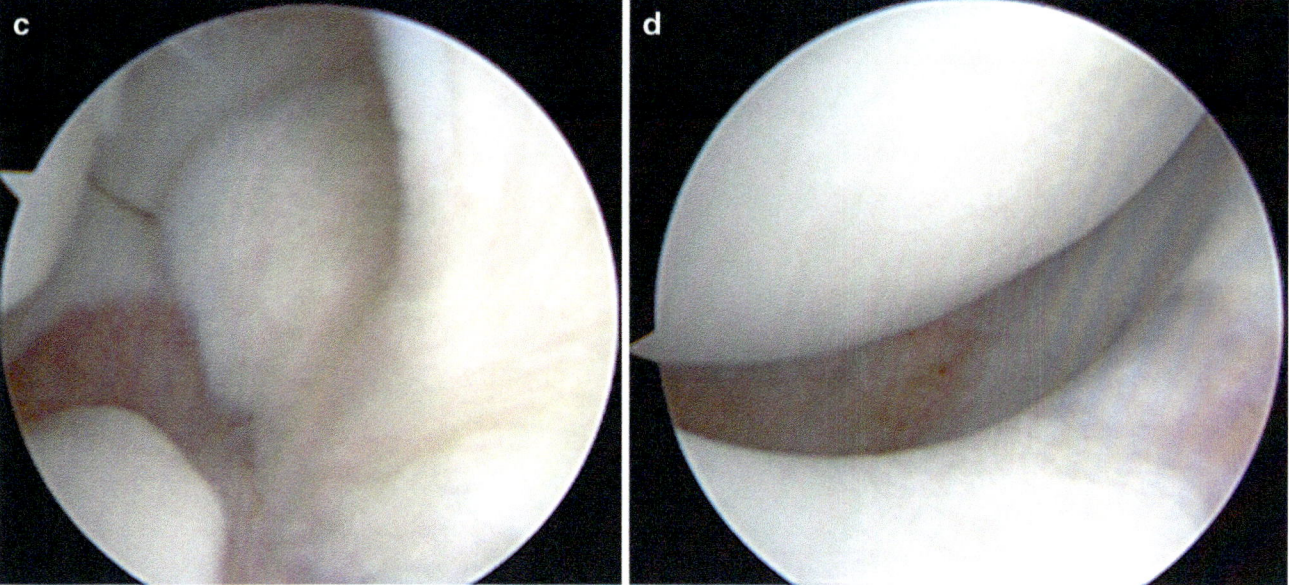

Fig. 22.9 (continued)

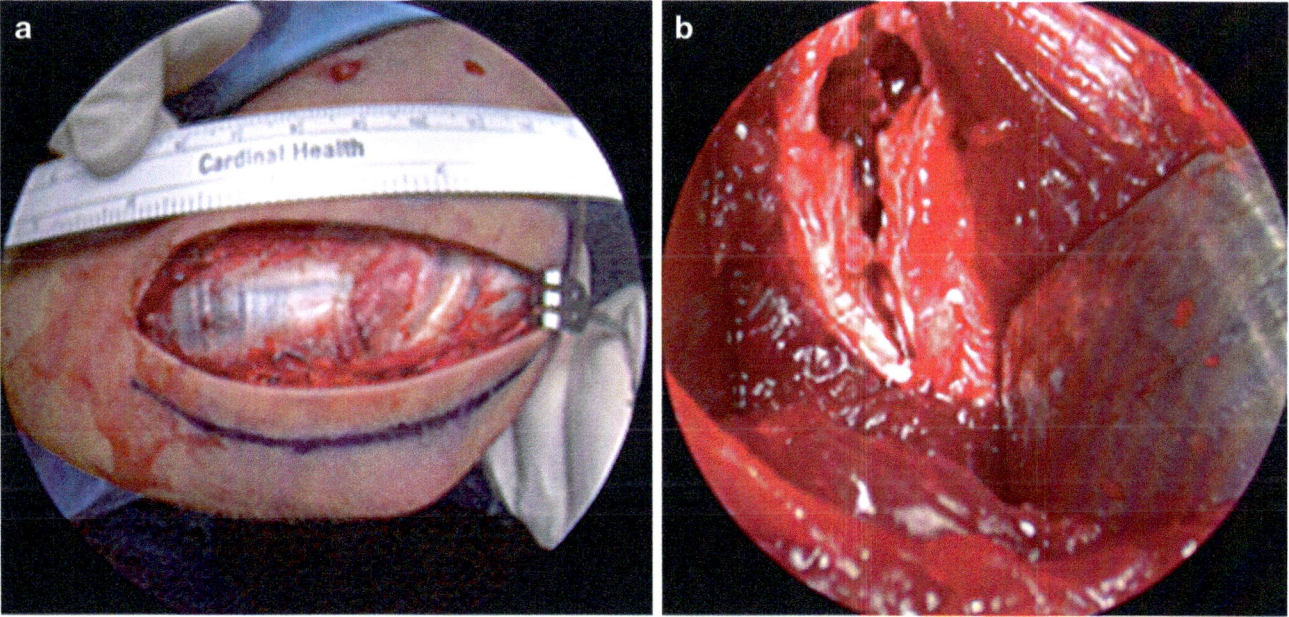

Fig. 22.10 (**a**) Initial incision and identification of the flexor mass and the ulnar nerve. (**b**) Initial identification of the torn UCL. (**c**) Excision of the small avulsion fragment from the medial epicondyle. (**d**) Placement of the palmaris graft (**a–d**: Published with kind permission. Copyright © Felix H. Savoie, III, MD)

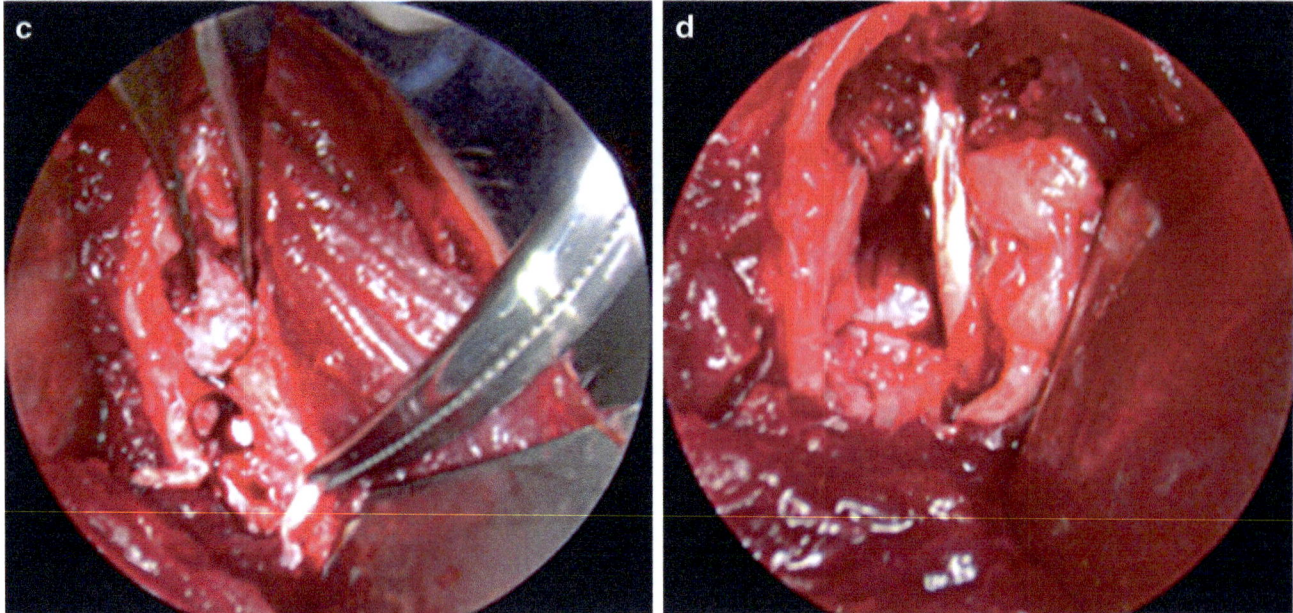

Fig. 22.10 (continued)

References

1. Feltner ME. Three-dimensional interactions in a two-segment kinetic chain, part II: application to the throwing arm in baseball pitching. Int J Sport Biomech. 1998;5:420–50.
2. Rettig AC, Sherrill C, Snead DS, Mendler JC, Mieling P. Nonoperative treatment of ulnar collateral ligament injuries in throwing athletes. Am J Sports Med. 2001;29(1):15–7.
3. Jobe FW, Stark H, Lombardo SJ. Reconstruction of the ulnar collateral ligament in athletes. J Bone Joint Surg Am. 1986;68(8):1158–63.
4. Dines JS, ElAttrache NS, Conway J, Smith W, Ahmad CS. Clinical outcomes of the DANE TJ technique to treat ulnar collateral ligament insufficiency of the elbow. Am J Sports Med. 2007;35:2039–44.
5. Dodson CC, Thomas A, Dines JS, Nho SJ, Williams III RJ, Altchek DW. Medial ulnar collateral ligament reconstruction of the elbow in throwing athletes. Am J Sports Med. 2006;34(12):1926–32.
6. Thompson WH, Jobe FW, Yocum LA, Pink MM. Ulnar collateral ligament reconstruction in athletes: muscle splitting approach without transposition of the ulnar nerve. J Shoulder Elbow Surg. 2001;10(2):152–7.
7. Bowers AI, Dines JS, Dines DM, Altchek DW. Elbow medial ulnar collateral ligament reconstruction: clinical relevance and the docking technique. J Shoulder Elbow Surg. 2010;19(2 suppl):110–7.
8. Savoie 3rd FH, Trenhaile SW, Roberts J, Field LD, Ramsey JR. Primary repair of ulnar collateral ligament injuries of the elbow in young athletes: a case series of injuries to the proximal and distal ends of the ligament. Am J Sports Med. 2008;36(6):1066–72.

OCD/Chondral Injuries of the Elbow

Jeffrey B. Witty, E. Rhett Hobgood, and Larry D. Field

Introduction

Osteochondritis dissecans (OCD) of the elbow is a localized lesion of the articular surface that most commonly involves the anterior capitellum. A variety of etiologies have been proposed including spontaneous osteonecrosis, vascular deficiency, genetics, and repetitive trauma. Inflammation has previously been hypothesized, but later studies revealed there to be no inflammatory cells at the lesion site. Repetitive trauma is now the most commonly accepted cause [1]. The histologic features of OCD lesions include the following [2]:

- Discontinuity of the articular surface. This includes fibrillations, clefts, and fissures which resemble that of degenerative change seen in osteoarthritis.
- Changes in the subchondral bone that include edema, fractures, loose bodies, and localized areas of necrosis. Subchondral fractures are often seen with adjacent callus.
- Areas of horizontal cleavage that may involve cartilage only just above the tidemark or deeper separation of the subchondral bone. Granulation, fibrocartilaginous, and fibrous tissue proliferation can be seen in these areas. These changes correlate with the International Cartilage Repair Society (ICRS) grading system.

Other lesions have been described in the trochlea where approximately 22 cases have been reported (Fig. 23.1a, b) [3]. A varus mechanical stress has been postulated as a potential cause. Medial lesions were typically smaller than lateral lesions [4–11]. OCD of the radial head has also been

J.B. Witty, MD
Acadiana Orthopaedic Center at Lafayette General,
1448 South College Road, Lafayette, LA 70503, USA
e-mail: jeffbwitty@gmail.com

E.R. Hobgood, MD • L.D. Field, MD (✉)
Mississippi Sports Medicine and Orthopedic Center,
Jackson, MS, USA
e-mail: rhetthobgood@msmoc.com; lfield@msmoc.com

described (Fig. 23.1c) [3]. Like OCD of the trochlea, it is more rare than capitellar lesions and has been associated with anterior atraumatic subluxation of the radial head resulting in a posteromedial lesion [12–14].

OCD has also been implicated in developmental instability of the elbow, the majority of which is posterolateral instability [15]. Lateral ligament injuries resulting in instability can cause posterior impaction of the capitellum that may be confused with OCD. It is also important not to confuse the normal pseudodefect on the posterior inferior capitellum with an actual lesion. This pseudodefect represents the normal transition of the capitellar cartilage with the nonarticular lateral epicondyle (Fig. 23.2) [3].

Diagnosis (Clinical/Imaging)

Although OCD lesions can be seen on plain radiography, they can be missed in up to 50 % of cases. To help increase the ability to detect OCD on plain radiographs, a view with the distal humerus in 45° of flexion and 30° of external rotation has been described [10, 16, 17]. Early lesions on radiographs can appear as a slight flattening and sclerosis and progress to radiolucent bone overlying the sclerotic area at approximately 4 months [18]. See Figs. 23.3a–d and 23.4a, b.

New bone continues to form over the flattened area and may have the appearance of a nondisplaced fragment which will begin to form and unite with the underlying bone at approximately 4 months for patients with an open growth plate and may take up to 8 months for those with a closed growth plate. This can continue until past a year. Complete healing can be expected at skeletal maturity [19, 20].

Takahara et al. have described a radiographic classification. Grade I lesions (Fig. 23.5a, b) show a translucent cystic shadow in the lateral or middle capitellum with or without localized flattening. Grade II lesions have a clear zone or split line between the lesion and the adjacent subchondral bone which represents a nondisplaced fragment (Fig. 23.6). Grade III lesions are a displaced or detached fragment, often associated with the presence of loose bodies (Fig. 23.7) [21]. Two

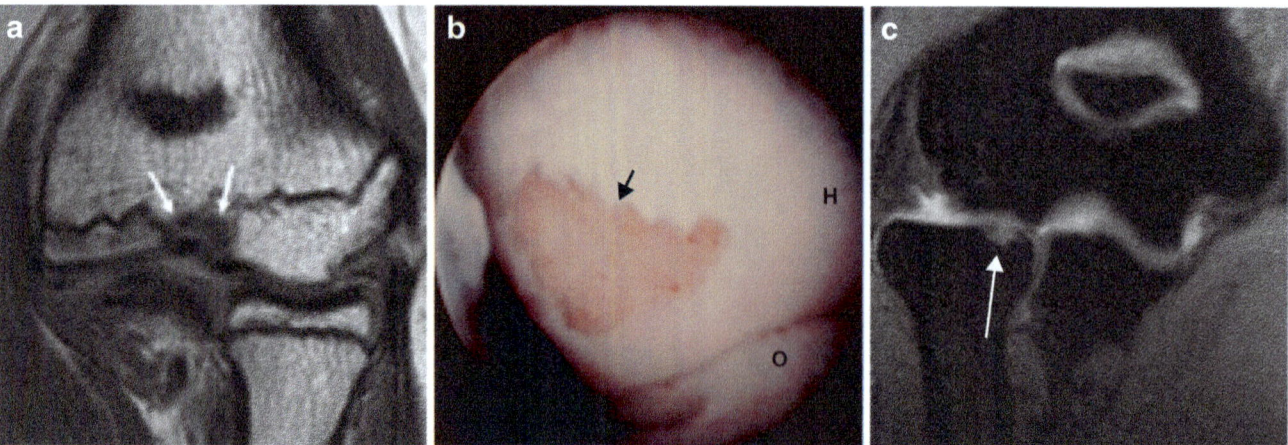

Fig. 23.1 (a–c) MRI and arthroscopic images demonstrating trochlear and radial head lesions (*arrows*) (**a**, **c**: Reprinted from Jans LBO et al. MR imaging findings and MR criteria for instability in osteochondritis dissecans of the elbow in children. Eur J Radiol. 2012;81:1306–10, with permission from Elsevier)

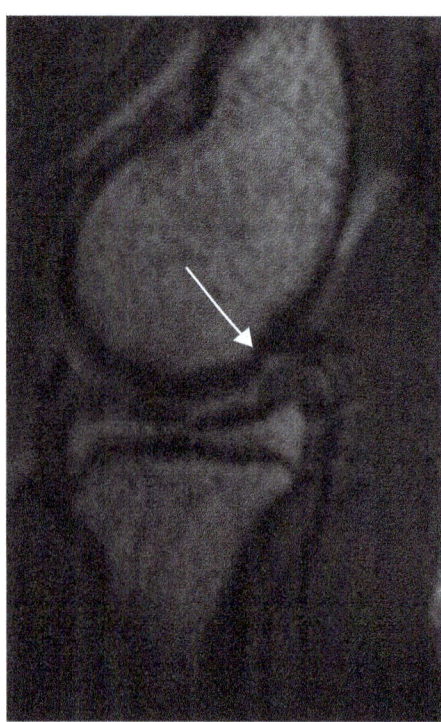

Fig. 23.2 Pseudodefect of posterior inferior capitellum (reprinted from Jans LBO et al. MR imaging findings and MR criteria for instability in osteochondritis dissecans of the elbow in children. Eur J Radiol. 2012;81:1306–10, with permission from Elsevier)

subgroups were added that divided grade II into IIA, which is a fragment not demarcated by sclerosis, and IIB which have a sclerotic rim [22]. These classifications have been used in studies to determine lesion stability as described below.

MRI can also provide information regarding the size, location, and stability of the lesion. MRI of the elbow is optimally performed with the arm at the patient's side,

supinated, and in full extension. This position maximizes the patient's comfort and image quality. Early lesions may demonstrate a low signal on T1 with more subtle abnormalities seen on T2 especially at the periphery [18]. See Figs. 23.8a, b and 23.9a, b.

Fast spin echo sequences can be used to emphasize cartilage, and fat suppression sequences will better show subchondral edema and small fluid/cystic collections [23]. T1 sequences appear similar when comparing stable and unstable lesions with variable low, intermediate, and heterogeneous low and intermediate signal intensity (Fig. 23.10a–c). However, on T2, there can be a high signal along the periphery of unstable lesions likely representing the interposition of synovial fluid (Fig. 23.11) [18, 24].

Histologically, diffuse enhancement on MRI at the subchondral junction may also indicate granulation tissue interposition and an unstable fragment [25]. There can be a lack of signal along the periphery of stable lesions which makes the lesion difficult to distinguish from the adjacent marrow. In addition, MRI may reveal surface flaps, early delamination, displacement of the lesion, and presence of loose bodies. Underlying cysts may also be seen (Fig. 23.12) [21, 23, 24].

Two systems by De Smet et al. [24, 26] and Dipaola et al. (Table 23.1) [27, 28] have utilized MRI findings to classify the stability of OCD lesions. However, both of these often cited studies surveyed lesions of the femoral condyles and talar dome. MRI signs as described by De Smet are summarized as follows:

- A thin, ill-defined or well-defined line of high signal intensity at the interface between the osteochondral lesion and underlying bone
- A discrete, round area of homogeneous high signal intensity beneath the lesion such as a cyst
- A focal defect in the articular surface of the lesion

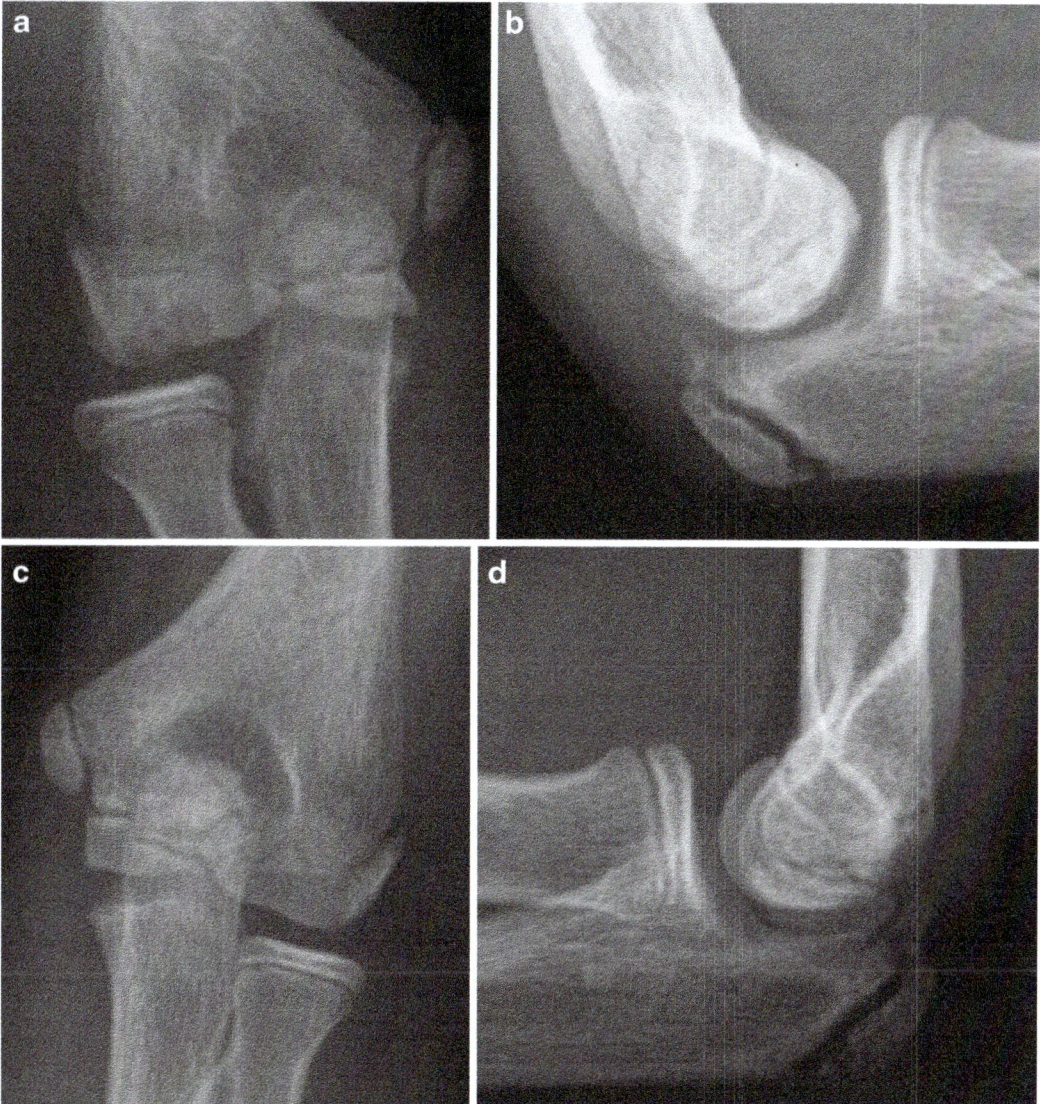

Fig. 23.3 (**a–d**) A 14-year-old baseball player with 2-month history of right elbow pain demonstrating cystic appearance and limited area of sclerosis. There is flattening of the capitellum most noticeable on the lateral view (**a, b**). Comparison views of the left elbow (**c, d**)

- A high-signal-intensity line penetrating the articular cartilage and subchondral bone into the lesion

In their study, they reviewed MRI reports and intraoperative assessments in an average patient population age of 25.7 years. They were able to correctly identify 97 % of unstable lesions and 100 % of stable lesions using their classification system. The most frequent sign of instability was a high-signal line at the junction between the lesion and subchondral bone seen in 72 % of cases. This line was not seen in any of the patients with stable lesions. The presence of at least one sign indicates fragment instability [26].

Dipaola et al. performed a double-blinded, prospective study of 12 patients with an average age of 26.5 years using a 0.35T MRI. They devised their own system, and the arthroscopic stages are not those of the ICRS classification. This staging system

originally used arthroscopic, MRI, and radiographic findings. However, more recent studies have only included the arthroscopic and MRI components [29]. MRI was able to correctly identify all stage I, III, and IV lesions. One patient with stage II lesion was incorrectly identified as a stage III lesion. Stages III and IV are considered unstable [27]. See Table 23.1 [27, 28].

The ICRS classification system has more recently been created for arthroscopic evaluation of OCD lesions which is summarized in Table 23.2 [30].

Even though MRI has been the standard for evaluating articular cartilage, it can have limitations. Theodoropoulous et al. looked at 31 patients with an average age of 38.7 years (range 15–63) with elbow articular cartilage defects that did not include OCD lesions diagnosed during arthroscopy and compared the findings with those of the MRI. The accuracy

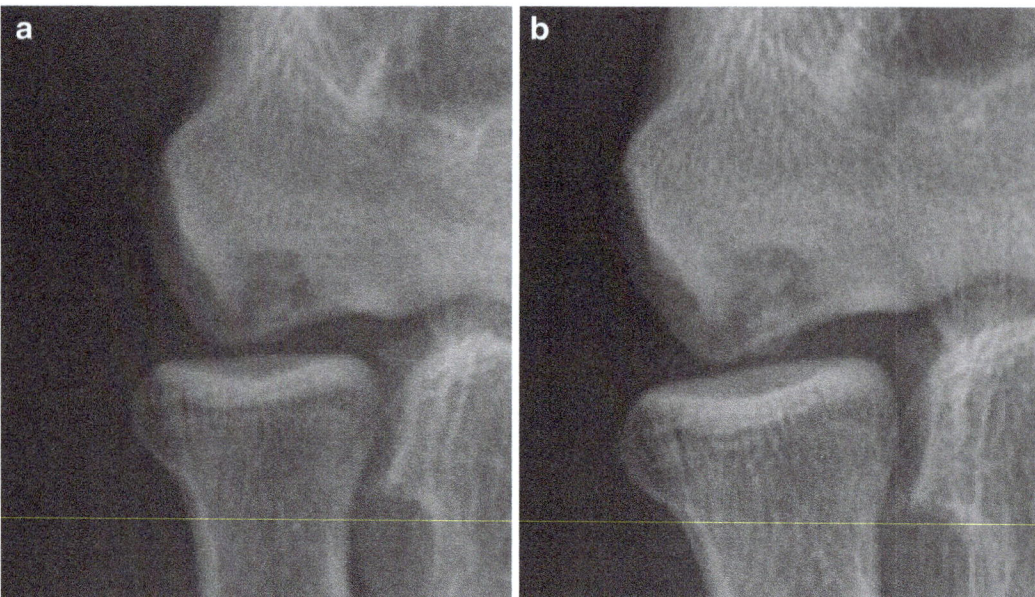

Fig. 23.4 (**a**, **b**) A 14-year-old quarterback treated nonoperatively. Initial presentation radiograph of lesion in capitellum (**a**). Radiograph 4 months (**b**) after initiation of treatment demonstrating progressive bony filling of capitellar defect

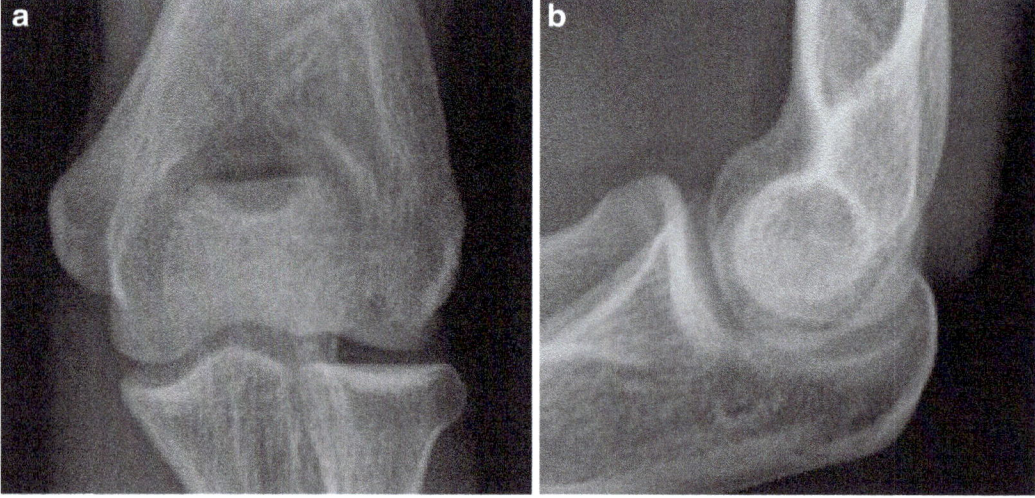

Fig. 23.5 (**a**, **b**) Grade I lesion with translucent cystic appearance on AP view (**a**) and flattening of capitellum noted on the lateral view (**b**)

was 45 %, 65 %, 20 %, and 30 % for the radius, capitellum, ulna, and trochlea, respectively. This study included ICRS grade II defects (not the ICRS OCD classification, lesion >50 % depth of cartilage) and used a 1.5T MRI and fast spin echo T2 sequences to highlight articular cartilage defects [31].

MRI also may have limitations predicting OCD stability especially in a younger, overhead athlete population. Using intraoperative assessment as the gold standard, Iwasaki et al. looked at 27 overhead athletes (average age of 14 years, range 11–30 years) and compared lesion stability between MRI using the classification systems of De Smet and Dipaola and the ICRS OCD classification system. The majority used a 1.5T MRI. For the De Smet system, sensitivity was 89 % and specificity was 44 % diagnosing fragment instability. The positive predictive value (PPV) and negative predictive value (NPV) were 76 % and 67 %, respectively. False negatives and false positives were 11 % and 56 %, respectively. For the Dipaola system, sensitivity was 83 % and specificity 44 %. PPV and NPV were 75 % and 57 %, respectively. False negative and false positives were 17 % and 56 %, respectively. Furthermore, all MRI predicted stable lesions but did not accurately predict the intraoperative/arthroscopic stage. It was able to predict 57 % of stage III and 64 % of stage IV unstable lesions. The

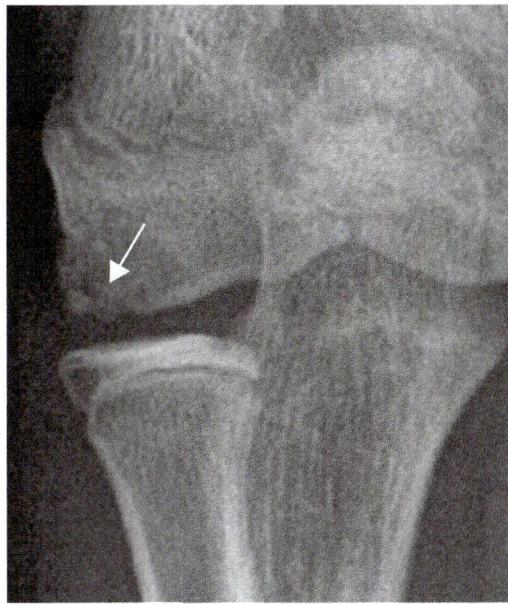

Fig. 23.6 Grade II lesion with cystic lesion of capitellum and linear lucency dividing the bone and nondisplaced fragment along the distal-lateral capitellum

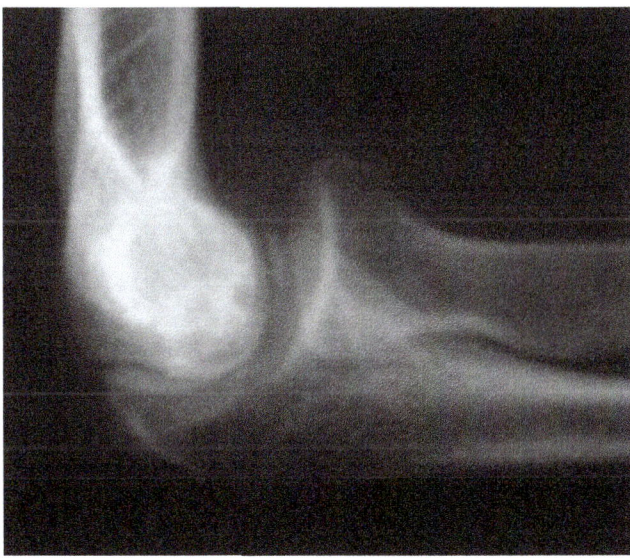

Fig. 23.7 Grade III lesion with loose fragments visible in the anterior compartment

authors stated that many patients with predicted stable lesions are unlikely to have a stable lesion once evaluated intraoperatively, especially in teenage patients who repetitively stress the radiocapitellar joint such as overhead athletes. Thus, these patients still have histopathological instability despite findings on MRI. MRI was better overall for predicting unstable lesions that were in fact unstable during arthroscopic evaluation [29].

Satake et al. [32] retrospectively reviewed 78 patients to determine signs of lesion instability. The average age between operatively and nonoperatively treated patients was 13.3 and 11.2 years. ICRS grading was used during intraoperative evaluation. Along with determining signs seen on MRI, the authors also used plain radiographs and CT scan. Their findings are summarized below.

Correspondence with intraoperative instability:
1. Minami grade III on plain radiographs
2. Closure of the epiphyseal line on the capitellum and lateral epicondyle
3. Articular irregularity on MRI
4. High signal intensity on T2 MRI at interface of lesion
5. Displaced fragment on CT scan

No correspondence with intraoperative instability:
1. Intralesional segmentation on CT
2. Signal line through articular surface on MRI
3. Articular defect (not irregularity) on MRI

Sensitivity >80 % to detect unstable lesion:
1. Epiphyseal closure of capitellum on radiographs
2. Segmentation on CT

Specificity >80 %:
1. Minami grade III
2. Epiphyseal closure of lateral epicondyle on radiograph
3. Articular irregularity
4. T2 high signal at interface
5. Displaced fragment on CT (may miss cartilaginous-only lesion)

The authors concluded that radiographic grade III lesions, closure of the epiphyseal line of the capitellum and lateral epicondyle, MRI findings of irregular articular contours, and high signal intensity at the lesion interface as well as a displaced fragment on CT were indicative of fragment instability.

Jans et al. retrospectively reviewed 25 patients with an average age of 14 years and found that using instability criteria for the knee described above by De Smet et al. (high T2 rim signal, surrounding/sublesional cysts, high-T2-signal fracture line, and a fluid-filled osteochondral defect). When all four criteria were combined, MRI was 100 % sensitive for unstable OCD of the elbow. Enhancement of the OCD fragment post-gadolinium contrast suggests that the lesion is viable [14].

Based on the studies described above, MRI findings suggestive of lesion instability are summarized below [17, 24, 26, 29, 32]:

- Articular cartilage breached and a thin, ill- or well-defined line of high signal intensity at the interface between the osteochondral lesion and underlying bone. See Fig. 23.17a–e.
- A discrete, round area of homogeneous high signal intensity beneath the lesion (cystic structure). See Fig. 23.18.

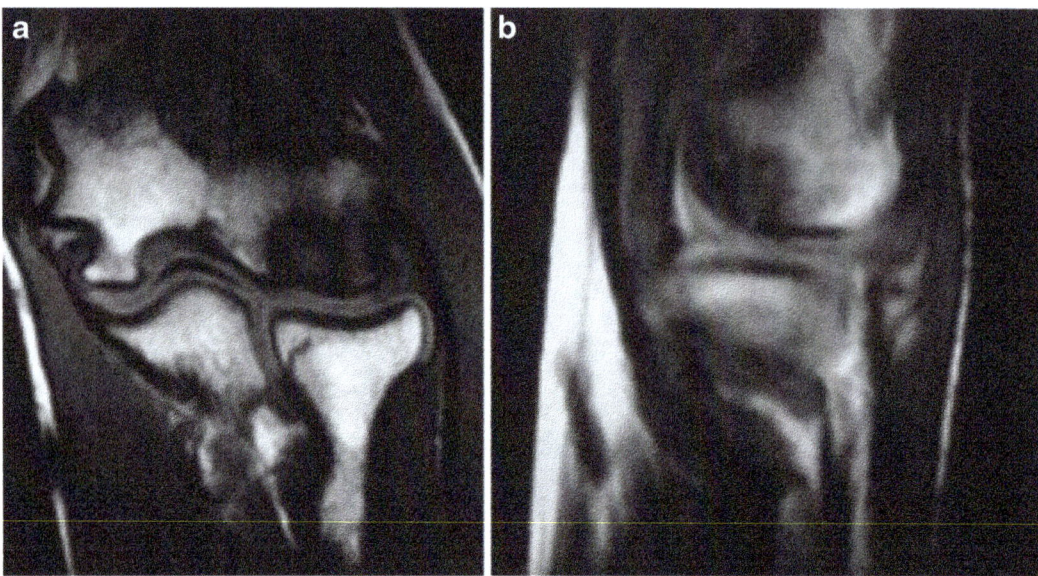

Fig. 23.8 Coronal (**a**) and sagittal (**b**) T1 MRI demonstrating low signal intensity in a stable capitellar lesion

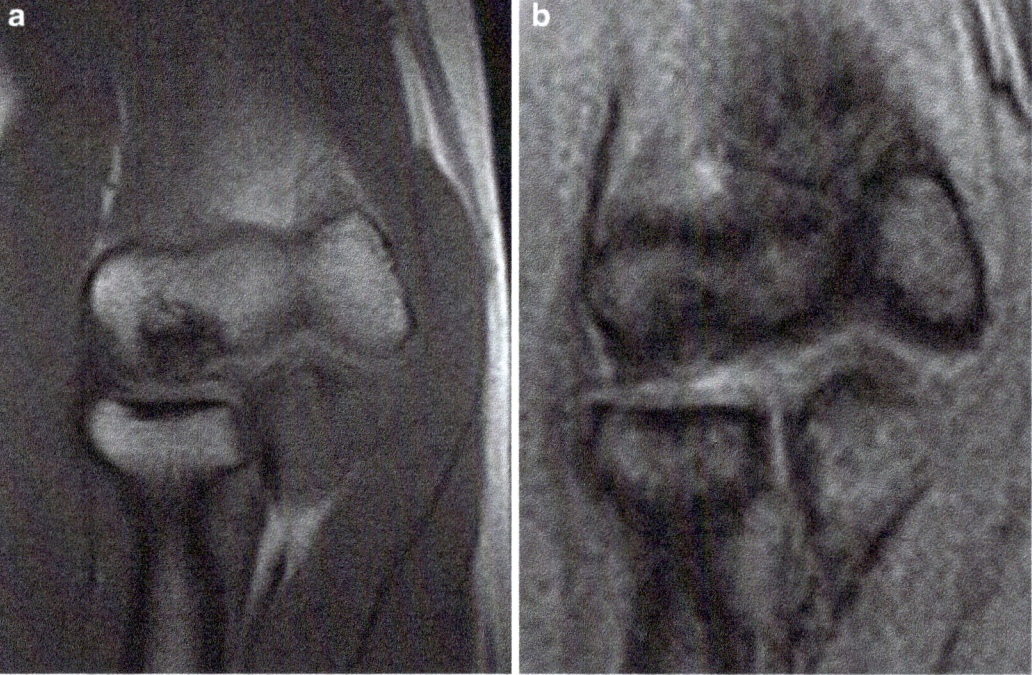

Fig. 23.9 Another example of a T1 MRI of a stable lesion (**a**) and the corresponding T2 (**b**). The periphery is indistinguishable from the surrounding marrow

- A focal defect in the articular surface of the lesion, multiple articular breaks, or high-signal-intensity line penetrating the articular cartilage and subchondral bone into the lesion. This is based on the criteria by De Smet et al. [24, 26]. This finding is not suggestive of lesion instability according to Satake et al. [32].
- Displaced or loose fragment. See Fig. 23.19a–e.
- Irregular articular contours.

It is essential to inspect the scan for any intra-articular loose bodies. They can block joint motion and are a common cause for operative treatment. MRI is better at picking up posterior fossa loose bodies than in the anterior compartment [33]. Other non-MRI signs of fragment instability are summarized below:

- All grade II lesions [21] or grade IIB [20, 34] and radiographic grade III

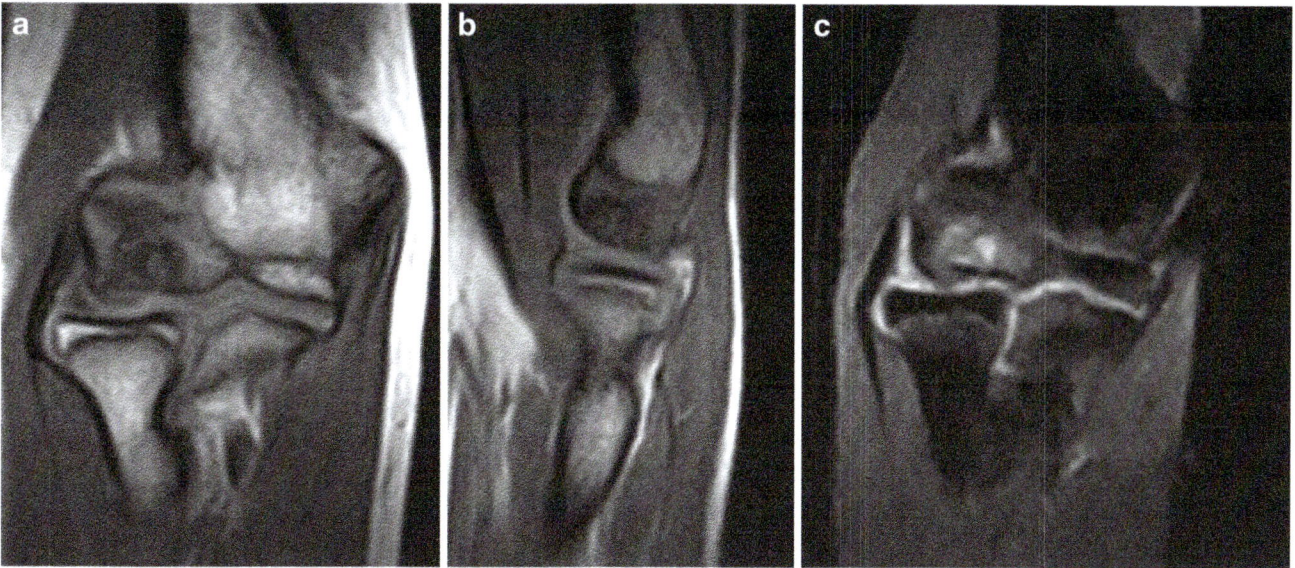

Fig. 23.10 T1 MRI with capitellar lesion with low peripheral signal and heterogeneous intermediate intensity in the central portion (**a**, **b**). T2 coronal image of the same lesion showing features consistent with an unstable lesion such as high-signal cystic and linear areas (**c**)

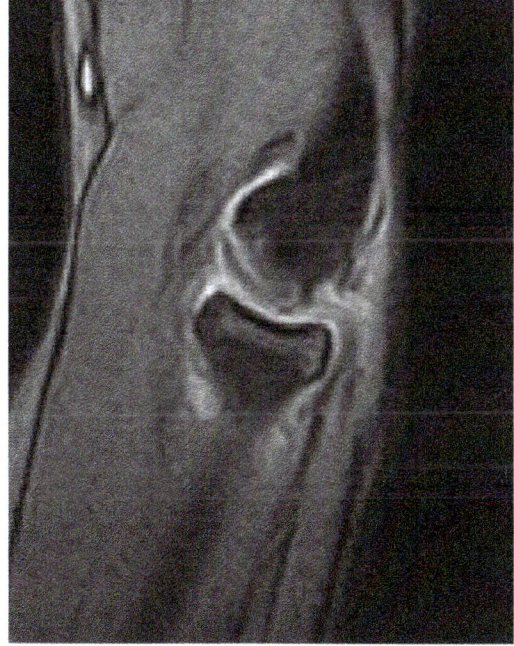

Fig. 23.11 T2 MRI demonstrating high-intensity signal at interface between the lesion and subchondral bone

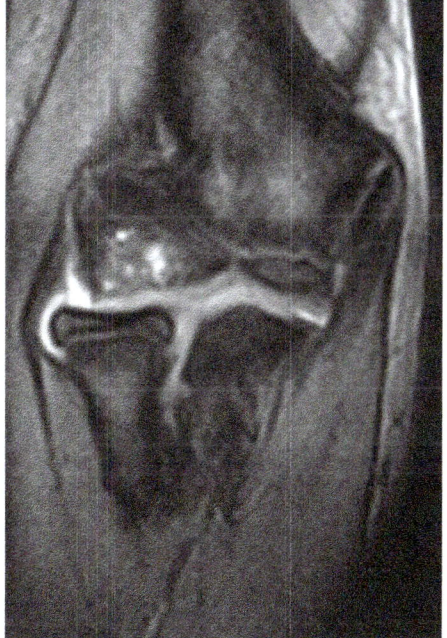

Fig. 23.12 Example of cystic area beneath lesion in the capitellum

- Closure of the epiphyseal line on the capitellum and lateral epicondyle [32]
- Displaced fragment on CT [32]
- Restriction of elbow motion >20° [21]

The lesion size can also be quantified. This is based on the description by Takahara et al. [28] and can be modified for use by MRI [35]. This measurement is taken from the coronal and sagittal images. The first parameter is the AP size determined as a percentage of the width of the capitellum (between the edge of the lateral epicondyle and the lateral edge of the trochlea), and the second is the defect angle made by the center of the capitellum on the sagittal view and the upper and lower ends of the defect. See Fig. 23.20a, b [28]. Defects can be classified based on the description by Takahara et al. (Table 23.3 [28]).

Table 23.1 OCD staging system

Stage	Arthroscopic findings	MRI
I	Irregularity and softening of articular cartilage. No definable fragment	Thickening of articular cartilage and low-signal changes. See Fig. 23.13
II	Articular cartilage breached, definable fragment, not displaceable	Articular cartilage breached, low-signal rim behind fragment indicating fibrous attachment. See Fig. 23.14
III	Articular cartilage breached, definable fragment, displaceable but attached by some overlying articular cartilage	Articular cartilage breached, high-signal changes behind fragment indicating synovial fluid between fragment and underlying subchondral bone. See Fig. 23.15a–d
IV	Loose body	Loose body. See Fig. 23.20a, b [28]

Data from Dipaola J, Nelson D, Colville M. Characterizing osteochondral lesions by magnetic resonance imaging. Arthroscopy. 1991;7(1):101–4

Table 23.2 International Cartilage Repair Society classification for OCD

ICRS OCD stage	Findings
I	Stable in continuity, softened area covered by intact cartilage
II	Partial discontinuity, stable on probing
III	Complete discontinuity, "dead in situ," not displaced
IV	Displaced fragment, loose within the bed or empty defect. See Fig. 23.16a, b
Subgroup B	>10 mm depth

Data from ICRS Cartilage Injury Evaluation Package [Internet] 2000 Jan. Available from: http://www.cartilage.org/_files/contentmanagement/ICRS_evaluation.pdf

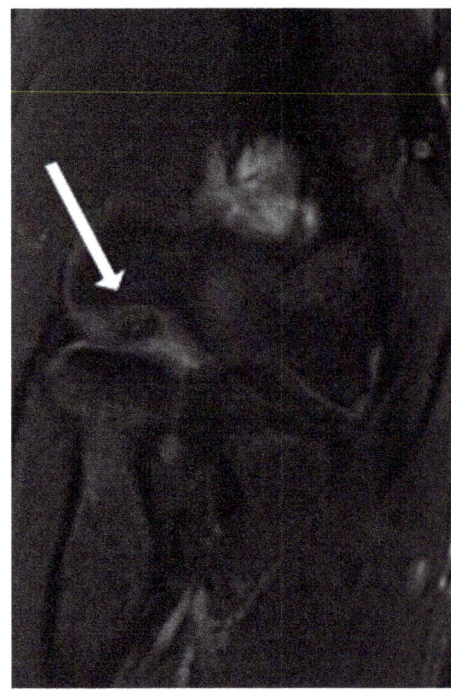

Fig. 23.14 Example of Dipaola stage II lesion. *White arrow* pointing to low-signal rim suggesting fibrous union of fragment

Management

Nonoperative treatment can be effective in appropriately selected patients. In the literature, this has usually consisted of discontinuation of throwing, batting, gymnastics, and other strenuous athletic activities as well as carrying heavy loads for 6 months. The younger the patient (skeletally immature), the more likely the lesion will be a lower radiographic grade/stage and the more likely healing will be achieved with nonoperative treatment. They can also be expected to have better pain levels and less restriction of elbow motion. Healing rates can be as high as 91 % and a return to overhead sport, including baseball as high as 87 %. Healing of grade/stage II lesions is less likely and the clinician can expect approximately half

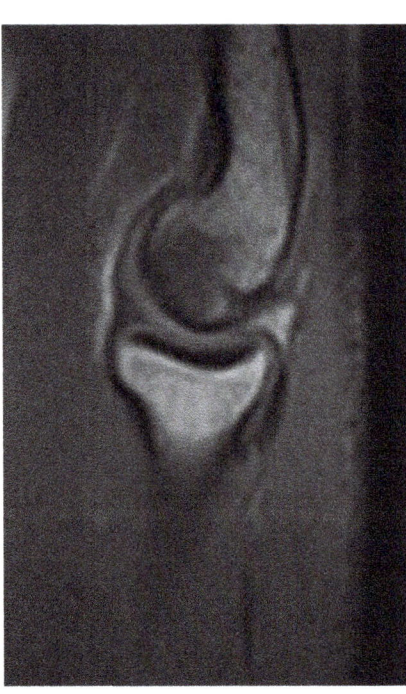

Fig. 23.13 Example of Dipaola stage I demonstrating low-signal changes in the capitellum

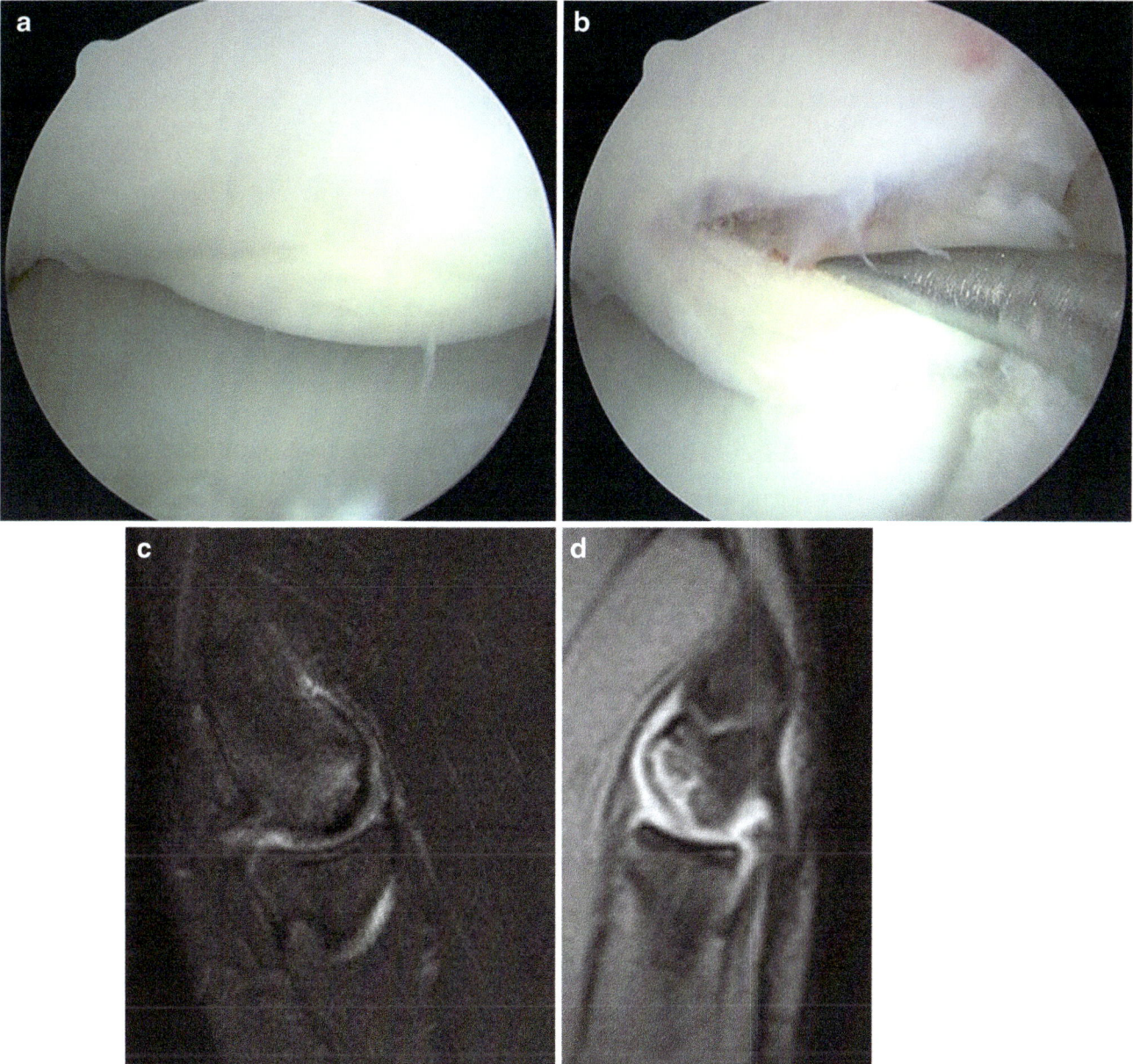

Fig. 23.15 Intraoperative images of Dipaola stage III lesion still attached to some overlying cartilage but still displaceable (**a, b**). MRI examples demonstrating a (**c**) thin and ill-defined line and (**d**) a more well-defined line dividing the lesion and underlying subchondral bone

of these to heal. If sclerosis is noted around the lesion (a grade IIB based on the study by Mihara et al. [20]), the healing rates noticeably drop off and are similar to grade III lesions. Grade/stage IIB and III lesions can be expected to have healing rates and return to sport as low as 11 % and 20 %, respectively. It is of paramount importance to stress to the patient and the family the need for strict adherence to the nonoperative plan. Failure to do so, even with early lesions, can result in progression to worsening OCD and the development of loose bodies [20, 21, 36–38].

Multiple surgical options have been described. These include drilling of the defect, fragment removal with or without curettage or drilling of the residual defect, fragment fixation, and reconstruction with osteochondral autograft from the knee or ribs. The appropriate treatment is based on a variety of factors that include the location of the lesion and size. Many articles do not describe the size of the lesion, which makes the decision of the type of operative treatment more difficult given the variety of options.

Simple fragment excision, loose-body removal, and debridement to a healthy, bleeding bone bed have produced good results in athletes. Up to 80 % of throwers and gymnasts are able to return to preinjury activity levels [39]. Better results are seen with defects less than 50 % and were similar to those achieved with fragment fixation or reconstruction [21]. Arthroscopic fragment removal and debridement do appear

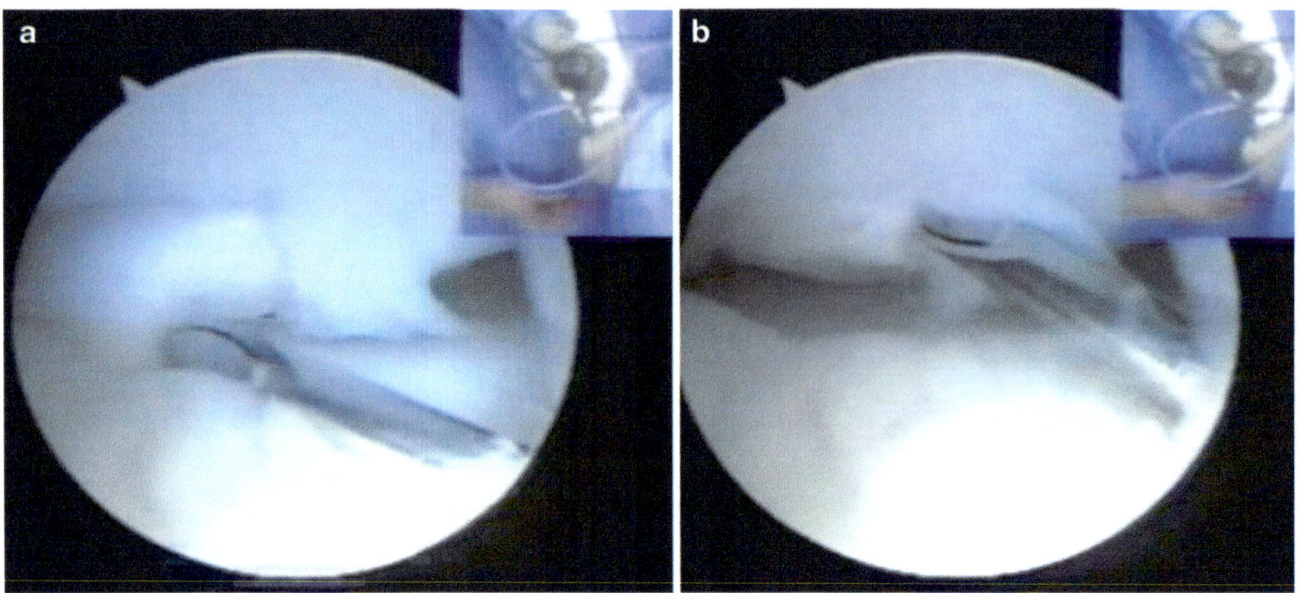

Fig. 23.16 Example of ICRS stage IV lesion. The spinal needle is manipulating a loose fragment within its bed in the capitellum (**a**, **b**)

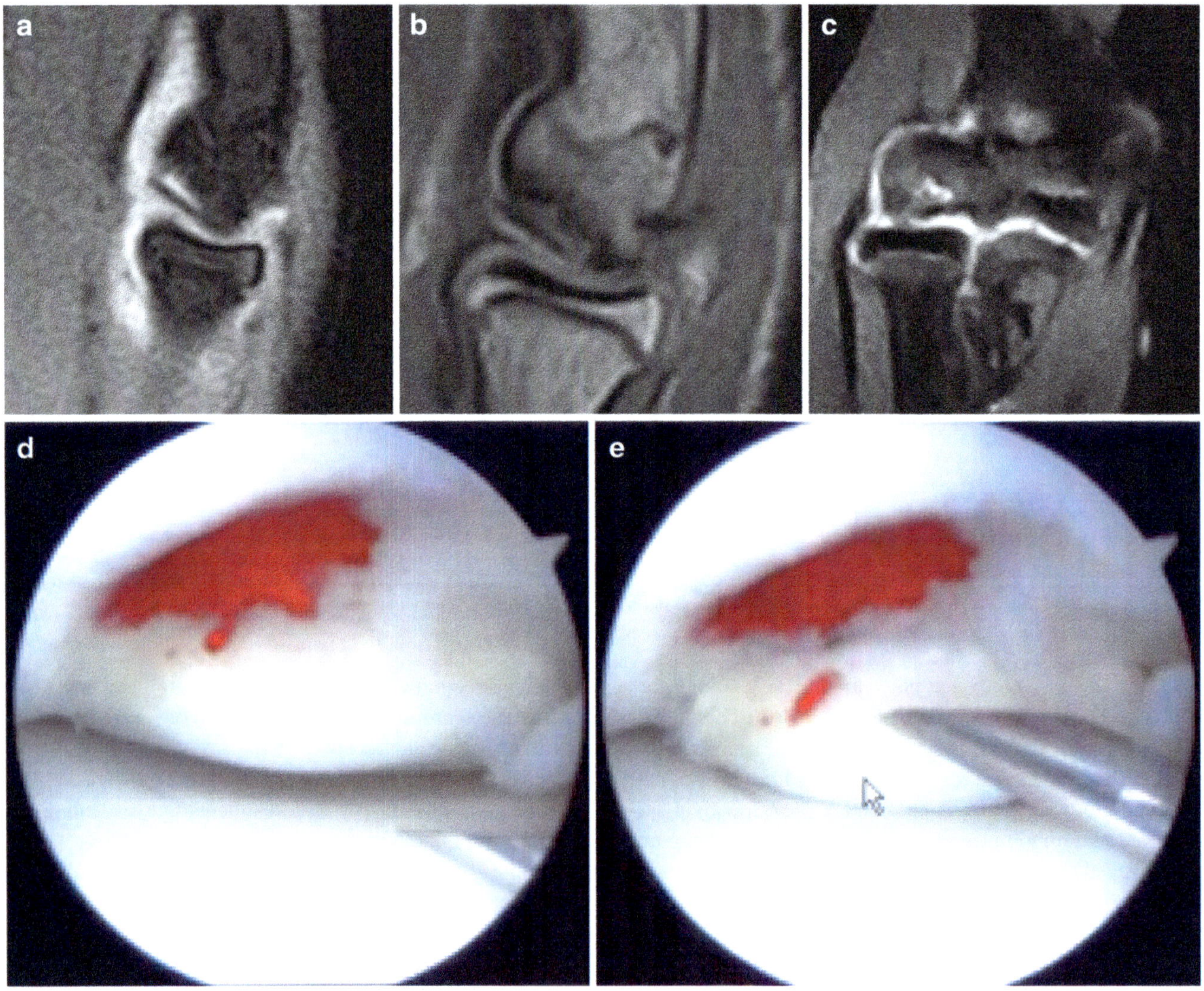

Fig. 23.17 MRI images illustrating a *thin line* demarcating the lesion from subchondral bone (**a–c**). Arthroscopic images demonstrating a similar lesion (**d**, **e**)

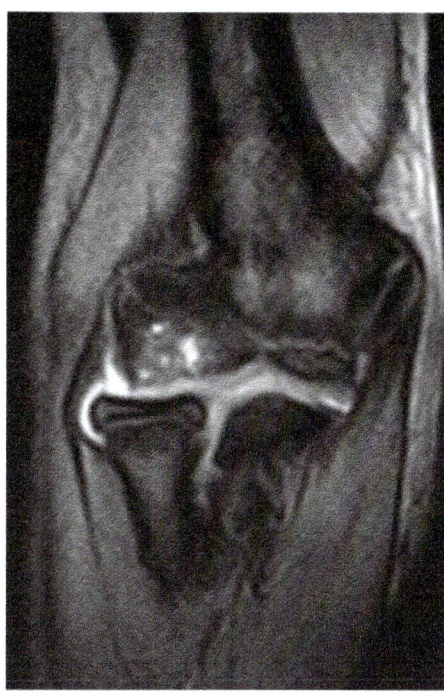

Fig. 23.18 Capitellar lesion with multiple cystic areas surrounding the lesion

to produce better results than open treatment. Residual symptoms have been seen in 42–65 % of patients treated with open techniques [25].

Open fixation of unstable fragments can provide resolution of pain as well as a return to throwing. In some studies, bone grafting of the defect was performed in addition to fixing the fragment. Return to throwing and baseball has ranged from 75 to 100 % of cases. Of note, in the majority of studies, the patients were on average skeletally immature. In addition, a clear description of the lesion and the underlying bony bed is often not provided, and this may make determining the best indications for internal fixation and/or bone grafting challenging [40–43].

Osteochondral autograft is another option. In some instances, the graft was used for fixation of a nondisplaced fragment. With advanced lesions (grades III and IV, complete discontinuity and dislocated fragments), approximately 67–89 % of cases returned to their previous sport as early as 6 months and usually within 1 year often with excellent functional scores. Pain relief is complete in up to 95 % of cases and range of motion restored to 90 % of the opposite extremity. These results were seen with a defect average size between 147 and 224.6 mm^2. Worse results can be expected when there is failure to achieve firm fixation and/or the lateral part of the capitellum is involved (Fig. 23.21a–c). Kosaka et al. described a 50 % reoperation rate in these cases [44–48].

To address these large and challenging lesions, Shimada et al. described a technique utilizing osteochondral grafts

and a wedge technique when a cleft remained on the lateral cortex. The minimum defect size was 15 mm with the smallest lesion being 11 × 16 mm and the largest being 20 × 18 mm. All patients returned to their previous daily activity within 4–6 weeks and returned to sport participation by 6 months. Baseball pitchers were started on a throwing program at 6 months. Release to full pitching occurred at approximately 9–12 months. Ninety-six percent of patients had excellent or good functional scores [46].

The cartilage of the graft from the knee is usually thicker than that of the elbow. When using this graft, shaving of the cartilage with a knife to contour the graft can be done. Radiographic union can be expected at 3 months, and follow-up MRI will typically demonstrate viability and integration of the graft [38]. See Figs. 23.22 [46] and 23.23a, b [38]. Slight incongruity, small cysts, and subchondral edema on long-term follow-up MRI may occur. However, this does not correlate with clinical findings, and patients can maintain full range of motion without extension deficits [38]. Subchondral irregularity seen on radiographs postoperatively has a propensity to remodel with time [46]. See Fig. 23.24a, b [46].

In larger lesions such as those described above, graft incorporation may not be as complete as in smaller lesions. In these cases, recurrent loose bodies, chondral flaps, and graft/cartilage hypertrophy may occur resulting in mechanical symptoms. About half of patients had low- and high-signal heterogeneity that was interpreted as remodeling. At 1 year, 77 % had congruent articular surfaces, but this decreased to 55 % by 2 years [49].

Arthroscopic treatment lends itself well to fragment removal and debridement like that described in Baumgarten et al. [39]. Brownlow et al. described an 81 % return to sport rate with arthroscopic debridement and removal of loose bodies. They did have a higher number of patients (38 %) that had recurrence of mechanical symptoms, and 15 % could not return to play. One factor may be the older age cohort in this group (average age of 22 years). Despite these findings, 94 % had good or excellent outcome scores [50]. Other studies report similar return-to-play numbers ranging between 80 and 86 % [51, 52].

There are more variable results regarding the return to play of baseball players with arthroscopic debridement, drilling, and loose-body removal. Studies have reported a return-to-play rate ranging from 40 to 92 %. Weaknesses of these studies are the lack of lesion description regarding size and location which appears to be an important determining factor [34, 35, 53]. A study by Miyake et al. on a cohort predominately made up of baseball players sheds some light on the size of the lesion as well as the influence of skeletal maturity on outcomes with arthroscopic treatment. See Table 23.3 for a description of sizes [28]. Patients with small- to medium-sized lesions had a return to play ranging between 75 and

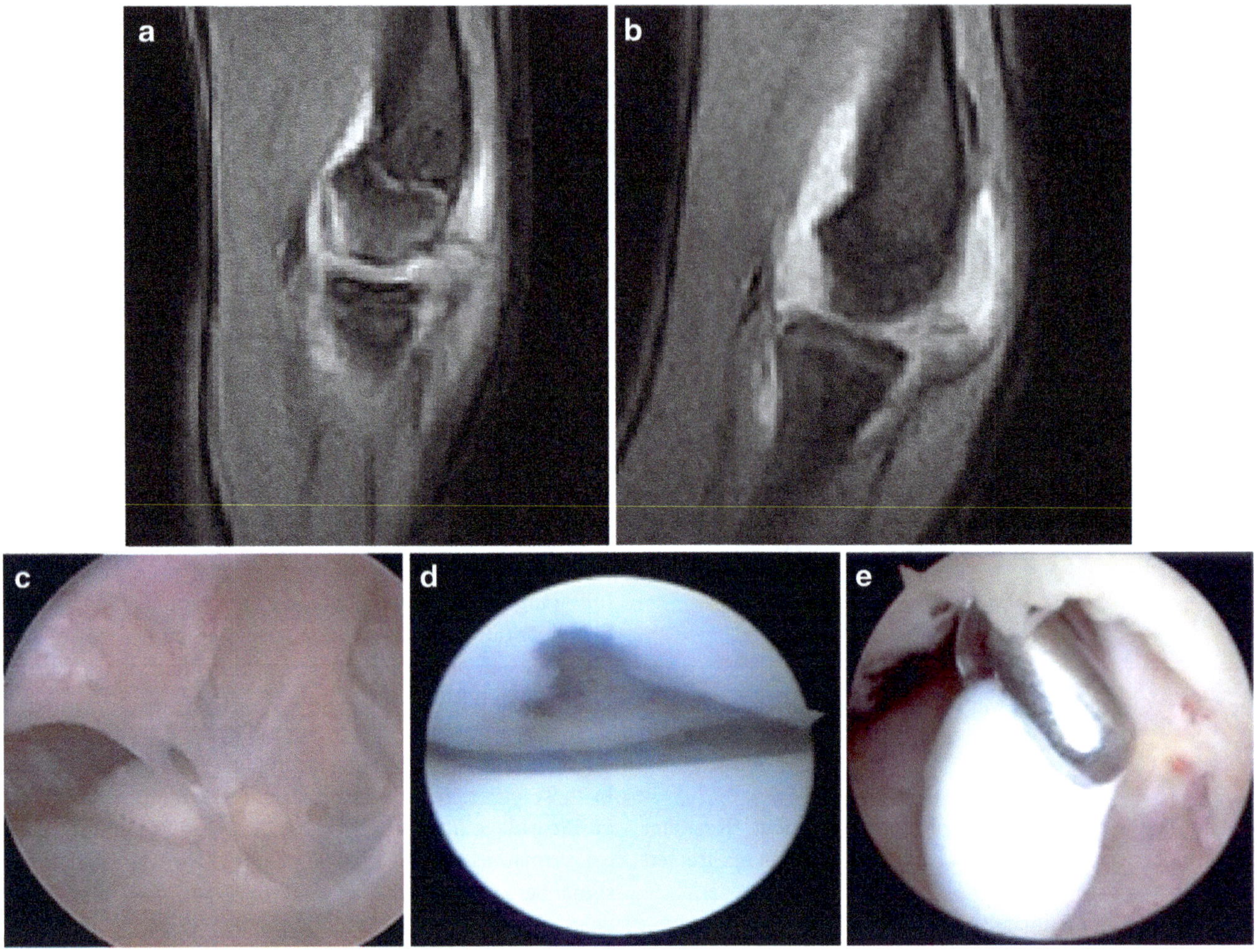

Fig. 23.19 Sagittal T2 MRI with high-signal line beneath the lesion in the capitellum (**a**) and repeat MRI of the same patient approximately 6 months later with empty bed and loose body in posterior compartment

(**b**). Arthroscopic image of adhesions and loose body (**c**). Other image examples of empty bed and loose-body removal (**d, e**)

Fig. 23.20 (**a, b**) Measurement of lesion size based on coronal and sagittal images (reprinted with permission from Takahara M et al. Long term outcome of osteochondritis dissecans of the humeral capitellum. Clin Orthop Relat Res. 1999;363:108–15)

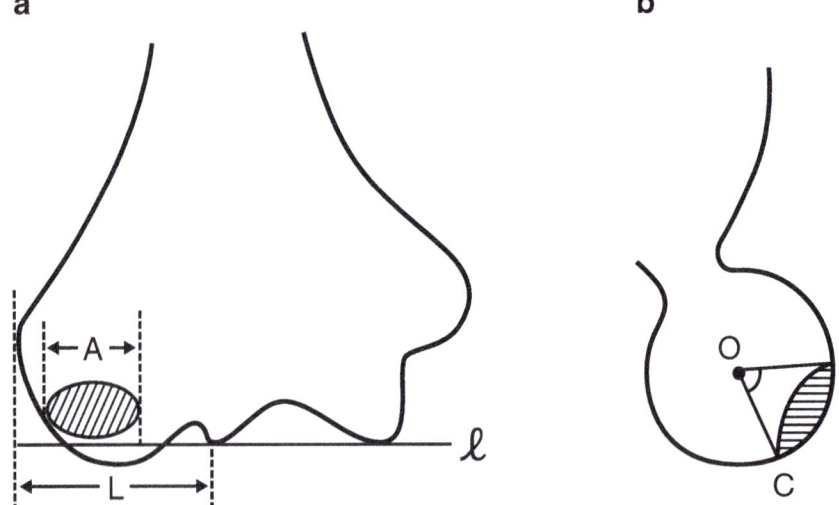

90 % regardless of the status of the physis. The larger open-physis lesion group had only a complete return in one patient (25 %) and incomplete return in two patients (50 %). Sixty-seven percent of the patients from the large closed-physis group returned to sport. The authors suggested arthroscopic debridement for all lesions except those with large and open physis [54].

Table 23.3 Classification of OCD defect size

Size	%/angle
Small	<55/60°
Medium	55–70/60–90°
Large	>70/90°

Data from Takahara M, Ogino T, Sasaki I, Kato H, Minami A, Kaneda K. Long term outcome of osteochondritis dissecans of the humeral capitellum. Clin Orthop Relat Res. 1999;363:108–15

Further clarifying the indications for arthroscopic micro-fracture treatment, Wulf et al. reported on ten patients (average age of 14 years), eight of which were throwers or gymnasts. The average lesion size was 98.1 mm^2 (50–180 mm^2). The authors found significant improvement in range of motion, and 75 % of competitive athletes were able to return to their previous level. The patients who did not return either switched positions or remained active as a coach in their sport. 80 % had a completely filled defect consistent with fibrocartilage and near-normal articular congruity [55].

Case Presentations

As done in the previous chapters, a case-based format will illustrate the correlation between MRI and arthroscopy for osteochondritis dissecans and other chondral lesions to the elbow. The cases to be discussed are as follows:

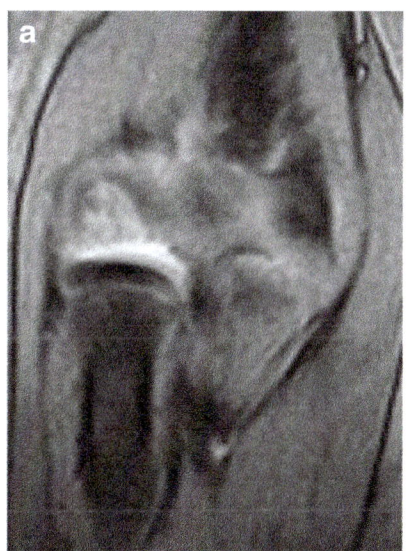

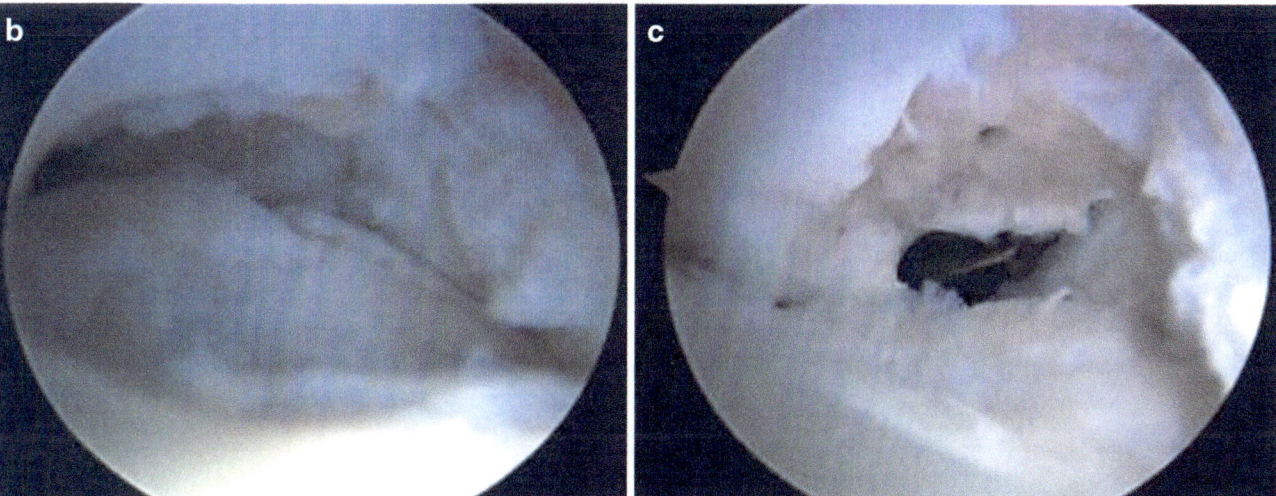

Fig. 23.21 Coronal MRI demonstrating large capitellar lesion abutting lateral column of capitellum (**a**). Arthroscopic images of the same lesion before and after debridement (**b, c**)

1. A 14-year-old baseball player with stable capitellar lesion treated nonoperatively
2. A 15-year-old baseball player with an unstable lesion and mechanical symptoms treated with arthroscopic loose-body removal, debridement, and microfracture of the lesion

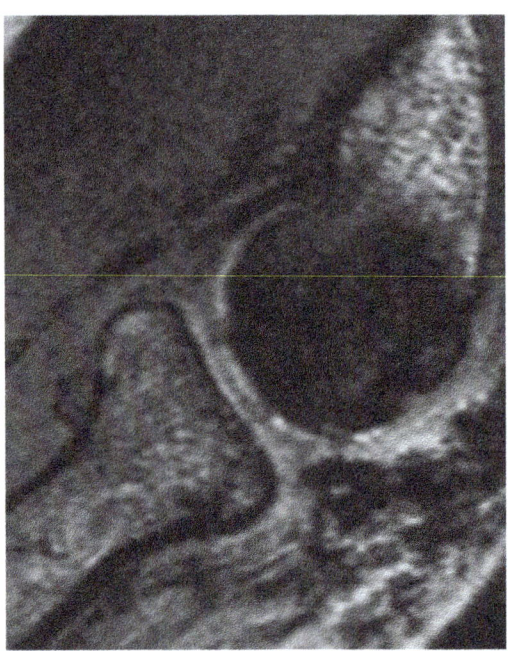

Fig. 23.22 MRI 3 months post-op demonstrating congruent articular surface (reprinted with permission from Shimada K et al. Reconstruction with an osteochondral autograft for advanced osteochondritis dissecans of the elbow. Clin Orthop Rel Res. 2005;435:140–7)

Case 1

The patient is a 14-year-old male baseball player with several-month history of lateral elbow pain with throwing a baseball. He describes occasional crepitus of the elbow during activity. On initial evaluation, he had no obvious effusion, tenderness over the radiocapitellar joint, and no ligamentous laxity. He had no flexion contracture with motion 0–140°. Plain radiographs were obtained at the initial evaluation, and the AP view is included in Fig. 23.25.

The radiograph demonstrates a lucent lesion in the central area of the capitellum in a skeletally mature individual. There are no sclerotic areas and no apparent loose bodies or fragments appreciated. This can be categorized as a Minami grade I lesion. An MRI was obtained approximately 2 weeks later. Selected images are shown in Fig. 23.26a–d.

On the coronal images, the lesion is seen in the central area of the capitellum. There are corresponding low-signal changes on the T1 and high signal on T2 images. The articular cartilage appears to be grossly intact without breach of the articular surface and, perhaps, mild, but mostly no, articular irregularity. There is no high-intensity subchondral line and no displaced or loose fragment. Based on these radiographic and MRI findings, the lesion was classified as stable and nonoperative treatment started.

The patient was placed in a hinged elbow brace to protect the elbow from any valgus stress. He was withheld from throwing and other strenuous activities on the elbow. Physical therapy was begun avoiding valgus stress. Therapy consisted of evaluation of posture, core, scapular stabilization for throwing mechanics, and elbow ROM.

Fig. 23.23 Complete graft incorporation and minimal (**a**) step-off (**b**) 9 years after surgery (reprinted from Vogt S et al. Osteochondral transplantation in the elbow leads to good clinical and radiologic long-term results: an 8 to 14 year follow-up examination. Am J Sports Med. 2011;39:2619–25, reprinted by permission of SAGE Publications)

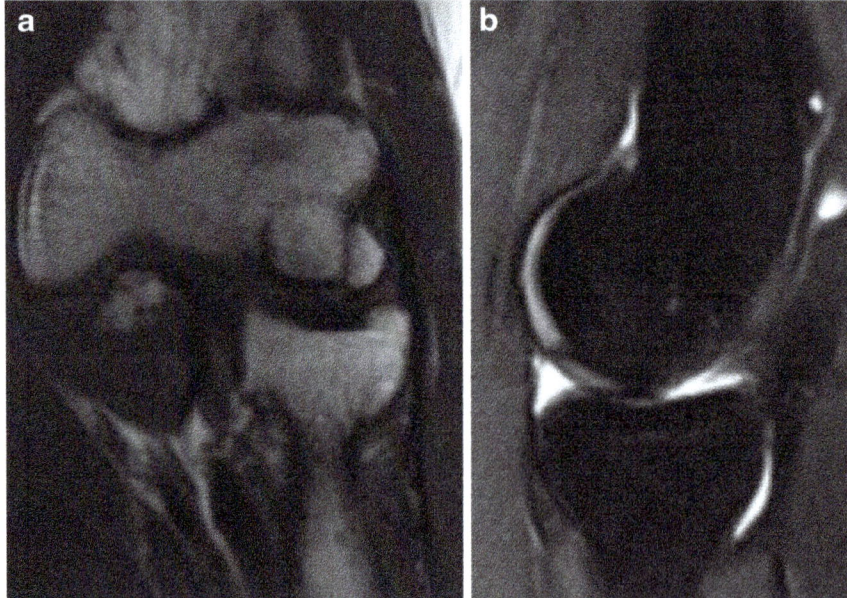

Fig. 23.24 Images showing progressive remodeling of graft at 12 months (**a**) and 45 months (**b**) (reprinted with permission from Shimada K et al. Reconstruction with an osteochondral autograft for advanced osteochondritis dissecans of the elbow. Clin Orthop Relat Res. 2005;435:140–7)

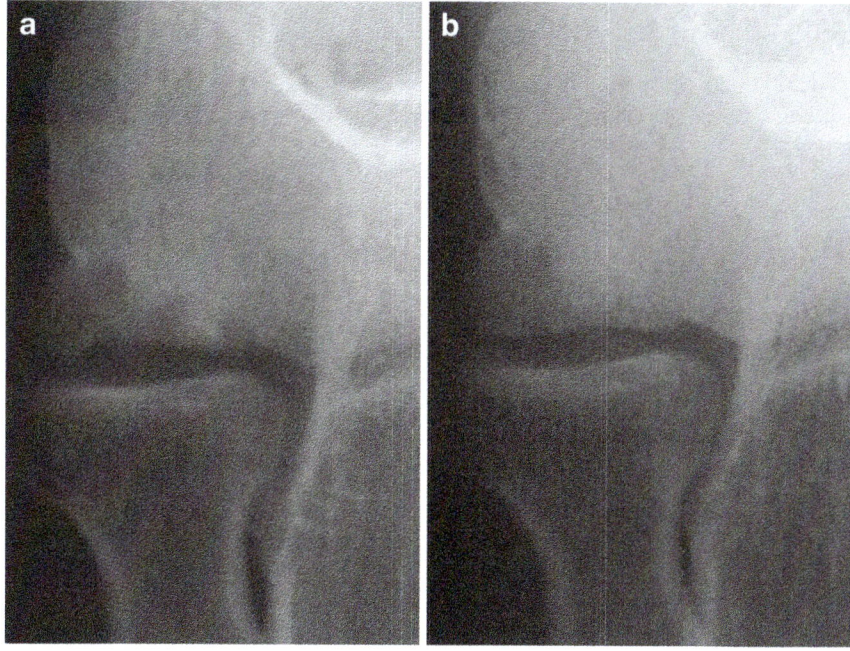

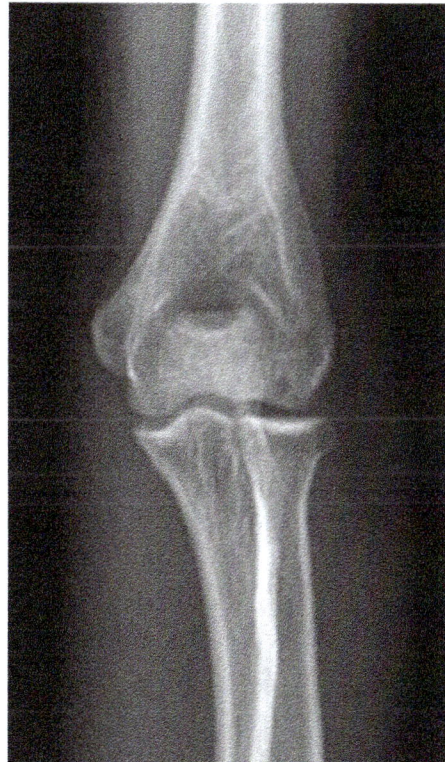

Fig. 23.25 AP radiograph demonstrating grade I OCD lesion of the capitellum

On his next follow-up, approximately 1 month later, his mechanical symptoms had improved. His pain was improved but still present with activity. He had a trace effusion and an intra-articular corticosteroid injection was performed. The

brace was continued, but therapy, which was thought to be contributing to his effusion and pain, was discontinued for the time being. He returned a month later with minimal, if any, pain and all mechanical symptoms resolved and was released to play baseball.

Case 2

The patient is a 17-year-old right-hand-dominant third base-man and fullback on the football team who presented within 1 week with a painful right elbow after a hyperextension-type injury during a football game. There was no dislocation. He denied a prior history of elbow pain. He denied any locking or catching with range of motion as well as any motion deficit. On initial examination, his elbow was mildly swollen with mild diffuse tenderness. There was no ecchymosis. He had a mild extensor lag of 5°, and he could flex his elbow approximately 90° before he began to have pain. He had no ligamentous instability. Plain radiographs were obtained on evaluation and are shown in Fig. 23.27a, b. They demonstrated evidence of a subchondral lucent area in the capitellum.

An MRI was obtained within a week of the injury. The scan demonstrated an OCD lesion of the capitellum approximately 7 mm×7 mm in size. The lesion exhibited signs of instability such as a breach in the articular cartilage with a high-signal line between the lesion and subchondral bone. A definable fragment that has not shifted from its bed is most notable on the sagittal images (Fig. 23.28a–d). There are no loose bodies.

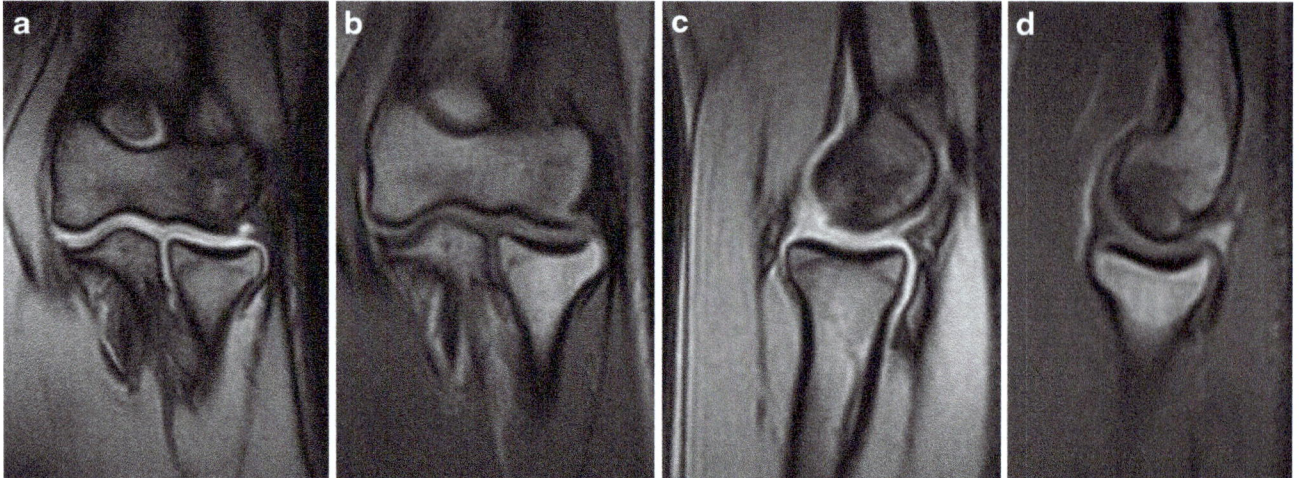

Fig. 23.26 Figures illustrate coronal (**a, b**) and sagittal (**c, d**) images, respectively

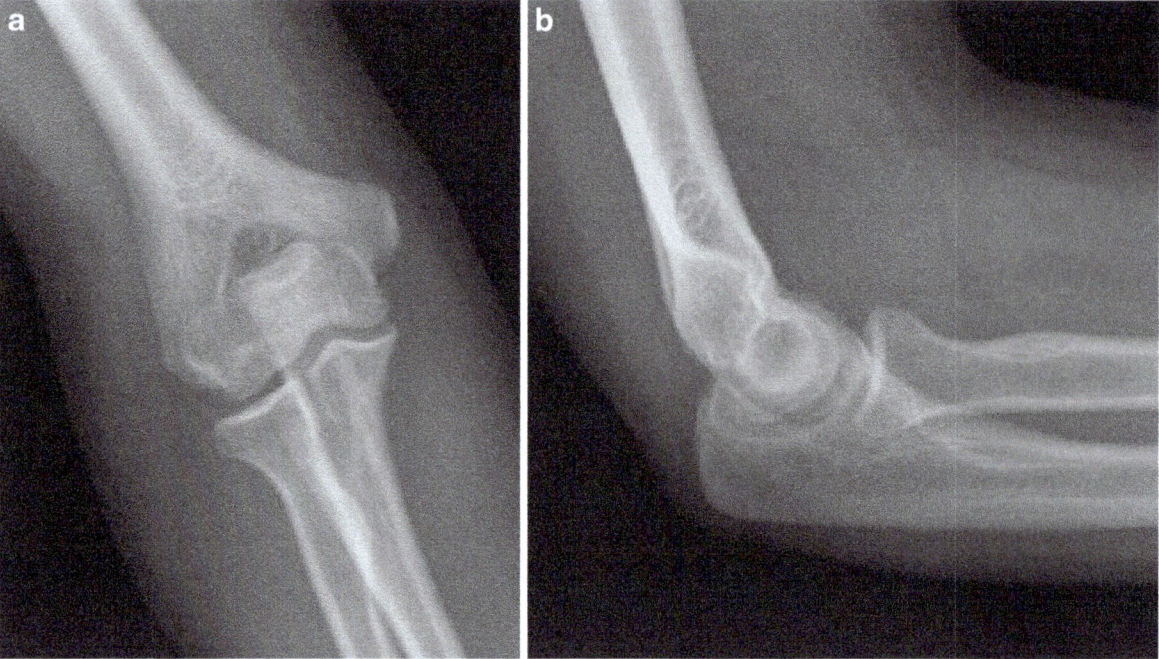

Fig. 23.27 (**a, b**) Radiographs demonstrating capitellar lesion on AP and lateral views

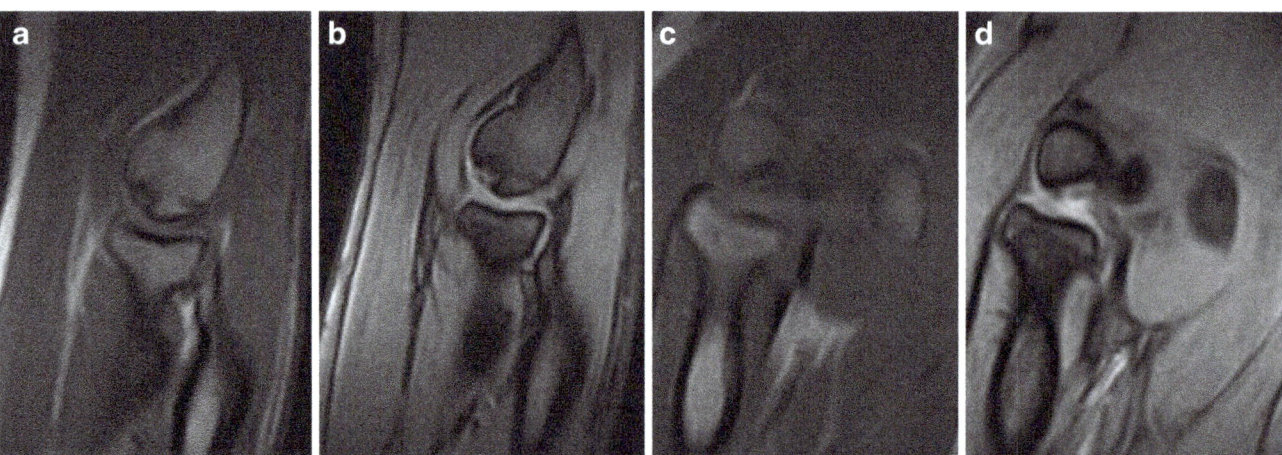

Fig. 23.28 (**a–d**) Selected MRI images demonstrating unstable capitellar lesion

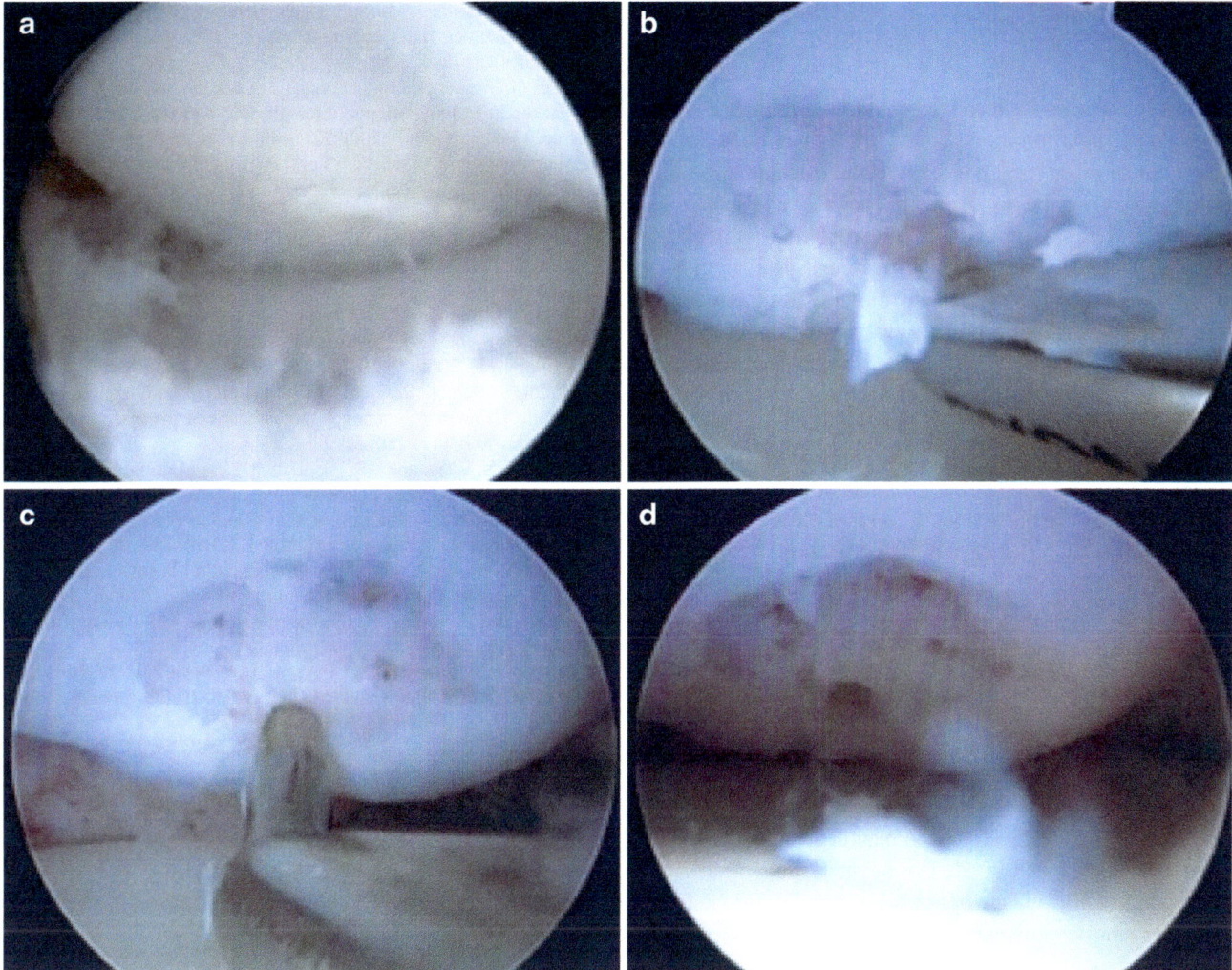

Fig. 23.29 Arthroscopic image showing unstable lesion prior to debridement (**a**). Unstable lesion undergoing debridement with a shaver (**b**). Lesion undergoing microfracture (**c**, **d**)

After treatment options were discussed with the patient and family, they elected to finish out the football season and a nonoperative treatment regimen was initiated. Within 3 weeks, he was able to regain all of his motion and finish out the football season without limitation. However, a year and a half later, he began to experience mechanical symptoms during baseball season and was unable to play third base. He described catching, popping, and grinding. His pain was localized to the radiocapitellar joint.

This time the patient proceeded with arthroscopic treatment. An unstable lesion was noted while visualizing from the anteromedial portal (Fig. 23.29a, b). A loose body was seen and removed from the posterior compartment. A posterolateral plica was identified and debrided through a posterolateral soft spot portal. The lesion was classified as stage IV and measured 1.0 cm×1.0 cm. The lesion was debrided and microfractured (Fig. 23.29b–d). All loose chondral flaps were debrided to stable edges.

One week postoperatively, he was placed in a hinged elbow brace to begin range-of-motion exercises in all planes as well as edema control. At 6 weeks, his range of motion was 5–135, and he had normal pronation and supination without any mechanical symptoms. His brace was discontinued at this time. He was released only for conditioning activity. Two months post-op, he had regained the remainder of his motion and was started on a strengthening program as comfort allowed. Three months post-op, he had maintained his motion and had been performing strengthening exercises without mechanical symptoms or other limitations and was released for full participation.

Summary

OCD of the elbow is a localized osteochondral lesion of the elbow that is most commonly found in the capitellum, but can also occur in other locations such as the trochlea and radial head. Lesions may be discovered in one of a variety of stages based on different radiographic, CT, MRI, and arthroscopic criteria. However, when deciding treatment, lesions may be simply classified into stable and unstable lesions each of which may be predicted based on a variety of findings seen on imaging. MRI is perhaps the best modality to determine staging preoperatively and has been shown to correlate with arthroscopic findings although it may not be as effective in younger/teenage patients. It is also effective at judging the size of the lesion, which also has implications on treatment.

Treatment of stable lesions is nonoperative which typically consists of strict activity modification for approximately 6 months. Healing and return to play after such treatment are approximately 90 %. Surgical treatment of OCD lesions is varied. Options include debridement of the defect and loose-body removal, microfracture or drilling, fixation of the fragment, and osteochondral grafting. Debridement, drilling, and microfracture appear to produce good results; however, analysis of the literature shows such results are more likely in smaller lesions (<50–60 % size and an average of 98 mm²). Return to play in such instances can range between 75 and 90 %. For larger lesions, fixation or osteochondral grafting are options. If the lesion can be fixed, outcomes can be similar to debridement and microfracture/drilling. Osteochondral grafting can achieve good pain relief in a high percentage of patients, but they and their families should be counseled that the return to play is often not as good as those with smaller lesions. Surgeons should pay close attention to whether the defect involves the lateral column of the capitellum and the amount of subchondral bone deficiency because these factors can influence the type of treatment and outcome.

References

1. Edmonds EW. A review of knowledge in osteochondritis dissecans: 123 years of minimal evolution from Konig to the ROCK study group. Clin Orthop Relat Res. 2013;471(4):1118–26.
2. Kusumi T, Ishibashi Y, Tsuda E, Kusumi A, Tanaka M, Sato F, Toh S, Kijima H. Osteochondritis dissecans of the elbow: histopathological assessment of the articular cartilage and subchondral bone with emphasis on their damage and repair. Pathol Int. 2006; 56(10):604–12.
3. Miyake J, Kataoka T, Murase T, Yoshikawa H. In-vivo biomechanical analysis of osteochondritis dissecans of the humeral trochlea: a case report. J Pediatr Orthop B. 2013;22:392–6.
4. Jans L, Ditchfield M, Anna G, Jaremko J, Verstraete K. MR imaging findings and MR criteria for instability in osteochondritis dissecans of the elbow in children. Eur J Radiol. 2012;81(6):1306–10.
5. Joji S, Murakami T, Murao T. Osteochondritis dissecans developing in the trochlea humeri: a case report. J Shoulder Elbow Surg. 2001;10(3):295–7.
6. Patel N, Weiner S. Osteochondritis dissecans involving the trochlea: report of two patients (three elbows) and review of the literature. J Pediatr Orthop. 2002;22(1):48–51.
7. Vanthournout I, Rudelli A, Valenti P, Montagne JP. Osteochondritis dissecans of the trochlea of the humerus. Pediatr Radiol. 1991; 21(8):600–1.
8. Marshall K, Marshall D, Busch M, Williams J. Osteochondral lesions of the humeral trochlea in the young athlete. Skelet Radiol. 2009;38:479–91.
9. Namba J, Shimada K, Akita S. Osteochondritis dissecans of the humeral trochlea with cubitus varus deformity. A case report. Acta Orthop Belg. 2009;75(2):265–9.
10. Pruthi S, Parnell S, Thapa M. Pseudointercondylar notch sign: manifestation of osteochondritis dissecans of the trochlea. Pediatr Radiol. 2009;39(2):180–3.
11. Iwsaki N, Yamane S, Ishikawa J, Majima T, Minami A. Osteochondritis dissecans involving the trochlea of the humerus treated with transplantation of tissue-engineered cartilage: a case report. J Shoulder Elbow Surg. 2008;17(5):e22–5.
12. Janarv P, Hesser U, Hirsch G. Osteochondral lesions in the radiocapitellar joint in the skeletally immature: radiographic, MRI, and arthroscopic findings in 13 consecutive cases. J Pediatr Orthop. 1997;17(3):311–4.
13. Dotzis A, Galissier B, Peyrou P, Longis B, Moulies D. Osteochondritis dissecans of the radial head: a case report. J Shoulder Elbow Surg. 2009;18(1):e18–21.
14. Tatebe M, Hirata H, Shinohara T, Yamamoto M, Morita A, Horri E. Pathomechanical significance of radial head subluxation in the onset of osteochondritis dissecans of the radial head. J Orthop Trauma. 2012;26(1):e4–6.
15. Klekamp J, Green N, Mencio G. Osteochondritis dissecans as a cause of developmental dislocation of the radial head. Clin Orthop Relat Res. 1997;338:36–41.
16. Rosenberg Z, Blutreich S, Schweitzer M, Zember J, Fillmore K. MRI features of posterior capitellar impaction injuries. AJR Am J Roentgenol. 2008;190(2):435–41.
17. Kijowski R, De Smet A. Radiography of the elbow for evaluation of patients with osteochondritis dissecans of the capitellum. Skelet Radiol. 2005;34:266–71.
18. Takahara M, Shundo M, Kondo M, Suzuki K, Nambu T, Ogino T. Early detection of osteochondritis dissecans of the capitellum in young baseball players. Report of three cases. J Bone Joint Surg Am. 1998;80(6):892–7.
19. Takahara M, Ogino T, Takagi M, Tsuchida H, Orui H, Nambu T. Natural progression of osteochondritis dissecans of the humeral capitellum: initial observations. Radiology. 2000;216(1):207–12.
20. Mihara K, Tsutsui H, Nishinaka N, Yamaguchi K. Nonoperative treatment for osteochondritis dissecans of the capitellum. Am J Sports Med. 2009;37(2):298–304.
21. Takahara M, Mura N, Sasaki J, Harada M, Ogino T. Classification, treatment, and outcome of osteochondritis dissecans of the humeral capitellum. J Bone Joint Surg Am. 2007;89(6):1205–14.
22. Iwase T, Igata T. Osteochondrosis of the humeral capitellum. Seikeigeka MOOK. 1988;54:26–44.
23. Potter H, Ho S, Altcheck D. Magnetic resonance imaging of the elbow. Semin Musculoskelet Radiol. 2004;8(1):5–16.
24. Kijowski R, De Smet A. MRI findings of osteochondritis dissecans of the capitellum with surgical correlation. AJR Am J Roentgenol. 2005;185(6):1453–9.
25. Baker III CL, Romeo A, Baker Jr CL. Osteochondritis dissecans of the capitellum. Am J Sports Med. 2010;38(9):1917–28.
26. De Smet A, Ilahi O, Graf B. Reassessment of the MR criteria for stability of osteochondritis dissecans in the knee and ankle. Skelet Radiol. 1996;25(2):159–63.

27. Dipaola J, Nelson D, Colville M. Characterizing osteochondral lesions by magnetic resonance imaging. Arthroscopy. 1991;7(1):101–4.
28. Takahara M, Ogino T, Sasaki I, Kato H, Minami A, Kaneda K. Long term outcome of osteochondritis dissecans of the humeral capitellum. Clin Orthop Relat Res. 1999;363:108–15.
29. Iwasaki N, Kamishima T, Kato H, Funakoshi T, Minami A. A retrospective evaluation of magnetic resonance imaging effectiveness on capitellar osteochondritis dissecans among overhead athletes. Am J Sports Med. 2012;40(3):624–30.
30. ICRS Cartilage Injury Evaluation Package [Internet]. 2000. Available from: http://www.cartilage.org/_files/contentmanagement/ICRS_evaluation.pdf
31. Theodoropoulous J, Dwyer T, Woline P. Correlation of preoperative MRI and MRA with arthroscopically proven articular cartilage lesions of the elbow. Clin J Sport Med. 2012;22(5):403–7.
32. Satake H, Takahara M, Harada M, Maruyama M. Preoperative imaging criteria for unstable osteochondritis dissecans of the capitellum. Clin Orthop Relat Res. 2013;471(4):1137–43.
33. Dubberley J, Faber KJ, Patterson SD, Bennett G, Romano W, MacDermid J, King G. The detection of loose bodies in the elbow: the value of MRI and CT arthrography. J Bone Joint Surg (Br). 2005;87(5):684–6.
34. Mihara K, Suzuki K, Makiuchi D, Nishinaka N, Yamaguchi K, Tsutsui H. Surgical treatment for osteochondritis dissecans of the humeral capitellum. J Shoulder Elbow Surg. 2010;19(1):31–7.
35. Tis J, Edmonds E, Bastrom T, Chambers H. Short-term results of arthroscopic treatment of osteochondritis dissecans in skeletally immature patients. J Pediatr Orthop. 2012;32(3):226–31.
36. Matsuura T, Kashiwaguchi S, Iwase T, Takeda Y, Yasui N. Conservative treatment for osteochondrosis of the humeral capitellum. Am J Sports Med. 2008;36(5):868–72.
37. Takahara M, Ogino T, Fukushima S, Tsuchida H, Kaneda K. Nonoperative treatment of osteochondritis dissecans of the humeral capitellum. Am J Sports Med. 1999;27(6):728–32.
38. Vogt S, Siebenlist S, Hensler D, Weigelt L, Ansah P, Woertler K, Imhoff A. Osteochondral transplantation in the elbow leads to good clinical and radiologic long-term results: an 8- to 14-year follow-up examination. Am J Sports Med. 2011;39(12):2619–25.
39. Baumgarten T, Andrews J, Satterwhite Y. The arthroscopic classification and treatment of osteochondritis dissecans of the capitellum. Am J Sports Med. 1998;26(4):520–3.
40. Harada M, Ogino T, Takahara M, Ishigaki D, Kashiwa H, Kanauchi Y. Fragment fixation with a bone graft and dynamic staples for osteochondritis dissecans of the humeral capitellum. J Shoulder Elbow Surg. 2002;11(4):368–72.
41. Kuwahata Y, Inoue G. Osteochondritis dissecans of the elbow managed by Herbert screw fixation. Orthopedics. 1998;21(4):449–51.
42. Nobuta S, Ogawa K, Sato K, Nakagawa T, Hatori M. Clinical outcome of fragment fixation for osteochondritis dissecans of the elbow. Ups J Med Sci. 2008;113(2):201–8.
43. Takeda H, Watarai K, Matsushita T, Saito T, Terashima Y. A surgical treatment for unstable osteochondritis dissecans lesions of the humeral capitellum in adolescent baseball players. Am J Sports Med. 2002;30(5):713–7.
44. Yamamoto Y, Ishibashi Y, Tsuda E, Sato H, Toh S. Osteochondral autograft transplantation for osteochondritis dissecans of the elbow in juvenile baseball players: minimum 2-year follow-up. Am J Sports Med. 2006;34(5):714–20.
45. Iwasaki N, Kato H, Ishikawa J, Masuko T, Funakoshi T, Minami A. Autologous osteochondral mosaicplasty for osteochondritis dissecans of the elbow in teenage athletes. J Bone Joint Surg Am. 2009;91(10):2359–66.
46. Shimada K, Yoshida T, Nakata K, Hamada M, Akita S. Reconstruction with an osteochondral autograft for advanced osteochondritis dissecans of the elbow. Clin Orthop Relat Res. 2005;435:140–7.
47. Kosaka M, Nakase J, Takahashi R, Toratani T, Ohashi Y, Kitaoka K, Tsuchiya H. Outcomes and failure factors in surgical treatment for osteochondritis dissecans of the capitellum. J Pediatr Orthop. 2013;33(7):719–24.
48. Ovesen J, Olsen B, Johannsen H. The clinical outcomes of mosaicplasty in the treatment of osteochondritis dissecans of the distal humeral capitellum of young athletes. J Shoulder Elbow Surg. 2011;20(5):813–8.
49. Shimada K, Tanaka H, Matsumoto T, Miyake J, Higuchi H, Gamo K, Fuji T. Cylindrical costal osteochondral autograft for reconstruction of large defects of the capitellum due to osteochondritis dissecans. J Bone Joint Surg Am. 2012;94(11):992–1002.
50. Brownlow H, O'Connor-Read L, Perko M. Arthroscopic treatment of osteochondritis dissecans of the capitellum. Knee Surg Sports Traumatol Arthrosc. 2006;14(2):198–202.
51. Rahusen F, Brinkman JM, Eygendaal D. Results of arthroscopic debridement for osteochondritis dissecans of the elbow. Br J Sports Med. 2006;40(12):966–9.
52. Jones KJ, Wiesel BB, Sankar WN, Ganley TJ. Arthroscopic management of osteochondritis dissecans of the capitellum: mid-term results in adolescent athletes. J Pediatr Orthop. 2010;30(1):8–13.
53. Byrd T, Jones K. Arthroscopic surgery for isolated capitellar osteochondritis dissecans in adolescent baseball players: minimum three-year follow-up. Am J Sports Med. 2002;30(4):474–8.
54. Miyake J, Masatomi T. Arthroscopic debridement of the humeral capitellum for osteochondritis dissecans: radiographic and clinical outcomes. J Hand Surg [Am]. 2011;36(8):1333–8.
55. Wulf C, Stone R, Giveans R, Lervick G. Magnetic resonance imaging after arthroscopic microfracture of capitellar osteochondritis dissecans. Am J Sports Med. 2012;40(11):2549–56.

The Elbow: Degenerative and Inflammatory Arthritis

Steven A. Giuseffi and Larry D. Field

Introduction

Traditionally, operative management of elbow arthritis and/or synovitis has been performed through an open approach. While satisfactory results were often obtained, open procedures were associated with relatively high complication rates and long recovery periods. As orthopedic surgeons have gained experience and familiarity with elbow arthroscopy, interest in addressing elbow pathology arthroscopically has increased [1, 2]. Potential advantages of an arthroscopic approach include improved articular visualization as well as decreased postoperative pain and accelerated recovery. Recent studies suggest that outcomes of arthroscopic management of elbow arthritis and synovitis are equivalent to those obtained via an open surgical approach [3–7].

Elbow arthroscopy is indicated for the evaluation and treatment of osteoarthritis and inflammatory arthritis. Patients often present with complaints of elbow pain, stiffness, and/or swelling. Pain at extremes of motion with loss of terminal extension is the hallmark of elbow osteoarthritis. Arthroscopic debridement of elbow osteoarthritis is particularly indicated for the patient who lacks significant mid-arc pain, but has pain at terminal flexion/extension secondary to impinging osteophytes.

Inflammatory arthritis of the elbow is most commonly caused by rheumatoid arthritis. Patients present with pain, swelling, and/or loss of motion. Boggy swelling of the elbow may be noted on physical examination, and bilateral involvement is common. Loss of elbow motion secondary to synovitis classically has a "soft" end point, while impinging

S.A. Giuseffi, MD
Department of Orthopedic Surgery, Mississippi Sports Medicine and Orthopedic Center, Jackson, MS, USA
e-mail: Steve.giuseffi@gmail.com

L.D. Field, MD (✉)
Mississippi Sports Medicine and Orthopedic Center, Jackson, MS, USA
e-mail: lfield@msmoc.com

osteophytes cause a "hard" end point. Advanced inflammatory disease can cause elbow instability secondary to ligamentous insufficiency and bone loss.

Case 1: Osteoarthritis

History/Exam

A 58-year-old male manual laborer presented for evaluation of progressive elbow pain and stiffness in his dominant arm. His symptoms had developed insidiously over a course of 2 years. He denied any history of trauma and had no locking or mechanical symptoms. The patient had no significant medical comorbidities.

On examination, the patient had markedly decreased range of motion, with a motion arc from 30° extension to 95° flexion. Pain was particularly noted in terminal flexion and extension. The patient did not have pain with forearm rotation. He was neurovascularly intact but did have pain in his posteromedial gutter with elbow flexion.

Imaging

Radiographs were obtained and are shown below. These X-rays showed prominent osteophyte formation about the olecranon tip posteriorly as well as the coronoid, radial head, and coronoid fossa anteriorly. A loose body was noted anteriorly. Moderate joint space narrowing was seen, but relative preservation of the articular space was noted on the anteroposterior (AP) view (Fig. 24.1a, b).

Treatment

Treatment options including nonsteroidal anti-inflammatory drugs (NSAIDs), physical therapy, steroid injections, and surgery were discussed with the patient. He elected to proceed

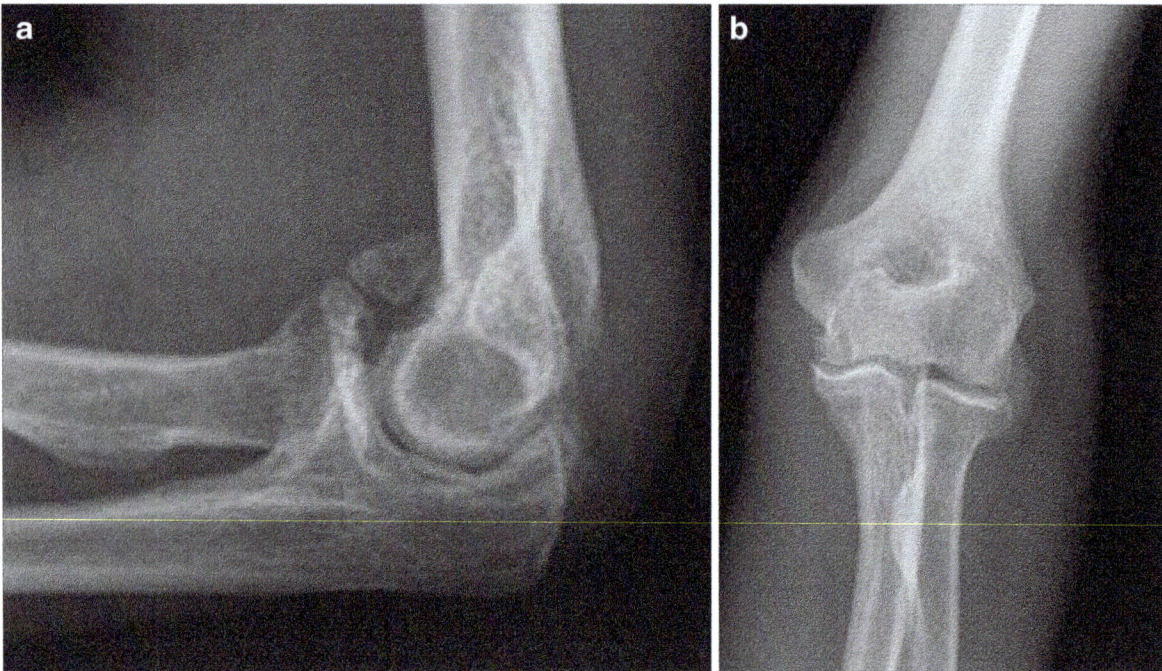

Fig. 24.1 (a, b) Anteroposterior (AP) and lateral elbow radiographs show posterior and anterior osteophytes as well as a loose body anteriorly. Relative preservation of the articular space is noted on the AP view

initially with conservative management including NSAIDs, an intra-articular corticosteroid injection, and an organized elbow exercise and range-of-motion program. However, the patient continued to experience significant symptoms after 3 months and did not have significant improvement in elbow range of motion.

Therefore, surgery was discussed with the patient. Surgical options considered included arthroscopic or open elbow capsular release and osteophyte excision, interposition arthroplasty, and implant arthroplasty. In this 58-year-old laborer with pain predominantly in terminal elbow flexion and extension, we felt that arthroscopic debridement and capsular release were promising surgical options.

We find advanced imaging helpful in formulating a surgical plan for osteophyte and loose-body removal. An MRI and a 3D CT scan were obtained for preoperative planning. In this case, imaging demonstrated a loose body in the coronoid fossa as well as prominent osteophytes in the coronoid process and olecranon tip. The prominent olecranon osteophytes seen in Fig. 24.2c exhibit the "Mickey Mouse ears" deformity, with osteophyte "ears" protruding from the posteromedial and posterolateral olecranon (Fig. 24.2a–c).

Surgery

The patient was taken to the operating room. A general anesthetic was provided, and the patient was placed in prone position with his operative arm in an arm holder.

Bony landmarks and the course of the ulnar nerve were identified and localized on the skin with a marker. The joint was insufflated with saline via the lateral soft spot portal. The standard proximal anteromedial and anterolateral portals were created. A loose body was seen in the coronoid fossa and was removed using an arthroscopic grabber via the proximal anterolateral portal. Prominent coronoid osteophytes were removed using a combination of the shaver and a small osteotome inserted through the arthroscopic cannulae.

Given the patient's marked elbow stiffness, anterior capsular release was performed using an arthroscopic biter. The plane between the brachialis and anterior capsule was carefully developed, allowing the brachialis to protect the anterior neurovascular structures. When performing the lateral portion of the anterior capsular release, care was taken to stay proximal to the radiocapitellar joint and anterior to the radial head to avoid iatrogenic injury to the radial nerve or lateral ulnar collateral ligament.

After work in the anterior compartment was completed, standard posterolateral viewing and posterior working portals were then created. As expected from preoperative imaging, large olecranon osteophytes were visualized. These were removed using an arthroscopic shaver and a small osteotome as demonstrated in the images below. After using the osteotome, a shaver was used to gently contour the olecranon tip and to resect posteromedial and posterolateral osteophytes as well as recontour the olecranon fossa to restore its normal anatomic architecture (Figs. 24.3a, b and 24.4a–c).

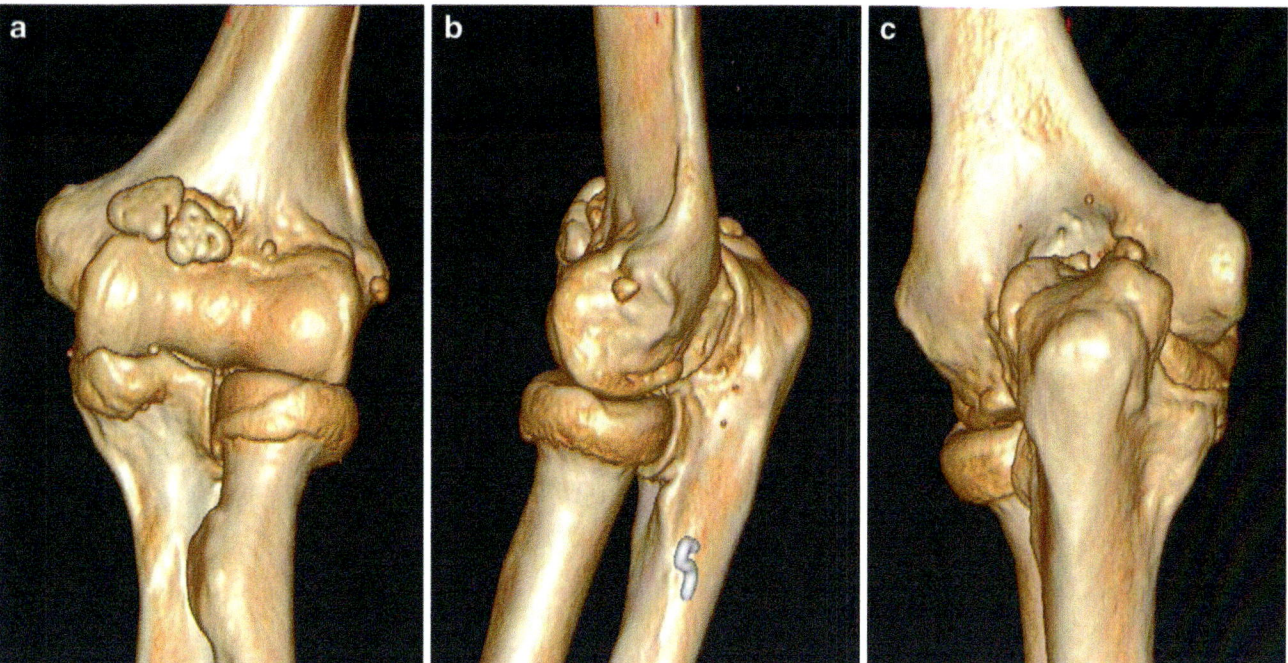

Fig. 24.2 (**a, b**) Three-dimensional CT images show coronoid and olecranon osteophytes as well as a loose body in the coronoid fossa. (**c**) Prominent posteromedial and posterolateral olecranon osteophytes create a "Mickey Mouse ears" deformity

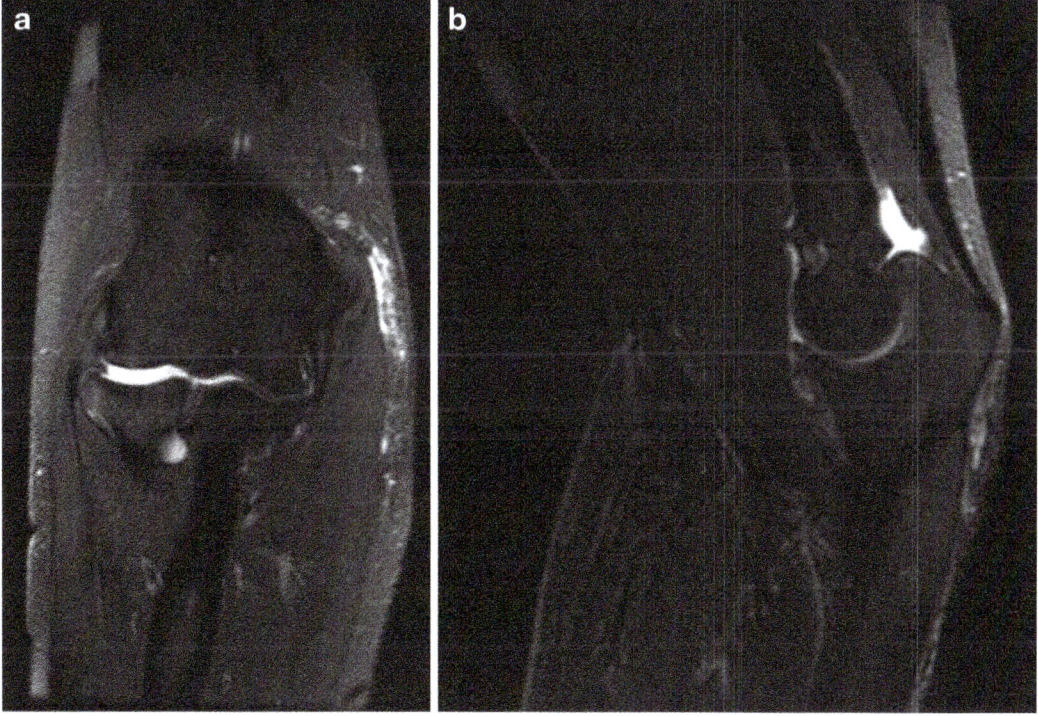

Fig. 24.3 (**a**) Coronal MRI demonstrating articular cartilage loss and subchondral edema. (**b**) Sagittal MRI demonstrating prominent coronoid and olecranon osteophytes. Hypertrophic degenerative changes in the coronoid and olecranon fossae are also noted

The elbow joint was then ranged while viewing the joint arthroscopically to demonstrate complete removal of all impinging osteophytes. While the elbow range of motion was improved after osteophyte resection and anterior capsular release, significant stiffness in elbow flexion remained.

Therefore, arthroscopic posterior capsular release was also performed. Great care was taken posteromedially to avoid iatrogenic ulnar nerve injury. Passive elbow range of motion improved to 5–125° after the completion of posterior osteophytectomy and capsular release.

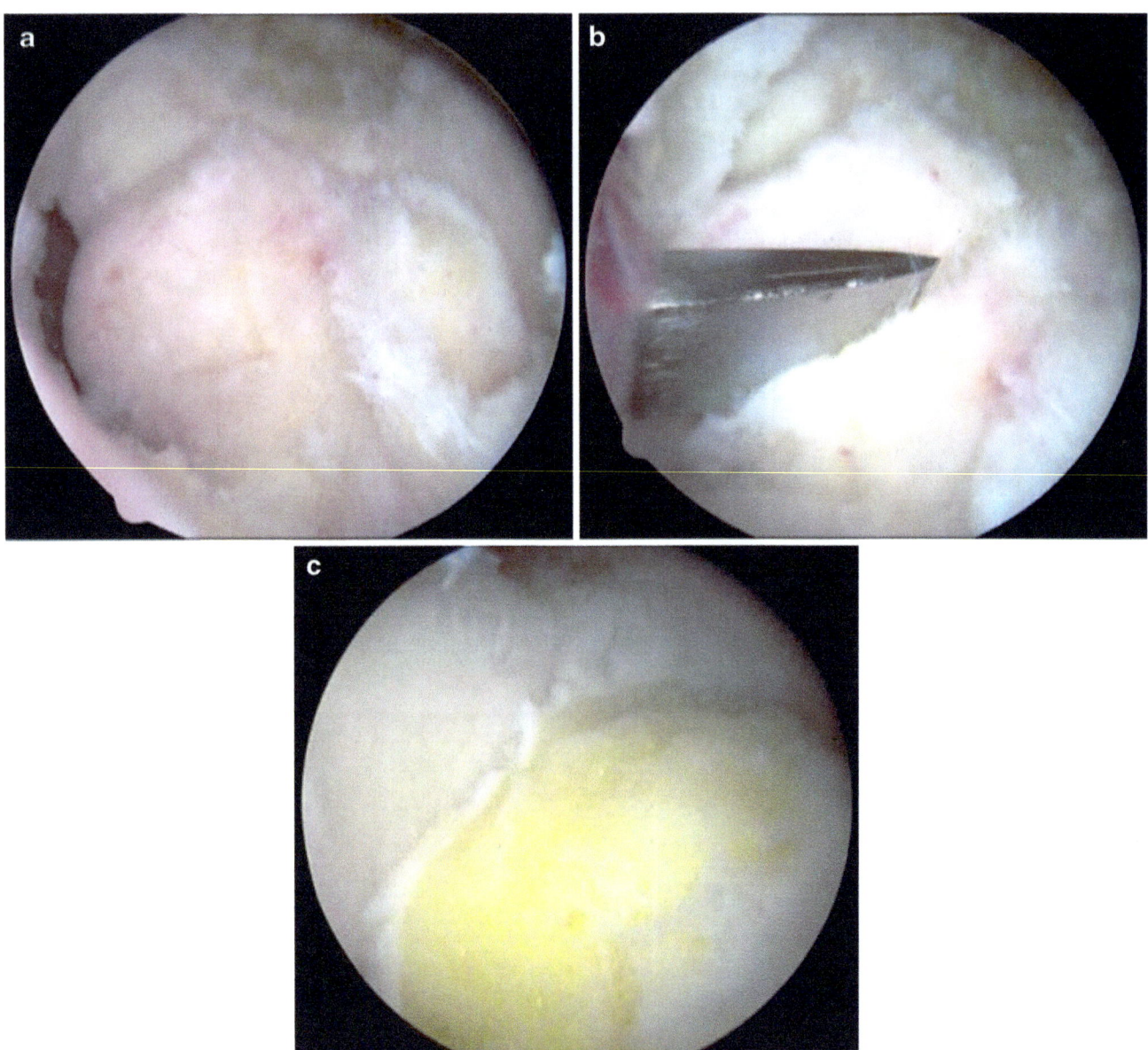

Fig. 24.4 (**a**) Corresponding arthroscopic view of posterior olecranon osteophytes. (**b**) Arthroscopic view of olecranon osteophyte removal with an osteotome. (**c**) Arthroscopic view of the smooth residual olecranon after osteophyte resection and final contouring

Additional procedures considered at the time of arthroscopy included radial head resection and ulnar nerve decompression and/or transposition. The patient did not have pain with forearm rotation preoperatively, and excellent outcomes after arthroscopic debridement without radial head resection have been reported [8]. Therefore, radial head resection was not performed in this case.

We did elect to decompress the ulnar nerve at the time of surgery. Ulnar nerve decompression was indicated in this case because of the patient's preoperative posteromedial elbow pain with flexion as well as the significant improvement in elbow flexion obtained at the time of surgery after osteophyte resection and capsular release (preoperative 95° flexion improved to 125° intraoperatively).

As the patient did not have evidence of ulnar nerve subluxation and had no prior ulnar nerve surgery, we performed a simple ulnar nerve decompression without transposition. This was performed at the conclusion of the surgical case by making a 3 cm incision directly over the cubital tunnel and decompressing the ulnar nerve under direct visualization.

Outcome

The patient was started on an outpatient physical therapy for elbow range of motion on postoperative day three. Continuous passive motion was not used. When seen at his

1-year postoperative appointment, the patient had active elbow range of motion from 10° to 115° and had minimal elbow pain. He was very pleased with his surgical outcome.

Case 2: Inflammatory Arthritis

History/Physical Exam

A 23-year-old female college student presented for evaluation of pain and swelling in her nondominant elbow. She described intermittent pain and occasional popping of her elbow for the last 2 years. Her elbow would often swell without apparent injury. Her symptoms were present more often than not and prevented her from playing intramural volleyball. The patient denied any fevers or rashes. She had intermittent swelling of her metacarpophalangeal joints as well. Her family history was significant for systemic lupus erythematosus in her aunt.

On examination, the patient had mild swelling and warmth in her elbow. Her elbow was mildly tender to palpation diffusely. She had elbow range of motion from 5° to 115°, with soft end points at terminal flexion and extension. She had pain throughout the elbow motion arc. Pronation and supination were not significantly decreased in comparison to her contralateral unaffected elbow. She had no evidence of elbow instability and was neurovascularly intact.

Imaging

X-ray imaging showed no evidence of fracture or degenerative changes. An effusion and mild soft tissue swelling were seen, but radiographs were otherwise unremarkable.

An MRI was obtained and demonstrated an effusion and diffuse synovitis. No loose bodies were identified, and there was no evidence of osteochondritis dissecans. Several small areas of chondromalacia were noted in both the radiocapitellar and ulnohumeral joints. Ligamentous structures were intact.

Treatment

The patient's clinical history and examination suggested inflammatory arthropathy. A trial of nonoperative management was undertaken, with the patient undergoing physical therapy and taking prescription anti-inflammatories. Her symptoms continued, and a steroid injection of her elbow provided good but only temporary relief.

Laboratory studies were obtained and were consistent with nonspecific inflammatory arthritis, and the patient was referred to a rheumatologist. She underwent a trial of various rheumatologic medications. These medications improved but did not resolve her elbow pain and swelling. The patient had elbow pain and swelling with activities of daily living. She remained unable to participate in intramural volleyball.

Various reports have documented reliable outcomes of arthroscopic synovectomy for inflammatory arthropathy [9–13]. Given the patient's continued pain and activity limitations, we offered her diagnostic elbow arthroscopy with the goal of removing any inflammatory synovitis as well as obtaining biopsy for pathologic diagnosis. The patient desired to proceed with operative intervention.

She underwent diagnostic elbow arthroscopy in prone position. After elbow exsanguination and joint insufflation, a standard proximal anteromedial portal was created. Moderate synovitis was noted in the anterior compartment. The proximal anterolateral portal was created under direct arthroscopic visualization. A shaver was introduced to debride the anterior synovitis. Great care was taken anteriorly, where the beefy red synovitic tissue can blend with the capsule and the similarly red brachialis muscle fibers. The shaver blade was always kept under direct arthroscopic visualization, and the blade was kept facing posteriorly to avoid neurovascular injury. Synovial biopsies were sent for microbiologic and pathologic examination.

Visualization was greatly improved after debridement of synovitic tissue. There were several small areas of superficial chondromalacia. There were no osteochondral lesions, and no loose bodies were seen. There was no evidence of elbow instability. We then turned our attention to the posterior compartment. Posterolateral and direct posterior portals were created. Inflammatory pannus and diffuse synovitis were again seen posteriorly. Careful debridement and evaluation of the posterolateral and posteromedial gutters were undertaken. After thorough synovectomy, the patient had passive elbow range of motion from 0° extension to 130° flexion. Therefore, capsulectomy was not performed (Figs. 24.5, 24.6, and 24.7).

Outcome

The patient's elbow pain and swelling were significantly improved after arthroscopic debridement. Synovial tissue biopsy showed synovial hyperplasia with a lymphocytic infiltrate, consistent with rheumatoid arthritis. The patient's rheumatologist placed her on a different targeted biologic antirheumatic medication, which provided more consistent control of her elbow synovitis. The patient was satisfied with her outcome and was able to return to volleyball for her senior year in college.

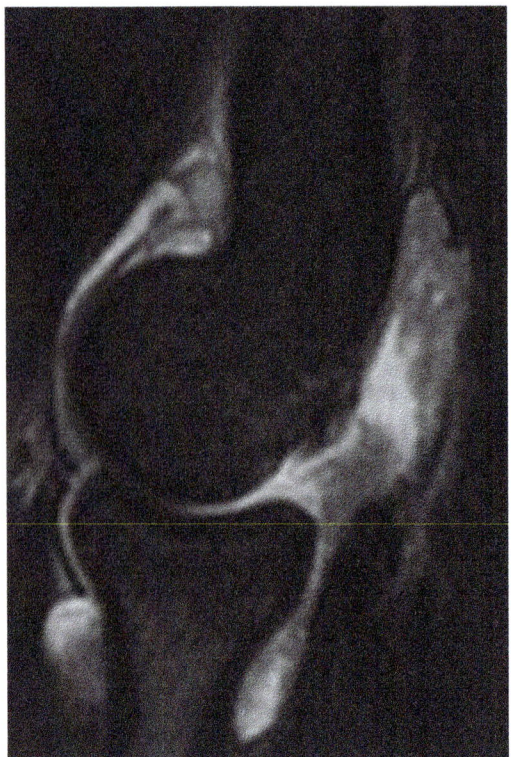

Fig. 24.5 Sagittal elbow MRI shows an elbow effusion and diffuse synovitis

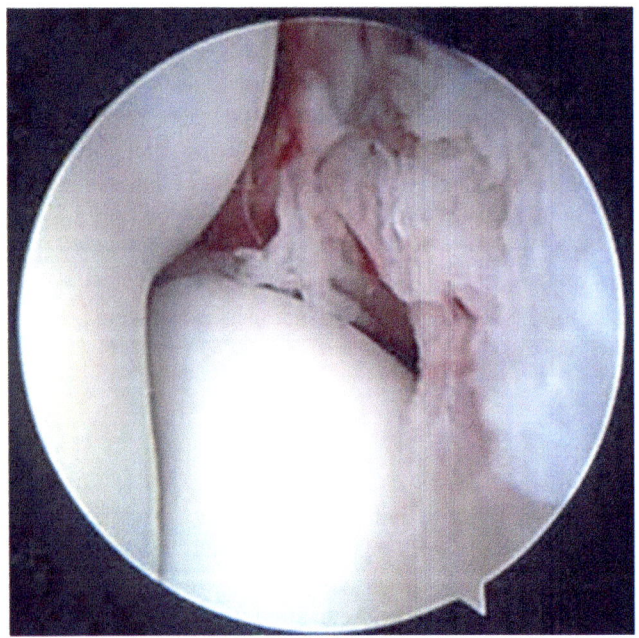

Fig. 24.6 Corresponding arthroscopic view of moderate synovitis in the anterior elbow near the radiocapitellar joint

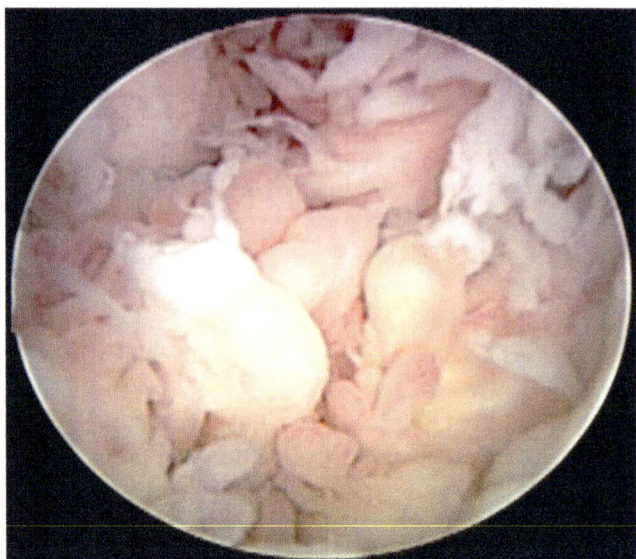

Fig. 24.7 Arthroscopic view of diffuse synovitis in the posterior compartment of the elbow

Conclusion

As orthopedic surgeons have gained experience with elbow arthroscopy, arthroscopic management of elbow arthritis and inflammatory synovitis has become common. Numerous studies have documented equivalent or improved outcomes with arthroscopic elbow debridement and synovectomy in comparison to open surgical techniques. With careful attention to surgical anatomy, arthroscopy is a safe and reliable surgical option for patients with degenerative or inflammatory arthritis of the elbow.

References

1. Kelly EW, Morrey BF, O'Driscoll SW. Complications of elbow arthroscopy. J Bone Joint Surg Am. 2001;83A:25–34.
2. Dodson CC, Nho SJ, Williams III RJ, Altchek DW. Elbow arthroscopy. J Am Acad Orthop Surg. 2008;16:574–85.
3. Savoie F, Nunley PD, Field LD. Arthroscopic management of the arthritis elbow: indications, technique, and results. J Shoulder Elbow Surg. 1999;8:214–9.
4. Cohen AP, Redden JF, Stanley D. Treatment of osteoarthritis of the elbow: a comparison of open and arthroscopic debridement. Arthroscopy. 2000;16:701–6.
5. Krishnan SG, Harkings DC, Pennington SD, et al. Arthroscopic ulnohumeral arthroplasty for degenerative arthritis of the elbow in patients under fifty years of age. J Shoulder Elbow Surg. 2007;16: 443–8.
6. DeGreef I, Samorjai N, DeSmet L. The outerbridge Kashiwagi procedure in elbow arthroscopy. Acta Orthop Belg. 2010;76(4):468–71.

7. Savoie III FH, O'Brien MJ, Field LD. Arthroscopy for arthritis of the elbow. Hand Clin. 2011;27(2):171–8.

8. Kelly E, Bryce R, Coghlan J, Bell SB. Arthroscopic debridement without radial head excision of the osteoarthritic elbow. Arthroscopy. 2007;23(2):151–6.

9. Lee BPH, Morrey BF. Arthroscopic synovectomy of the elbow for rheumatoid arthritis. J Bone Joint Surg Br. 1997;79B:770–2.

10. Horiuchi K, Momohara S, Tomatsu T, et al. Arthroscopic synovectomy of the elbow in rheumatoid arthritis. J Bone Joint Surg Am. 2002;84A:342–7.

11. Kauffman JI, Chen AL, Stuchin S, Di Cesare PE. Surgical management of the rheumatoid elbow. J Am Acad Orthop Surg. 2003;11:100–8.

12. Nemoto K, Arino H, Yoshihara Y, Fujikawa K. Arthroscopic synovectomy for the rheumatoid elbow: a short-term outcome. J Shoulder Elbow Surg. 2004;13:652–5.

13. Tanaka N, Sakahashi H, Hirose K, et al. Arthroscopic and open synovectomy of the elbow in rheumatoid arthritis. J Bone Joint Surg Am. 2006;88:521–5.

Elbow Trauma and Arthrofibrosis

25

Wendell M.R. Heard, Michael J. O'Brien,
and Felix H. Savoie III

Introduction

Range-of-motion loss is a common complication of elbow trauma. Decreased range of motion can be caused by the trauma itself, by a mechanical block from a displaced fracture fragment, or by arthrofibrosis caused by treatment of the primary injury, whether that treatment is surgical or nonsurgical. Three of the factors that make the elbow particularly susceptible to arthrofibrosis include the intrinsic congruity of the ulnohumeral joint, the presence of three articulations within the joint, and the close relationship of the capsule to the intracapsular ligaments and extracapsular muscles [1]. Studies have shown that the majority of activities of daily living can be performed within a functional arc of 100° (30–130°) of elbow flexion and extension and 100° of forearm rotation (50° of supination and 50° of pronation) [2]. Some patients may find these parameters to be acceptable, while others may put demands on their elbow that requires additional range of motion.

Nonoperative treatment modalities for the stiff elbow are most successful for up to 6–12 months after injury and include physical therapy and static splinting. An adequate amount of motion may be different for different patients because of unique lifestyle or work demands. It is important to tailor treatment based on individual patient needs. If an adequate amount of motion cannot be regained through nonoperative means, arthroscopic debridement can be offered to assist in the restoration of elbow motion. Arthroscopic treatment is particularly useful for elbow stiffness caused by pathology within the joint such as a contracted capsule, scar tissue, loose body, and osteophyte.

A complete history and physical examination is needed to formulate an effective treatment plan. The extent to which the motion loss affects the patient's abilities to perform tasks must be determined, as this will set the motion goals of surgical intervention. The mechanism of injury and the nature of the trauma are important. Any previous surgical interventions must be investigated and operative notes should be reviewed.

The physical examination begins with inspection of the extremity. Special note should be made of any soft tissue injuries or previous operative incisions. The range-of-motion assessment should include the hand, wrist, forearm, and elbow and should be compared to the contralateral arm. A careful neurovascular examination must be well documented. The ulnar nerve lies in close proximity to the medial joint capsule and may become entrapped in scar tissue causing an ulnar neuropathy that could be improved with an ulnar nerve transposition at the time of surgery. The elbow must also be examined for stability. In some cases, a posterolateral rotatory instability can be the underlying cause of the patient's complaints of stiffness.

Imaging includes standard elbow radiographs to include anteroposterior, lateral, and oblique views. If instability is suspected, stress radiographs can be helpful. Computed tomography (CT) can give information about a bony structure including heterotopic ossification, loose bodies, or deformity from previous fracture. Magnetic resonance imaging (MRI) is helpful in diagnosing cartilage defects, loose bodies, or ligamentous injuries causing instability.

This chapter will present two cases to help illustrate the appearance of pathology seen arthroscopically and correlate it to MRI. The first case is one in which trauma caused decreased range of motion because of a displaced fracture fragment. The second case illustrates a postsurgical arthrofibrosis with ligamentous instability.

W.M.R. Heard, MD (✉) • M.J. O'Brien, MD
F.H. Savoie III, MD
Department of Orthopedic Surgery, Division of Sports Medicine,
Tulane Medical Center, Tulane University School of Medicine,
New Orleans, LA, USA
e-mail: wheard@tulane.edu; mobrien@tulane.edu;
fsavoie@tulane.edu

S.F. Brockmeier (ed.), *MRI-Arthroscopy Correlations: A Case-Based Atlas of the Knee, Shoulder, Elbow and Hip*,
DOI 10.1007/978-1-4939-2645-9_25, © Springer Science+Business Media New York 2015

Case 1

A 10-year-old left-hand-dominant boy presented with loss of motion of his right elbow after a fall at school. He was diagnosed with a non-displaced supracondylar fracture and treated in a cast for 3 weeks. Upon removal of the cast, he was noted to be quite stiff, and therapy was initiated. He remained stiff but complained that his elbow was "going out of place" with stretching. The persistent complaints prompted his mother to seek further treatment approximately 5 weeks after the injury. When he presented to the office, radiographs showed an anterior ossific density (Fig. 25.1). An MRI was obtained and confirmed a large capitellar fracture fragment (Figs. 25.2 and 25.3). After a discussion of risks, benefits, and alternatives with the family, an operative course was planned to regain motion of the elbow.

The patient was brought to the operating room and placed in the prone position after placement of an interscalene block and induction of general anesthesia. Examination under anesthesia showed posterolateral instability with stable medial structures. The range of motion showed poor pronation and supination with −30° of extension and flexion to 90°.

Arthroscopy was initiated with formation of a proximal anteromedial portal. A large, loose fragment of articular car-

tilage was seen in front of the radiocapitellar joint. A lateral portal was established to assist in evaluation. The cartilage piece was approximately 1.5 cm × 1.0 cm (Fig. 25.4), but unfortunately, there was no bone on the backside of the car-

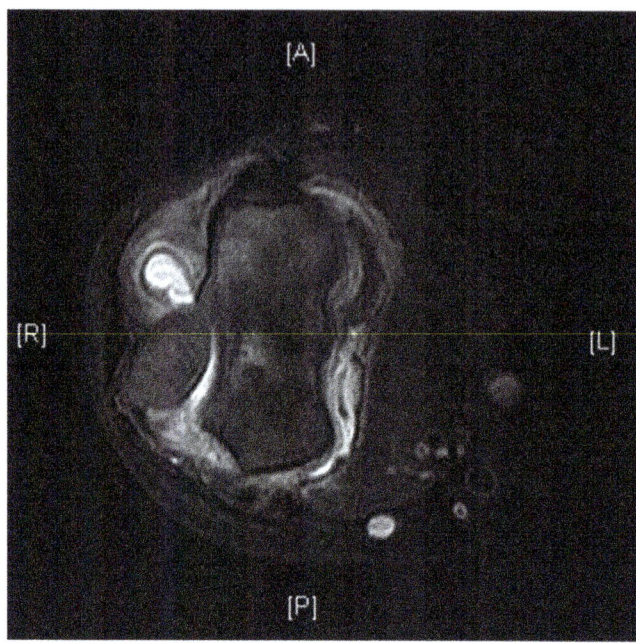

Fig. 25.2 Axial MRI view showing a large displaced capitellar fragment (published with kind permission. Copyright © Felix H. Savoie, III, MD)

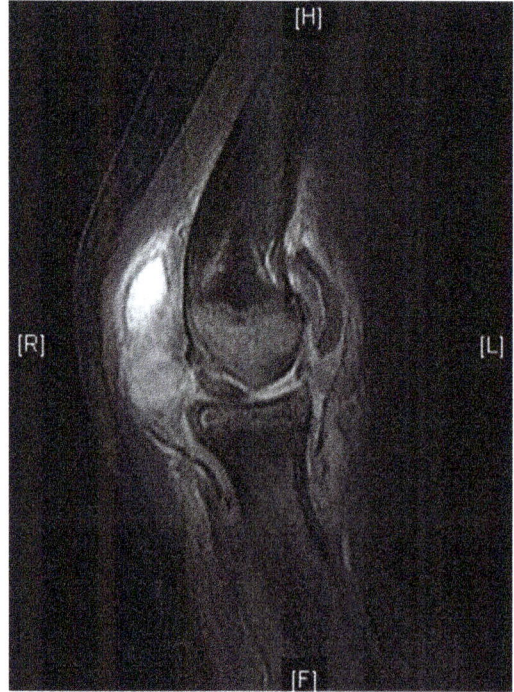

Fig. 25.3 Sagittal MRI view of the displaced capitellar fragment (published with kind permission. Copyright © Felix H. Savoie, III, MD)

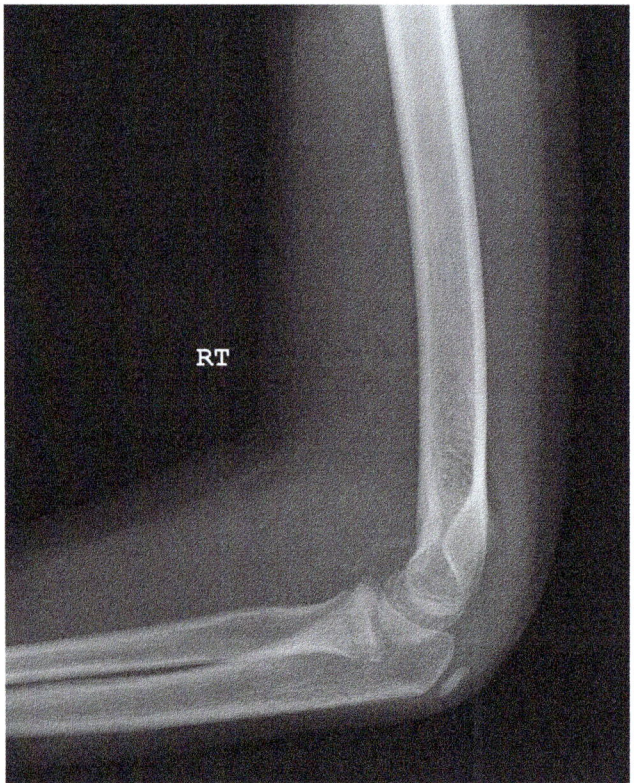

Fig. 25.1 Lateral radiograph showing ossific density anterior to the distal humerus (published with kind permission. Copyright © Felix H. Savoie, III, MD)

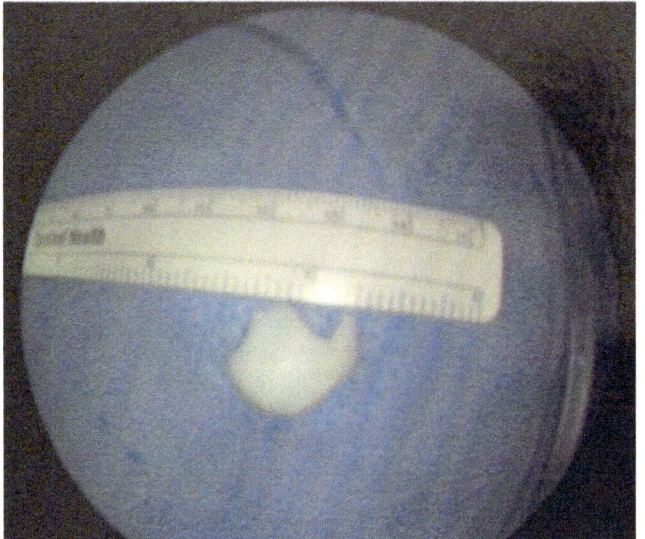

Fig. 25.4 Arthroscopic view of the capitellar cartilage fragment. The fragment did not have any bone on its backside and was deemed to be irreparable (published with kind permission. Copyright © Felix H. Savoie, III, MD)

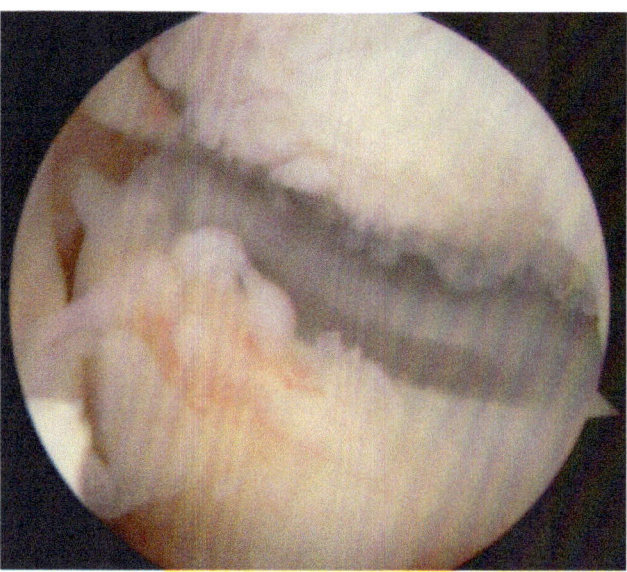

Fig. 25.6 Arthroscopic view again showing the bare capitellum and the central portion of the radial head without cartilage coverage (published with kind permission. Copyright © Felix H. Savoie, III, MD)

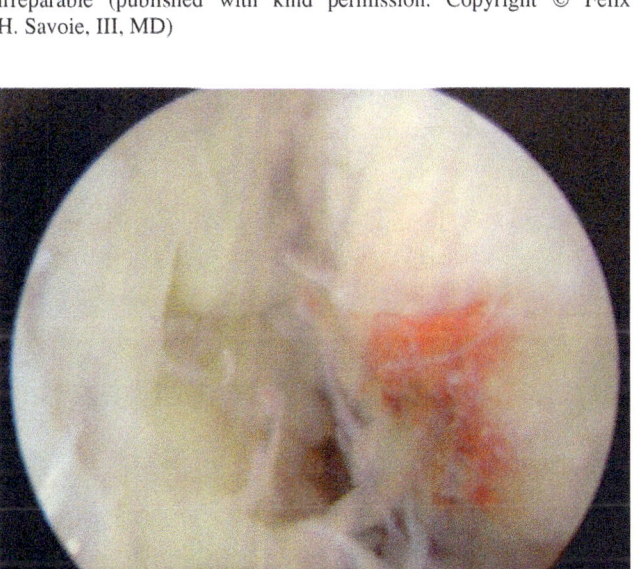

Fig. 25.5 Arthroscopic view of the capitellum devoid of cartilage (published with kind permission. Copyright © Felix H. Savoie, III, MD)

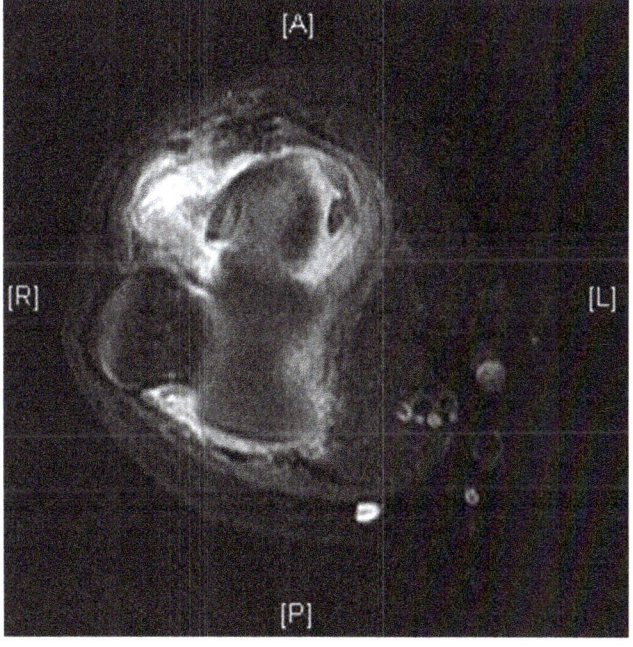

Fig. 25.7 Axial MRI view of the smaller capitellar fragment that had the lateral ligaments attached to it (published with kind permission. Copyright © Felix H. Savoie, III, MD)

tilage fragment. The piece was deemed irreparable and removed. Further arthroscopic evaluation showed arthrofibrosis involving the capsule. The capsule was incised from lateral to medial and resected. The capitellum was devoid of cartilage (Fig. 25.5) as was the central portion of the radial head (Fig. 25.6). These two areas were microfractured. Range-of-motion assessment now showed extension of 0°, flexion of 145°, and full pronation and supination. No pathology was seen posteriorly in the olecranon fossa. The medial gutter showed evidence of previous injury to the medial

ulnar collateral ligament (MUCL) that appeared to be healing well. A positive "drive-through sign" on the lateral side confirmed lateral instability. In the lateral gutter, there was a second large osteochondral fragment of capitellum with ligaments attached that was separated from its base without evidence of healing. This piece can be seen on the MRI (Figs. 25.7 and 25.8). It was felt that this fragment warranted fixation. The area was debrided and microfractured. A bioab-

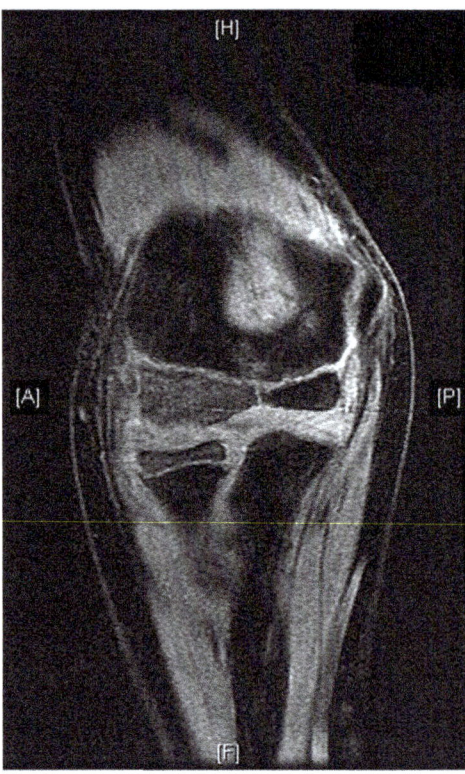

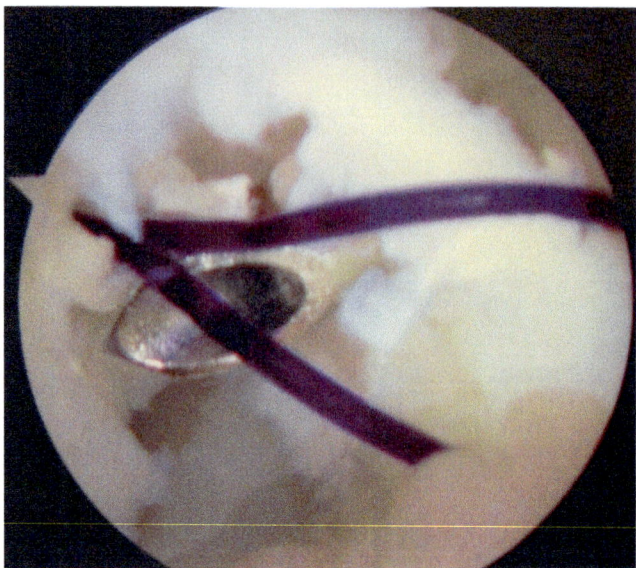

sorbable anchor with PDS® suture (Ethicon, Somerville, NJ) was placed. The PDS® was passed through the fragment and tied, securing the piece in its bed (Figs. 25.9, 25.10, and 25.11). A test of range of motion confirmed stable fragment fixation with maintenance of range of motion. The patient was placed into a splint in full extension and awoken from anesthesia.

The patient's last follow-up was 9 months after surgery. He had no pain and range of motion showing full extension, full pronation/supination, and 110° of flexion. The most recent radiograph is shown (Fig. 25.12).

This case represents a loss of elbow range of motion because of both arthrofibrosis and a mechanical block from a displaced osteochondral fragment, both of which were successfully treated arthroscopically. Fixation of the smaller piece was critical to regaining elbow stability as it included the attachment of the lateral ligaments.

Case 2

A 26-year-old baseball player presented with right elbow pain and decreased range of motion. He had undergone a MUCL reconstruction with transposition of the ulnar nerve

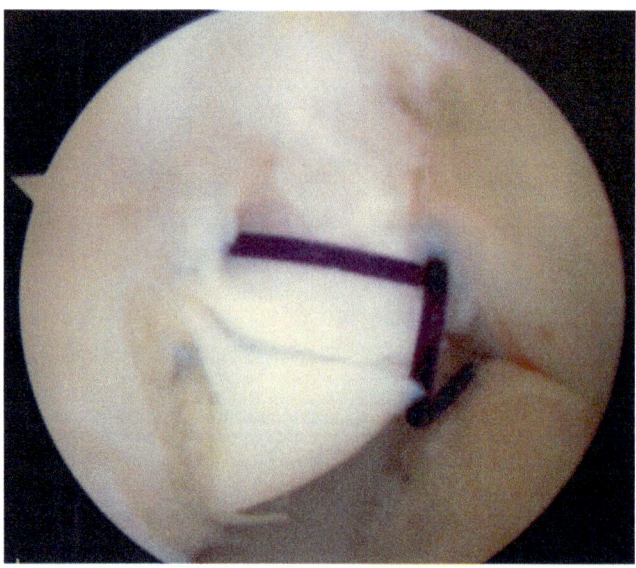

2 years prior and a second surgery for arthroscopic debridement 1 year prior to presentation.

Physical examination in the office showed that he lacked 45° of extension and he had a flexion of 90°. He displayed 2+ valgus instability and 2+ posterolateral instability.

After full evaluation and discussion with the patient, it was determined that surgical treatment would be undertaken to consist of an open exploration of the ulnar nerve followed

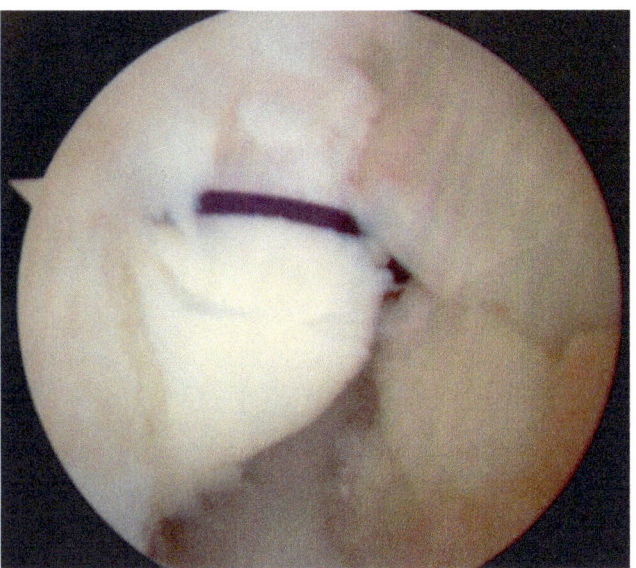

Fig. 25.11 Arthroscopic view of the final repair (published with kind permission. Copyright © Felix H. Savoie, III, MD)

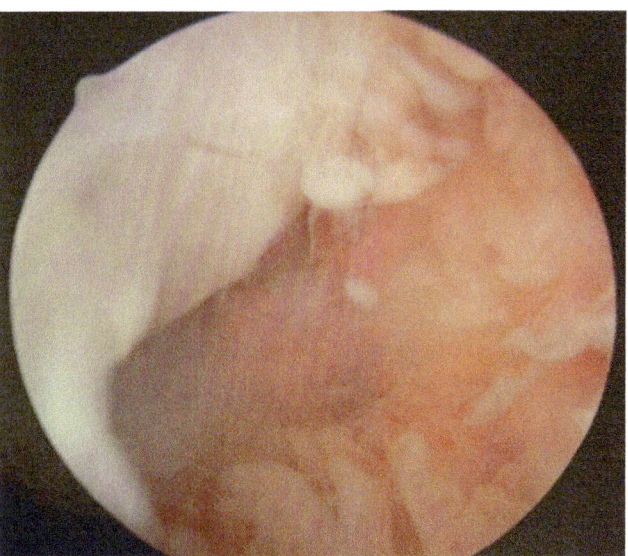

Fig. 25.13 A proliferative synovitis was encountered during arthroscopy that appeared postinfectious; however, cultures were negative (published with kind permission. Copyright © Felix H. Savoie, III, MD)

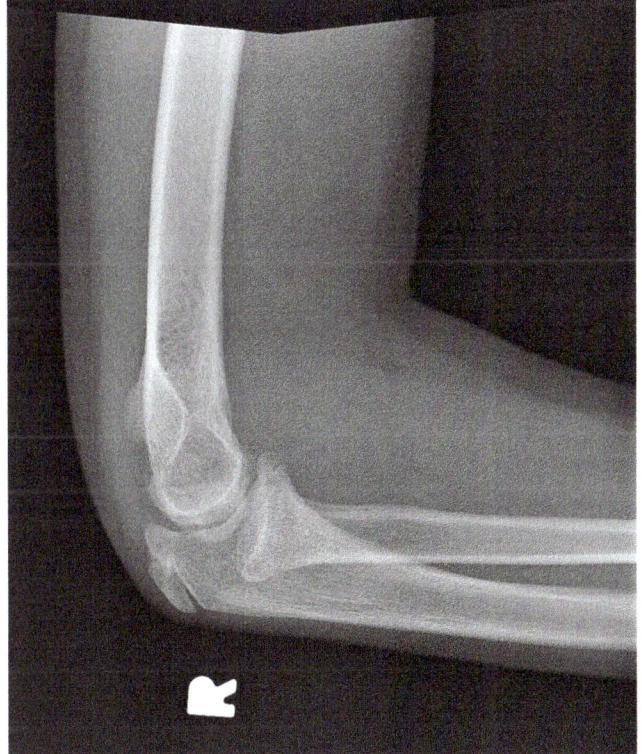

Fig. 25.12 Lateral radiograph 9 months postoperatively (published with kind permission. Copyright © Felix H. Savoie, III, MD)

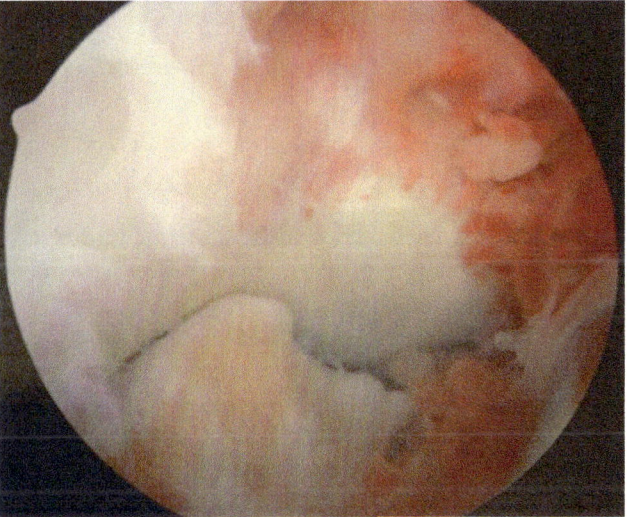

Fig. 25.14 Coronoid after osteophyte removal (published with kind permission. Copyright © Felix H. Savoie, III, MD)

by an arthroscopic debridement, synovectomy, arthrofibrosis takedown, and spur excision. The MUCL reconstruction would be left alone.

The patient was brought to the operating room and placed in the prone position after induction of general anesthesia and placement of an interscalene nerve block. An open approach was performed and the ulnar nerve identified in its anteriorly transposed position. It was released from a significant amount of scar tissue that surrounded it.

Anteromedial and anterolateral portals were established for the arthroscopic procedure. A proliferative synovitis that appeared postinfectious was encountered (Fig. 25.13) and cultures were taken, but did not show evidence of active infection. A synovectomy was performed anteriorly, and the capsule was released from the humerus and completely excised from medial to lateral. Osteophytes were removed from the coronoid tip (Fig. 25.14) and from the coronoid fossa.

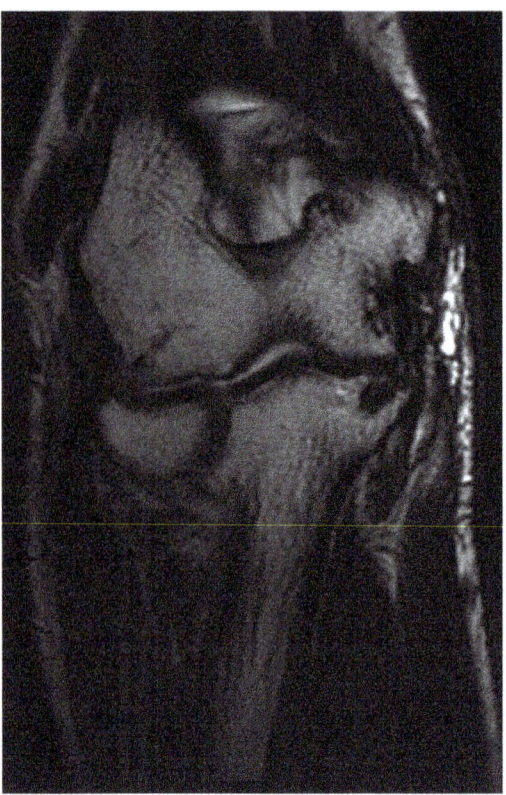

Fig. 25.15 Coronal MRI view showing the initial MUCL reconstruction with increased signal within the graft (published with kind permission. Copyright © Felix H. Savoie, III, MD)

With the inflow left anteriorly, the posterior central and posterolateral portals were made. More proliferative synovitis was encountered and resected. The olecranon fossa was filled with heterotopic bone and was removed. An arthroscopic Outerbridge–Kashiwagi fossa fenestration was then made. Range-of-motion assessment showed full extension, full flexion, and normal pronation and supination. A drain was placed anteriorly and a splint in full extension was applied. Aggressive physical therapy for range of motion was begun the next day.

On postoperative day number 9, range-of-motion assessment showed 0° of extension and 140° of flexion. Two months postoperatively, extension lacked 30° and flexion was 145° with normal pronation and supination. As expected, he continued to show valgus laxity.

An MRI was repeated and showed increased signal intensity within the mid-MUCL and proximal MUCL (Fig. 25.15), arthritis, and osteophytes (Fig. 25.16). At the time of MRI review, the patient's range of motion lacked 30° of extension with 120° of flexion. He was functionally impaired because of MUCL laxity. The decision was made to proceed with MUCL revision reconstruction with arthroscopic debridement and ulnar nerve transposition.

The patient was brought to the operating room for an open exploration of the medial elbow, complete capsular excision,

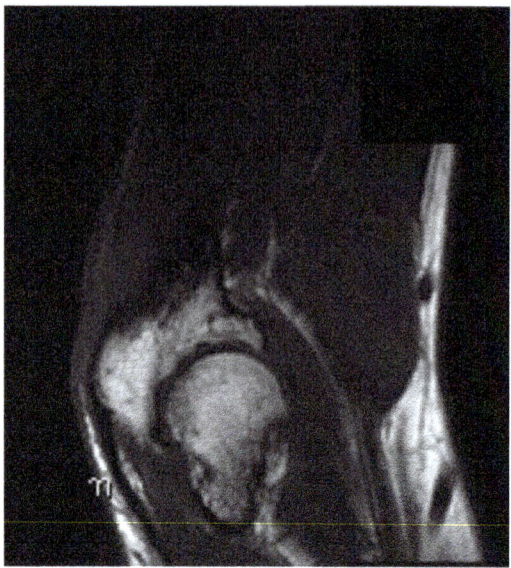

Fig. 25.16 Sagittal MRI view of the ulnohumeral joint showing osteophytes on the coronoid and olecranon (published with kind permission. Copyright © Felix H. Savoie, III, MD)

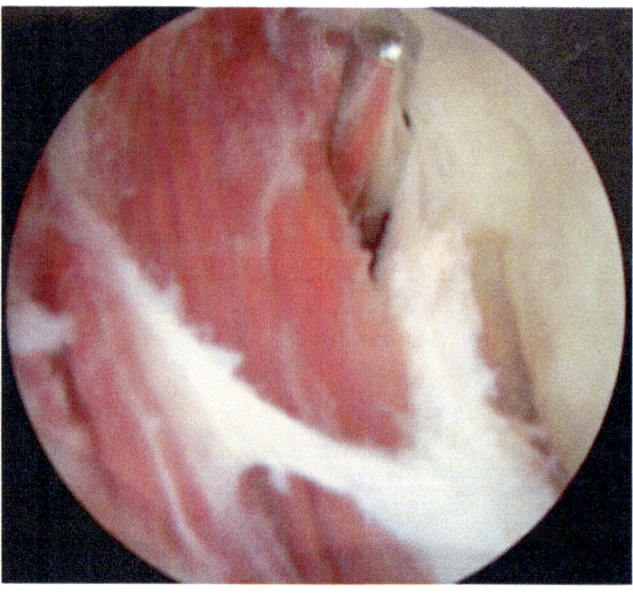

Fig. 25.17 Arthroscopic view after capsulectomy (published with kind permission. Copyright © Felix H. Savoie, III, MD)

and revision MUCL reconstruction with gracilis allograft. He was placed in the prone position after placement of an interscalene block and induction of general anesthesia. An incision was made and the ulnar nerve was found and isolated. A proximal anteromedial portal and proximal anterior lower lateral portal were established, and the anterior capsule was excised (Fig. 25.17). This resulted in an improvement in extension from −30 to −5° and flexion improving from 120 to 140°. The previously made Outerbridge–Kashiwagi fenestration was reopened (Fig. 25.18), and some scar tissue in the back of the elbow was removed. Attention was then directed

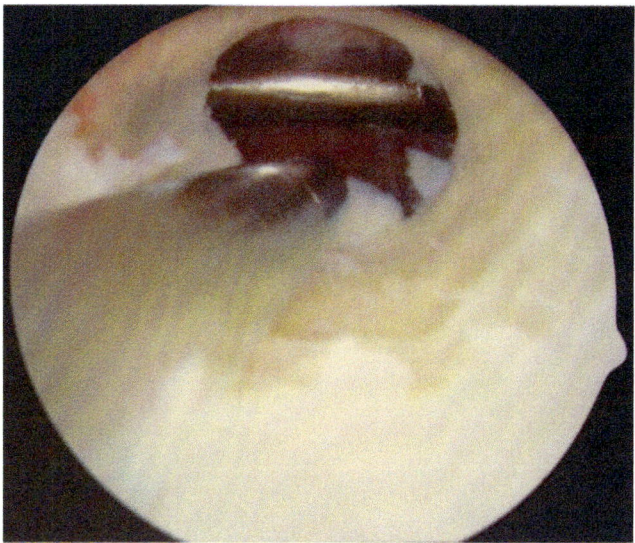

Fig. 25.18 Arthroscopic view of the revised Outerbridge–Kashiwagi fenestration (published with kind permission. Copyright © Felix H. Savoie, III, MD)

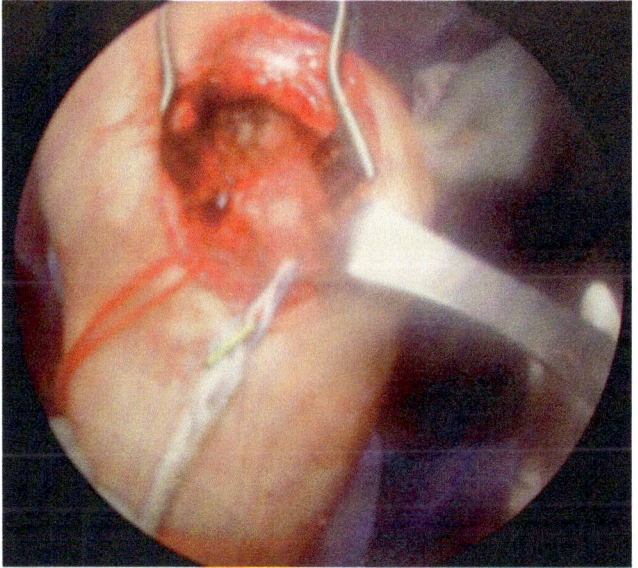

Fig. 25.19 The gracilis allograft was attached to an EndoButton (Smith and Nephew, Andover, MA) which was used for ulnar-sided fixation for the revision MUCL reconstruction (published with kind permission. Copyright © Felix H. Savoie, III, MD)

to the revision MUCL reconstruction. The ulnar nerve was again identified and dissection was taken down to the flexor/pronator mass, which was found to be detached from the medial condyle. Dissection revealed the epicondyle and the sublime tubercle. The graft was attached to an EndoButton (Smith and Nephew, Andover, MA) which was placed through the sublime tubercle (Fig. 25.19). Proximally, a hole was drilled at the normal site of the origin of the MUCL at the more lateral portion of the inferior aspect of the medial epicondyle exiting in the olecranon fossa. The graft was pulled

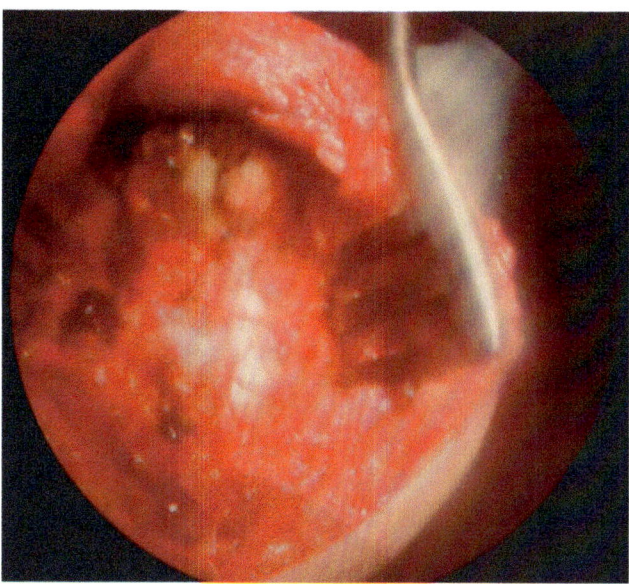

Fig. 25.20 View of the revised MUCL reconstruction after final graft passage and fixation (published with kind permission. Copyright © Felix H. Savoie, III, MD)

through this tunnel and an interference screw was placed (Fig. 25.20). The flexor/pronator mass was reattached using a suture anchor. The ulnar nerve was left in its anteriorly transposed position.

At his last follow-up, the patient was approximately 6 months postsurgery. He had a stable elbow and range of motion from 10 to 130°. He could throw a baseball and a football but not at the level prior to his first injury.

This case illustrates a postsurgical arthrofibrosis with ulnar neuropathy and medial-sided instability, all of which had to be addressed in a stepwise manner to improve elbow function.

Conclusions

Elbow trauma leading to decreased elbow range of motion is a difficult problem. It can occur after operative or nonoperative treatment of elbow trauma. A thorough evaluation and determination of the cause of the motion loss is essential to formulate an operative plan. Advancements in elbow arthroscopy have made it possible to expand the indications for its use as an effective way to treat the elbow suffering from decreased range of motion.

References

1. Cohen MS, Schimmel DR, Masuda K, et al. Structural and biochemical evaluation of the elbow capsule after trauma. J Shoulder Elbow Surg. 2007;16(4):484–90.
2. Morrey BF, Askew LJ, Chao EY. A biomechanical study of normal functional elbow motion. J Bone Joint Surg Am. 1981; 63(6):872–7.

Other Entities: PLRI, HO, Triceps, and Plica

26

Wade C. VanSice, Michael J. O'Brien, and Felix H. Savoie III

Posterolateral Rotatory Instability

Introduction

Posterolateral rotatory instability (PLRI) of the elbow is a well-defined instability pattern, originally described by O'Driscoll in 1991 [1]. PLRI results from an incompetent radial ulnohumeral ligament (RUHL), also known as the lateral ulnar collateral ligament (LUCL). When the RUHL is nonfunctional, the radial head subluxates posterolaterally off of the capitellum during forearm supination, and the ulnohumeral joint begins to gap. As the pattern of instability continues the entire, elbow joint may dislocate [1].

PLRI is identified through a combination of history and physical examination. The most common etiology is trauma, such as falling onto an outstretched hand or a simple elbow dislocation, but it may also result from iatrogenic injury. PLRI resulting from cortisone injections or surgery for lateral epicondylitis has been described [2, 3].

Patients with PLRI will complain of lateral-sided elbow pain and discomfort with activities. They will frequently report mechanical symptoms of locking, catching, and clicking or a palpable "clunk" with certain activities [1]. This is typically noted at mid-flexion as the elbow goes into extension, especially with the forearm supinated. Lateral-sided elbow instability can be very debilitating. Activities of daily living, such as opening doors or lifting objects in front of

them with the elbow extended, become painful and difficult [4, 5]. Pushing up from a chair or a seated position can cause pain and feelings of instability, as the combination of supination, valgus force, and axial load causes the radial head to subluxate posterolaterally.

The diagnosis of PLRI is best demonstrated clinically with the *lateral pivot shift test* of the elbow. This test, first described by O'Driscoll [1], can be performed in the supine or prone position and will elicit gross instability or simply pain and apprehension. Two additional clinical tests have been described by Regan and colleagues [6] and are also useful in the diagnosis of PLRI. The *chair push-up test* is performed with the patient pushing up from an arm chair with the palms facing inward and forearms supinated. The *table-top relocation test* requires the patient to push up from a prone or wall-leaning position first with the forearms maximally pronated and then repeat the test with the forearms maximally supinated. The tests are considered positive when they reproduce the patient's pain, instability, or both [6].

The diagnosis is confirmed with magnetic resonance imaging (MRI) arthrography. In the acute setting, injection of contrast is not necessary as blood in the joint from the traumatic injury serves as contrast medium. The RUHL is usually avulsed from its origin on the posterior aspect of the lateral epicondyle of the humerus. In the chronic setting, laxity of the lateral collateral ligament complex will be evident, with posterolateral subluxation of the radial head from the capitellum.

Once diagnosed, surgery is necessary to correct persistent instability. In most instances, the ligament has failed to heal with conservative treatment. Instability can be confirmed arthroscopically through several findings, including subluxation of the radial head on the capitellum and the arthroscopic "drive through sign" of the elbow, where the arthroscope in the posterior portal can be driven from the lateral gutter across the ulnohumeral articulation into the medial gutter. This maneuver is not possible in the stable elbow. Acute repairs, both open and arthroscopic, heal with excellent

W.C. VanSice, MD, MPH (✉) • F.H. Savoie III, MD
Department of Orthopedic Surgery, Tulane University School of Medicine, Tulane Medical Center, New Orleans, LA, USA
e-mail: wvansice@tulane.edu; fsavoie@tulane.edu

M.J. O'Brien, MD
Department of Orthopedic Surgery, Division of Sports Medicine, Tulane University School of Medicine, Tulane Medical Center, New Orleans, LA, USA
e-mail: mobrien@tulane.edu

S.F. Brockmeier (ed.), *MRI-Arthroscopy Correlations: A Case-Based Atlas of the Knee, Shoulder, Elbow and Hip,*
DOI 10.1007/978-1-4939-2645-9_26, © Springer Science+Business Media New York 2015

patient outcomes [2]. In the chronic setting, graft reconstruction may be required.

This report describes cases of arthroscopic repair of the RUHL in the acute and chronic setting. A high index of suspicion is necessary to correctly diagnose this condition in patients with lateral elbow pain and feelings of instability.

Case 1: Acute Elbow Dislocation

History/Exam

A 17-year-old high school football running back presented to the orthopedic clinic 1 day following a traumatic elbow dislocation to his nondominant arm. He fell onto his outstretched left hand while being tackled and sustained a closed posterolateral elbow dislocation, which was reduced on the field of play. He had no history of previous injury to the elbow. At presentation, his left elbow was immobilized in a posterior long arm splint. He complained of diffuse pain and swelling in the elbow on both the medial and lateral sides.

Physical examination revealed swelling on both sides of the elbow with skin intact. Range of motion was stable from 30 to 120° of flexion with full rotation and feelings of instability at terminal extension. He had tenderness over both medial and lateral collateral ligaments, instability to valgus stress, and evidence of posterolateral rotatory instability with lateral pivot shift testing. Neurologic testing was intact distally in the extremity.

Imaging

Radiographs were obtained with four views of the elbow including anteroposterior (AP), lateral, and oblique projections. Radiographs revealed a concentric reduction of the ulnohumeral joint with no fractures or subluxations. In some cases, radiographs may reveal an avulsion fragment from the posterior aspect of the lateral epicondyle of the humerus. An MRI without contrast was obtained the following day. Injection of contrast was not necessary in the acute period. A complete sequence of images was obtained, including axial T1 and fat-saturated T2 sequences, oblique coronal fat-saturated T1 and T2 sequences, and oblique sagittal T1 and fat-saturated T2 sequences. Coronal T2-weighted images are demonstrated in Fig. 26.1a, b, sagittal T2-weighted images in Fig. 26.2a, b, and axial T2-weighted image in Fig. 26.3.

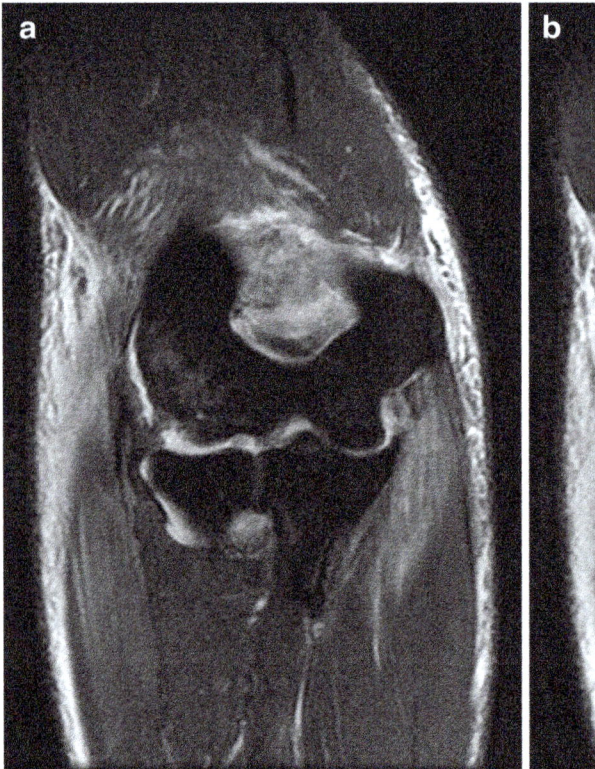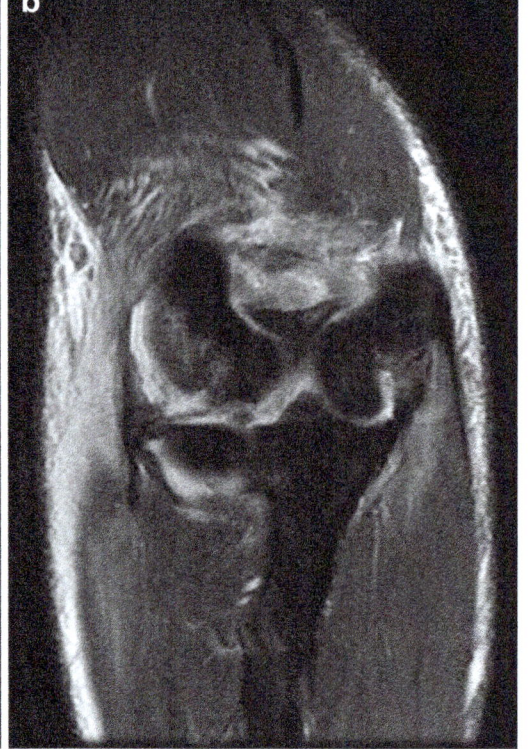

Fig. 26.1 (**a**, **b**) T2-weighted coronal oblique MRI images demonstrate tearing of the RUHL and LCL complex off the posterior aspect of the lateral epicondyle of the humerus, laxity in the annular ligament around the radial head, and edema in the bone of the lateral epicondyle and surrounding musculature. **a** also shows tearing in the mid-substance of the MUCL with avulsion distally off the sublime tubercle of the ulna (**a**, **b**: Published with kind permission. Copyright © Felix H. Savoie, III, MD)

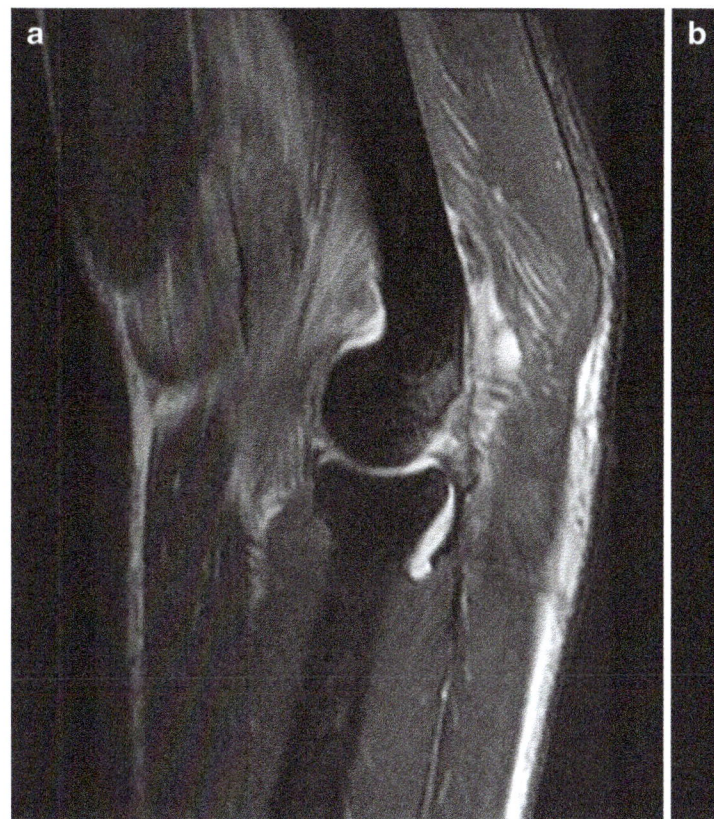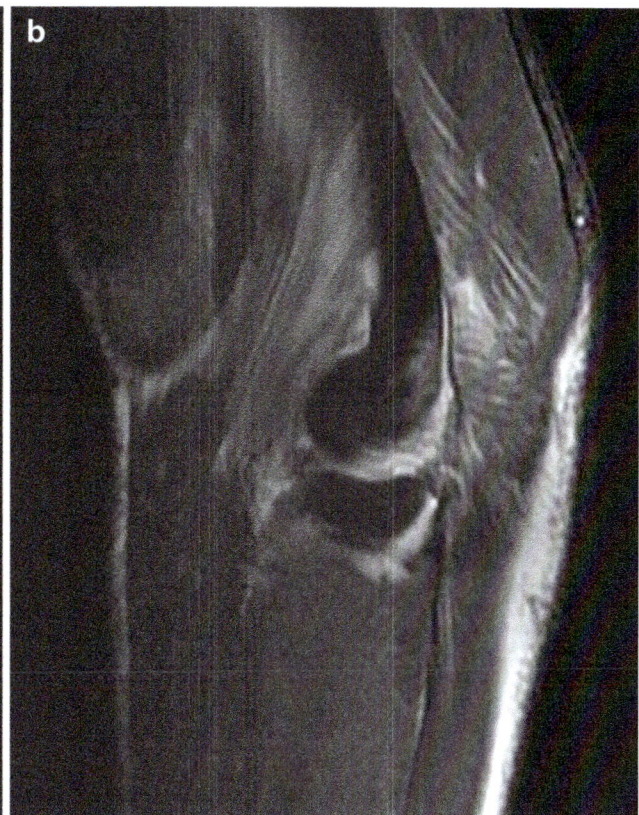

Fig. 26.2 (**a, b**) T2-weighted sagittal oblique MRI images demonstrate tearing of the RUHL and LCL complex off the posterior aspect of the lateral epicondyle of the humerus, laxity in the annular ligament, edema in the bone posteriorly, and edema in the brachialis muscle anteriorly and triceps muscle posteriorly (**a, b**: Published with kind permission. Copyright © Felix H. Savoie, III, MD)

MRI revealed concentric reduction of the ulnohumeral joint with no interposed soft tissues. On the lateral side, the RUHL complex is avulsed from the posterior aspect of the lateral epicondyle of the humerus (Fig. 26.1a, b) with edema seen in the bone at the avulsion site. On the medial side, mid-substance tearing of the medial ulnar collateral ligament (MUCL) and avulsion from the sublime tubercle on the ulna are demonstrated in Fig. 26.1a. Surrounding edema with increased signal intensity is visualized in the common flexor/pronator muscle origin in Fig. 26.1a. Sagittal oblique T2 sequences (Fig. 26.2a, b) also demonstrate avulsion of the RUHL complex from the posterior aspect of the lateral epicondyle, with edema in the brachialis anteriorly and triceps muscle posteriorly. Axial T2 image (Fig. 26.3) demonstrates avulsion of the RUHL in the upper right corner of the image. The left side of Fig. 26.3 shows tearing of the anterior capsule, edema in the brachialis muscle, and hematoma in the anterior compartment of the elbow joint.

Given the identified RUHL avulsion on MRI consistent with the patient's history and clinical examination of elbow dislocation, risks and benefits of operative intervention were discussed with the patient. He was the starting senior run-

ning back for his high school football team and had verbally committed to a college program. His team was the #1 seed, favored to play in the state championship game, and had already earned a first-round bye in the play-offs. He had one regular season game remaining, with 2 weeks before the team's first play-off game. Surgery was offered as a possible treatment for arthroscopic repair of the RUHL to stabilize the elbow and potentially return him to play faster in a brace. After an extensive discussion with the family of both operative and nonoperative treatment options, he elected to proceed with the proposed surgical intervention.

Arthroscopy

The patient was taken to the operating room and placed in the prone position with the operative arm placed on a bump over an arm board. A pneumatic tourniquet was used for the case. A standard diagnostic arthroscopy of the left elbow was completed. A standard proximal anteromedial viewing portal was established for the arthroscope and a working anterolateral portal established for the shaver. Hematoma in the anterior compartment was evacuated with the shaver, and tearing of the anterior capsule was evident with exposed muscle

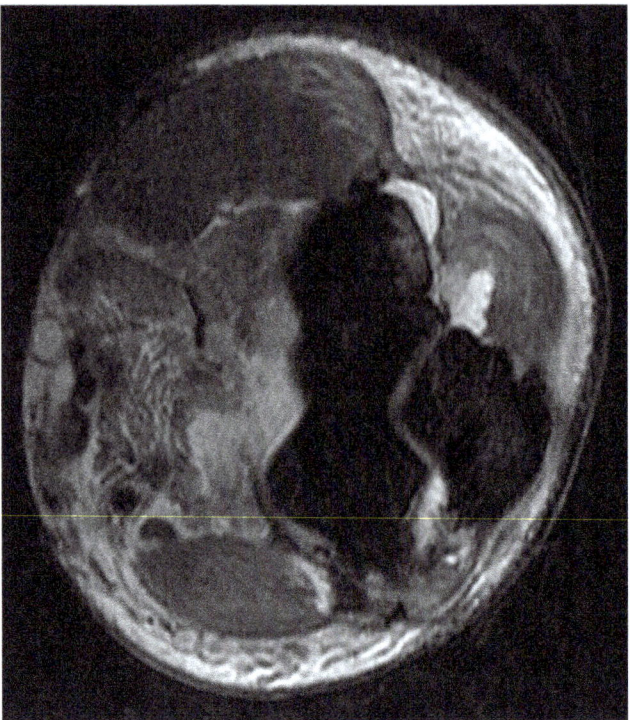

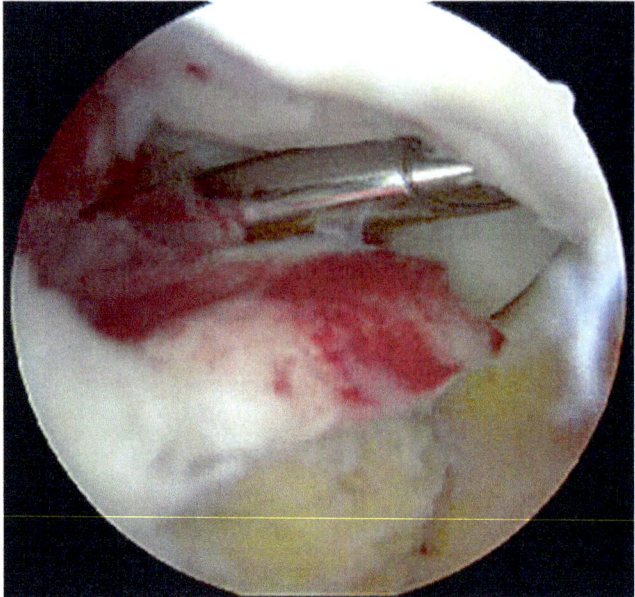

Fig. 26.3 A T2-weighted axial MRI image shows tearing of the RUHL off the posterior aspect of the lateral epicondyle in the *upper right corner* of the image. The *left side* of the image demonstrates tearing in the anterior capsule, edema in the brachialis, and hematoma in the anterior compartment of the elbow (Published with kind permission. Copyright © Felix H. Savoie, III, MD)

Fig. 26.4 An arthroscopic view of the posterolateral gutter in a left elbow, with the arthroscope in a posterior trans-tendon portal. The shaver is entering the posterior radiocapitellar joint through a lateral soft spot portal. The radial head is visible beyond the shaver. The stump of the RUHL is viewed in the center of the image, avulsed off the posterior aspect of the lateral epicondyle (Published with kind permission. Copyright © Felix H. Savoie, III, MD)

fibers of the brachialis. Inspection of the radiocapitellar joint showed laxity in the annular ligament. Rotation of the forearm demonstrated posterolateral subluxation of the radial off the capitellum, indicative of posterolateral rotatory instability.

The arthroscope was then placed into the posterior compartment through a posterior trans-tendon portal. Hematoma in the olecranon fossa was evacuated with a shaver in a posterolateral portal. The site of avulsion of the RUHL off the posterior aspect of the lateral epicondyle was visualized just lateral and distal to the olecranon fossa. The arthroscope was easily advanced down the posterolateral gutter due to laxity in the lateral collateral ligament (LCL) complex. The avulsed RUHL was visualized distally in the posterolateral gutter near the level of the radiocapitellar joint (Fig. 26.4). The arthroscope could be advanced from the lateral gutter across the ulnohumeral joint and into the medial gutter, with a positive arthroscopic "drive through sign" of the elbow (Fig. 26.5).

The site of origin of the RUHL was roughened with a shaver, and a double-loaded 2.9 mm suture anchor was inserted percutaneously into the humerus at the origin of the ligament (Fig. 26.6). The sutures were placed down the lateral gutter with a suture retriever. Utilizing a lateral soft spot

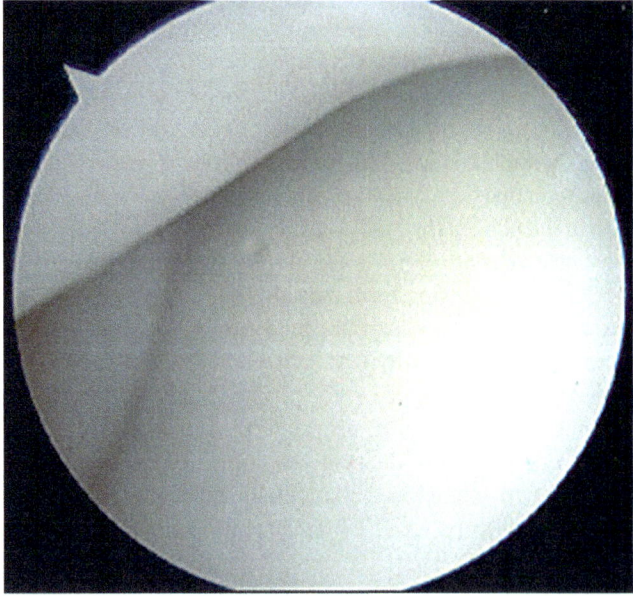

Fig. 26.5 The "drive through sign" of the elbow is demonstrated in this arthroscopic view of the ulnohumeral joint of a left elbow. The arthroscope is in the ulnohumeral joint, viewing from a posterior trans-tendon portal. The articular cartilage of the distal humerus is at the *top* of the image, with the articular cartilage of the ulna and proximal radioulnar joint at the *bottom* of the image (Published with kind permission. Copyright © Felix H. Savoie, III, MD)

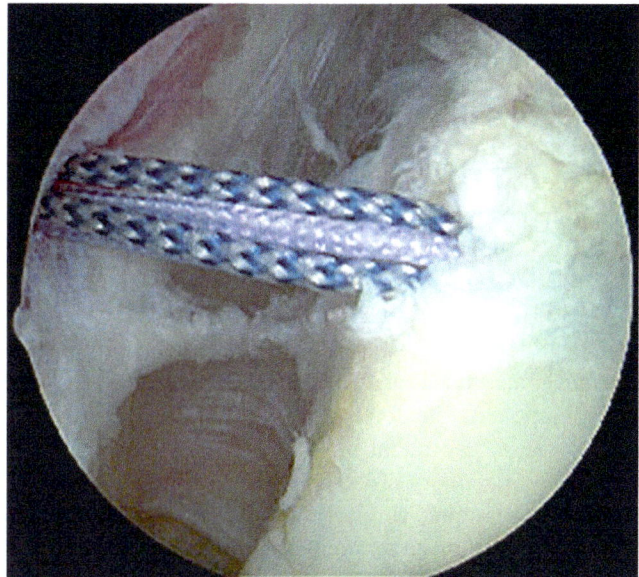

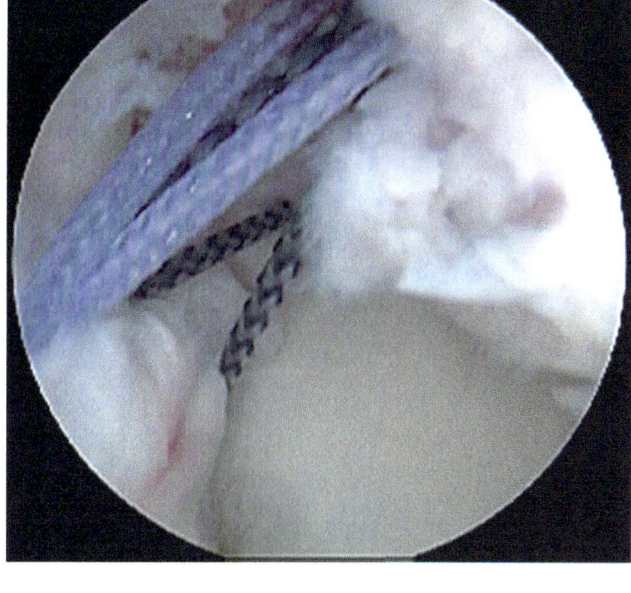

Fig. 26.6 An arthroscopic view of the posterolateral gutter in a left elbow with the arthroscope in a posterior trans-tendon portal. A double-loaded suture anchor has been inserted at the anatomic humeral origin of the RUHL just lateral and distal to the olecranon fossa on the posterior aspect of the lateral epicondyle (Published with kind permission. Copyright © Felix H. Savoie, III, MD)

Fig. 26.7 An arthroscopic view of the posterolateral gutter in a left elbow with the arthroscope in a posterior trans-tendon portal. Mattress sutures have been placed through the healthy portion of the RUHL. The sutures have not yet been tied (Published with kind permission. Copyright © Felix H. Savoie, III, MD)

portal and a percutaneous antegrade suture passer, two mattress sutures were placed in the healthy portion of the ligament. A second suture anchor was placed more distally with a mattress suture placed at the distal aspect of the ligament (Fig. 26.7). The sutures were retrieved and tied, placing the knots deep to the anconeus muscle. As the sutures were tied, tension was restored to the lateral collateral ligament complex, which had the effect of pushing the arthroscope out of the posterolateral gutter. The arthroscopic "drive through sign" could no longer be performed, indicating that adequate tension was restored to the lateral side of the elbow. The arthroscope was then placed back into the anterior compartment. Tension was restored to the annular ligament around the radial head, and the radial head no longer subluxated off the capitellum with forearm supination.

The patient was splinted for a week and then started physical therapy in a protective brace. The patient returned to play in the brace at 3 weeks, participation in the semifinals and finals. The brace was eliminated at 4 weeks and progress in rehabilitation continued. The patient is currently in his third year of collegiate competition, with no subsequent elbow problems.

Case 2: Chronic PLRI

History/Exam

A 30-year-old, right-hand-dominant, male carpenter presented to the orthopedic clinic complaining of left elbow pain. He had fallen off a roof 3 months prior, landing on his outstretched left arm, and sustained a closed left elbow dislocation. The elbow was reduced in the emergency department, and he was treated conservatively in a hinged elbow brace for 6 weeks. He complained of lateral-sided left elbow pain, feelings of instability, and a palpable clunk with certain activities, especially lifting objects with the left elbow extended.

Physical examination of the left elbow revealed prominence of the radial head and intact skin with no swelling. Range of motion was 10 to 135° of flexion with full rotation. He had tenderness over the radial head and lateral epicondyle, especially posteriorly. He had no gross instability to varus or valgus stress, a positive lateral pivot shift test, and a positive chair push-up test. His wrist exam was normal, and he was neurologically intact distally.

Imaging

Radiographs were obtained with four views of the elbow including AP, lateral, and oblique projections. Radiographs revealed an oval, opaque density on the lateral side of the elbow at the level of the radiocapitellar joint (Fig. 26.8), a concentric reduction of the ulnohumeral joint, and no fractures or subluxations. An MRI arthrogram was ordered with a complete sequence of images; the MRI was ordered with intra-articular contrast, as this was a chronic case. Coronal T2-weighted images are demonstrated in Fig. 26.9a–c, coronal T1-weighted image in Fig. 26.10, sagittal T2-weighted image in Fig. 26.11, and axial T2-weighted image in Fig. 26.12.

MRI revealed concentric reduction of the ulnohumeral joint. On the lateral side, there were indistinctness and heterogeneity of the RUHL complex as it neared the humeral attachment

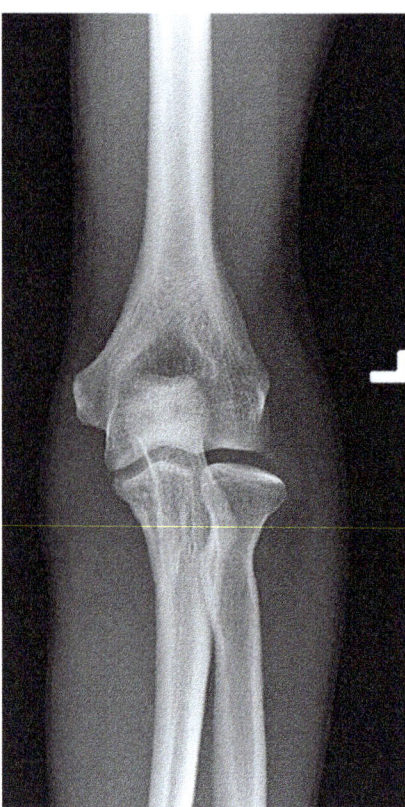

Fig. 26.8 An anteroposterior (AP) radiograph of a left elbow. A small oval density at the level of the radiocapitellar joint represents the avulsed RUHL off the humerus. The ulnohumeral joint is concentrically reduced, and there is slight lateral subluxation of the radial head off the capitellum (Published with kind permission. Copyright © Felix H. Savoie, III, MD)

(Fig. 26.9a–c) and lateral subluxation of the radial head. Figure 26.9a shows the stump of the RUHL and a void near the humeral attachment. Figure 26.9b shows heterogeneity and thickening of the RUHL and LCL complex, with an intact MUCL on the medial side. Figures 26.9c and 26.10 show the stump of the RUHL in the radiocapitellar joint, with a small avulsed piece of bone on the most proximal aspect of the ligament. The sagittal oblique image (Fig. 26.11) demonstrates the torn RUHL at the level of the radiocapitellar joint. The radial head is subluxated posterior, and the bare area on the posterior aspect of the lateral epicondyle represents the humeral origin of the RUHL. Figure 26.12 also shows avulsion of the RUHL off the posterior aspect of the lateral epicondyle in the axial plane. There is no soft tissue or bony edema on any image sequence, confirming that this represents a remote injury.

The MRI findings of an avulsed RUHL were consistent with the clinical exam of PLRI. Due to the appearance of the RUHL on MRI sequences with a grossly intact ligament avulsed off the humerus with an attached small piece of bone, an arthroscopic repair was offered, with the possible need for open reconstruction. The risks and benefits of the surgery were discussed with the patient. He had failed nonoperative management with clinical instability of the elbow. After an extensive discussion with the patient, he elected to proceed with the proposed surgical intervention.

Arthroscopy

The patient was taken to the operating room and placed in the prone position. Examination under anesthesia demonstrated a positive lateral pivot shift test (Fig. 26.13a, b). A standard diagnostic arthroscopy of the left elbow was completed. As in the first case, laxity of the annular ligament was identified (Fig. 26.14). There was no hematoma in the anterior compartment as this was a case of chronic instability. Rotation of the forearm demonstrated posterolateral subluxation of the radial off the capitellum, indicative of posterolateral rotatory instability.

The arthroscope was placed into the posterior compartment through a posterior trans-tendon portal. The arthroscope was again easily advanced down the posterolateral gutter, due to laxity in the LCL complex. The RUHL with attached bone fragment was visualized distally at the level of the radiocapitellar joint. The synovium had a yellowish appearance due to the chronic nature of the injury (Fig. 26.15).

The site of origin of the RUHL was roughened with a shaver, and a double-loaded 2.9 mm suture anchor was inserted percutaneously into the humerus at the origin of the ligament. Using a percutaneous antegrade suture passer (Fig. 26.16), two mattress sutures were placed into the healthy portion of the ligament, incorporating the lateral capsule (Fig. 26.17). The sutures were retrieved and tied in the same manner as the first case, and tension was restored to the lateral collateral ligament complex.

Heterotopic Ossification

Introduction

Heterotopic ossification (HO) is the formation of bone in nonskeletal tissue, usually in muscle or outside the joint capsule. It most commonly affects the elbow and the hip [7] and presents following trauma, significant brain injury, or major burns with symptoms of stiffness or complete ankylosis [8]. Although the exact etiology is unknown, predisposing factors have been proposed that include increased prostaglandin activity, tissue hypoxia, alterations in the sympathetic nervous system, and immobilization [9].

Diagnosis is made with history and physical exam, specifically severe pain, stiffness, joint swelling, warmth, and lack of motion, and confirmed with radiographs. Lack of understanding limits the ability to treat heterotopic bone formation both before and after it has occurred [10]. Range of motion exercises and stretching [11–13], medical interventions such as indomethacin and disphosphonates [14, 15], and radiation

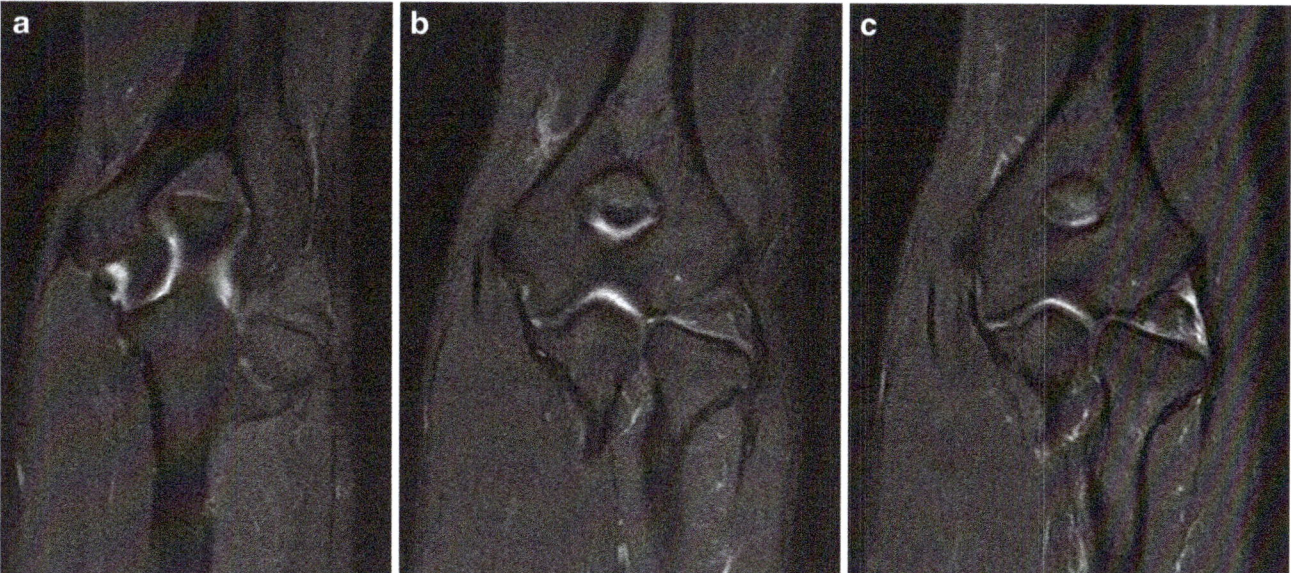

Fig. 26.9 (**a–c**) T2-weighted coronal oblique MRI images demonstrate tearing of the RUHL and LCL complex off the posterior aspect of the lateral epicondyle of the humerus. **a** shows the stump of the RUHL on the *right* of the image with a void of tissue at the humeral origin of the ligament. **b** shows heterogeneity in the LCL complex with an intact MUCL on the *left side* of the image. **c** shows the stump of the RUHL in the radiocapitellar joint and lateral subluxation of the radial head. The lack of edema in the bone and soft tissues confirms that this is a chronic injury (**a–c**: Published with kind permission. Copyright © Felix H. Savoie, III, MD)

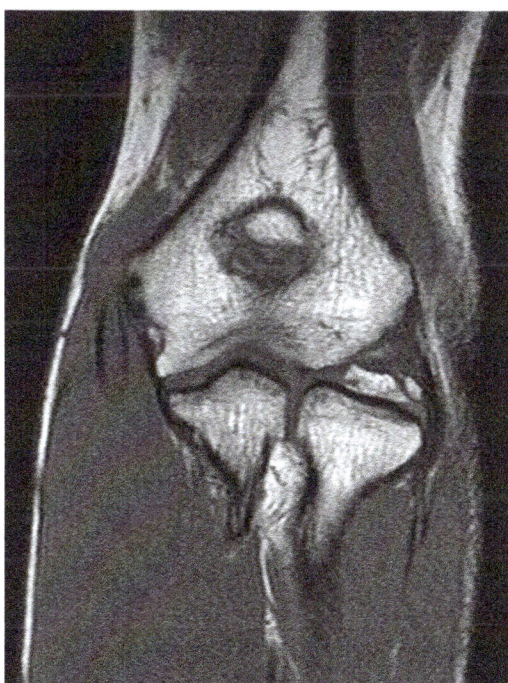

Fig. 26.10 A T1-weighted coronal oblique MRI image demonstrates heterogeneity of the RUHL and LCL complex on the *right side* of the image with a small oval of avulsed bone in the stump of the RUHL (Published with kind permission. Copyright © Felix H. Savoie, III, MD)

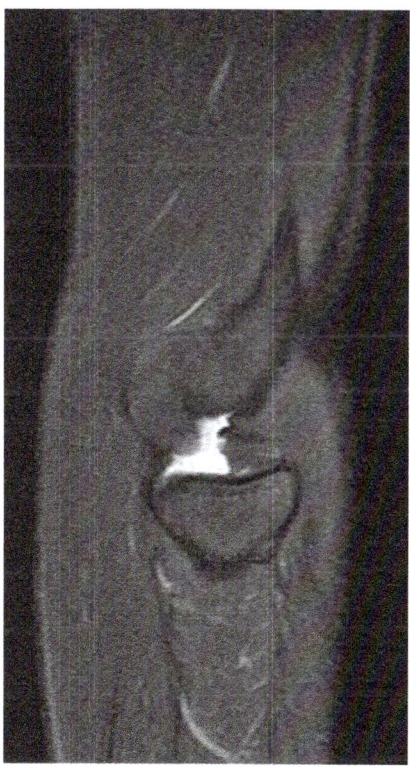

Fig. 26.11 A T2-weighted sagittal oblique MRI image shows tearing of the RUHL off the posterior aspect of the lateral epicondyle of the humerus, with posterior subluxation of the radial head off the capitellum (Published with kind permission. Copyright © Felix H. Savoie, III, MD)

therapy [16] have all been proposed as potential treatment options for the prevention of HO.

When HO about the elbow does occur, open surgical procedures incorporating ectopic bone removal and contracture release are practical options for regaining elbow motion. Traditionally, open excision is recommended at approximately 6–12 months after diagnosis to ensure that the rapid growth phase is complete and the bone has matured [17]. However, arthroscopic excision is possible and has recently shown to be effective early in the process.

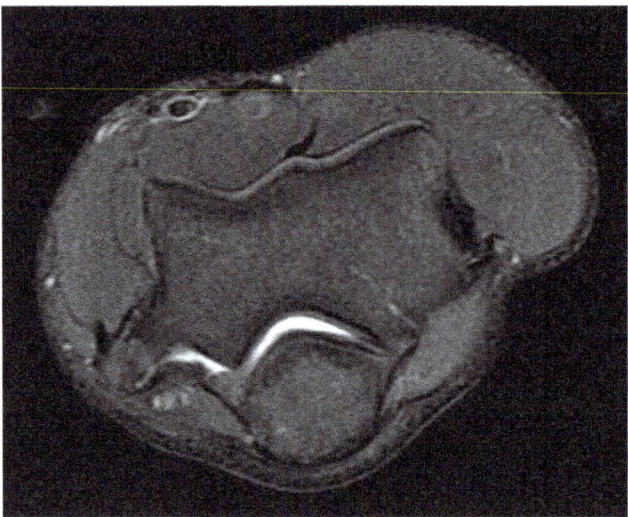

Fig. 26.12 A T2-weighted axial MRI image shows tearing of the RUHL off the posterior aspect of the lateral epicondyle of the humerus. There is no edema in the soft tissues and no hematoma in the anterior compartment of the elbow joint (Published with kind permission. Copyright © Felix H. Savoie, III, MD)

Case 1: Heterotopic Ossification

History/Exam

A 52-year-old, right-hand-dominant female presented to the orthopedic clinic with a chief complaint of left elbow pain. She sustained an elbow dislocation and previously underwent arthroscopic elbow surgery with medial and lateral ligament repairs. Approximately 2 months following surgery, she began to develop worsening pain and stiffness in the left elbow, with loss of motion despite appropriate physical therapy. Examination of the elbow revealed healed incisions with no signs of infection, fullness posteriorly in the olecranon fossa with tenderness to palpation, and a flexion contracture with approximately 30–40° loss of full extension.

Imaging

Radiographs (Fig. 26.18a, b) obtained showed heterotopic ossification in the posterior compartment. An MRI without contrast was obtained with a complete sequence of images. Sagittal T1, T2, and T2-fat-saturated images (Fig. 26.19a–c) and an axial image (Fig. 26.20) demonstrate heterotopic bone in the posterior compartment deep to the triceps filling the olecranon fossa. Increased signal intensity in the bone and surrounding musculature shows that this is an active process with acute inflammation. The lack of cortical edges surrounding the developing bone demonstrates that the bone is still immature and soft.

Arthroscopy

She failed to progress in physical therapy, including aggressive stretching and dynamic bracing at home, and continued to have pain and a progressive loss of motion.

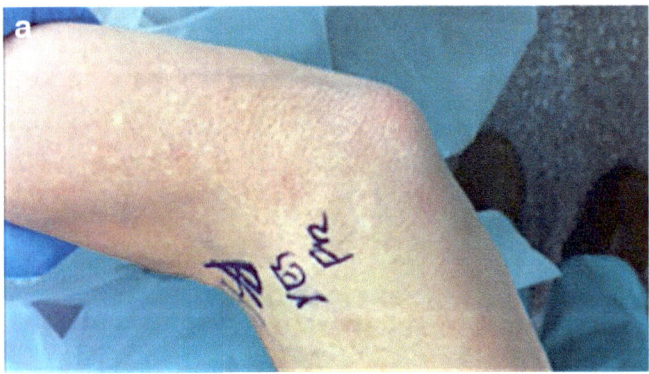
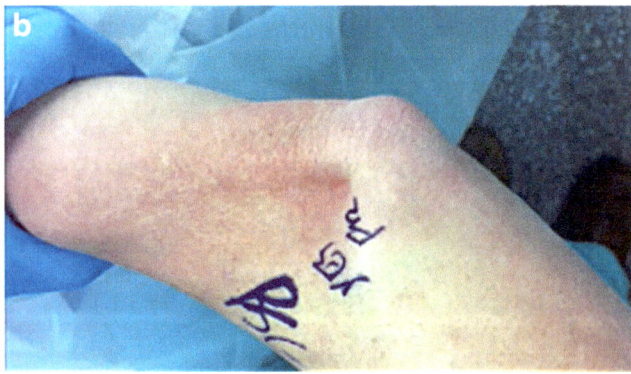

Fig. 26.13 (**a**, **b**) Photographs of the lateral pivot shift test in a left elbow. In **a**, the elbow is reduced. With axial load, valgus force, and supination, the radial head subluxates posterolaterally, and the ulnohu-meral joint begins to dislocate (**b**). The dimple appears proximal to the radial head as the radial head dislocates (**a**, **b**: Published with kind permission. Copyright © Felix H. Savoie, III, MD)

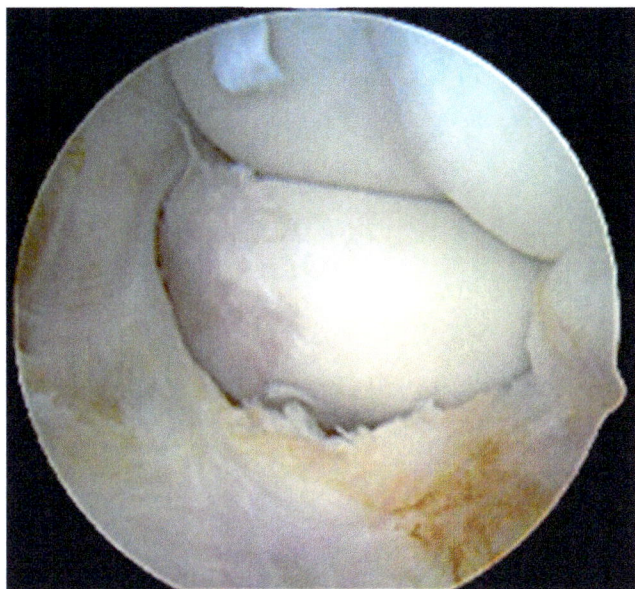

Fig. 26.14 An arthroscopic view of the anterior compartment of a left elbow, viewed from a proximal anteromedial viewing portal. Inspection of the radiocapitellar joint shows laxity in the annular ligament and chronic synovitis in the anterior compartment (Published with kind permission. Copyright © Felix H. Savoie, III, MD)

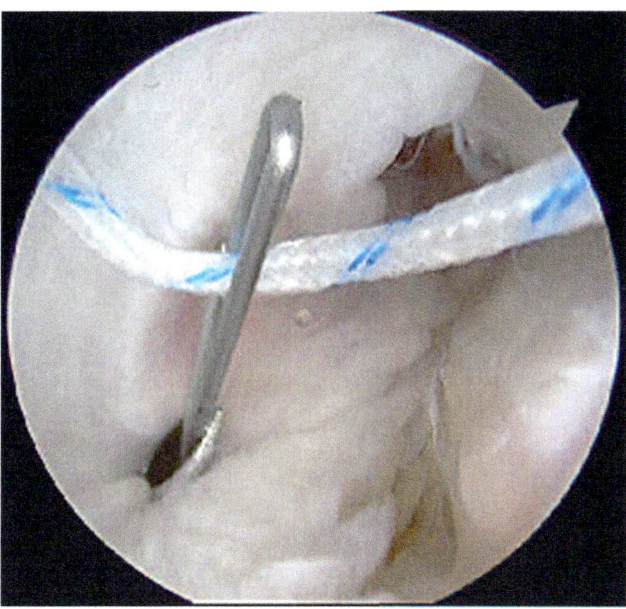

Fig. 26.16 An arthroscopic view of the posterolateral gutter in a left elbow. A suture has been placed down the lateral gutter. A percutaneous suture passer enters through a lateral soft spot portal to retrieve the suture through a healthy portion of the ligament (Published with kind permission. Copyright © Felix H. Savoie, III, MD)

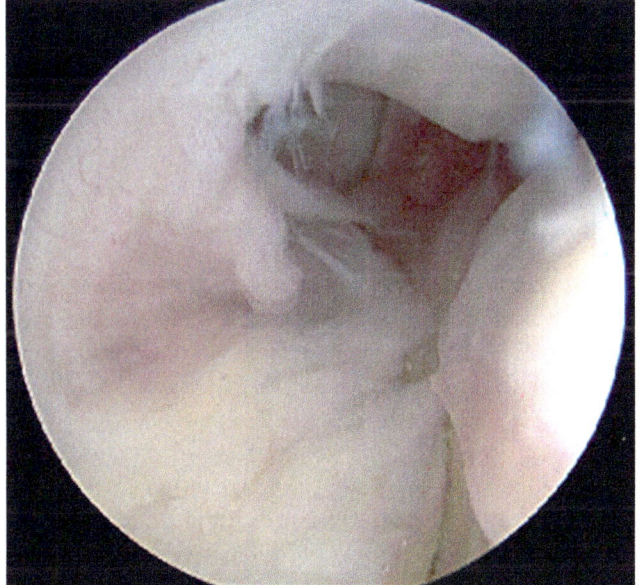

Fig. 26.15 An arthroscopic view of the posterolateral gutter in a left elbow with the arthroscope in a posterior trans-tendon portal. The avulsed RUHL is on the *left* of the image, sitting in the radiocapitellar joint. The posterior radiocapitellar joint is at the *top* of the image. The *yellowish* appearance of the ligament confirms the chronic nature of the injury (Published with kind permission. Copyright © Felix H. Savoie, III, MD)

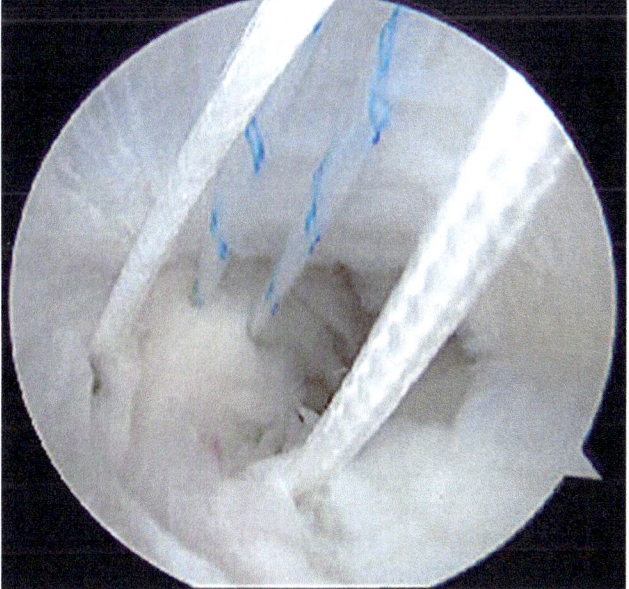

Fig. 26.17 An arthroscopic view of the posterolateral gutter in a left elbow. Two mattress sutures have been placed in the healthy portion of the RUHL (Published with kind permission. Copyright © Felix H. Savoie, III, MD)

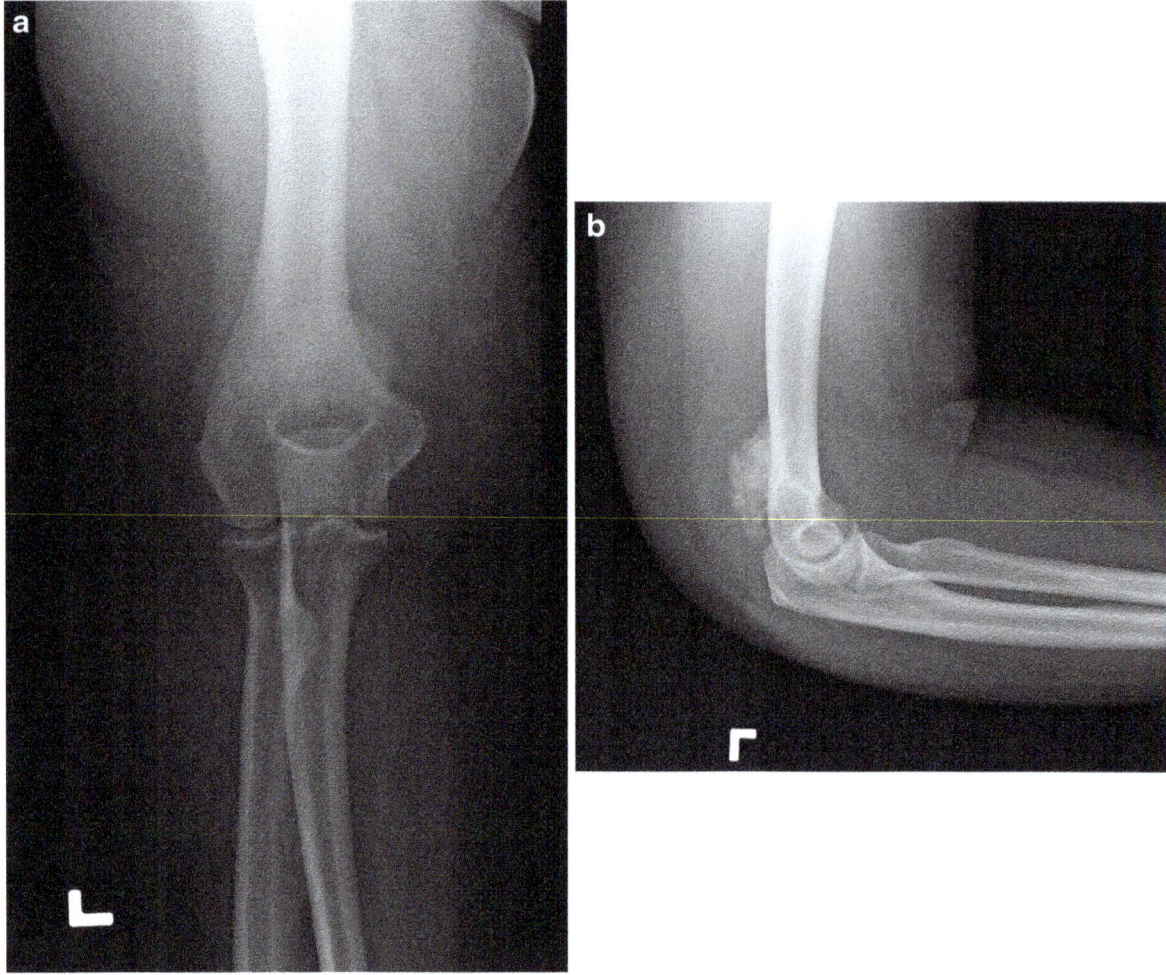

Fig. 26.18 (**a**, **b**) AP and lateral radiographs of the left elbow demonstrating the development of heterotopic ossification in the posterior aspect of the elbow. The lack of cortical edges to the bone shows that this is an immature bone (**a**, **b**: Published with kind permission. Copyright © Felix H. Savoie, III, MD)

Therefore, surgery was offered for arthroscopic debridement and resection of the HO. She was informed of risks and benefits of surgery, particularly neurovascular injury and recurrence of the HO, and informed consent was obtained.

Arthroscopic elbow surgery was performed in the prone position with the use of a pneumatic tourniquet and the operative arm positioned on an arm board with a bolster. Standard diagnostic arthroscopy was performed. Inspection of the anterior compartment revealed scar tissue with thickening of the anterior capsule, and an anterior capsulectomy was performed.

The arthroscope was then placed in the posterior compartment through a posterior trans-tendon portal. Using the blunt trocar, the arthroscope was driven through the distal extent of the heterotopic bone and into the olecranon fossa; the hard cortical bone at the base of the fossa stops advancement of the trocar. Next, a motorized shaver was placed into the center of the olecranon fossa through a posterolateral portal, and the heterotopic bone was excised. The immature spongy

bone is very soft at this stage; it easily fragments and can be removed with the shaver (Fig. 26.21). The bone was excised until the tip of the olecranon could be viewed, and excision was continued proximally under the triceps tendon. A plane can be developed between the heterotopic bone and overlying triceps muscle. The resection was continued both medially and laterally, taking great care to protect the ulnar nerve on the medial side. The entire area of HO was excised (Fig. 26.22), using fluoroscopic images to confirm a full resection had been performed.

The patient was admitted overnight for pain control. A continuous passive motion (CPM) was initiated immediately postoperative. She received a single dose of radiation therapy to the elbow on postoperative day 1, prior to discharge, for the prevention of HO recurrence. She began aggressive physical therapy on postoperative day 2. Radiographs obtained 2 months postoperative (Fig. 26.23a, b) show that the HO did not recur.

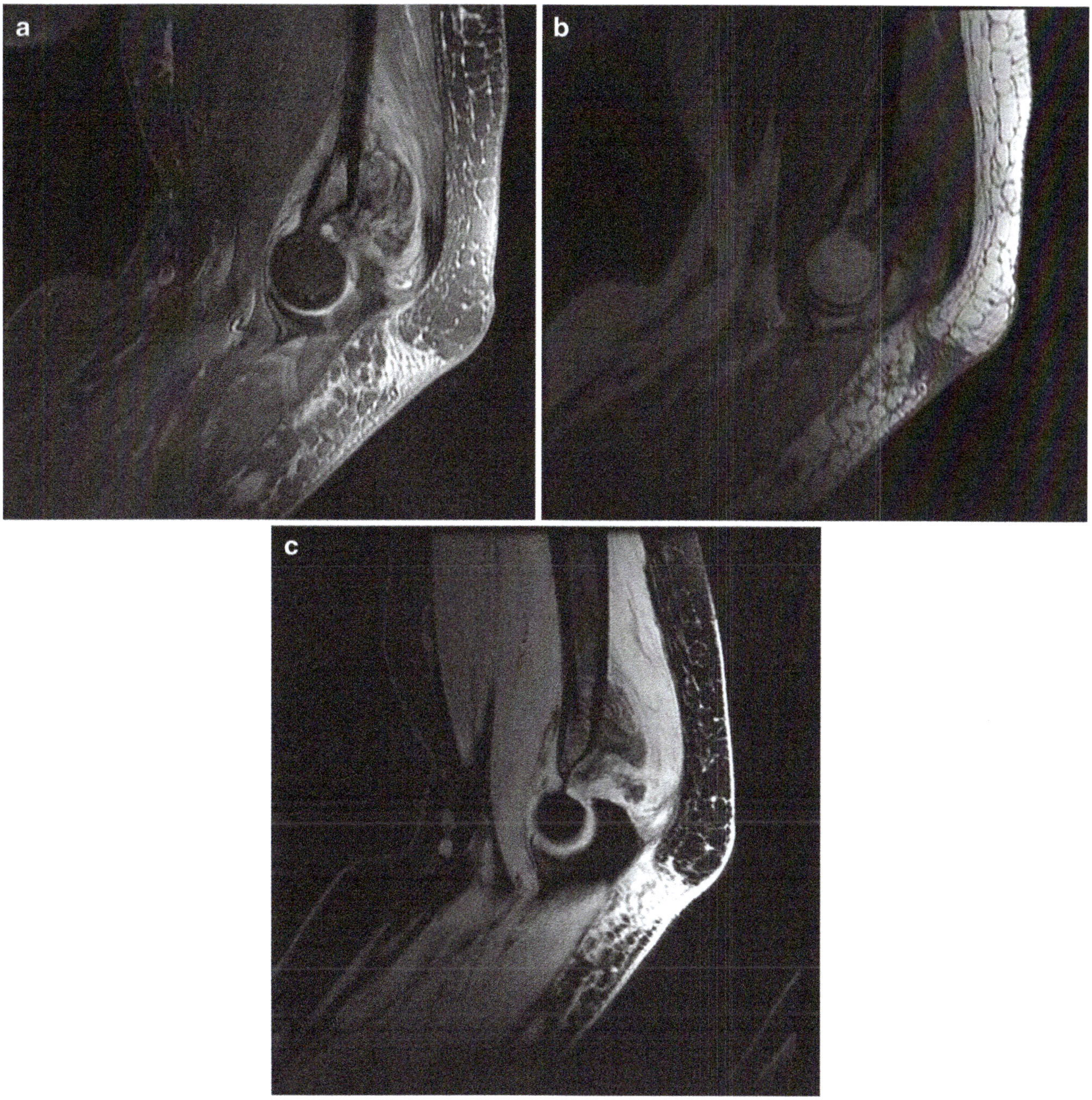

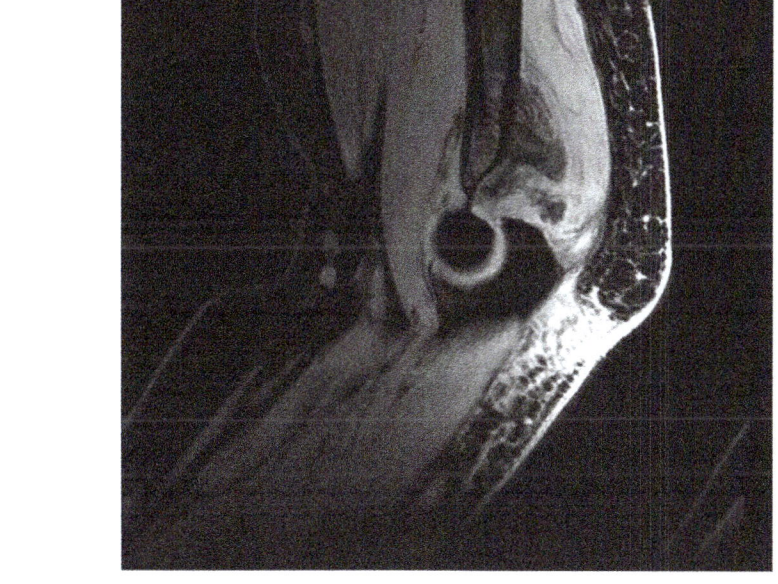

Fig. 26.19 (**a–c**) Sagittal T1, T2, and T2-fat-saturated MRI images showing the formation of HO in the posterior aspect of the elbow. The HO is deep to the triceps tendon, filling the olecranon fossa. This is an active process, with the development of spongy immature bone, as evidenced by edema in the bone and surrounding musculature (**a–c**: Published with kind permission. Copyright © Felix H. Savoie, III, MD)

Triceps Repair

Introduction

Distal triceps rupture is a rare injury, among the least frequent of tendon injuries. It is most commonly associated with anabolic steroid use, weight lifting, and traumatic laceration [18].

An eccentric load applied to a contracting triceps is the most common mechanism of injury. Ruptures can also occur spontaneously or after surgical release and reattachment [19]. Injuries to the triceps include partial and complete avulsions from the bone, intrasubstance tears, and muscle tendon junction tears. The mean age of occurrence is the fourth decade of life; however, the spectrum is wide as people continue to be more active later in life [20, 21].

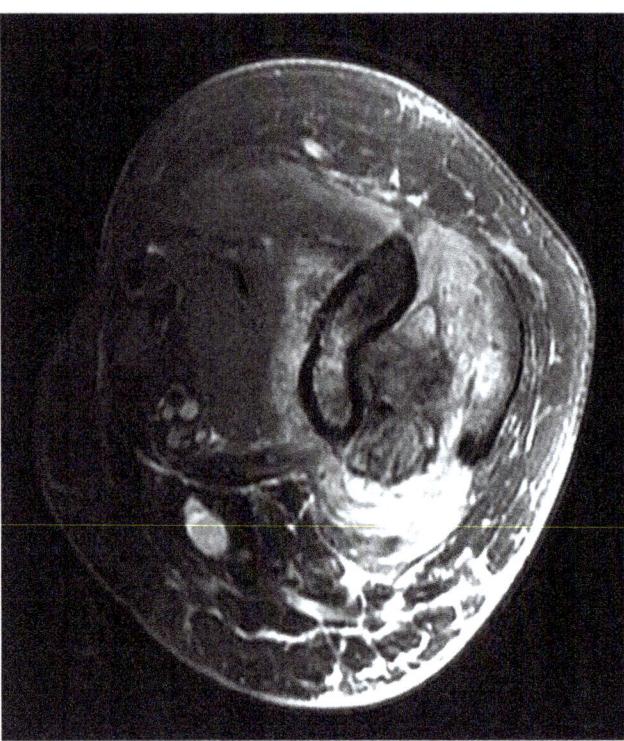

Fig. 26.20 Axial MRI image showing heterotopic bone in the posterior compartment. The HO is deep to the triceps, filling the olecranon fossa, with edema in the bone and surrounding musculature (Published with kind permission. Copyright © Felix H. Savoie, III, MD)

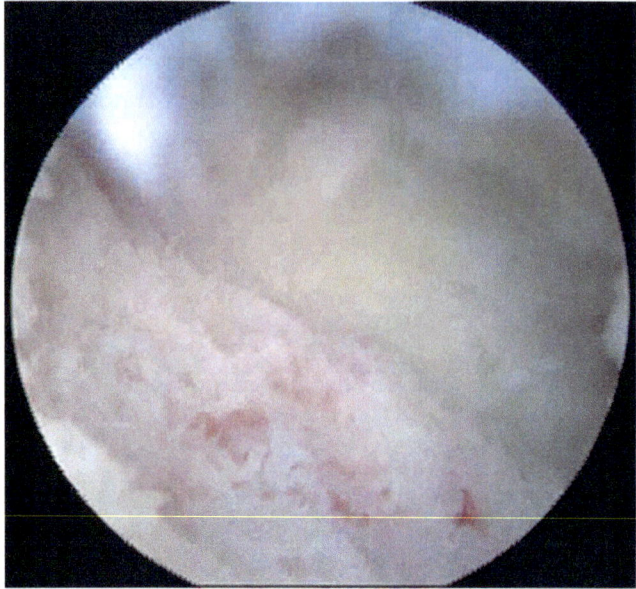

Fig. 26.22 Arthroscopic image after resection of the heterotopic bone in the posterior compartment of the elbow. The arthroscope is in a posterior trans-tendon portal. The HO has been resected, with cortical bone of the humerus at the *top* of the image (Published with kind permission. Copyright © Felix H. Savoie, III, MD)

The history will usually describe a fall onto an outstretched arm or injury during weight lifting. Physical examination may reveal a palpable defect at the insertion of the triceps. Also, a "Thompson squeeze test" of the elbow has been described where compression of the triceps fails to create extension of a flexed elbow [20]. Partial tears may not demonstrate such a defect or positive compression test and may only be suspected when a patient has weakness in elbow extension. One of the key exam findings is a + triceps stress test. In this examination, the elbow is fully flexed, and the patient is asked to extend against resistance while the examiner palpates the distal triceps tendon. A positive test occurs when there is pain and/or a palpable defect with this maneuver. All exam findings should be compared to the contralateral side.

Imaging can be helpful in the diagnosis of distal triceps rupture. Simple radiographs may demonstrate a fleck of bone from the olecranon. MRI and ultrasound are also useful. The sagittal MRI is useful to identify the extent and location of the tear. It is important to describe the tear based on the degree of the tear (complete or partial) and/or location of the tear (muscle belly, musculotendinous junction, tendonous insertion, or avulsion). It is also important to note the integrity of the lateral expansion (intact versus torn) [18]. An intact lateral expansion in conjunction with the anconeus may be able to compensate for an otherwise torn triceps tendon.

In general, partial tears less than 50% can be treated nonoperatively with satisfactory results [22]. Partial tears greater

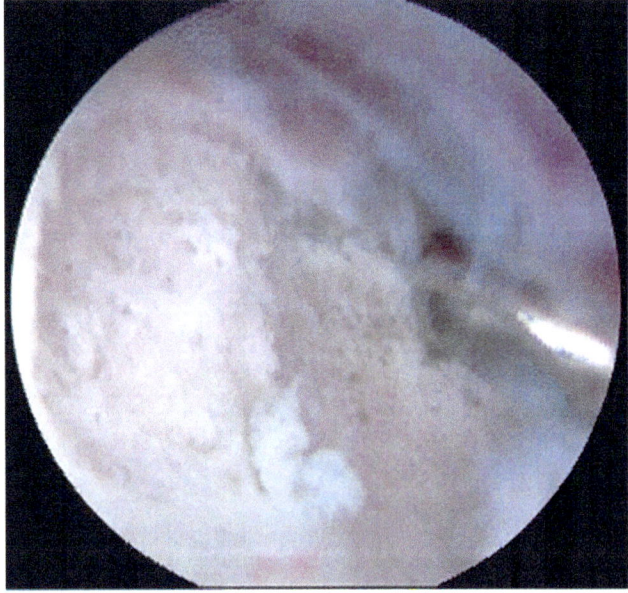

Fig. 26.21 Arthroscopic image of heterotopic bone in the posterior compartment of a left elbow. The arthroscope is viewing from a posterior trans-tendon portal. The HO fills the olecranon fossa with the triceps muscle on the *upper right* of the image. The bone is very soft and spongy. It easily fragments and can be removed with a motorized shaver (Published with kind permission. Copyright © Felix H. Savoie, III, MD)

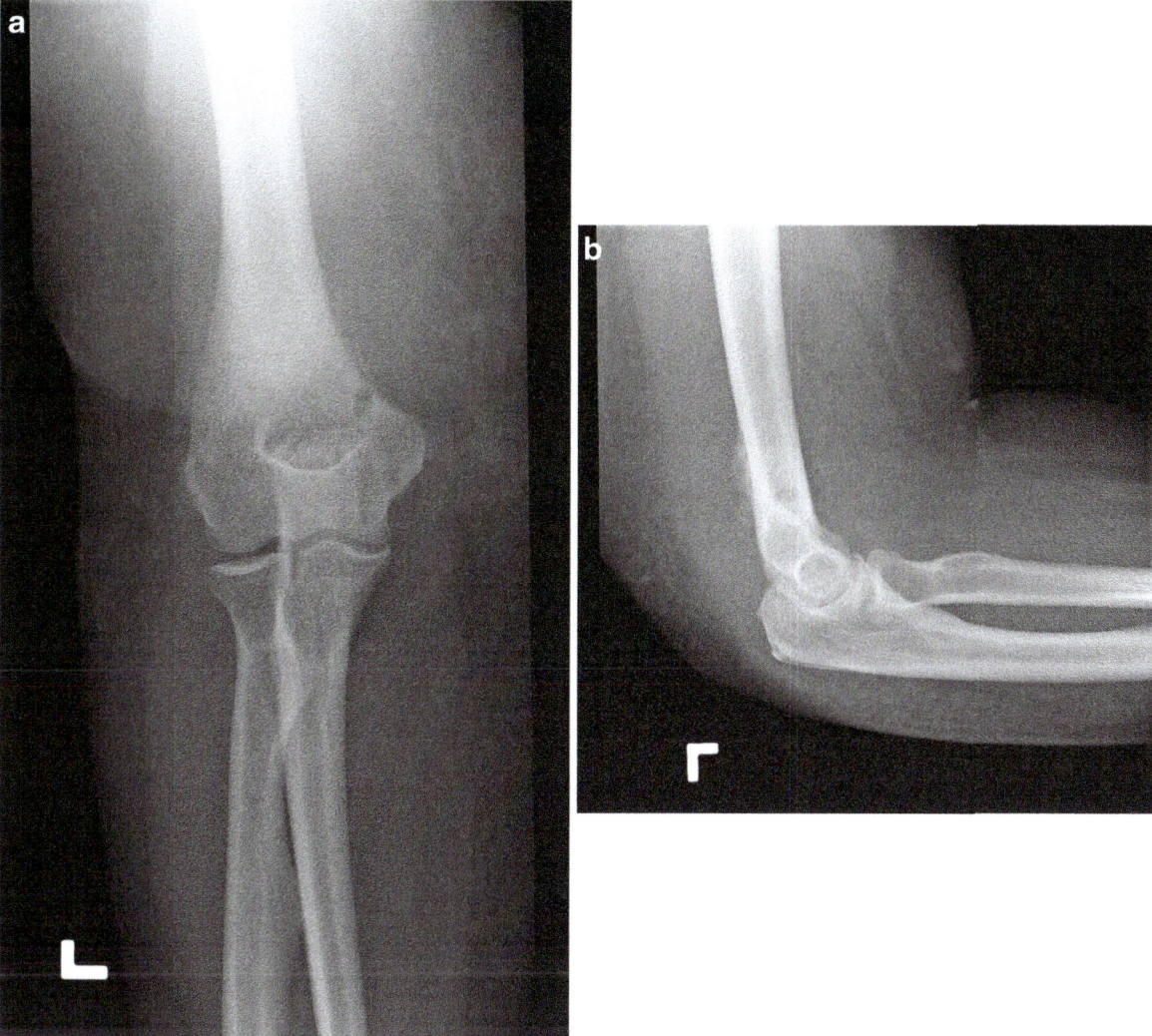

Fig. 26.23 (**a, b**) Postoperative AP and lateral radiograph 2 months postoperative. The HO in the posterior compartment has not recurred (Published with kind permission. Copyright © Felix H. Savoie, III, MD)

than 50% can be treated non-operatively in sedentary individuals but may require surgery in highly active individuals [23, 24]. Complete tears are treated surgically [25].

Case 1: Distal Triceps Tear

History/Exam

A 70-year-old male who is a very active physical therapist and weightlifter presented to the clinic complaining of left elbow pain and weakness. He has a history of chronic olecranon bursitis undergoing multiple corticosteroid injections in the past. He reported a specific event where he felt a "pop" during weight lifting that prompted him to come to the clinic.

Physical examination revealed a large effusion over the olecranon. He had no erythema, full passive range of motion of the elbow, and a positive triceps stress test. Motor strength testing revealed 1/5 motor strength in elbow extension.

Imaging

Imaging, including X-ray and MRI, was performed. Figure 26.24a–c (a plain lateral radiograph and corresponding arthroscopic images) shows a fleck of bone off the tip of the olecranon and what appears to be chronic calcification of the tendon. MRI demonstrated a complete avulsion of the central portion of the tendon with intact medial and lateral bands (Figs. 26.24a–c, 26.25, 26.26, 26.27, 26.28, 26.29, 26.30, and 26.31).

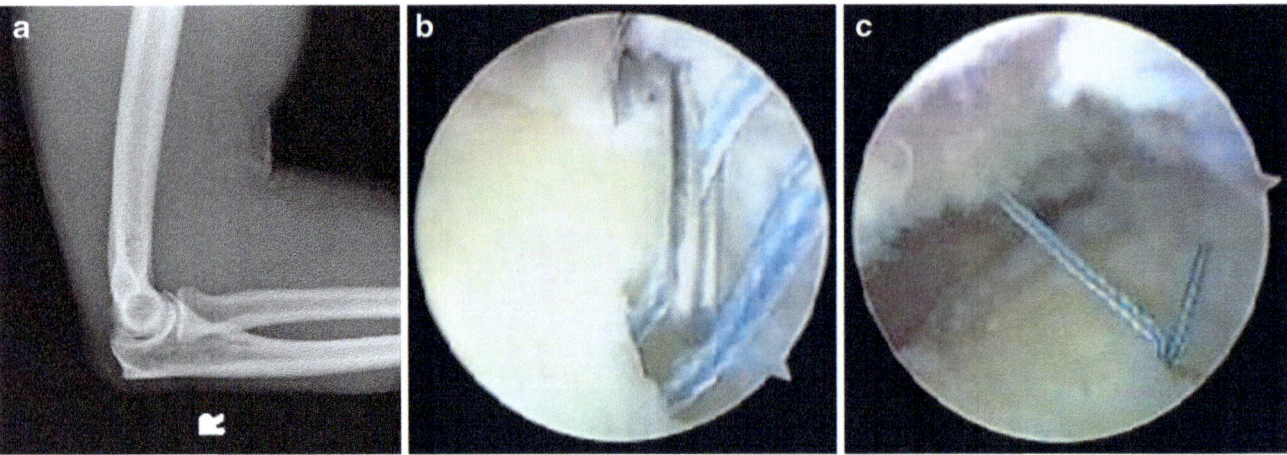

Fig. 26.24 (**a–c**) Lateral radiograph and corresponding arthroscopic images demonstrating mild soft tissue swelling over the olecranon and small calcific densities near the insertion of the triceps tendon (**a–c**: Published with kind permission. Copyright © Felix H. Savoie, III, MD)

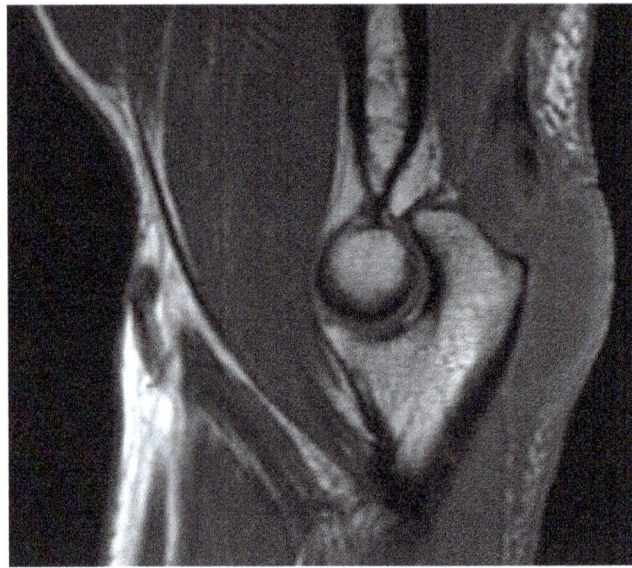

Fig. 26.25 T1-weighted sagittal view of a complete distal triceps tear (Published with kind permission. Copyright © Felix H. Savoie, III, MD)

The patient failed conservative treatments including injections and therapy and was unable to return to his previous activity level. Despite his older age, he was still very active and demonstrated functional limitations. Therefore, arthroscopic surgery to repair the torn triceps tendon was offered. After a lengthy discussion of treatment options and the risks and benefits of surgery, the patient consented to have the procedure performed.

Arthroscopy

The patient was placed in the prone position, and standard diagnostic arthroscopy of the anterior compartment revealed synovitis but no other pathology. The arthroscope was placed

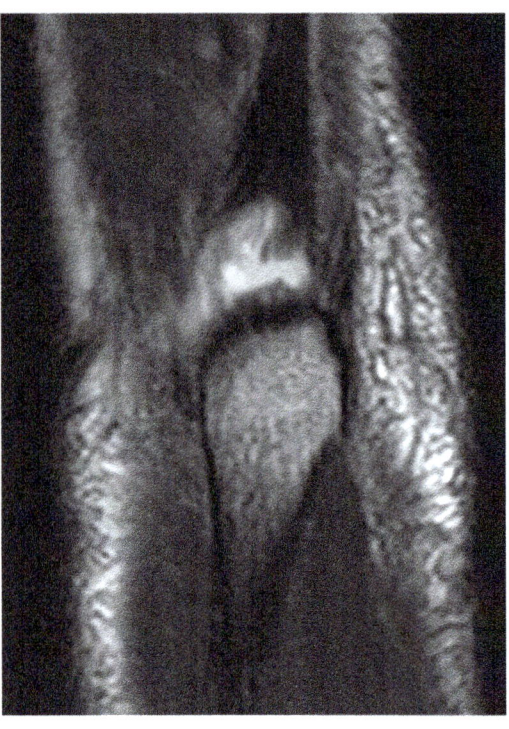

Fig. 26.26 Coronal T2-weighted MRI demonstrating complete distal triceps tear (Published with kind permission. Copyright © Felix H. Savoie, III, MD)

in the posterior compartment through a posterior trans-tendon portal, with motorized shaver placed through a posterolateral portal. The central portion of the triceps tendon was visualized avulsed from the tip of the olecranon. The triceps tendon was lightly debrided as well as the bone of the olecranon. A double-row triceps repair was performed, with the initial anchor placed into the tip of the olecranon. The sutures were retrieved through the triceps proximal to the tear and tied

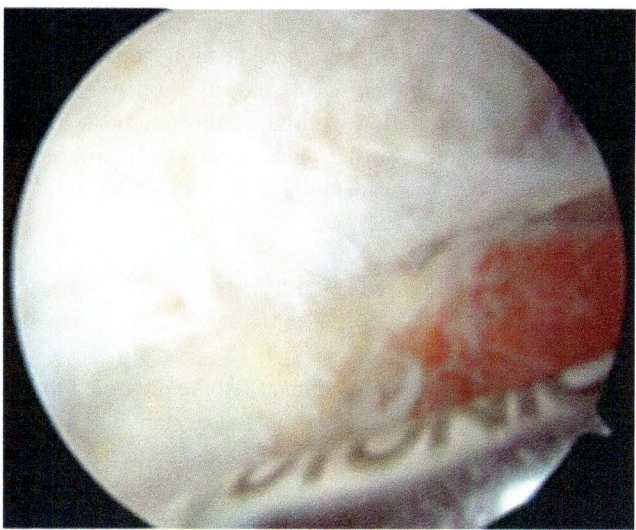

Fig. 26.27 View from the posterior portal showing the tip of the olecranon without the normal triceps attachment (Published with kind permission. Copyright © Felix H. Savoie, III, MD)

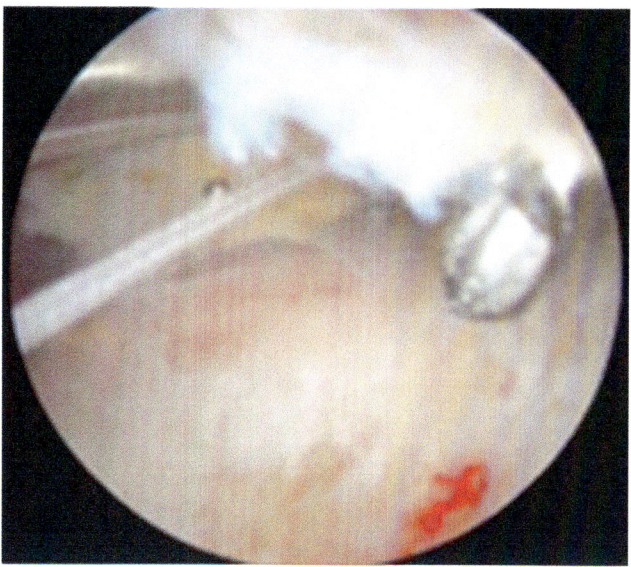

Fig. 26.29 In this view from the posterolateral portal, one suture is being retrieved proximal to the tear (Published with kind permission. Copyright © Felix H. Savoie, III, MD)

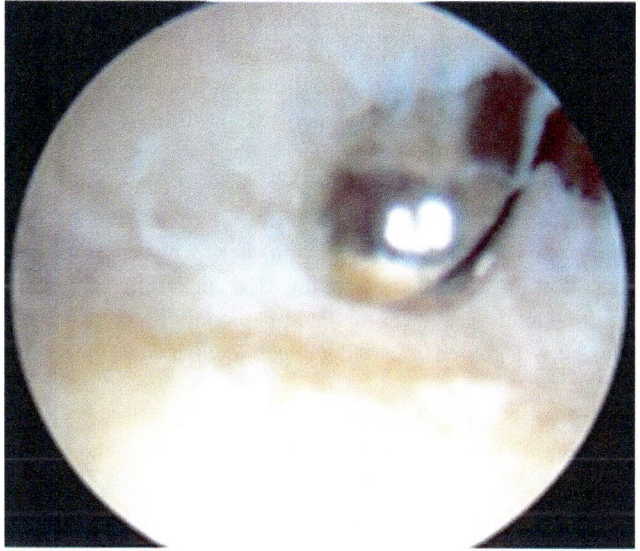

Fig. 26.28 In this view from the proximal posterolateral portal, the shaver is seen entering the elbow through the tear in the triceps. The olecranon is at the *bottom* of the picture (Published with kind permission. Copyright © Felix H. Savoie, III, MD)

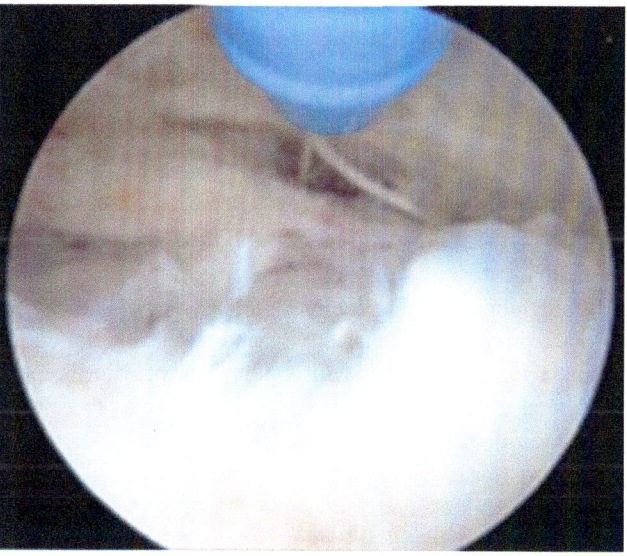

Fig. 26.30 In this view from the distal olecranon bursa portal, the tip of the olecranon is covered by proximal row repair, and the proximal sutures are seen entering the cannula (Published with kind permission. Copyright © Felix H. Savoie, III, MD)

down in mattress fashion, repairing the tear to the proximal olecranon. The arthroscope was then placed into the olecranon bursa through a more distal central portal. The bursa was excised with the shaver. The limbs of the sutures were placed into a smaller knotless anchor, and the anchor was impacted into the dorsal aspect of the olecranon to complete the double-row repair. See Figs. 26.28, 26.29, 26.30, and 26.31.

The patient was placed in an elbow brace in full extension. At 1 week, the brace was set to allow 0–30 degrees of motion.

Ten degrees was added to the flexion each week until 90° of pain-free motion was achieved at 7 weeks postoperative. The brace was discontinued and strengthening/exercise initiated. Ten weeks postoperatively, the patient achieved a full range of motion with 80% strength recovery and had resumed both work and working out. Biodex test at 6 months showed no side-to-side strength difference.

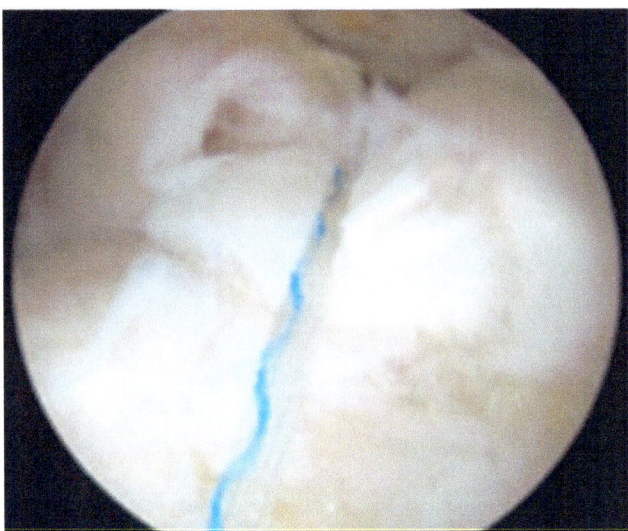

Fig. 26.31 Final view of the second part of the repair from the distal olecranon bursa portal showing the suture bridge in the center of the tendon (Published with kind permission. Copyright © Felix H. Savoie, III, MD)

Posterolateral Plica Excision

Introduction

Posterolateral plica syndrome of the elbow is a relatively rare cause of persistent pain in the posterior and lateral aspects of the elbow. The plica is a normal synovial fold found in most elbows, but it may become inflamed and painful in certain cases. The hypertrophic synovial plica can be associated with localized synovitis and radiocapitellar chondromalacia [26]. Patients will complain of pain in the posterolateral aspect of the elbow, usually worse as the elbow goes into full extension and supination, and may experience symptoms of snapping. It is common in baseball players, gymnasts, golfers, and tennis players [27], where elbow extension, axial load, and valgus force may compress the plica and lead to synovial irritation. It has also been described as a possible pain source in the setting of recalcitrant lateral epicondylitis [28].

Physical exam may demonstrate fullness in the posterolateral gutter. Range of motion is usually full, but loss of terminal extension can occur with a 10° flexion contracture. The plica is usually palpable and tender in the posterior radiocapitellar joint. Pain with forced terminal extension is common. The lateral compression test is performed with forced terminal extension and supination, which pinches the inflamed plica between the radial head and capitellum and recreates the pain. The flexion-pronation test reproduces a snapping sensation by passively flexing a pronated arm in the range of 90–110° of flexion [26].

Conservative treatment is usually successful, beginning with rest, oral anti-inflammatory medication, activity modification, and a possible corticosteroid injection. When conservative treatment fails to provide relief, surgery for an arthroscopic resection of the plica is an option, with complete relief of symptoms in 71–92% of cases [26, 27].

Case 1: Posterolateral Plica Syndrome

History/Exam

A 41-year-old, right-hand-dominant female presented to the orthopedic clinic with a chief complaint of right elbow pain. She was an avid golfer and referred for evaluation of lateral epicondylitis. She complained of posterolateral pain in the right elbow. It initially bothered her while swinging a golf club, and she described a sharp pain with snapping on the outside of the elbow during follow-through of her golf swing. The pain became more consistent and now bothered her during activities of daily living and occasionally at night. It was exacerbated by reaching to the side and lifting objects with the forearm supinated. She was diagnosed with lateral epicondylitis and treated with three cortisone injections into the lateral epicondylar region with limited relief.

Physical examination revealed a slight fullness in the posterolateral gutter of the right elbow. She had tenderness over a palpable synovial fold in the posterior radiocapitellar joint which recreated her pain. She had full active range of motion, pain with forced elbow extension, and a positive flexion-pronation test. She had no ligamentous instability on exam, minimal tenderness over the lateral epicondyle, no pain with resisted wrist extension, and a negative Cozen's test.

Imaging

Radiographs were obtained with four views of the elbow including AP, lateral, and oblique projections. Radiographs were normal with a concentric ulnohumeral joint and no fractures or subluxations. She presented with an MRI of the right elbow without contrast. A complete sequence of images was obtained, including axial T1 and fat-saturated T2 sequences, oblique coronal fat-saturated T1 and T2 sequences, and oblique sagittal T1 and fat-saturated T2 sequences. A fat-saturated sagittal T2-weighted image is demonstrated in Fig. 26.32.

MRI revealed an inflamed posterolateral plica that extended into the posterior radiocapitellar joint with increased signal on T2-weighted images (Fig. 26.32). There was no signal intensity in the common extensor origin at the lateral epicondyle, no ligament tears, and no cartilage defects in the radial head or capitellum.

The MRI findings demonstrated an inflamed posterolateral plica, which was consistent with her physical exam. At her initial visit, she was given a corticosteroid injection directly into the posterolateral plica. This eliminated her pain

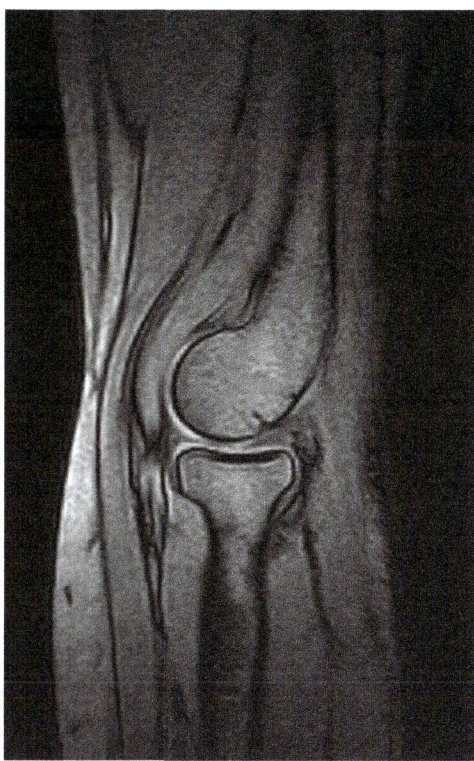

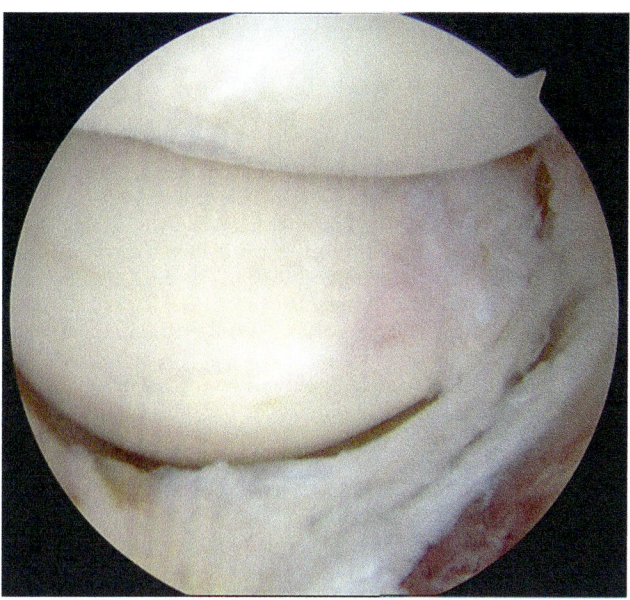

Fig. 26.33 An arthroscopic view of the posterolateral gutter in a right elbow with the arthroscope in a posterior trans-tendon portal. An enlarged posterolateral plica is visualized on the *right* of the image, projecting into the radiocapitellar joint (Published with kind permission. Copyright © Felix H. Savoie, III, MD)

Fig. 26.32 A T2-weighted sagittal oblique MRI image demonstrates an enlarged posterolateral plica in the posterior radiocapitellar joint. Increased signal in the plica signifies inflammation and swelling (Published with kind permission. Copyright © Felix H. Savoie, III, MD)

for 8 weeks. When the pain returned, she was offered an additional cortisone injection or surgery for an arthroscopic excision of the posterolateral plica. After an extensive discussion with the patient, she elected to proceed with the proposed surgical intervention.

Arthroscopy

The patient was taken to the operating room and placed in the prone position with the operative arm placed on a bump over an arm board. A pneumatic tourniquet was used for the case. A standard diagnostic arthroscopy of the anterior compartment was completed with no pathologic findings. The arthroscope was then placed into the posterior compartment through a posterior trans-tendon portal. The arthroscope was advanced down the posterolateral gutter. An inflamed plica was visualized in the posterolateral gutter (Fig. 26.33). A lateral soft portal was established with a spinal needle, and the plica was excised with a motorized shaver. After plica excision, she was noted to have a small area of chondromalacia on the posterior aspect of the radial head (Fig. 26.34). No full thickness cartilage defects were identified, and a microfracture was not performed.

The patient began therapy at 1 week postoperatively and had regained full motion by 3 weeks postoperatively.

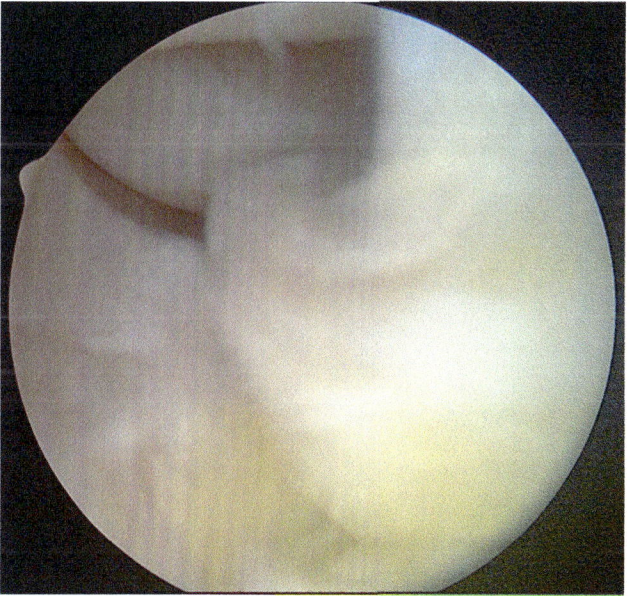

Fig. 26.34 The same view after resection of the plica. The annular ligament is intact coursing around the radial head. There is chondromalacia on the posterior aspect of the radial head (Published with kind permission. Copyright © Felix H. Savoie, III, MD)

Physical therapy was initiated, along with return to golf program. The patient resumed play at 6 weeks post-surgery with no limitations.

References

1. O'Driscoll SW, Bell DF, Morrey BF. Posterolateral rotatory instability of the elbow. J Bone Joint Surg Am. 1991;73(3):440–6.
2. Smith JP, Savoie FH, Field LD. Posterolateral rotatory instability of the elbow. Clin Sports Med. 2001;20(1):47–58.
3. Kalainov DM, Cohen MS. Posterolateral rotatory instability of the elbow in association with lateral epicondylitis. A report of three cases. J Bone Joint Surg Am. 2005;87(5):1120–5.
4. Melhoff TL, Noble PC, Bennett JB, Tullos HS. Simple dislocation of the elbow in the adult: results after closed treatment. J Bone Joint Surg. 1988;70:244–9.
5. Stoneback JW, Owens BD, Sykes J, Athwal GS, Pointer L, Wolf JM. Incidence of elbow dislocations in the United States population. J Bone Joint Surg Am. 2012;94:240–5.
6. Regan W, Lapner PC. Prospective evaluation of two diagnostic apprehension signs for posterolateral instability of the elbow. J Shoulder Elbow Surg. 2006;15(3):344–6.
7. Hardy AG, Dickson JW. Pathological ossification in traumatic paraplegia. J Bone Joint Surg Br. 1963;45:76–87.
8. Viola RW, Hastings H, 2nd. Treatment of ectopic ossification about the elbow. Clin Orthop Relat Res. 2000;(370):65–86.
9. Baird EO, Kang QK. Prophylaxis of heterotopic ossification—an updated review. J Orthop Surg Res. 2009;4:12.
10. Dodds SD, Hanel DP. Heterotopic ossification of the elbow. In: Tumble TE, Budoff JE, editors. Master skills: wrist and elbow arthroscopy and reconstruction. Rosemont, IL: American Society for Surgery of the Hand; 2006. p. 425–38.
11. Crawford CM, Barghese G, Mani MM, et al. Heterotopic ossification: are range of motion exercises contraindicated? J Burn Care Rehabil. 1986;7(4):323–4.
12. Peterson SL, Mani MM, Crawrord JR, et al. Post-burn heterotopic ossification: insights for management decision making. J Trauma. 1989;29(3):365–9.
13. Evan EB. Heterotopic bone formation in thermal burns. Clin Orthop Relat Res. 1991;263:94–101.
14. Nollen AJ. Effects of ethylhydroxydiphosphonate (EHDP) on heterotopic ossification. Acta Orthop Scand. 1986;57(4):358–61.
15. Hurvitz EA, Mandac BR, Davidoff G, et al. Risk factors for heterotopic ossification in children and adolescents with severe traumatic brain injury. Arch Phys Med Rehabil. 1992;73(5):459–62.
16. Stein DA, Patel R, Egol KA, et al. Prevention of heterotopic ossification at the elbow following trauma using radiation therapy. Bull Hosp Jt Dis. 2003;61(3–4):151–4.
17. Garland D. A clinical perspective on common forms of acquired heterotopic ossification. Clin Orthop Relat Res. 1991;263:13–29.
18. Yeh P, Dodds S, Smart L, Mazzocca A, Sethi P. Distal triceps rupture. J Am Acad Orthop Surg. 2010;18:31–40.
19. Bauman GI. Triceps tendon rupture. J Bone Joint Surg. 1934;16:966–7.
20. Viegas SF. Avulsion of the triceps tendon. Orthop Rev. 1990;19(6):533–6.
21. Clayton ML, Thirupathi RG. Rupture of the triceps tendon with olecranon bursitis: A case report with a new method of repair. Clin Orthop. 1984;184:183–5.
22. Vidal AF, Drakos MC, Allen AA. Biceps tendon and triceps tendon injuries. Clin Sports Med. 2004;23:707–22.
23. Mair SD, Isbell WM, Gill TL, Schegel TF, Hawkins RJ. Triceps tendon ruptures in professional football players. Am J Sports Med. 2004;32:431–4.
24. Straunch RJ. Biceps and triceps injuries of the elbow. Orthop Clin North Am. 1999;30:95–107.
25. Van Riet RP, Morrey BF, Ho E, O'Driscoll SW. Surgical treatment of distal triceps ruptures. J Bone Joint Surg Am. 2003;85:1961–967.
26. Antuna SA, O'Driscoll SW. Snapping plicae associated with radiocapitellar chondromalacia. Arthroscopy. 2001;17(5):491–5.
27. Kim DH, Gambardella RA, Elattrache NS, Yocum LA, Jobe FW. Arthroscopic treatment of posterolateral elbow impingement from lateral synovial plicae in throwing athletes and golfers. Am J Sports Med. 2006;34(3):438–44.
28. Ruch DS, Papadonikolakis A, Campolattaro RM. The posterolateral plica: a cause of refractory lateral elbow pain. J Shoulder Elbow Surg. 2006;15(3):367–70.

Part IV

The Hip

Section Editor: John J. Christoforetti

Diagnostic Hip Arthroscopy

27

F. Winston Gwathmey and J.W. Thomas Byrd

Introduction

The evolution of hip arthroscopy over the past quarter century is among the great advances in the treatment of hip injuries and conditions [1]. Improvements in techniques and instrumentation have helped overcome the anatomical obstacles inherent the tightly congruent femoroacetabular articulation and have established a wide array of interventions for a variety of hip pathology, both within the joint and in the adjacent extraarticular spaces [1–3]. Pathology that previously required extensive open surgery may now be effectively treated through a minimally invasive approach that spares exposure-related morbidity and accelerates recovery [4]. Hip arthroscopy has also elucidated previously misunderstood or unrecognized problems within the joint and has become the gold standard for the diagnosis of intraarticular hip pathology [3].

The ability to correlate arthroscopic findings with diagnostic imaging has greatly enhanced the overall understanding of hip anatomy and has improved the ability to diagnose pathology [5]. Magnetic resonance imaging (MRI) is the imaging modality of choice for the characterization of musculoskeletal anatomy around the hip and the diagnosis of injuries to soft tissue structures including muscle, tendons, ligaments, articular cartilage, and fibrocartilage. MR arthrography utilizes gadolinium injected into the joint to distend the joint capsule and better delineate intraarticular structures such as the labrum [6–9]. While arthrography improves the sensitivity and specificity of MR, important findings such as a joint effusion or subchondral edema may be obscured

by the high signal from the contrast [6]. Stronger magnets (1.5 and 3.0 Tesla) and surface coils have also improved the capabilities of MRI for evaluation of the hip [10].

The hip joint, however, presents diagnostic imaging challenges given its oblique orientation, spherical shape, and the anatomical variability among patients [9]. The close coaptation of the articular surfaces of the acetabulum and femoral head may obscure labral or cartilage pathology. Additionally, unlike the shoulder and knee in which decades of arthroscopic experience have allowed for systematic documentation and MR correlation of normal and variant anatomy as well as pathological entities, the comparatively shorter hip arthroscopy experience has not enabled an equivalent accumulation of information. The recent proliferation of hip arthroscopy, however, has propagated an expansion of the arthroscopic database of hip anatomy and pathology and has contributed to a concurrent evolution of hip imaging. This chapter will introduce hip arthroscopy and correlate arthroscopic anatomy with MR anatomy.

Hip Arthroscopy

Difficulty gaining operational access to the femoroacetabular articulation has historically restricted the ability to effectively apply arthroscopic techniques to the hip joint. The depth, orientation, and shape of the joint create additional instrumentation obstacles. Surgeons have developed strategies to overcome these obstacles and continue to expand the field of hip arthroscopy. Axial and lateral traction provided by a specialized operative table are used to pull the femoral head out of the acetabular socket, thus establishing a working space to diagnose and treat intraarticular pathology (Fig. 27.1). Alternating use of arthroscopes with 70 and 30° lenses is frequently necessary to adequately visualize and navigate the spaces within the hip joint. Cannulated systems permit safer and more efficient insertion of equipment, and specialized long and/or curved instruments allow intricate procedures to be carried out deep within the joint (Fig. 27.2).

F.W. Gwathmey, MD (✉)
Department of Orthopedic Surgery, University of Virginia Health System, Charlottesville, VA, USA
e-mail: Fwg7d@hscmail.mcc.virginia.edu

J.W.T. Byrd, MD
Department of Orthopedics and Rehabilitation,
Vanderbilt University School of Medicine, Nashville, TN, USA
e-mail: byrd@nsmfoundation.org

Fig. 27.1 The patient is positioned on a specialized table that can apply traction to the leg to distract the femoral head from the acetabulum to facilitate intraarticular visualization and instrumentation. The table attachment also allows manipulation of the leg so that the hip can be rotated and flexed as needed. Fluoroscopy can be brought in between the legs or from the contralateral side of the table

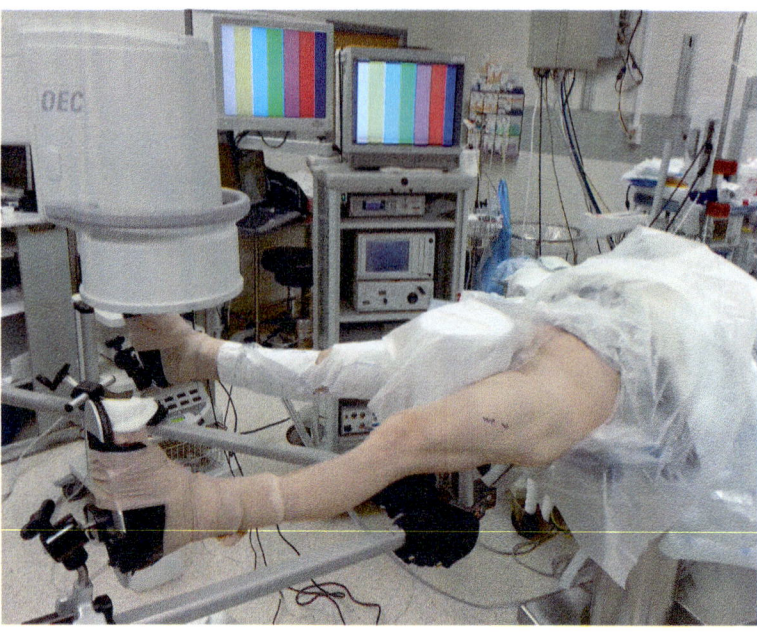

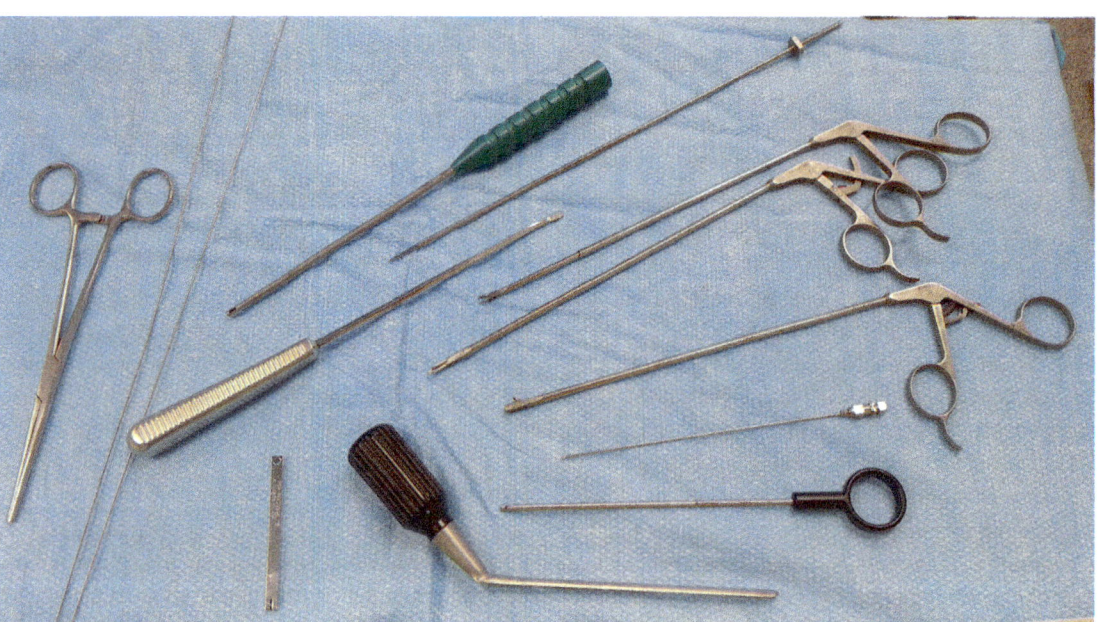

Fig. 27.2 Cannulated systems are commonly used for hip arthroscopy to safely establish portals and efficiently pass equipment into the joint. Hip arthroscopic instruments are longer than standard arthroscopic instruments to permit intricate procedures to be performed deep within the body. Some surgeons use curved instruments to navigate the spherical and concave structures within the hip joint

Two distinct arthroscopic spaces are recognized within the hip joint, the central compartment between the femoral head and acetabulum and the peripheral compartment within the hip capsule but outside the femoroacetabular articulation (Fig. 27.3). In general, traction affords access to the central compartment, while the peripheral compartment is accessed out of traction and with some degree of hip flexion to relax the anterior capsule.

Depending on the planned procedure, two to five portals are used during hip arthroscopy. The neurovascular anatomy surrounding the hip joint has been well studied and safe zones for portal placement have been described [11]. Standard portals include an anterolateral portal (just anterior to the tip of the greater trochanter), posterolateral portal (posterior to the tip of the greater trochanter), and an anterior portal (lateral and distal to the intersection of a line drawn transversely from the greater trochanter and a line drawn distally from the ASIS) [2] (Fig. 27.4). Modifications of these portals and additional portals have been introduced as techniques and instrumentation have evolved [12].

Coronal plane

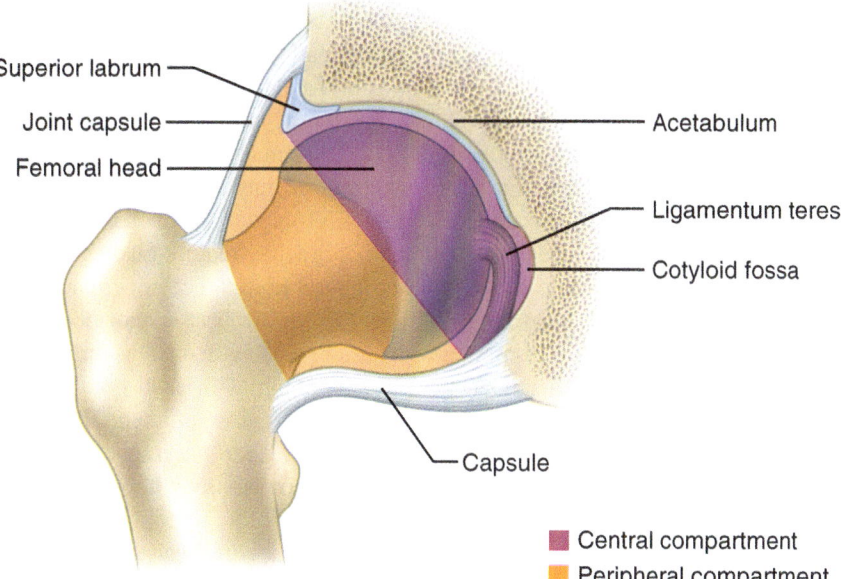

Superior labrum

Joint capsule

Femoral head

Acetabulum

Ligamentum teres

Cotyloid fossa

Capsule

■ Central compartment
■ Peripheral compartment

Fig. 27.3 During arthroscopy, two distinct compartments within the hip are recognized, the central and peripheral compartments. The central compartment comprises the space within joint encompassed by the acetabular labrum. Traction is required to pull the femoral head out of the acetabular fossa for access to the central compartment. Structures within the central compartment include the acetabular labrum, the artic-ular cartilage surfaces of the femoral head and acetabulum, the cotyloid fossa, and the ligamentum teres. The peripheral compartment is accessed out of traction and with the hip in some flexion to relax the anterior capsule. Structures within the peripheral compartment include the femoral head/neck junction, femoral neck, medial and lateral synovial folds, zona orbicularis, and hip joint capsule

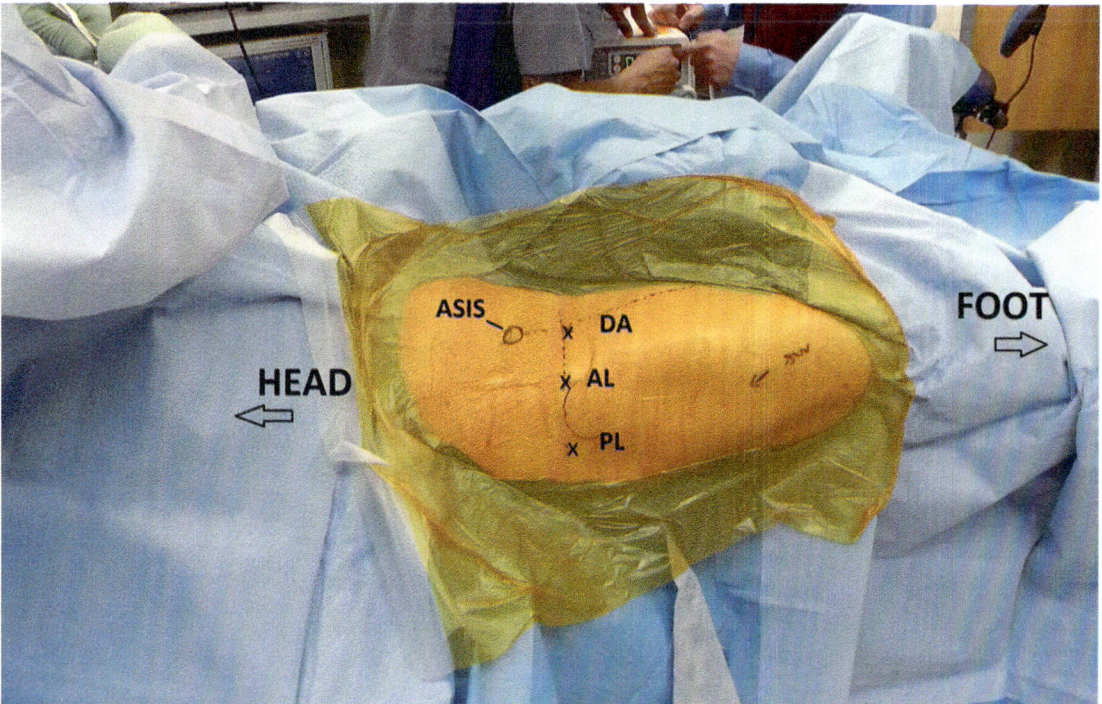

ASIS   × DA

× AL

× PL

HEAD

FOOT

Fig. 27.4 Standard portals described for hip arthroscopy include the anterolateral (AL), anterior (DA), and posterolateral (PL) portals. Modifications of these portals and additional portals are commonly used depending on the procedure. The ASIS and greater trochanter are the key surface landmarks for portal placement. The anterolateral (AL) and posterolateral (PL) portals are adjacent the anterior and posterior aspect of the greater trochanter. The direct anterior (DA) portal is positioned lateral and distal to the intersection between a line drawn distally from the ASIS and medially from the tip of the greater trochanter. Fluoroscopy may be used to verify position

Arthroscopic Anatomy

Central Compartment

Most hip arthroscopic procedures start with gaining access to the central compartment. Traction is applied to the leg to open the femoroacetabular articulation, and fluoroscopy is used to verify adequate distraction and guide the initial portal placement. The anterolateral portal is established under fluoroscopic guidance and the 70° scope is inserted into the joint. Through the anterolateral portal, a cursory initial inspection of the joint may be performed. An anterior portal for instrumentation may then be made under arthroscopic visualization.

Orientation within the joint may be confusing given the round concave configuration of the acetabulum and the spherical femoral head. A clockface applied to the acetabulum centered on the cotyloid fossa can be used for a systematic assessment of the joint and documentation of findings (Fig. 27.5). The clockface is positioned so that 6 o'clock marks the center of the transverse acetabular ligament and the apex of the cotyloid fossa is at the 12 o'clock position. On a right hip, the anterior joint is at the 3 o'clock position, while 9 o'clock references the posterior joint. On a left hip, some surgeons keep the clock facing forward and assign the 9 o'clock position to the anterior joint, while others invert the clockface to maintain consistency. An alternative geographic zone method has also been described [13].

Once the viewing and instrumentation portals have been established, the joint is inspected for pathology. With the arthroscope in the anterolateral portal, the structures of the superior, anterior, and medial joint are examined. A probe inserted in the anterior portal is helpful to palpate and manipulate intraarticular structures (Fig. 27.6a–e). Most chondrolabral pathology tends to be anterior to the 12 o'clock position and this area should be emphasized in the diagnostic arthroscopy. Rotating the 70° scope in the anterolateral portal 180° brings the posterior labrum into view. A posterolateral portal may be established for access to the posterior joint. Visualization of far posterior and posteroinferior pathology may require placing the arthroscope into the posterolateral portal. The superolateral and lateral labrum and acetabulum are best visualized with the arthroscope in the anterior portal with the lens directed laterally (Fig. 27.7a–c). Use of cannulas in each portal that can accommodate the arthroscope aids efficient movement between portals. Capsulotomies of varying sizes and orientations also facilitate maneuverability within the joint.

Similar to the glenoid labrum in the shoulder, a variety of acetabular labral variants have been observed in the hip. Sublabral sulci or recesses may be present in up to 20 % of patients and can be found at all anatomic positions around the acetabular labrum [14, 15]. On MRI, several features of a sublabral sulcus help differentiate it from a tear. A linear MR appearance and lack of secondary findings including cysts, chondral damage, or edema are suggestive of a normal anatomic variant [16]. The location on the acetabulum of the finding is also important. Sublabral sulci frequently occur posteriorly or inferomedially [14, 16] (Fig. 27.8a, b). Additionally, at the junction between the labrum and the transverse acetabular ligament, contrast may appear to penetrate the labrum. While labral variants

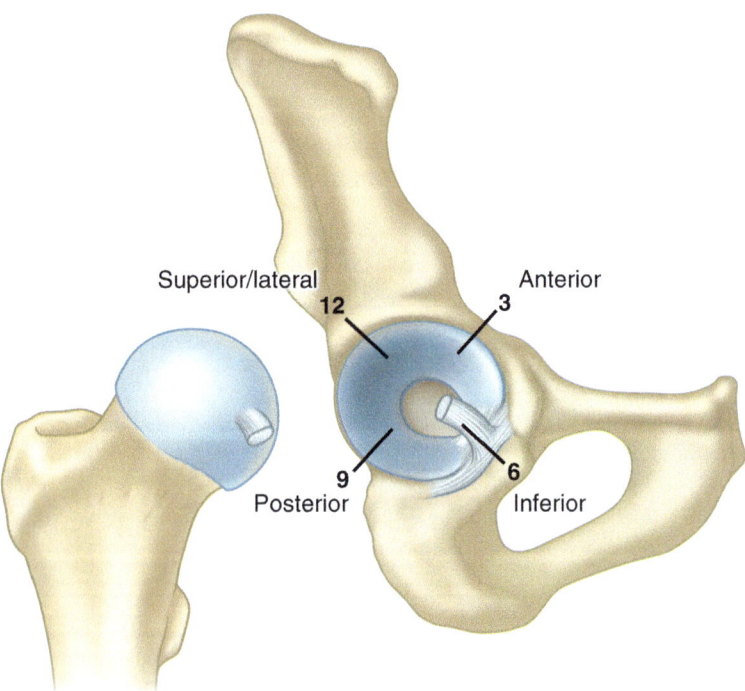

Fig. 27.5 For orientation and documentation, a clockface is often applied to the acetabular fossa. The 6 o'clock position is set at the transverse acetabular ligament with the 12 o'clock position directly opposite at the apex of the cotyloid fossa

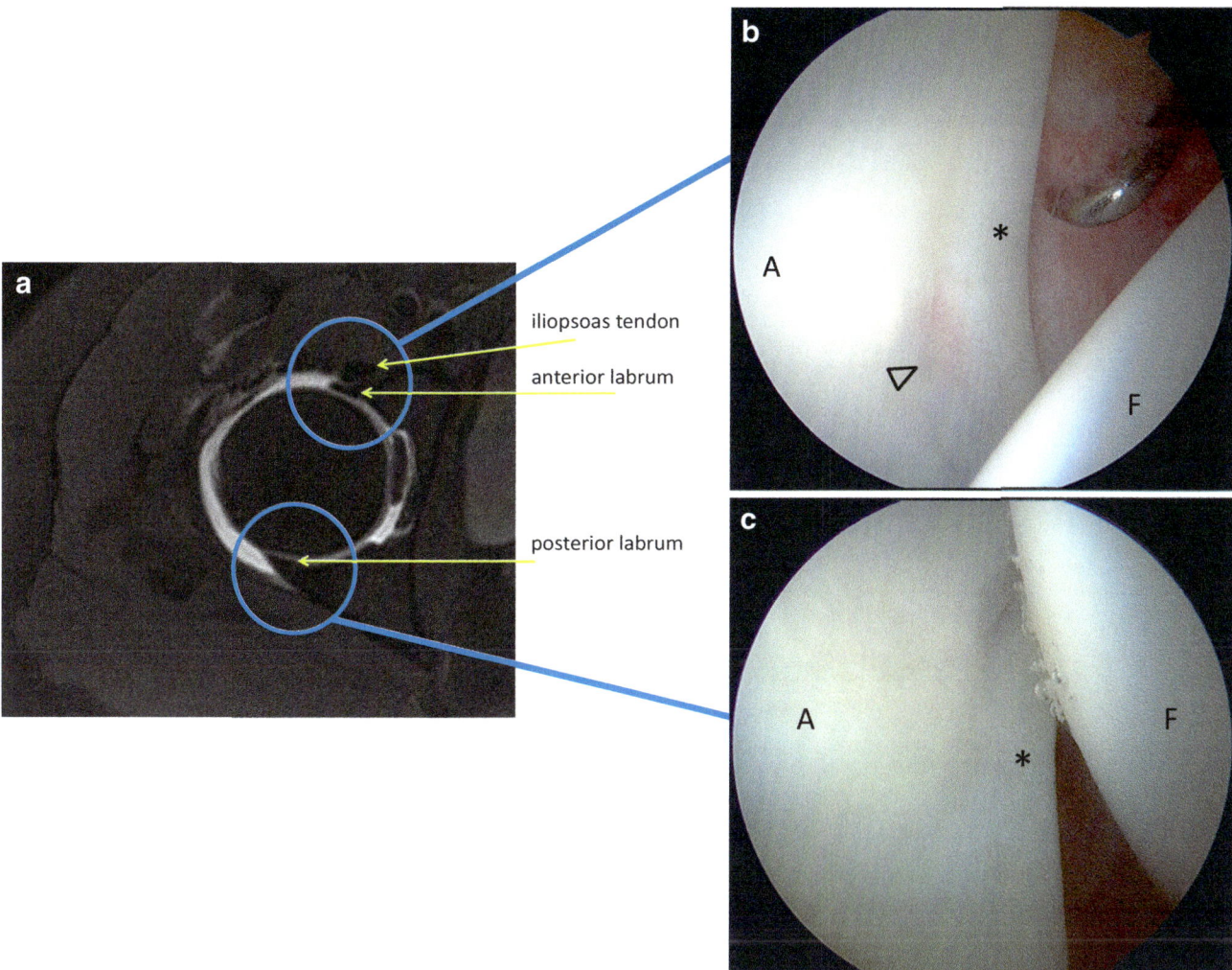

Fig. 27.6 (**a**) Axial T2 MR-arthrogram of the right hip. The outline of the anterior and posterior labrum may be seen on this sequence. The labrum conforms to the femoral head and the articular aspect blends into the articular cartilage. (**b**) Arthroscopic photograph of the anterior labrum (*asterisk*) at approximately the 3 o'clock position. The arthroscope is positioned in the anterolateral portal and the lens is directed anteriorly. The acetabulum (A) is on the *left* of the picture and the femoral head (F) on the *right*. The probe is inserted through the anterior portal and is used to examine the structure of the anterior labrum and adjacent cartilage. A normal smooth transition is evident between the labrum and articular cartilage. The recess in the acetabular rim here (*arrowhead*) corresponds to the approximate position of the iliopsoas tendon as it crosses the joint. (**c**) Arthroscopic photo of the posterior labrum (*asterisk*). The arthroscope is in the anterolateral portal and the lens is directed posteriorly. (**d**) Anatomical rendering of the anterior labrum viewed from the anterolateral portal with the 70° arthroscope. (**e**) Anatomical rendering of the posterior labrum viewed from the anterolateral portal by rotating the 70° arthroscope 180° and directing it posteriorly. Further visualization of the posteroinferior joint is afforded by moving the arthroscope to the posterolateral portal

d

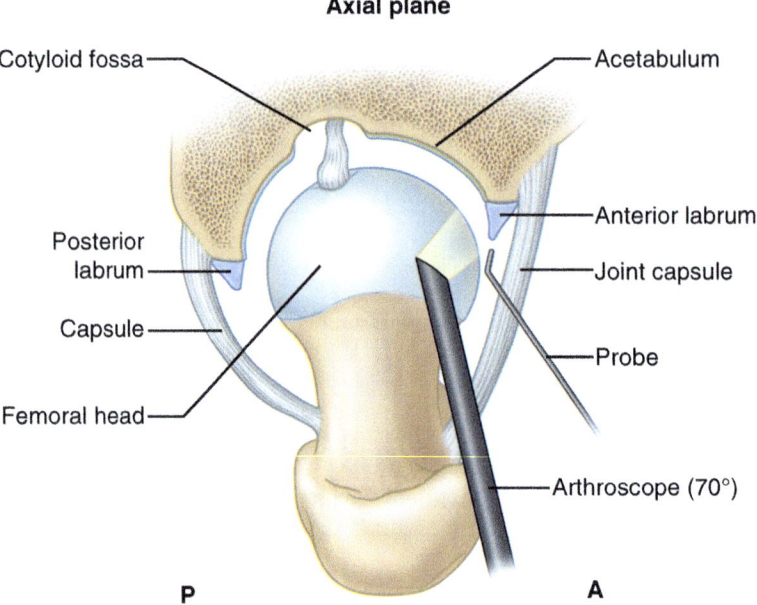

e

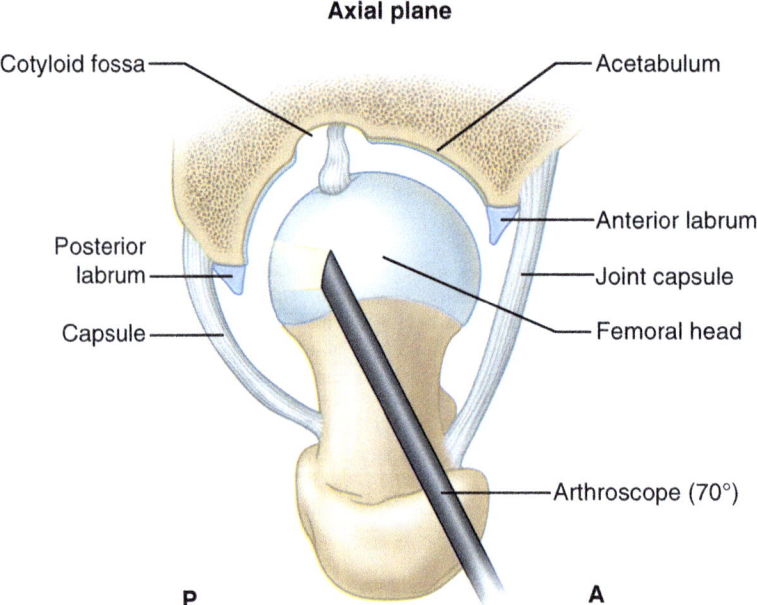

Fig. 27.6 (continued)

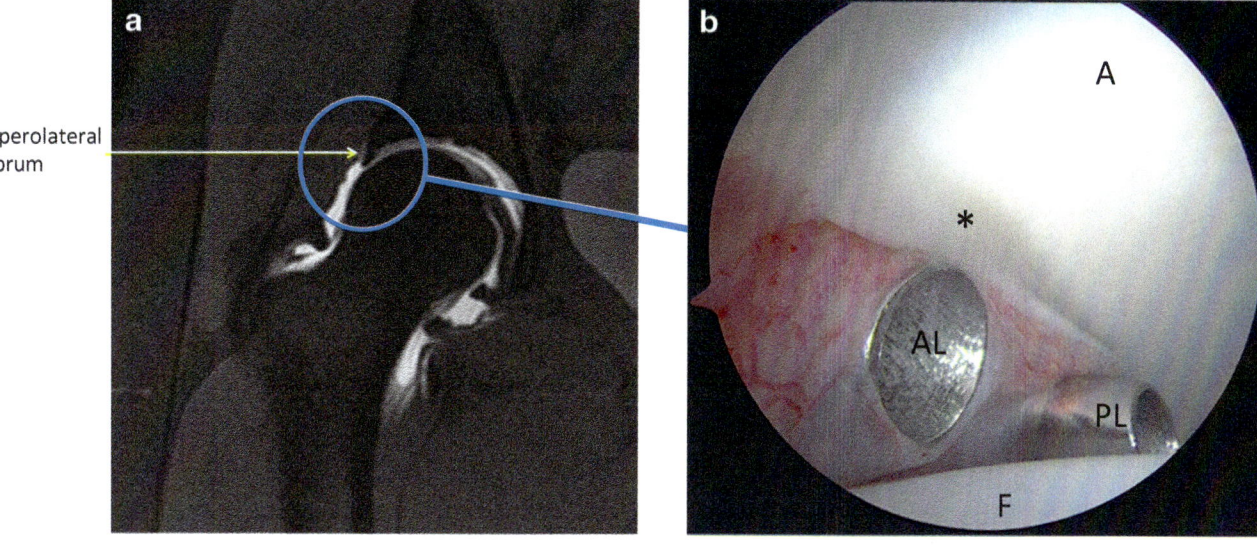

superolateral
labrum

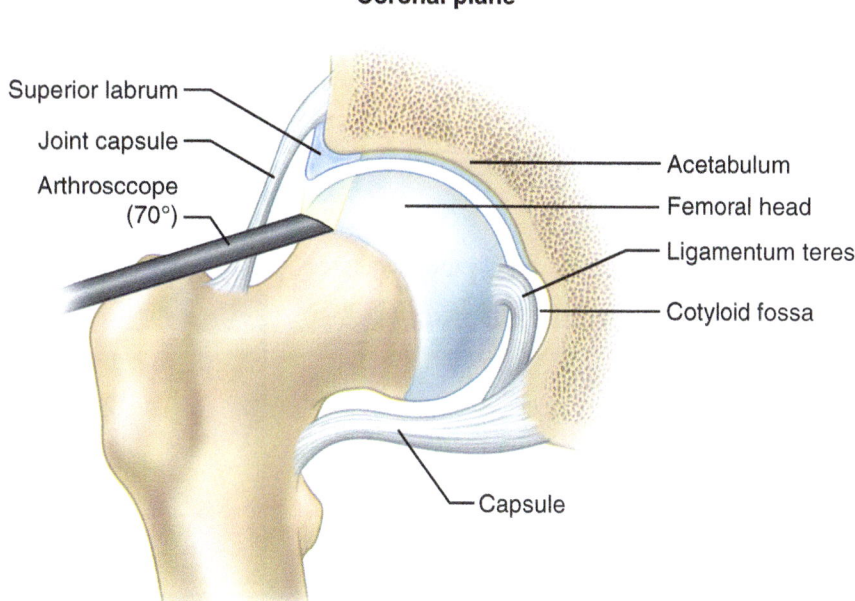

Coronal plane

Superior labrum
Joint capsule
Arthrosccope
(70°)

Acetabulum
Femoral head
Ligamentum teres
Cotyloid fossa

Capsule

Fig. 27.7 (**a**) Coronal T2 MR-arthrogram of the right hip demonstrating the superolateral labrum (*arrow*). (**b**) Arthroscopic photograph of the lateral labrum. The arthroscope is in the anterior portal and the lens is directed laterally. The acetabulum (A) is at the *top right* of the picture and the femoral head (F) is at the *bottom*. Metal cannulas are positioned in the anterolateral (AL) and posterolateral portals (PL). (**c**) Anatomical rendering showing that moving the 70° arthroscope into the anterior portal allows visualization of the superolateral labrum

may also occur anteriorly or superiorly, a higher index of suspicion for pathologic labral tear should be maintained in these locations. Underlying pincer morphology or acetabular dysplasia warrants consideration of true labral pathology [17].

The cotyloid fossa is situated at the most medial aspect of the acetabulum. This location cannot be accessed without traction and special care must be taken to avoid the femoral head as the arthroscope is moved into position. While the acetabular rim is best visualized by the 70° arthroscope, changing to a 30°

arthroscope improves visualization of the medial joint. The cotyloid fossa contains the ligamentum teres and the accompanying fat pad (Fig. 27.9a, b). The femoral head often presents a navigation obstacle and alternating among the portals may be necessary for complete inspection. Internal and external rotation of the hip may also be necessary for a thorough evaluation of the structures within the cotyloid fossa. Petechiae within the fat pad are often seen with the negative intraarticular pressure generated by the traction and should not be confused with a traumatic injury to the ligamentum teres (Fig. 27.9c).

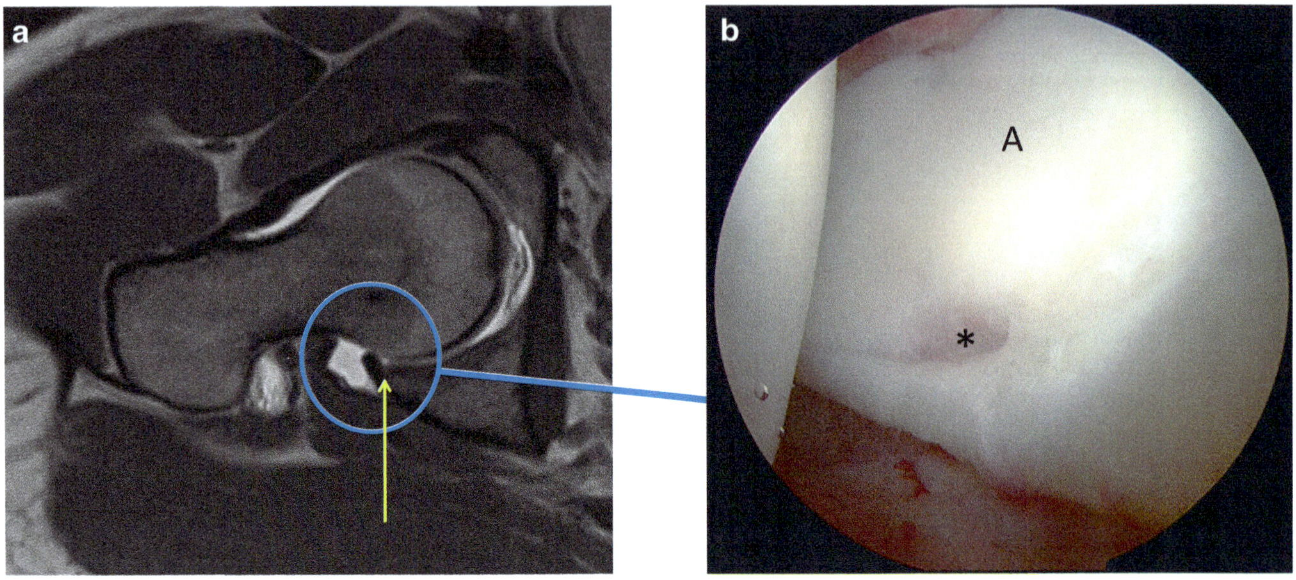

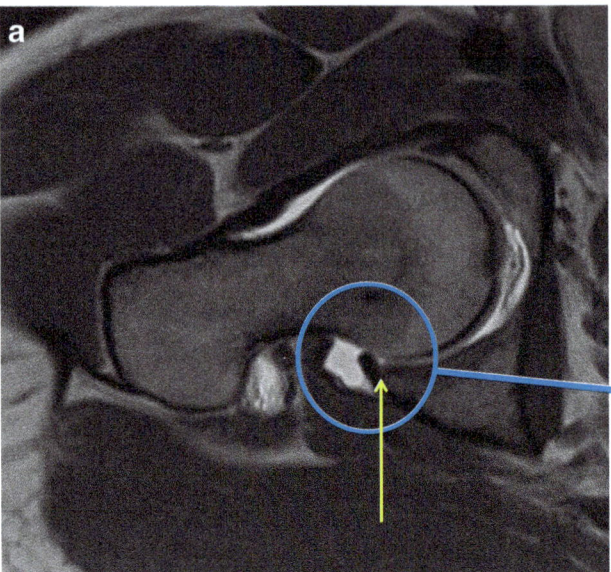

Fig. 27.8 (**a**) Coronal T1 MR-arthrogram of the right hip demonstrating a posterior labral recess (*arrow*). The contrast is visible penetrating the articular interface between the labrum and articular cartilage. The lack of signal within the substance of the labrum, the absence of secondary findings, and the posterior location suggest that this finding is not pathological. (**b**) Arthroscopic photograph of the posterior labral recess. A cleft is visible between the labrum (*asterisk*) and acetabular cartilage (A). This is a common labral variant and does not represent a tear.

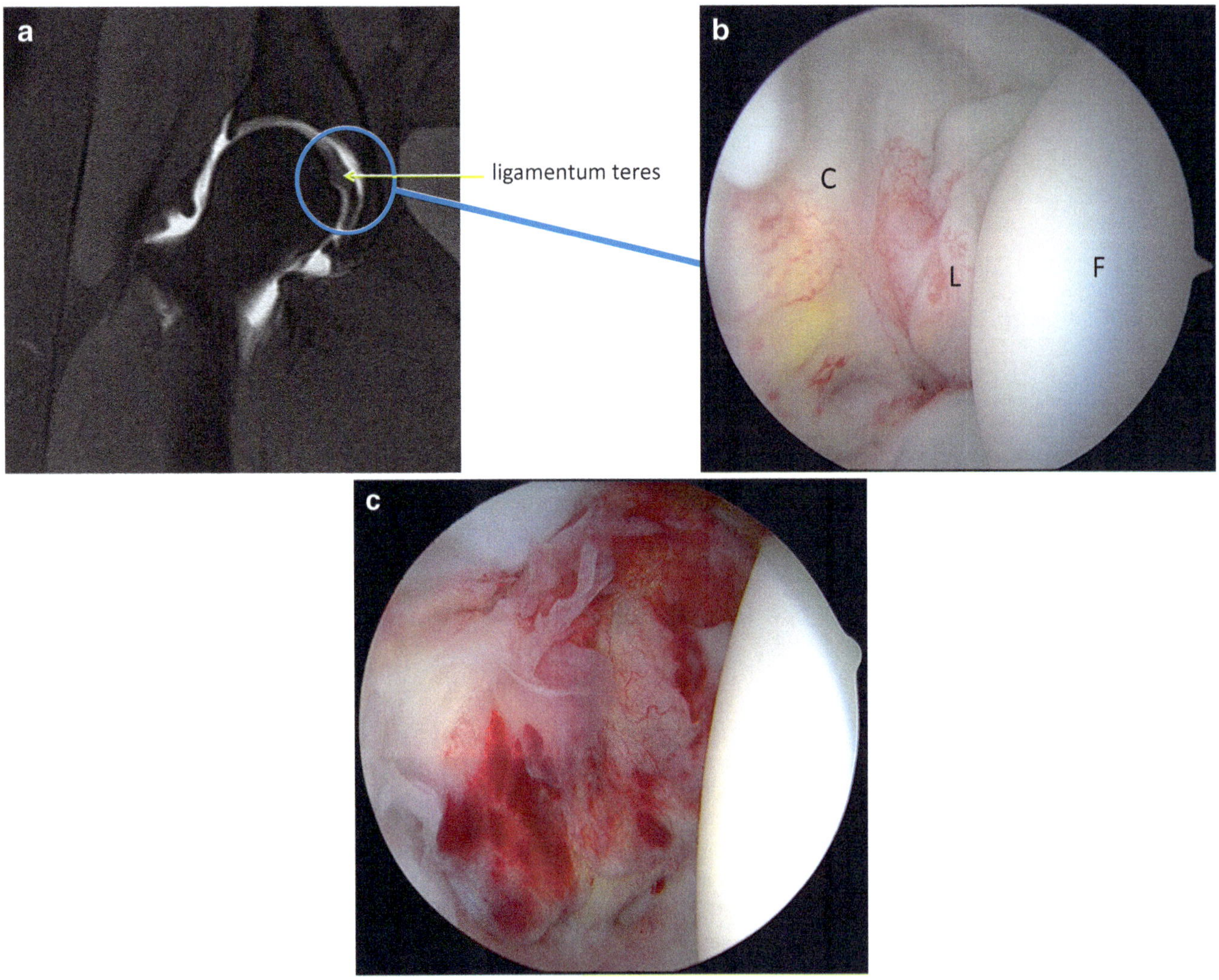

ligamentum teres

Fig. 27.9 (**a**) Coronal MR-arthrogram of the right hip demonstrating the acetabular fossa and ligamentum teres (*arrow*). (**b**) Arthroscopic photograph of the cotyloid fossa (C) and ligamentum teres (L) attaching to the femoral head (F). For adequate evaluation, an arthroscope with a 30° lens may be needed as well as visualization through multiple portals. (**c**) The negative intraarticular pressure created by applying traction to the hip may cause petechiae and localized hemorrhage within the fat pad and synovium within the fossa

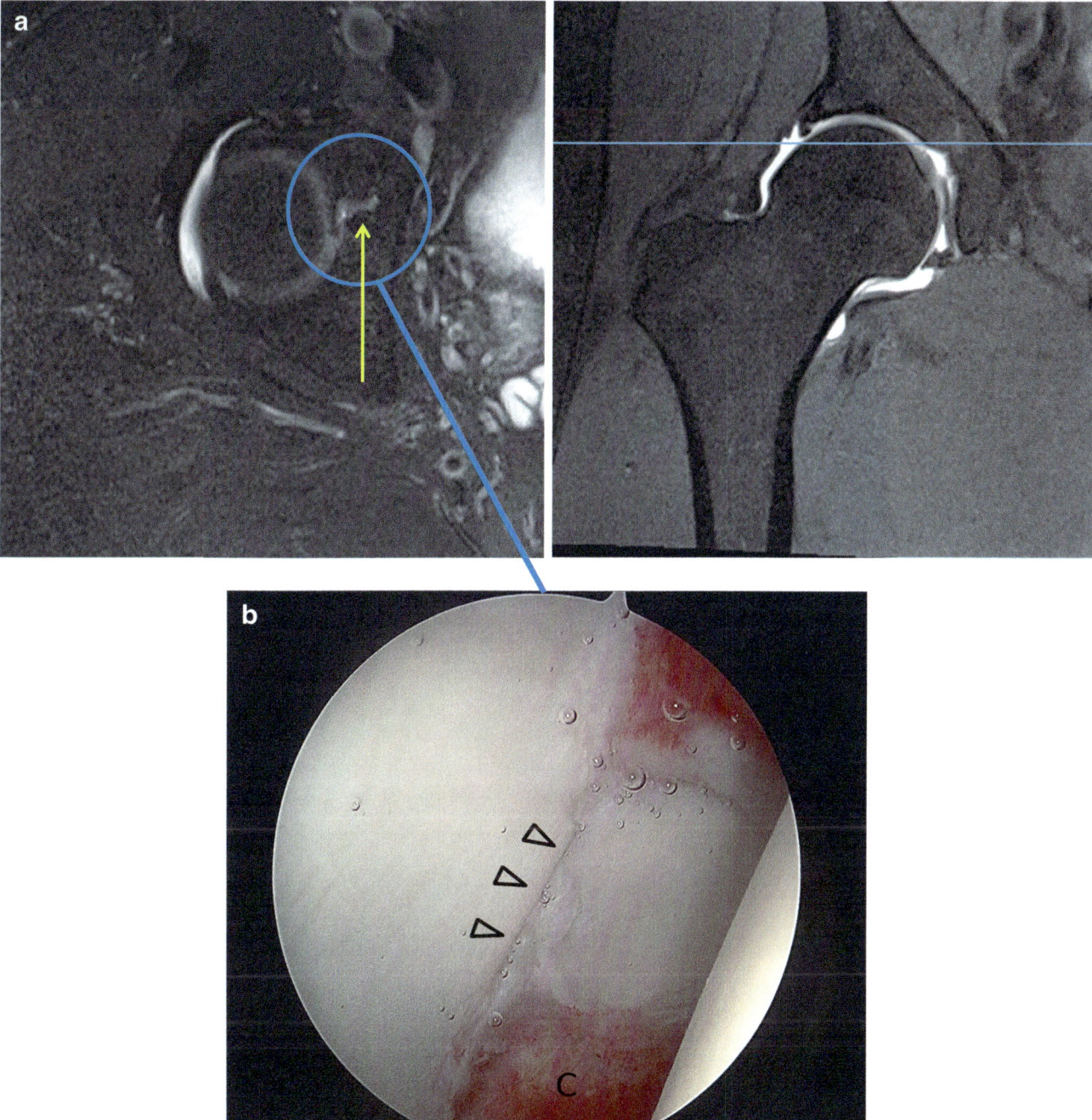

Fig. 27.10 (**a**) Linked axial and coronal T2 MR-arthrogram images of a physeal scar between the ilium and pubis (*arrow*). The scar is seen as a linear defect in the anteromedial aspect of the articular cartilage but may not be readily apparent on imaging. (**b**) Arthroscopic appearance of the physeal scar (*arrowheads*) extending radially from the cotyloid fossa (C) to the medial acetabular rim

The adult acetabulum is made up of three bones, the pubis, ilium, and ischium, which normally fuse at the triradiate cartilage during adolescence. Persistence of a physeal scar anteriorly between the ilium and pubis or posteriorly between the ilium and ischium has been described [18]. These anatomical variants are difficult to identify on MR but may appear as a linear signal extending radially from the cotyloid fossa at the confluence between the two ossification centers (Fig. 27.10a, b).

Another developmental variant seen commonly in the central compartment during hip arthroscopy is a supraacetabular fossa [19]. Located in the acetabular roof at the apex of the cotyloid fossa, a supraacetabular fossa has been found in up to 10 % of normal adult hips and most likely represents a focal delay in skeletal maturation [20] (Fig. 27.11a, b). Sometimes mislabeled a focal cartilage defect or an osteochondritis dissecans lesion on MR, the supraacetabular fossa is found mostly

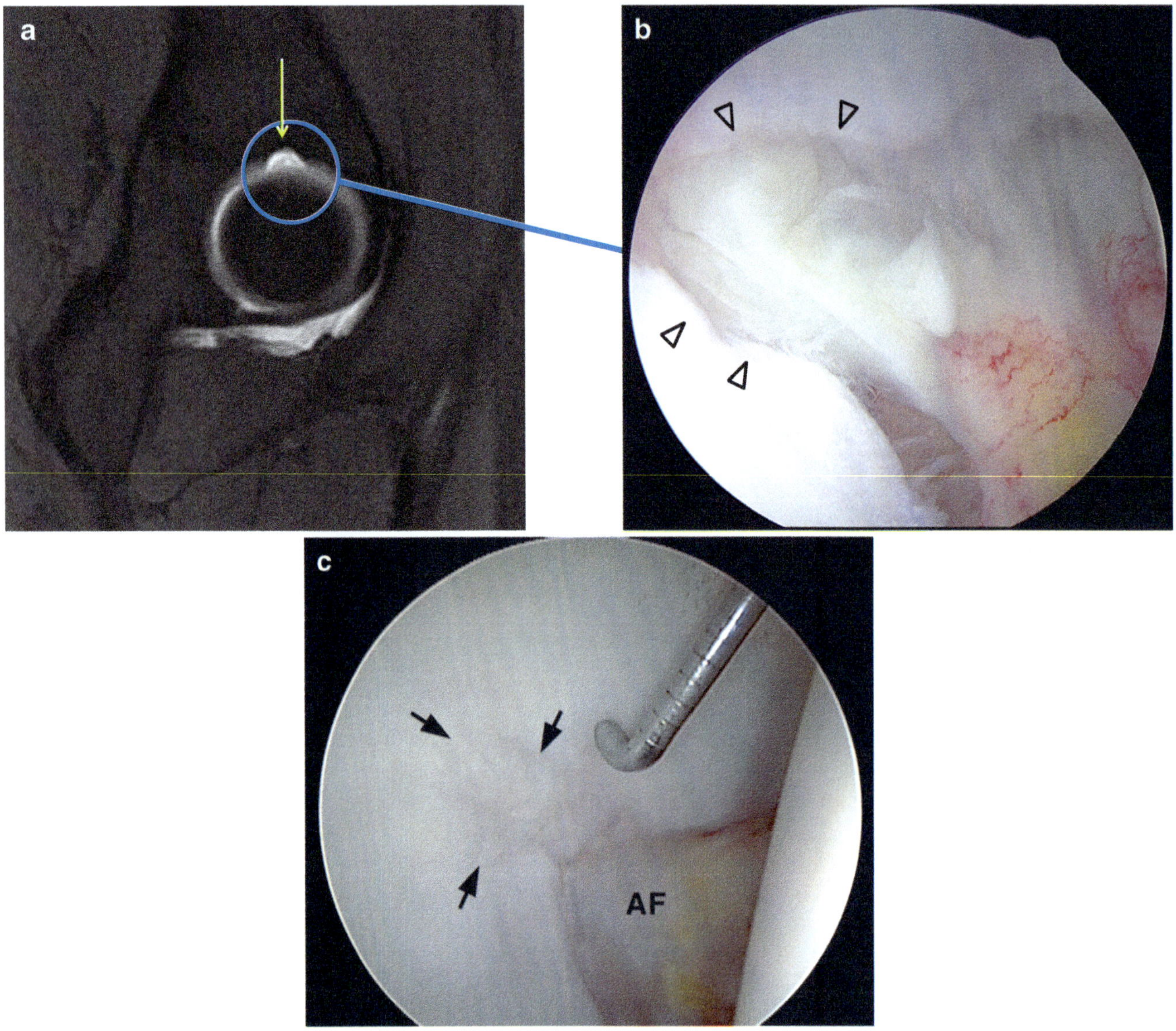

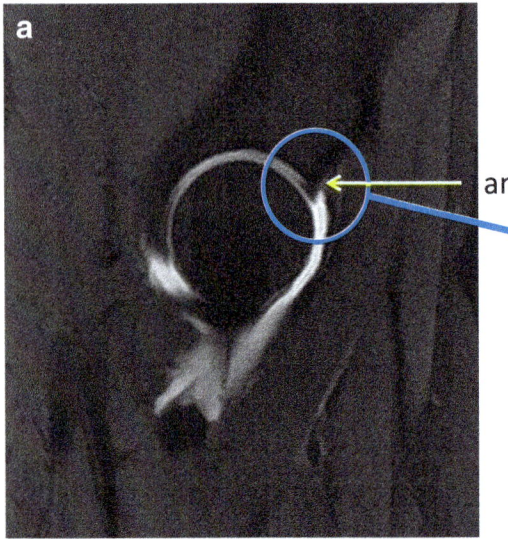

Fig. 27.11 (**a**) Sagittal T2 MR-arthrogram demonstrating a defect in the acetabular roof consistent with a supraacetabular fossa (*arrow*). (**b**) Arthroscopic appearance of the supraacetabular fossa (*arrowheads*) filled with fibrous tissue. (**c**) Arthroscopic appearance of the stellate crease (*arrowheads*) which appears to be a remnant of the filled in supraacetabular fossa (**c**: published with kind permission. Copyright © J.W. Thomas Byrd, MD)

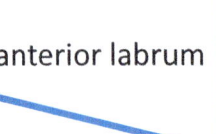

anterior labrum

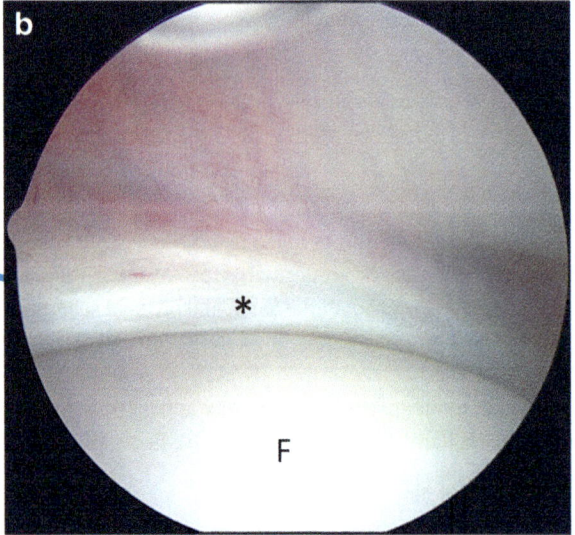

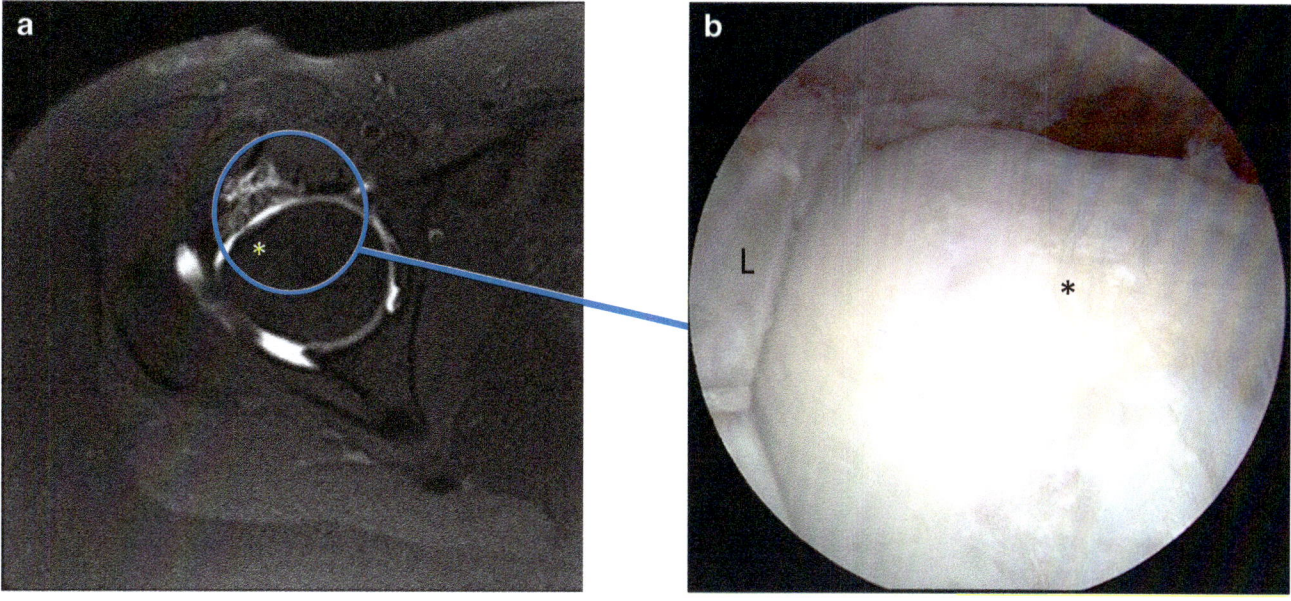

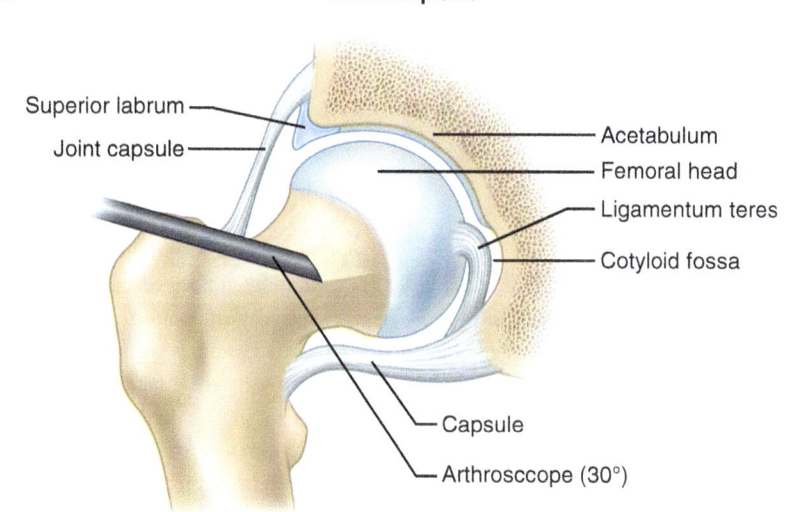

c   **Coronal plane**

Superior labrum ———

Joint capsule ———

——— Acetabulum

——— Femoral head

——— Ligamentum teres

——— Cotyloid fossa

——— Capsule

——— Arthrosccope (30°)

Fig. 27.13 (**a**) Axial T2 MR-arthrogram demonstrating the femoral head/neck junction (*asterisk*). Analysis of multiple cuts from cross-sectional imaging is essential to characterize the femoral head/neck junction to identify cam morphology. (**b**) Arthroscopic appearance of the femoral head/neck junction (*asterisk*). A capsulotomy connecting the anterior and anterolateral portals has been made and the hip is flexed to 35° to improve visualization of the entire anterior femoral neck. The repaired acetabular labrum (L) in on the *left* of the picture. In general, the cam deformity of the femoral head/neck junction is adjacent the area of chondrolabral damage seen in the central compartment. Rotation of the hip aids in visualization of the medial and lateral aspects of the femoral neck. (**c**) Anatomical rendering showing that removing traction and flexing the hip to 40° permits access to the peripheral compartment and visualization of the femoral neck and head/neck junction. Switching to a 30° arthroscope may facilitate visualization within this space

Fig. 27.12 (**a**) Sagittal T2 MR-arthrogram demonstrating the relationship between the anterior labrum (*arrow*) and the femoral head. The labrum conforms circumferentially around the femoral head creating a seal that facilitates fluid joint motion, enhances joint stability through negative intraarticular pressure, and maintains lubrication of the articular surfaces. (**b**) Arthroscopic appearance of the labral seal (*asterisk*). Traction has been released to locate the femoral head (F) within the acetabular vault. The arthroscope is positioned within the peripheral compartment. Arthroscopic intervention in the joint must not compromise the labral seal so that the biomechanics of the labrum are maintained

Fig. 27.14 Intraoperative fluoroscopic image of a right hip during femoroplasty. Rotation of the hip under fluoroscopy helps to characterize deformities of the femoral head/neck junction and guides correction

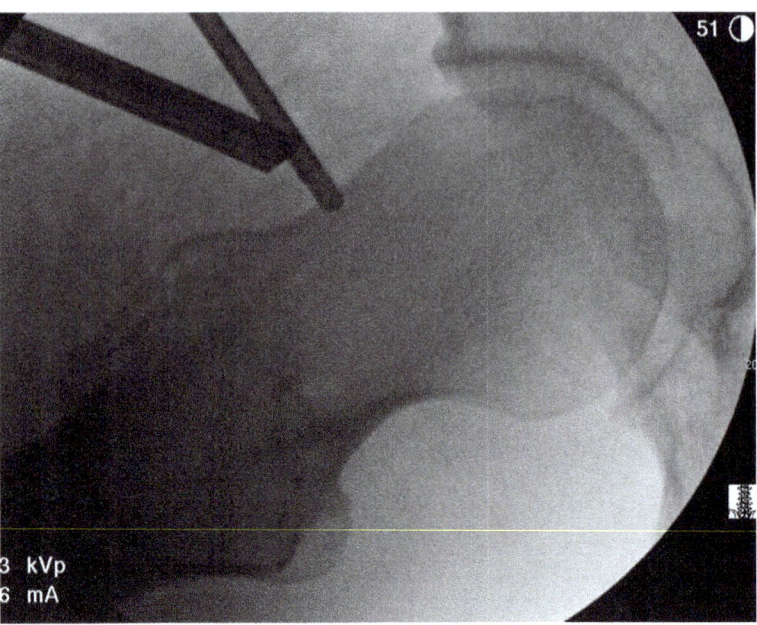

in young adults and usually fills in over time. It has been proposed that the stellate crease represents a residual scar left after obliteration of the supraacetabular fossa [21–23] (Fig. 27.11c).

Peripheral Compartment

The peripheral compartment comprises the space within the joint capsule outside of the femoroacetabular articulation. Once traction is released and the femoral head returns to its position within the acetabular vault, the peripheral compartment is accessed by flexing the hip until the anterior capsule is sufficiently relaxed to permit navigation. While the previously made anterolateral or anterior portals generally allow access to peripheral compartment, adequate visualization and instrumentation are permitted by either expanding or extending the central compartment capsulotomy or by penetrating the anterolateral capsule distally from the central compartment capsulotomy. While some surgeons continue to use the 70° arthroscope in the peripheral compartment, the anatomy of the peripheral compartment is conducive to visualization with a 30° arthroscope.

The hip joint capsule has a proximal attachment circumferentially along the periphery of the acetabular rim and attaches distally at the intertrochanteric line anteriorly and on the femoral neck posteriorly. The femoroacetabular labral seal can be inspected proximally within the peripheral compartment (Fig. 27.12a, b). The labrum should fit snugly against the cartilage of the femoral head circumferentially around the joint and maintain contact throughout hip flexion and rotation. The quality of a pincer correction and labral refixation or repair may be assessed from this view.

An excessive or asymmetrical acetabuloplasty or femoroplasty may compromise the sealing function of the labrum.

The morphology of the femoral head/neck junction and femoral neck is evaluated in the peripheral compartment (Fig. 27.13a–c). While preoperative imaging is critical for demonstrating proximal femoral morphology, the pathological features of femoroacetabular impingement are best characterized during arthroscopy by the pattern of articular cartilage damage within the acetabular vault as well as the arthroscopic appearance of the femoral head/neck junction. Arthroscopic observation of the femoroacetabular articulation while the hip is taken through increasing flexion and internal and external rotation demonstrates the dynamic biomechanics underlying potential impingement. Intraoperative fluoroscopy helps to localize position on the femoral neck and helps define the femoroplasty (Fig. 27.14).

The medial and lateral arthroscopic borders of the peripheral compartment are the medial and lateral synovial folds, respectively. These folds contain the terminal retinacular branches of medial and lateral circumflex arteries and must be protected during arthroscopy of the peripheral compartment. Improved access to the medial and lateral gutters is afforded by external and internal rotation of the hip, respectively. The lateral epiphyseal vessels along the posterosuperior neck constitute the major blood supply to the femoral head [24–26]. These folds are frequently well demonstrated on MR arthrography as linear structures coursing parallel to the femoral neck (Fig. 27.15a–c). The zona orbicularis is a thickening of the joint capsule that runs circumferentially around the femoral neck resisting axial distraction of the joint [27]. This is seen arthroscopically running perpendicular to the retinacular vessels.

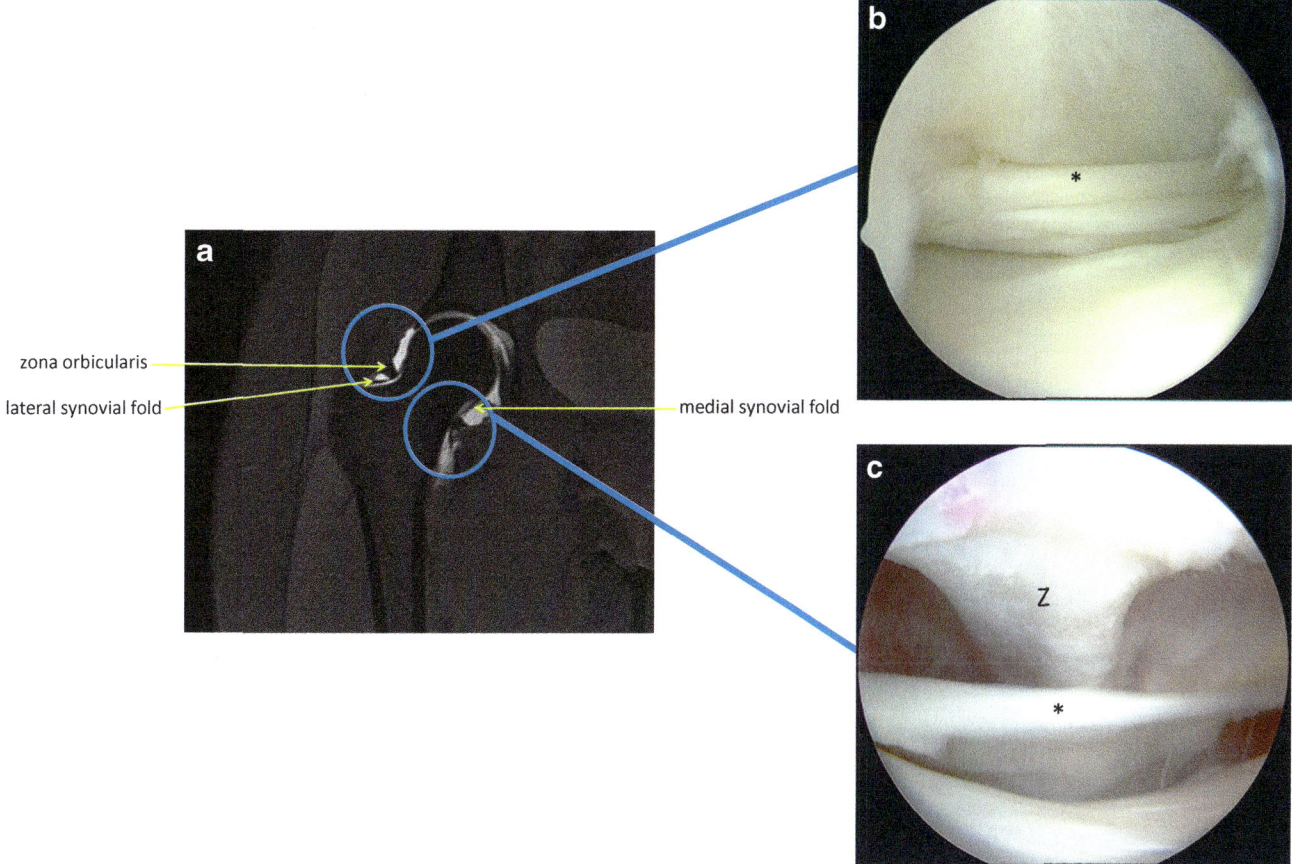

zona orbicularis

lateral synovial fold

medial synovial fold

Fig. 27.15 (**a**) Coronal T2 MR-arthrogram of a right hip demonstrating the zona orbicularis and lateral and medial synovial folds. (**b**) The arthroscope is maneuvered into the lateral gutter of the peripheral compartment and the lens is directed posteromedially to visualize the lateral synovial fold (*asterisk*) and lateral retinacular vessels. These vessels provide critical blood flow to the femoral head and must be protected during femoroplasty. (**c**) Arthroscopic appearance of the medial synovial fold (*asterisk*) passing under the zona orbicularis (Z). The arthroscope is maneuvered across the anterior femoral neck into the medial gutter to visualize this structure

The rectus femoris and iliopsoas tendons traverse the hip joint superficial to capsule. The origin of the rectus femoris consists of a direct head off of the anterior inferior iliac spine and an indirect head off of the posterolateral acetabular rim. The rectus femoris may be visualized from the central compartment in the extraarticular space through an extended anterior capsulotomy running perpendicular to the anterior acetabular rim (Fig. 27.16). The iliopsoas tendon may be seen as a linear indentation in the anteromedial capsule as it courses toward its insertion on the lesser trochanter of the femur (Fig. 27.17a, b). It may be exposed through an anteromedial capsulotomy from the central or peripheral compartment (Fig. 27.17c).

Conclusion

Treating a patient with a painful hip is challenging due to the complexities of the hip joint and the broad differential diagnosis of pathology in this region. Making an accurate diagnosis requires a systematic algorithm and incorporates elements of the history, examination, and preoperative imaging. MRI of the hip may be difficult to interpret given the anatomical complexity, variability, and orientation of the joint.

Hip arthroscopy has revolutionized the approach to the non-arthritic hip. The advancement of the technique is self-perpetuated as arthroscopy allows the development of innovative ways to treat hip pathology and continues to reveal newly understood hip pathology amenable to arthroscopic intervention. As our collective arthroscopic experience in the hip grows, our understanding of the complex anatomy and biomechanics of hip joint will also expand. Analysis of the variables inherent the morphology of the femoroacetabular articulation and systematic cataloguing of the anatomical variants and pathological entities of the hip joint will promote the continued evolution of hip arthroscopy. Correlation of arthroscopic findings to MR findings and collaboration with colleagues in musculoskeletal radiology will fuel a concomitant evolution of MR imaging of the hip joint. These

Fig. 27.16 Arthroscopic appearance of the tendon of the rectus femoris during left hip arthroscopy. The arthroscope is positioned in the anterolateral portal with the lens directed anteriorly. A capsulotomy has been made that connects the anterolateral to the anterior portal. The tendon is visualized traveling perpendicular to the anterior labrum (L) and should be protected while extending the capsulotomy

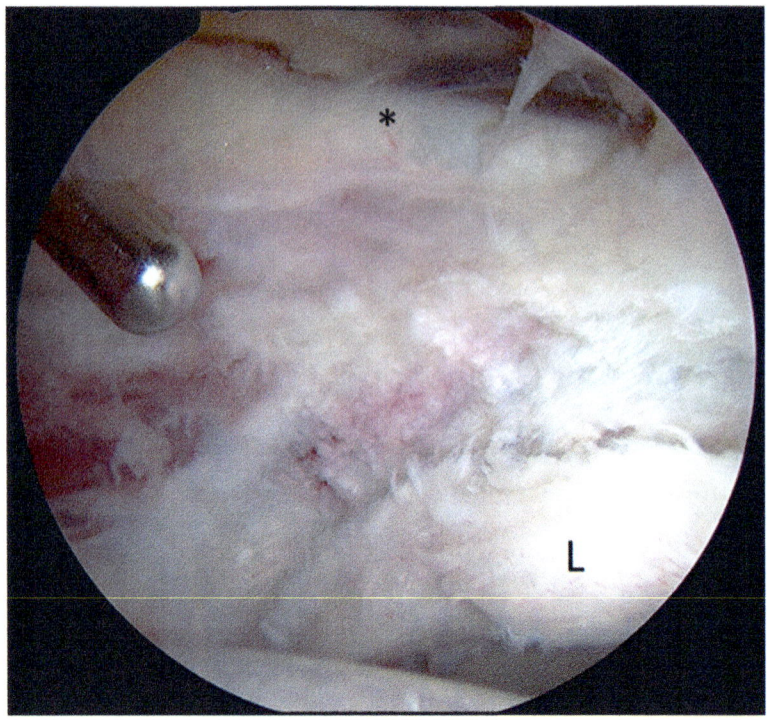

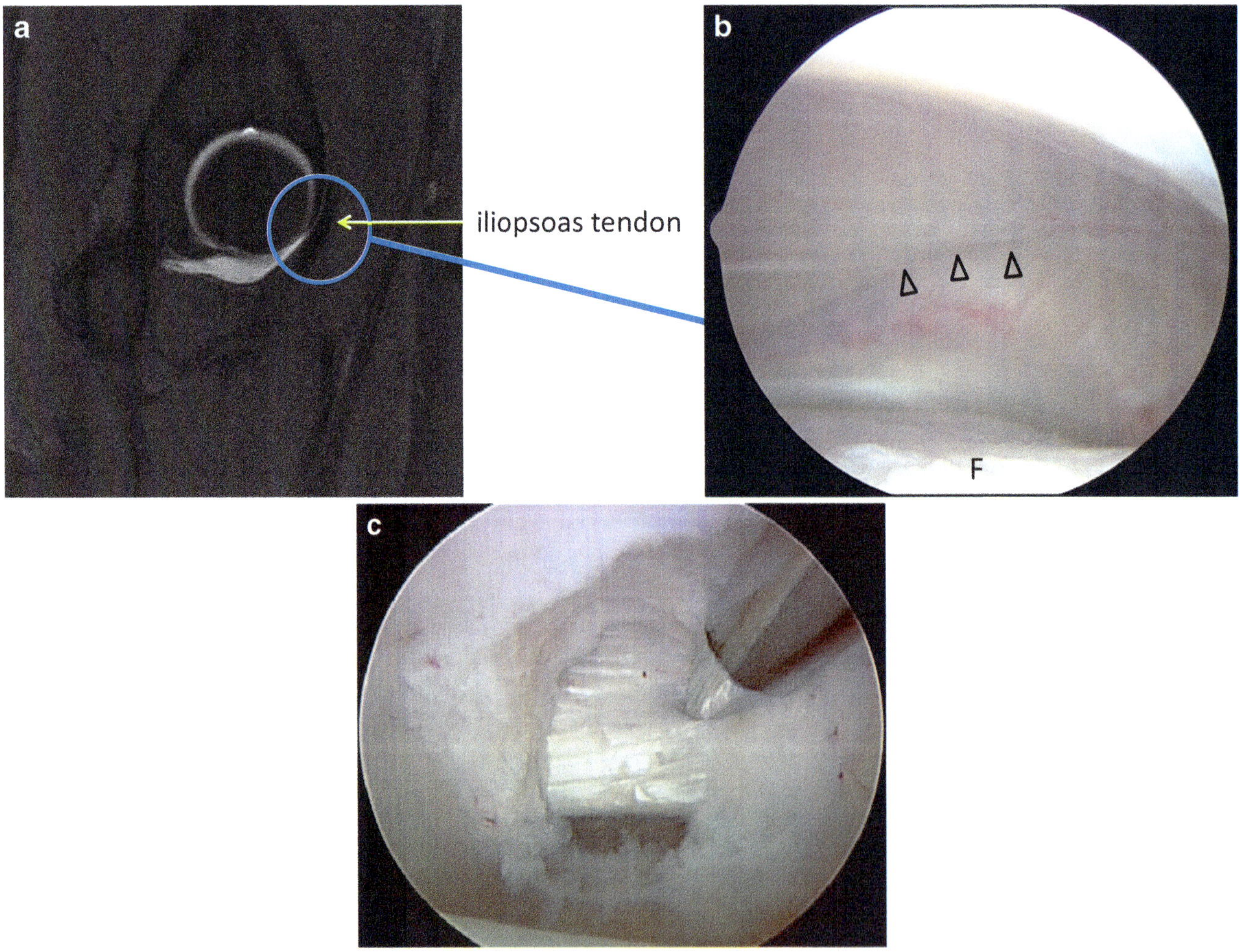

iliopsoas tendon

Fig. 27.17 (**a**) Sagittal MR-arthrogram demonstrating the iliopsoas tendon (*arrow*) coursing just anterior to the anteromedial acetabulum. Note the intimate relationship between the anterior rim and the tendon. (**b**) Arthroscopic appearance of the indentation made in the capsule from the extraarticular iliopsoas tendon (*arrowheads*). The arthroscope is in the peripheral compartment aimed anteriorly. The femoral neck (F) is at the *bottom* of the picture and the iliopsoas is seen coursing obliquely across the medial joint toward its insertion on the iliopsoas. (**c**) A small capsulotomy in the anteromedial capsule demonstrates the tendon of the iliopsoas (**c**: published with kind permission. Copyright © J.W. Thomas Byrd, MD)

advances promoted by hip arthroscopy will refine the diagnostic algorithm and improve our ability to deliver superior care to patients with hip problems.

References

1. McCarthy JC, Lee J-A. History of hip arthroscopy: challenges and opportunities. Clin Sports Med. 2011;30(2):217–24.
2. Byrd JWT. Hip arthroscopy. J Am Acad Orthop Surg. 2006;14(7): 433–44.
3. Kelly BT, Williams RJ, Philippon MJ. Hip arthroscopy: current indications, treatment options, and management issues. Am J Sports Med. 2003;31(6):1020–37.
4. Matsuda DK, Carlisle JC, Arthurs SC, Wierks CH, Philippon MJ. Comparative systematic review of the open dislocation, mini-open, and arthroscopic surgeries for femoroacetabular impingement. Arthroscopy. 2011;27(2):252–69.
5. Keeney JA, Peelle MW, Jackson J, Rubin D, Maloney WJ, Clohisy JC. Magnetic resonance arthrography versus arthroscopy in the evaluation of articular hip pathology. Clin Orthop Relat Res. 2004;429:163–9.
6. Byrd JWT. Diagnostic accuracy of clinical assessment, magnetic resonance imaging, magnetic resonance arthrography, and intra-articular injection in hip arthroscopy patients. Am J Sports Med. 2004;32(7):1668–74.
7. Toomayan GA, Holman WR, Major NM, Kozlowicz SM, Vail TP. Sensitivity of MR arthrography in the evaluation of acetabular labral tears. AJR Am J Roentgenol. 2006;186(2):449–53.
8. Freedman BA, Potter BK, Dinauer PA, Giuliani JR, Kuklo TR, Murphy KP. Prognostic value of magnetic resonance arthrography for Czerny stage II and III acetabular labral tears. Arthroscopy. 2006;22(7):742–7.
9. Chang CY, Huang AJ. MR imaging of normal hip anatomy. Magn Reson Imaging Clin N Am. 2013;21(1):1–19.
10. Sundberg TP, Toomayan GA, Major NM. Evaluation of the acetabular labrum at 3.0-T MR imaging compared with 1.5-T MR arthrography: preliminary experience. Radiology. 2006;238(2):706–11.
11. Byrd JW, Pappas JN, Pedley MJ. Hip arthroscopy: an anatomic study of portal placement and relationship to the extra-articular structures. Arthroscopy. 1995;11(4):418–23.
12. Robertson WJ, Kelly BT. The safe zone for hip arthroscopy: a cadaveric assessment of central, peripheral, and lateral compartment portal placement. Arthroscopy. 2008;24(9):1019–26.
13. Ilizaliturri VM, Byrd JWT, Sampson TG, et al. A geographic zone method to describe intra-articular pathology in hip arthroscopy: cadaveric study and preliminary report. Arthroscopy. 2008;24(5): 534–9.
14. Saddik D, Troupis J, Tirman P, O'Donnell J, Howells R. Prevalence and location of acetabular sublabral sulci at hip arthroscopy with retrospective MRI review. AJR Am J Roentgenol. 2006;187(5): W507–11.
15. Nguyen MS, Kheyfits V, Giordano BD, Dieudonne G, Monu JUV. Hip anatomic variants that may mimic abnormalities at MRI: labral variants. AJR Am J Roentgenol. 2013;201(3): W394–400.
16. Studler U, Kalberer F, Leunig M, et al. MR arthrography of the hip: differentiation between an anterior sublabral recess as a normal variant and a labral tear. Radiology. 2008;249(3):947–54.
17. Wenger DE, Kendell KR, Miner MR, Trousdale RT. Acetabular labral tears rarely occur in the absence of bony abnormalities. Clin Orthop Relat Res. 2004;426(426):145–50.
18. Paliobeis CP, Villar RN. Arthroscopic identification of iliopubic and ilioischial grooves in a single adult acetabulum. BMJ Case Rep. 2010;2010:1–3.
19. Byrd JWT. [Hip arthroscopy. Portal technique and arthroscopic anatomy]. Orthopade. 2006;35(1):41–2, 44–50, 52–3.
20. Dietrich TJ, Suter A, Pfirrmann CWA, Dora C, Fucentese SF, Zanetti M. Supraacetabular fossa (pseudodefect of acetabular cartilage): frequency at MR arthrography and comparison of findings at MR arthrography and arthroscopy. Radiology. 2012;263(2):484–91.
21. Keene GS, Villar RN. Arthroscopic anatomy of the hip: an in vivo study. Arthroscopy. 1994;10(4):392–9.
22. Byrd JWT. Hip arthroscopy in athletes. In: Byrd JWT, editor. Operative hip arthroscopy. New York: Springer; 2012.
23. Byrd JWT. Supraacetabular fossa. Radiology. 2012;265(2):648. Author reply 648.
24. Gautier E, Ganz K, Krügel N, Gill T, Ganz R. Anatomy of the medial femoral circumflex artery and its surgical implications. J Bone Joint Surg Br. 2000;82(5):679–83.
25. Anderson K, Strickland SM, Warren R. Hip and groin injuries in athletes. Am J Sports Med. 2001;29(4):521–33.
26. Kalhor M, Beck M, Huff TW, Ganz R. Capsular and pericapsular contributions to acetabular and femoral head perfusion. J Bone Joint Surg Am. 2009;91(2):409–18.
27. Ito H, Song Y, Lindsey DP, Safran MR, Giori NJ. The proximal hip joint capsule and the zona orbicularis contribute to hip joint stability in distraction. J Orthop Res. 2009;27(8):989–95.

Femoroacetabular Impingement: Labrum, Articular Cartilage

28

Gary Salvador, John J. Christoforetti, and Bojan Zoric

Introduction

Osteoarthritis (OA) of the hip is a very common problem. While there are many different etiologies for OA of the hip, often a specific cause cannot be determined. Recently, Femoroacetabular Impingement (FAI) has been found to be a possible cause of progressive degenerative changes leading to early OA of the hip in younger patients [1, 2]. In FAI, morphologic abnormalities of the proximal femur, acetabulum, or both cause abnormal contact between the femur and acetabulum during motion of the hip joint. This most commonly occurs during flexion combined with internal rotation. Impingement can occur in normal hips in extreme flexion and internal rotation or may be from morphologic changes that cause undesired contact between the structures during normal ranges of motion. This contact causes abnormal stress on the acetabular labrum and articular cartilage. The resulting microtrauma from recurrent impingement can lead to tearing of the labrum and degeneration of the adjacent acetabular cartilage [1–6].

Chronic impingement leads to acetabular labral tears and breakdown of the articular cartilage potentially resulting in global hip osteoarthritis. The morphologic abnormalities of FAI have been suggested to be one of the main causes in idiopathic or primary osteoarthritis [7]. Timely diagnosis is therefore of utmost importance. Surgical intervention can give pain relief, remove bony impingement, and potentially slow down the progression of further cartilage degeneration.

Intra-articular hip impingement can occur from abnormal morphology on the femoral head–neck junction, acetabular rim, or both. Impingement secondary to abnormalities of the proximal femur is referred to as *cam impingement*, while impingement secondary to acetabular rim/neck contact is described as *pincer impingement*. While the two types of FAI are described as two separate, distinct entities, often a combination of factors can lead to the development of FAI [1].

Cam impingement lesions are the result of morphologic bone growth on the anterolateral head–neck junction leading to impingement against the articular acetabular cartilage during hip motion [1, 3–6, 8]. A classic cam deformity is a pistol grip appearance of the femoral head–neck junction often recognizable on plain radiographs (Fig. 28.1a, b). This type of deformity has an association with childhood hip disorders, including slipped capital femoral epiphysis (SCFE) and Legg-Calve' Perthes disease. However, cam impingement can occur in the absence of childhood hip disorders. The cam lesion alters the spherical shape of the femoral head and results in reduced rotational range of motion before incongruent contact occurs. Because of the cam lesion's typical location on the anterolateral aspect of the femoral head–neck junction, the abutment will most often occur in hip flexion, internal rotation, and adduction. Consequences of a cam lesion are shearing forces to the acetabular articular cartilage and/or abutment on the acetabular labrum. This, in turn, may cause destabilization of the chondrolabral junction and progressive degenerative changes to the articular cartilage or separation of the articular cartilage from the subchondral bone.

A reduced femoral head–neck offset is best assessed on MRI using dedicated oblique axial images that are obtained parallel to the long axis of the femoral neck. Methods of quantitatively evaluating the femoral head–neck offset have been described with the "alpha" angle [9]. The alpha angle is calculated on the abovementioned oblique axial MR images of the hip. The angle is measured between a line drawn from the center of the femoral head through the central axis of the femoral neck and a second line drawn from the center of the femoral head to the anterior point where the distance from

G. Salvador, MS, PA-C (✉) • B. Zoric, MD
Sports Medicine North, Peabody, MA, USA
e-mail: gary@sportsmednorth.com; Bzoric7@gmail.com

J.J. Christoforetti, MD
Department of Orthopedic Surgery, Sports Medicine Division,
Allegheny Health Network, West Penn Hospital,
Pittsburgh, PA, USA
e-mail: John.christoforetti@gmail.com

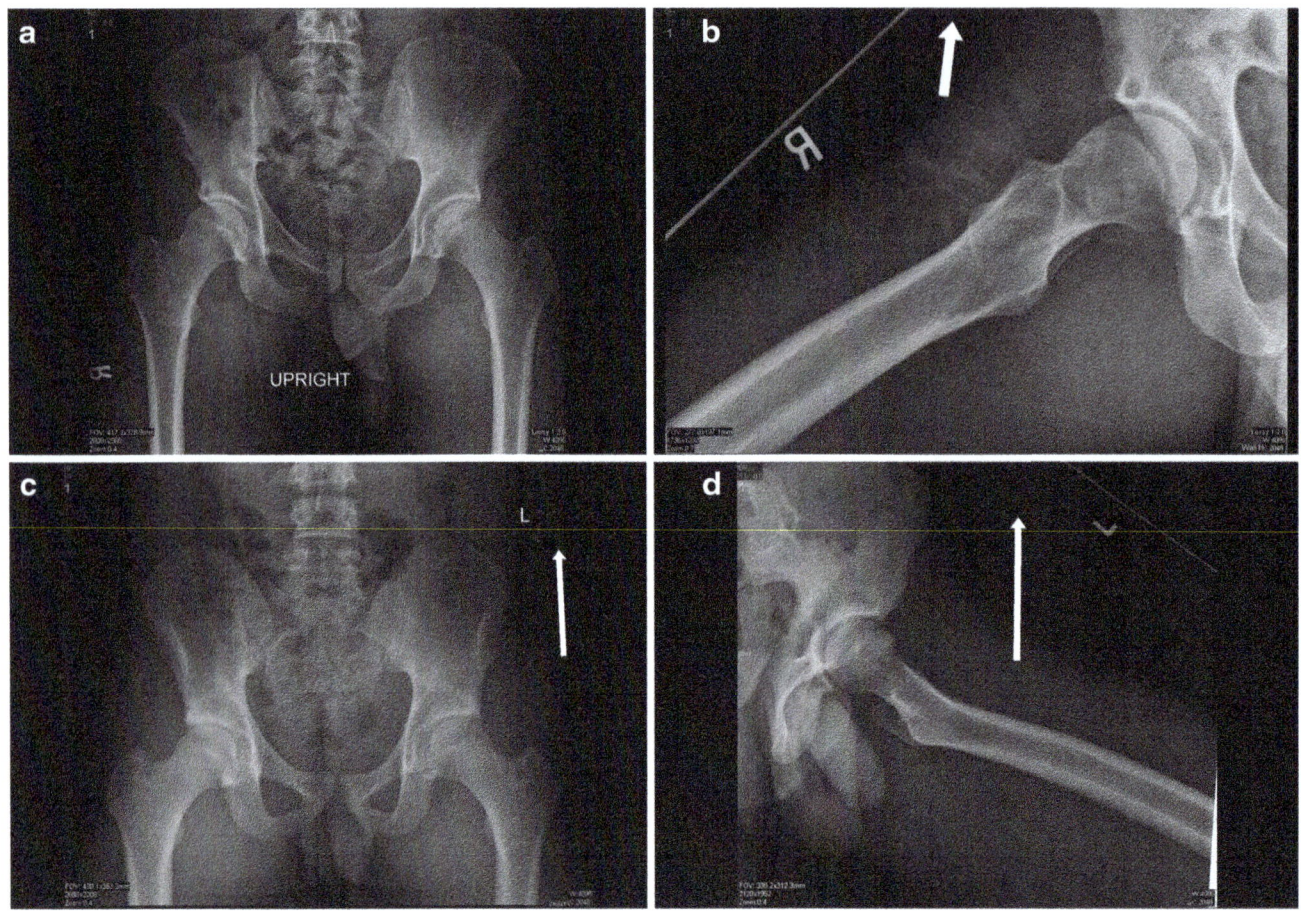

Fig. 28.1 (a–d) Radiographs of cam and pincer lesions. (a, b) AP (a) and lateral (b) X-rays demonstrating CAM lesion of right hip. (c, d) AP (c) and lateral (d) X-rays demonstrating periacetabular ossicle effec-tively creating pincer-type lesion of left hip. Also note adjacent CAM lesion on left femoral neck

the center of the head exceeds the radius of the subchondral femoral head. It has been proposed that an alpha angle >55° predisposes a patient to cam FAI [9].

Pincer Impingement

Pincer impingement is caused by abnormal contact between the acetabular rim and the femoral neck as a result of acetab-ular abnormalities [1, 8, 10–12]. Hip joint abnormalities such as coxa profunda (deep socket), protrusio acetabula (acetab-ular fossa medial to the pelvic border, or acetabular retrover-sion (backward facing acetabular opening) can predispose patients to pincer impingement (Fig. 28.1c, d). In pincer-type impingement, during hip flexion, the femoral neck abuts against the acetabular labrum, resulting in compression and tearing of the labrum. Because pincer impingement involves often the entire acetabulum, as in protusio, damage to the femoral head can be seen in both the anterolateral femo-ral head as well as the posterior inferior femoral head.

The bony acetabulum and pincer lesion act like a snowplow, skiving into the femoral articular cartilage as the hip is brought through a range of motion, especially hip flexion and internal rotation. Protrusio acetabuli and acetabular ret-roversion can be seen on oblique axial MRI of the hip. Acetabular retroversion results in an increase in coverage of the anterior aspect of the femoral head [13]. Acetabular depth can be quantified on the same oblique axial images that are used to calculate the alpha angle. The depth is calcu-lated by drawing a line connecting the anterior and posterior acetabular rims and a parallel line that passes through the center of the femoral head. The distance between these two lines is the acetabular depth, with the value being positive if the center of the femoral head is lateral to the acetabular rim [14]. As would be expected, the acetabulum is significantly deeper in patients with pincer FAI. In patients with cam FAI, acetabular depth is often normal. Future research may recognize a specific value for the acetabular depth that puts a patient at increased risk for the development of pincer FAI.

Clinical Diagnosis

A thorough history should be taken from the patient with special attention focused on any history of trauma, childhood hip disorders, or previous surgery. The activity level of the patient can vary with respect to provocative maneuvers. Symptoms are common in activities that require repetitive hip flexion, but symptoms may also occur at rest, especially with periods of prolonged sitting. Recreational sports and exercise may also be provocative. Mechanical symptoms (popping, snapping, clicking) should be differentiated from snapping psoas syndrome or a snapping iliotibial band syndrome.

Classically, patients present with deep anterior hip or groin pain and potentially radiation of pain to the anterior thigh. Commonly, this pain is localized deep, and patients are unable to reproduce it with tactile pressure. Less commonly, patients may also present with lateral hip pain or pain radiating to the buttocks. The patient experiences hip or groin pain exacerbated by walking, prolonged sitting, or deep squatting. Mechanical symptoms, such as locking, catching, or clicking may be present but are fairly rare. Provocative testing elicits symptoms when the hip is passively flexed, adducted, and internally rotated (positive Anterior Impingement test) or flexed, abducted, and externally rotated (positive FABER test) [1, 3, 8].

Imaging Principles

As this text concerns itself with MRI and arthroscopy correlations, the cases will focus specifically on those aspects. The diagnosis of impingement, however, currently relies heavily on the clinical context, exam findings, and plain radiographic imaging. MRI findings are viewed by most expert clinicians as confirmatory of the diagnosis and as essential for ruling out alternative diagnoses.

Patients undergo a standard series of plain radiographs: Standing AP pelvis, long neck lateral view, and False profile view of the hip. The main purpose of the X-rays is to evaluate the bony structures for FAI or other mechanical deformity. X-rays can also be used to evaluate the presence of acetabular dysplasia as well as other pain producing pathology such as fractures and early degenerative joint disease. If the patient has failed conservative management and there is evidence of FAI in the absence of alternate diagnosis, we routinely order an MRI arthrogram.

Magnetic resonance imaging (MRI) and MR arthrography are excellent imaging modalities for showing the morphologic abnormalities of the proximal femur and acetabulum as well as the various changes seen in the hip secondary to FAI. The normal anatomy of the hip allows for a wide range of motion. The morphologic abnormalities that predispose a patient to the development of FAI result in decreased joint clearance between the femoral neck and acetabulum. MRI arthrograms can evaluate any evidence of abnormal contact, or impingement, between the femoral neck and acetabulum. Associated degenerative changes in the acetabular labrum and/or adjacent articular cartilage can also be evaluated simultaneously [2, 8, 15, 16].

MRI findings of changes secondary to FAI within the acetabulum can be seen involving the acetabular bone, labrum, and articular cartilage. Studies suggest that a majority of the abnormalities are located peripherally at the chondrolabral transition zone [17]. The cases that follow will illustrate these characteristic MRI and (if applicable) arthroscopy findings.

Case 1

A 34-year-old female presented with a 10-month history of anterior hip pain, which occurred acutely during a boot camp exercise class. She had been treated previously with physical therapy, activity modification, and rest for a lumbar spine etiology and piriformis syndrome. Diagnostic steroid and local anesthetic injection in the femoral-acetabular joint gave excellent short-term relief. See Figs. 28.2a, b and 28.3.

Discussion

This case is shown to highlight the early findings of Cam impingement in the region of shear injury at the chondrolabrum juncture in a non-arthritic patient. The articular cartilage in FAI cases can show a variety of changes. Chondral damage occurs commonly first on the acetabular side of the joint with FAI. Progression to involve the femoral head occurs only late in the degenerative process. Cartilage damage is located anterosuperiorly with cam-type FAI, due to local compression by the cam. Areas of signal hyper-intensity on MR that represent areas of chondral softening manifest early damage. Arthroscopically, this is seen as focal delamination or a "wave sign." Eventually, this softening progresses from articular cartilage fissures to chondral fragmentation and resultant full-thickness chondral defects seen on MRI/MRA. This can be visualized arthroscopically as a partial thickness or full-thickness chondral flap. These changes are classically described as appearing in the anterosuperior aspect of the acetabulum.

Case 2

A 19-year-old Division 1 female college soccer player presents with a 5-year history of anterior left hip and groin pain. Her symptoms became progressively more painful 1 month prior to the presentation in the office. The pain was

a   b

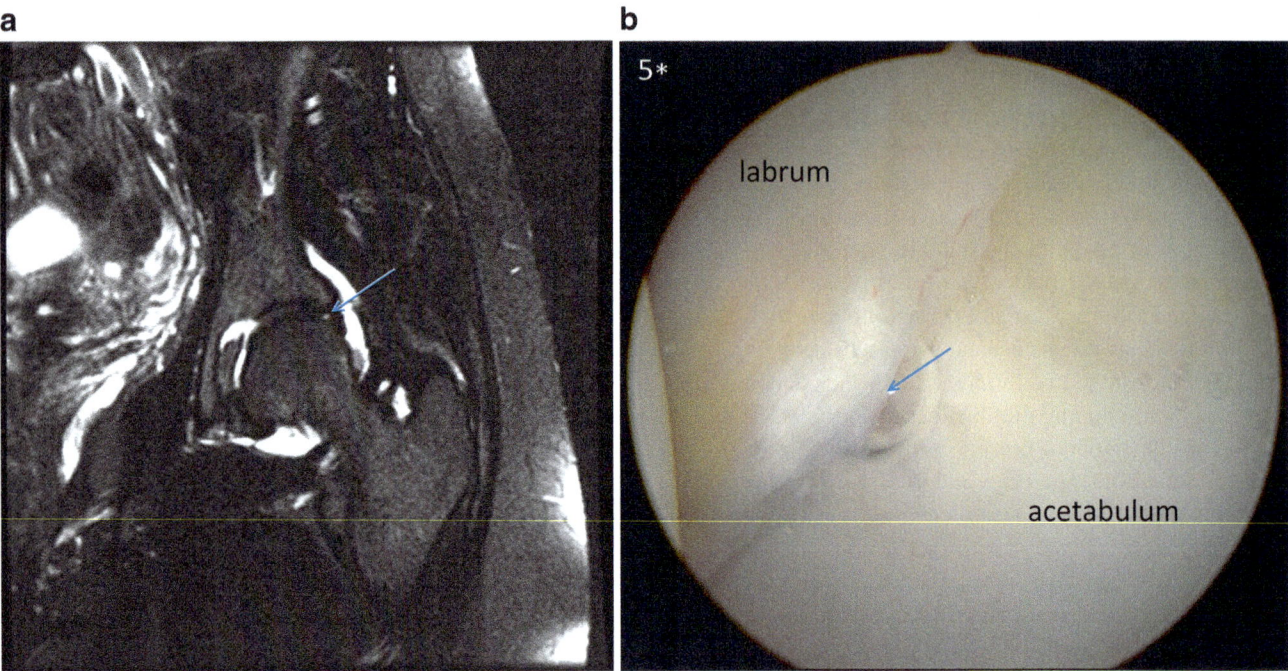

Fig. 28.2 (**a**, **b**) MRI arthrogram T2-weighted coronal image (**a**) demonstrating chondro-labrum separation (*blue arrow*) and arthroscopy image of same area (**b**)

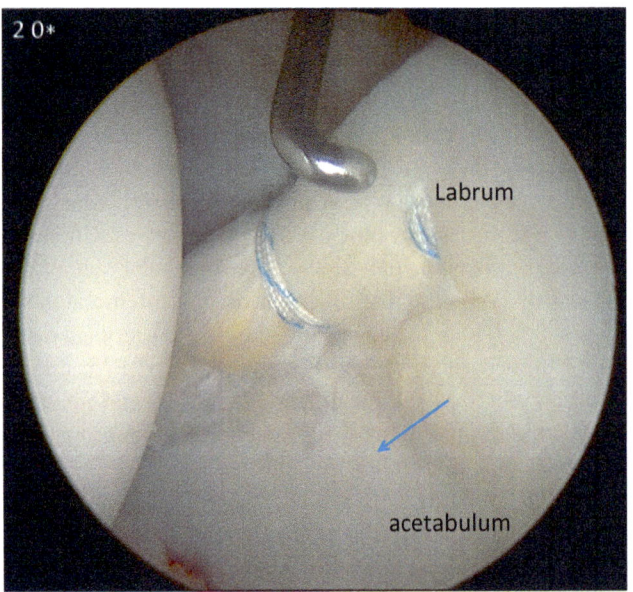

Fig. 28.3 Arthroscopy image showing repair of the labrum damage with persistent articular acetabular chondral damage due to Cam-delamination (*arrow*)

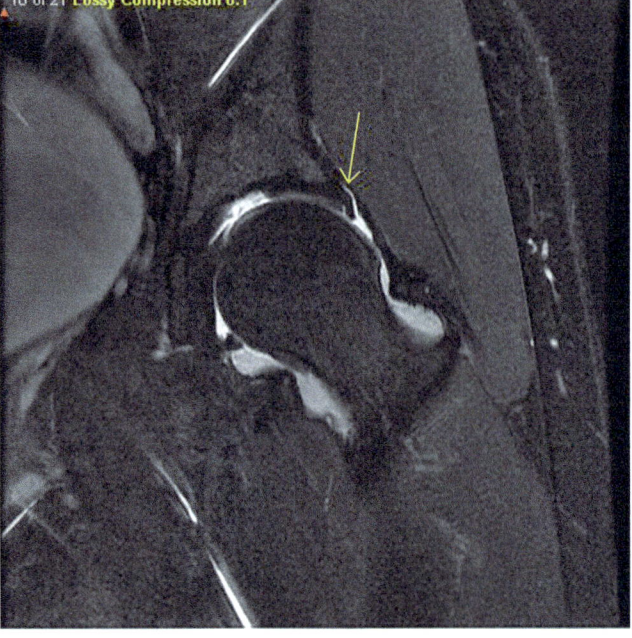

Fig. 28.4 T2-weighted MRI arthrogram image of affected hip. Note the light signal tracking between the articular cartilage and subchondral bone and the contrast signal penetrating the chondrolabral juncture (*yellow arrow*)

exacerbated by running and soccer performance. The team trainers diagnosed psoas tendinitis and FAI. Activity modification, sports cessation, and physical therapeutic exercise failed to relieve her pain. After physical exam and plain radiographs confirmed impingement, MRI arthrogram confirmed chondrolabral injury. Arthroscopy with correction of

Cam impingement through femoral osteochondroplasty and labrum repair was performed. She returned to play 1 year following the procedure shown. See Figs. 28.4, 28.5, and 28.6.

Discussion

This case illustrates the progressive and combined findings of mixed pattern FAI at the articular cartilage. The typically visible carpet-chondral detachment and chondro-labrum

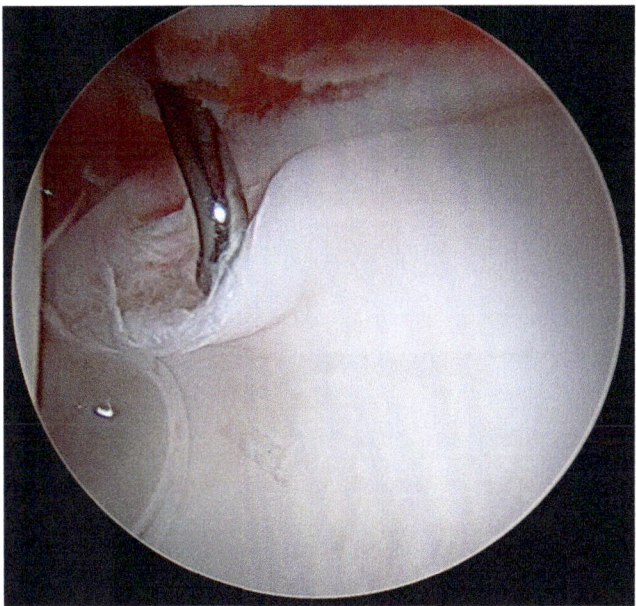

Fig. 28.5 Arthroscopy image with probe exposing the chondrolabral separation due to the Cam impingement in the same region as MRI arthrogram demonstrated signal abnormalities

separation are clear on MRI arthrogram. Arthroscopy was required to appreciate the bruising within the substance of the intact labrum caused by pincer pattern conflict.

Recent research suggests that patients with cam FAI tend to have articular cartilage lesions in the anterosuperior portion of the acetabulum, while patients with pincer FAI tend to have cartilage lesions in the posteroinferior aspect of the acetabulum [14]. With pincer-type FAI, chondral injury seems to be more common posteroinferiorly or diffusely [14, 18]. MR arthrography can allow better delineation of chondral defects than standard MRI, though intra-articular contrast will not always outline early delamination lesions. These can be assessed on T2-weighted images but still remain a challenge to identify.

Case 3

A 21-year-old male collegiate golfer presents to the office with increasing pain in the groin and inability to perform over a semester of conservative care. Physical exam is significant for limited internal rotation at 90° hip flexion and reproduction of his pain with passive flexion, adduction, and internal rotation of the hip. Plain radiographs show mixed pattern femoroacetabular impingement.

MRI arthrogram reveals chondrolabral injury as well as large ossicle within the labrum, presumably due to persistent femoral neck-acetabular rim conflict (pincer impingement). Arthroscopy was performed for removal of ossicle, labrum

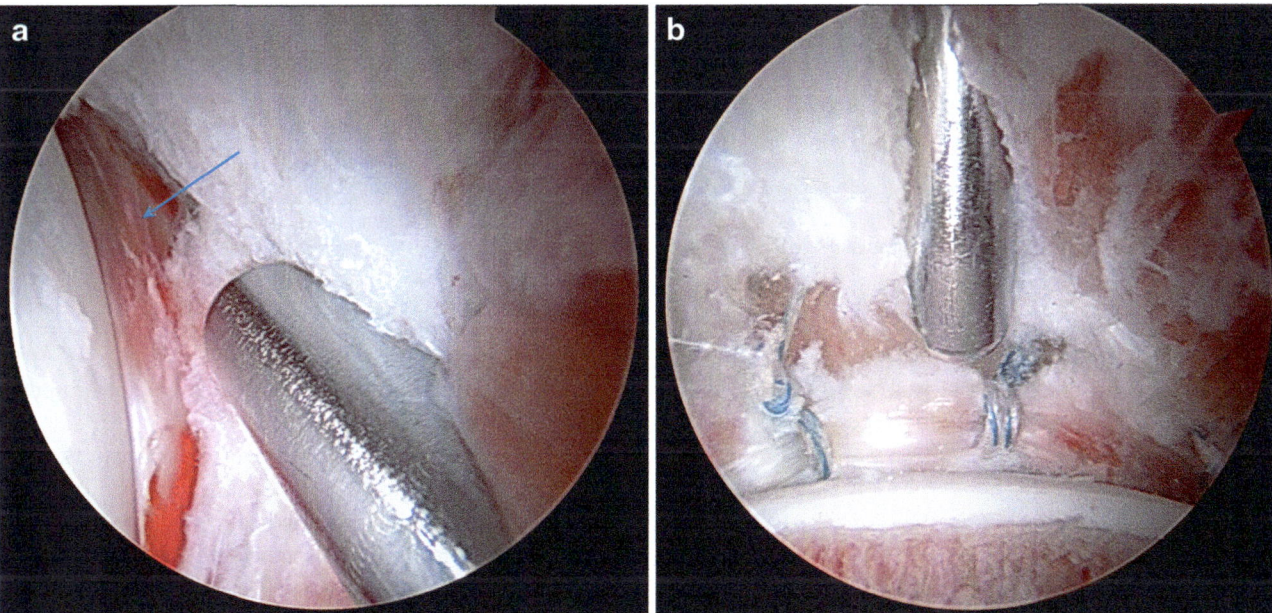

Fig. 28.6 (**a, b**) Arthroscopy images of the hip reduced following labrum repair and Cam decompression. **a** demonstrates bruising in the labrum (*arrow*) consistent with pincer pattern damage. This type of injury is frequently not appreciable on MRI

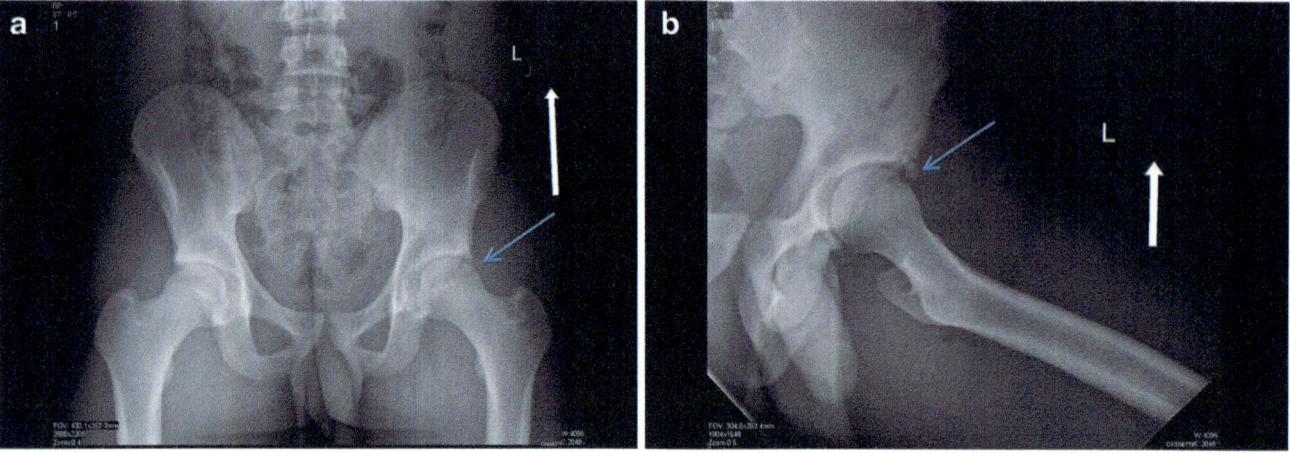

Fig. 28.7 (**a, b**) Plain radiographs demonstrating mixed pattern FAI and os acetabuli on symptomatic left side (*blue arrow*)

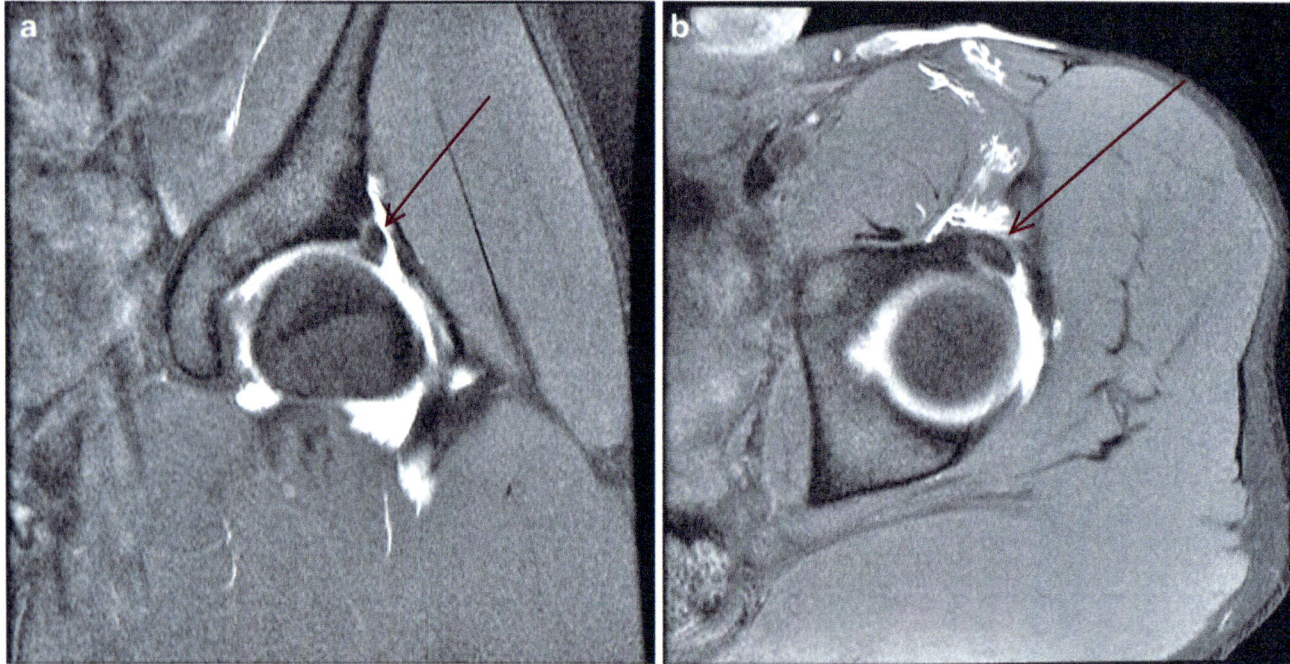

Fig. 28.8 Coronal (**a**) and axial (**b**) T2-weighted MRI arthrogram images showing large ossicle (*arrow*) at the area of mixed pattern impingement

repair, and femoral neck osteoplasty. The patient returned to competitive golf 6 months following surgery. See Figs. 28.7, 28.8, and 28.9a–c.

Discussion

This case illustrates the extreme example of pincer pattern acetabular damage in mixed pattern impingement. Both bone and chondral causes and effects of impingement contribute to the clinical picture and were correlated well arthroscopically to exist in the zone of dysfunction.

Labral degeneration and tears are important abnormalities that can lead to hip instability and faster hyaline cartilage breakdown. They are increased in patients with FAI, particularly anterosuperiorly. Labral pathology can be associated with both cam and pincer types of FAI. Tears are usually best seen on sagittal or oblique sagittal imaging sequences, followed by coronal images. Changes in the acetabular labrum include degenerative signal manifested as increased signal in

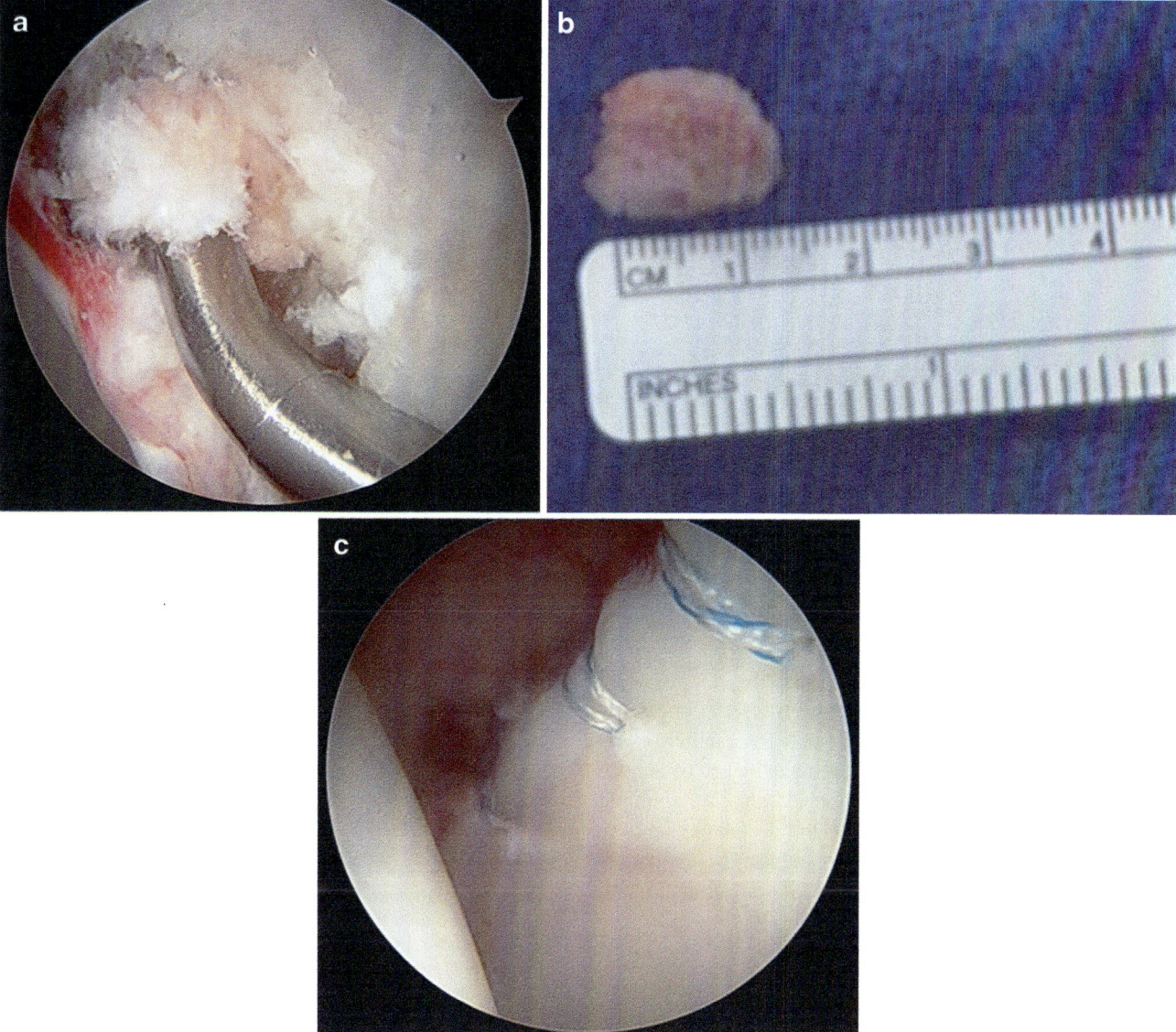

Fig. 28.9 (**a**) Arthroscopic image of supraacetabular space and ossicle with subjacent labrum rim erythema. (**b**) Explanted ossicle. (**c**) Arthroscopic image post repair of labrum in the region of ossicle detachment

the normally dark labrum on fluid-sensitive sequences as well as labral tears and complete labral detachments [15, 19, 20]. A useful indicator for a labral tear is that of a paralabral cyst (Fig. 28.10a, b). This is frequently more conspicuous than the tear itself and may be very large, very small, or non-existent. They are usually located in the soft tissues adjacent to the labrum, frequently projecting superiorly. They also frequently have an intraosseous component, which may be difficult to distinguish from subchondral cystic changes associated with hyaline cartilage damage. It is important to distinguish between tears and a normal anteroinferior and posteroinferior labral sulcus or sublabral recess. This recess should be distinguished from a labral tear and is often localized away from the usual anterosuperior labral pathology.

Summary

Magnetic resonance imaging (MRI) and MR arthrography are excellent imaging modalities for showing the morphologic abnormalities of the proximal femur and acetabulum as well as the various changes seen in the hip secondary to hip impingement. The morphologic abnormalities that predispose a patient to the development of FAI result in decreased joint clearance between the femoral neck and acetabulum. The pathologic process of FAI results in mechanical abutment of the femoral head–neck junction on the acetabulum. Labral tears, chondral degeneration and delamination, paralabral cysts, femoral neck herniation pits, and periacetabular

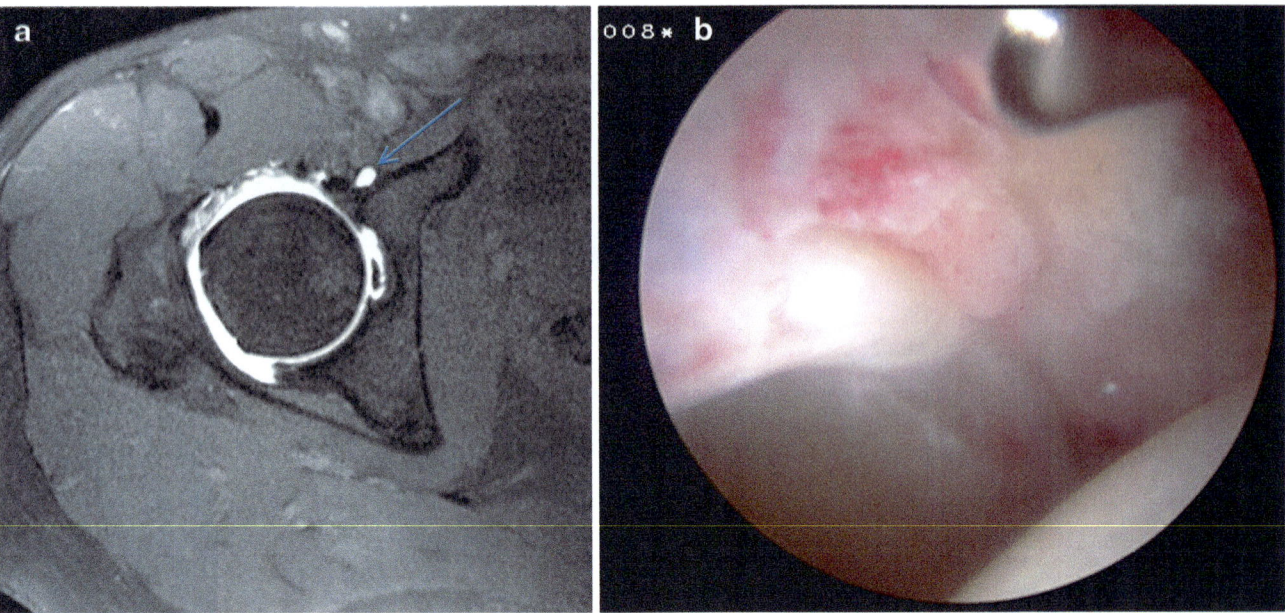

Fig. 28.10 (**a, b**) MR Arthrogram and arthroscopic findings in a 33-year-old male with CAM-type FAI, labral tear, and mild DJD. (**a**) Note the paralabral cyst noted on MRA. (**b**) Same paralabral cyst identified on arthroscopic evaluation

ossicles are all part of the pathologic process. Along with regular radiographic evaluation, MRI or MRA can help evaluate the bony architecture as well as any evidence of abnormal contact between the femoral neck and acetabulum. Associated degenerative changes of the acetabular labrum and/or adjacent articular cartilage can also be evaluated simultaneously [2, 8, 15, 16] and used for preoperative planning in treating patients with symptomatic FAI.

References

1. Ganz R, Parvizi J, Beck M, et al. Femoroacetabular impingement: a cause for osteoarthritis of the hip. Clin Orthop Relat Res. 2003;417:112–20.
2. Tanzer M, Noiseux N. Osseous abnormalities and early osteoarthritis: the role of hip impingement. Clin Orthop Relat Res. 2004; 429:170–7.
3. Beck M, Leunig M, Parvizi J, et al. Anterior femoroacetabular impingement: Part II. Midterm results of surgical treatment. Clin Orthop Relat Res. 2004;418:67–73.
4. Ito K, Leunig M, Ganz R. Histopathologic features of the acetabular labrum in femoroacetabular impingement. Clin Orthop Relat Res. 2004;429:262–71.
5. Ito K, Minka 2nd MA, Leunig M, et al. Femoroacetabular impingement and the cam-effect. A MRI-based quantitative anatomical study of the femoral head-neck offset. J Bone Joint Surg Br. 2001;83:171–6.
6. Jäger M, Wild A, Westhoff B, Krauspe R. Femoroacetabular impingement caused by a femoral osseous head-neck bump deformity: clinical, radiological, and experimental results. J Orthop Sci. 2004;9:256–63.
7. Ganz R, Leunig M, Leunig-Ganz K, Harris WH. The etiology of osteoarthritis of the hip, an integrated mechanical concept. Clin Orthop Relat Res. 2008;466(2):264–72.
8. Lavigne M, Parvizi J, Beck M, et al. Anterior femoroacetabular impingement: Part I. Techniques of joint preserving surgery. Clin Orthop Relat Res. 2004;418:61–6.
9. Nötzli HP, Wyss TF, Stoecklin CH, et al. The contour of the femoral head-neck junction as a predictor for the risk of anterior impingement. J Bone Joint Surg Br. 2002;84:556–60.
10. Reynolds D, Lucas J, Klaue K. Retroversion of the acetabulum. A cause of hip pain. J Bone Joint Surg Br. 1999;81:281–8.
11. Ferguson SJ, Bryant JT, Ganz R, Ito K. The acetabular labrum seal: a poroelastic finite element model. Clin Biomech (Bristol, Avon). 2000;15:463–8.
12. Ferguson SJ, Bryant JT, Ganz R, Ito K. An in vitro investigation of the acetabular labral seal in hip joint mechanics. J Biomech. 2003;36:171–8.
13. Reynolds D, Lucas J, Klaue K. Retroversion of the acetabulum. A cause of hip pain. J Bone Joint Surg Br. 1999;81:281–8. Comment in: J Bone Joint Surg Br. 1999;81:743–4.
14. Pfirrmann CW, Mengiardi B, Dora C, et al. Cam and pincer femoroacetabular impingement: characteristic MR arthrographic findings in 50 patients. Radiology. 2006;240:778–85.
15. Leunig M, Podeszwa D, Beck M, et al. Magnetic resonance arthrography of labral disorders in hips with dysplasia and impingement. Clin Orthop Relat Res. 2004;418:74–80.
16. Beck M, Leunig M, Clarke E, Ganz R. Femoroacetabular impingement as a factor in the development of nonunion of the femoral neck: a report of three cases. J Orthop Trauma. 2004;18: 425–30.
17. Erratum in: Radiology. 2007;244:626. Comment in Radiology. 2007;244:625–6; author reply 626.
18. Bittersohl B, Steppacher S, Haamberg T, Kim YJ, Werlen S, Beck M, Siebenrock KA, Mamisch TC. Cartilage damage in femoroacetabular impingement (FAI): preliminary results on comparison of standard diagnostic vs delayed gadolinium-enhanced magnetic resonance imaging of cartilage (dGEMRIC). Osteoarthritis Cartilage. 2009;17(10):1297–306.
19. Kassarjian A, Yoon LS, Belzile E, et al. Triad of MR arthrographic findings in patients with cam-type femoroacetabular impingement. Radiology. 2005;236:588–92.

20. Stoller DW, Tirman PFJ, Bredella MA. Femoroacetabular impingement. In: Diagnostic imaging: orthopaedics. Salt Lake City, UT: Amirsys; 2004.

Bibliography

Eijer H, Myers SR, Ganz R. Anterior femoro-acetabular impingement after femoral neck fractures. J Orthop Trauma. 2001;15: 475–81.

James SL, Ali K, Malara F, et al. MRI findings of femoroacetabular impingement. AJR Am J Roentgenol. 2006;187:1412–9.

Klaue K, Durnin CW, Ganz R. The acetabular rim syndrome. A clinical presentation of dysplasia of the hip. J Bone Joint Surg Br. 1991;73:423–9.

Leunig M, Beck M, Kalhor M, et al. Fibrocystic changes at anterosuperior femoral neck: prevalence in hips with femoroacetabular impingement. Radiology. 2005;236:237–46.

Leunig M, Beck M, Woo A, et al. Acetabular rim degeneration: a constant finding in the aged hip. Clin Orthop Relat Res. 2003;413:201–7.

Leunig M, Casillas MM, Hamlet M, et al. Slipped capital femoral epiphysis: early mechanical damage to the acetabular cartilage by a prominent femoral metaphysics. Acta Orthop Scand. 2000;71:370–5.

Myers SR, Eijer H, Ganz R. Anterior femoro-acetabular impingement after periacetabular osteotomy. Clin Orthop Relat Res. 1999;363:93–9.

Pitto RP, Klaue K, Ganz R, Ceppatelli S. Acetabular rim pathology secondary to congenital hip dysplasia in the adult. A radiographic study. Chir Organi Mov. 1995;80:361–8.

Sadro C. Current concepts in magnetic resonance imaging of the adult hip and pelvis. Semin Roentgenol. 2000;35:231–48.

Siebenrock KA, Schoeniger R, Ganz R. Anterior femoroacetabular impingement due to acetabular retroversion. Treatment with periacetabular osteotomy. J Bone Joint Surg Am. 2003;85-A(2):278–86.

Stulberg SD, Cordell, LD, Harris WH, et al. Unrecognized childhood hip disease: a major cause of idiopathic osteoarthritis of the hip. In: Proceedings of the third open scientific meeting of the Hip Society. The Hip. St Louis, MO: CV Mosby; 1975. p. 2112–228.

Femoroacetabular Impingement: Femoral Morphology and Correction

29

Misty Suri, John J. Christoforetti, Rami Joseph Elkhechen, and Shawn Evette Johnson

Introduction

There has been an explosion of interest in treating hip pathology arthroscopically recently. One of those entities, femoroacetabular impingement (FAI), has received much of this attention. FAI encompasses both cam-type and pincer-type impingement, both of which need to be addressed for successful management. Harris and colleagues first observed asphericity of the femoral head, referring to its morphology as a "pistol grip deformity" [1]. They discovered a high correlation of early-onset osteoarthritis occurring in patients with this deformity. Ganz and colleagues coined and popularized the theory behind "femoroacetabular impingement," categorizing it into two types: cam and pincer impingement [2]. They felt this entity, and with great foresight, was a precursor for early-onset osteoarthritis. In the late 1990s, safe surgical correction of this type of impingement was described allowing open treatment of this condition in attempt to decelerate the degenerative changes felt to be initiated by this process [3]. As early results of surgical management appeared to be promising, surgeons explored arthroscopic ways to effectively treat FAI minimally invasive [4].

The scope of this chapter will focus on the femoral-sided contribution to FAI, including its diagnosis and surgical

M. Suri, MD (✉) • S.E. Johnson, MD
Department of Sports Medicine, Ochsner Clinic,
Jefferson, LA, USA
e-mail: msuri@ochsner.org; Swtdst96_2@me.com

J.J. Christoforetti, MD
Department of Orthopedic Surgery, Sports Medicine Division,
Allegheny Health Network, West Penn Hospital,
Pittsburgh, PA, USA
e-mail: John.christoforetti@gmail.com

R.J. Elkhechen, MD
Orthopedic Care Specialists of North Palm Beach,
North Palm Beach, FL, USA
e-mail: Rami.joseph.elkhechen@gmail.com

management. After a brief introduction, a case-based format will demonstrate the correlation between imaging studies and surgery for correction of femoroacetabular impingement. Femoral morphology and its correction arthroscopically will be the focus. Review of diagnosis and management will be performed with the aid of three cases:

1. Conventional anterolateral cam lesion in the middle-aged working male
2. Atypical anterior and posterior cam lesions in the younger male athlete
3. Conventional anterolateral cam lesion in the younger female dancer

Pathoanatomy

Cam-type impingement occurs secondarily to an aspherical femoral head rotating into the acetabulum. This morphologic variant in itself may not primarily cause pain, but predisposes the joint to intra-articular pathology that can become symptomatic. For instance, it can lead to delamination of cartilage from subchondral bone as well as tearing of the labrum. These pathologic conditions have most commonly been found on the anterosuperior aspect of the acetabulum correlating to between 1 and 2 o'clock [5]. Acetabular contributions to impingement exist including coxa profunda, protrusio, and retroversion, but their discussion is beyond the scope of this chapter [6]. Many different theories exist to explain the etiology of the asphericity of the femoral head with most focusing on the physis. They include a subtle, subclinical slipped capital femoral epiphysis or a premature asymmetrical closure of the physis [7].

A bimodal distribution of patients has been elucidated, including the middle-aged patient and the younger athletic patient [8]. Both have demonstrated a male predilection and similar cam-related pathology. The difference in timing of presentation is likely due to a higher physiologic demand placed on the hips of the younger patients by their participation in athletic activities.

History and Physical Examination

FAI commonly presents in an insidious and intermittent manner mirroring the repetitive and progressive nature of its development. Many times the patient places higher demands on the hip joint through lifestyle or athletics than it is possible given structural limitations defined by the patient's morphology. Thus, our history taking includes but is not limited to duration of symptoms, daily activities producing symptoms, prolonged positional symptoms, athletic involvement, and lifestyle activities.

Our hip examination is comprehensive including assessment of gait, leg lengths, and noting areas significant for tenderness and/or crepitus. Pertaining specifically to patients with impingement, they can present with reduced range of motion with secondary compensatory mechanisms. Thus, they are assessed for mechanical limitations as well as pain during specific periods in arc of motion and at terminal ranges of motion. To better understand the patient's clinical entity, we attempt to reproduce the patient's symptoms with provocative maneuvers in the office setting. Provocative exams include dynamic internal rotatory impingement (DIRIT) and posteroinferior impingement tests [9]. These maneuvers aid in localizing location of cam lesions when involved in the process of FAI. Weakness of core and hip musculature is demonstrated with our assessment of stepdown and bridge testing [10].

Stand-alone fluoroscopic intra-articular injections of 4–6 mL of 0.25 % bupivacaine and/or corticosteroids provide diagnostic and prognostic value and are performed occasionally to aid in surgical decision making and address patient's expectation of surgical intervention [11]. To ascertain diagnostic value, the percentage relief should be quantified by patient in the hours after injection. Corticosteroids are usually limited to the older population.

Imaging

Imaging modalities play a confirmatory diagnostic role as well as preparation for surgical planning. Complete radiographs are obtained with good techniques including standing AP, Dunn, and cross-table lateral and frog lateral views [12]. Meyer et al. were able to demonstrate that the radiograph that best demonstrates the location of maximal cam deformity is the 45° Dunn view [13]. Although measuring alpha angles remains popular in quantifying cam lesions, there is substantial overlap between measurements between asymptomatic volunteers and symptomatic FAI patients [14]. Thus, the presence of a cam lesion must be viewed in context of the patient's clinical presentation and recreational activities. Appreciating the presence of a cam lesion on radiographs in

the appropriate clinical context provides more importance than accurately assigning a maximum alpha angle value in the diagnosis of symptomatic cam-type impingement. It can be difficult to accurately measure a true peak alpha angle on two-dimensional imaging, demonstrated by Milone et al. [15].

Magnetic resonance arthrography (MRA) with 5–20 mL of gadolinium–DTPA injected fluoroscopically provides very sensitive and specific detection of the presence of cam lesions and soft tissue pathology related to their impingement, such as chondral or labral injury [16]. MRA provides another modality to measure alpha angles on reformats, but with three-dimensional surface renderings unavailable, they do not provide the most accurate method to spatially localize and quantify bony anatomy associated with cam lesions.

Computed tomography (CT) with three-dimensional static renderings and simulation for motion analysis does provide a precise definition of bony anatomy for surgical planning. CT more accurately localizes and quantifies the amount of bony resection needed to relieve impingement in order to best avoid revision surgery as a result of under resection [17]. This is of course at the expense of substantial radiation exposure as novel protocols are not yet routinely available to limit exposure.

Preferred Operative Technique

Hip arthroscopy most frequently is performed in the supine position. Traction is performed and confirmed via fluoroscopy. A standard anterolateral (AL) portal is established followed by a mid-anterior (MA) portal at a 45° angle to the longitudinal axis, 7-cm distal and medial to AL portal [18]. Dry capsulotomy is performed connecting the two portals. At this time, diagnostic arthroscopy of the central compartment is performed, and pathologies secondary to cam lesion are evaluated and addressed. Traction is released and the hip is flexed to approximately 30°. Dimensions of the cam lesion are identified, and a line of demarcation occurring at the junction between normal articular cartilage and abnormal fibrocartilage covering the cam lesion is produced. To facilitate assessment of the cam lesion and its resection, limited 1–1.5-cm "T-capsulotomy" can be performed at this time. Resection of cam lesion is initiated, viewing from the AL portal and working through the MA portal. Femoroplasty is performed by 5-mm spherical burr with goal to recreate the concavity at this junction with a smooth, gradual transition at the chondral-bone interface. Alternating viewing and working portals allow full appreciation of the dimensions of the cam lesion, especially the lateral aspect of an anterosuperior lesion. This is a critical step as incomplete resection to restore the offset remains one of the leading causes of revision surgery [15]. Generally speaking, the MA portal is used to address the medial and anterior aspect of the cam lesion,

Fig. 29.1 After cam lesions have been resected arthroscopically, adequacy of the resection is checked via direct arthroscopic visualization on dynamic examination. Hip is flexed to 90° in neutral rotation

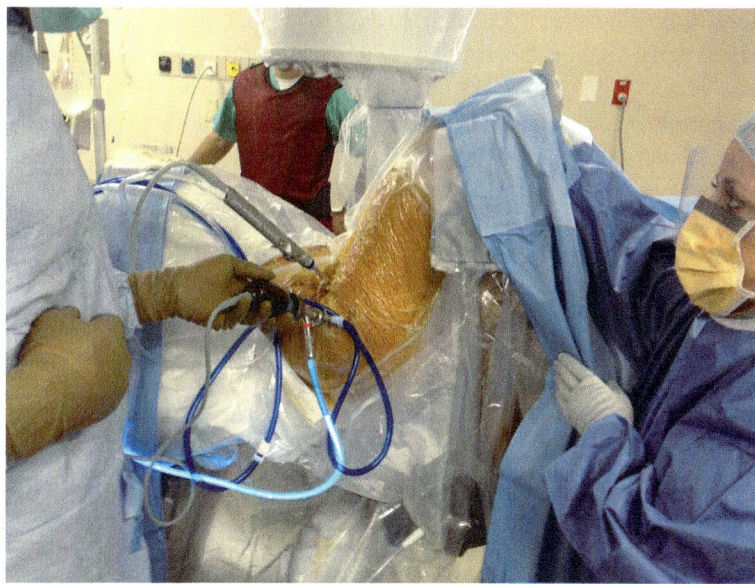

Fig. 29.2 Afterward, hip is rotated internally and externally to confirm no areas of impingement remain

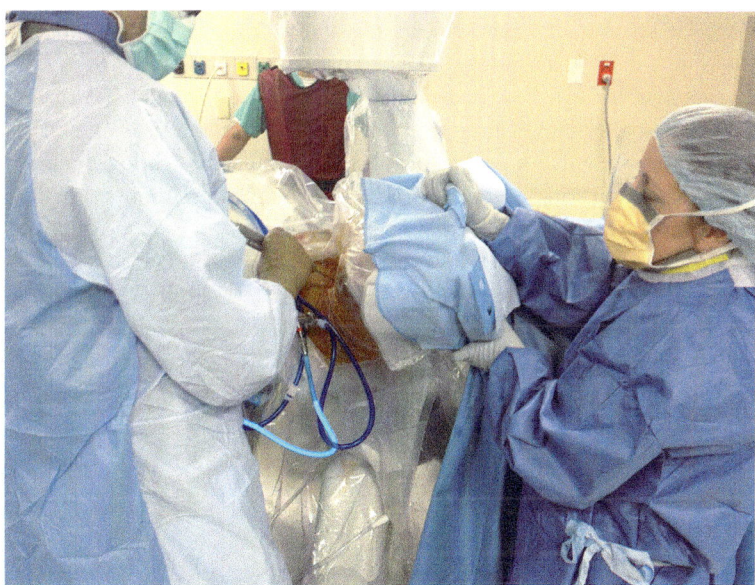

while the anterolateral portal is utilized to treat the lateral and posterior-most extent of the lesion. Strong emphasis is placed on preserving the lateral retinacular vessels and avoidance of notching on the tension side of the femoral neck [19]. All bone debris from femoroplasty is removed to diminish risk of heterotopic ossification.

Periodic arthroscopic dynamic examination cannot be overemphasized at this time to confirm adequate resection. This is performed with the hip flexed to approximately 90° (Fig. 29.1) with visualization of the head-labral junction during internal and external rotation (Fig. 29.2). Goals of the test include demonstration of no remaining impingement between femoral neck and labrum and preservation of seal or

contract between labrum and area of previously resected cam lesion. "T-capsulotomy" closure is performed with one (sometimes two) nonabsorbable high-strength sutures passed with a 90° suture-passing device and tied in a simple fashion.

Rehabilitation

An orthotic hip brace set for 0–90° flexion is utilized postoperatively while awake for 2 weeks, with formal physical therapy beginning on the first postoperative day. In addition, patient is instructed on the use of rotation precaution hip boots and pillow during sleep for 10 days to prevent inadvertent external rotation. Toe-touch weight bearing with crutches is implemented for 3 weeks after a formal femoral osteochondroplasty is performed in order to protect against torsion at the site of resection and femoral neck fracture. Protocol is modified for concomitant procedures such as microfracture by toe-touch weight bearing for 8 weeks, along with continuous passive motion for 6 h daily, lasting 4–6 weeks [20].

Case 1: Classic FAI in the Middle-Aged Working Male

History/Exam

A 49-year-old male, who works as a production supervisor, presented to the orthopedic sports clinic reporting 3 months of left hip pain when ascending stairs and doing computer work, requiring prolonged sitting. His pain measures 5/10 on VAS. He also reports pain with driving and getting into and out of his car. He has a history of right hip arthroscopy for FAI 2 years ago, for which he underwent labral debridement and femoroplasty for large cam lesion. His symptoms improved greater than 80 %. He states that pain is similar in nature to his contralateral hip prior to surgery, and it is preventing him from doing yard work; it requires him to bend down.

His physical examination revealed a positive flexion impingement test and pain with circumduction of the hip. It also demonstrated FABER asymmetry and weakness in hip musculature manifested by positive step-down and bridge tests. Passive range of motion was limited to flexion of 100°, IR 20°, ER 40°, abduction of 45°, and adduction of 20°. Due to the fact that he had failed extensive nonsurgical options and was unable to perform his ADLs, decision was made to proceed with imaging and surgical intervention. He also received 90 % effective, but temporary relief from an intra-articular cortisone injection lasting only a few weeks.

Imaging

Radiographs in Figs. 29.3 and 29.4 reveal extensive asphericity of his femoral head with significant cam lesion. His head–neck offset was significantly diminished and a minimal cross over sign. Lateral center-edge angle was measured at 24° with minimal joint space narrowing. Magnetic resonance imaging with contrast arthrography exhibited a manifestation of impingement via herniation pit on the lateral aspect of the femoral neck on the coronal images (Fig. 29.5). The axial images made it evident that the patient had a labral tear extending from anterior to superior (Fig. 29.6). Some mild adjacent chondral shearing was evident. Significant asphericity was again noted with decreased head–neck offset. Alpha angle was high and evidence of impingement was noted on the lateral aspect of head–neck junction.

Arthroscopy

Patient was taken to the operating room for hip arthroscopy via technique stated above. After capsulotomy and labral repair were performed under distraction, arthroscopy of the peripheral compartment with the hip reduced revealed significant cam

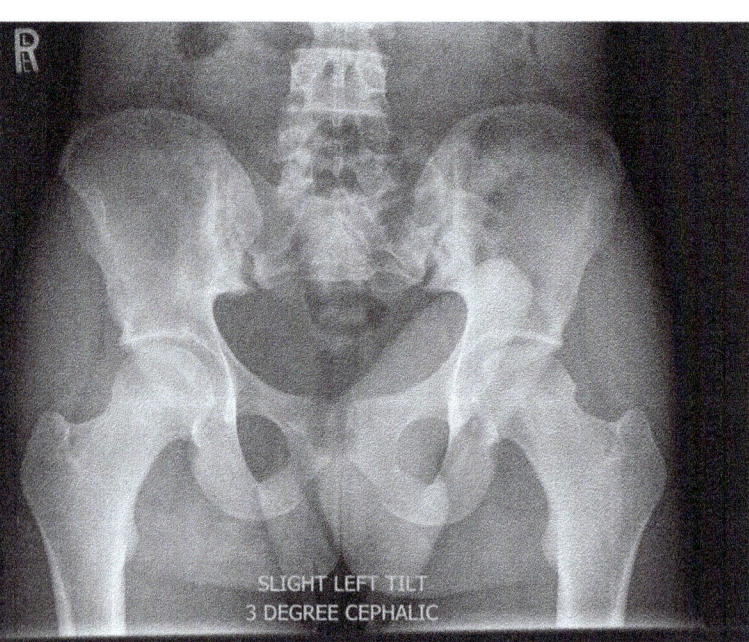

Fig. 29.3 AP pelvis demonstrates anterolateral cam lesion of left hip and loss of asphericity manifested by decrease in femoral head–neck offset when compared to contralateral hip

Fig. 29.4 Dunn view radiographs confirm this loss of femoral head–neck offset when compared to contralateral hip which has undergone previous hip arthroscopy, femoroplasty

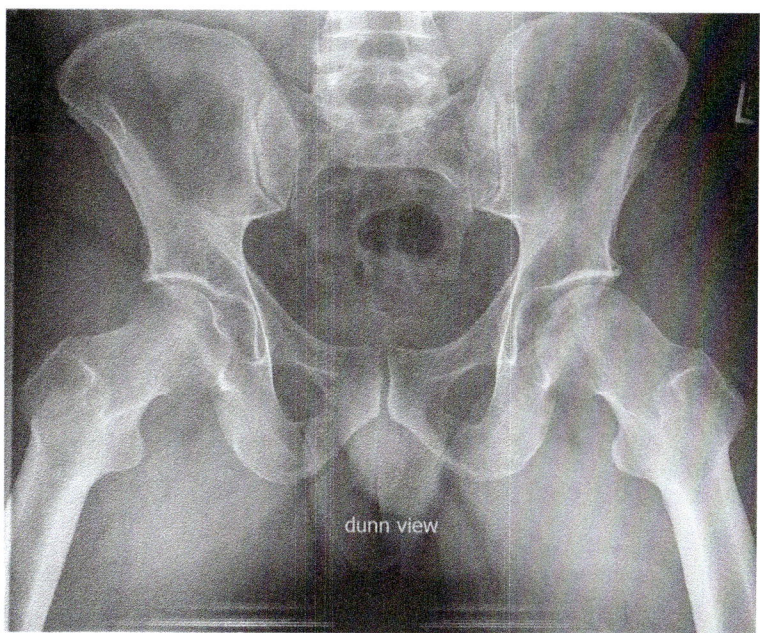

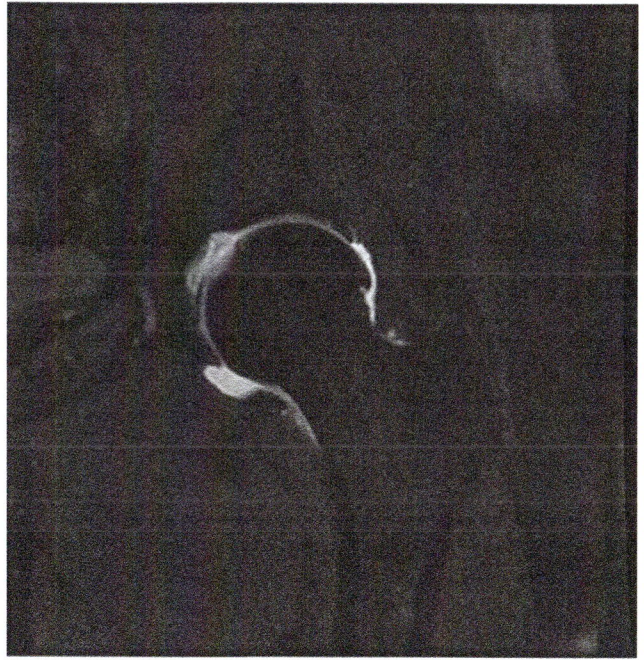

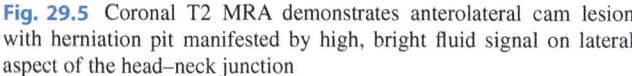

Fig. 29.5 Coronal T2 MRA demonstrates anterolateral cam lesion with herniation pit manifested by high, bright fluid signal on lateral aspect of the head–neck junction

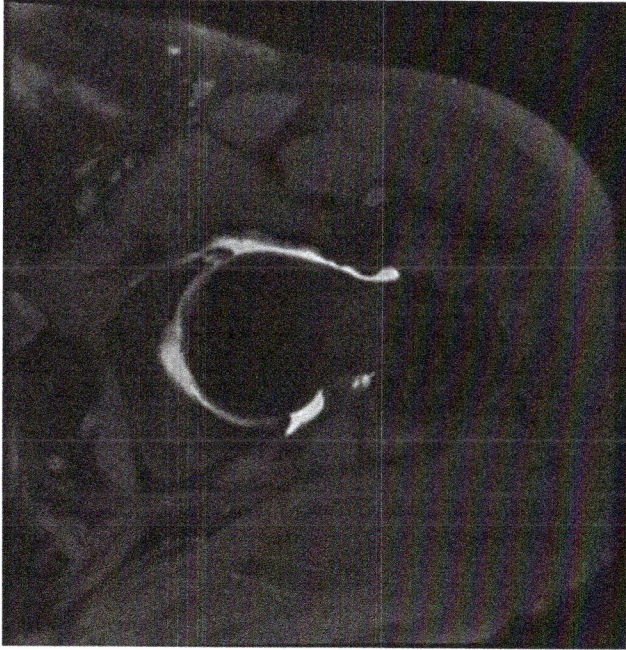

Fig. 29.6 Axial T2 MRA demonstrates same anterior cam lesion with adjacent anterior labral tear suggested by high, bright fluid signal at the labral–chondral junction

lesion on the anterolateral aspect of the head–neck junction seen in Fig. 29.7. Areas of impingement were noted and quantified in this area on arthroscopic impingement test. Thus, cam lesion was removed utilizing a 5-mm-round burr while viewing from the anterolateral portal and working through the mid-anterior portal (Fig. 29.8). A critical step in fully appreciating and adequately resecting the entire lesion is to switch the viewing and working portals in order to obtain a different vantage point.

Figure 29.9 demonstrates this and allows complete resection of the lateral gutter. Cam resection measured 5-mm deep and 35-mm wide from a medial 6 o'clock position to a lateral 12 o'clock position. Periodic dynamic examination was performed to indicate sufficient resection with no impingement.

After completion of femoroplasty, hip flexion is removed in neutral rotation and "T-capsulotomy" closure is performed with one nonabsorbable high-strength suture passed with a

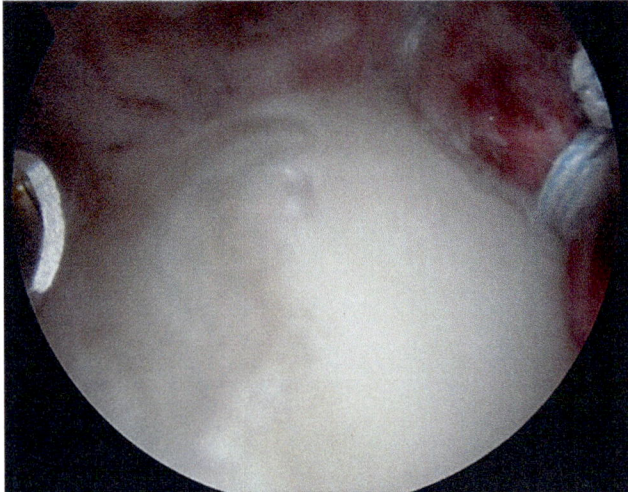

Fig. 29.7 Anterolateral cam lesion apparent during visualization of peripheral compartment via standard anterolateral portal after capsulotomy and labral repair seen in the background

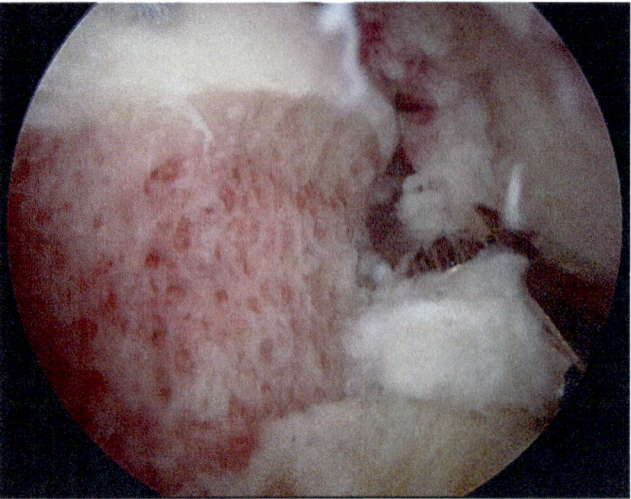

Fig. 29.9 Critical step in relieving entire cam lesion involves moving arthroscope to the distal anterior portal in order to adequately visualize and resect the lateral-most aspect of the lesion

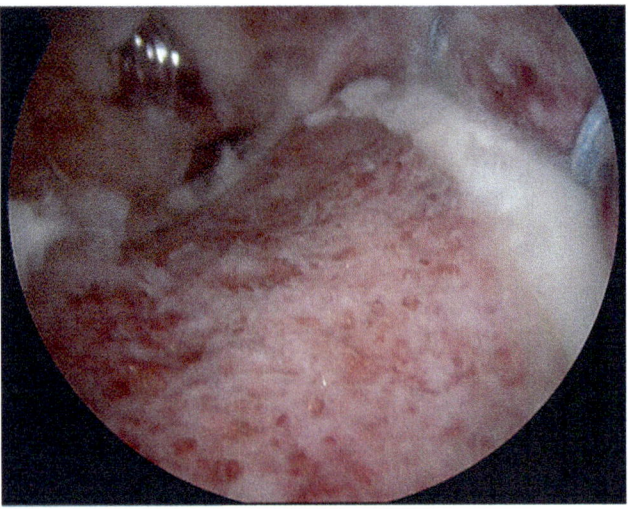

Fig. 29.8 Combination of electrocautery and high-speed burr is utilized to resect the cam lesion to reestablish the femoral head–neck offset and relieve source of impingement

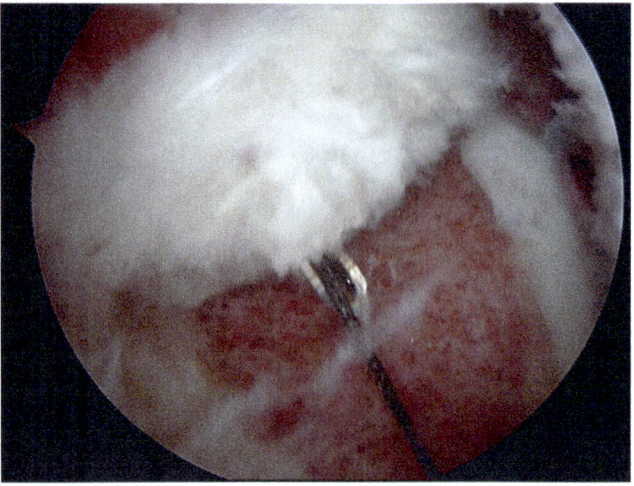

Fig. 29.10 A 90° suture-passing device is used via cannula in the mid-anterior portal to pass a nonabsorbable high-strength suture, aiding to close "T-capsulotomy"

90° suture-passing device and tied in a simple fashion (Figs. 29.10, 29.11, and 29.12).

Discussion

The clinical history of reduced hip motion and increasing pain with deep-flexion activity coupled with prior success with contralateral side correction indicated imaging with MRI for this case. The MRI signs of articular chondral and labrum tearing in the anterior superior regions of the hip along with the femoral head asphericity were pertinent positives. Pertinent negatives included absence of severe subchondral cystic change and bone edema within the femoral head or acetabulum. The intraoperative decision making describes the importance of correlating preoperative imaging and exam findings with arthroscopic exam to adequately correct impingement.

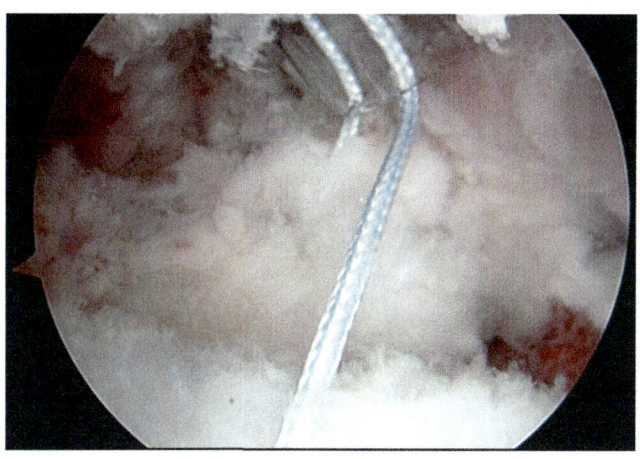

Fig. 29.11 Nonabsorbable high-strength suture visible passed through each limb of the "T-capsulotomy," exiting cannula via the mid-anterior portal

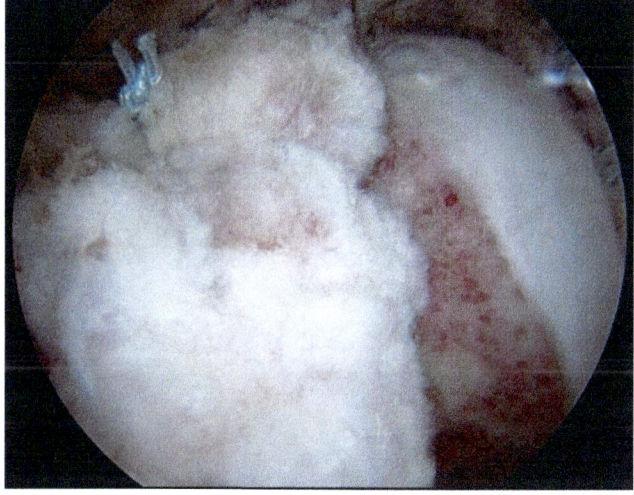

Fig. 29.12 One nonabsorbable high-strength suture tied in a simple fashion demonstrating closure of "T-capsulotomy" and good coverage of femoral neck and femoroplasty region

Case 2: Atypical FAI in the Younger Male Athlete

History/Exam

A 17-year-old high school baseball player presented with bilateral hip pain, L>R, for the last 5 years that worsened with sports activity and twisting motions. He rated the pain as a 5/10 on a daily basis on the VAS. He had recently stopped participating in baseball due to his hip pain. The only relief from pain was rest from activities and anti-inflammatory medication.

On physical examination, there was no tenderness to palpation or crepitus. Both flexion impingement and posterior

rim impingement tests were markedly positive. He also demonstrated a positive posterior rim impingement test. There was pain with circumduction of the hip. Patient also demonstrated weakness in hip musculature manifested by positive step-down and bridge tests. Patient's passive range of motion was limited to flexion of 110°, IR 30°, ER 40°, abduction of 45°, and adduction of 20°. These symptoms with prolonged duration and recent regression in his chosen sport facilitated the decision to proceed with imaging studies and subsequent intervention.

Imaging

Radiographs demonstrated asphericity of the femoral head in bilateral hips. When examining the left hip, it was evident in Fig. 29.13 on the frog leg radiograph that there was a large posterior cam lesion in addition to the standard anterolateral lesion causing classic FAI. The lateral center-edge angle was measured at 35° with maintained joint space [21]. Magnetic resonance imaging with contrast arthrography confirmed the presence of anterior and posterior cam lesions. It also suggested a large labral tear manifested by significant contrast visualized medial to the labrum (Figs. 29.14 and 29.15). Enhancement of the tear is secondary to the use of contrast to improve sensitivity and specificity.

In addition, fine 2-mm-cut CT scan of the hip joints was performed to characterize detailed bony anatomy of cam lesions in order for surgical planning. On axial CT scan in Fig. 29.16, posterior impingement is evident by a posterior cam lesion and herniation pit as a result of impingement episodes. Three-dimensional reconstruction aids in full appreciation, spatial anatomical localization, and quantification of the cam lesion size. Figure 29.17 exhibits the large anterolateral lesion with loss of femoral sphericity.

Surgery

Given the presence of posterior cam lesions, a decision was made to perform surgical hip dislocation in order to effectively and safely resect them (Fig. 29.18). The procedure is performed utilizing a technique described by Ganz et al. [22], with the patient in the lateral decubitus position. A straight incision is made centered over the anterior border of the greater trochanter. Dissection is carried through the subcutaneous tissue down to the deep fascia. Gibson's interval was identified and used between the tensor fascia lata and gluteus maximus. Care needs to be taken when performing trochanteric osteotomy, preserving insertions of the gluteus medius/minimus and vastus lateralis tendons. Incomplete osteotomy is performed after which the fragment is levered anteriorly, allowing controlled fracture of the anterior cortex. Z-shaped

Fig. 29.13 Frog leg radiograph demonstrates bilateral anterior cam lesion with suspicion of posterior cam lesion and impingement in the left hip

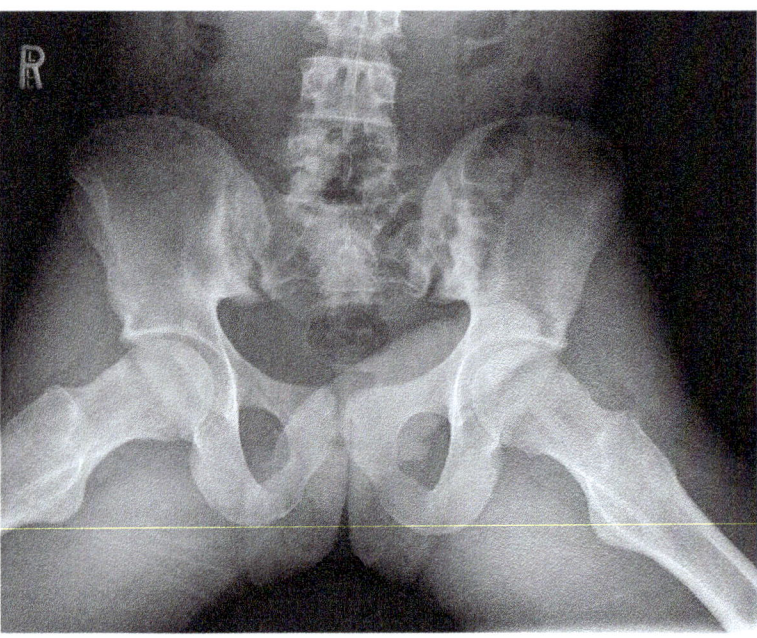

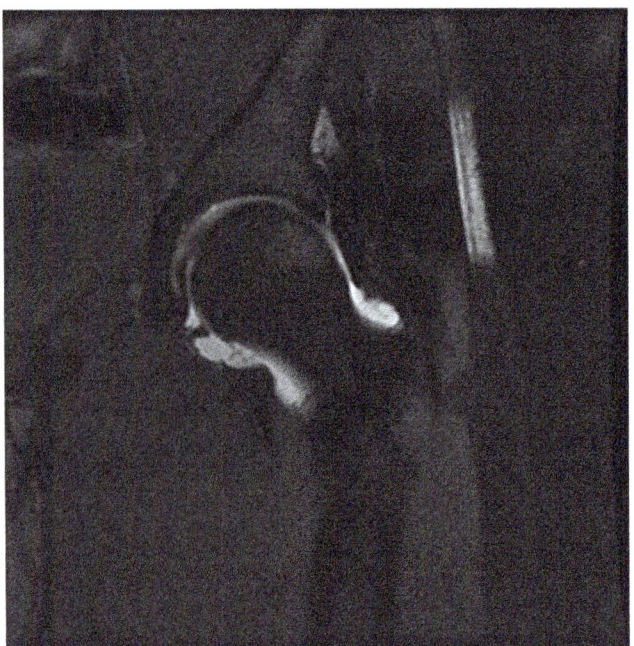

Fig. 29.14 Coronal T2 MRA demonstrates asphericity of femoral head with evidence of a large anterior cam lesion and loss of femoral head–neck offset. A labral tear is suggested by a bright fluid signal medial to the labral tissue

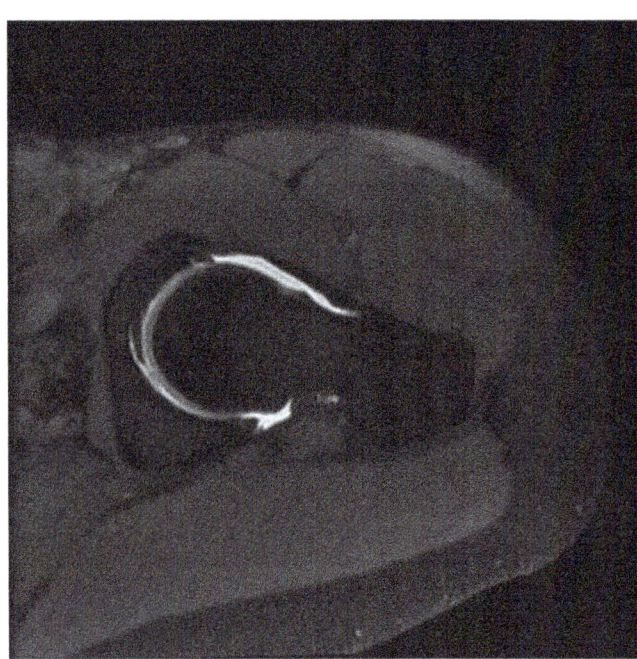

Fig. 29.15 Axial T2 MRA identifies anterior and posterior cam lesions with evidence of a labral tear suggested by a bright fluid signal medial to the labrum

capsulotomy is performed for visualization followed by incising of the ligamentum teres, utilizing ligamentum teres skid knife or curved Mayo scissors.

Flexion and external rotation allows for controlled anterior dislocation of the femoral head and assessment of chondral surfaces, cam lesions, and labral pathology. Figure 29.19 reveals the posterior cam lesion well by tangentially viewing the posterior aspect of the femoral head. Resection of the lesion is performed via rongeur and high-speed burr reestablishing the sphericity of the femoral head posteriorly (Fig. 29.20). Attention is turned to the anterolateral cam lesion in Fig. 29.21. There is obvious loss of femoral head–neck offset at the site of the forceps. A semicircular plastic template can be used to mark out the osteotomy site for the

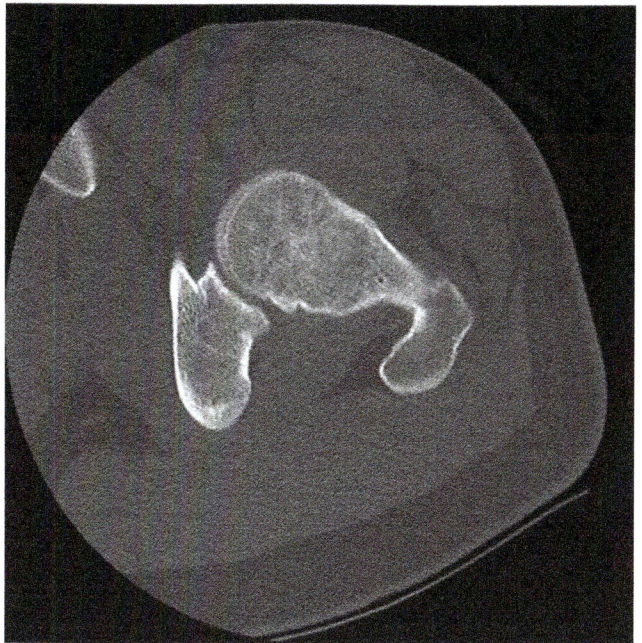

Fig. 29.16 Axial CT scan clearly demonstrates anterior and posterior cam lesions. Herniation pit is demonstrated adjacent to the posterior lesion

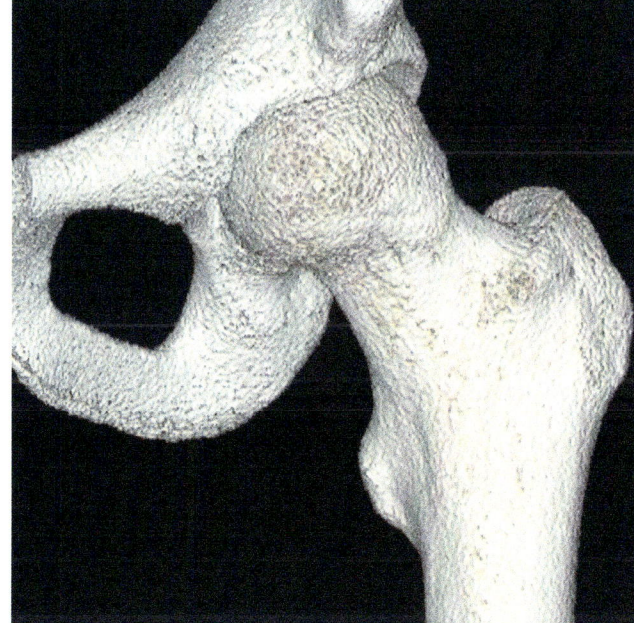

Fig. 29.17 CT scan was reconstructed to produce this three-dimensional image to aid the understanding of the anterior cam lesion's spatial relationship

cam lesion. An osteotome in Fig. 29.22 is used in a controlled manner to perform the resection. Reevaluation of the sphericity with the semicircular plastic template and the use of a high speed burr and rongeur to fine-tune resection is

performed (Fig. 29.23). Final resection of femoral head and reestablishment of femoral head–neck offset is evident in Fig. 29.24.

After completion of the cam resections, the labral tear is addressed. Unlike in arthroscopy where traction is being performed via hip table while addressing central compartment and labral pathology, open surgery precludes this. Thus, these pathologies are addressed while the hip is dislocated for access. Discussion of these is beyond the scope of this chapter and will be discussed in another chapter. Upon completion of central compartment and labral pathology, the hip is subsequently reduced and a dynamic open impingement test is performed as in Fig. 29.25. Goals of the test include demonstration of no remaining impingement between femoral neck and labrum and preservation of seal or contract between labrum and area of previously resected cam lesion.

Discussion

The MRI findings in this case confirmed the severity of the posterior femoral deformity suggested by plain radiography. Expert understanding of the anatomical limitations of arthroscopic correction of aspherical femoral head includes the knowledge that limitations exist. This case highlights the appropriateness of considering open surgical dislocation when MRI and radiographs significant offset abnormality or proximity of femoral deformity to the lateral epiphyseal vessels.

Case 3: Classic FAI in the Younger Female Dancer

History/Exam

A 21-year-old college student, working as a dancer, presented with right hip pain that began 4 months previously after attempting to perform a dance move at work involving a quick squat and external rotation of both hips. She described her symptoms as a deep-seated groin pain exacerbated by hip flexion and abduction activities. She denied any snapping episodes. She was unable to continue dancing for work as well as difficulty getting into and out of her car.

On physical examination, she had no tenderness to palpation or snapping appreciated when ranging the hip joint. She had a classically positive flexion impingement test as well as pain on pure abduction of the hip. She demonstrated mild weakness with step-down and bridge testing. Her range of motion was limited in flexion to 110°, IR to 20°, ER to 50°, abduction to 35° with pain, and adduction of 20°. Patient presented with an MRI already performed at an outside institution.

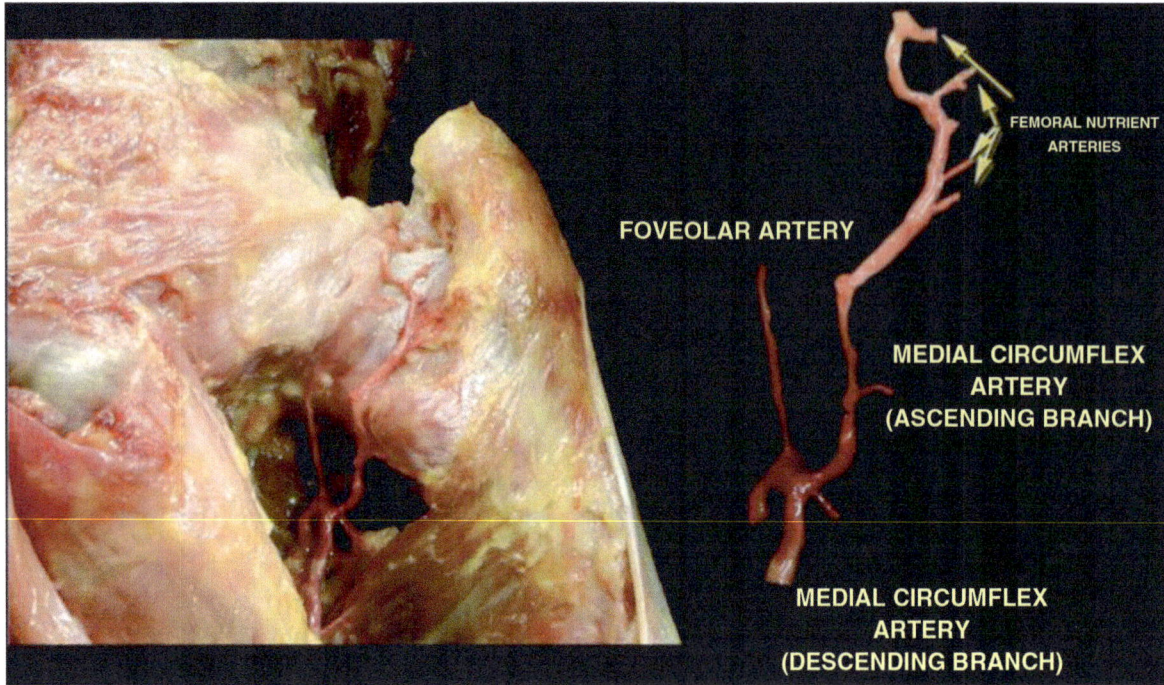

Fig. 29.18 Anatomical study of the hip demonstrates that the main blood supply of the adult femoral head or medial femoral circumflex artery courses along the posteromedial aspect of the femoral neck

Fig. 29.19 Tips of forceps demonstrate posterior cam lesion after surgical anterior hip dislocation of left hip

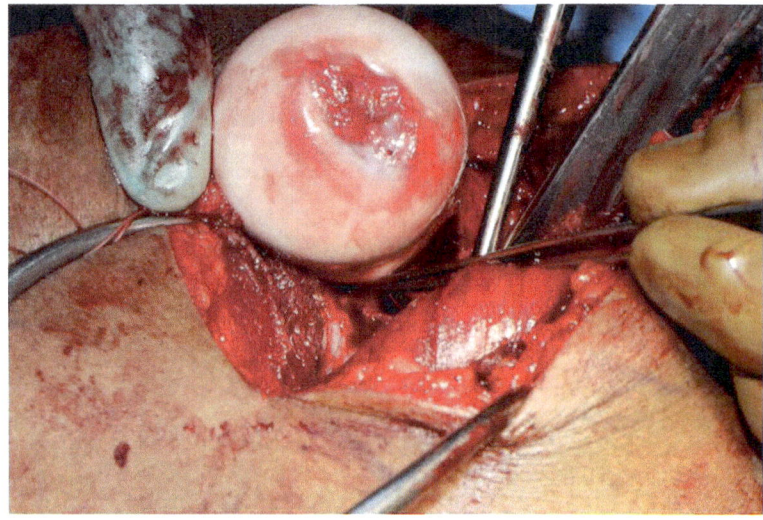

Imaging

Radiographs demonstrated mild asphericity of the femoral heads in the right hip. There was no crossover sign present and the lateral center-edge angle measured 31° without narrowing of the joint space. Magnetic resonance imaging had been performed without contrast at an outside facility but confirmed the presence of a cam lesion on the anterolateral aspect of the neck more conspicuous on the lateral aspect of the T2 coronal images (Figs. 29.26 and 29.27). Also present was a likely disruption of the labrum at its junction with the chondral surface. She was sent for an intra-articular bupivacaine to confirm diagnosis as well as predict success of surgical intervention. She received 100 % relief for 48 h, and pain had regressed back to baseline by two weeks postinjection. Thus, she was indicated for hip arthroscopy.

Arthroscopy

Patient was taken to the operating room for hip arthroscopy via preferred technique. After capsulotomy and labral repair were performed, arthroscopy of the peripheral compartment with distraction removed revealed significant cam lesion on

Fig. 29.20 Tips of forceps demonstrate area where posterior cam lesion had been excised using combination of rongeur and high-speed burr technique

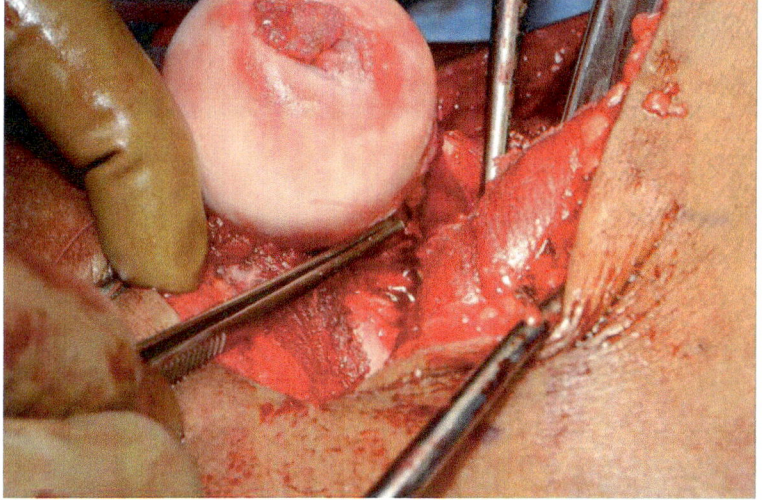

Fig. 29.21 Tips of forceps demonstrate a large anterior cam lesion with significant asphericity of femoral head

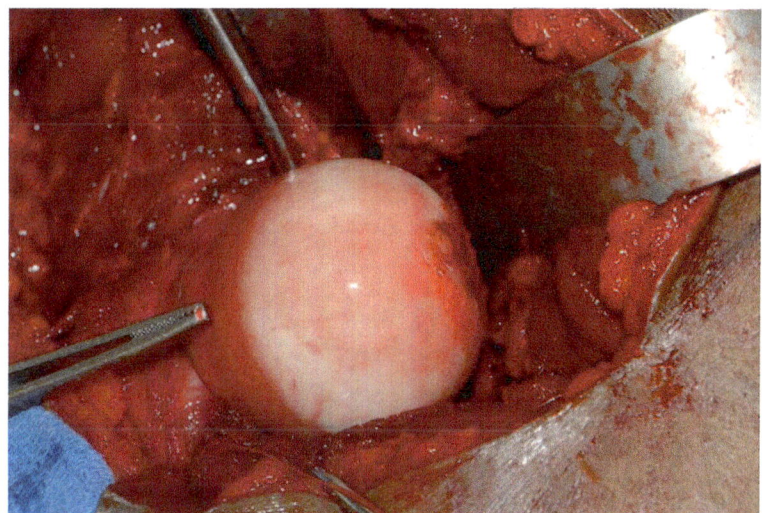

Fig. 29.22 Osteotome being used at the fibrocartilage-articular cartilage junction of the femoral head in order to remove anterior cam lesion

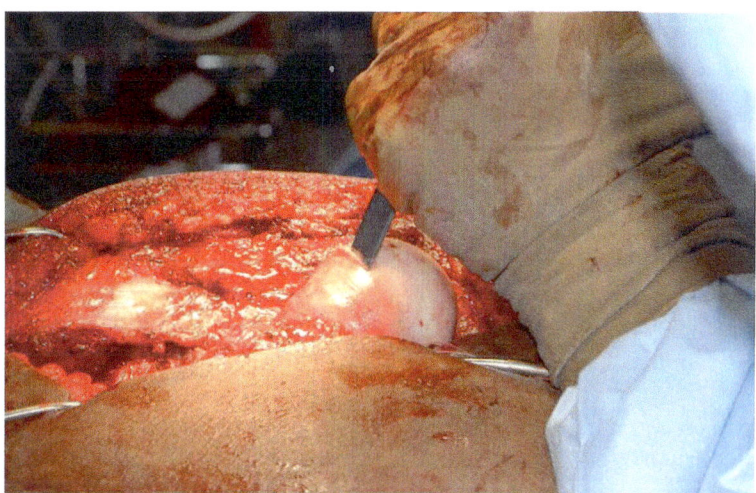

Fig. 29.23 Completed resections of both anterior and posterior cam lesions causing impingement

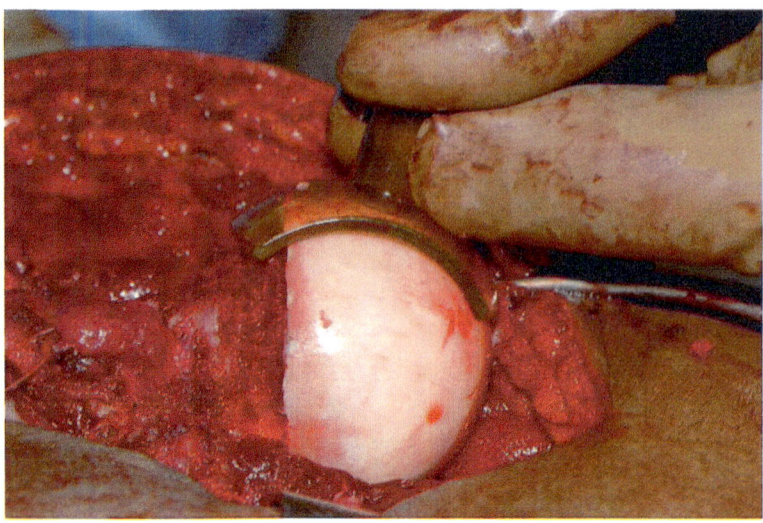

Fig. 29.24 Semicircular plastic template is used to confirm adequate resection of cam lesions

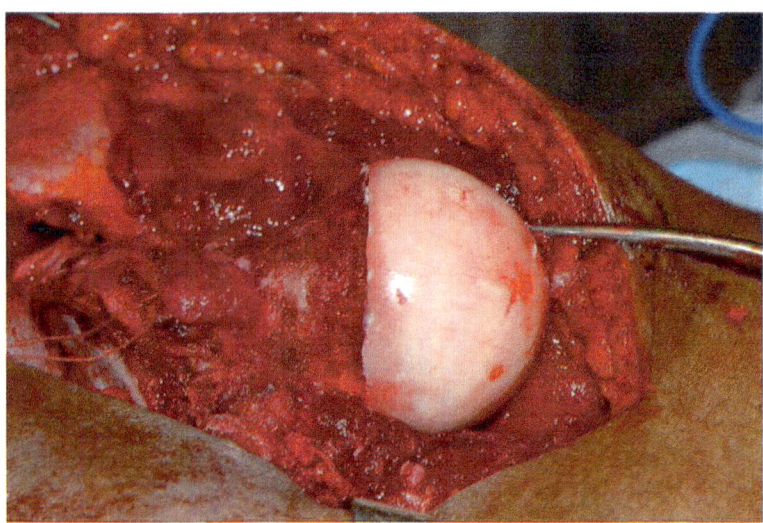

Fig. 29.25 Hip is subsequently reduced and final check is performed under direct visualization with a dynamic examination. Labral repair can be visualized here with cam resections

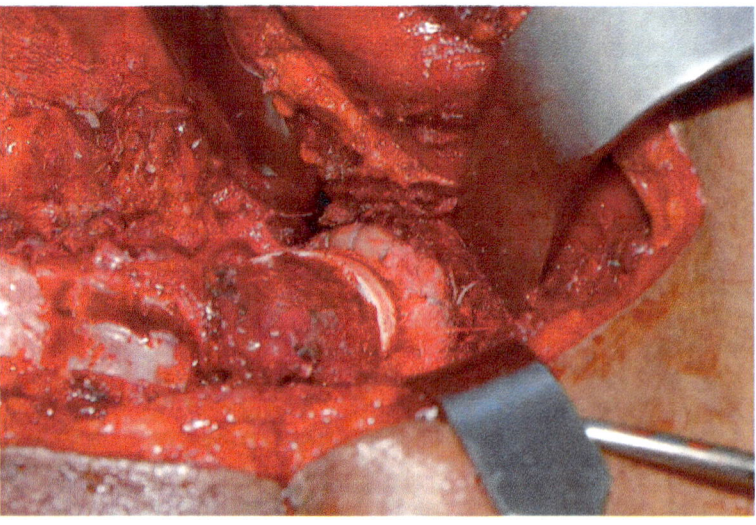

Fig. 29.26 Coronal T2 MRI sequence shows asphericity of the femoral head on lateral margin of head–neck junction with possible disruption at the chondral–labral junction laterally

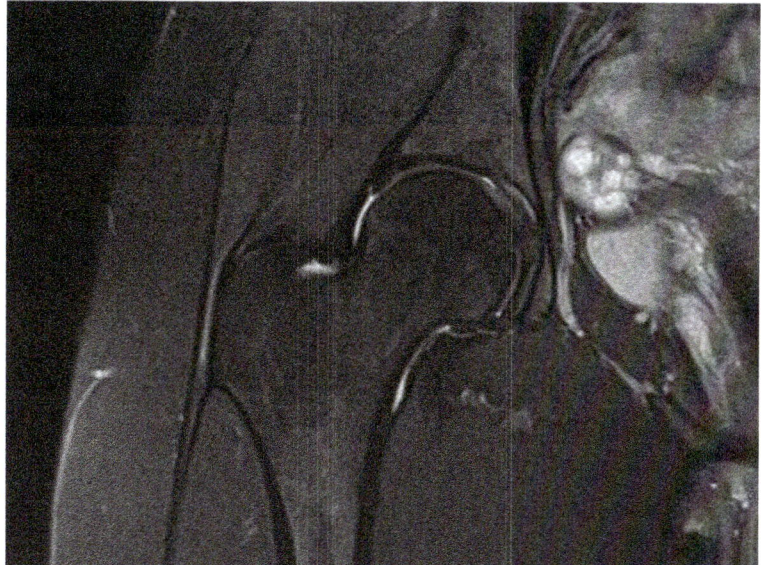

Fig. 29.27 Axial T2 MRI appears relatively normal with mild loss in head–neck offset anteriorly

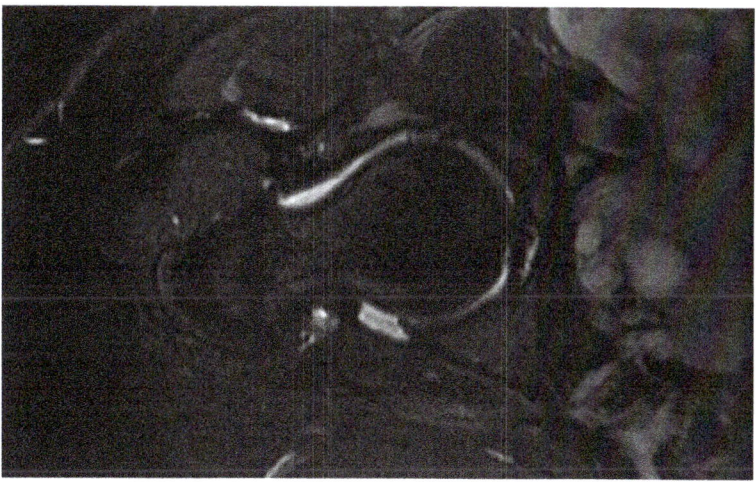

anterolateral aspect of the head–neck junction seen in Fig. 29.28. Areas of impingement were noted and quantified in this area on arthroscopic impingement test. Thus, cam lesion was removed utilizing a 5-mm-round burr while viewing from the anterolateral portal and working through the mid-anterior portal (Fig. 29.29). Again, to fully appreciate and adequately resect the entire lesion, we switch to the mid-anterior portal for viewing in order to visualize the lateral aspect of her lesion. Figure 29.30 demonstrates this and allows complete resection of the lateral gutter. Cam resection measured 3-mm deep and 30-mm wide from a medial 6 o'clock position to a lateral 12 o'clock position. Periodic

dynamic examination was performed to indicate sufficient resection with no impingement.

Discussion

This case reinforces the role for understanding isolated mild femoral deformity and activity in treating labrum tears. The MRI again instructs awareness of chondrolabrum tearing being the typical variation of labrum tearing in the hip. The mechanism of sheer force disrupting the articular

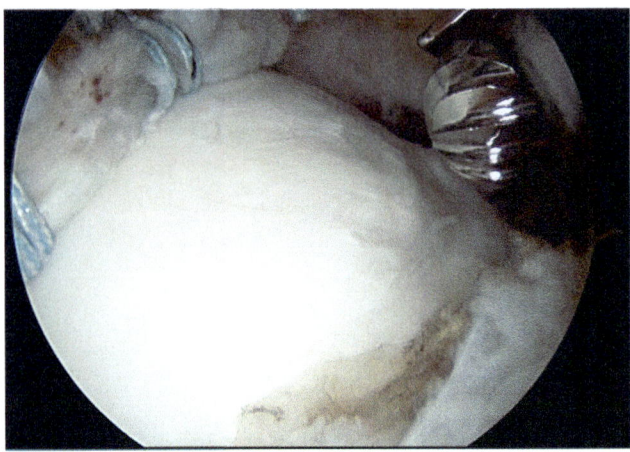

Fig. 29.28 Viewing via anterolateral portal, cam lesion visualized adjacent to the newly repaired labrum. Appearance of cam lesion is different from articular cartilage in color and texture

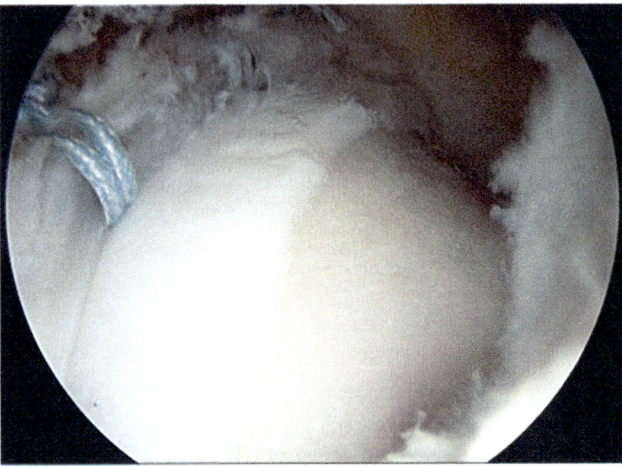

Fig. 29.29 Viewing from the anterolateral portal., femoral head–neck junction has been contoured by high-speed burr to reestablish head–neck offset anteriorly

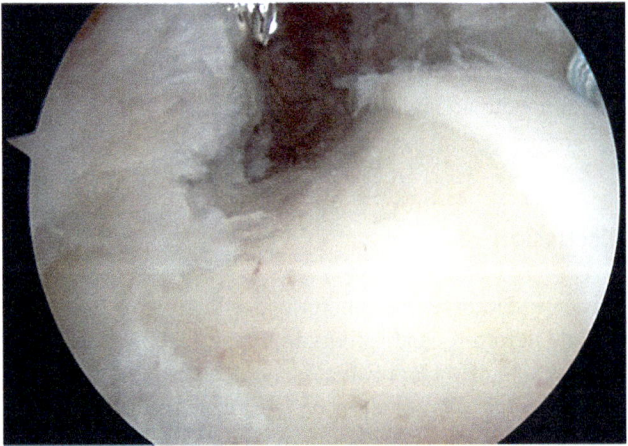

Fig. 29.30 Viewing from the mid-anterior portal, lateral aspect of the lesion is resected to the 12 o'clock position

cartilage/labrum juncture due to femoral asphericity leads to the articular surface tearing from the labrum, rather than the labrum tearing away from the acetabular rim.

Conclusions

The interaction between morphologically abnormal femur and acetabulum combined with extensive, vigorous demands placed on the hip joint culminates in FAI, manifesting as repetitive and progressive intra-articular soft tissue injury. Although cam impingement itself is not painful, it may contribute and lead to pathology that becomes symptomatic over time, including chondral delamination and labral tears. While most cam lesions can be comfortably treated arthroscopically, posterior lesions are difficult to access and thus can safely be treated utilizing an open surgical hip dislocation popularized by Ganz. The key lies in detection and treatment of symptomatic patients prior to the secondary arthritic-disease process becoming too advanced to reasonably benefit from hip preservation surgery. Principles for evaluation of patients presenting with the appropriate clinical picture and lifestyle activities presented in this chapter along with correlation to appropriate imaging modalities allow for appropriate intervention and halt progression of a deleterious process.

References

1. Harris WH. Etiology of osteoarthritis of the hip. Clin Orthop Relat Res. 1986;213:20–33.
2. Ganz R, Parvizi J, Beck M, Leunig M, Notzli H, Siebenrock KA. Femoroacetabular impingement: a cause for osteoarthritis of the hip. Clin Orthop Relat Res. 2003;417:112–20.
3. Ganz R, Gill TJ, Gautier E, Ganz K, Krugel N, Berlemann U. Surgical dislocation of the adult hip a technique with full access to the femoral head and acetabulum without the risk of avascular necrosis. J Bone Joint Surg. 2001;83(8):1119–24.
4. Byrd JW. The role of hip arthroscopy in the athletic hip. Clin Sports Med. 2006;25(2):255–78, viii.
5. Ito K, Minka 2nd MA, Leunig M, Werlen S, Ganz R. Femoroacetabular impingement and the cam-effect. A MRI-based quantitative anatomical study of the femoral head-neck offset. J Bone Joint Surg Br. 2001;83(2):171–6.
6. Audenaert EA, Peeters I, Vigneron L, Baelde N, Pattyn C. Hip morphological characteristics and range of internal rotation in femoroacetabular impingement. Am J Sports Med. 2012;40(6):1329–36.
7. Leunig M, Casillas MM, Hamlet M, Hersche O, Notzli H, Slongo T, et al. Slipped capital femoral epiphysis: early mechanical damage to the acetabular cartilage by a prominent femoral metaphysis. Acta Orthop Scand. 2000;71(4):370–5.
8. Byrd JW, Jones KS. Arthroscopic femoroplasty in the management of cam-type femoroacetabular impingement. Clin Orthop Relat Res. 2009;467(3):739–46.
9. Martin HD, Kelly BT, Leunig M, Philippon MJ, Clohisy JC, Martin RL, et al. The pattern and technique in the clinical evaluation of the adult hip: the common physical examination tests of hip specialists. Arthroscopy. 2010;26(2):161–72.

10. Chinkulprasert C, Vachalathiti R, Powers CM. Patellofemoral joint forces and stress during forward step-up, lateral step-up, and forward step-down exercises. J Orthop Sports Phys Ther. 2011;41(4): 241–8.
11. Nepple JJ, Prather H, Trousdale RT, Clohisy JC, Beaule PE, Glyn-Jones S, et al. Clinical diagnosis of femoroacetabular impingement. J Am Acad Orthop Surg. 2013;21 Suppl 1:S16–9.
12. Clohisy JC, Carlisle JC, Beaulé PE, Kim Y-J, Trousdale RT, Sierra RJ, et al. A systematic approach to the plain radiographic evaluation of the young adult hip. J Bone Joint Surg. 2008;90 Suppl 4:47–66.
13. Meyer DC, Beck M, Ellis T, Ganz R, Leunig M. Comparison of six radiographic projections to assess femoral head/neck asphericity. Clin Orthop Relat Res. 2006;445:181–5.
14. Sutter R, Dietrich TJ, Zingg PO, Pfirrmann CW. How useful is the alpha angle for discriminating between symptomatic patients with cam-type femoroacetabular impingement and asymptomatic volunteers? Radiology. 2012;264(2):514–21.
15. Milone MT, Bedi A, Poultsides L, Magennis E, Byrd JW, Larson CM, et al. Novel CT-based three-dimensional software improves the characterization of cam morphology. Clin Orthop Relat Res. 2013;471(8):2484–91.
16. Leunig M, Podeszwa D, Beck M, Werlen S, Ganz R. Magnetic resonance arthrography of labral disorders in hips with dysplasia and impingement. Clin Orthop Relat Res. 2004;418:74–80.
17. Bedi A, Dolan M, Magennis E, Lipman J, Buly R, Kelly BT. Computer-assisted modeling of osseous impingement and resection in femoroacetabular impingement. Arthroscopy. 2012;28(2):204–10.
18. Skendzel JG, Philippon MJ. Management of labral tears of the hip in young patients. Orthop Clin North Am. 2013;44(4):477–87.
19. McCormick F, Kleweno CP, Kim YJ, Martin SD. Vascular safe zones in hip arthroscopy. Am J Sports Med. 2011;39 Suppl:64s–71.
20. Steadman JR, Rodkey WG, Rodrigo JJ. Microfracture: surgical technique and rehabilitation to treat chondral defects. Clin Orthop Relat Res. 2001;391(Suppl):S362–9.
21. Philippon MJ, Briggs KK, Yen YM, Kuppersmith DA. Outcomes following hip arthroscopy for femoroacetabular impingement with associated chondrolabral dysfunction: minimum two-year follow-up. J Bone Joint Surg. 2009;91(1):16–23.
22. Espinosa N, Beck M, Rothenfluh DA, Ganz R, Leunig M. Treatment of femoro-acetabular impingement: preliminary results of labral refixation. Surgical technique. J Bone Joint Surg Am. 2007;89 Suppl 2 Pt.1:36–53.

Acetabular Fossa, Femoral Fovea, and the Ligamentum Teres

Jason W. Folk, Fernando Portilho Ferro, Marc J. Philippon, and Bryan Whitfield

Introduction

While pathology of the acetabular labrum and chondrolabral junction is often studied, lesions and pathology associated with the ligamentum teres and acetabular cotyloid fossa have been clearly elucidated as an important and perhaps overlooked source of nonarthritic hip pain and mechanical symptoms. Tears of the ligamentum teres, synovial disorders such as synovial chondromatosis, and stenosis of the cotyloid fossa are representative of the more commonly encountered pathologies in this area. Although recently defined physical examination tests exist, imaging and arthroscopy remain essential for diagnosis and management of these injuries.

The precise function of the ligamentum teres (LT) remains unclear and multiple theories exist. Some authors' work demonstrated evidence of a role as a static stabilizer of the hip joint with contributions to force and fluid distribution. Other sources diverge from this view, characterizing the LT as a functionless remnant of embryonic tissue [1–3]. Most recently, theories propose the LT as a possible source of proprioceptive and somatosensory feedback [4] and also as a stabilizer of the hip joint. Basic science evidence has shown that the LT resists dislocation and microinstability with

J.W. Folk, MD (✉) • B. Whitfield, MD
Department of Orthopedic Surgery and Sports Medicine, Greenville Health System—Steadman Hawkins Clinic of the Carolinas, University of South Carolina School of Medicine, Greenville, SC, USA
e-mail: jfolk@ghs.org; bwhitfield@ghs.org

F.P. Ferro, MD
Department of Orthopedic Surgery,
Hospital de Acidentados, Goiânia, Brazil
e-mail: fpferro@gmail.com

M.J. Philippon, MD
The Steadman Clinic and Steadman Philippon Research Institute, Vail, CO, USA
e-mail: drphilippon@sprivail.org

tensile strength comparable to the anterior cruciate ligament (ACL) in a porcine model [1]. This stabilization role seems to be even more pronounced in dysplastic hips [5]. Some have established its role as an important static stabilizer of the joint and have advocated reconstruction in the setting of symptomatic insufficiency [6]. The role of the LT as a source of hip pain is more well established [5–11].

Pathology of the LT includes both traumatic and nontraumatic tears. Gray and Villar introduced a classification of LT tears that is comprised of a type I full-thickness tear, a type II partial-thickness tear, and a type III degenerative tear [12]. Botser et al. proposed a descriptive classification that quantifies the degree of tearing. It includes a type I <50 % partial-thickness tear, a type II >50 % but <100 % partial-thickness tear, and a type III full-thickness tear [13]. Nontraumatic tears of the LT have been associated with developmental dislocation of the hip, Legg–Calve–Perthes disease, and osteoarthritis/degenerative signs [13–16]. Domb et al. have also established associations between acetabular bony morphology and patient age to the presence of LT tears. Tears of the LT were more frequent in those with a diminished lateral acetabular coverage as defined by a decreased lateral center-edge angle of Wiberg in conjunction with an elevated Tonnis acetabular inclination angle. An increased prevalence of LT tears was also associated with age >30 years [17]. Traumatic rupture of the LT secondary to hip dislocation is a well-recognized cause of tears as well, and it is not known how much this may contribute to recurrent instability in these patients [5–7, 9–11].

Clinically, patients with a clear injury mechanism resulting in acute rupture may subsequently report symptoms of instability and pain [7, 18–20]. Diagnosis otherwise may be elusive and challenging as patients will likely describe nonspecific symptoms of groin pain, catching, and giving way. Physical examination will often reveal painful range of motion consistent with intra-articular pathology. More specific tests such as the posterior impingement test, the dial test, the apprehension with distraction test, and the LT test as described by O'Donnell et al. have been described [20–23]. The incidence of LT tears is varied ranging from as low as 4–17 % [5, 19] in earlier reports to as high as 49–65 % in more recent reports [13, 17, 18]. This variation may be a result of observation bias in some groups with heightened awareness of this pathology and recognition of less severe lesions.

Persistent symptoms of pain or mechanical symptoms following appropriate conservative care constitute potential surgical candidacy. Literature support exists for arthroscopic mechanical and/or radiofrequency debridement when evidence of intra-articular pathology amenable to arthroscopic treatment exists [8, 10, 11, 13, 17, 21]. In those patients with symptomatic instability and both subjective and positive clinical exam findings who have failed prior surgical procedures, LT reconstruction using varying techniques and graft sources has shown promising early results [6, 23–25]. Further study is required to validate the exact role for this procedure.

Synovial chondromatosis (SC) is an uncommon, benign, often monoarticular disease characterized by the formation of sessile or pedunculated collections of cartilage nodules [26]. Histology shows metaplasia of the synovial mesenchymal cells [27]. This can result in cartilaginous loose bodies which can ossify or undergo endochondral ossification [27]. The hip is the second most commonly involved joint after the knee [28]. The main consequence is chondral damage secondary to mechanical abrasion from the loose bodies. Small, cartilaginous loose bodies may result in minimal articular damage, whereas larger and/or ossified bodies may result in more severe, irreversible damage.

Clinically, an early diagnosis is important as a poor prognosis has been associated with retained intra-articular loose bodies [29, 30]. The severity of osteoarthritic changes at the time of treatment is the main predictor of successful clinical outcome [27]. Plain radiographs may show loose bodies in the joint or peripheral compartment but would fail to show noncalcified loose bodies. CT and especially MRI has aided in earlier and more accurate diagnosis [27].

Recommended treatment consists of surgical removal. Conventional open surgery has shown good results but with recurrence rates as high as 15 % with arthrotomy alone versus the morbidity and prolonged rehab associated with surgical dislocation [31, 32]. By contrast, arthroscopic removal of loose bodies and synovectomy has shown satisfactory results with a shortened recovery time and fewer complications [27, 33, 34].

A stenotic cotyloid fossa can be secondary to marginal heterotopic bone formation in the fossa and also abnormal amounts of fibrous and fatty tissue. A theory proposes that this can lead to incarceration of the LT. The space-occupying effect of this can perhaps lead to lateral subluxation of the femoral head and may have implications to chondrolabral pathology secondary to edge/rim loading [35]. Philippon et al. reported a 7 % rate of cheilectomy for a stenotic cotyloid fossa in a report on 45 professional athletes with femoroacetabular impingement (FAI) and their associated pathologies [18]. Plain radiographic and MRI evaluation can show bony projection into the fossa that is contiguous with the medial margin of the acetabular sourcil [1]. The goal of treatment is to remove any space-occupying tissue from the cotyloid fossa, decompress the constriction upon the LT, and perhaps improve joint congruence [35].

This chapter demonstrates the correlation between MRI and arthroscopic findings for lesions and pathology associated with the LT and cotyloid fossa and their associated diagnosis and management. Three cases will be presented, including:

1. Decompression of a stenotic cotyloid fossa
2. A ligamentum teres reconstruction for symptomatic deficiency
3. Arthroscopic treatment of synovial chondromatosis with associated FAI pathology

Case 1: Cotyloid Fossa Stenosis

History

Male, 39 years old, snowboarder. Patient has had left hip pain for several years. He recalls first feeling hip pain while surfing, which made him limp for a few days. The pain progressed slowly and now prevents him from performing any kind of exercise. He can walk up to four blocks before starting to limp. He also noticed some loss in range of motion and difficulty to put on shoes. His pain is 5/10 at rest and 8/10 at its worst.

Exam

Hip flexion 0–110°. Internal rotation 5°. Abduction 30°. Flexion abduction and external rotation (FABER) 20 cm, knee to table distance. Positive anterior impingement sign. Negative posterior impingement sign. Negative dial test. Thomas test was positive. Ober's test was negative.

Imaging

Radiographs

Decreased joint space (<2 mm), bilateral mild hip arthritis, pistol grip deformity with mild osteophytes; false profile view shows ossified anterior labrum (Fig. 30.1a, b).

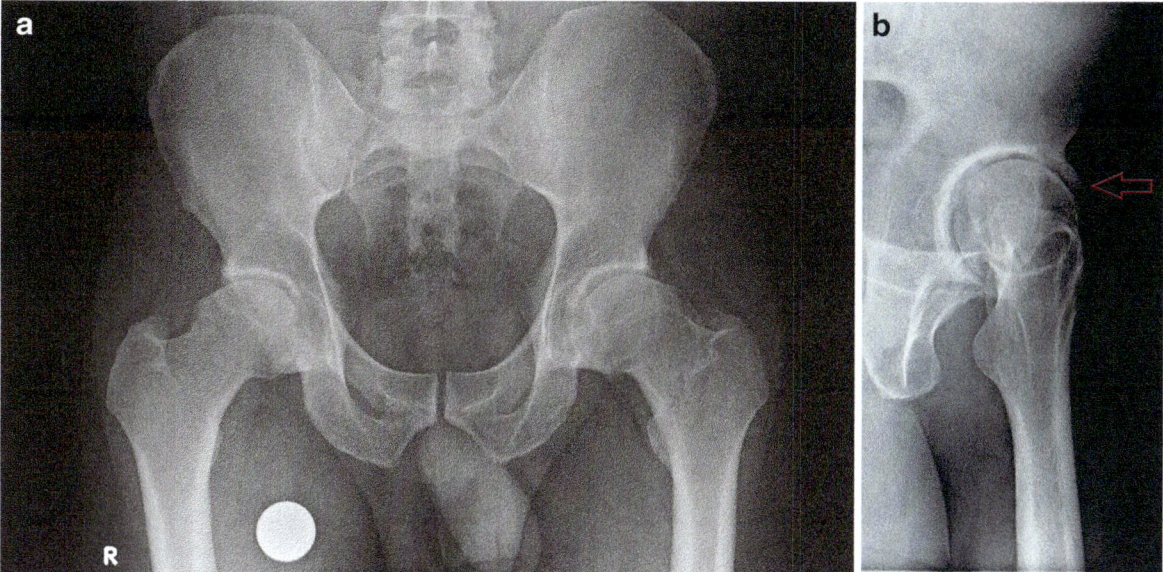

Fig. 30.1 (**a**) Pre-op anteroposterior radiograph; note reduced joint space in the left hip. (**b**) False profile view: *arrow* shows ossified labrum anteriorly

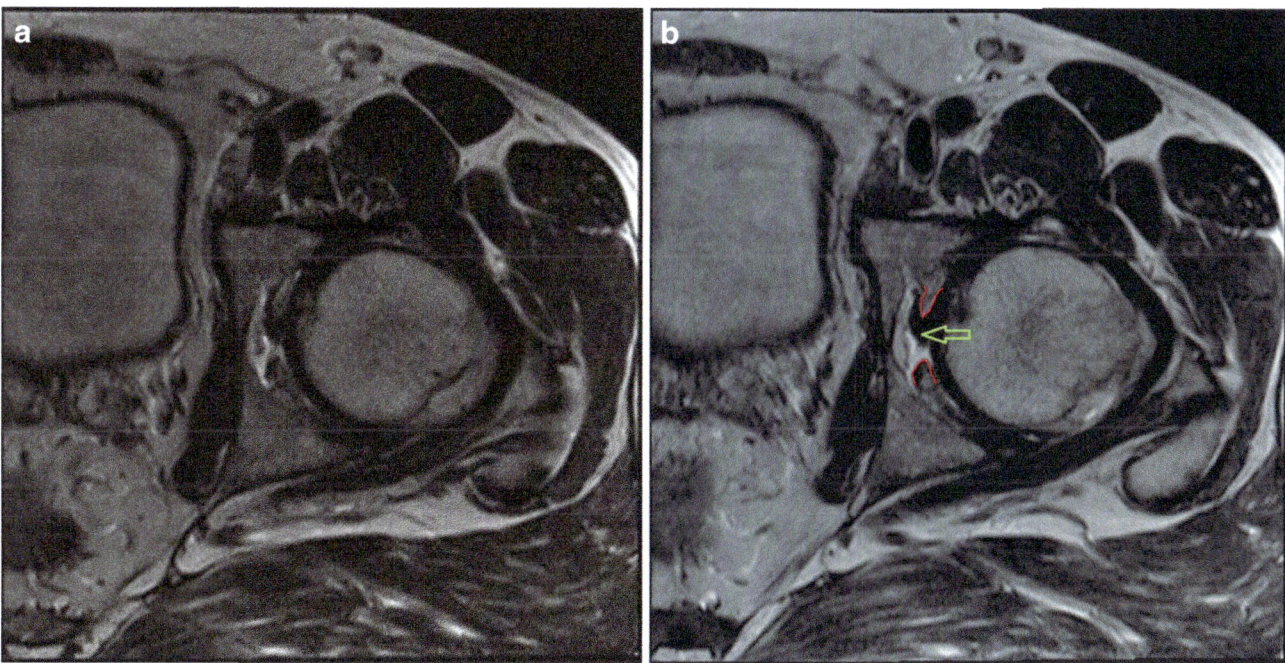

Fig. 30.2 (**a**, **b**) MRI of cotyloid fossa stenosis—axial view. *Red lines*: border of osteophytes causing the cotyloid fossa stenosis. *Yellow arrow*: ligamentum teres

MRI

Labral tearing of the anterior and lateral portions of the labrum. Chondral thinning and fissuring; lateral center-edge angle is 23°; alpha angle is 76°; femoral retroversion is 4°. Moderate effusion with capsular scarring and extensive synovitis, debris, and possible loose bodies. A prominent osteophyte was observed around the cotyloid fossa (Fig. 30.2a, b).

Arthroscopy

The patient underwent a left hip arthroscopy, synovectomy, rim trimming, neck osteoplasty, removal of loose bodies, cartilage debridement, and chondroplasty,

An ossification of the acetabular labrum from 8:00 to 2:00 position was observed. This was removed with an osteotome

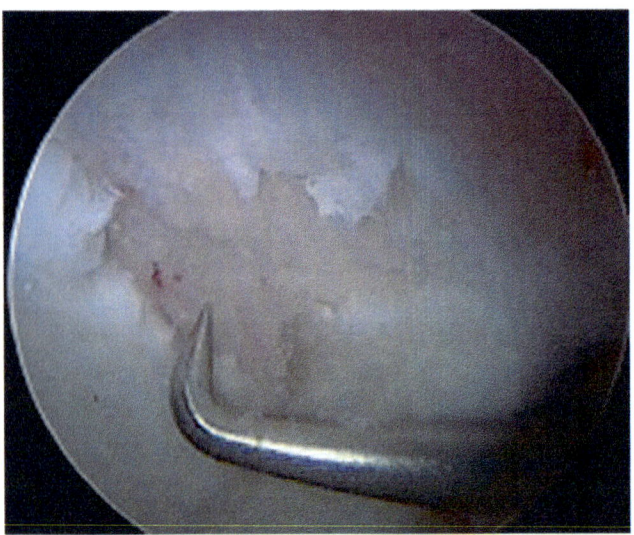

Fig. 30.3 Microfracture using an arthroscopic awl

and a burr. A labral reconstruction was performed with a 50 mm IT band graft and six suture anchors.

There was a grade 4 acetabular chondral defect of roughly 30×15 mm. Microfracture was used to treat this lesion (Fig. 30.3).

With the hip in distraction, the cotyloid fossa was inspected, and osteophytes were removed from this area to allow the femoral head to be well seated within the acetabular cup and to release the ligamentum teres entrapment. To accomplish this, we utilized different instruments such as an osteotome, burr, chisel, and basket punch (Fig. 30.4a–e).

After this, we debrided the ligamentum teres with the RF device, removing the inflamed synovium around it so it would sit better inside the cotyloid fossa (Fig. 30.5).

After the cotyloid fossa stenosis and LT debridement, we observed a better congruence between the femoral head and the cotyloid fossa. Traction was released so a dynamic assessment could be performed, and the femoral head could glide freely inside the acetabulum with restoration of the fluid seal.

Discussion

This case reveals the multifactorial nature of hip dysfunction in the active patient with moderate osteoarthritis. The acetabular rim, sclerotic and with ossified labrum, was a component of lost joint motion. The large cam-style femoral osteophyte also contributed. The theoretical contribution of space-occupying degenerative acetabular fossa contents also appeared to contribute. Attention to the deep central hip compartment arthroscopically was guided by clinical suspicion and the MRI findings of synovitis, effusion, and acetabular fossa stenosis. Further study is required to advocate global acceptance of this type of debridement, but preliminary case-based evidence is promising.

Case 2: Ligamentum Teres Reconstruction

History

Female, 25 years old, softball coach. Patient had already undergone two prior right hip arthroscopies and two left hip arthroscopies.

The last left hip surgery (1 year before) included labral debridement, lysis of adhesions, chondroplasty, synovectomy, psoas lengthening, and a labral reconstruction using an IT band autograft.

The patient complains of left hip pain that continues to bother her daily. She has signs of hip instability. She complains of her left hip giving out multiple times a day, preventing her from performing daily activities. Sometimes she has the feeling that the hip "pops out."

Past surgical history: positive for multiple surgeries on both hips, both shoulders, and left foot.

Exam

Normal strength of the muscles surrounding the hip joint, including hip flexors bilaterally. Normal sensation throughout lower extremities. Positive anterior impingement sign. Physical exam is consistent with generalized laxity. ROM: flexion 126°, abduction 45°, and adduction 30°. Grossly positive left hip manual distraction test.

Imaging

Radiographs
Joint space was preserved (>2 mm). Sourcil measuring 2–3 mm, anterior sourcil 3 mm. Tonnis angle is 5.5°. Lateral center-edge angle is 29°. Alpha angle is 43°. Sharp angle is 42°. See Fig. 30.6.

MRI
Labral reconstruction appears stable, without any gross separation identified. Diminutive ligamentum teres with signs of scarring and possible prior debridement. A complete LT tear could be present. See Fig. 30.7a, b.

Arthroscopy

Before putting the leg into table traction, a physical exam was performed under anesthesia. The joint could be distracted with manual traction alone, confirming severe hip laxity (Fig. 30.8).

Initial arthroscopic inspection: significant synovitis throughout the joint, significant adhesions especially at the

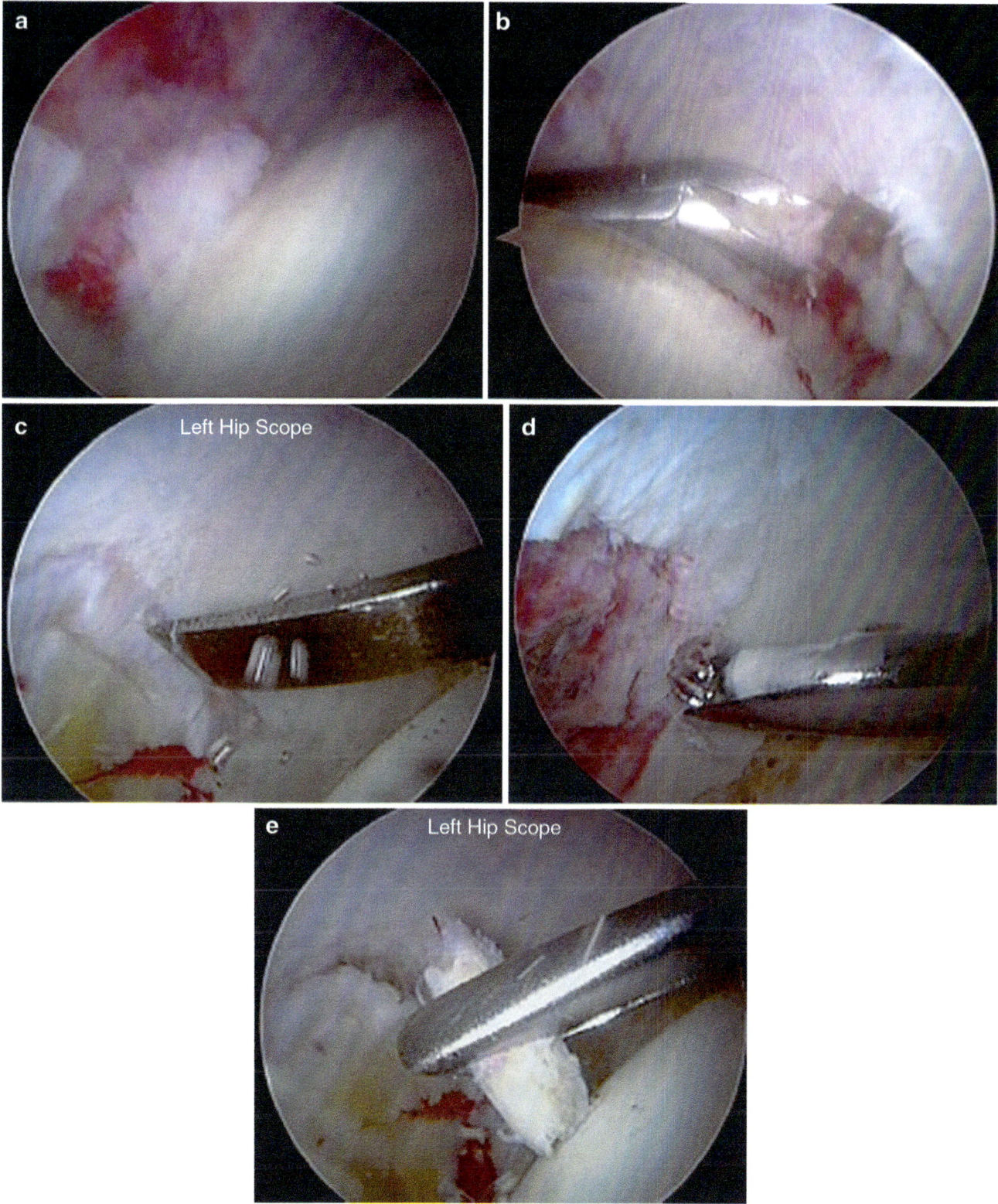

Fig. 30.4 (**a**) Fossa stenosis; ligamentum teres entrapment. (**b**) Osteophyte removal with a basket punch. (**c**) Chisel used for osteophyte removal. (**d**) Fossa stenosis decompression with burr. (**e**) Osteophyte removed with grasper

capsulolabral recess, and a visible ligamentum teres tear (Fig. 30.9).

Synovectomy was done using a combination of the electrocautery wand, ablator, and shaver. Hemostasis was assured with the RF device.

We then removed the adhesions by using the RF ablator and shaver, clearing up the capsulolabral recess. The labral reconstruction was intact and the suction seal was restored once the adhesions were removed.

Ligamentum teres: the LT was torn and grossly insufficient. The scar tissue surrounding it was debrided.

To begin the LT reconstruction, the arthroscopic shaver and burr were used to debride the cotyloid fossa, partially removing the pulvinar fat, and to expose the footprint of the ligamentum teres.

Then, using the C-arm, a K-wire was inserted from the lateral cortex of the femur, in line with the femoral neck. The trajectory was 1 cm below the center of the neck, so the tip of the K-wire would exit at the femoral fovea. The correct position of the K-wire was confirmed at both lateral and AP views (Fig. 30.10).

We then drilled a hole using a cannulated 6 mm reamer over this K-wire. This was then enlarged to 7 mm and finally to 8 mm. The tunnel went all the way to the femoral fovea, and a curette was placed inside the joint to protect the acetabular joint surface from damage by the reamer and the K-wire (Fig. 30.11a–c).

The anchor guide was placed through this hole on the femoral neck; a hole was drilled on the cotyloid fossa for insertion of a 2.9 mm anchor loaded with a #2 suture.

This #2 suture was retrieved arthroscopically through the anterolateral portal. One of the suture limbs was passed through a tibialis anterior allograft using a free needle. Then an arthroscopic knot was used to push the graft into the joint through a cannula, until it was compressed against the fossa. A sequence of knots secured this end of the graft at this position (Fig. 30.12a, b).

Then an arthroscopic grasper was inserted through the femoral neck hole to pull the allograft into the femoral neck tunnel. About 2.5 cm of the graft remained between the fovea and the fossa, with the leg in extension and external rotation (Fig. 30.13a, b). This is critical to avoid loss of movement.

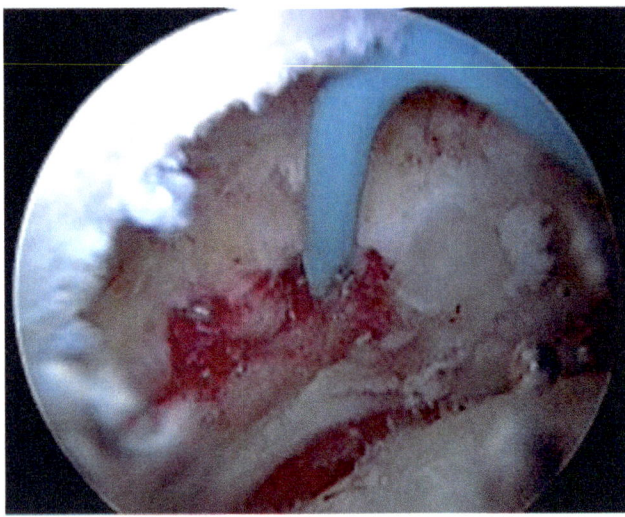

Fig. 30.5 LT debridement

Fig. 30.6 AP pelvis before surgery

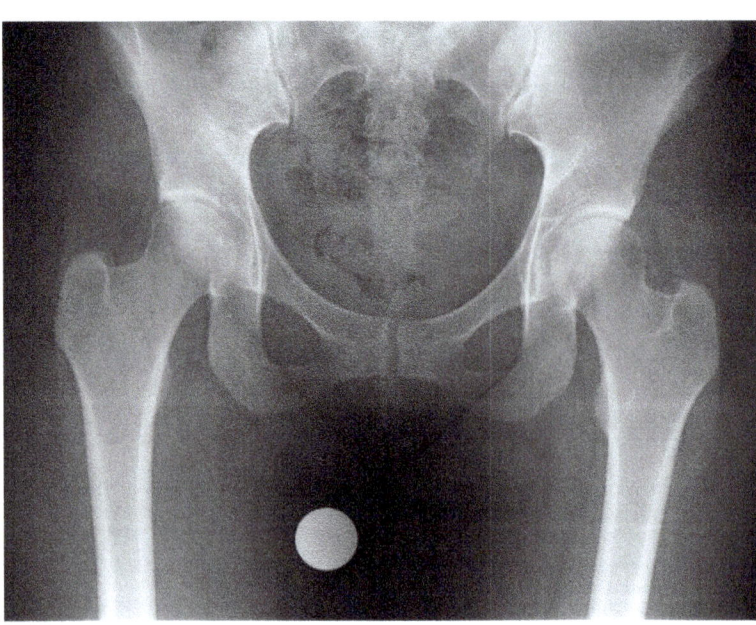

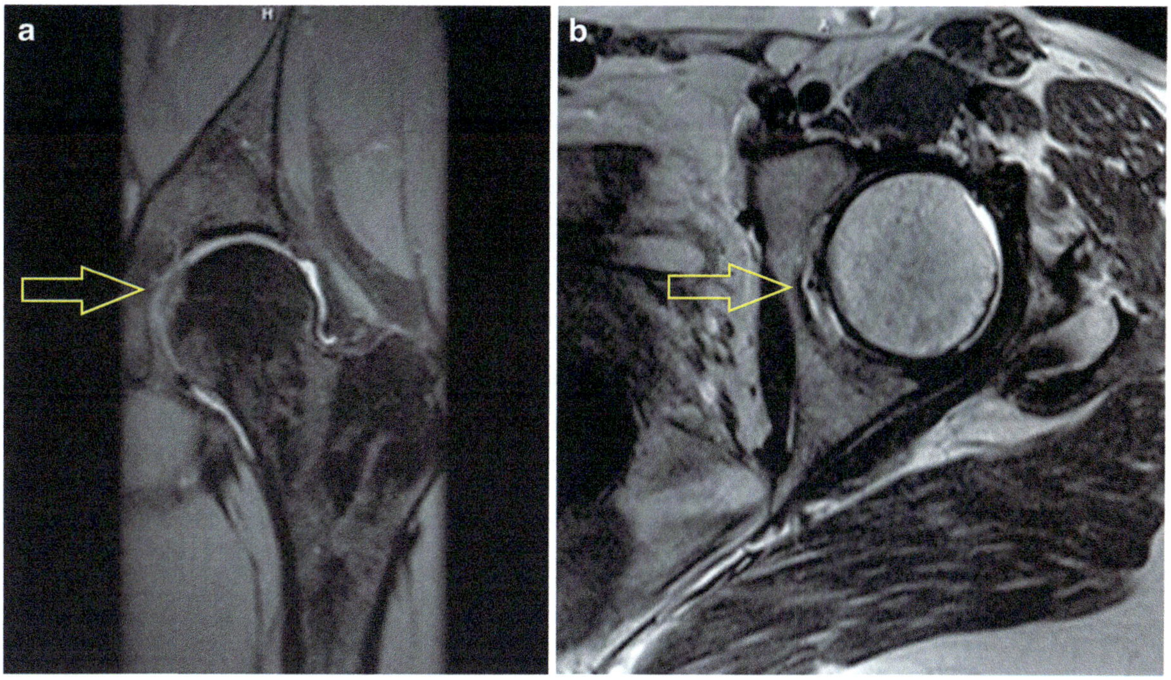

Fig. 30.7 (**a, b**) MRI pre-op: ligamentum teres is frayed and cannot be precisely outlined, which could be due to a complete tear

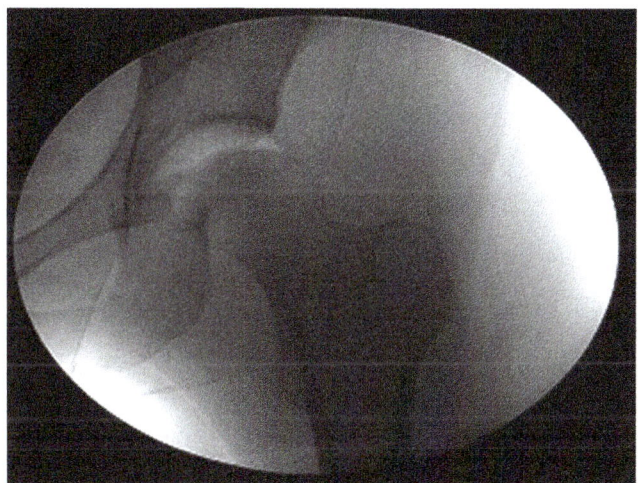

Fig. 30.8 Effortless manual distraction of the hip joint, under anesthesia

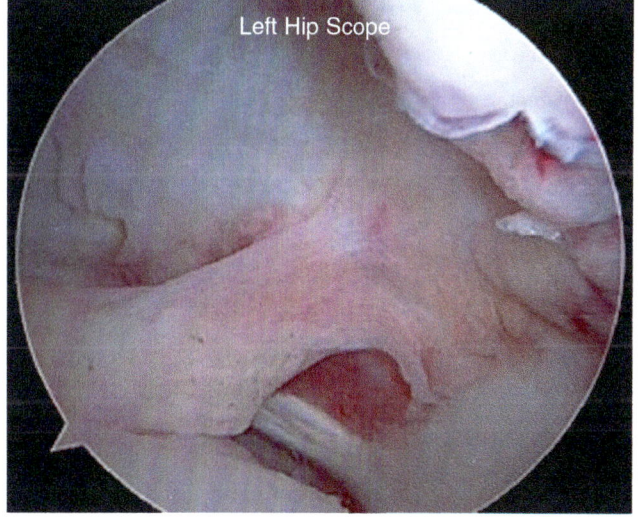

Fig. 30.9 Torn insufficient ligamentum teres

Tension level was verified by checking the hip's range of motion and graft excursion. After reaching the desired tension, an 8×35 mm interference screw was placed to assure fixation of the graft inside the tunnel. After fixation, the hip range of motion was again verified to be satisfactory.

To end the case, we performed a capsular plication to make sure that the capsule would heal with an appropriate amount of tension, restoring its function as a secondary stabilizer.

Discussion

There are conceptual and technical points to consider upon review of this case. Conceptually, we believe that hip microinstability is multifactorial. The ligamentum teres is a secondary stabilizer of the hip joint. LT insufficiency may become symptomatic in patients with dysplasia and/or following surgical LT debridement. Technically, the LT reconstruction with an allograft needs to be associated with other

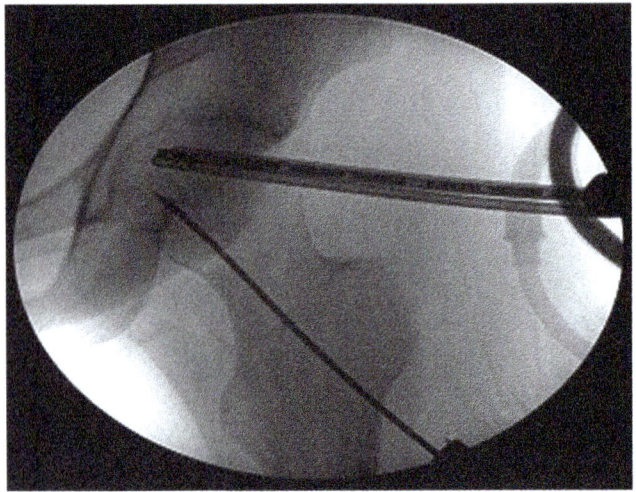

Fig. 30.10 K-wire is drilled into the femoral neck with c-arm and arthroscopic guidance

procedures to address microinstability, such as capsular plication. Meticulous attention should be given to correct allograft length and tension. Reduced length may impair full range of motion. This procedure requires mastery of all advanced hip arthroscopy techniques prior to performance and is presented here as an example of the frontier of treatment in the salvage setting.

Case 3: Synovial Chondromatosis

History/Exam

A 35-year-old male with a desk job who recreationally plays golf and attends spinning classes presented to the orthopedic clinic with 6 months of insidious onset mild, intermittent left groin and lateral hip pain with stiffness as he began undertaking

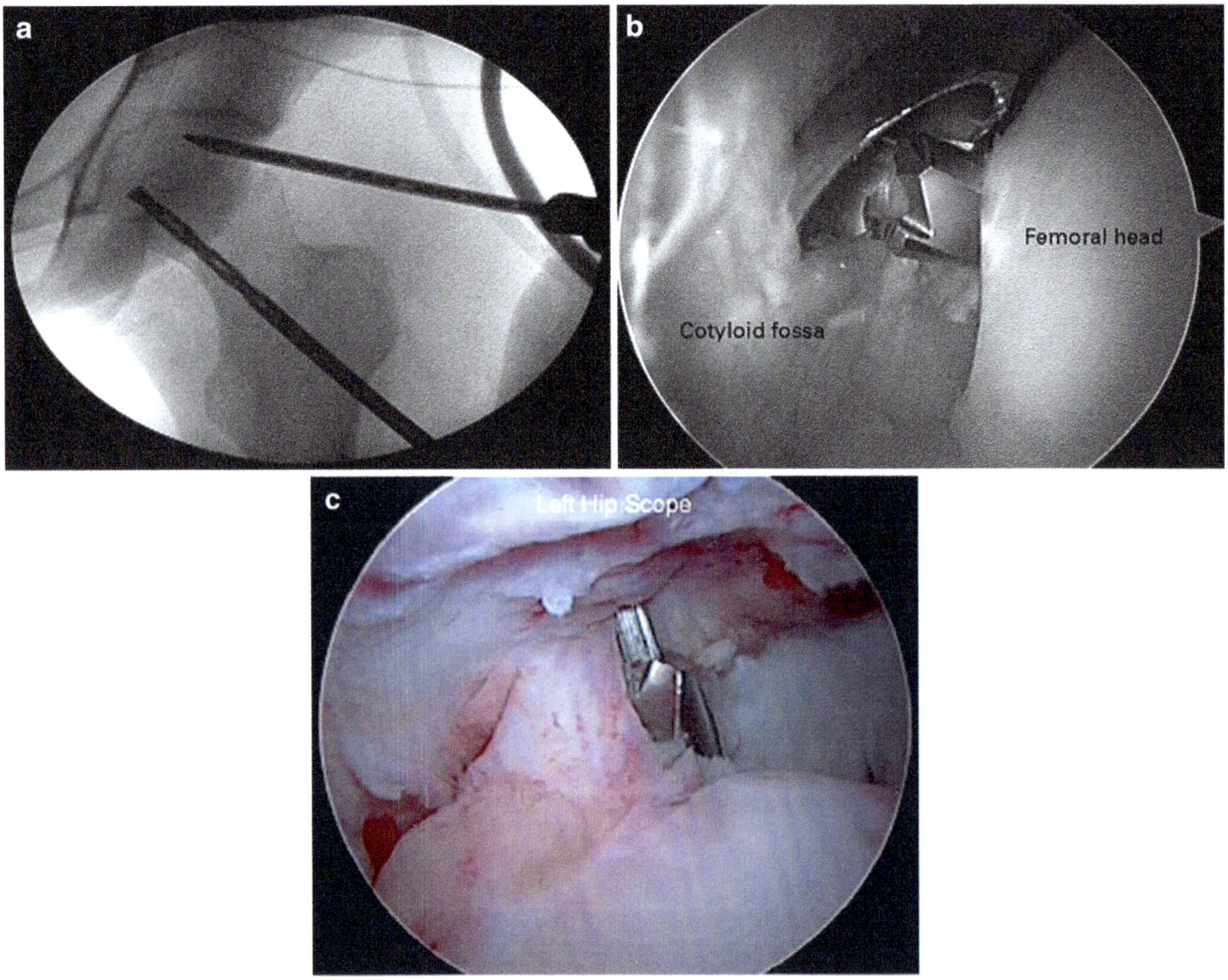

Fig. 30.11 (a) The 8 mm tunnel is made with a reamer. (b) A curette is used to protect the acetabular surface. (c) Drill bit exiting through the fovea

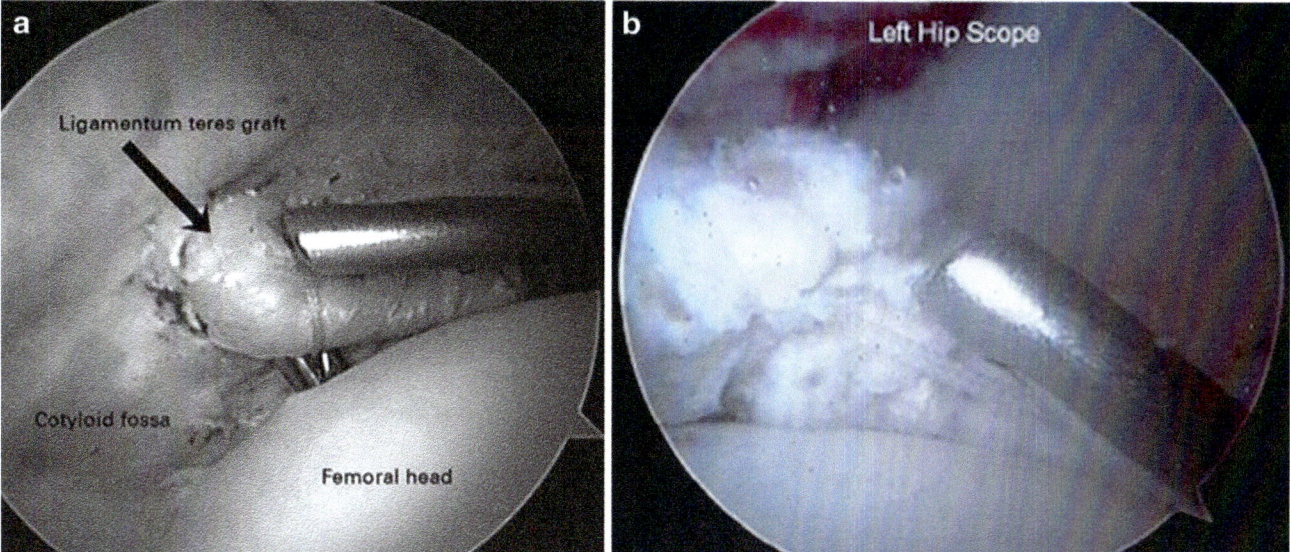

Fig. 30.12 (**a, b**) Graft is pushed into position with a knot pusher

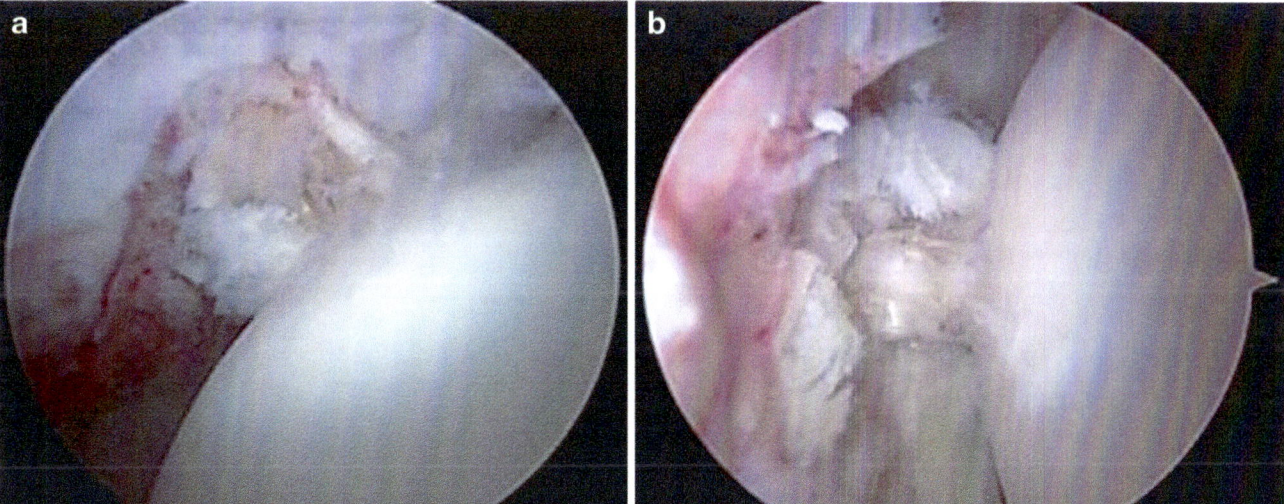

Fig. 30.13 (**a, b**) Status post fixation of the allograft in position

his spinning classes. He denied any symptoms 6 months ago. The pain was worse with lying on his back, deep hip flexion activity such as putting on his shoes, and twisting or rotation of the hip such as getting in and out of the car.

On physical exam, the patient was found to have full and symmetric range of motion of the hip with pain at the extremes of motion and a positive anterior impingement sign, positive Stinchfield test, and positive FABER test for reproduction of anteriorly based pain. He had no areas of tenderness and no appreciable weakness compared to the contralateral side. He was neurovascularly intact distally.

Imaging

Plain radiographs (Fig. 30.14a, b) revealed maintained joint space with findings of femoroacetabular impingement. Magnetic resonance imaging was obtained to further characterize the extent and character of any chondral or labral pathology and to look for other attendant signs of femoroacetabular impingement given the long-standing symptoms.

A complete exam was obtained and key images are shown. Figure 30.15a, b reveals an effusion with an acetabular labral tear as well as pincer pitting at the femoral head–neck junction.

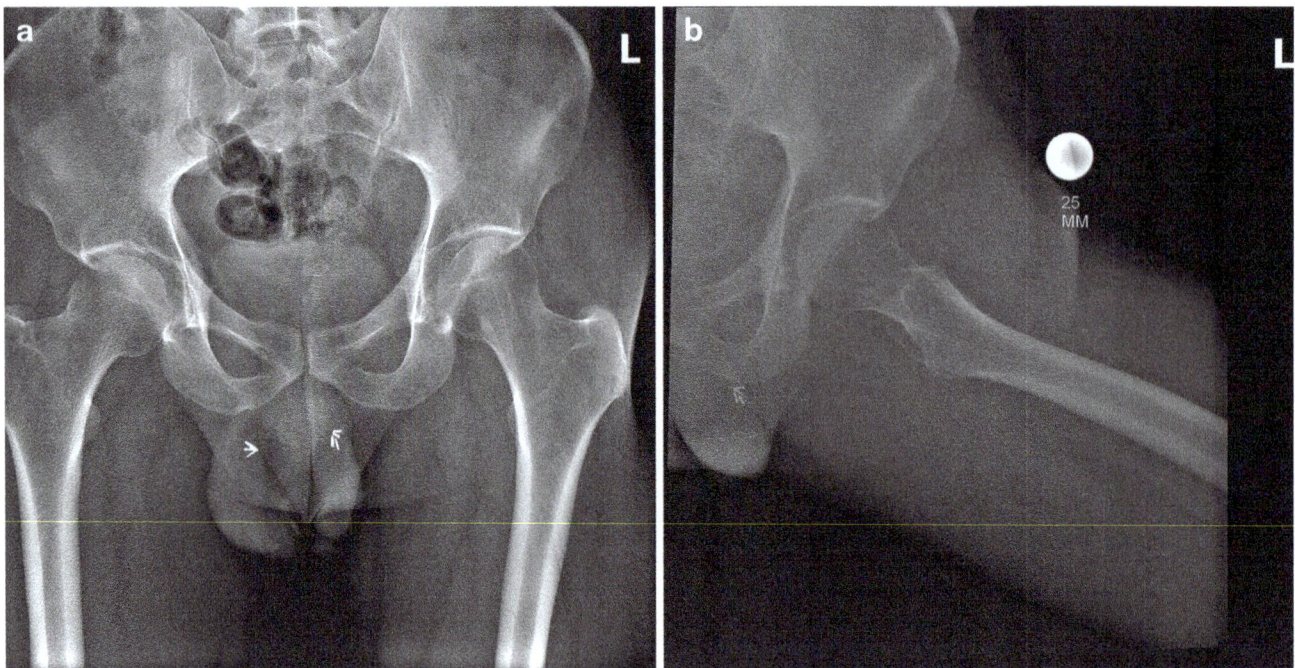

Fig. 30.14 (**a, b**) AP pelvis and frog leg lateral of the pathologic hip, pre-op

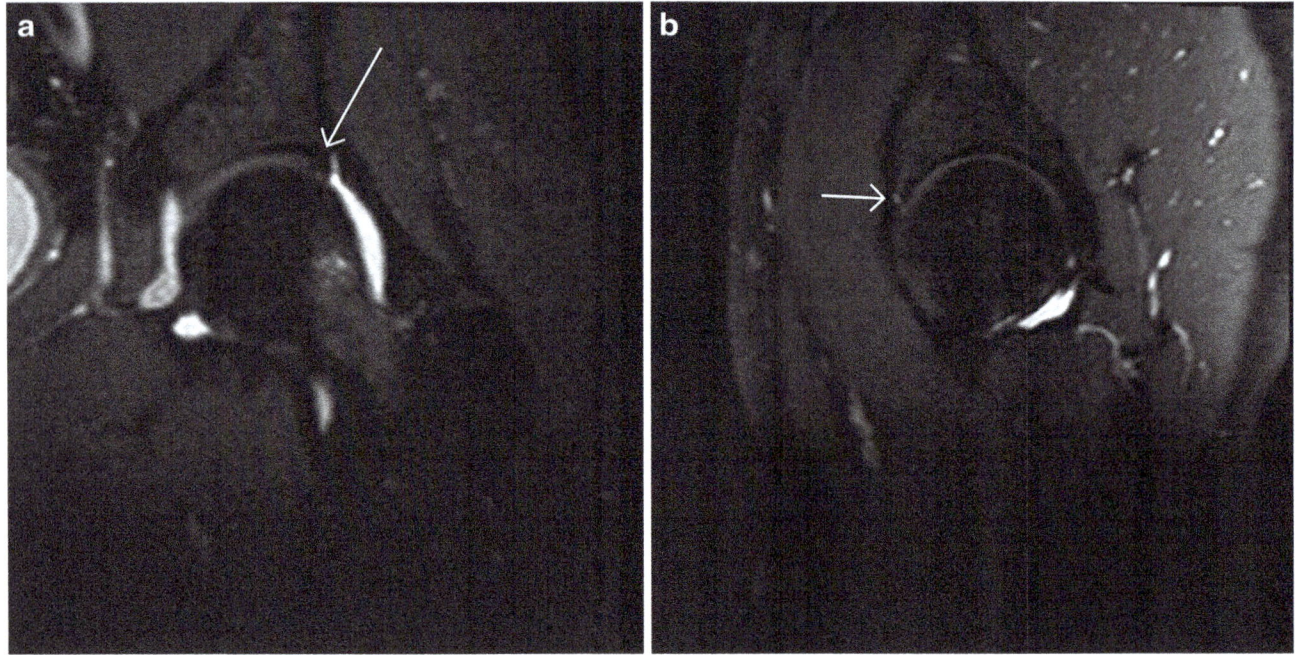

Fig. 30.15 (**a**) T2 coronal MRI image of the left hip, pincer lesion with labral tear. (**b**) T2 sagittal MRI image of the left hip, pincer lesion with labral tear

Although at first underappreciated, the imaging clearly shows many intermediate signal loose bodies within the acetabular fossa (Fig. 30.16a, b).

Despite nonoperative management including nonsteroidal anti-inflammatory medications, rest, physical therapy including low-impact activity and core strengthening, and beneficial, albeit transient, responses to intra-articular corticosteroid injections, his symptoms persisted and worsened slowly over the course of 2 years. Surgical intervention with the intention of treating the femoroacetabular impingement and associated

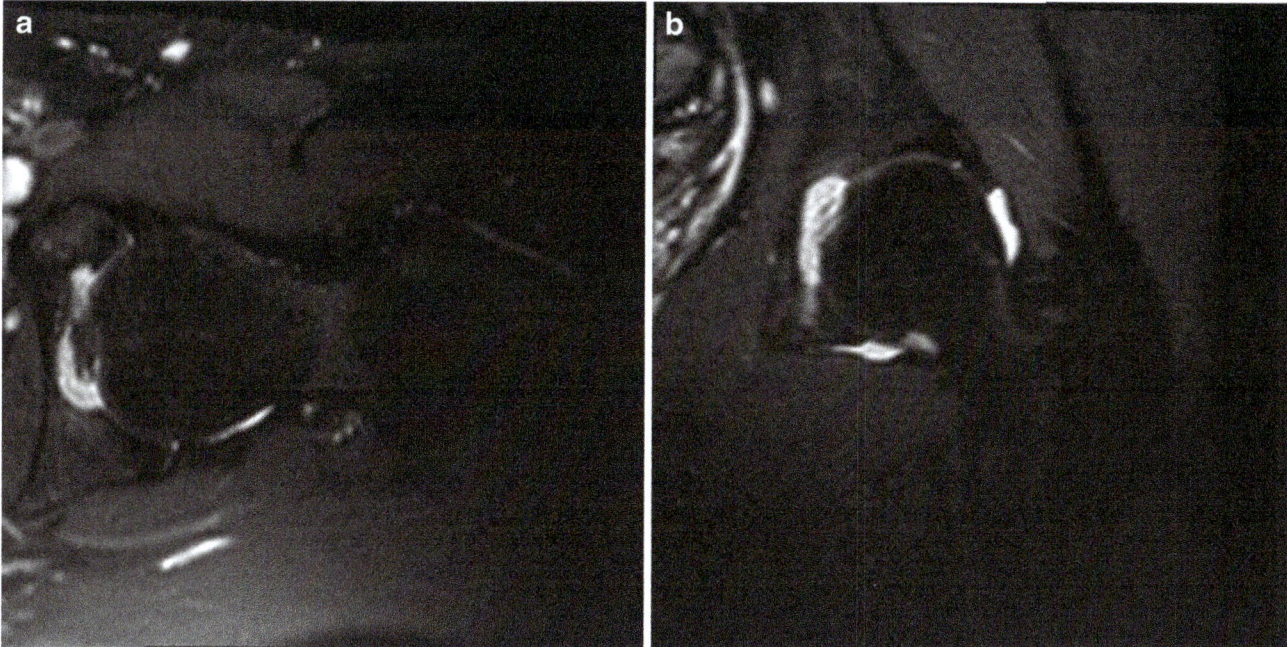

Fig. 30.16 (**a**) T2 axial MRI images, effusion, and loose bodies in the fossa. (**b**) T2 coronal MRI images, effusion, and loose bodies in the fossa (gray signal)

chondrolabral pathology was recommended, and the risks and benefits were discussed. He elected to proceed with arthroscopic evaluation of the hip joint with a plan for labral repair, acetabuloplasty, and femoroplasty.

Arthroscopy

The patient was taken to the operating room and placed supine on a Hana traction table. A standard diagnostic arthroscopy of the left hip was completed. The patient had moderate synovitis peripherally. The chondrolabral junction was also found to have high-grade chondrolabral instability with labral detachment from the acetabular margin with junctional attrition and marginal contusion of the labral tissue from about 9:30 to 12 o'clock position (Fig. 30.17). In addition, there was a margin of softened, unstable articular cartilage but no areas of unstable delamination. The femoral head articular cartilage was normal. The ligamentum had some synovitis but otherwise the fovea itself was normal. The fossa on the other hand had accretions of multiple cartilaginous loose bodies completely incarcerating the entirety of the acetabular fossa (Fig. 30.18a–c).

A capsulotomy was then performed and a synovectomy was performed with a shaver. A labral takedown was performed meticulously in a retrograde fashion to maintain the bulk of the labral tissue. The unstable marginal articular cartilage was then debrided with a shaver. After labral takedown and debridement of the unstable marginal articular cartilage,

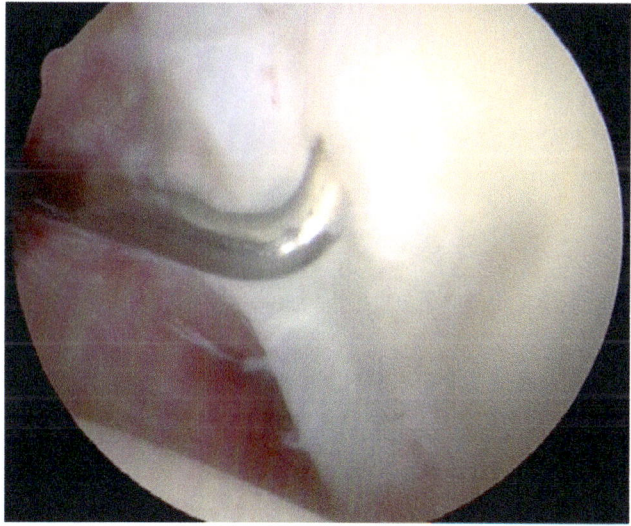

Fig. 30.17 Labral tear

the full extent of the pincer lesion was visualized, and a burr was used to perform an acetabuloplasty negating the anterior crossover sign seen fluoroscopically and removing the grossly visualized pincer lesion. The labrum was then repaired with two #2 nonabsorbable sutures placed circumferentially in a baggage tag fashion and then secured to the acetabular margin via two 2.9 mm-knotless anchors (Fig. 30.19). The chondrolabral stability and suction seal of the joint were confirmed to be reestablished through direct palpation and dynamic evaluation.

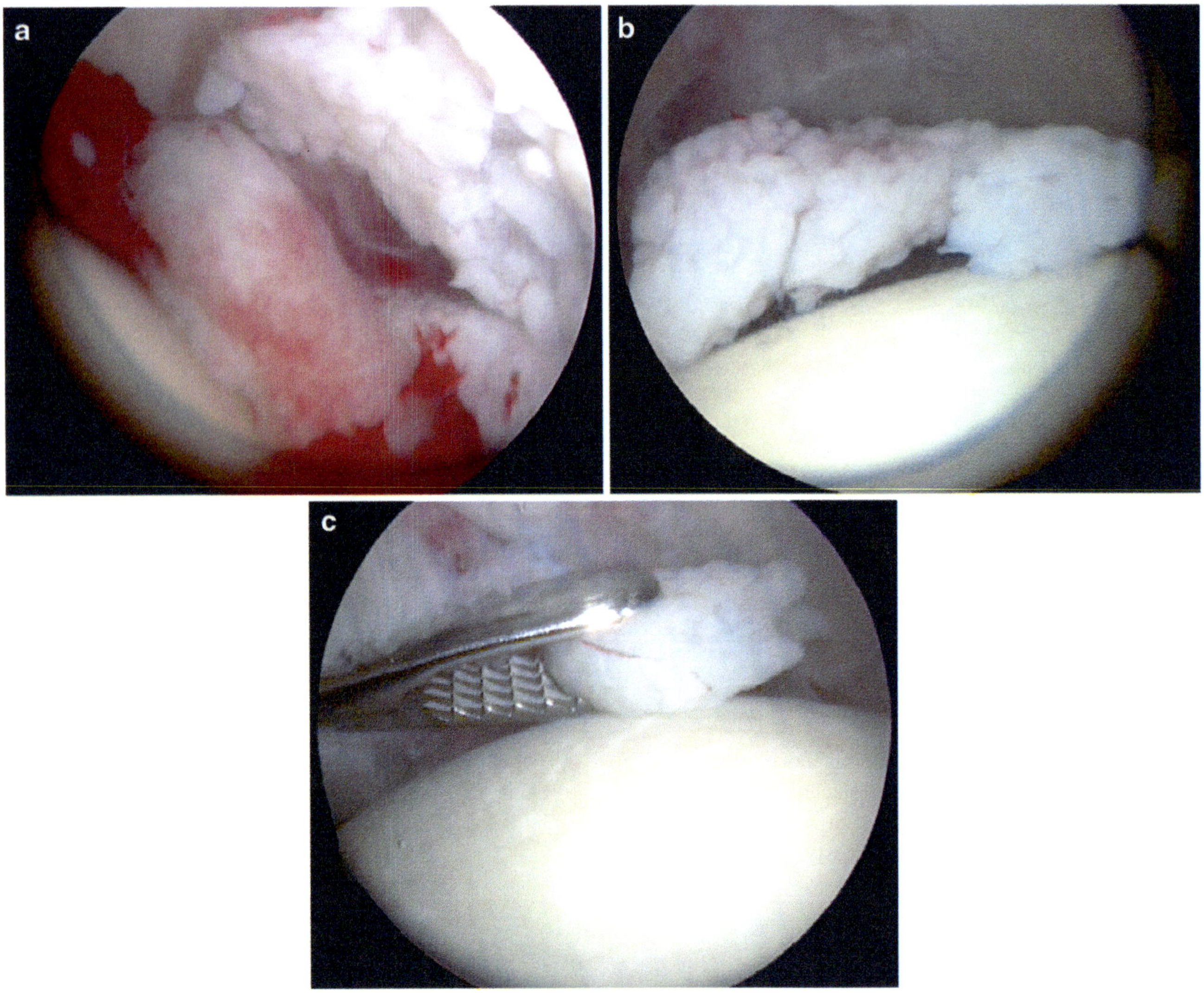

Fig. 30.18 (**a–c**) Loose bodies in the cotyloid fossa and central compartment; removal of loose body with grasper

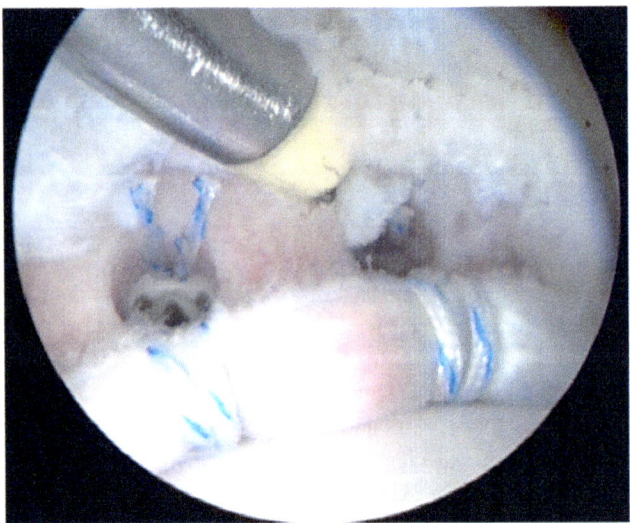

Fig. 30.19 Labral repair with luggage handle fixation through knotless suture anchors

Once the pincer lesion had been debrided and the chondrolabral junction was restored, the loose bodies were removed from the acetabular fossa. The removal was meticulous and required the use of multiple instruments in concert including graspers, the motorized shaver, and intra-articular suction. Some could be retrieved in whole, but others required debridement and suction irrigation (Fig. 30.18a–c).

At the completion of the evaluation and treatment of the pathology in the central compartment, the gross traction was relieved and the peripheral compartment was then examined arthroscopically. Dynamic evaluation revealed residual bony conflict with the acetabulum and pincer pitting with reactive cam lesion at the head–neck junction anteriorly. A T-capsulotomy was performed, and the fibrocartilage was removed from the head–neck junction down to the bony cam lesion with electrocautery. There was also appreciated a loss of head–neck offset down to the area of the cam lesion. A motorized burr was used to perform femoroplasty, therefore restoring the normal head–neck offset and removing the cam lesion. Further exploration was done to confirm the absence of any more loose bodies. A dynamic exam revealed the successful resolution of the bony conflict.

Discussion

This case illustrates the requirement for thorough consideration of the possibility that loose bodies may contribute to hip complaints. MRI findings of low-signal areas in the acetabular fossa, particularly when arthrogram contrast is added, should raise clinical suspicion. This case being a clear case of secondary chondromatosis, the primary pathology was treated as well in the form of osteochondroplasty and impingement correction. There is little evidence to support or reject the concern that osteoplasty would lead to recurrence of synovial chondroma formation.

References

1. Wenger D, Miyanji F, Mahar A, Oka R. The mechanical properties of the ligamentum teres: a pilot study to assess its potential for improving stability in children's hip surgery. J Pediatr Orthop. 2007;27:408–10.
2. Savory W. The use of the ligamentum teres of the hip-joint. J Anat Physiol. 1874;8:291–6.
3. Sutton JB. The ligamentum teres. J Anat Physiol. 1883;17:190–3.
4. Leunig M, Beck M, Stauffer E, Hertel R, Ganz R. Free nerve endings in the ligamentum capitis femoris. Acta Orthop Scand. 2000;71:452–4.
5. Bardakos N, Villar R. The ligamentum teres of the adult hip. J Bone Joint Surg Br. 2009;91:8–15.
6. Simpson JM, Field RE, Villar RN. Arthroscopic reconstruction of the ligamentum teres. Arthroscopy. 2011;27:436–41.
7. Wettstein M, Garofalo R, Borens O, Mouhsine E. Traumatic rupture of the ligamentum teres as a source of hip pain. Arthroscopy. 2005;21:382.
8. Kusma M, Jung J, Dienst M, Goedde S, Kohn D, Seil R. Arthroscopic treatment of an avulsion fracture of the ligamentum teres of the hip in an 18-year-old horse rider. Arthroscopy. 2004;20 Suppl 2:64–6.
9. Cerezal L, Kassarjian A. Anatomy, biomechanics, imaging, and management of ligamentum teres injuries. Radiographics. 2010;30:1637–51.
10. Haviv B, O'Donnell J. Arthroscopic debridement of the isolated Ligamentum Teres rupture. Knee Surg Sports Traumatol Arthrosc. 2011;19:1510–3.
11. Yamamoto Y, Usui I. Arthroscopic surgery for degenerative rupture of the ligamentum teres femoris. Arthroscopy. 2006;22:689.e1–3.
12. Gray A, Villar RN. The ligamentum teres of the hip: an arthroscopic classification of its pathology. Arthroscopy. 1997;13:575–8.
13. Botser IB, Martin DE, Stout CE, Domb BG. Tears of the ligamentum teres: prevalence in hip arthroscopy using 2 classification systems. Am J Sports Med. 2011;39(Suppl):117S–25.
14. Roy DR. Arthroscopic findings of the hip in new onset hip pain in adolescents with previous Legg-Calve-Perthes disease. J Pediatr Orthop B. 2005;14:151–5.
15. Bulut O, Oztürk H, Tezeren G, Bulut S. Arthroscopic-assisted surgical treatment for developmental dislocation of the hip. Arthroscopy. 2005;21:574–9.
16. Philippon MJ, Kuppersmith DA, Wolff AB, Briggs KK. Arthroscopic findings following traumatic hip dislocation in 14 professional athletes. Arthroscopy. 2009;25:169–74.
17. Domb BG, Martin DE, Botser IB. Risk factors for ligamentum teres tears. Arthroscopy. 2013;29:64–73.
18. Philippon M, Schenker M, Briggs K, Kuppersmith D. Femoroacetabular impingement in 45 professional athletes: associated pathologies and return to sport following arthroscopic decompression. Knee Surg Sports Traumatol Arthrosc. 2007;15:908–14.
19. Byrd JWT, Jones KS. Traumatic rupture of the ligamentum teres as a source of hip pain. Arthroscopy. 2004;20:385–91.
20. Kelly BTB, Williams RRJ, Philippon MMJ. Hip arthroscopy: current indications, treatment options, and management issues. Am J Sports Med. 2003;31:1020–37.
21. O'Donnell J, Economopoulos K, Singh P, Bates D, Pritchard M. The ligamentum teres test: a novel and effective test in diagnosing tears of the ligamentum teres. Am J Sports Med. 2014;42:138–43.
22. Lynch TS, Terry M, Bedi A, Kelly BT. Hip arthroscopic surgery: patient evaluation, current indications, and outcomes. Am J Sports Med. 2013;41:1174–89.
23. Philippon MJ, Pennock A, Gaskill TR. Arthroscopic reconstruction of the ligamentum teres: technique and early outcomes. J Bone Joint Surg Br. 2012;94:1494–8.
24. Amenabar T, O'Donnell J. Arthroscopic ligamentum teres reconstruction using semitendinosus tendon: surgical technique and an unusual outcome. Arthrosc Tech. 2012;1:e169–74.
25. Lindner D, Sharp KG, Trenga AP, Stone J, Stake CE, Domb BG. Arthroscopic ligamentum teres reconstruction. Arthrosc Tech. 2013;2:e21–5.
26. Mussey R, Henderson M. Osteochondromatosis. J Bone Joint Surg Am. 1949;31:619–27.
27. Boyer T, Dorfmann H. Arthroscopy in primary synovial chondromatosis of the hip: description and outcome of treatment. J Bone Joint Surg Br. 2008;90:314–8.
28. Murphey M, Vidal J. Imaging of synovial chondromatosis with radiologic-pathologic correlation. Radiographics. 2007;27:1465–89.
29. Epstein H. Posterior fracture-dislocations of the hip: long-term follow-up. J Bone Joint Surg Am. 1974;56:1103–27.
30. Thompson V, Epstein H. Traumatic dislocation of the hip: a survey of two hundred and four cases covering a period of twenty-one years. J Bone Joint Surg Am. 1951;33-A:746–78.
31. Schoeniger R, Naudie DDR, Siebenrock K, Trousdale RT, Ganz R. Modified complete synovectomy prevents recurrence in synovial chondromatosis of the hip. Clin Orthop Relat Res. 2006;451:195–200.
32. Lim S, Chung H, Choi Y, Moon Y, Seo J, Park Y. Operative treatment of primary synovial osteochondromatosis of the hip. J Bone Joint Surg Am. 2006;88:2456–64.
33. Marchie A, Panuncialman I, McCarthy JC. Efficacy of hip arthroscopy in the management of synovial chondromatosis. Am J Sports Med. 2011;39(Suppl):126S–31.
34. Zini R, Longo U, de Benedetto M, et al. Arthroscopic management of primary synovial chondromatosis of the hip. Arthroscopy. 2013;29:420–6.
35. Brannon JK. Hip arthroscopy: intra-articular saucerization of the acetabular cotyloid fossa. Orthopedics. 2012;35:e262–6.

Traumatic and Atraumatic Hip Instability

Marc J. Philippon, Ryan J. Warth, and Karen K. Briggs

Introduction

The hip is an inherently stable joint as a result of its characteristic osseous topology that allows the femoral head to sit deeply within the highly congruent acetabular fossa. However, despite its bony architecture, recent evidence suggests that maintenance of hip stability throughout the various planes of motion requires intact surrounding capsuloligamentous structures [1–3].

The hip capsule is composed of several ligamentous structures that resist abnormal femoral head translation throughout the entire range of motion. The iliofemoral ligament, the strongest of the capsular ligaments, spans an area covering the anterior aspect of the femoral head and prevents anterior translation during motions that involve hip extension and external rotation. The pubofemoral ligament travels from the pubis to the femoral neck and prevents excessive abduction and extension of the hip. The ischiofemoral ligament comprises a portion of the posterior capsule and resists posterior translation during adduction and internal rotation of the hip (Fig. 31.1). The deep arcuate ligament is another component of the posterior capsule that prevents abnormal translation with extension and deep flexion. The zona orbicularis makes up the inferior portion of the hip capsule and has been found to primarily resist inferior femoral head translation [3]. The ligamentum teres, an intra-articular and extracapsular ligament which is

taught in adduction, flexion, and external rotation, has also been suggested as a potential contributor to hip stability [4–7]. Evidence suggests that the acetabular labrum may also be involved in maintaining stability of the hip by both increasing acetabular depth and generating a negative intra-articular pressure that each help to prevent abnormal femoral head translation [8, 9] (Fig. 31.2). Disruption of any of these soft tissue structures, including the surrounding musculature, can result in extraphysiologic hip motion ranging from transient subluxation to frank dislocation.

The etiologies of hip instability are most often conceptually divided into traumatic and atraumatic causes.

Most cases of acute traumatic dislocation occur when a sudden, excessive axial load is applied to the femur with the hip in a flexed position—this type of injury may or may not result in fracture of the posterior wall of the acetabulum [10, 11]. Some athletes may be predisposed to have an acute dislocation as a manifestation of chronic overuse [12, 13]. Although specific injury patterns following acute dislocations have not been well described, concomitant injuries to the articular surface, ligamentum teres, acetabular labrum, and capsuloligamentous structures may result in symptoms of recurrent, painful microinstability [11].

Atraumatic hip instability has numerous potential etiologies. Congenital defects involving bone or soft tissues, multiligamentous laxity, certain systemic diseases, or any one of several acquired causes such as previous open or arthroscopic hip surgery may predispose an individual to develop chronic, atraumatic hip instability which can be debilitating [14]. In most adults, true hip dislocations are uncommon without significant trauma or previous surgery. On the other hand, dislocations in children are more often associated with congenital malformations, such as torticollis and talipes equinovarus [15], that may lead to developmental abnormalities of the hip with a high potential for long-term sequelae including degenerative osteoarthritis and/or femoroacetabular impingement.

Developmental dysplasia of the hip (DDH) is a frequently cited entity associated with atraumatic hip instability that has

M.J. Philippon, MD (✉)
The Steadman Clinic and Steadman Philippon Research Institute, Vail, CO, USA
e-mail: drphilippon@sprivail.org

R.J. Warth, MD
Department of Orthopedic Surgery, University of Texas Health Sciences Center, Houston, TX, USA
e-mail: Ryan.j.warth@uth.tmc.edu

K.K. Briggs, MPH
Steadman Philippon Research Institute, Vail, CO, USA
e-mail: Karen.briggs@sprivail.org

S.F. Brockmeier (ed.), *MRI-Arthroscopy Correlations: A Case-Based Atlas of the Knee, Shoulder, Elbow and Hip*,
DOI 10.1007/978-1-4939-2645-9_31, © Springer Science+Business Media New York 2015

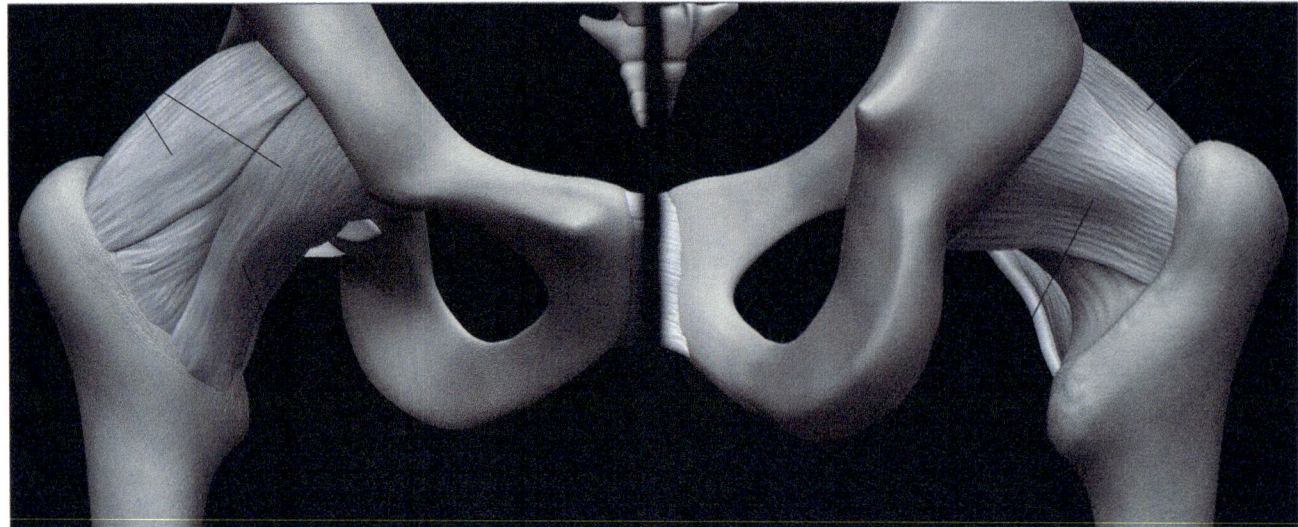

Fig. 31.1 Illustration depicting *anterior* and *posterior* views of the ligamentous constraints of the hip. The iliofemoral and pubofemoral ligaments can be seen anteriorly, and the ischiofemoral ligament can be seen posteriorly

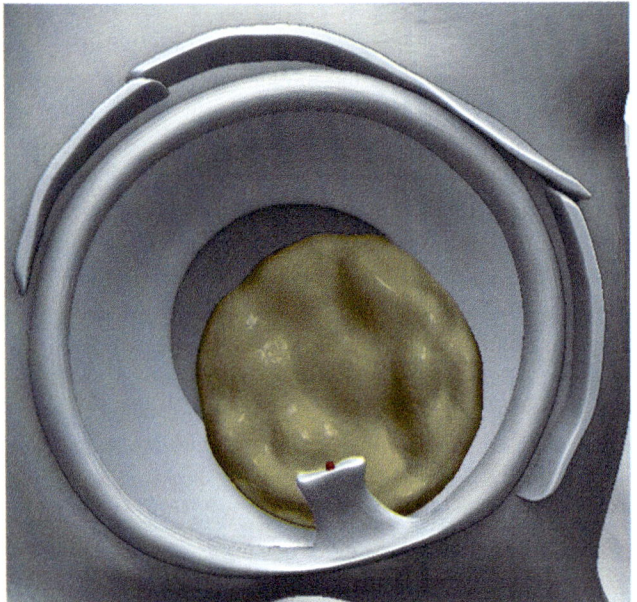

Fig. 31.2 Illustration showing the orientation of the ligamentum teres relative to the acetabular labrum. Note the significant increase in acetabular depth produced by the labrum

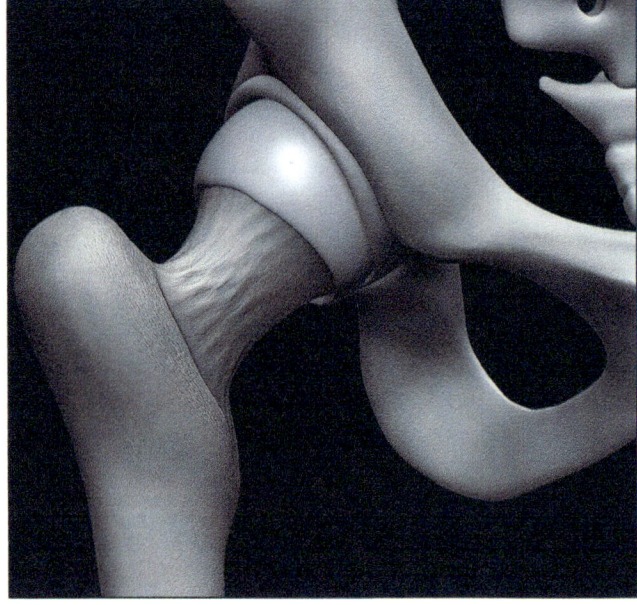

Fig. 31.3 Illustration depicting a dysplastic hip with a decreased head–neck offset and shallow acetabulum

yet to be clearly defined in the literature. As a result, published research related to DDH can be confusing and often conflicting. Nevertheless, DDH is generally considered to be a continuum of pathologies with various morphologic features ranging from normal hip development to gross abnormalities that can result in significant instability. Some of these features may include a shallow or underdeveloped acetabular fossa (a cause and effect of recurrent hip dislocations in children), an abnormally small head–neck offset, and an excessive chondral wear as a result of altered biomechanical shear

forces across the articular surfaces (Fig. 31.3). The development of ultrasonographic screening programs for the detection of hip subluxations and dislocations in young children has provided a cost-effective avenue for early recognition and treatment of DDH, thus significantly reducing the morbidity and cost associated with known long-term sequelae.

In all patients, a thorough history is necessary to determine the circumstances associated with their reasons for seeking medical treatment and to develop a succinct, yet thoughtful, differential diagnosis that can be used to guide

Table 31.1 Radiographic signs of dysplasia

Signs of dysplasia	Measurement	Definition
Tonnis angle >10° (Tonnis 1999)	Acetabular inclination	Angle of the horizontal line of the pelvis and the line connecting the most lateral and most medial parts of the acetabular weight-bearing sourcil
<25° (Wiberg 1939)	CE angle	Angle of a vertical line (in relation to the pelvis) and a line connecting the femoral head center
>42° (Sharp 1961)	Sharp's acetabular angle	Angle of a horizontal line of the pelvis connecting both teardrop signs and the line of the teardrop to the most lateral point of the acetabular articular surface
<20° (Lequesne 1961)	Anterior center-edge angle (VCA)	Angle of a line connecting the center of both femoral heads and the one between the center of the femoral head and the anteriormost edge of the acetabulum articular surface

further management decisions. During the patient encounter, it is also important to obtain information regarding hip pathologies throughout the family history, especially inquiring about those pathologies that may be involved with the development of hip instability such as Ehlers–Danlos syndrome and Marfan syndrome. A documented history of instability involving other appendicular joints, such as the shoulder, may also be important in the diagnosis of multiligamentous laxity.

A complete assessment of gait, posture, and neurovascular function should be performed in all patients presenting with signs and/or symptoms of hip instability. In addition, palpation of relevant landmarks should also be undertaken to identify potential sources of pain. Range of motion should always be tested bilaterally to assess capsular laxity and to potentially reproduce the patient's symptoms. Mechanical crepitation, snapping, or popping with range-of-motion testing may suggest the presence of a labral tear or flap, a chondral defect with or without an intra-articular loose body or snapping hip, especially when these sounds are associated with pain and apprehension.

There are numerous provocative maneuvers that can be performed to help solidify the differential diagnosis. For capsular laxity, the posterior impingement test and dial test are particularly useful. The posterior impingement test is performed by gently extending and externally rotating the hip with the patient supine. Reproduction of pain or apprehension with this maneuver suggests that posterosuperior osseous impingement may be the result of anterior capsular laxity [16]. Safran et al. demonstrated that the posterior impingement test may also be helpful in identifying abnormal stresses across the anterolateral labrum [17]. A positive test can also occur in patients with normal joint laxity; however, these patients often have abnormal skeletal morphology (e.g., coxa profunda). The dial test is performed by first passively internally rotating the affected hip. The limb is then released which allows the hip to externally rotate back toward the neutral position. Capsular laxity may be suspected when the extremity passively externally rotates >45° from the midline in the axial plane and/or lacks a definitive end point [7]. Pain or apprehension with gentle limb traction

and/or hyperexternal rotation may also be suggestive of capsular laxity.

Standard radiographic analysis includes an anteroposterior (AP) view of the pelvis and a lateral view of the affected hip. An additional Judet view and/or a false-profile view may be helpful to assess acetabular coverage in cases where clinical instability is suspected. The center-edge angle is used to objectively measure femoral head coverage by the acetabulum. Additional measurement can be made to assess the presence of dysplasia (Table 31.1). In some cases, a traction view may be necessary to identify a "vacuum sign" which is often indicative of increased inferior capsular distraction.

Magnetic resonance imaging (MRI) is used to evaluate the patency of surrounding soft tissue structures such as the acetabular labrum, joint capsule, and associated ligaments in cases of either traumatic or atraumatic hip instability. MRI with or without arthrography also plays an important role in locating chondral defects and labral tears that may require surgical treatment. In addition, the alpha angle is measured on MRI to assess abnormal bony growth on the femoral head–neck junction. Femoroacetabular impingement related to capsular laxity can lead to secondary chondral injury [18].

Computed tomography (CT) is routinely performed after reduction of traumatic hip dislocations (1) to assess the adequacy of reduction, (2) to identify acetabular fractures that may not have been visible on initial radiographs, (3) to identify intra-articular loose bodies, and (4) to plan the subsequent surgical approach (if indicated). CT scanning is not often indicated in patients with atraumatic instability due to the lack of significant clinical benefit coupled with the risks associated with exposure to excessive radiation.

Case 1: Traumatic Hip Instability

History/Exam

A 16-year-old high school student with no previous surgical history was playing football after school when he was tackled from behind and suffered an acute posterior dislocation of his left hip. The patient was taken to the emergency room

Fig. 31.4 AP radiograph
following left hip dislocation
showing posterior wall fracture
on the left hip and an avulsion
fracture of the right ischial
tuberosity

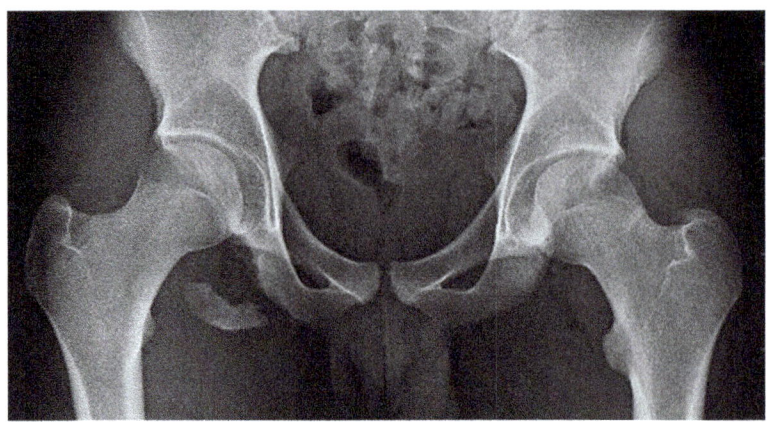

where the hip was immediately reduced approximately 1 h after the initial incident. After being sent home on crutches, the patient presented to our clinic several days later for further evaluation of the injury. On physical examination of his left hip, there were no signs of abrasions, open wounds, ecchymoses, or neurovascular injuries. Only limited range-of-motion testing was performed given the nature of the injury and his level of pain at the time of examination.

Imaging

Following reduction in the emergency room, standard AP and lateral radiographs of the left hip revealed intra-articular loose bodies and fractures of both the posterior wall of the acetabulum and the right ischial tuberosity (Fig. 31.4). CT scanning was then performed which confirmed the diagnosis of a posterior wall fracture with lateral displacement (size, 2.2 cm anteroposteriorly×0.6 cm mediolaterally×2.6 cm superoinferiorly). An osseous fragment of approximately 1.5 cm in diameter was also noted adjacent to the anterior aspect of the femoral head. An MRI scan was also obtained (Fig. 31.5a–d) in which an avulsion fracture of the right ischial tuberosity was discovered with 3.0 cm of inferior displacement. Additionally, posterior labral tear, large joint effusion, and extensive soft tissue edema were identified (Fig. 31.5a, b). Given the findings on history, physical examination, and diagnostic imaging, left hip arthroscopy with possible open reduction and internal fixation was performed the following day.

Arthroscopy

The patient was positioned in the modified supine position on a traction table with a well-padded perineal post. Three loose bodies were discovered within the joint and were subsequently removed with an arthroscopic grasper and pitu-itary rongeur (Fig. 31.6a). Diagnostic arthroscopy revealed a posterior acetabular fracture between the 2 o'clock and 5 o'clock positions which involved approximately 10 % of the acetabulum (Fig. 31.6b). Tearing of the posterior labrum was found; however, the labrum was still firmly attached to the fracture fragment. Bruising of the anterosuperior labrum suggestive of CAM-type femoroacetabular impingement was found (Fig. 31.6c). The ligamentum teres was also completely torn (Fig. 31.6d).

Fragment fixation was undertaken given the increased risk of postoperative instability when a fracture fragment of this size is removed. Two 2.3 mm suture anchors were placed into the fracture site and the suture limbs were passed around the fracture fragment and firmly attached labrum. This method sufficiently reduced the fracture and restored the anatomy of the posterior acetabulum (Fig. 31.6e). The area of grade 4 chondromalacia was sufficiently debrided with a motorized arthroscopic shaver. Debridement of the labrum was then performed using a combination of radiofrequency ablation and arthroscopic shaving between the 2 o'clock and 5 o'clock positions. Debridement of the inflamed synovium and the completely torn ligamentum teres was also performed using the same instrumentation.

Traction was then removed and osteoplasty of the femoral head and neck was performed. After dynamic examination confirmed the site of the CAM lesion and labral impingement, an arthroscopic bur was used to resect excess bone from the 12 o'clock to the 6 o'clock position, thus reestablishing a normal femoral head–neck offset. The lateral epiphyseal vessels were identified and protected throughout the procedure. Dynamic examination was performed once again to confirm adequate osteoplasty, acetabuloplasty, and fracture fixation. The central and peripheral compartments were copiously lavaged with arthroscopic fluid. The capsulotomy was closed using two #2 sutures in a double-limb fashion and secured with a racking half-hitch knot. The arthroscopic instruments were removed and the portal sites were closed using 3-0 nylon sutures in a vertical mattress configuration.

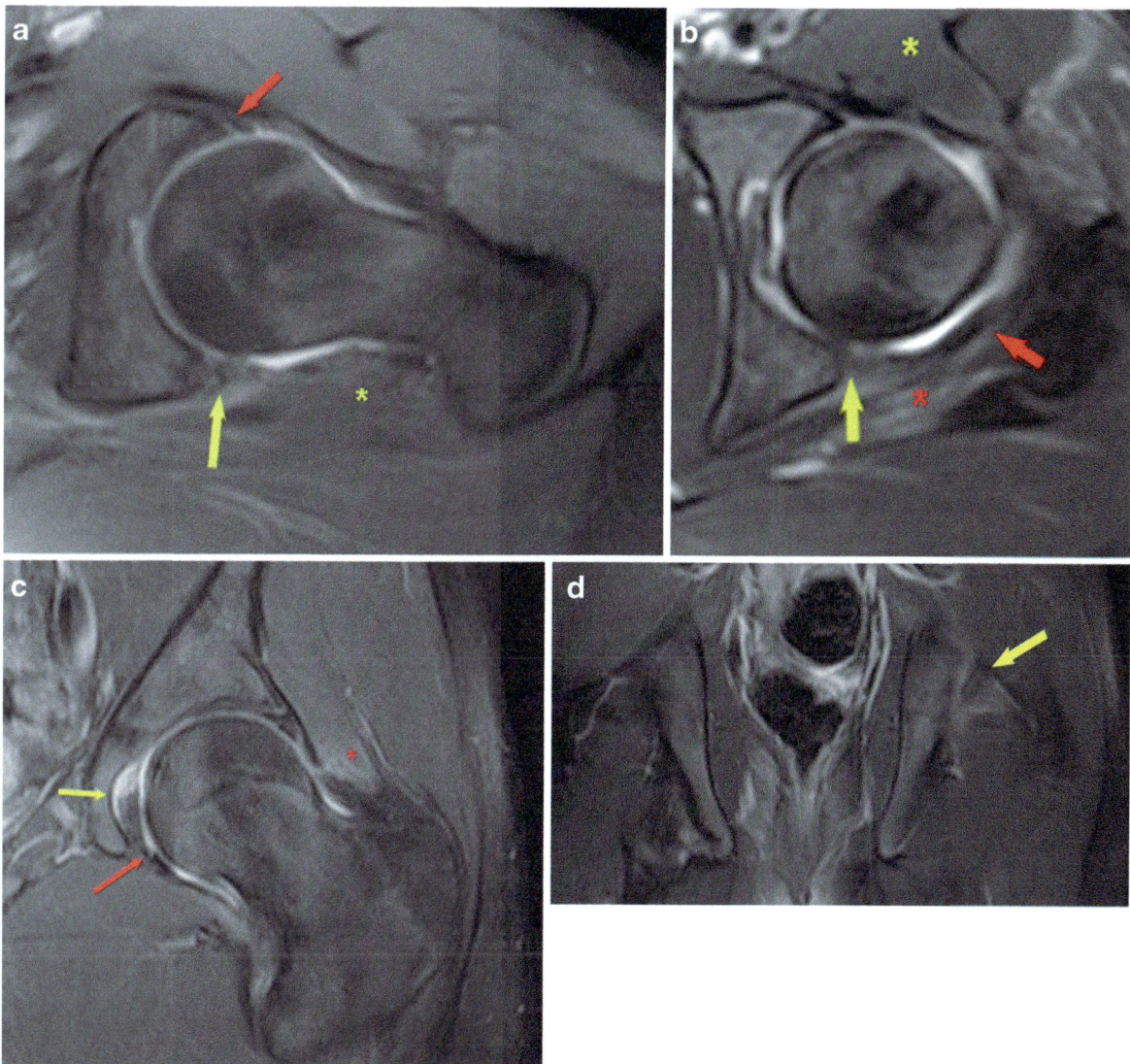

Fig. 31.5 (**a–d**) 3T MRI scan following left hip dislocation. (**a**) This image demonstrates a posterior labral tear with possible avulsion of the posterior acetabular wall (*yellow arrow*) along with increased soft tissue edema posteriorly (*yellow asterisk*). Partial detachment of the anterior labrum can also be seen (*red arrow*). (**b**) In this image, truncation of the posterior labrum can be seen along with irregularity or strain of the posterior capsule. Increased soft tissue edema can also be seen anteriorly and posteriorly (*red* and *yellow asterisks*) with the addition of a muscle strain (*red asterisk*). (**c**) This image demonstrates a high-grade partial tear or full-thickness tear of the ligamentum teres (*yellow arrow*). Strain of the gluteus minimus (*red asterisk*) and a mild joint effusion (*red arrow*) can also be seen. (**d**) Avulsion fracture involving the posterior acetabular wall of the left hip (*yellow arrow*)

Discussion

The femoral head should be immediately reduced in all cases of acute traumatic hip dislocations to prevent the development of avascular necrosis (AVN) [19]. Following reduction, stability should be assessed through an evaluation of passive range of motion. Stress radiography and/or fluoroscopic examination under anesthesia may be necessary in cases where physical examination reveals residual instability despite adequate closed reduction. In all patients, a postreduction CT scan of the pelvis is necessary to rule out the presence of an acetabular wall fracture, intra-articular loose bodies, and other injuries to the femoral head and/or neck. Aspiration of the joint may be necessary when significant hemarthrosis is visible on imaging studies to prevent femoral head osteonecrosis and to provide symptomatic relief [20, 21].

Following closed reduction of an acute hip dislocation, early arthroscopic intervention may also be indicated in select patients to remove intra-articular loose bodies and address other hip pathologies. However, caution should be exercised in patients with acetabular wall fractures due to the potential for leakage of arthroscopic fluid through the fracture crevasse

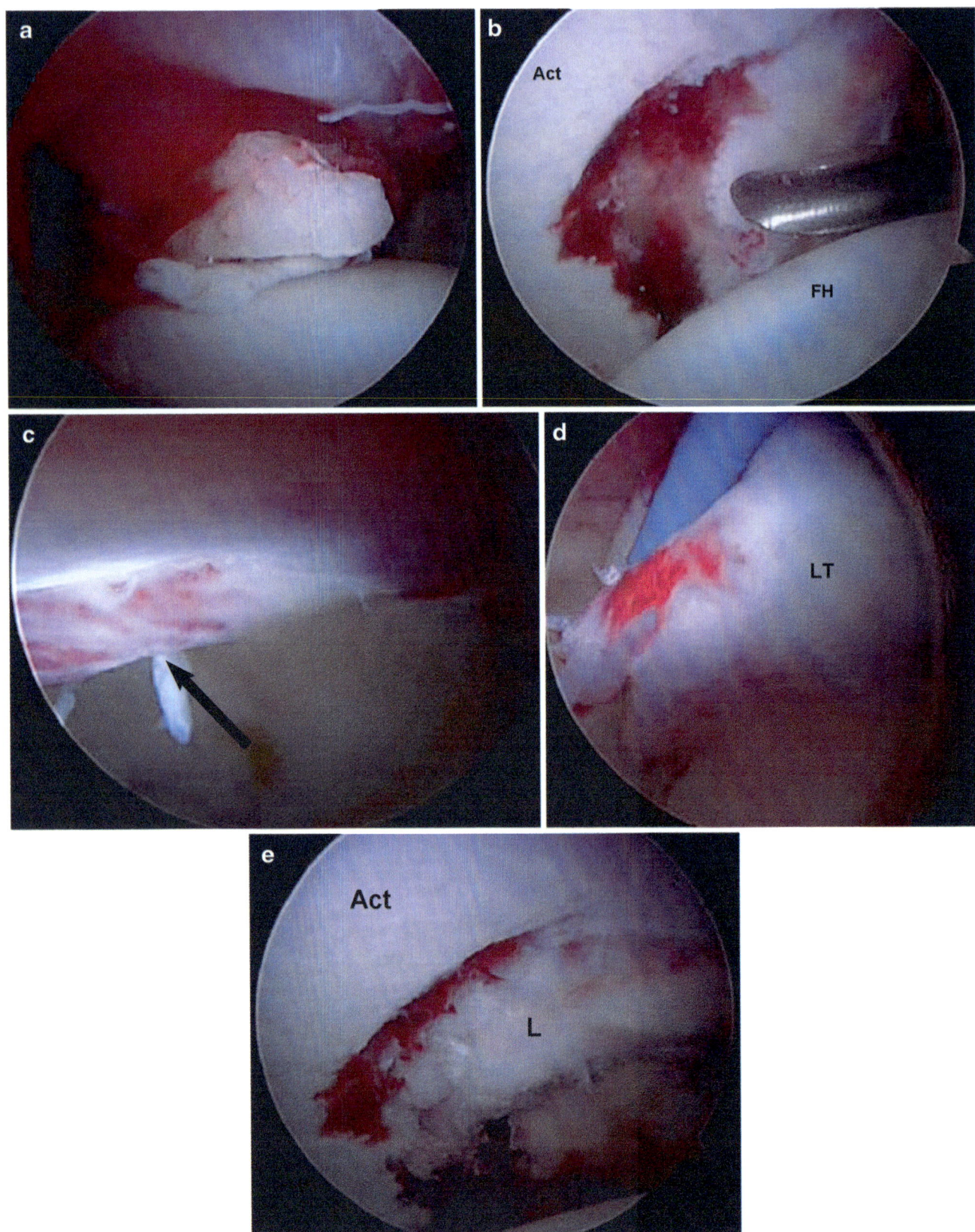

Fig. 31.6 (**a–e**) Arthroscopic images. (**a**) Loose bodies in the joint at the time of arthroscopy. (**b**) Cartilage damage associated with posterior acetabular rim fracture (*Act* acetabulum, *FH* femoral head). (**c**) Bruising of the anterosuperior labrum suggestive of CAM-type femoroacetabular impingement. (**d**) Torn ligamentum teres (LT). (**e**) View of acetabular rim fracture following fixation (*Act* acetabulum, *L* labrum)

and into the abdomen, especially after release of the iliopsoas tendon [22].

Open or arthroscopic suture plication techniques have been described as viable methods for the treatment of acute traumatic hip instability [23, 24]. Arthroscopic thermal capsulorrhaphy is thought to stimulate the inflammatory cascade which may enhance the volume and quality of newly formed collagen within the hip capsule, potentially improving clinical outcomes [23, 25, 26]. However, care must be taken to avoid thermal injury to articular cartilage when using this technique. In addition, acute injuries to the acetabular labrum or the ligamentum teres may also require early arthroscopic management (repair or reconstruction) to prevent painful microinstability which can lead to increased labral stress and chondral defects of the femoral head and/or acetabulum.

Cases 2 and 3: Atraumatic Hip Instability

Case 2: History/Exam

A 21-year-old female elite-level skier presented with complaints of gradually intensifying right hip pain which had begun approximately 1.5 years prior. As a result, she was forced to modify her training program in an effort to alleviate her discomfort. She eventually sought treatment by an orthopedic surgeon in her hometown who initially suggested the possibility of periacetabular osteotomy at the end of the competitive ski season. She was able to control her symptoms well enough to complete the ski season and was subsequently evaluated at our clinic. Upon physical examination, her hip was not tender to palpation and range of motion was adequate; however, flexion and adduction of the hip produced mild pain with an audible click. In addition, there was no firm end point to external rotation of her affected hip (positive dial test).

Case 2: Imaging

Standard radiographs demonstrated a center-edge angle of approximately 23° with normal joint space (Fig. 31.7). An MRI obtained 1 year prior to presentation revealed a bone marrow edema, subchondral cystic changes along the roof of the acetabulum, a mild joint effusion, and a possible labral tear, all of which appeared to be related to concomitant femoroacetabular impingement and mild acetabular dysplasia. Upon presentation to our clinic, we obtained an MR arthrogram which revealed scarring of the iliofemoral ligament, synovitis, mild trochanteric bursitis, and subcortical bone marrow edema along the anterolateral femoral head suggestive of femoroacetabular impingement (Fig. 31.8a, b). We could not definitively rule out the presence of a concomitant labral tear. The relevant findings on history, physical examination, and diagnostic imaging suggest the presence of acetabular dysplasia, capsular laxity with associated femoroacetabular impingement, and possible labral tear within the right hip.

Case 2: Arthroscopy

After the induction of general anesthesia, the right lower extremity was gently distracted to approximately 10 mm. The extremity was prepared and draped using a standard technique. Anterior and lateral viewing portals were established,

Fig. 31.7 AP radiograph showing center-edge angle of 23° and normal joint space

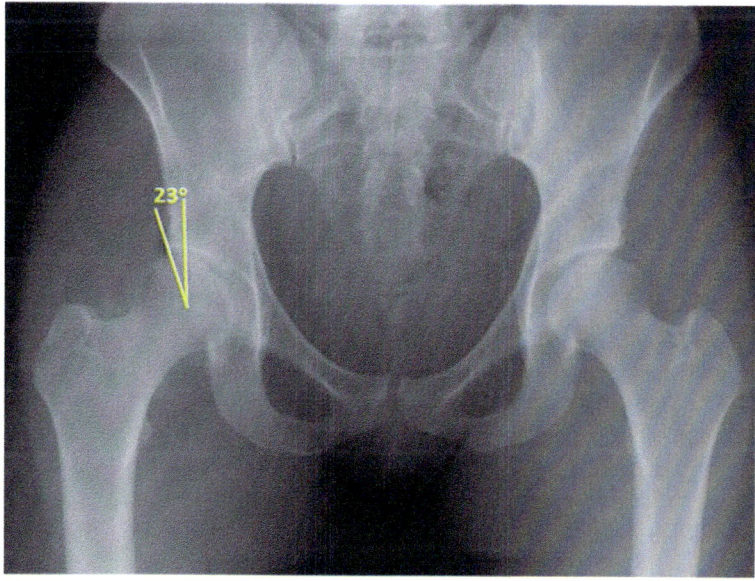

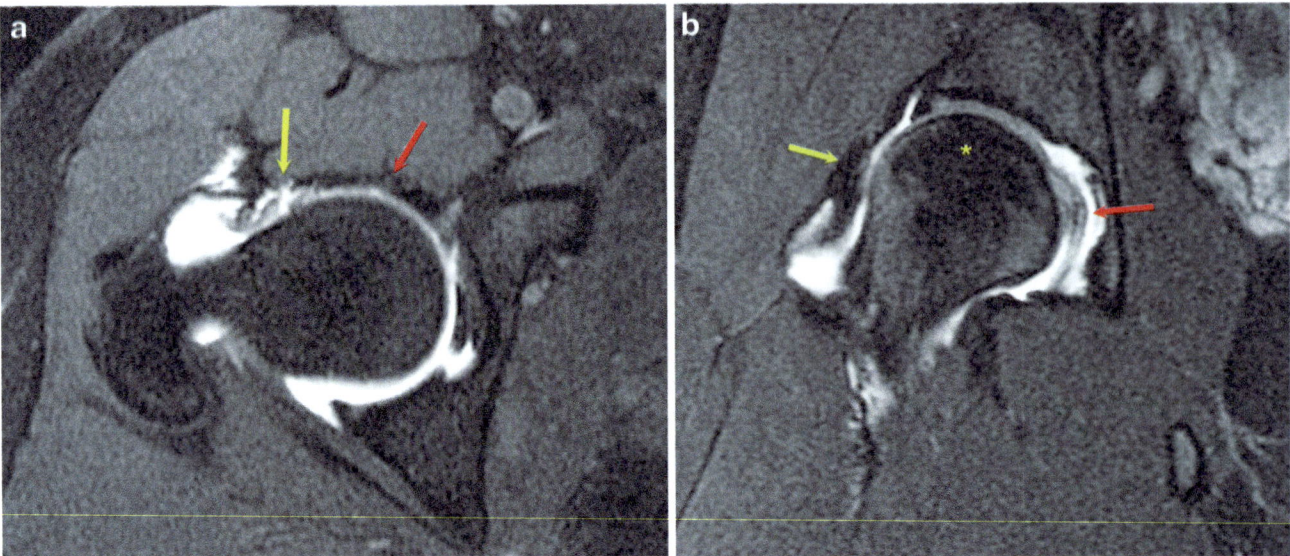

Fig. 31.8 (**a**, **b**) MRI arthrogram. (**a**) This image demonstrates irregular synovial margins consistent with synovitis (*yellow arrow*). Thickening or scarring of the anterior capsule is also visible (*red arrow*). (**b**) In this image, thickening or scarring of the iliofemoral ligament (*yellow arrow*), thickening and irregularity of synovial tissue (*red arrow*), and subchondral bone edema (*yellow asterisk*) are present

a 70° arthroscope was inserted into the joint, and diagnostic arthroscopy was performed. The anterosuperior labrum was found to be patulous with an intra-substance degenerative tear and associated synovitis. Early delamination of articular cartilage was also found near the anterior chondrolabral junction. Consistent with preoperative MRI scans, the anterior wall of the acetabulum appeared to be slightly hypoplastic with labral tearing and bruising (Fig. 31.9a, b) between the 11 o'clock and 2 o'clock positions. An additional partial-thickness tear of the ligamentum teres was found (Fig. 31.9c).

Using the combination of an arthroscopic bur and an osteotome, minimal resection of the anterosuperior acetabular rim was performed to alleviate the previously identified pincer-type impingement resulting in labral delamination and intra-substance tearing. Reattachment of the anterosuperior labrum was performed using three suture anchors. The partial-thickness tear of the ligamentum teres was debrided back to healthy, stable ligament tissue.

Attention was then turned to the peripheral compartment where an obvious bump was identified at the head–neck junction (Fig. 31.9d). After identification and protection of the lateral vessels, an osteoplasty was performed using an arthroscopic bur between the 8 o'clock and 12 o'clock positions at the location of the pincer lesion. Additional bruising and early chondral changes were noted on the femoral head at the site of impingement, and debridement was performed when possible.

At this point, dynamic examination was performed under direct visualization which revealed excellent seal in flexion, extension, abduction, adduction, and internal and external rotation. However, there was some joint laxity with deep flexion. Due to this finding, subsequent suture plication with two #2 high-strength sutures was performed. Dynamic examination was again performed which demonstrated a good end point to external rotation at 45° and excellent labral fixation both before and after the release of traction. Despite the presence of a hypoplastic anterior acetabulum, the femoral head was found to be well contained within the acetabulum after labral repair. The arthroscopic instruments were removed and the portal sites were closed using a standard technique.

Case 3: History/Exam

A 20-year-old female with a history of multiple previous surgeries related to ligamentous laxity presented with a continuation of her right hip pain and loss of motion. She had been diagnosed with Ehlers–Danlos syndrome type III. During the previous year, she underwent arthroscopic debridement of the anterosuperior labrum and an open iliopsoas tendon lengthening procedure on her affected hip at another institution. None of these interventions had provided symptomatic relief, and therefore, the patient sought further treatment at our clinic. On physical examination, passive flexion of her unaffected left hip was approximately 140°, abduction was 70°, adduction was 30°, internal rotation was 20°, and external rotation was 50°. Her right hip had decreased range of motion when compared to the unaffected side. Specifically, passive flexion was 105°, abduction was 45°, adduction was 30°, internal rotation was 20°, and external rotation was 40°. She has pain with flexion, abduction, and adduction. The dial test was negative; however, she had positive impingement signs.

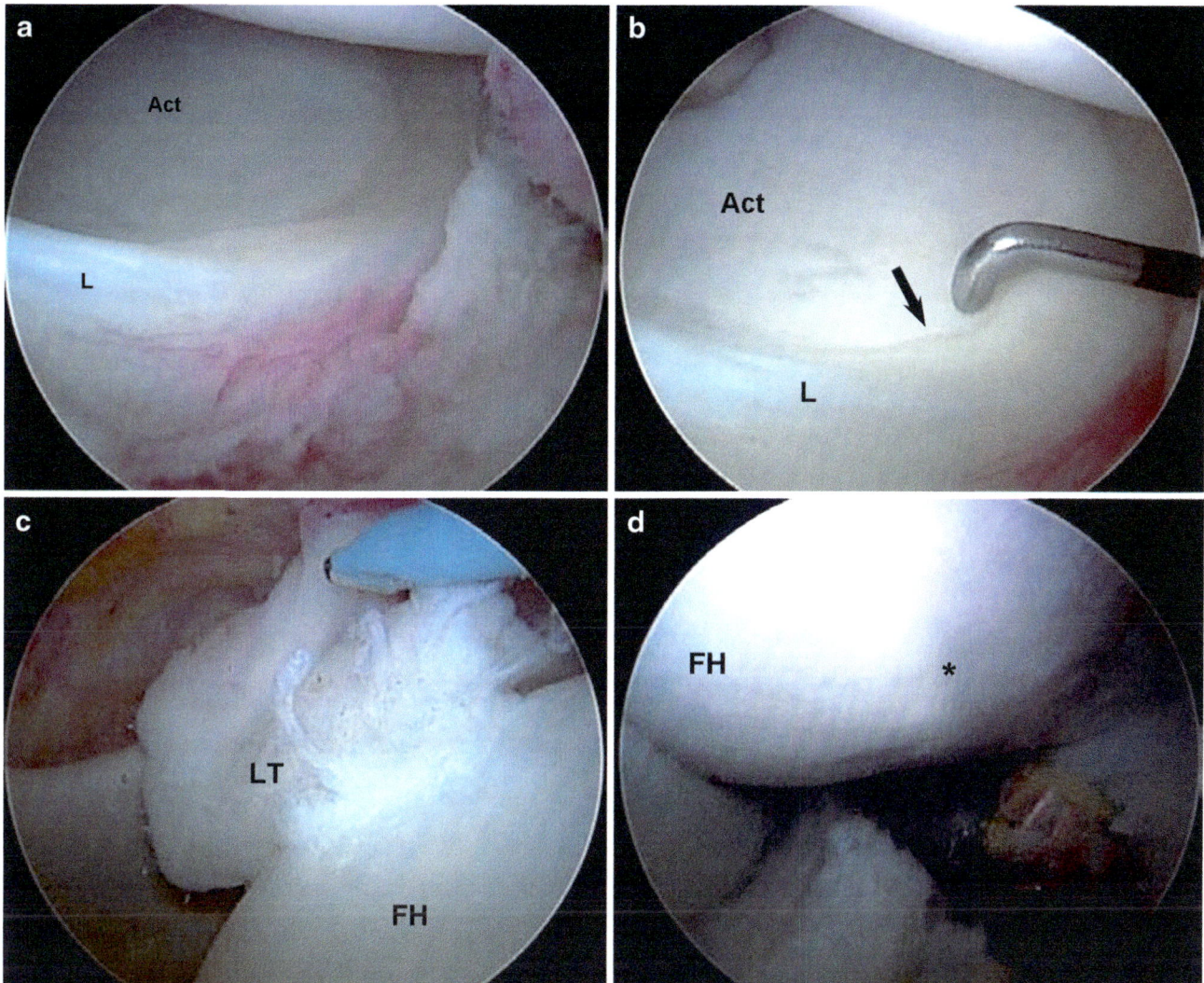

Fig. 31.9 (**a–d**) Arthroscopic images. (**a**) Labral bruising associated with FAI (*L* labrum, *Act* acetabulum). (**b**) Labral tear (*arrow*) at the chondrolabral junction (*Act* acetabulum, *L* labrum). (**c**) Torn ligamentum teres (LT) (*FH* femoral head). (**d**) "Bump" (*asterisk*) on femoral head (FH)–neck junction causing cam impingement

Case 3: Imaging

AP and lateral radiographs of the pelvis and right hip, respectively, demonstrated joint space preservation, a center-edge angle of 31° and an alpha angle of 54° (Fig. 31.10a, b). Subsequent MR arthrogram revealed partial detachment of the lateral and posterolateral chondrolabral junction and mild trochanteric bursitis (Fig. 31.11a–c).

The relevant findings on history, physical examination, and diagnostic imaging suggested the presence of a clinically significant posterolateral labral tear and femoroacetabular impingement in the setting of multiligamentous laxity.

Case 3: Arthroscopy

Following the induction of general anesthesia, the patient was placed supine on the operating table, the operative extremity was prepared and draped using standard technique, and the hip was distracted to approximately 10 mm. Anterior and lateral portals were established, and a 70° arthroscope was introduced into the joint. Diagnostic arthroscopy revealed evidence of capsular adhesions (Fig. 31.12a), severe posterosuperior labral deficiency (Fig. 31.12b), and a partial-thickness tear of the ligamentum teres (Fig. 31.12c). Following debridement of the capsular adhesions, it was

Fig. 31.10 (**a**) AP radiograph of the right hip demonstrates a center-edge angle of 31° and an alpha angle of 54°. (**b**) Cross-table lateral radiograph of the right hip shows maintenance of adequate joint space

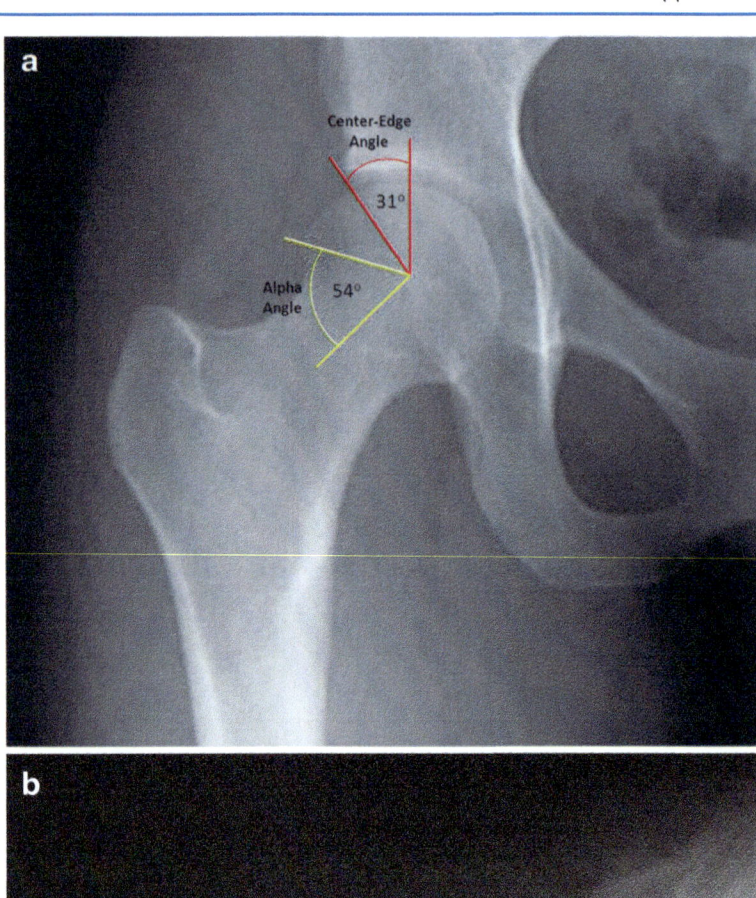

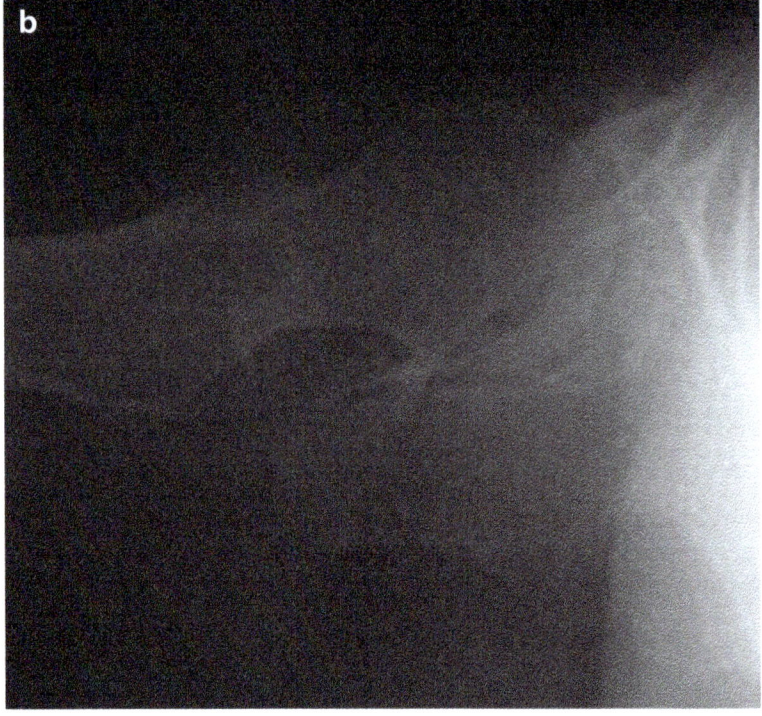

decided that labral reconstruction with autograft was necessary. The ITB graft was prepared and was approximately 4 cm in length and 8 mm in width. An osteochondroplasty was performed at the site of cam impingement, and resection of a pincer lesion was performed using a motorized bur.

The autograft was then inserted, positioned, and secured within the joint using six suture anchors (Fig. 31.12d).

A single 2-0 suture was additionally placed at each graft–labrum junction. This recreated an excellent seal between the femoral head and acetabulum (Fig. 31.12e). Using a motorized shaver and gliding probe, chondroplasty was performed at the location of a grade 3 chondral lesion. Synovectomy was also performed anteriorly, centrally, and peripherally while protecting the lateral vessels.

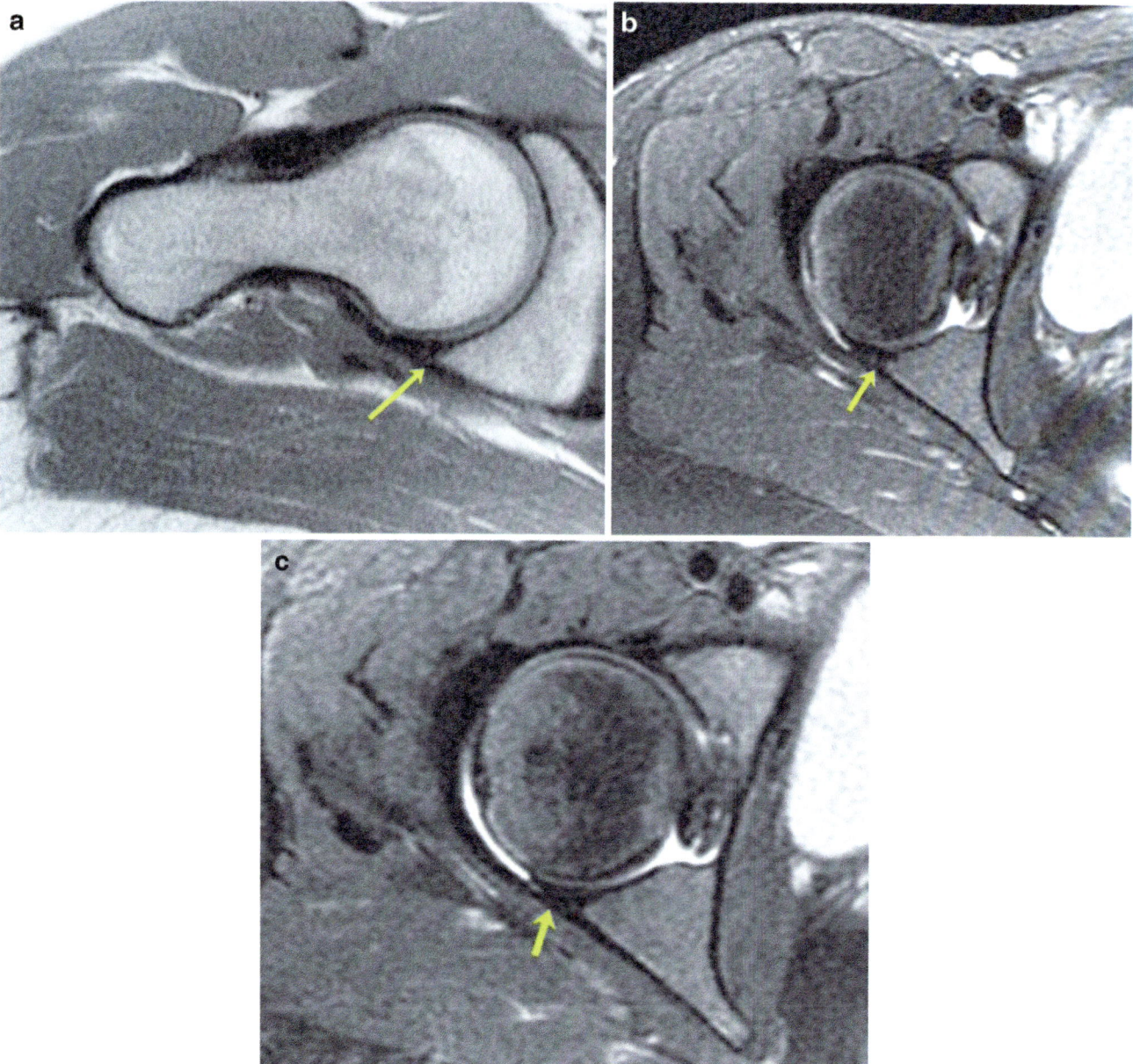

Fig. 31.11 (**a**) This *image* shows mild irregularity of the posterior labrum suggesting a possible tear (*yellow arrow*). (**b**) This axial image demonstrates detachment of the posterior labrum near the chondro-labral junction (*yellow arrow*). (**c**) Subsequent axial image also shows posterior chondrolabral detachment (*yellow arrow*)

Dynamic examination was then performed under direct visualization which demonstrated relief of impingement with adequate range of motion; however, there was still evidence of significant capsular laxity. Due to this, thermal capsulorrhaphy was performed medially followed by anterior capsular plication with interrupted 2-0 sutures. The arthroscopic instruments were then removed and the portal sites were closed using a standard technique.

Cases 2 and 3: Discussion

In most patients with atraumatic instability, initial nonoperative treatment is typically undertaken which includes activity modification and a course of supervised physical therapy to strengthen surrounding musculature. An intra-articular injection of local anesthetic using fluoroscopic or ultrasonographic guidance may also provide some symptomatic relief [27, 28].

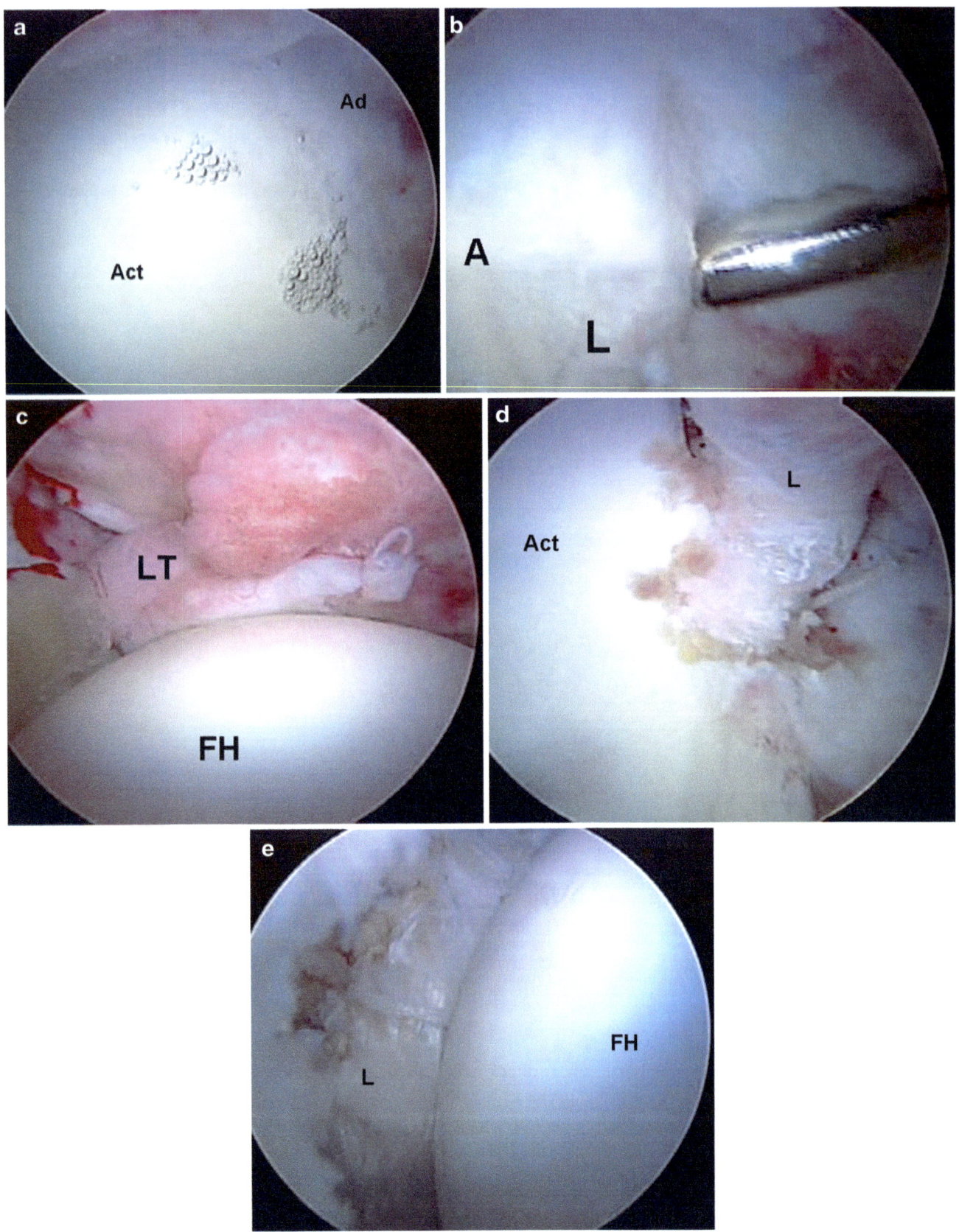

Fig. 31.12 (a–e) Arthroscopic images. (a) Capsulolabral adhesions (Ad) (*Act* acetabulum). (b) Small labrum (L) with capsulolabral adhesions (*A* acetabulum). (c) Torn ligamentum teres (LT) (*FH* femoral head). (d) Labral ITB graft inserted into a joint and attached to the acetabular rim. (e) On dynamic exam, the seal is recreated between the labrum (L) and the femoral head (FH)

Surgical intervention may be performed when conservative measures fail to provide symptomatic relief, especially in cases where genetic predisposition for capsular laxity is present or in cases where clinical evidence of joint hypermobility exists. Additionally, relief of symptoms following intra-articular injection of local anesthetic may also be an indication for surgical treatment [22]. Patients with labral pathology are also likely to benefit from arthroscopic debridement, repair or reconstruction with or without suture plication, or thermal capsulorrhaphy [22, 29].

The role of arthroscopic management in patients with evidence of acetabular dysplasia is currently under debate. Current evidence suggests that arthroscopy may be preferable in cases of borderline dysplasia owing to satisfactory clinical outcomes [30–32], whereas open periacetabular osteotomy or proximal femoral osteotomy may be preferable in cases of severe dysplasia with a low center-edge angle [33–35].

Conclusion

Despite its osseous congruity and inherently stable architecture, the hip joint can become unstable as a result of numerous potential etiologies, most of which are categorized as either traumatic or atraumatic. Early arthroscopic management is often indicated in cases of traumatic instability where intra-articular loose bodies, fractures of the acetabulum, and/or labral tears are visible on initial diagnostic imaging studies. In contrast, arthroscopy in patients with atraumatic instability is most often indicated after an appropriate course of nonoperative therapy fails to result in symptomatic improvement. Regardless of the etiology, preliminary clinical outcomes following hip arthroscopy have been favorable and its role in the management of patients with instability is becoming more clearly defined.

References

1. Fuss FK, Bacher A. New aspects of the morphology and function of the human hip joint ligaments. Am J Anat. 1991;192:1–13.
2. Hewitt JD, Glisson RR, Guilak F, et al. The mechanical properties of the human hip capsule ligaments. J Arthroplasty. 2002;17(1):82–9.
3. Ito H, Song Y, Lindsey DP, et al. The proximal hip joint capsule and the zona orbicularis contribute to the hip joint stability in distraction. J Orthop Res. 2009;27:989–95.
4. Kivlan BR, Richard Clemente F, Martin RL, Martin HD. Function of the ligamentum teres during multi-planar movement of the hip joint. Knee Surg Sports Traumatol Arthrosc. 2013;21(7):1664–8.
5. Martin RL, Kivlan BR, Clemente FR. A cadaveric model for ligamentum teres function: a pilot study. Knee Surg Sports Traumatol Arthrosc. 2013;21(7):1689–93.
6. Philippon MJ, Pennock A, Gaskill TR. Arthroscopic reconstruction of the ligamentum teres: technique and early outcomes. J Bone Joint Surg (Br). 2012;94(11):1494–8.
7. Philippon MJ, Zehms CT, Briggs KK, Manchester DJ, Kuppersmith DA. Hip instability in the athlete. Oper Tech Sports Med. 2007;15:189–94.
8. Cadet ER, Chan AK, Vorys GC, Gardner T, Yin B. Investigation of the preservation of the fluid seal effect in the repair, partially resected, and reconstructed acetabular labrum in a cadaveric hip model. Am J Sports Med. 2012;40(10):2218–23.
9. Myers CA, Register BC, Lertwanich P, Ejnisman L, Pennington WW, Giphart JE, LaPrade RF, Philippon MJ. Role of the acetabular labrum and the iliofemoral ligament in hip stability: an in vitro biplane fluoroscopy study. Am J Sports Med. 2011;39(Suppl):85S–91.
10. Foulk DM, Mullis BH. Hip dislocation: evaluation and management. J Am Acad Orthop Surg. 2010;18(4):199–209.
11. Philippon MJ, Kuppersmith DA, Wolff AB, Briggs KK. Arthroscopic findings following traumatic hip dislocation in 14 professional athletes. Arthroscopy. 2009;25(2):169–74.
12. Berkes MB, Cross MB, Shindle MK, Beda A, Kelly BT. Traumatic posterior hip instability and femoroacetabular impingement in athletes. Am J Orthop (Belle Mead NJ). 2012;41(4):166–71.
13. Krych AJ, Thompson M, Larson CM, Byrd JW, Kelly BT. Is posterior hip instability associated with cam and pincer deformity? Clin Orthop Relat Res. 2012;470:3390–7.
14. Domb BG, Philippon MJ, Giordano BD. Arthroscopic capsulotomy, capsular repair, and capsular plication of the hip: relation to atraumatic instability. Arthroscopy. 2013;29(1):162–73.
15. Bracken J, Tran T, Ditchfield M. Developmental dysplasia of the hip: controversies and current concepts. J Paediatr Child Health. 2012;48(11):963–72.
16. Signorelli C, Lopomo N, Bonanzinga T, Marcheggiani Muccioli GM, Safran MR, Marcacci M, Zaffagnini S. Relationship between femoroacetabular contact areas and hip position in the normal joint: an in vitro evaluation. Knee Surg Sports Traumatol Arthrosc. 2013;21(2):408–14.
17. Safran MR, Giordano G, Lindsey DP, Gold GE, Rosenberg J, Zaffagnini S, Giori NJ. Strains across the acetabular labrum during hip motion: a cadaveric model. Am J Sports Med. 2011;39(Suppl):92S–102.
18. Johnston TL, Schenker ML, Briggs KK, Philippon MJ. Relationship between offset angle alpha and hip chondral injury in femoroacetabular impingement. Arthroscopy. 2008;24(6):669–75.
19. Zlotorowicz M, Czubak J, Caban A, Kozinski P, Boguslawska-Walecka R. The blood supply to the femoral head after posterior fracture/dislocation of the hip, assessed by CT angiography. Bone Joint J. 2013;95-B(11):1453–7.
20. Moorman 3rd CT, Warren RF, Hershman EB, Crowe JF, Potter HG, Barnes R, O'Brien SJ, Guettler JH. Traumatic posterior hip subluxation in American football. J Bone Joint Surg Am. 2003;85-A(7):1190–6.
21. Soto-Hall R, Johnson LJ, Johnson RA. Variation sin the intra-articular pressure of the hip joint in injury and disease: a probable factor in avascular necrosis. J Bone Joint Surg Am. 1964;46:509–16.
22. Kocher MS, Frank JS, Nasreddine AY, Safran MF, Philippon MJ, Sekiya JK, Kelly BT, Byrd JW, Guanche CA, Martin HD, Clohisy JC, Mohtadi NG, Griffin DR, Sampson TG, Leunig M, Larson CM, Ilizaliturri Jr VM, McCarthy JC, Gambacorta PG. Intra-abdominal fluid extravasation during hip arthroscopy: a survey of the MAHORN group. Arthroscopy. 2012;28(11):1654–60.e2.
23. Philippon MJ. The role of arthroscopic thermal capsulorrhaphy in the hip. Clin Sports Med. 2001;20(4):817–29.
24. Graham B, Lapp RA. Recurrent posttraumatic dislocation of the hip: a report of two cases and review of the literature. Clin Orthop Relat Res. 1990;256:115–9.
25. Hayashi K, Hecht P, Thabit 3rd G, Peters DM, Vanderby Jr R, Cooley AJ, Fanton GS, Orwin JF, Markel MD. The biologic response to laser thermal modification in an in vivo sheep model. Clin Orthop Relat Res. 2000;373:265–76.

26. Hayashi K, Peters DM, Thabit 3rd G, Hecth P, Vanderby Jr R, Fanton GS, Markel MD. The mechanism of joint capsule thermal modification in an in-vitro sheep model. Clin Orthop Relat Res. 2000;370:236–49.

27. Furtado RN, Pereira DF, Luz KR, Santos MF, Konai MS, Mitraud SD, Rosenfeld A, Fernandes AD, Natour J. Effectiveness of imaging-guided intra-articular injection: a comparison study between fluoroscopy and ultrasound. Rev Bras Reumatol. 2013;53(6):476–82.

28. Mathews J, Alshameeri Z, Loveday D, Khandiju V. The role of fluoroscopically guided intra-articular hip injections in potential candidates for hip arthroscopy: experience at a UK tertiary referral center over 34 months. Arthroscopy. 2014;30(2):153–5.

29. Geyer MR, Philippon MJ, Fagrelius TS, Briggs KK. Acetabular labral reconstruction with an iliotibial band autograft: outcome and survivorship analysis at minimum 3-year follow-up. Am J Sports Med. 2013;41(8):1750–6.

30. Byrd JW, Jones KS. Hip arthroscopy in the presence of dysplasia. Arthroscopy. 2003;19(10):1055–60.

31. Yamamoto Y, Ide T, Nakamura M, Hamada Y, Usui I. Arthroscopic partial limbectomy in hip joints with acetabular hypoplasia. Arthroscopy. 2005;21(5):586–91.

32. Domb BG, Stake CE, Lindner D, El-Bitar Y, Jackson TJ. Arthroscopic capsular plication and labral preservation in borderline hip dysplasia: two-year clinical outcomes of a surgical approach to a challenging problem. Am J Sports Med. 2013;41(11): 2591–8.

33. Ganz R, Klaue K, Vinh TS, Mast JW. A new periacetabular osteotomy for the treatment of hip dysplasias: technique and preliminary results. Clin Orthop Relat Res. 1988;232:26–36.

34. Clohisy JC, Barrett SE, Gordon JE, Delgado ED, Schoenecker PL. Periacetabular osteotomy for the treatment of severe acetabular dysplasia. J Bone Joint Surg Am. 2005;87(2):254–9.

35. Clohisy JC, Nunley RM, Curry MC, Schoenecker PL. Periacetabular osteotomy for the treatment of acetabular dysplasia associated with major aspherical femoral head deformities. J Bone Joint Surg Am. 2007;89(7):1417–23.

Peritrochanteric Space Disorders: Anatomy and Management

32

Austin W. Chen, John M. Redmond, Kevin F. Dunne, and Benjamin G. Domb

Introduction

The peritrochanteric space is an important area to be considered in the differential diagnosis of hip pain. Classically, trochanteric bursitis has been defined as "tenderness to palpation over the greater trochanter with the patient in the side-lying position" [1–3]. However, recent studies have shown that adjacent structures are also involved, and bursal inflammation itself is rare [4–6]. The term, greater trochanteric pain syndrome (GTPS), encompasses all involved pathology in this region. Improved knowledge of the anatomy, pathology, advances in magnetic resonance imaging (MRI), evolution of hip arthroscopy and endoscopy, and more specific diagnostic criteria has led to better recognition and understanding of this disease process [7].

Greater trochanteric bursitis, external coxa saltans (snapping hip), and gluteus medius and minimus pathology are distinct etiologies of GTPS [8, 9]. GTPS is a very common clinical entity with an incidence ranging from 10 to 25 % of the general population and a prevalence of 17.6 % [9, 10]. Patients usually present with a dull pain on the lateral aspect of the hip, occasionally with radiation posteriorly and into the thigh. Pain is typically exacerbated by excessive activity and direct pressure over the greater trochanter. Patients may have an antalgic gait or limp; however, range of motion is usually preserved.

A.W. Chen, MD
Department of Orthopedic Surgery, University of Illinois Hospital at Chicago, Chicago, IL, USA
e-mail: Achen9@uic.edu

J.M. Redmond, MD • K.F. Dunne, BS
American Hip Institute, Westmont, IL, USA
e-mail: John.redmond@live.com; Kfdunne11@gmail.com

B.G. Domb, MD (✉)
American Hip Institute, Westmont, IL, USA

Adventist Hinsdale Hospital, Hinsdale, IL, USA
e-mail: drdomb@americanhipinstitute.org

Multiple risk factors for GTPS have been identified. The most commonly affected age groups are those in the fourth to sixth decade of life. Gender appears to play a role, as women are affected three to four times more frequently than men [10]. It has been associated with ipsilateral knee osteoarthritis, obesity, and low back pain among many others [9, 10]. A trochanter further lateral than the lateral border of the iliac crest has been shown to be a predisposing risk factor for GTPS [11].

The etiology of GTPS is frequently due to overuse or acute direct trauma, especially falls [10]. Rarely, it may be due to crystal deposition or infection, especially tuberculosis [12, 13]. Although a significant portion of patients with trochanteric pain will respond to conservative management, with success rates reported at 60–90 %, a portion of patients will continue to experience disabling symptoms despite treatment directed at the trochanteric bursa [14]. Those afflicted with GTPS confer levels of disability and quality of life similar to those with end-stage hip osteoarthritis and are even less likely to be in full-time work [7]. Thus, an accurate diagnosis and timely treatment are of the utmost importance [15].

Anatomy

The anatomy of the peritrochanteric space has been well described [9, 16]. The precise anatomy of the tendon insertions, bursae, and bony facets of the greater trochanter can be seen in Fig. 32.1a–c. Most individuals have three bursae peripheral to the greater trochanter, though four have been consistently described. The function of these fluid-filled sacs is to provide cushion and aid in smooth motion of the gluteus tendons, iliotibial band (ITB), and tensor fascia lata [17]. The subgluteus maximus bursa is the largest. Located between the gluteus maximus muscle and gluteus medius tendon, lateral to the greater trochanter, it is most frequently implicated in GTPS and referred to as the "trochanteric bursa" [18].

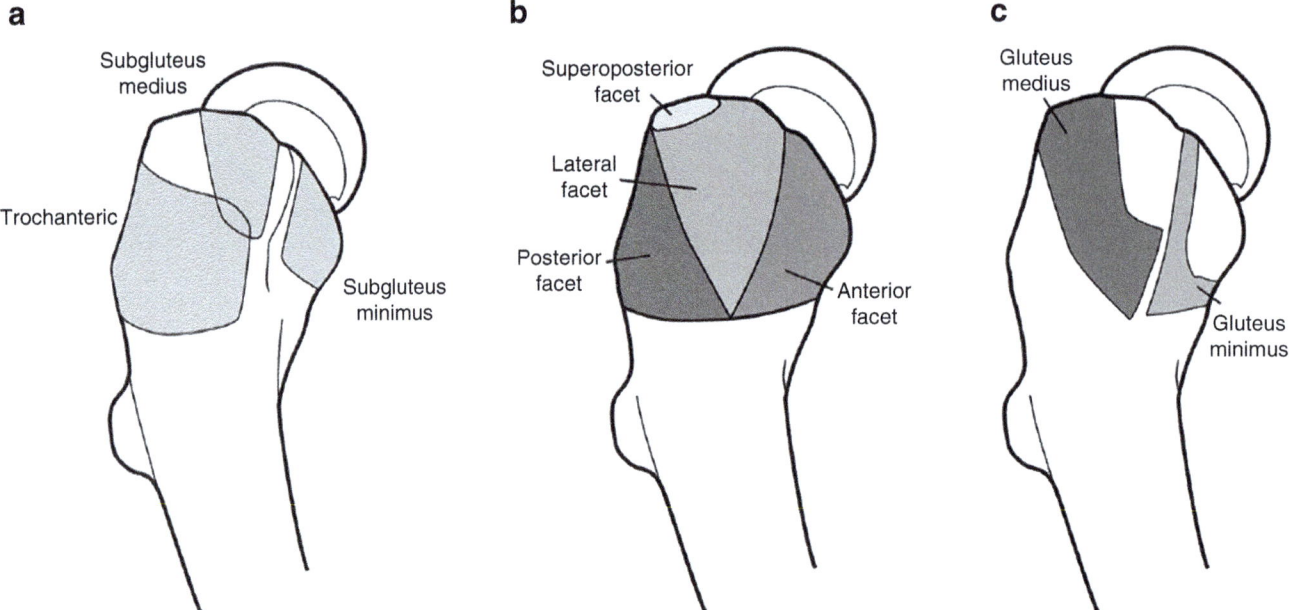

Fig. 32.1 (**a–c**) Anatomy of greater trochanter with tendinous insertion sites and bursae. (**a**) The three main bursae and their positions. (**b**) Geometry of greater trochanter with different facets. (**c**) Footprints of gluteus medius and minimus tendon insertions (**a–c**: Used with permission from Domb BG, Nasser RM, Botser IB. Partial-thickness tears of the gluteus medius: rationale and technique for trans-tendinous endoscopic repair. Arthroscopy. 2010; 26(12):1697–1705)

Table 32.1 Similarities and differences between shoulder and hip rotator cuffs

	Shoulder rotator cuff	Hip rotator cuff
Functional anatomy		
Internal rotator	Subscapularis	Iliopsoas
Stabilizers and rotators, initiation and assistance in abduction	Supraspinatus and infraspinatus	Gluteus medius and minimus
Abduction	Deltoid	Tensor fascia lata
Clinical presentation	Pain with motion	Tenderness over lateral aspect of hip
	Tenderness	Weakness in abduction
	Weakness in abduction	
MRI/ultrasound	Visualized on MRI and ultrasound	Visualized on MRI and ultrasound
Mechanism	Degenerative tearing	Degenerative tearing
	Acute trauma	Acute trauma
Arthroscopic evaluation	Articular tears can be visualized as either exposed footprint or delamination	Undersurface tears cannot be easily visualized

Used with permission from Domb BG, Nasser RM, Botser IB. Partial-thickness tears of the gluteus medius: rationale and technique for trans-tendinous endoscopic repair. Arthroscopy. 2010; 26(12):1697–1705

The most superficial structure of the peritrochanteric space is a fibromuscular sheath composed of the gluteus maximus, tensor fascia lata, and ITB. The gluteus maximus inserts into the posterior aspect, while the tensor fascia lata inserts into the superior and anterior aspects of the ITB. The fascia lata that encloses these structures extends superiorly without muscle attachment to the tubercle of the iliac crest. Just distal to the hip joint, the ITB has a thick expansion—the gluteus maximus sling—that inserts on the posterolateral femur. The ITB crosses the knee joint distally and inserts onto Gerdy's tubercle on the anterolateral aspect of the proximal tibia.

The hip abductors consisting of the gluteus medius and minimus have been referred to as the "rotator cuff tears of the hip" [14, 19]. Table 32.1 shows similarities and differences between shoulder and hip rotator cuffs. The smaller gluteus minimus originates from the anterior inferior iliac spine (AIIS) to the posterior inferior iliac spine (PIIS), runs parallel to the femoral neck, and inserts into both the hip capsule and lateral facet beneath the gluteus medius [20]. The fan-shaped gluteus medius originates from the anterior superior iliac spine (ASIS), outer edge of the iliac crest, and back to the posterior superior iliac spine (PSIS). Depending on the source, it has two or three insertion points on the greater trochanter: the superoposterior facet has a thick insertion from the central posterior portion of the muscle, a thin, broad lateral component inserts onto the lateral facet, and a continuation onto the anterior facet that is not visible macroscopically [16, 21, 22].

Using electromyography (EMG), Gottschalk et al. describe the primary function of the gluteus minimus and posterior gluteus medius as a stabilizer of the femoral head in the acetabulum during motion and gait [23]. The anterior and middle portions of the gluteus medius have a vertical pull and help initiate abduction, whereas the tensor fascia lata is the major abductor of the hip.

Differential Diagnosis

The diagnosis of GTPS can be complicated due to the multiple possible sources of pain surrounding the hip girdle. The differential diagnosis includes intra-articular hip pathology, extra-articular hip pathology, and sources outside of the hip. Intra-articular sources include labral tears, loose bodies, femoroacetabular impingement, capsular laxity, ligamentum teres rupture, and chondral damage. Extra-articular sources include stress fractures, piriformis syndrome, and neoplasm [24]. Sources of hip pain that are outside the hip include pathology of the superior gluteal nerve, meralgia paresthetica, lumbar spondylosis, and lumbar radiculopathy [20]. In regard to the latter two, a limp and hip abductor weakness may be present along with radiating pain, similar to GTPS. Also, patients with a history of total hip arthroplasty, especially through an anterolateral approach, may have iatrogenic injury to the abductor mechanism or its innervations [20]. A detailed history, physical exam, and the appropriate imaging will help to narrow the differential.

Imaging

Imaging has long been thought to be largely unnecessary for the diagnosis of GTPS. However, with cases refractory to standard conservative management, imaging can be very helpful. The most common imaging modalities include plain radiographs, ultrasound, and MRI.

Radiographs do not typically show specific abnormalities with regard to GTPS. A trochanter further lateral than the lateral border of the iliac crest has been shown to be a predisposing risk factor for GTPS [11]. Intrabursal calcifications, abductor calcific tendinosis, or enthesophytes of the greater trochanter may be seen but are not specific. Radiographs are also useful to rule out fracture or osteoarthritis of the hip.

Ultrasound can also aid in the diagnosis of GTPS. It can be especially useful in diagnosing abductor tendon pathology, as

it has been shown to have a sensitivity of 79 % and positive predictive value of 100 %, rivaling that of MRI [25]. Dynamic ultrasound can be used to visually confirm the diagnosis of external snapping hip [26].

MRI is currently considered the gold standard for diagnosing GTPS [9, 27]. In the setting of GTPS, patients with abnormalities seen in T2-weighted images are significantly more likely to have abductor tendinopathy [28]. Kingzett-Taylor et al. reviewed 250 hip MRIs for pain involving the buttock, lateral hip, and groin [29]. Gluteus medius and minimus tears were seen in 35 studies. They concluded that tendinopathy is a frequent cause of GTPS and likely associated with trochanteric bursitis. However, another study cautioned that MRI might have a false-positive rate as high as 88 % when evaluating abductor tendon tears [30].

Treatment

Conservative management is effective for the great majority of greater trochanteric pain syndrome cases. Treatment begins with rest, refraining from pain exacerbating activities, ice, nonsteroidal anti-inflammatory medications (NSAIDs), and physical therapy. Therapy focuses on stretching and strengthening of the iliotibial band (ITB) and gluteal muscles. Independent or a combination of these measures can have a cure rate of greater than 90 % [31]. For refractory cases, glucocorticoid injections have been shown to return patients to their baseline activity level 49–100 % of the time [32]. Low-energy shock-wave therapy has also been shown to have superior improvement in visual analog scale and Harris hip scores compared with the primary outcome of other conservative measures [33, 34]. All of these options should be exhausted before surgical options are considered.

As with many surgical procedures, open techniques have given way to arthroscopic and endoscopic solutions. Hip arthroscopy has made significant advances since its introduction in 1931 and popularization during the late 1980s and early 1990s [35–37]. These surgical techniques and other technological achievements have helped expand hip arthroscopy to extra-articular anatomic regions, which is considered peritrochanteric endoscopy. The peritrochanteric endoscopic borders are the tensor fascia lata and ITB laterally, the abductor tendons superomedially, the vastus lateralis inferomedially, and the gluteus maximus muscle superiorly and its tendon posteriorly [8].

Hip arthroscopy and peritrochanteric endoscopy can be utilized based on surgical goals; however, portal placement, visualization pearls, and other procedural nuances have been described. Voos et al. suggest using the same portals used for evaluation of central and peripheral compartment disorders with the anterior portal offering best access to the peritrochanteric space [38]. This portal is made 1 cm lateral to the anterior superior iliac spine within the interval of the tensor fascia lata and sartorius. For optimal access, safety, and hemostasis, balloon dissection has been shown to be superior to blunt dissection [39]. A standard 30° or 70° arthroscope is sufficient for peritrochanteric endoscopy.

Case-based examples of common causes of greater trochanteric pain syndrome will be outlined in this chapter. Multiple figures will be utilized to reveal the relationship between MRI imaging and intraoperative arthroscopy for each case. The three cases include:

1. Recalcitrant trochanteric bursitis
2. External snapping hip
3. Gluteus medius tear

Case 1: Recalcitrant Trochanteric Bursitis

History/Exam

A 45-year-old female presented to orthopedic clinic with an 18-month history of right hip pain. The patient stated that the pain began while running. Initially, running was the only activity that bothered her; however, she began to experience pain with prolonged standing, sitting with the affected leg crossed, or lying on the affected side. She had an active lifestyle that included running 2 miles 6 days per week but has since stopped. She located the pain to the lateral aspect of her hip and noted that it radiated down the lateral aspect of the thigh. She quantified her pain as a 5 on a scale of 0–10. The pain was intermittent in nature.

She was initially seen by a chiropractor and was prescribed a course of physical therapy that included range of motion and strengthening exercises. This, however, exacerbated the patient's pain to a 9 out of 10, and she discontinued physical therapy after 1 month. She subsequently sought treatment by her primary care physician who again recommended physical therapy with the addition of NSAIDs. However, due to the prior failure of physical therapy and an allergy to NSAIDs, she could not complete her recommendations.

On physical examination, her gait was normal without signs of Trendelenburg. The skin was normal—no ecchymosis, erythema, or swelling. There was point tenderness to palpation over the greater trochanter. Her hip range of motion was as follows: 120° of flexion, 10° of internal rotation with pain, 30° of external rotation, and 30° of abduction. She experienced pain with resisted abduction and internal rotation, but there were no signs of weakness. She had a positive FABER test and Ober's test. Anterior impingement and internal snapping were also evident. She was otherwise neurovascularly intact throughout the lower extremity.

After failing physical therapy and other conservative measures, the patient was offered a corticosteroid injection with local anesthetic into her right trochanteric bursa. The injection was conducted under ultrasound guidance. Within 30 min, the patient's pain had substantially improved. The injection provided 3–4 weeks of pain relief before symptoms began to return.

Imaging

Standard X-rays were obtained. Views including anterior/posterior pelvis, right hip false profile, bilateral Dunn views, and a right hip cross-table lateral. The joint spaces were well preserved. The patient did have a mild femoral cam lesion and a small crossover sign. There was no sign of antecedent trauma to the trochanter.

Typically, the diagnosis of trochanteric bursitis is clinical; however, due to the recalcitrant nature of the problem and signs of both intra- and extra-articular pathology, an MRI arthrogram was obtained to delineate other possible pathology. Coronal fat-saturated T2-weighted images are shown in Fig. 32.2a–d, and axial fat-saturated T2-weighted images are shown in Fig. 32.3a–d.

Figure 32.2a denotes the anatomic structures being scrutinized. A moderate amount of fluid and edema is seen lateral to the greater trochanter suggesting bursitis as shown by the long thin arrow in Figs. 32.2a–d and 32.3b–d. In addition to bursitis, mild signal heterogeneity can be seen in the substance and at the insertion of the abductor tendons indicating tendinosis without evidence of tear evidenced by the short fat arrow in Fig. 32.2b–d. A labral tear was also identified.

The patient's clinical and radiographic presentation was consistent with trochanteric bursitis, although she also had mild signs and symptoms of femoroacetabular impingement. Given her failure to improve with conservative treatment, the patient elected to proceed with surgery and was consented for right hip arthroscopy with labral treatment, femoral osteoplasty, acetabuloplasty, and peritrochanteric endoscopy with trochanteric bursectomy and debridement. The patient was counseled that if a gluteus medius tear was identified, it would be repaired.

Arthroscopy

The patient was brought to operating room placed in the supine position on a traction table extension with a well-padded perineal post. Traction was applied to the hip under fluoroscopy. An anterolateral portal was created first, followed by a more distal lateral accessory portal. A capsulotomy was made parallel to the acetabular rim connecting the two portals. Diagnostic arthroscopy and intra-articular procedures were completed first.

A blunt obturator was used to reinsert the arthroscope into the peritrochanteric compartment through the mid-anterior portal. A thickened band of bursa is seen being probed in Fig. 32.4. The shaver was introduced via the anterolateral portal and trochanteric bursectomy, and peritrochanteric debridement was performed. The remainder of the peritrochanteric space was examined, including the gluteus medius and maximus tendon insertions, which were found to be intact.

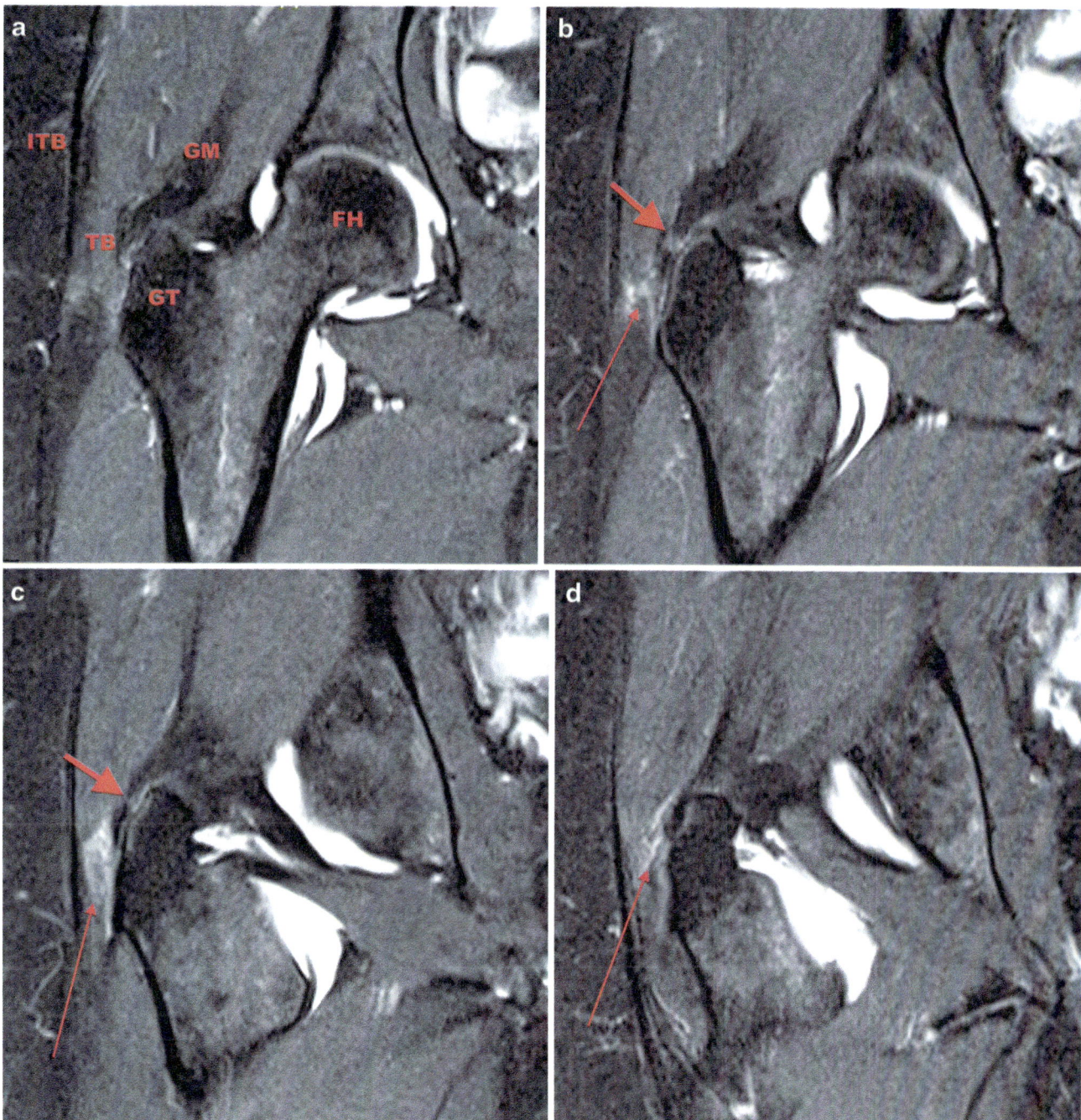

Fig. 32.2 (**a**) Coronal fat-saturated T2-weighted image. The anatomic structures being scrutinized: *GM* gluteus medius, *FH* femoral head, *GT* greater trochanter, *TB* trochanteric bursa, *ITB* iliotibial band. (**b, c**) Mild signal heterogeneity can be seen in the substance and at the insertion of the abductor tendons indicating tendinosis without evidence of tear evidenced by the *short fat arrow*. (**b–d**) A moderate amount of fluid and edema is seen lateral to the GT suggesting bursitis as shown by the *long thin arrow*

Discussion

Trochanteric bursitis is usually self-limited and responds well to conservative treatment [2, 40]. Open or arthroscopic surgical management of this condition is effective but rarely necessary lending to a paucity of high-level research. Fox et al. retrospectively reported on 27 patients treated with arthroscopic bursectomy for recalcitrant trochanteric bursitis.

At a minimum of 1 year, 23 out of 27 patients had "good or excellent" results immediately postoperative with no complications. Symptoms recurred in one patient at 1 year and two patients at 5 years.

A tight ITB rubbing over the greater trochanter is a documented etiology of trochanteric bursitis [41]. Thus, there are reports of modifying the ITB in addition to trochanteric bursectomy during arthroscopic surgery. Farr et al. performed

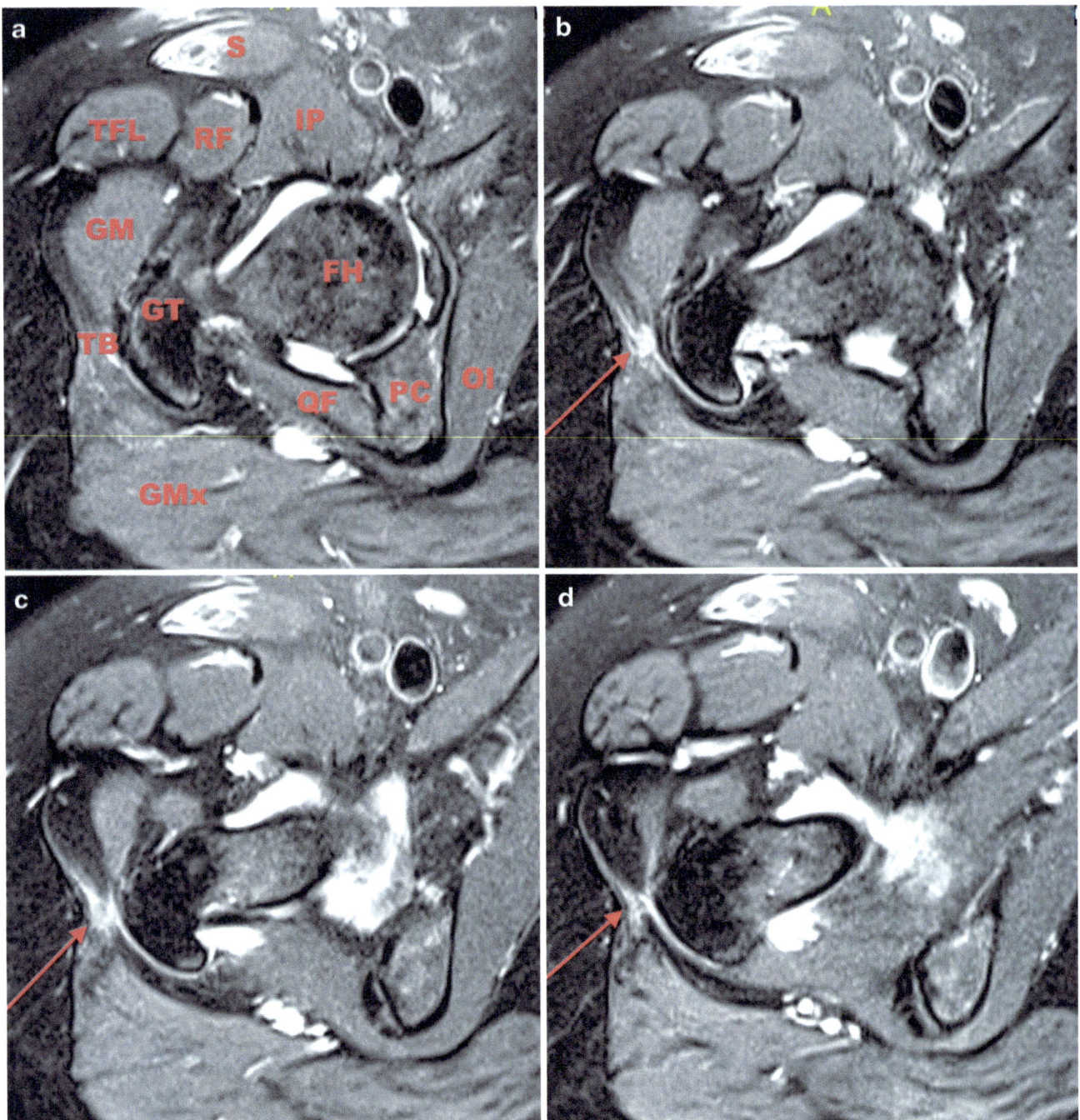

Fig. 32.3 (**a**) Sagittal fat-saturated T2-weighted image. Surrounding anatomic structures in clockwise direction: *S* sartorius, *IP* iliopsoas, *FH* femoral head, *OI* obturator internus, *PC* posterior column, *QF* quadratus femoris, *GMx* gluteus maximus, *TB* trochanteric bursa, *GT* greater trochanter, *GM* gluteus medius, *TFL* tensor fascia lata, *RF* rectus femoris. (**b–d**) A moderate amount of fluid and edema is seen lateral to the GT suggesting bursitis as shown by the *long thin arrow*

arthroscopic bursectomy along with an ITB release in two patients. They reported that both had complete relief of symptoms and returned to their preoperative occupational and recreational activities without recurrence. Govaert et al. also advocated for release of the ITB during surgical management of GTPS [42]. They treated five patients with a follow-up of 6 weeks in which three were "satisfied" and two were "very satisfied." One patient, however, developed a large hematoma that required open evacuation. Weinrauch et al. describe ultrasound-assisted arthroscopy to ensure adequate decompression of the peritrochanteric space [43]. Strauss et al. believe releasing the posterior one third of the

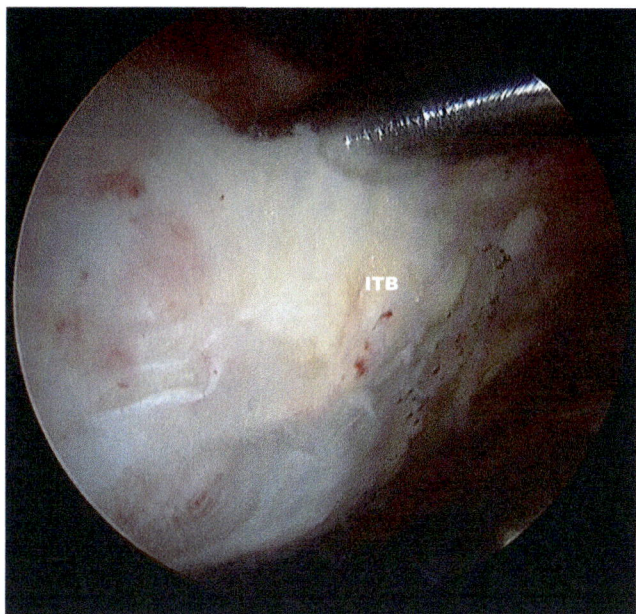

Fig. 32.4 Thickened band of bursa is seen being probed

ITB is only necessary when there is clinical evidence of external snapping or ITB tightness (positive Ober's test); otherwise, bursectomy alone is sufficient [8].

Baker et al. prospectively evaluated 30 patients with recalcitrant trochanteric bursitis following arthroscopic bursectomy for a mean of 26.1 months [44]. Significant improvements in pain scores (7.2 preoperatively versus 3.1 postoperatively) and Harris hip scores (51 preoperatively versus 77 postoperatively) were noted in the 25 patients available for follow-up. Of note, the authors "often noted scuffing or irritation of the gluteus medius and minimus tendons and, occasionally frank tears of their insertions…that were treated with debridement of the edges and decompression of the area." The precise number of patients with these findings was not mentioned; therefore, it is difficult to apply their results to recalcitrant trochanteric bursitis, specifically. Their results should more appropriately be applied to patients with the general diagnosis of GTPS. In addition, the diagnostic criteria used in this study were mainly clinical. MRIs were not routinely obtained. Of those that were available, "no attempt to correlate the MRI results with the findings at the time of surgery" was made.

An isolated diagnosis of recalcitrant trochanteric bursitis is likely rare. Bird et al. reviewed the MRIs of 24 women with GTPS finding that 62.5 % had evidence of gluteus medius tendonitis, 45.8 % with gluteus medius tears, but only 8.3 % had objective evidence of trochanteric bursitis [4]. Additionally, Long et al. retrospectively reviewed the ultrasound findings of 877 patients with GTPS [5]. Nearly 80 % (700 patients) did not have bursitis on ultrasound, while 50 % (438 patients) had abductor tendinosis, and 28.5 % (250 patients) had a thickened ITB. The case presented here had concomitant abductor tendinosis and femoroacetabular impingement with labral damage, in addition to the trochanteric bursitis. Therefore, when preoperatively planning for surgical management of recalcitrant trochanteric bursitis, there should be a high degree of suspicion for coexisting pathology in the peritrochanteric space as well as intra-articularly.

Case 2: External Snapping Hip

History/Exam

A 23-year-old female presents to the orthopedic clinic with long-standing bilateral hip pain, left side greater than the right. She states that since childhood, she has been able to "take her hip out of its socket" referring to a snapping/clunking sensation. As an adult, her pain has been increasing and is associated with same snapping during the last 4 years. Of recent, it has also begun to affect her knees. The hip pain is located on the lateral aspect of the hip, is intermittent, and is rated at 8 out of 10. She locates her knee pain to the anterolateral aspect of the knee just inferior to the joint line. Both her hip and knee pains increase with activity level. The only relieving factor she has found is ice. She has completed three courses of physical therapy of 6–8 weeks each without relief of symptoms. She has also had corticosteroid injections into bilateral greater trochanteric bursas and knee joints without improvement.

On physical examination, she appears healthy. Examination of her gait and overall alignment reveals mild genu valgum but a normal heel-to-toe gait. Her bilateral hip range of motion is as follows: 120° of flexion, 30° of internal rotation with pain, 50° of external rotation with pain, and 50° of abduction. She denies pain directly over the greater trochanters, however, does admit to tenderness over the piriformis. With the patient lying on her side, affected side up, flexing the hip while palpating the greater trochanter reveals a snapping sensation of the IT band over the trochanter. Applying a firm pressure relieves the snapping. The patient also exhibits a positive Ober's test. Of note, the patient did also exhibit signs of internal impingement and internal snapping.

Examination of the patient's knees does not show any effusion or erythema. Bilateral knee range of motion is 130° flexion with pain to −5° extension. She is tender to palpation over Gerdy's tubercle of the bilateral tibias. There is no patellar instability, but there is crepitus and mild tenderness to palpation at the inferior pole of the patella. Muscle testing of the lower extremities reveals 5/5 strength bilaterally. Additionally, bilateral lower extremities are neurovascularly intact.

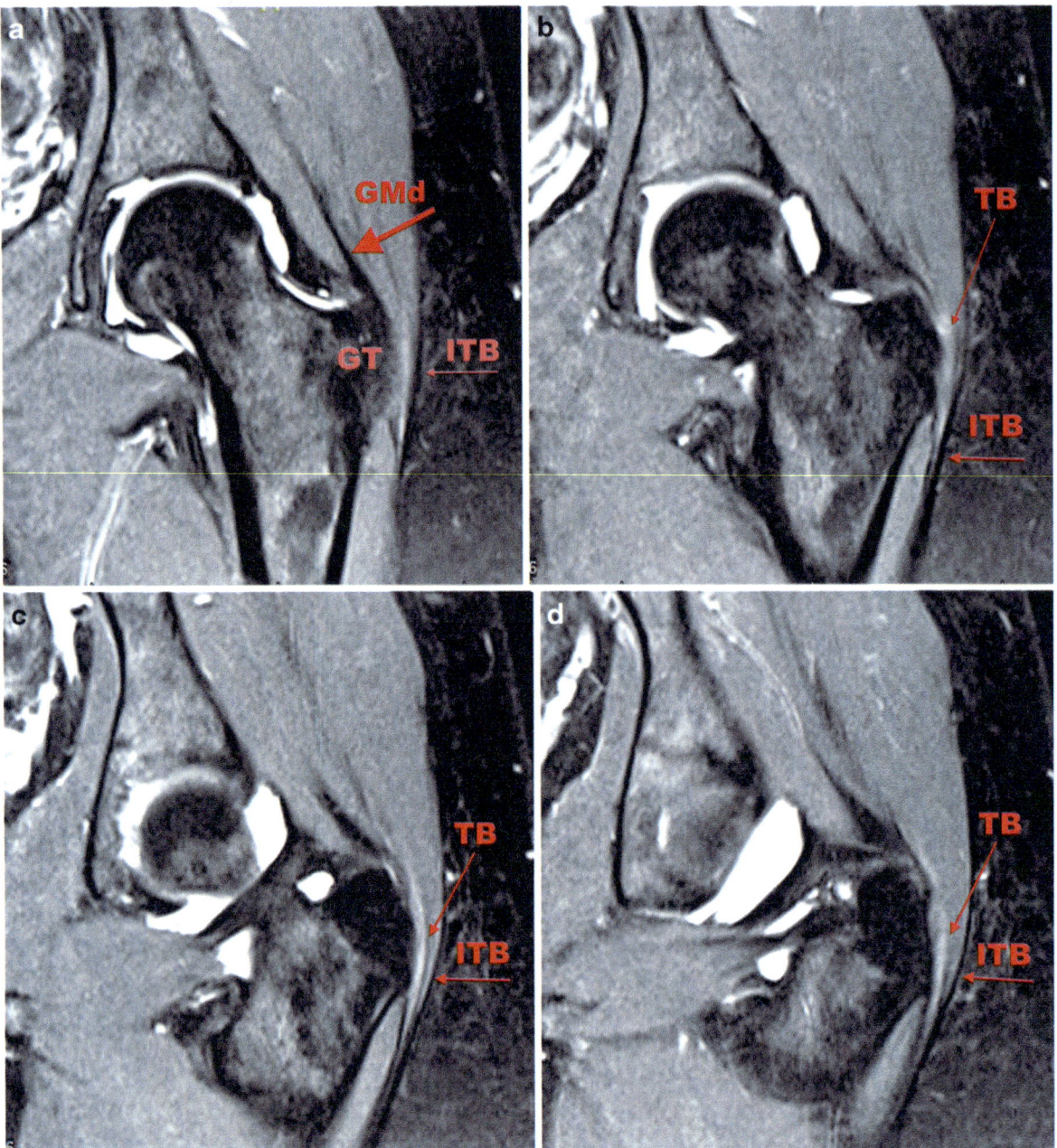

Fig. 32.5 (**a**) Coronal T2 fat-saturated weighted MRI. A *thin black line* lateral to the greater trochanter (GT) represents the iliotibial band (ITB). The gluteus medius tendon is also identified (GMd). (**b–d**) Coronal T2 fat-saturated weighted MRI. There is slight thickening of the trochanteric bursa (TB) with mild increase in signal intensity between the GT and ITB

Imaging

X-rays included a supine AP view of the pelvis, bilateral false profile and Dunn views, and a cross-table lateral view. Joint spaces are preserved bilaterally. There is a 20 % crossover sign bilaterally.

An MRI arthrogram was conducted due to the patient's anterior impingement symptoms in order to further delineate a labral tear—the pathology and treatment of the labral tear will not be discussed in this chapter. Figures 32.5a–d and

32.6a–d depicts coronal and axial T2 fat-saturated weighted MRI cuts moving from anterior to posterior and inferior to superior, respectively. A thin black line lateral to the greater trochanter (GT) represents the iliotibial band (ITB). The gluteus medius tendon is also identified (GMd) in Fig. 32.5a. Figure 32.5b–d depict slight thickening of the trochanteric bursa (TB) with a very mild increase in signal intensity. The iliotibial band (ITB) does not demonstrate significant abnormalities in these cuts. The axial sequences, however, are more useful to show areas of thickening of the iliotibial band

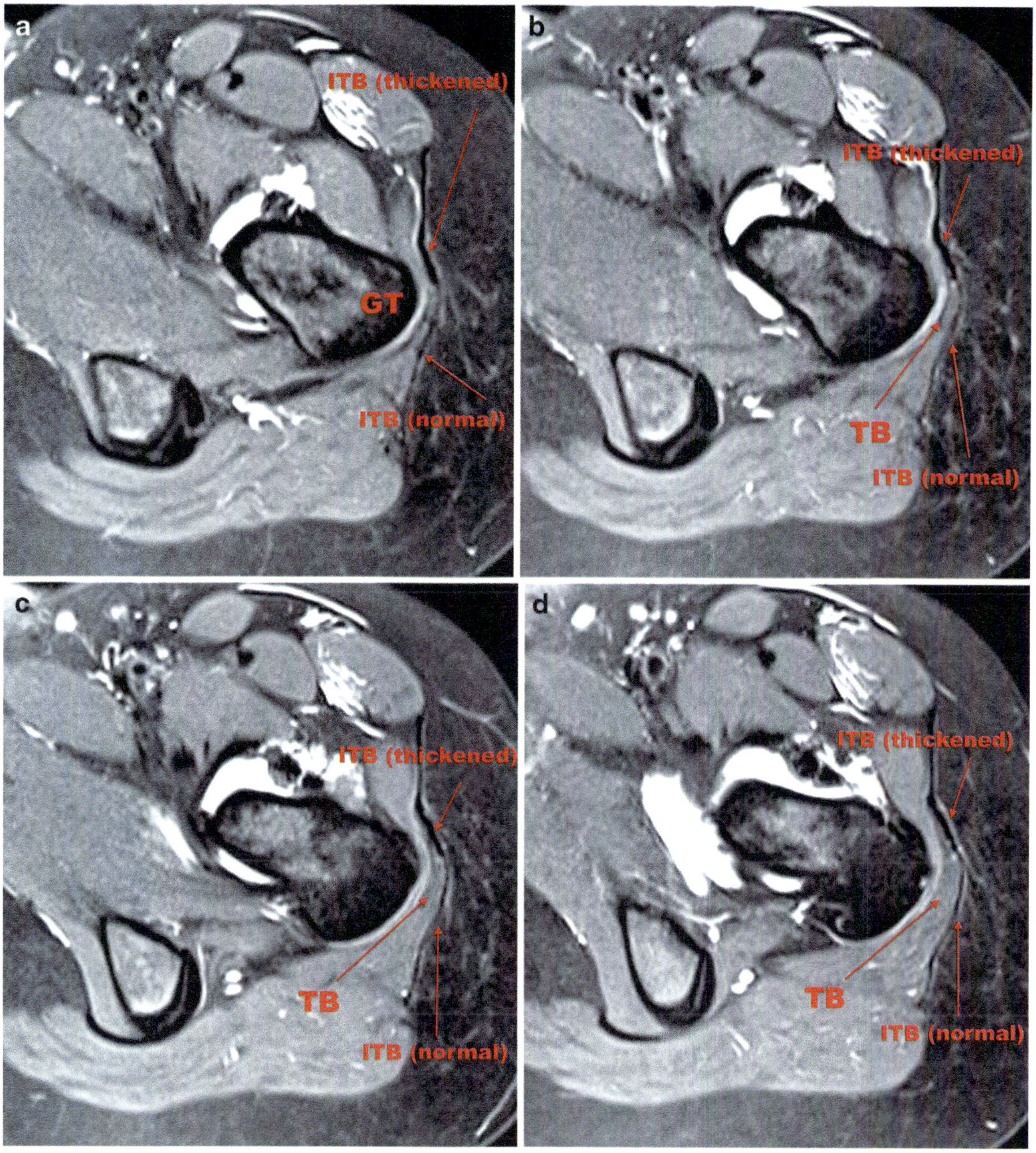

Fig. 32.6 (**a**) Axial T2 fat-saturated weighted MRI. An area of thickened ITB can be seen just anterolateral to the GT in contrast to the normal appearing posterolateral ITB. (**b–d**) Axial T2 fat-saturated weighted MRI. An area of thickened ITB can be seen just anterolateral to the GT in contrast to the normal appearing posterolateral ITB. There is slight thickening of the trochanteric bursa (TB) with mild increase in signal intensity between the GT and ITB

in the sagittal plane. An area of thickened ITB can be seen just anterolateral to the greater trochanter in contrast to the posterolateral ITB seen in Fig. 32.6a–d.

The patient failed all conservative management of the external snapping hip related to a contracted ITB. The decision was then made to proceed with surgery. The patient was informed of the risks, benefits, and alternatives of trochanteric bursectomy, IT band release, with possible labral repair, debridement, or reconstruction. The patient understood and agreed to proceed with surgery.

Arthroscopy

The patient was brought to operating room placed in the supine position on a traction table extension with a well-padded perineal post. Traction was applied to the hip under fluoroscopy. An anterolateral portal was created first, followed by a more distal lateral accessory portal. A capsulotomy was made parallel to the acetabular rim connecting the two portals. Diagnostic arthroscopy and intra-articular procedures were completed first. A capsular plication was

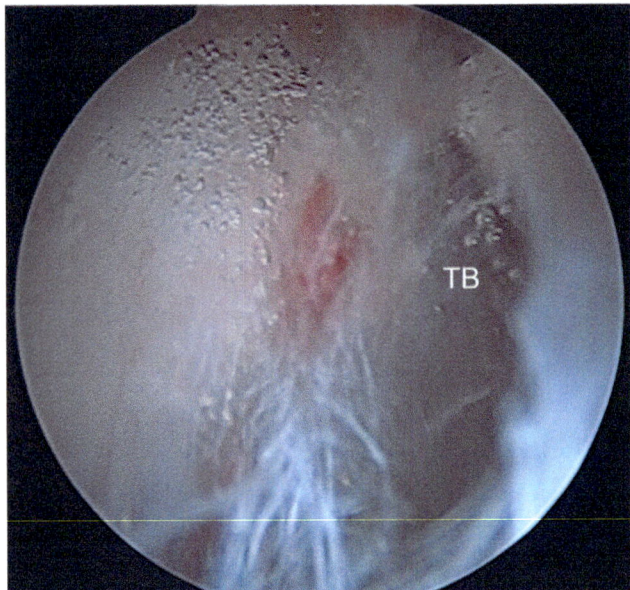

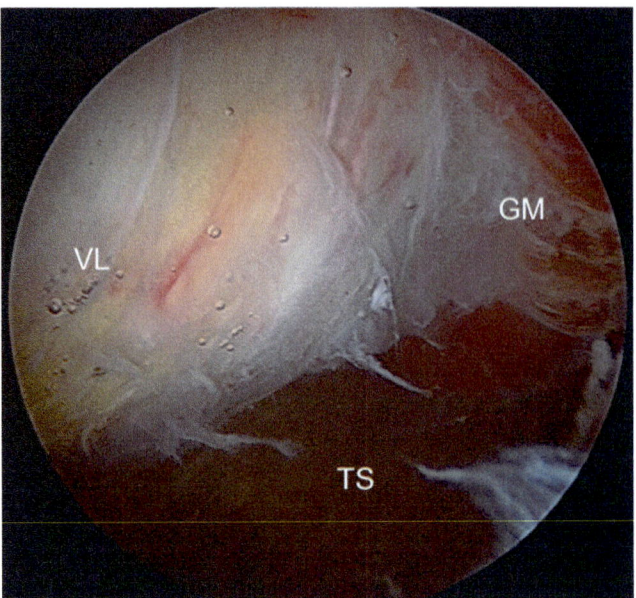

Fig. 32.7 Peritrochanteric endoscopy of the left hip. The arthroscope is inserted in the distal mid-anterior portal viewing cephalad. Note the trochanteric bursa (TB) present prior to shaver insertion and bursectomy

Fig. 32.8 Peritrochanteric endoscopy of the left hip. The arthroscope is inserted in the distal mid-anterior portal viewing cephalad. With the bursal tissue removed, the gluteus medius (GM), vastus lateralis (VL), and trochanteric space (TS) can be identified. No tears of the gluteus medius tendon are identified

completed prior to turning attention to the peritrochanteric space.

The arthroscope was placed into the peritrochanteric compartment via a mid-anterior portal and the shaver through the anterolateral portal (Fig. 32.7). Trochanteric bursectomy and debridement were performed (Fig. 32.8). The entire peritrochanteric space was examined, including the gluteus medius and maximus tendon insertions. No abductor pathology could be identified. Next, a radiofrequency wand was used to perform a cruciform-shaped incision in the IT band in the area overlying the greater trochanter to address the external snapping hip (Figs. 32.9, 32.10 and 32.11).

Discussion

External coxa saltans, or external snapping hip, is most commonly due to thickened portions of the posterior ITB or the anterior border of the gluteus maximus sliding over the greater trochanter [45]. Flexing the hip causes the posterior thickened band to snap anteriorly in relation to the greater trochanter. Asymptomatic snapping should be considered a normal occurrence [46]. The main cause for increased tension in the ITB is still unknown as the biomechanical repercussions of its modification [47].

Though modifying the ITB is an accepted treatment for refractory external snapping hip, the manner in which it is modified has various descriptions in the literature. Open Z-lengthening of the ITB was first described in 1983 with several modifications and reported outcomes in the following

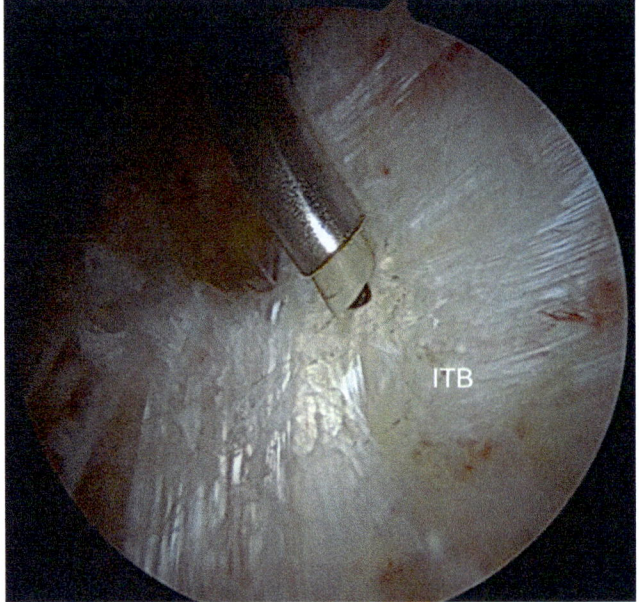

Fig. 32.9 Peritrochanteric endoscopy of the left hip. The arthroscope is inserted in the distal mid-anterior portal viewing cephalad and lateral. The electrocautery is being used to divide the iliotibial band (ITB) overlying the trochanter

years [46, 48–50]. Until recently, only open procedures had been described.

Ilizaliturri et al. was first to describe an all-endoscopic technique in 2006 [51]. They prospectively reported on a consecutive series of 11 hips. All were clinically diagnosed with

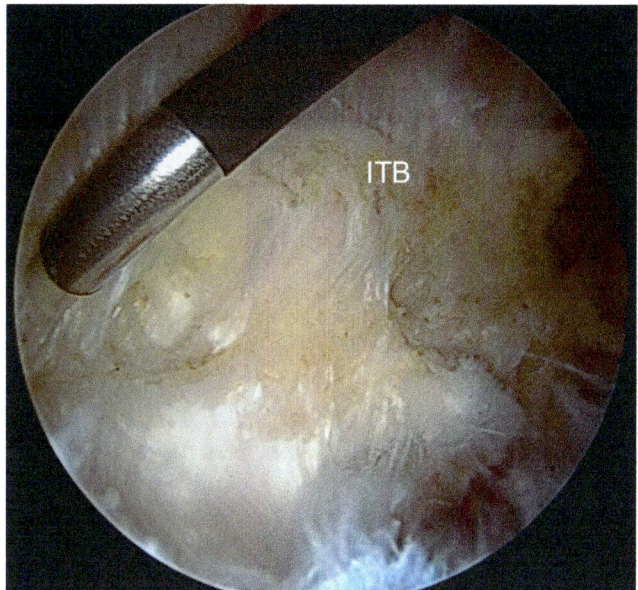

Fig. 32.10 Peritrochanteric endoscopy of the left hip. The arthroscope is inserted in the distal mid-anterior portal viewing cephalad and lateral. The electrocautery is being used to divide the iliotibial band (ITB) overlying the trochanter

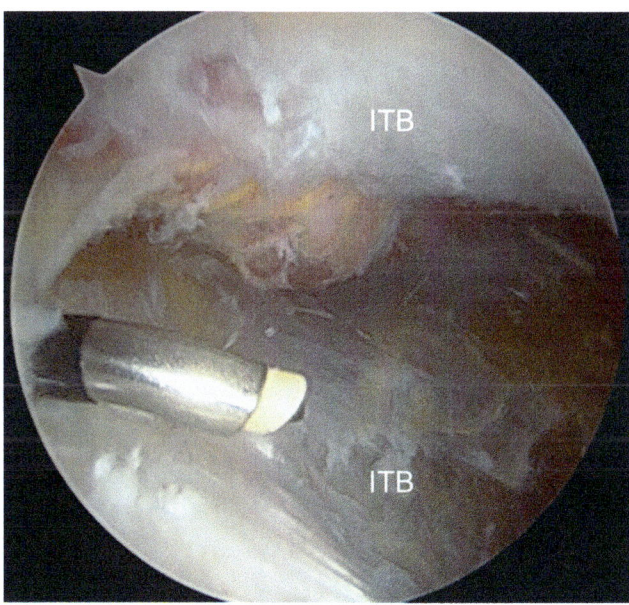

Fig. 32.11 Peritrochanteric endoscopy of the left hip. The arthroscope is inserted in the distal mid-anterior portal viewing cephalad and lateral. The electrocautery has divided the iliotibial band (ITB)

external snapping hip, had failed conservative management, and were treated with a diamond-shaped partial resection of ITB directly overlying the greater trochanter along with trochanteric bursectomy. At an average follow-up of 2 years, one patient had painless snapping, while the remainder had no complaints and returned to a preoperative level of activity. Zini et al. reported similar results on 15 retrospectively reviewed patients [52]. In contrast to Ilizaturi et al., the ITB

was transversally released [51]. They report significant improvements in visual analog scale (VAS) scores. All patients returned to preoperative levels of activity without revisions or complications; however, 40 % did admit to "very slight" pain with strenuous sporting activities.

Polsello et al. hypothesized that endoscopic release of the gluteus maximus tendon (GMT) near its insertion at the linea aspera would have a similar effect on ITB tension and provide similar results for treating symptomatic external snapping hip [47]. Eight patients (nine hips) were treated with endoscopic GMT release and retrospectively reviewed with an average follow-up of 22 months. Seven of the eight patients achieved resolution of the pain and snapping after the initial procedure. One patient required a revision procedure for complete relief. All eight patients returned to their previous level of activity.

Voos et al. give a detailed description with specific dimensions of an ITB release [38]. They state it should be performed along the posterolateral portion of the greater trochanter, beginning at the vastus tubercle insertion extending to the tip of the greater trochanter. The release should be a Z-type of 1 cm anterior, 3 cm distal, and 1 cm posterior with slight variation based on the fibers under the greatest amount of tension.

The senior author (B.G.D.) prefers a cruciform incision of the ITB for external snapping hip along with trochanteric bursectomy. Though evidence is sparse regarding endoscopic modifications for treatment of external snapping hip, our early experience has demonstrated this to be a safe and effective treatment option.

Case 3: Gluteus Medius Tear

History/Physical

A 66-year-old female was referred by an orthopedic surgeon for evaluation of left lateral hip pain. The patient reports pain for 2 years that has progressively worsened. It is aggravated by bending to and sleeping on the left side as well as prolonged sitting. She has completed a 4-week course of physical therapy that exacerbated her pain. She received a corticosteroid injection into her trochanteric bursa that did help relieve her pain temporarily.

Physical examination reveals a left-sided Trendelenburg gait. Left hip range of motion is 120° of flexion, 30° of internal rotation, 50° of external rotation with pain, and 50° of abduction. She has significant tenderness to palpation over her greater trochanter, but the remainder of her bony landmarks is asymptomatic. She has a positive FABER sign but no signs of impingement or snapping. Ober's test is negative. Her strength is 5/5 throughout the right lower extremity with the exception of her abductors, which are 4/5 with pain. She is otherwise neurovascularly intact.

Imaging

Multiple X-ray views of the patient's pelvis and hips were obtained. Joint spaces are intact bilaterally; however, there is mild osteophyte formation on the lateral aspect of bilateral acetabulums. In addition, bilateral greater trochanters exhibit enthesophyte changes. Using the Tonnis classification of grading hip osteoarthritis, the patient's radiographic changes are consistent with grade 1.

MRI was obtained for suspicion of an abductor tendon tear. Osseous structures are without bony edema or abnormalities. Figures 32.12a–d and 32.13a–e depict coronal and

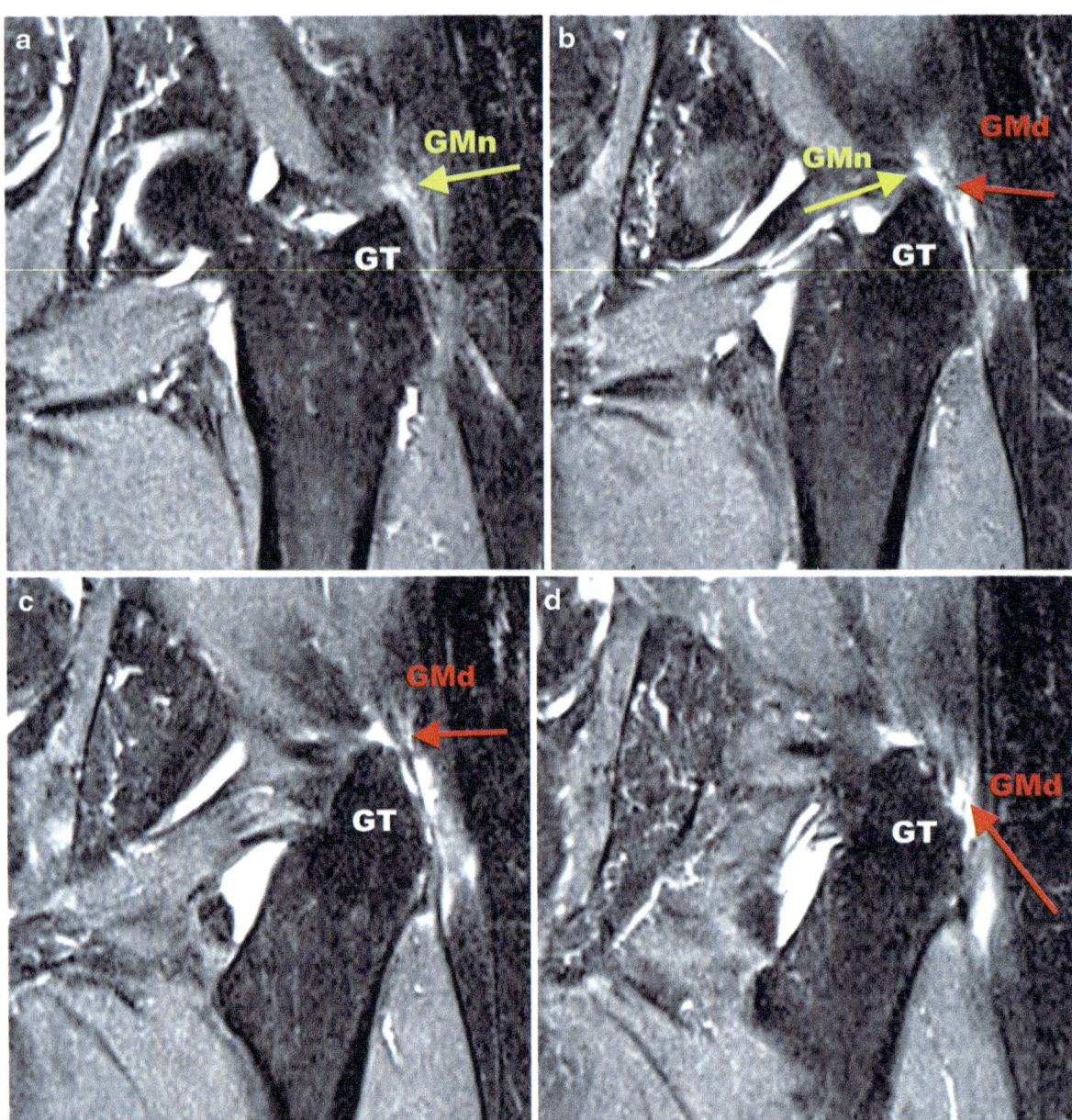

Fig. 32.12 (**a**) Coronal T2 fat-saturated weighted MRI. A high-grade partial-thickness tear of the gluteus minimus (GMn) is seen. (**b**) Coronal T2 fat-saturated weighted MRI. A high-grade partial-thickness tear of the gluteus minimus (GMn) and a full-thickness tear of the gluteus medius (GMd) tendon from its greater trochanteric (GT) insertion are seen. (**c**, **d**) Coronal T2 fat-saturated weighted MRI. A full-thickness tear of the gluteus medius (GMd) tendon from its greater trochanteric (GT) insertion is seen. Because the gluteus inserts onto the anterior facet of the greater trochanter, it is no longer seen as sequences progress posteriorly

Fig. 32.13 (**a**, **b**) Axial T2 fat-saturated weighted MRI. Increased signal intensity lateral to the greater trochanter can be attributed to tearing/tendinosis of the gluteus medius (GMd) tendon at its insertion as well as trochanteric bursitis. (**c**–**e**) Axial T2 fat-saturated weighted MRI. As sequences move superiorly, more of the femoral head (FH) and less of the GT are visible. Increased signal intensity superior to the greater trochanter can be attributed to intra-substance tearing/tendinosis of the gluteus medius (GMd) tendon

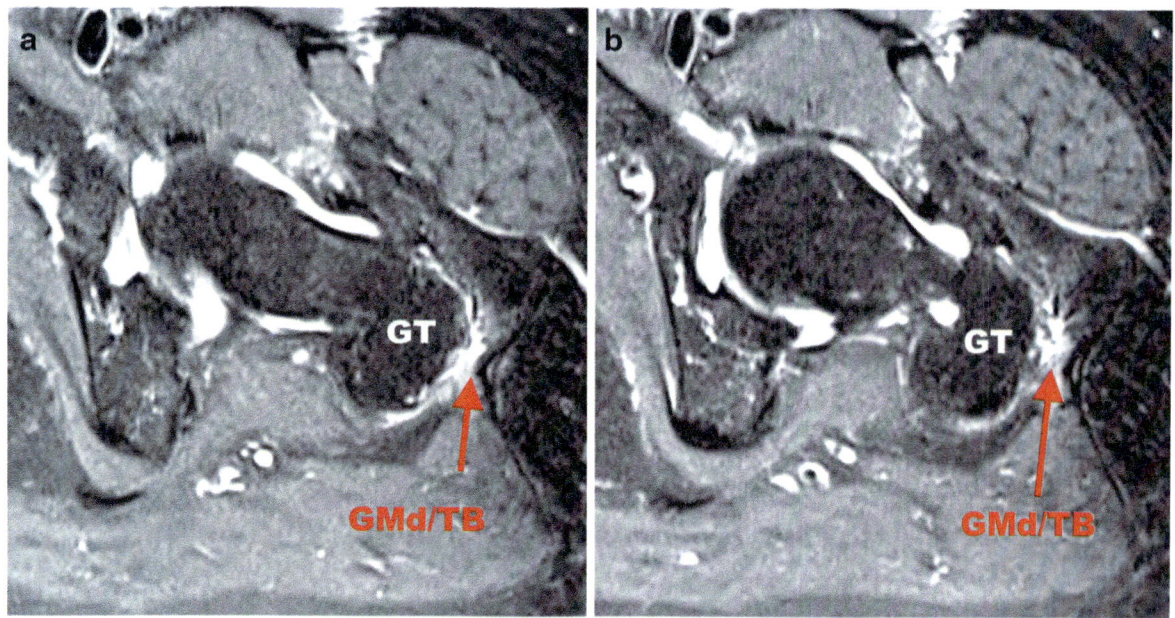

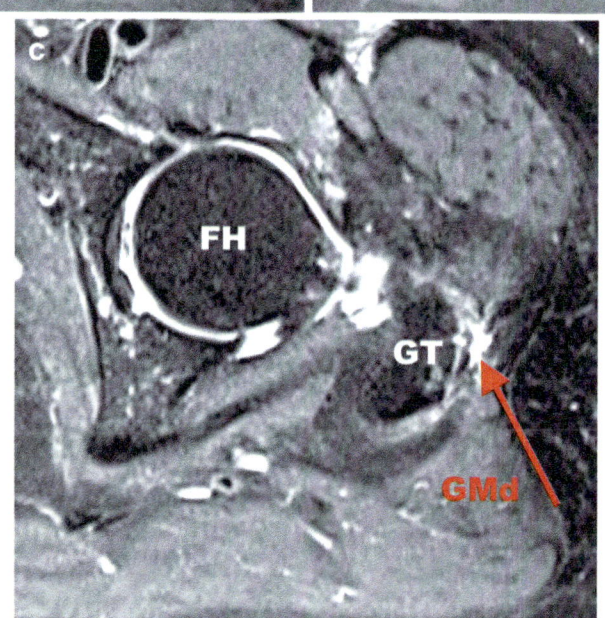

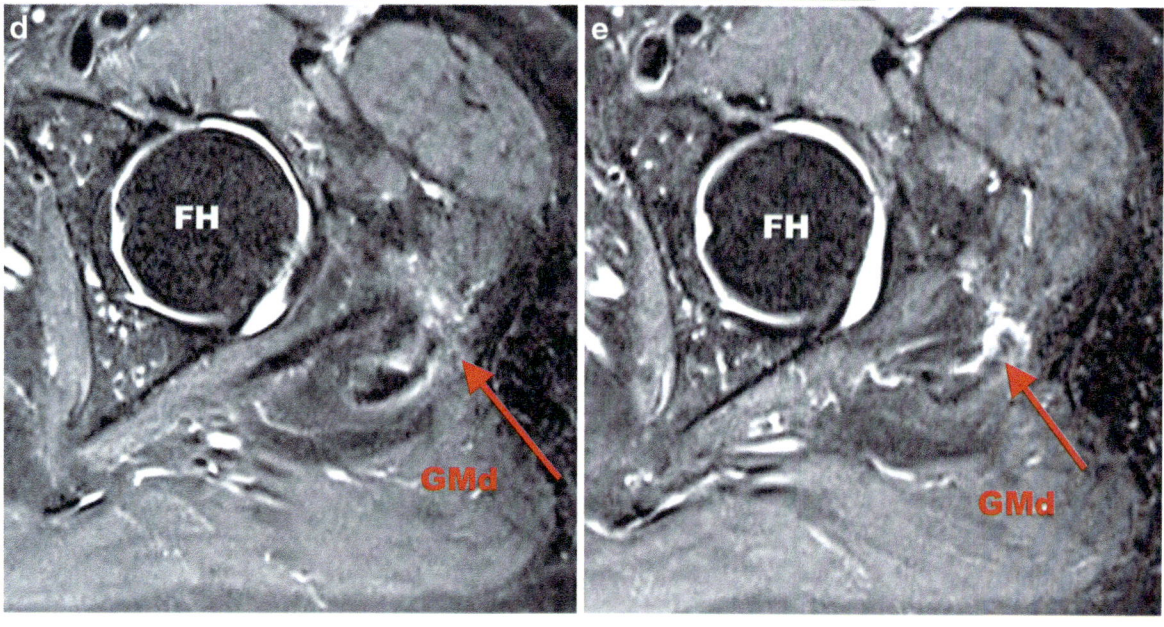

axial T2 fat-saturated weighted MRI cuts, respectively. A high-grade partial-thickness tear of the gluteus minimus (GMn) is seen in Fig. 32.12a–b, and a full-thickness tear of the gluteus medius (GMd) tendon from its greater trochanteric insertion is seen in Figs. 32.12b–d and 32.13b–e. Fraying of the acetabular labrum was noted with a small superior tear. Chondral surfaces were thinned but intact.

Arthroscopy

The patient continued to have debilitating pain despite conservative management of her abductor tendon tears. A decision was made to proceed with left hip peritrochanteric endoscopy with gluteus medius repair and trochanteric bursectomy. The plan also included diagnostic hip arthroscopy with treatment as indicated. The patient was made aware that the arthritis currently seen in her hip would not be treated by the procedure nor was there any evidence that it would slow the progression of arthritis.

Positioning, set-up, and portal placement were performed in a similar fashion as the previous cases in this chapter. The labral tear was found to be stable and was therefore selectively debrided. The peritrochanteric space was then entered. An additional posterolateral portal was also created in this case.

As in the previous cases, trochanteric bursectomy and debridement were carried out in a similar fashion with the arthroscope in the mid-anterior portal and shaver in the anterolateral portal. Examination of the gluteus medius tendon insertion confirmed a full-thickness tear (Fig. 32.14). In preparation for reinsertion, the lateral facet of the greater trochanter was decorticated to create a bleeding bed of bone for healing using the burr (Fig. 32.15). To complete the repair, an anchor was placed in the lateral facet under fluoroscopy, and two horizontal mattress sutures were passed through the tendon (Fig. 32.16). This was repeated with a second anchor for better tissue approximation (Fig. 32.17). The sutures were then tied down with standard arthroscopic knot-tying technique, achieving excellent closure of the tendon over the lateral facet (Fig. 32.18).

Discussion

Once thought of as a rare clinical entity, it is likely that the prevalence of gluteus medius and minimus tendon tear has been underdiagnosed [53]. The ever-increasing interest and possibilities in hip arthroscopy and endoscopy have teased this diagnosis out from under the broad category of GTPS and the mislabeling of it as "trochanteric bursitis." Many cases are labeled as "recalcitrant trochanteric bursitis" that have failed to improve with extensive conservative measures.

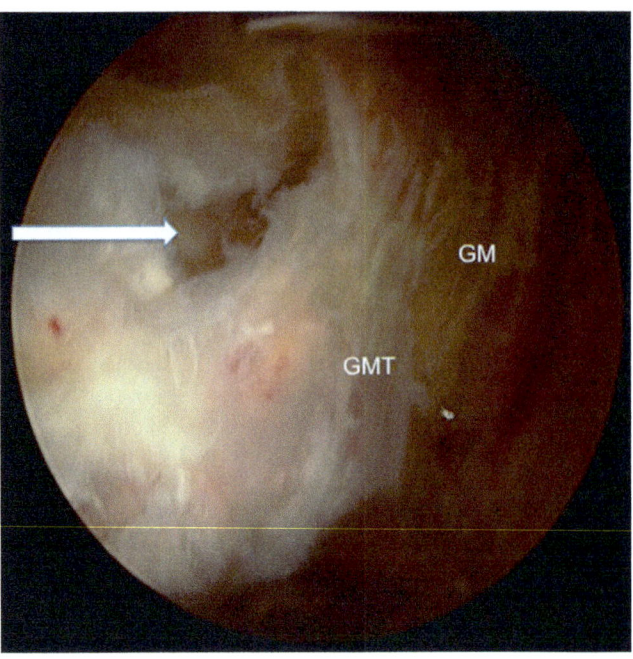

Fig. 32.14 Left hip peritrochanteric endoscopy viewing cephalad and medial from the distal mid-anterior portal. The gluteus medius (GM) muscle and tendon (GMT) are visible. Note the full-thickness tear (*arrow*) involving the gluteus medius tendon

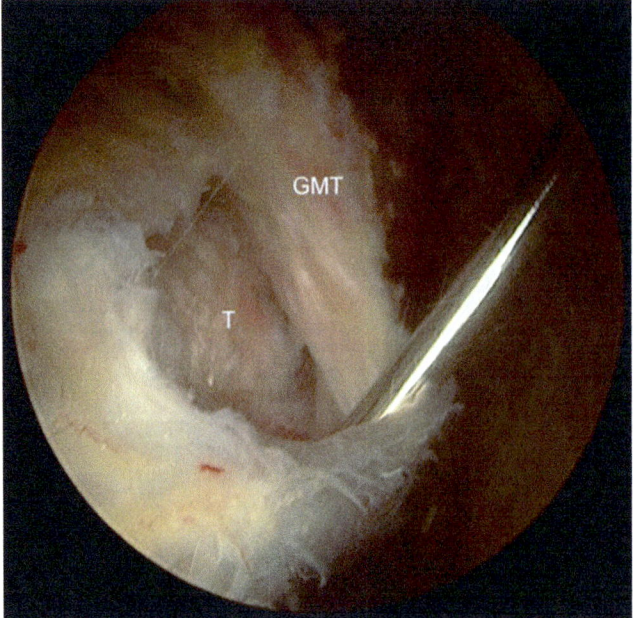

Fig. 32.15 Left hip peritrochanteric endoscopy viewing cephalad and medial from the distal mid-anterior portal. The underlying trochanter (T) can be visualized. The probe is elevating the fibers of the gluteus medius tendon (GMT)

While literature surrounding the treatment of gluteus medius tendon tears is lacking in comparison to the rotator cuff of the shoulder, indications for treatment may be similar [38].

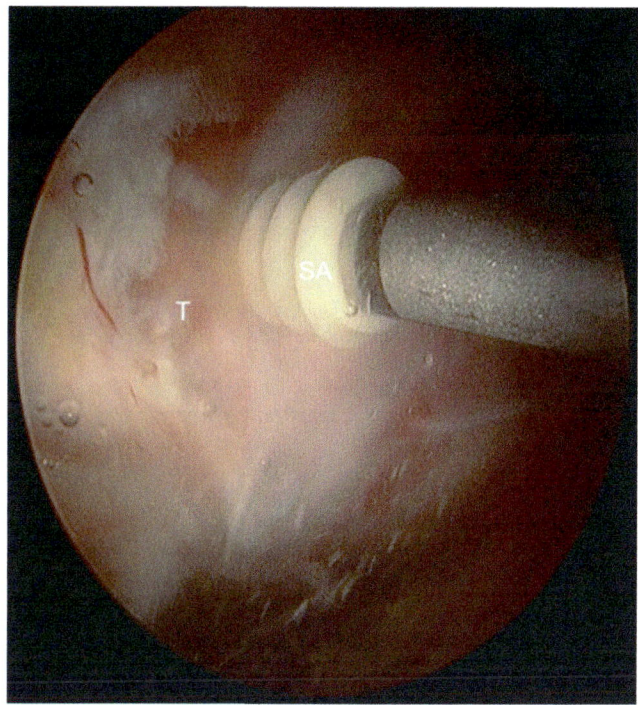

Fig. 32.16 Left hip peritrochanteric endoscopy viewing cephalad and medial from the distal mid-anterior portal. A suture anchor (SA) is being placed in the underlying trochanter (T)

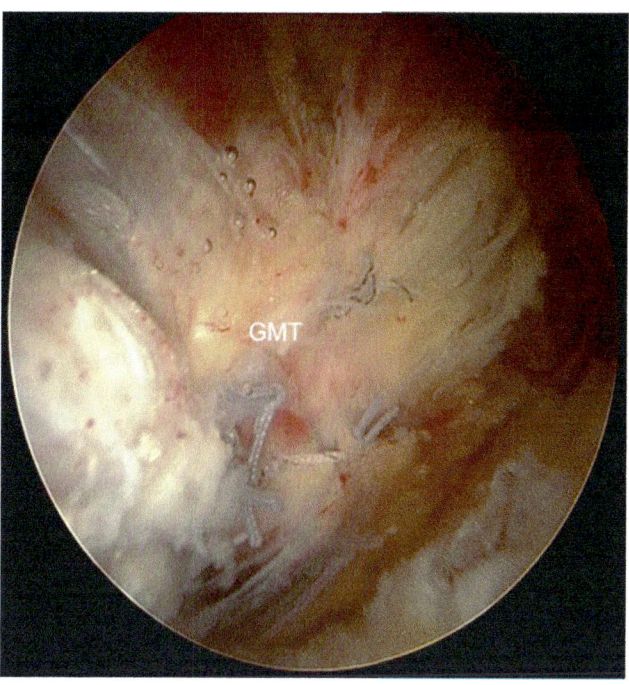

Fig. 32.18 Left hip peritrochanteric endoscopy viewing cephalad and medial from the distal mid-anterior portal after insertion of two double-loaded suture anchors and suture passage. The sutures are now tied which approximates the gluteus medius tendon (GMT) to the trochanter

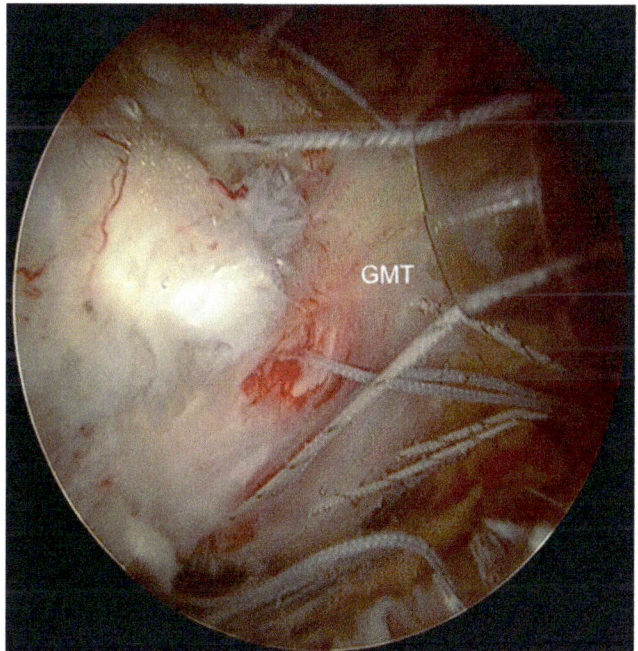

Fig. 32.17 Left hip peritrochanteric endoscopy viewing cephalad and medial from the distal mid-anterior portal after insertion of two double-loaded suture anchors and suture passage. Gluteus medius tendon (GMT)

Endoscopic treatment of these tears has only been described within the last decade. Voos et al. were the first to describe an endoscopic repair of the gluteus medius in 2007

[38]. Their technique mirrors that of an arthroscopic rotator cuff repair of the shoulder: the tendon edges and its attachment site were debrided. Suture anchors were placed into the tendon footprint (with or without fluoroscopic guidance). The sutures were then retrieved and passed through the tendon edges and tied under arthroscopic visualization. Voos et al. later reported outcomes of the procedure in 2009 [54]. They prospectively evaluated ten patients with gluteus medius tears diagnosed by physical exam and MRI that had failed extensive conservative measures. At a mean follow-up of 25 months, all ten patients had complete resolution of pain and regained 5 out of 5 motor strength with hip abduction.

Three other studies published in 2013 have shown comparable results (level IV evidence case series). Domb et al. identified 15 patients—six with partial-thickness and nine with full-thickness tears [55]. At an average f/u of 27.9 months, 14/15 patients had postoperative improvement of 30 or more points in four hip-specific scores, and satisfaction rated from good to excellent. It should be noted, however, that all patients had labral procedures (10 debridements, 4 repairs, 1 reconstruction), and nearly half of them were treated for femoroacetabular impingement (3 acetabuloplasty, 4 femoroplasty) as well. Thaunat et al. describe partial-thickness undersurface tears repaired in four patients [56]. At 6 months follow-up, the mean modified Harris hip score (mHHS) rose from 36.75 to 72.25. Finally, McCormick et al. reported the endoscopic treatment of ten patients with a mean follow-up of 23 months [57]. Average mHHS, hip outcome scores (HOS)—activities of daily living, and HOS—sports were 84.7, 89.1, and 76.8. All patients rated their level of activity as "normal or near normal," and 9 out of 10 said they would undergo the procedure again.

Surgical techniques, tear patterns, and biomechanical studies are all in their infancy. Byrd describes techniques for access to the peritrochanteric space, tear-specific gluteus medius repair akin to rotator cuff repair, and repair with double-row fixation [58]. Domb et al. describe a trans-tendinous approach for partial-thickness tears and the creation of an optional iliotibial window [59]. Yanke et al. also report a case of a musculotendinous junction tear repaired endoscopically [60].

Dishkin-Paset et al. compared biomechanical fixation stability of two specific gluteus medius arthroscopic repair techniques in cadaveric specimens [61]. The double-row repair with massive cuff stitches was not significantly different from the double-row repair with knotless lateral anchors.

Conclusion

Diagnosing lateral hip pain that is tender to palpation has become more sophisticated than "trochanteric bursitis." A careful history, physical exam, and appropriate imaging are crucial to initiate the proper treatment. The vast majority of cases of GTPS will resolve with appropriate conservative management. For refractory cases, endoscopic treatment has become a viable, safe, and effective method of treating these patients.

References

1. Anderson TP. Trochanteric bursitis: diagnostic criteria and clinical significance. Arch Phys Med Rehabil. 1958;39(10):617–22.
2. Gordon EJ. Trochanteric bursitis and tendinitis. Clin Orthop. 1961;20:193–202.
3. Karpinski MR, Piggott H. Greater trochanteric pain syndrome. A report of 15 cases. J Bone Joint Surg (Br). 1985;67(5):762–3.
4. Bird PA, et al. Prospective evaluation of magnetic resonance imaging and physical examination findings in patients with greater trochanteric pain syndrome. Arthritis Rheum. 2001;44(9): 2138–45.
5. Long SS, Surrey DE, Nazarian NL. Sonography of greater trochanteric pain syndrome and the rarity of primary bursitis. AJR Am J Roentgenol. 2013;201(5):1083–6.
6. Silva F, et al. Trochanteric bursitis: refuting the myth of inflammation. J Clin Rheumatol. 2008;14(2):82–6.
7. Fearon AM, et al. Greater trochanteric pain syndrome negatively affects work, physical activity and quality of life: a case control study. J Arthroplasty. 2014;29(2):383–6.
8. Strauss EJ, Nho SJ, Kelly BT. Greater trochanteric pain syndrome. Sports Med Arthrosc. 2010;18(2):113–9.
9. Williams BS, Cohen SP. Greater trochanteric pain syndrome: a review of anatomy, diagnosis and treatment. Anesth Analg. 2009; 108(5):1662–70.
10. Segal NA, et al. Greater trochanteric pain syndrome: epidemiology and associated factors. Arch Phys Med Rehabil. 2007;88(8): 988–92.
11. Viradia NK, Berger AA, Dahners LE. Relationship between width of greater trochanters and width of iliac wings in trochanteric bursitis. Am J Orthop (Belle Mead NJ). 2011;40(9):E159–62.
12. Abdelwahab IF, et al. Atypical extraspinal musculoskeletal tuberculosis in immunocompetent patients: Part II, tuberculous myositis, tuberculous bursitis, and tuberculous tenosynovitis. Can Assoc Radiol J. 2006;57(5):278–86.
13. Butcher JD, Salzman KL, Lillegard WA. Lower extremity bursitis. Am Fam Physician. 1996;53(7):2317–24.
14. Kagan 2nd A. Rotator cuff tears of the hip. Clin Orthop Relat Res. 1999;368:135–40.
15. Craig RA, et al. Iliotibial band Z-lengthening for refractory trochanteric bursitis (greater trochanteric pain syndrome). ANZ J Surg. 2007;77(11):996–8.
16. Robertson WJ, et al. Anatomy and dimensions of the gluteus medius tendon insertion. Arthroscopy. 2008;24(2):130–6.
17. Shbeeb MI, Matteson EL. Trochanteric bursitis (greater trochanter pain syndrome). Mayo Clin Proc. 1996;71(6):565–9.
18. Woodley SJ, Mercer SR, Nicholson HD. Morphology of the bursae associated with the greater trochanter of the femur. J Bone Joint Surg Am. 2008;90(2):284–94.
19. Bunker TD, Esler CN, Leach WJ. Rotator-cuff tear of the hip. J Bone Joint Surg (Br). 1997;79(4):618–20.
20. Lachiewicz PF. Abductor tendon tears of the hip: evaluation and management. J Am Acad Orthop Surg. 2011;19(7):385–91.
21. Dwek J, et al. MR imaging of the hip abductors: normal anatomy and commonly encountered pathology at the greater trochanter. Magn Reson Imaging Clin N Am. 2005;13(4):691–704, vii.
22. Pfirrmann CW, et al. Greater trochanter of the hip: attachment of the abductor mechanism and a complex of three bursae—MR imaging and MR bursography in cadavers and MR imaging in asymptomatic volunteers. Radiology. 2001;221(2):469–77.
23. Gottschalk F, Kourosh S, Leveau B. The functional anatomy of tensor fasciae latae and gluteus medius and minimus. J Anat. 1989; 166:179–89.
24. Tibor LM, Sekiya JK. Differential diagnosis of pain around the hip joint. Arthroscopy. 2008;24(12):1407–21.
25. Westacott DJ, Minns JI, Foguet P. The diagnostic accuracy of magnetic resonance imaging and ultrasonography in gluteal tendon tears—a systematic review. Hip Int. 2011;21(6):637–45.
26. Reich MS. Hip arthroscopy for extra-articular hip disease. Curr Rev Musculoskelet Med. 2013;6(3):250–7.
27. McMahon S, Fleury J. External validity of physical activity interventions for community-dwelling older adults with fall risk: a quantitative systematic literature review. J Adv Nurs. 2012;68(10): 2140–54.
28. Blankenbaker DG. Correlation of MRI findings with clinical findings of trochanteric pain syndrome. Skelet Radiol. 2008;37(10):903–9.
29. Kingzett-Taylor A, et al. Tendinosis and tears of gluteus medius and minimus muscles as a cause of hip pain: MR imaging findings. AJR Am J Roentgenol. 1999;173(4):1123–6.
30. Kong A, Van der Vliet A, Zadow S. MRI and US of gluteal tendinopathy in greater trochanteric pain syndrome. Eur Radiol. 2007;17(7):1772–83.
31. Brooker Jr AF. The surgical approach to refractory trochanteric bursitis. Johns Hopkins Med J. 1979;145(3):98–100.
32. Lustenberger DP, et al. Efficacy of treatment of trochanteric bursitis: a systematic review. Clin J Sport Med. 2011;21(5):447–53.
33. Furia JP, Rompe JD, Maffulli N. Low-energy extracorporeal shock wave therapy as a treatment for greater trochanteric pain syndrome. Am J Sports Med. 2009;37(9):1806–13.
34. Rompe JD, et al. Home training, local corticosteroid injection, or radial shock wave therapy for greater trochanter pain syndrome. Am J Sports Med. 2009;37(10):1981–90.

35. Burman MS. Arthroscopy or the direct visualization of joints: an experimental cadaver study. 1931. Clin Orthop Relat Res. 2001;390:5–9.

36. Byrd JW. Hip arthroscopy utilizing the supine position. Arthroscopy. 1994;10(3):275–80.

37. Glick JM, et al. Hip arthroscopy by the lateral approach. Arthroscopy. 1987;3(1):4–12.

38. Voos JE, et al. Arthroscopic anatomy and surgical techniques for peritrochanteric space disorders in the hip. Arthroscopy. 2007;23(11):1246e1–5.

39. Audenaert E, Pattyn C. Balloon dissection for improved access to the peritrochanteric compartment. Arthroscopy. 2009;25(11):1349–53.

40. Schapira D, Nahir M, Scharf Y. Trochanteric bursitis: a common clinical problem. Arch Phys Med Rehabil. 1986;67(11):815–7.

41. Clancy WG. Runners' injuries. Part two. Evaluation and treatment of specific injuries. Am J Sports Med. 1980;8(4):287–9.

42. Govaert LH, et al. Endoscopic bursectomy and iliotibial tract release as a treatment for refractory greater trochanteric pain syndrome: a new endoscopic approach with early results. Arthrosc Tech. 2012;1(2):e161–4.

43. Weinrauch P, Kermeci S. Ultrasonography-assisted arthroscopic proximal iliotibial band release and trochanteric bursectomy. Arthrosc Tech. 2013;2(4):e433–5.

44. Baker Jr CL, et al. Arthroscopic bursectomy for recalcitrant trochanteric bursitis. Arthroscopy. 2007;23(8):827–32.

45. Allen WC, Cope R, Saltans C. The snapping hip revisited. J Am Acad Orthop Surg. 1995;3(5):303–8.

46. Provencher MT, Hofmeister EP, Muldoon MP. The surgical treatment of external coxa saltans (the snapping hip) by Z-plasty of the iliotibial band. Am J Sports Med. 2004;32(2):470–6.

47. Polesello GC, et al. Surgical technique: endoscopic gluteus maximus tendon release for external snapping hip syndrome. Clin Orthop Relat Res. 2013;471(8):2471–6.

48. Brignall CG, Stainsby GD. The snapping hip. Treatment by Z-plasty. J Bone Joint Surg (Br). 1991;73(2):253–4.

49. Dederich R. [The snapping hip. Enlargement of the iliotibial tract by Z-plasty]. Z Orthop Ihre Grenzgeb. 1983;121(2):168–70.

50. Nam KW, et al. A modified Z-plasty technique for severe tightness of the gluteus maximus. Scand J Med Sci Sports. 2011;21(1):85–9.

51. Ilizaliturri Jr VM, et al. Endoscopic iliotibial band release for external snapping hip syndrome. Arthroscopy. 2006;22(5):505–10.

52. Zini R, et al. Endoscopic iliotibial band release in snapping hip. Hip Int. 2013;23(2):225–32.

53. Davies JF, et al. Surgical treatment of hip abductor tendon tears. J Bone Joint Surg Am. 2013;95(15):1420–5.

54. Voos JE, et al. Endoscopic repair of gluteus medius tendon tears of the hip. Am J Sports Med. 2009;37(4):743–7.

55. Domb BG, Botser I, Giordano BD. Outcomes of endoscopic gluteus medius repair with minimum 2-year follow-up. Am J Sports Med. 2013;41(5):988–97.

56. Thaunat M, et al. Endoscopic repair of partial-thickness undersurface tears of the gluteus medius tendon. Orthop Traumatol Surg Res. 2013;99(7):853–7.

57. McCormick F, et al. Endoscopic repair of full-thickness abductor tendon tears: surgical technique and outcome at minimum of 1-year follow-up. Arthroscopy. 2013;29(12):1941–7.

58. Byrd JW. Gluteus medius repair with double-row fixation. Arthrosc Tech. 2013;2(3):e247–50.

59. Domb BG, Nasser RM, Botser IB. Partial-thickness tears of the gluteus medius: rationale and technique for trans-tendinous endoscopic repair. Arthroscopy. 2010;26(12):1697–705.

60. Yanke AB, et al. Endoscopic repair of a gluteus medius tear at the musculotendinous junction. Arthrosc Tech. 2013;2(2):e69–72.

61. Dishkin-Paset JG, et al. A biomechanical comparison of repair techniques for complete gluteus medius tears. Arthroscopy. 2012;28(10):1410–6.

Proximal Hamstring Pathology and Endoscopic Management

Michael B. Gerhardt and David L. Schub

Introduction

Rupture of the proximal origin of the hamstring tendons is a relatively uncommon injury classically described as a water-skier injury that occurs with violent eccentric contraction of the hamstring in a position of knee extension and hip flexion [1]. While hamstring strains at the muscle belly or myotendinous junction account for 25–30 % of all strains and, in fact, are the most commonly strained muscle group in the athlete [2, 3], true proximal hamstring ruptures account for just 9–12 % of all hamstring injuries [4]. It is important to recognize these proximal injuries promptly as delays in diagnosis can affect the overall outcome.

The mechanism of injury in acute ruptures most commonly involves a sudden and unexpected flexion of the hip with the knee in an extended position. Proximal hamstring injuries were coined as the "waterskier injury" as the novice water skier was pulled suddenly by the tow rope leading to a rapid flexion moment at the hip with the knees locked in an extended position, while the waterskis provided tremendous counterforce to the pull of the boat. One could imagine how the proximal hamstring may rupture under such tremendous tension and load.

While water skiing certainly accounts for many of these injuries, in reality, a wide variety of activities can result in proximal hamstring rupture (Fig. 33.1). The most common mechanism of injury in our clinic involves the patient's foot slipping on a wet surface. The patient's stable leg remains anchored in one position, while the unstable leg juts violently in front of the body creating an inadvertent "splits" maneuver resulting in damage to the proximal hamstring complex.

Oftentimes, the patient reports a history of a "pop" or a series of "pops" and when asked to localize the pain points to the proximal lower gluteus and proximal posterior thigh. Initially the injury can seem innocuous, and the inexperienced clinician may falsely diagnose these injuries as a hamstring muscle strain. However, with a suspicious mechanism of injury, such as a slip on a wet floor and a history of a pop, the clinician should error on the side of caution and order an MRI to assess the level and severity of the injury.

Usually within 48–72 h, a significant ecchymosis is apparent in the midthigh region, which quickly darkens and extends distally sometimes all the way to the foot (Fig. 33.2). While some mild ecchymosis may occur in a mid hamstring muscle strain, it is nowhere near the severity and size of the ecchymotic changes seen in a proximal hamstring avulsion injury.

Although hamstring strains reliably heal after a period of rest and dedicated physiotherapy, nonoperative management of complete ruptures and high-grade partial ruptures may result in low return to sports, persistent pain, weakness, and instability [5–9]. While the natural history of partial tears is not clearly defined, certain partial tears, particularly those with retraction greater than 2 cm and tendinous detachment greater than 50 %, have also been shown to do poorly with nonoperative management [9–11].

Given the unreliable results with nonoperative management, the trend has been toward open repair with suture anchor fixation as the surgical method of choice [2, 5, 9, 10, 12–17]. This can be performed through either a transverse or vertical incision. Whereas open repair leads to high rates of good and excellent outcomes in both the acute and chronic setting [18, 19]; complications include wound dehiscence 2.4 % [20], wound infection 1–2.4 % [16, 20, 21], seroma 2.4 % [20], posterior cutaneous neuralgia 9.8–40 % [15, 20], hypertrophic scar formation 2.0 % [16], wound fistula 1.1 % [11], incisional numbness 60.9 % [12], and cosmetic deformity 60.9 % [12].

M.B. Gerhardt, MD (✉)
Institute for Sports Science, Cedars-Sinai Medical Center, Santa Monica, CA, USA
e-mail: mgerhardt@smog-ortho.net

D.L. Schub, MD
Department of Orthopedic Surgery, Kaiser Permanente Hospital—San Diego, San Diego, CA, USA
e-mail: davidschub@gmail.com

S.F. Brockmeier (ed.), *MRI-Arthroscopy Correlations: A Case-Based Atlas of the Knee, Shoulder, Elbow and Hip*, DOI 10.1007/978-1-4939-2645-9_33, © Springer Science+Business Media New York 2015

Fig. 33.1 A variety of activities, such as a water skier being pulled forward, can result in proximal hamstring rupture

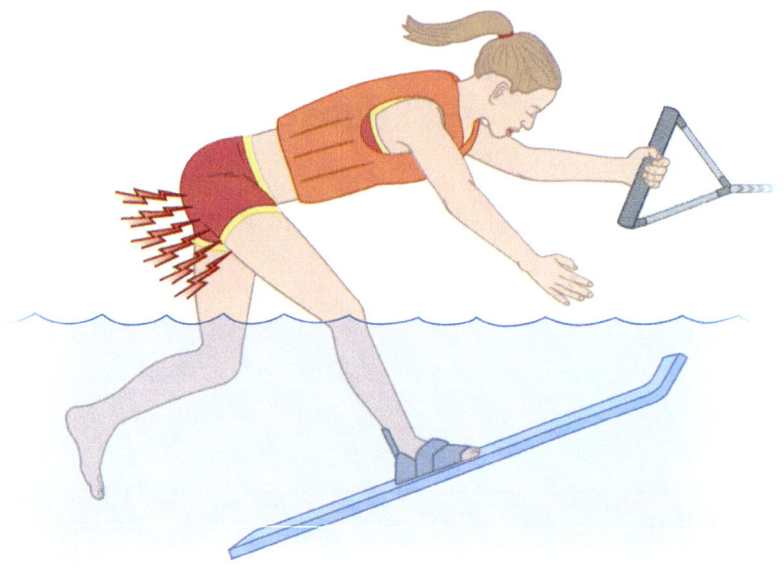

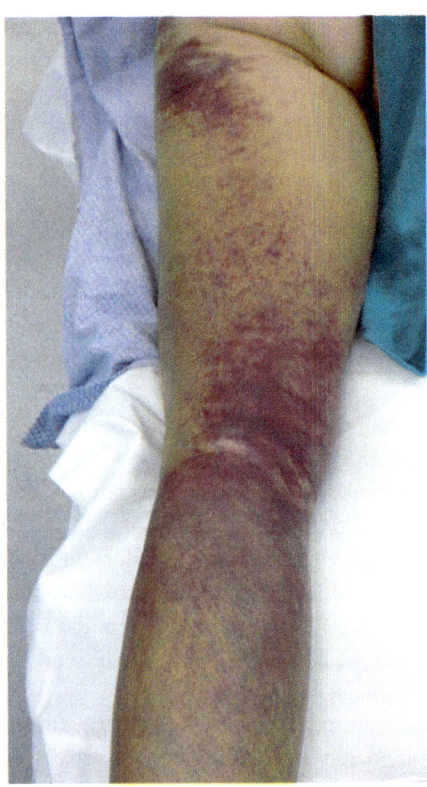

Fig. 33.2 Ecchymosis following a complete proximal hamstring avulsion

Arthroscopic and endoscopic techniques have been used throughout sports medicine in an effort to minimize surgical incisions, decrease morbidity, and speed recovery. In an effort to mitigate the potential morbidity of an open repair, advanced surgical techniques have allowed us to endoscopically treat some of these injuries to the proximal hamstring. Here we present a case example of one of our patients treated with endoscopic repair of a proximal hamstring injury.

Case Description

The patient is a very active 53-year-old female who presented 6 weeks months after sustaining an injury to her right hamstring while sprinting during a soccer match. She attempted rest and rehabilitation but complained of persistent pain, weakness, and inability to return to explosive acceleration required in sports that she enjoyed including recreational soccer. The exertional symptoms included cramping of the mid-substance hamstring musculature as well as sharp pain and sitting intolerance at the ischial tuberosity region. On physical examination, she had tenderness over the ischial tuberosity with a small palpable defect over the proximal hamstring origin. She had pain with resisted knee flexion and slightly decreased sensation in the sciatic nerve distribution. MRI revealed a high-grade partial avulsion with approximately 2 cm of retraction (Fig. 33.3a, b). Given that she had failed conservative management and desired to return to soccer, she elected to undergo proximal hamstring repair, and an endoscopic approach was discussed as an option.

Under general endotracheal tube anesthesia, the patient was placed in the prone position with the gluteal and posterior thigh prepped and draped. The first portal, the direct posterior portal, was made in the gluteal crease over the proximal hamstrings. The arthroscope was placed into the subgluteal space and, using a low-pressure pump, the space was insufflated with fluid; the subgluteal is defined as the space between the gluteus maximus and proximal hamstring fascia. Under direct visualization, a second portal, the posterolateral portal, was made in the gluteal crease just lateral to the first portal, directly over the lateral facet of the ischial tuberosity. An arthroscopic shaver was carefully used to

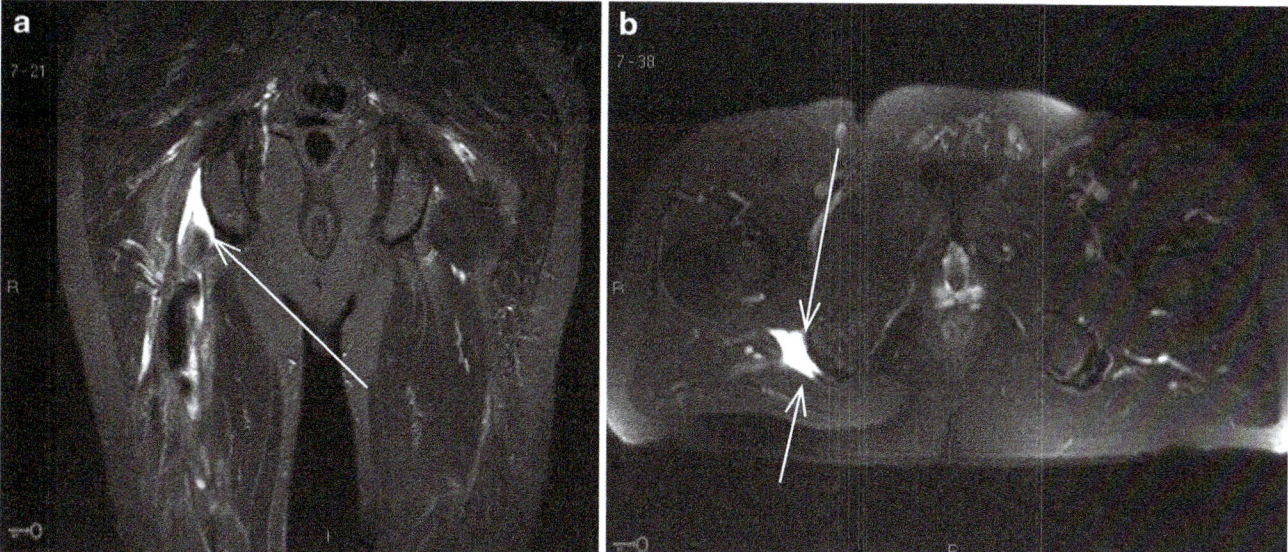

Fig. 33.3 (**a**, **b**) MRI of proximal hamstring avulsion: coronal and axial views

Fig. 33.4 Subgluteal space. Potential space between the gluteus maximus and proximal hamstring fascia

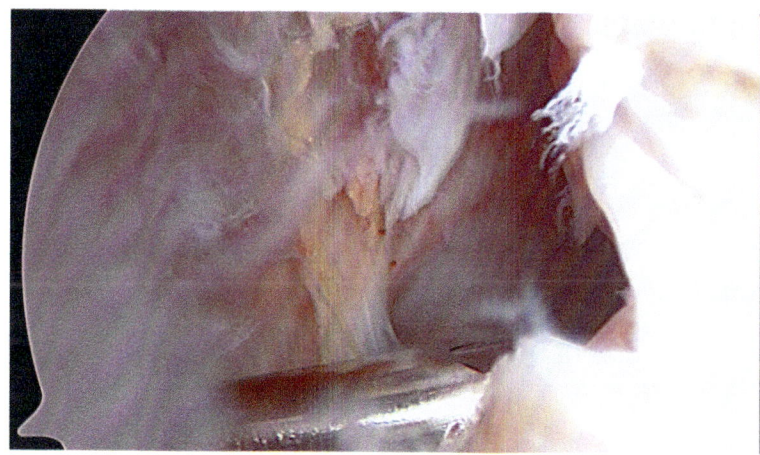

debride the ischial bursa and develop the subgluteal space (Fig. 33.4). Working laterally, the shaver was used bluntly to identify the sciatic nerve. Several adhesions were bluntly dissected from the sciatic nerve. Care was taken to avoid damage to the sciatic nerve throughout the remainder of the case. Next, the ischial tuberosity and proximal hamstring ruptured fibers were visualized (Fig. 33.5). Approximately 60 % of the tendon footprint was detached and retracted. All scar tissues were debrided. The torn and retracted fibers were thoroughly debrided and "freshened" in an effort to enhance healing upon refixation. A combination of clear cannulas and Passport cannulas was placed into each of the portals. The dissection using the motorized shaver was carried distally 4–5 cm which was helpful in mobilizing the tendon stump and would allow easier reduction to the footprint. An arthroscopic grasper was used to assess mobilization of the

tendon (Fig. 33.6). Next, a single 4.5 mm double-loaded poly-ether-ether-ketone (PEEK) corkscrew anchor was used (Arthrex, Naples, FL), and sutures were passed using a combination of angled crescent suture passers and the Scorpion Fastpass suture passer device (Arthrex, Naples, FL). A horizontal mattress configuration was made. A second anchor was placed, and similar suture passing through the proximal hamstring tendon was performed. With the knee flexed, the tendon was easily reduced to the bone using standard arthroscopic suture technique and then tied in place (Fig. 33.7). Solid reduction and fixation were confirmed while flexing and extending the knee.

The patient was discharged home the same day. Aspirin 325 mg was used for 1 month for DVT prophylaxis. A hinged knee brace initially locked in 70° of flexion was progressively brought into full extension over the next 10–14 days.

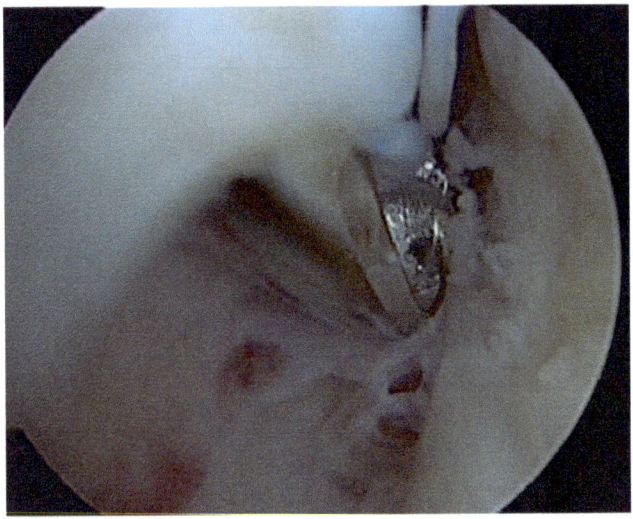

Fig. 33.5 Arthroscopic shaver debriding the empty footprint of the ischial tuberosity at site of avulsed proximal hamstring fibers

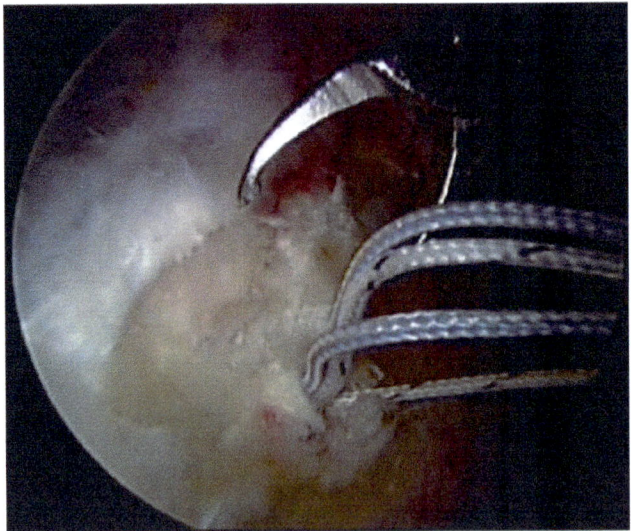

Fig. 33.6 Mobilization of avulsed proximal hamstring tendon

Fig. 33.7 Repaired proximal hamstring fibers reduced to anatomic footprint of ischium

The patient was kept non-weight bearing until full extension was achieved. Weight bearing was then gradually progressed to full by 6 weeks, and crutches were abandoned. Physical therapy and range of motion exercises were initiated at this point. Strengthening exercises began at 12 weeks with progressive return to sport at 4–6 months. Final follow-up was 1 year after the surgery. The patient had normal muscular contour, full strength, and range of motion and had returned to competitive recreational soccer at the same level as prior to the injury. The numbness that was experienced preoperatively had resolved.

Discussion Points

Anatomic Considerations of the Proximal Hamstring Region

The anatomy of the proximal hamstring is important to review as it has significant implications particularly when attempting surgical intervention whether in an acute or chronic setting. The two most important anatomic considerations involve the sciatic nerve and the true anatomic footprint of the proximal hamstring tendon.

The sciatic nerve courses in close approximation to the proximal hamstring origin at the ischial tuberosity. The sciatic nerve is located just lateral to the proximal hamstring and proceeds to course distally before arborizing and sending branches to each of the muscle bellies of the hamstring complex. The sciatic nerve has two distinct bundles at the proximal level called the tibial branch and the peroneal branch. The tibial branch supplies innervation to the three main muscles of the hamstring complex including the semimembranosus, semitendinosus, and the long head of the biceps femoris. The short head of the biceps femoris muscle is innervated by the peroneal branch of the sciatic nerve, but it is important to note that the short head of the biceps femoris does not contribute to the proximal hamstring tendon.

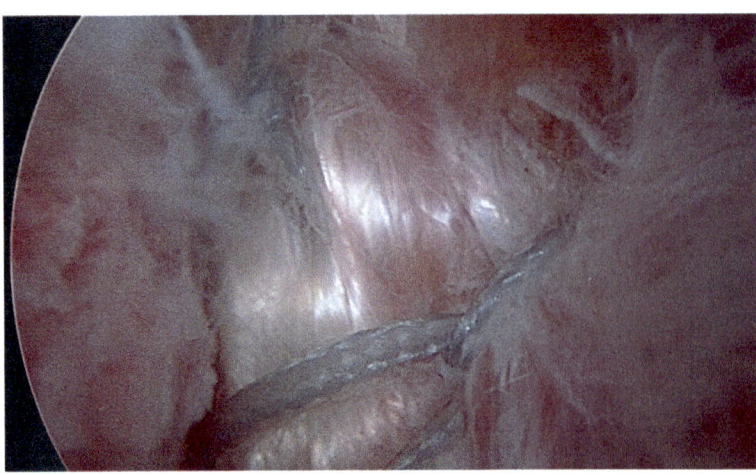

Important neurovascular structures lurk proximally as well. The inferior gluteal neurovascular bundle lies just 5.0 cm proximal to the inferior border of the ischial tuberosity [22]. Whether the approach to the area is performed endoscopically or in an open fashion, care must be taken not to place retractors or instruments into this zone.

Proximally the sciatic nerve also gives off a purely sensory branch called the posterior femoral cutaneous nerve (PFCN). This nerve branch supplies sensation to a large portion of the posterior thigh skin. It takes off from the sciatic nerve just proximal to the level of the ischium and darts superficially through the gluteus maximus and into the subcutaneous layer of the skin of the posterior thigh. The PFCN is particularly vulnerable to injury when making the approach to the proximal hamstring. Injury can occur as a direct transection of the PFCN or one of its branches or more commonly as a neuropraxia while retracting the gluteus maximus muscle.

The sciatic nerve is at risk during the surgical dissection and approach to the proximal hamstring region. In its native state, the sciatic nerve lies in close approximation to the ischial footprint of the proximal hamstring attachment. In an injured state following rupture, the disrupted hamstring fibers are avulsed violently and retract distally away from the bone and oftentimes come to rest in even closer apposition to the course of the sciatic nerve. As part of the normal healing response, scar tissue formation inevitably occurs between the ruptured tendinous fibers and the sciatic nerve. Patients may develop a significant sciatic neuritis, which can become a chronic situation in some instances. The typical complaints of sciatica occur with attempted contraction of the hamstring musculature; as the muscle contracts, if the sciatic nerve is tethered to the contracting musculotendinous complex, the result is a painful tug on the nerve resulting in sciatic pain. One of the arguments for early proximal hamstring repair is to ensure that the proximal hamstring tendon is carefully dissected away from the nearby sciatic nerve, thus mitigating the risk of future sciatic neuritis.

Review of Literature of Proximal Hamstring Repair

Excellent results can be expected with open repair of proximal hamstring tendon avulsions. Sarimo et al. [20] reported on 41 patients (average age, 46 years) with complete ruptures of the proximal hamstring. Seventy-one percent had good-to-excellent results with repair. Those with moderate-to-poor results had a mean time to surgery of 11.7 months, suggesting that early surgical intervention is ideal.

Birmingham et al. [12] followed 23 patients with an average age of 46 years who underwent surgical repair for complete rupture of the proximal hamstring. Ninety-one percent

returned to their sport at the same level within 10 months. Isokinetic testing revealed hamstring strength of 90 % compared to the contralateral side.

Wood et al. [9] reported on 72 proximal hamstring ruptures with an average age of 40 years that underwent surgical repair. Forty cases, including seven incomplete ruptures, were chronic cases that had failed nonoperative management. Postoperative hamstring strength and endurance were 84 % and 89 %, respectively, compared to the contralateral extremity. Patients with preoperative sciatic nerve symptoms from retracted ruptures were significantly weaker than those without. Eighty percent of patients returned to sport at their pre-injury level by 6 months.

Lempainen et al. [16] reported their results on surgical repair of 48 partial tears of the proximal hamstring tendons. Forty-two patients had failed conservative management. All patients were athletes (average age, 33 years) including 13 professional and 15 competitive athletes. Eight-eight percent had a good-to-excellent outcome and returned to pre-injury level of sports after an average of 5 months.

While results with open repair of the proximal hamstring ruptures are good, complications have been described. Wound complications include dehiscence, infection, fistula, seroma, hypertrophic scar formation, and cosmetic deformity. Neurologic complications include posterior cutaneous nerve numbness or hyperesthesia, neuroma, and incisional numbness [11, 12, 15, 16, 20].

Additionally, while the open technique is straightforward, gluteus maximus retraction can be difficult, particularly with larger or more muscular individuals. Care must be taken with prolonged retraction as the inferior gluteal neurovascular bundle lies just 5.0 cm proximal to the inferior border of the ischial tuberosity [22]. Deep retractors and a head lamp are necessary as are 1–2 assistants, thus making this procedure cumbersome in general.

The current literature regarding endoscopic proximal hamstring is limited. A technical report on endoscopic proximal hamstring technique including a case presentation was published by Domb and Gerhardt [23]. Another case report on endoscopic proximal hamstring repair was published by Guanche et al. [24] There are no current studies comparing open versus endoscopic proximal hamstring repair.

Despite the lack of comparative studies, it appears that endoscopic repair of proximal hamstring rupture provides potential advantages over the traditional open technique. Endoscopic repair avoids larger incisions, avoids risk of excessive gluteus maximus retraction, and inflicts minimal disruption of normal anatomy. This may result in decreased incidence of neurovascular complications.

Visualization can prove challenging in the open approach, and this can lead to a nonanatomic repair. Sitting pain is a known side effect following open proximal hamstring repair, and it is likely secondary to imprecise attachment of the tendon to the incorrect region of the ischial footprint. The endoscopic approach clearly allows for superior visualization of the ischial tuberosity, which is crucial for anatomic recreation of the proximal hamstring footprint on the lateral facet of the ischium.

Endoscopy also allows for improved evaluation of partial thickness tears; this becomes increasingly valuable as evidence mounts on the poor outcomes seen with nonoperative management of partial tears.

While these factors may lead to decreased complications, faster recovery, and improved results, endoscopic proximal hamstring repair is technically challenging. The sciatic nerve must be respected during portal placement and endoscopic dissection. Operative times can be longer than the open approach, particularly at the beginning of the learning curve. Due to the endoscopic nature of the procedure, the authors recommend working in a low-pressure environment to minimize the risk of extravasation into the local soft tissue planes. If significant swelling occurs at any point, it is recommended that conversion to a traditional open approach be performed to complete the repair. In our experience, conversion to an open procedure after a failed endoscopic attempt causes no deleterious effects in outcomes and therefore a low threshold to conversion if any untoward events occur during attempted endoscopic repair.

References

1. Blasier RB, Morawa LG. Complete rupture of the hamstring origin from a water skiing injury. Am J Sports Med. 1990;18:435–7.
2. Chalal J, Bush-Joseph CA, Chow A, Zelazny A, Mather RC, Lin E, Gupta D, Verma NN. Clinical and magnetic resonance imaging outcomes after surgical repair of complete proximal hamstring ruptures. Does the tendon heal? Am J Sports Med. 2012;40: 2325–30.
3. Clanton TO, Coupe KJ. Hamstring strains in athletes: diagnosis and treatment. J Am Acad Orthop Surg. 1998;6:237–48.
4. Koulouris G, Connell D. Evaluation of the hamstring muscle complex following acute injury. Skeletal Radiol. 2003;32:582–9.
5. Harris JD, Griesser MJ, Best TM, Ellis TJ. Treatment of proximal hamstring ruptures—a systematic review. Int J Sports Med. 2011;32:490–5.
6. Kurosawa H, Nakasita K, Nakasita H, Sasaki S, Takeda S. Complete avulsion of the hamstring tendons from the ischial tuberosity: a report of two cases sustained in judo. Br J Sports Med. 1996;30:72–4.
7. Orava S, Kujala UM. Rupture of the ischial origin of the hamstring muscles. Am J Sports Med. 1995;23:702–5.
8. Sallay PI, Friedman RL, Coogan PG, Garrett WE. Hamstring muscle injuries among water skiers. Functional outcome and prevention. Am J Sports Med. 1996;24:130–6.
9. Wood DG, et al. Avulsion of the proximal hamstring origin. J Bone Joint Surg Am. 2008;90:2365–74.
10. Cohen S, Bradley J. Acute proximal hamstring rupture. J Am Acad Orthop Surg. 2007;15:350–5.
11. Lempainen L, Sarimo J, Mattila K, Vaittinen S, Orava S. Proximal hamstring tendinopathy: results of surgical management and histopathologic findings. Am J Sports Med. 2009;37:727–34.
12. Birmingham P, Muller M, Wickiewicz T, Cavanaugh J, Rodeo S, Warren R. Functional outcome after repair of proximal hamstring avulsions. J Bone Joint Surg Am. 2011;93:1819–26.
13. Brucker PU, Imhoff AB. Functional assessment after acute and chronic complete ruptures of the proximal hamstring tendons. Knee Surg Sports Traumatol Arthrosc. 2005;13:411–8.
14. Klingele KE, Sallay PI. Surgical repair of complete proximal hamstring tendon rupture. Am J Sports Med. 2002;30:742–7.
15. Konan S, Haddad F. Successful return to high level sports following early surgical repair of complete tears of the proximal hamstring tendons. Int Orthop. 2010;34:119–23.
16. Lempainen L, Sarimo J, Heikkila J, Mattila K, Orava S. Surgical treatment of partial tears of the proximal origin of the hamstring muscles. Br J Sports Med. 2006;40:688–91.
17. Miller SL, Webb GR. The proximal origin of the hamstrings and surrounding anatomy encountered during repair. A surgical technique. J Bone Joint Surg Am. 2008;90 Suppl 2(Part 1):108–16.
18. Folsom GJ, Larson CM. Surgical treatment of acute versus chronic proximal hamstring ruptures. Am J Sports Med. 2008;36:104–9.
19. Sallay PJ, et al. Subjective and functional outcome following surgical repair of complete ruptures of the proximal hamstring complex. Orthopedics. 2008;31:1092.
20. Sarimo J, Lempainen L, Mattila K, Orava S. Complete proximal hamstring avulsions: a series of 41 patients with operative treatment. Am J Sports Med. 2008;36:1110–5.
21. Carmichael F, et al. Avulsion of the proximal hamstring origin: surgical technique. J Bone Joint Surg Am. 2009;91 Suppl 2:250–6.
22. Miller SL, Gill J, Webb GR. The proximal origin of the hamstrings and surrounding anatomy encountered during repair. A cadaveric study. J Bone Joint Surg Am. 2007;89:44–8.
23. Domb BG, Linder D, Sharp KG, Sadik A, Gerhardt MB. Endoscopic repair of proximal hamstring avulsion. Arthrosc Tech. 2013;2(1): e35–9.
24. Dierckman BD, Guanche CA. Endoscopic proximal hamstring repair and ischial bursectomy. Arthrosc Tech. 2012;1(2):e201–7.

Athletic Pubalgia and Sports Hernia: Evaluation and Management

Scott T. King, Joshua A. Tuck, Craig M. Roberto, and Brian Busconi

Introduction

Athletic pubalgia, or "sports hernia," is a condition characterized by lower abdominal and inguinal pain. It is defined as weakness or tearing of the rectus abdominus insertion to the superior pubic ramus, in the absence of an obvious mass or abdominal wall defect. This condition can occur in athletes or nonathletes, although it is often encountered in the male athletic community, with a particular preponderance for sports involving repetitive and powerful hip flexion, such as soccer and ice hockey [1]. Most lower abdomen and groin injuries are self-limited and usually will heal in a 3-to 4-week time period.

The pathophysiology of this condition is not completely understood, and multiple theories have been described in the literature. It has been described as an overuse injury leading to muscular imbalance of the musculature surrounding the hip joint [2], specifically between the proximal pull of the rectus abdominus and the distal pull of the adductors through their insertion sites upon the pubic bone. This imbalance may lead to relative muscular overload with subsequent increased stresses and eventual attenuation noted within the rectus abdominus insertion site. The chronic pain associated

S.T. King, DO (✉)
Orthopedic and Spine Specialists, York, PA, USA
e-mail: sking@osshealth.com

J.A. Tuck, DO, MS
Department of Orthopedic Surgery, LECOM Wellness Center, LECOM Orthopedic and Sports Medicine, Lake Erie College of Osteopathic Medicine, Erie, PA, USA
e-mail: Physh22@yahoo.com

C.M. Roberto, DO
Williamsville, NY, USA
e-mail: Crobo21@gmail.com

B. Busconi, MD
Department of Orthopedics, UMass Memorial Medical Center, Worcester, MA, USA
e-mail: Brian.busconi@umassmemorial.org

with athletic pubalgia is likely secondary to a large tear, or multiple small tears (microtears), involving one or several muscles in the region, which includes the external oblique aponeurosis, rectus abdominis, and conjoined tendon (internal oblique or transversus abdominis) [3].

The presentation of athletic pubalgia may be vague, consisting of lower abdomen and groin pain and can often be confused with other diagnoses. Disorders of the hip joint, injury to the muscles of the thigh and or abdominal wall, and genitourinary or intraabdominal disease may cause similar patient symptoms as are seen in athletic pubalgia [4, 5]. Generalized, vague lower abdominal and groin pain may be caused by myriad pathologies, and the pain associated with athletic pubalgia may involve discomfort through the perineum, adductor origin, rectus insertion, inguinal ligament, or testicular region. The pain associated with athletic pubalgia is often most pronounced at the insertion of the rectus abdominus upon the pubic crest and symphysis of the involved side, and is typically asymptomatic at rest [6, 7].

Further complicating the diagnosis and successful treatment of athletic pubalgia is the possible overlap of this condition with other causes of hip and groin pain within the young athletic population [7]. Given the multiple layers of overlying structures in the area of the lower abdomen, pubic bone, and hip, there are many clinical entities that should be considered as the cause of pain and symptoms. Anterior groin pain caused mainly by intra-articular pathologies should be differentiated from anterior mid-line pain resulting from pathology at the pubic symphysis/rami, pubalgia, and the adductors.

Generally, the athletic pubalgia patient will have either pinpoint or generalized pain in the area of the distal rectus abdominus, at its insertion upon the pubis. Although this pain may radiate into the adductor region, perineum, rectus muscles, inguinal ligament, or testicular area, the most consistent and confirmatory physical exam finding is the insertional rectus pain at the pubis. There is accentuation of this pain achieved with having the patient perform a sit-up while the examiner applies pressure to the distal rectus abdominus

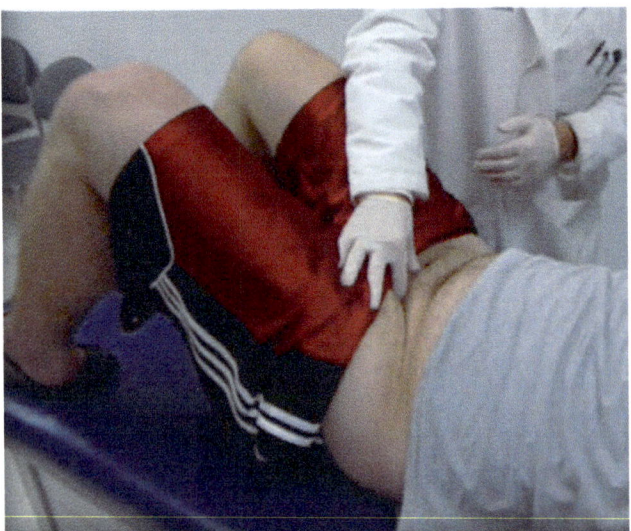

Fig. 34.1 Sit-up test with pressure at the inferior rectus abdominus

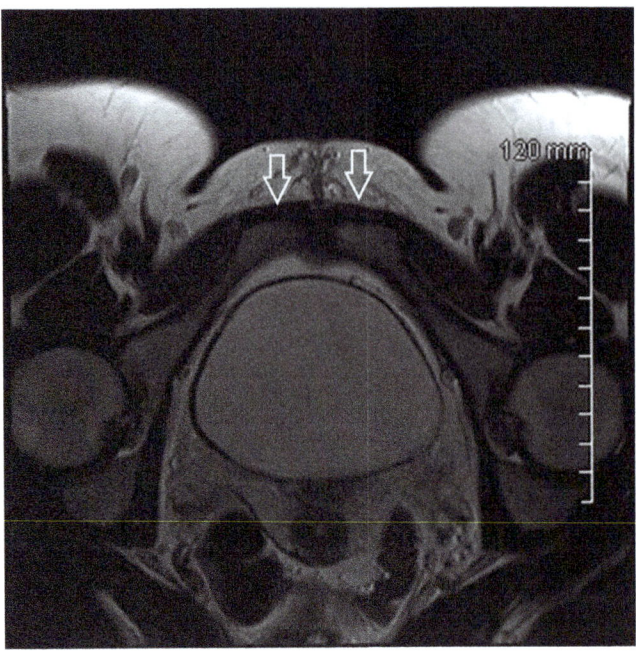

Fig. 34.2 MRI T2 sequence, axial oblique plane. *Arrows* represent normal appearing rectus abdominus–adductor longus aponeurosis

insertion (Fig. 34.1). This provocative maneuver most often reproduces the patient's pain over the pubic insertion site of the rectus abdominus. It is important to determine what makes it better or worse, if there is any pain at rest, and if there are any associated bowel or bladder changes or testicular pain.

In addition to this examination, a thorough bilateral hip examination is preformed, focusing on passive range of motion, asymmetry, and any pain production with hip motion. Impingement testing of the hip should be included in the physical examination to evaluate for femoroacetabular impingement.

The role of imaging modalities in the diagnosis of hip and groin pain, and specifically for athletic pubalgia, continues to evolve. We typically obtain an AP pelvis, AP and lateral hip, and 45° Dunn view, which has previously been shown to accurately diagnose cam FAI [8]. The Dunn view is particularly useful in detecting femoral neck lesions consistent with cam-type FAI. Several studies have demonstrated the improved accuracy of MRI over plain radiographs alone for establishing hip and groin diagnoses [9–14] and have even recommended that it be considered the "gold standard" for imaging of athletic pubalgia [10]. Other studies, however, have shown a high false-positive rate for this modality, with Silvis et al. reporting a rate of 77 % of pathologic hip or groin MRI findings in asymptomatic collegiate and professional ice hockey players [15].

For various reasons, including coexisting pathology, and the considerable anatomic overlap of anterior structures, diagnostic imaging is often required to obtain a definitive diagnosis. Magnetic resonance imaging (MRI) should be obtained to confirm the diagnosis of athletic pubalgia. If other coexisting pathology is visualized on MRI, then information collected from the history and physical exam, as well as other diagnostic tools such as diagnostic injections, should be utilized to confirm the diagnosis of athletic pubalgia.

MRI is important for both the diagnosis of athletic pubalgia, as well as to evaluate for other conditions that may be causing the patient's groin pain, including hip joint pathology, strains, labral tears, osteitis pubis, iliopsoas bursitis, and occult stress fractures. Fluid-sensitive sequences should be done in three orthogonal planes [16]. A key sequence is the axial oblique, which shows the aponeurosis of the adductor longus and rectus abdominis (Fig. 34.2). The plane of the axial oblique MRI should parallel the arcuate line of the pelvic inlet [17]. A secondary cleft sign is an indication of an aponeurotic tear. The secondary cleft sign is seen on the axial oblique MRI as a curvilinear region of high signal intensity adjoining the pubic symphysis, on the side of the groin pain. This is believed to represent a microtear at the origin of the adductor longus and gracilis tendons [18].

Fluid-sensitive sequences allow direct visualization of increased signal intensity, indicating a tear of the rectus abdominis–adductor longus aponeurosis, or a tear/avulsion of the adductor longus. Tears of rectus abdominis–adductor longus aponeurosis appear as fluid or increased signal intensity undermining the aponeurosis, indicative of a tenoperiosteal disruption [16]. MRI sagittal and axial fluid-sensitive images acquired approximately 1–2 cm lateral to the pubic symphysis display the tenoperiosteal disruption at the aponeurosis [16].

T2-weighted fat-suppressed sagittal images obtained 1 cm lateral to the pubic symphysis visualize the rectus abdominis muscle/tendon, the adductor longus muscle/tendon, and the aponeurosis (Fig. 34.3).

Beyond the lack of consensus in diagnostic techniques and modalities, there also currently exists a multitude of both

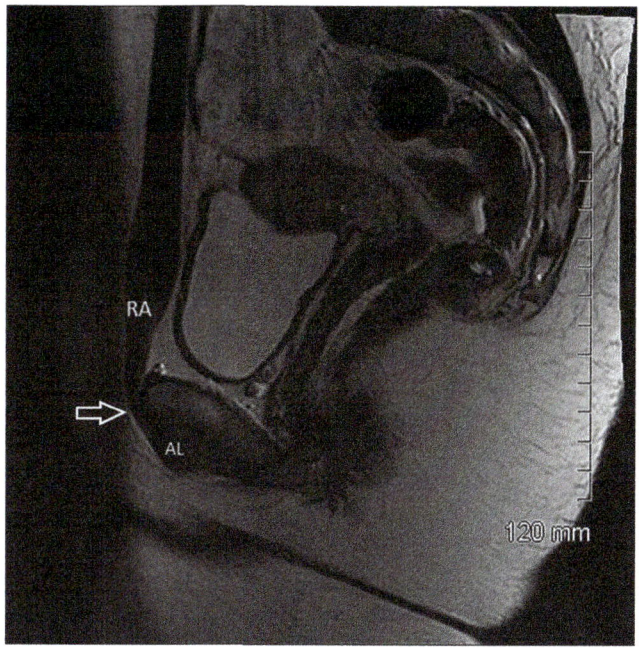

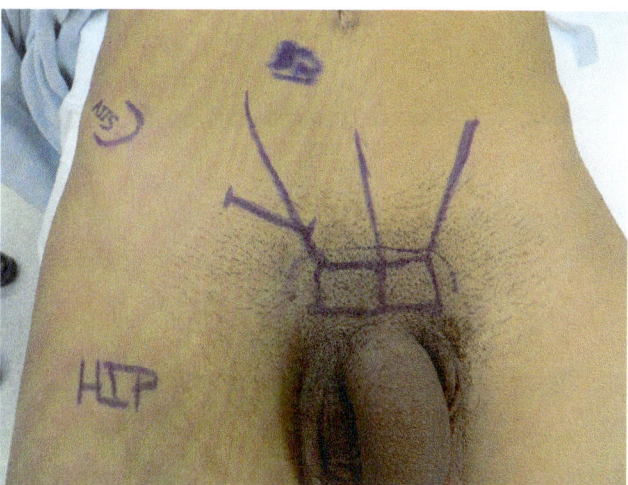

Fig. 34.4 Surface anatomy of rectus abdominus insertion and planned skin incision

Fig. 34.3 MRI T2 sequence, sagittal plane. The rectus abdominus is marked, which continues to the aponeurosis (*open arrow*) anterior to the pubis, and transitions to the adductor longus tendon

conservative [19, 20] and operative [21–25] indications and techniques, with a wide array of reported outcomes. Furthermore, much controversy exists in regard to the treatment of those patients who present with physical exam and/ or radiographic findings consistent with both athletic pubalgia and femoroacetabular impingement.

The chief muscular injury involved in athletic pubalgia is the insertion of the rectus abdominus. It has been our experience that this region is most often attenuated, and that direct reinsertion of the tendon back to its pubic insertion site appears to achieve excellent and consistent results. One of the most critical steps in our open repair technique involves the diligent bony preparation of the pubic insertion site and widened reinsertion area of the rectus tendon. We believe that the success we have encountered with this repair is the result of spreading these muscular forces over a wider insertion point, thus creating a relative decrease in the concentrated forces applied through the tendon attachment.

Operative Technique

As previously described by Litwin et al. [3], operative treatment at our institution is based on the theory of either gross tears, or more commonly microtears, within the muscles of the lower abdominal region. This region of pathology involves the external oblique aponeurosis, rectus abdominus, interface of the rectus abdominus and conjoined tendon, internal oblique, or transversus abdominus. Muscular attenuation in

the aforementioned regions may predispose the transversalis fascia of the posterior wall of the inguinal canal to further injury, creating a subsequent defect and resultant bulge when present [3]. The pain associated with athletic pubalgia is believed to arise from the muscle injury, and not the resultant posterior wall defect, which may or may not be present in any given case [3].

Our technique focuses primarily on the insertion of the rectus abdominus to the pubis, along with stabilization of the interface between the rectus and conjoined tendon, with reinforcement of the posterior wall of the inguinal canal [3]. Figure 34.4 demonstrates the surface anatomy of the rectus abdominus insertion and site for skin incision.

Appropriate preoperative antibiotic prophylaxis is administered unless contraindicated. The patient is placed in a supine position and prepped and draped to allow access to the lower abdomen on the side of pathology. A small 5 cm skin incision is made just above the external inguinal ring (Fig. 34.5). Dissection is carried down through the subcutaneous fat and Scarpa's fascia, exposing the underlying external oblique aponeurosis (Fig. 34.6).

Next, the external oblique is carefully incised in the direction of its fibers into the external inguinal ring, with care to avoid adjacent nerves (Fig. 34.7). The muscle is then elevated from the underlying structures, and the spermatic cord is identified and encircled with a penrose drain (Fig. 34.8). At this point in the operation, specific anatomic landmarks are evaluated, including the lateral edge of the rectus, the conjoined tendon, the pubic tubercle, the shelving portion of the ilioinguinal ligament, and the posterior wall of the inguinal canal [3]. The cord is elevated from the posterior wall and retracted inferiorly. The posterior wall is inspected for any defects (Fig. 34.9). In addition, the rectus abdominus insertion is carefully inspected for the presence of any tearing, laxity, or attenuation.

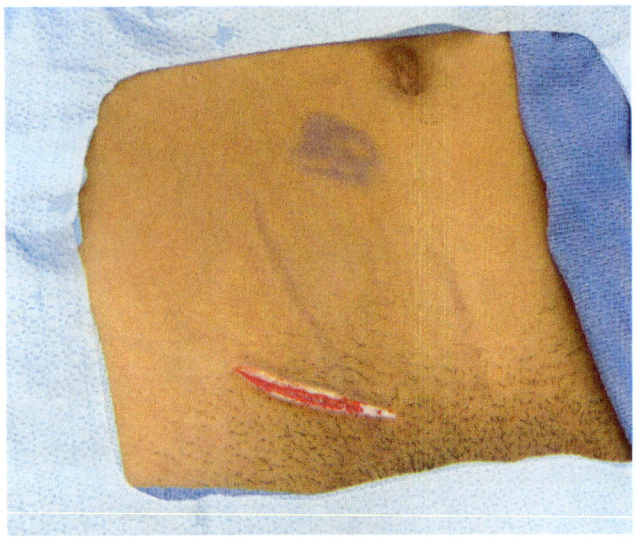

Fig. 34.5 Incision along skin crease just proximal to external inguinal ring

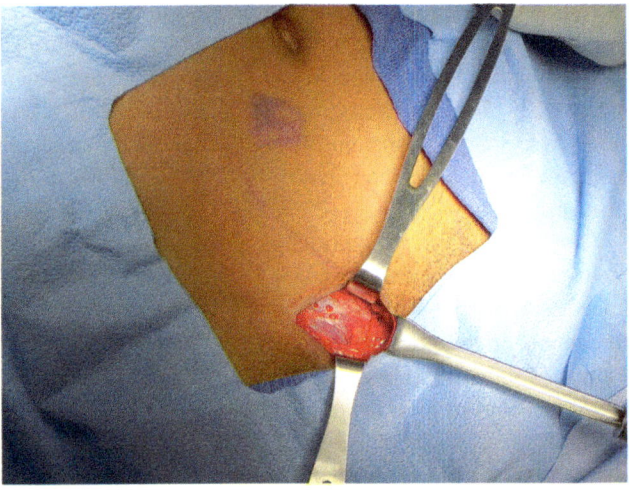

Fig. 34.6 Exposed external oblique aponeurosis

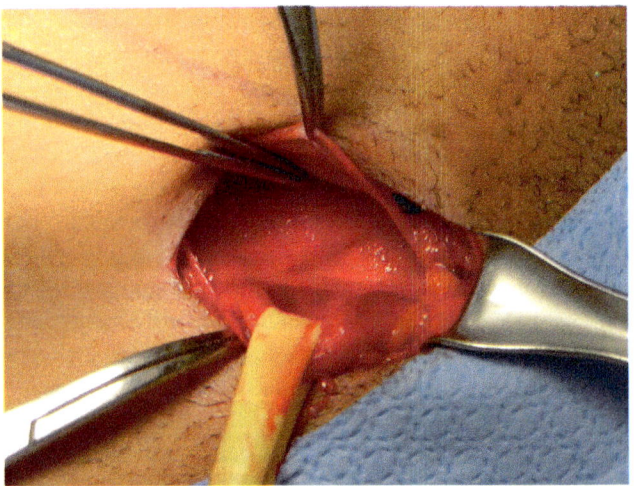

Fig. 34.7 Penrose around spermatic cord. Integrity of posterior wall and rectus insertion evaluated

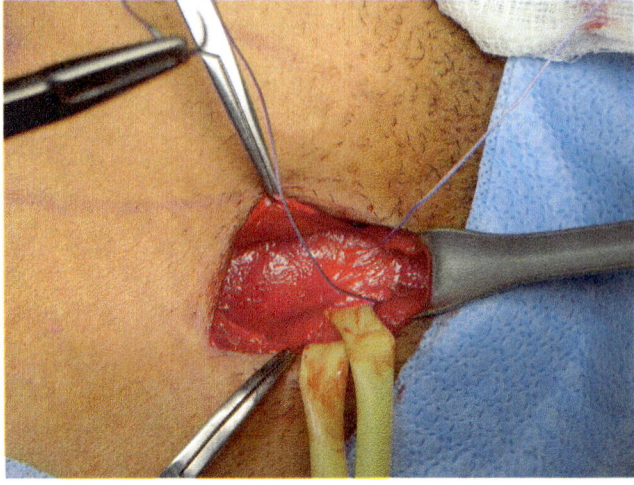

Fig. 34.8 Suture approximating rectus abdominus to the pubic tubercle periosteum

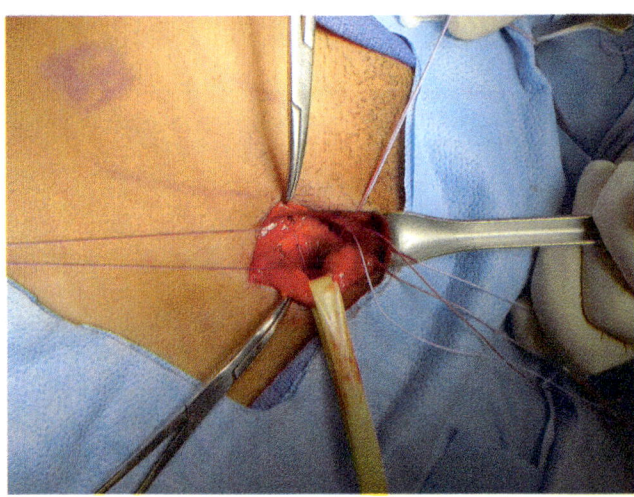

Fig. 34.9 Rectus approximated to Cooper's ligament, and interface of conjoined tendon/rectus brought to shelving portion of ilioinguinal ligament, with reinforcing sutures laterally from conjoined tendon to shelving portion

The insertion site of the rectus abdominus on the pubic tubercle is prepared to a bleeding bony bed. The inferolateral edge of the rectus is then brought down to the tubercle periosteum with 1–2 stitches of Orthocord (Depuy Orthopaedics, Warsaw, IN, USA) (Fig. 34.9). The tendon edge is next approximated to Cooper's ligament with another stitch, followed by a third stitch brining the interface of the conjoined tendon and rectus down to the shelving portion of the ilioinguinal ligament. Finally, one to two additional stitches are placed laterally and used to reinforce the conjoined tendon to the shelving portion (Fig. 34.10). Typically, a total of five stitches are used and once in place are sequentially tied down. Once the sutures are tied, appropriate re-tensioning of the rectus is appreciated through palpation.

The spermatic cord is allowed to resume its native position, and the aponeurosis of the external oblique is closed with running 2-0 Vicryl (Ethicon Inc, Somerville, NJ), followed by closure of the subcutaneous tissues with 2-0 Vicryl in an interrupted fashion. The skin is re-approximated with a 4-0 monofilament, using a running subcuticular technique. Local anesthetic is used on the incision site and also to perform an ilioinguinal nerve block to help decrease postoperative pain. Sterile dressings are then applied.

Our surgical procedure is performed as an outpatient procedure. Postoperatively, patients are immediately weight-bearing as tolerated. Patients return for their initial postoperative visit and wound check approximately 10 days postoperative. At this time, gentle hip range of motion and closed-chain exercises are encouraged, followed by gradual progression to core exercises by week 4. Return to sporting activity is anticipated by postoperative week 6.

Our institution's multidisciplinary team treatment approach is based on the belief that the chief pathology involved in athletic pubalgia is the insertion of the rectus abdominus. It has been our experience that this region is most often attenuated, and that direct reinsertion of the tendon back to its pubic insertion site has provided excellent and consistent results. Another important aspect of our surgical technique is the widened reinsertion of the rectus tendon. We believe that the success of operative treatment is a result of spreading of the muscular forces of the rectus insertion over a wider insertion area on the pubic bone, thereby decreasing the concentrated forces applied through the tendon attachment.

Cases

Case 1: Athletic Pubalgia, Rectus Abdominus Tear

History/Exam

A 48-year-old male hockey centerman presented to the orthopedic clinic with a history of intermittent right groin and hip pain for 5 years, occurring during hockey season. It typically resolved with rest and physical therapy. Despite extensive conservative treatment, including rest and physical therapy, he underwent bilateral laparoscopic inguinal direct wall hernia repair, utilizing mesh. He continued to have right groin pain, despite postoperative physical therapy. Postoperatively, he underwent a diagnostic/therapeutic injection ultrasound-guided injection along the right side of the pubic symphysis, utilizing a peppering technique. He reported minimal improvement following this injection. He was referred to the orthopedic clinic.

On physical examination, the patient is noted to have a non-antalgic gait. The patient is noted to have tenderness to palpation at the pubic symphysis area and in the lower right rectus region. He has full range of motion of his right hip. He has no pain elicited with passive right hip flexion/adduction/internal rotation (FADIR test). The patient's right lower

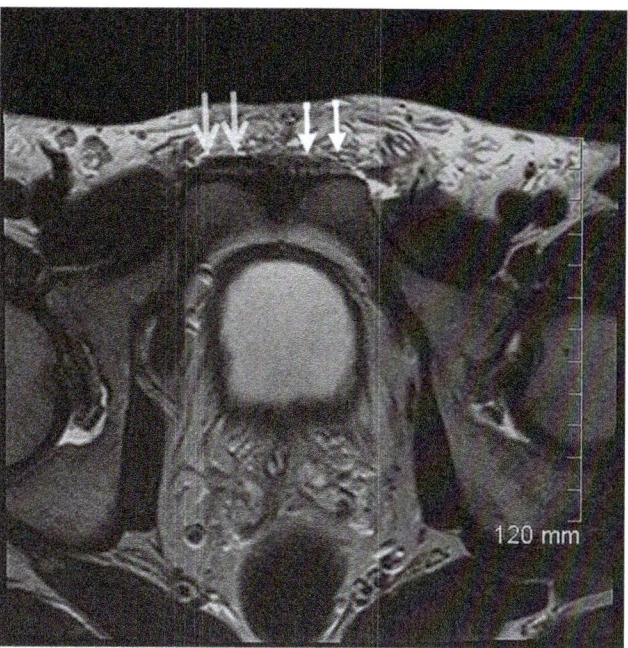

Fig. 34.10 The axial oblique T2-weighted sequence shows the increased signal intensity at the left rectus abdominus–adductor longus aponeurosis consistent with a tear

abdominal pain is worsened with resisted right hip flexion as well as with performing a sit-up. He has no palpable direct or indirect hernias present.

Imaging

Plain radiography did not demonstrate any significant pathology. Specifically, there was no evidence of right hip degenerative changes or evidence of findings consistent with femoroacetabular impingement.

MRI of the pelvis was then obtained. The axial oblique T2-weighted sequence (Fig. 34.10) shows the increased signal intensity at the left rectus abdominus–adductor longus aponeurosis consistent with a tear. In addition, the tear at the aponeurosis was visualized on the sagittal T2-weighted fat-suppressed image (Fig. 34.11).

Surgery

The patient was placed in a supine position. A right inguinal skin incision approach was utilized. The posterior abdominal wall was intact secondary to the previous laparoscopic repair. The lateral edge of the rectus abdominus was found to be torn at the insertion site of the pubis. The insertion site on the pubic bone just lateral to the pubic symphysis was prepared to formulate a bleeding bed. The rectus abdominus tendon was then repaired to its insertion site.

Discussion

This case highlights the distinct nature of rectus abdominus tendon insertional tearing (core muscle injury). The patient demonstrated no signs of hip pathology, had prior surgical

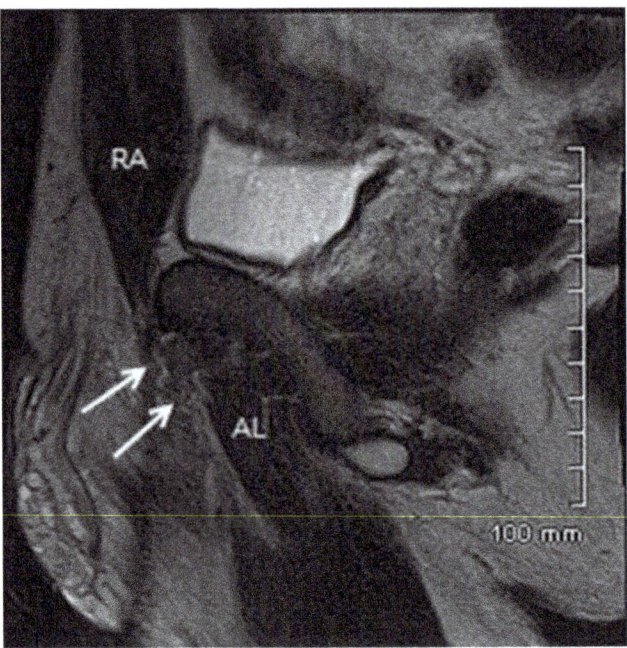

Fig. 34.11 MRI of the pelvis, T2-weighted image in the sagittal plane illustrates the tear at the aponeurosis (*arrows*)

correction of standard inguinal hernia pathology, and remained symptomatic. MRI findings were restricted to images obtained at the rectus insertion to the pelvis. Centers endeavoring to manage this patient population should carefully review with radiology staff and technicians the importance of including the rectus abdominis insertion in the standard hip and abdominal MRI sequences. The findings of increased signal or absent tendon on these multiplanar cuts suggest the diagnosis, and the clinical exam plus response to diagnostic injection confirms it.

Case 2: Athletic Pubalgia, Rectus Abdominus Tear

History/Exam

A 20-year-old male reports right hip and groin pain for 6 months. He first noticed the pain during football camp, following an insidious onset. He continued to play wide receiver at the Division I collegiate level, although his pain continued to worsen. Anti-inflammatory medication did improve his pain. He underwent a core strengthening program, as well as a stretching and hip strengthening program. He was unable to finish the season secondary to the pain. He rested for 6 weeks and had improvement in his right groin pain. He had immediate return of his right groin pain upon return to running program after a period of rest.

On physical examination, the patient is found to have a non-antalgic gait. He has tenderness to palpation at the right proximal adductor region. He reports pain in his right lower abdomen with resisted sit-ups. He has mild pain with flexion/adduction/internal rotation, FADIR test. He has no palpable direct or indirect hernias present.

Imaging

Radiographs obtained included an AP pelvis, an AP of the right hip, a cross table lateral, and a Dunn view. Radiographs demonstrated a mild CAM lesion, with a small cyst located at the head/neck junction of the proximal femur. There were no other osseous abnormalities noted.

An MRI of the pelvis and MR arthrogram of the right hip were performed. A diagnostic injection in the right hip was done at the time of the arthrogram and did not provide any relief of pain. The MRI findings were consistent with a right rectus abdominus–adductor longus aponeurosis tear (Figs. 34.12 and 34.13).

Surgery

The patient was placed in a supine position. A standard incision was made from the ASIS to the pubic tubercle area. Dissection was taken down to the fascia to reveal the internal and external rings. Dissection was taken down through the fascia. Inspection revealed a significant tear of the rectus abdominus tendon of the pubis with retraction. A delamination type of defect was visualized in the posterior wall. The insertion site on the pubic bone just lateral to the pubic symphysis was prepared to formulate a bleeding bed. Three nonabsorbable, braided sutures were used to repair the rectus tendon to the pubis. A small relaxing incision was made in the rectus tendon in order to mobilize the tendon for reattachment. Two nonabsorbable, braided sutures were then placed between the external oblique reflected edge down to the ilioinguinal ligament and the shelving portion. The rectus abdominus and the posterior wall were approximated to create a repair of the posterior wall of the inguinal canal.

Discussion

This case demonstrates the distinct character of pain associated with core muscle injury in the setting of coexistent femoroacetabular impingement. By performing intra-articular hip joint injection and noting no subjective symptom relief, the common adductor/rectus abdominis area was implicated in pain generation. The MRI confirmed abnormal signal at this area, and exam confirmed provocative testing reproduced pain.

Theories concerning limited hip motion or excessive sport motion as causative factors for the core muscle injury exist. This case illustrates the importance of addressing the actual pain generator once MRI signs of tissue level damage exist at the core insertion. Longitudinal follow-up of larger patient populations is required to determine if reinjury is inevitable in the absence of correction of hip impingement or sport cessation.

Fig. 34.12 The axial oblique T2-weighted sequence shows the increased signal intensity at the right rectus abdominus–adductor longus aponeurosis consistent with a tear (*arrows*)

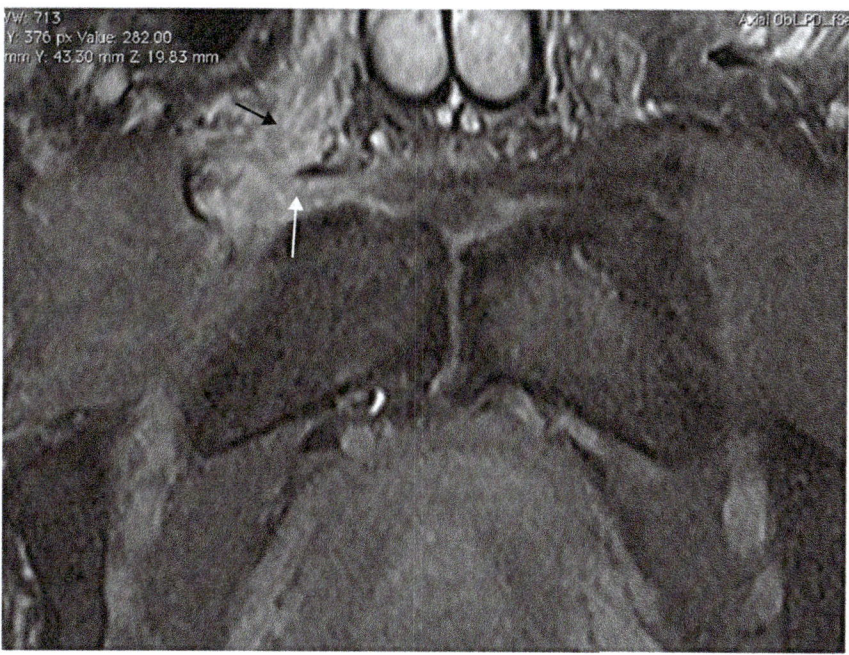

Case 3: Athletic Pubalgia, Rectus Abdominus/Adductor Longus Tear

History/Examination

A 27-year-old male presented to the orthopedic clinic for evaluation of left lower abdominal and groin pain. He is a former Division I collegiate basketball player who then went on to play professionally in Europe. He has not been playing for the last 6 months secondary to his left lower abdominal and groin pain. He was previously seen by an Urologist for evaluation of his left groin pain. The patient was diagnosed with prostatitis and treated with antibiotics with minimal improvement. He has minimal discomfort with straightforward jogging but increased pain with any lateral movements or cutting. He underwent an ultrasound-guided diagnostic/therapeutic injection into his left proximal adductor longus tendon sheath. This provided significant relief of his pain. He then underwent physical therapy and eventually returned to playing basketball. Following resuming cutting movements in basketball, he had recurrence of his pain.

Physical examination revealed a non-antalgic gait. The patient has full and symmetric range of motion of his bilateral hips. He has no tenderness to palpation at the distal aspect of his left rectus abdominus, in the area of the left pubis. He has a negative FADIR test. The patient does have tenderness to palpation at the origin of the adductor longus. He has no palpable direct or indirect hernias present.

Imaging

Radiographs were obtained, including an AP pelvis, AP left hip, cross table lateral, and Dunn view. The X-rays showed a

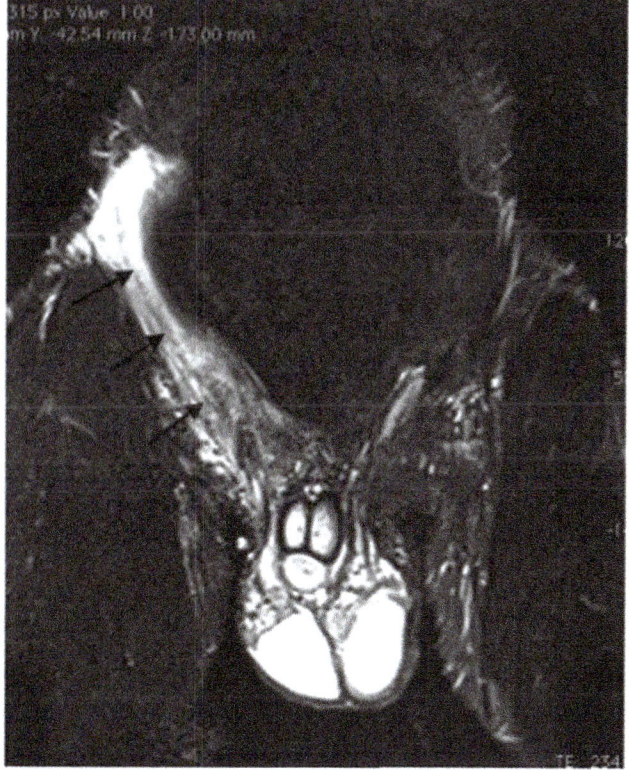

Fig. 34.13 MRI T2 sequence in the coronal plane shows edema in the rectus abdominus, aponeurosis, and adductor longus (*arrows*)

mild, small CAM lesion. There are no other osseous abnormalities, including no evidence of degenerative joint disease of the left hip. An MRI of the pelvis was obtained and is detailed in Figs. 34.14, 34.15, 34.16, 34.17, and 34.18.

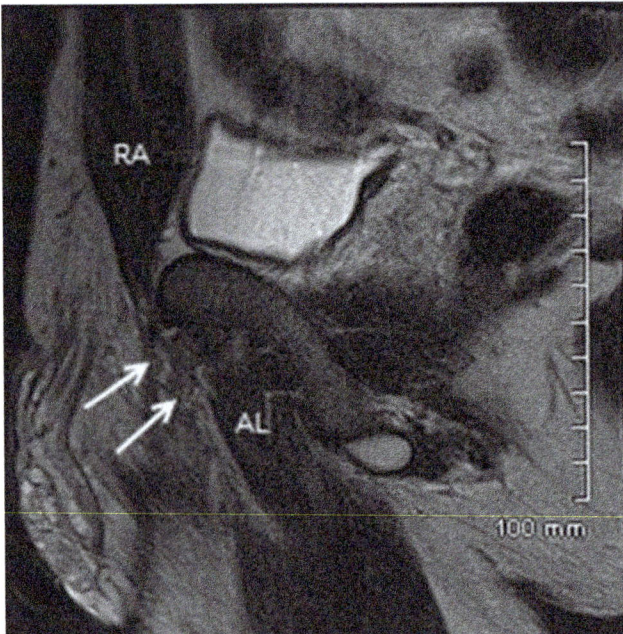

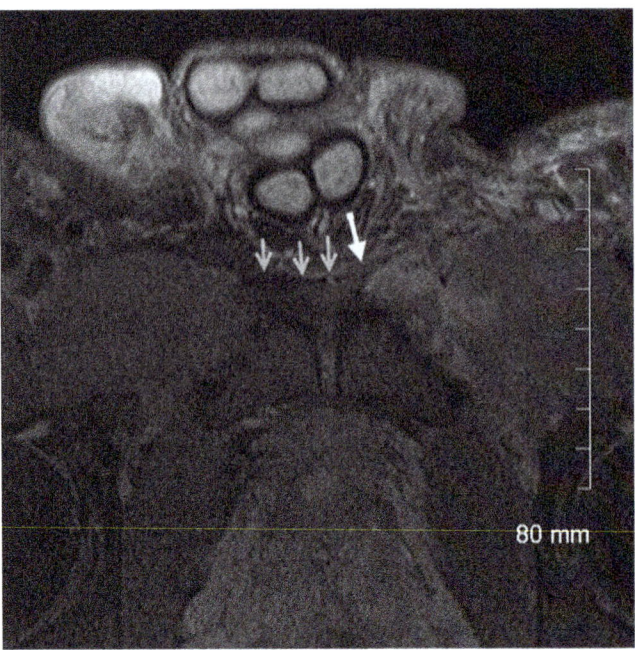

Fig. 34.14 MRI T2 sequence in the sagittal plane 1 cm lateral to the pubic symphysis. Increased signal intensity is at the rectus abdominus–adductor longus aponeurosis, indicating a tear at this location (*arrows*)

Fig. 34.15 MRI T2 sequence in the axial oblique plane. *Open arrows* indicate normal appearance of aponeurosis, indicated by a *transverse line* of decreased signal intensity just anterior to the pubic symphysis. The *block arrow* on the *left side*, just lateral to the pubic symphysis, indicates increased signal and injury to the aponeurosis. There is edema present

Fig. 34.16 MRI T1 sequence in the axial oblique plane. *Open arrows* indicate area of decreased signal intensity at the inferior/medial aspect of the left pubis. This finding is the so-called secondary cleft sign, indicating injury to the abdominus–adductor longus aponeurosis

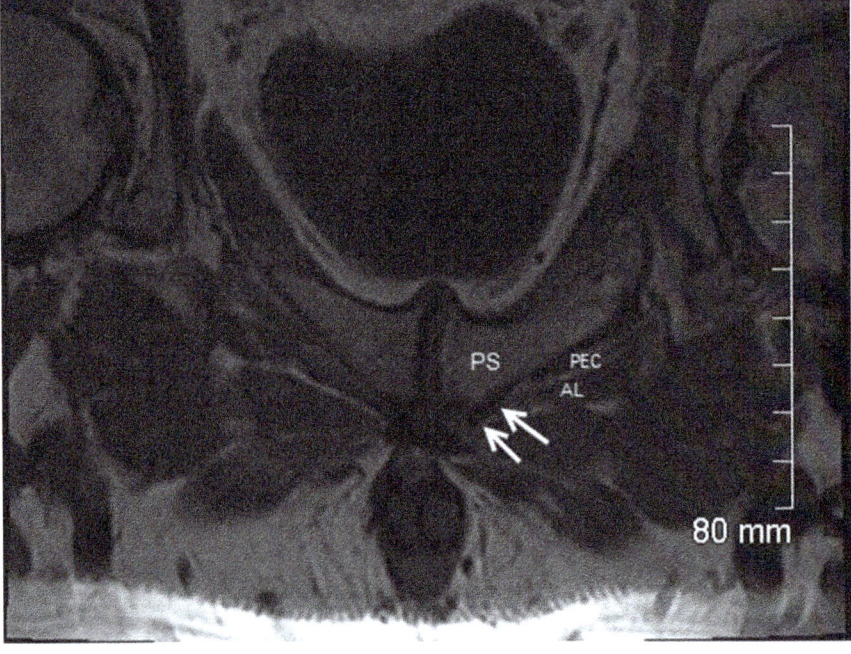

Fig. 34.17 MRI T2 sequence in the axial oblique plane. *Open arrow* indicates area of subtle increase in signal intensity at the inferior/medial aspect of the left pubis. This finding is the so-called secondary cleft sign, indicating injury to the abdominus–adductor longus aponeurosis

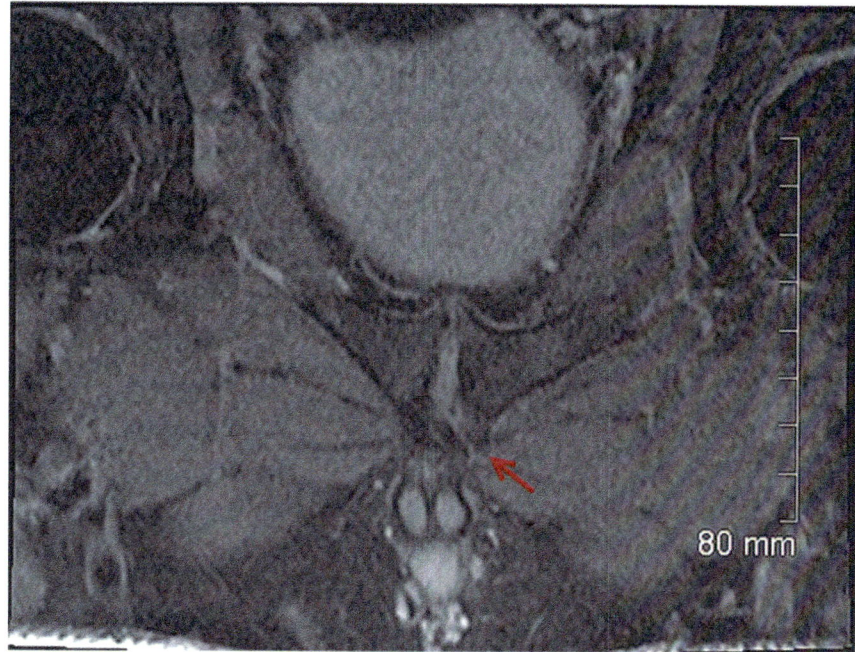

Fig. 34.18 MRI T2 sequence in the coronal plane shows edema in the rectus abdominus, aponeurosis, and adductor longus

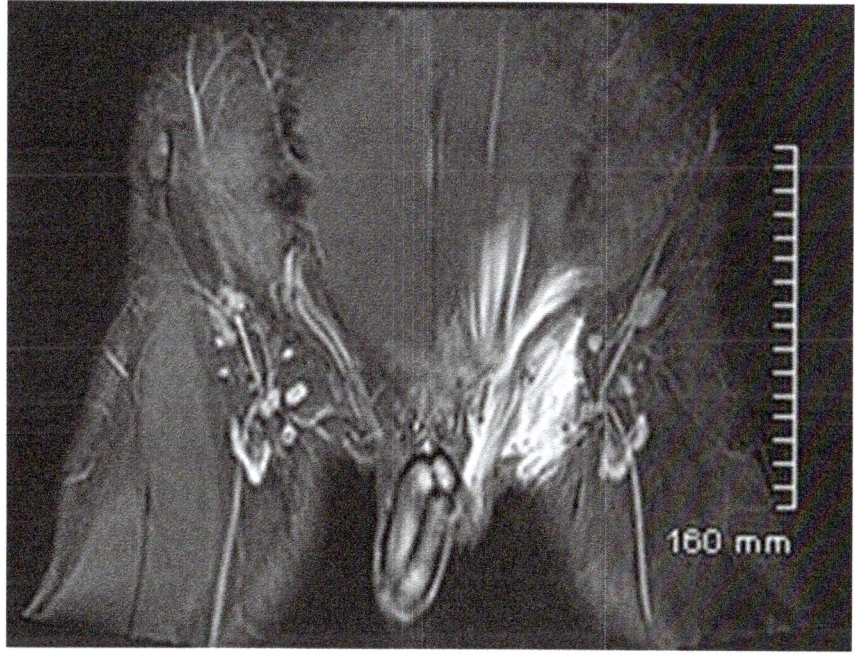

Surgery

The patient was placed in a supine position. A standard inguinal incision was made and dissection was taken down through the fascia. Inspection revealed a tear of the rectus abdominus tendon of the pubis. A defect was visualized in the posterior inguinal wall. The insertion site on the pubic bone just lateral to the pubic symphysis was prepared to formulate a bleeding bed. Two nonabsorbable, braided sutures were used to repair the rectus tendon to the pubis. A primary medial to lateral repair of the posterior wall of the inguinal canal was performed. The soft tissue and skin were then closed in the usual fashion. The left leg was then brought into abduction, and the adductor longus origin at the pubic bone was identified. An incision was made at the proximal aspect of the adductor longus tendon region. Careful dissection revealed the adductor longus tendon. The tendinous portion of the adductor longus tendon was incised. The wound was then closed in the usual fashion.

Discussion

This case illustrates the importance of examination of the posterior extent of the inguinal canal. While the athlete did respond to conservative care resulting in pain-free activities of daily living, return to sport resulted in return of symptoms. Again, coexistent pathology was shown to be unrelated to his pain pattern. Surgical care of the abdominal region resulted in successful return.

Case 4: Athletic Pubalgia, Rectus Abdominus/ Adductor Longus Tear

History/Examination

A 21-year-old male collegiate soccer player presented to the orthopedic clinic for evaluation of left lower quadrant abdominal pain that radiates to the left groin. Approximately 5 months ago, he had a spontaneous onset of left lower quadrant abdominal pain that worsened over the next 3–4 weeks. He then underwent physical therapy and rest for 6 weeks. He returned to playing soccer and continued to have similar pain without improvement. He reports increased left lower abdominal and left groin pain with core exercises, as well as with explosive movements such as pivoting or sprinting.

Physical examination reveals a normal gait. He has full and symmetric bilateral hip range of motion. There is not an internal or external hernia present. He has tenderness to palpation about the location of the rectus abdominus attachment to the pubis. He has pain in the area of his left lower abdomen when performing sit-ups. The patient has a negative FADIR test.

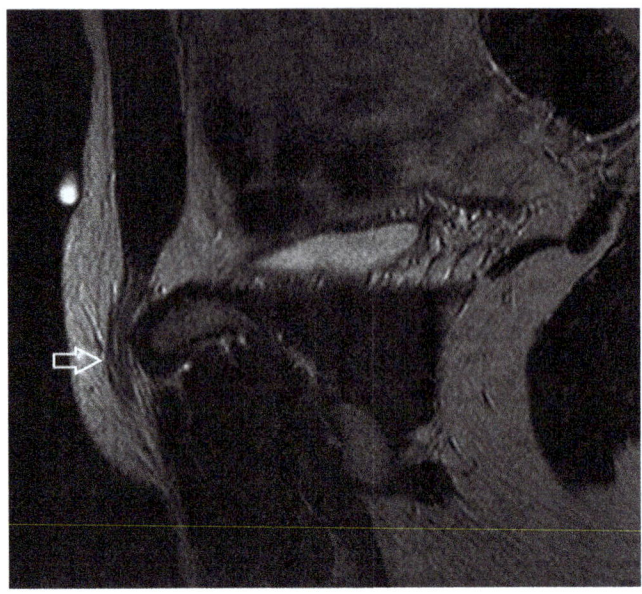

Fig. 34.19 MRI T2 sequence in the sagittal plane 1 cm lateral to the pubic symphysis. Increased signal intensity is at the rectus abdominus–adductor longus aponeurosis, indicating a tear at this location (*arrow*)

Imaging

Radiographs were obtained, including an AP pelvis, AP left hip, cross table lateral, and Dunn view. The X-rays showed a small CAM lesion. There are no other osseous abnormalities, including no evidence of degenerative joint disease of the right hip. An MRI of the pelvis was obtained and is detailed in Figs. 34.19, 34.20, and 34.21.

Surgery

The patient was placed in a supine position. The left proximal adductor region was then identified. A therapeutic steroid injection was performed into the left adductor longus tendon sheath. The left hip and groin were then prepped and draped. A standard inguinal incision was made and dissection was taken down through the fascia. Inspection revealed no evidence of an inguinal hernia. A tear of the rectus abdominus tendon at the pubic attachment was identified. The insertion site on the pubic bone just lateral to the pubic symphysis was prepared to formulate a bleeding bed. Two nonabsorbable, braided sutures were used to repair the rectus tendon to the pubis. This was performed by reattaching the lateral edge of the rectus abdominus to the pubis, utilizing two nonabsorbable, braided sutures. The fascia of the posterior wall was indentified. Using three nonabsorbable, braided sutures, the external oblique aponeurosis was re-approximated to the inguinal ligament, in a lateral to medial fashion.

Discussion

This final case provides another set of images and a vignette that seems to support the relevance of athletic pubalgia and core injury treatment. As in prior examples, MRI sequences

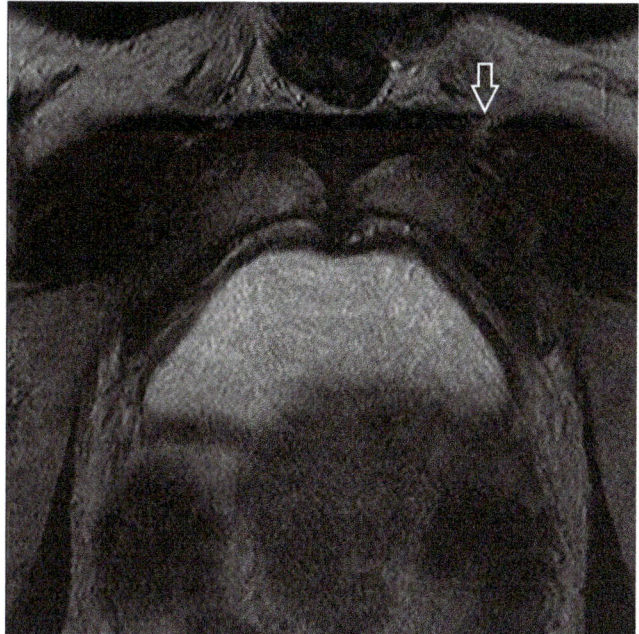

Fig. 34.20 MRI T2 sequence in the axial oblique plane. Normal appearance of aponeurosis, indicated by a *transverse line* of decreased signal intensity just anterior to the pubic symphysis, is seen at the right aponeurosis. The *block arrow* on the *left side*, just lateral to the pubic symphysis, indicates increased injury to the aponeurosis. There is edema present

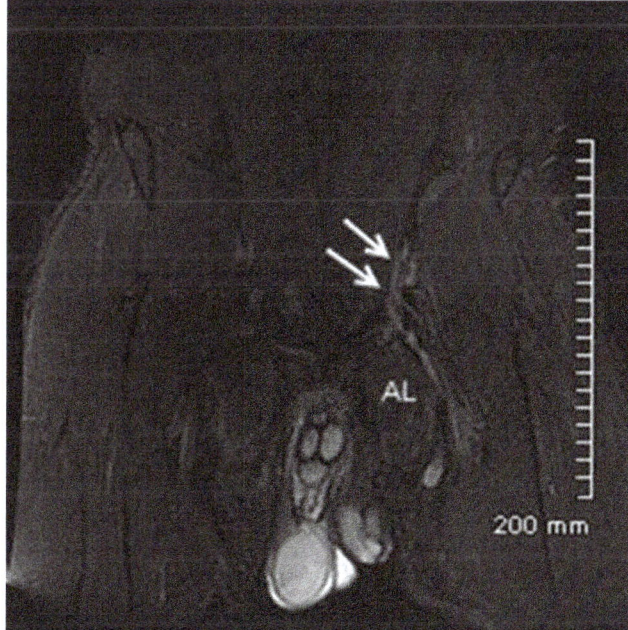

Fig. 34.21 MRI T2 sequence in the coronal plane shows edema in the rectus abdominus, aponeurosis, and adductor longus

were critical in identifying side by side asymmetry at the core insertional area. Without appropriate in-plane sequence acquisition, this would be impossible pathology to identify prior to surgery. While many questions exist related to the appropriate timing, recovery, and indications for surgery, these cases hope to illustrate for the reader the importance of inclusion of athletic pubalgia in the differential diagnosis of hip area dysfunction.

References

1. Taylor DC, Meyers WC, Moylan JA, Lohnes J, Bassett FH, Garrett Jr WE. Abdominal musculature abnormalities as a cause of groin pain in athletes. Inguinal hernias and pubalgia. Am J Sports Med. 1991;19(3):239–42.
2. Puig PL, Trouve P, Savalli L. Pubalgia: from diagnosis to return to the sports field. Ann Readapt Med Phys. 2004;47(6):356–64.
3. Litwin DE, Sneider EB, McEnaney PM, Busconi BD. Athletic pubalgia (sports hernia). Clin Sports Med. 2011;30(2):417–34.
4. Nam A, Brody F. Management and therapy for sports hernia. J Am Coll Surg. 2008;206(1):154–64.
5. LeBlanc KE, LeBlanc KA. Groin pain in athletes. Hernia. 2003;7:68–71.
6. Farber AJ, Wilckens JH. Sports hernia: diagnosis and therapeutic approach. J Am Acad Orthop Surg. 2007;15(8):507–14.
7. Hackney RG. The sports hernia: a cause of chronic groin pain. Br J Sports Med. 1993;27:58–62.
8. Barton C, Salineros MJ, Rakhra KS, Beaule PE. Validity of the alpha angle measurement on plain radiographs in the evaluation of cam-type femoroacetabular impingement. Clin Orthop Relat Res. 2011;469(2):464–9.
9. Albers SL, Spritzer CE, Garrett Jr WE, Meyers WC. MR findings in athletes with pubalgia. Skelet Radiol. 2001;30(5):270–7.
10. Lischuk AW, Dorantes TM, Wong W, Haims AH. Imaging of sports-related hip and groin injuries. Sports Health. 2010;2(3):252–61.
11. Patel K, Wallace R, Busconi BD. Radiology. Clin Sports Med. 2011;30(2):239–83.
12. Robinson P, Bhat V, English B. Imaging in the assessment and management of athletic pubalgia. Semin Musculoskelet Radiol. 2011;15(1):14–26.
13. Zoga AC, Meyers WC. Magnetic resonance imaging for pain after surgical treatment for athletic pubalgia and the "sports hernia". Semin Musculoskelet Radiol. 2011;15(4):372–82.
14. Zoga AC, Mullens FE, Meyers WC. The spectrum of MR imaging in athletic pubalgia. Radiol Clin N Am. 2010;48(6):1179–97.
15. Silvis ML, Mosher TJ, Smetana BS, Chinchilli VM, Flemming DJ, Walker EA, Black KP. High prevalence of pelvic and hip magnetic resonance imaging findings in asymptomatic collegiate and professional hockey players. Am J Sports Med. 2011;39(4):715–21.
16. Omar IM, Zoga AC, Kavanagh MD, Koulouris G, Bergin D, Gopez AG, Morrison WB, Meyers WC. Athletic pubalgia and "sports hernia": optimal MR imaging technique and findings. Radiographics. 2008;28:1415–38.
17. Robinson P, Barron DA, Parsons W, Grainger AJ, Schilders EM, O'Connor PJ. Adductor-related groin pain in athletes: correlation of MR imaging with clinical findings. Skelet Radiol. 2004;33:451–7.
18. Cunningham PM, Brennan D, O'Connell M, MacMahon P, O'Neill P, Eustace S. Patterns of bone and soft-tissue injury at the symphysis

pubic in soccer players: observations at MRI. AJR J Roentgenol. 2007;188:W291–6.

19. Hegedus EJ, Stern B, Reiman MP, Tarara D, Wright AA. A suggested model for physical examination and conservative treatment of athletic pubalgia. Phys Ther Sport. 2013;14(1):3–16.

20. Kachingwe AF, Grech S. Proposed algorithm for the management of athletes with athletic pubalgia (sports hernia): a case series. J Orthop Sports Phys Ther. 2008;38(12):768–81.

21. Ahumada LA, Ashruf S, Espinosa-de-los-Monteros A, Long JN, de la Torre JI, Garth WP, Vasconez LO. Athletic pubalgia: definition and surgical treatment. Ann Plast Surg. 2005;55(4):393–6.

22. Meyers WC, Foley DP, Garrett WE, Lohnes JH, Mandlebaum BR. Management of severe lower abdominal or inguinal pain in high-performance athletes. PAIN (Performing Athletes with Abdominal or Inguinal Neuromuscular Pain Study Group). Am J Sports Med. 2000;28(1):2–8.

23. Muschaweck U, Berger L. Minimal repair technique of sportsmen's groin: an innovative open-suture repair to treat chronic inguinal pain. Hernia. 2010;14(1):27–33.

24. Paajanen H, Brinck T, Hermunen H, Airo I. Laparoscopic surgery for chronic groin pain in athletes is more effective than nonoperative treatment: a randomized clinical trial with magnetic resonance imaging of 60 patients with sportsman's hernia (athletic pubalgia). Surgery. 2011;150(1):99–107.

25. Srinivasan A, Schuricht A. Long-term follow-up of laparoscopic preperitoneal hernia repair in professional athletes. J Laparoendosc Adv Surg Tech A. 2002;12(2):101–6.

Revision Hip Arthroscopy

John J. Christoforetti, Michael J. Palmer, Bojan Zoric, and Marc J. Philippon

Introduction

Every year, the indications for arthroscopic hip surgery expand, leading to increased volumes of arthroscopic hip surgery performed yearly [1–6]. This has also created a need for treating physicians to understand and care for patients who have failed arthroscopic hip surgery [7]. There is a paucity of literature focused on failed arthroscopic hip surgery and/or revision arthroscopic hip surgery, and further study is warranted. This chapter will first briefly review current evidence for revision hip arthroscopy indications and outcomes. Next, it will present the authors' strategy for use of MRI technology in the evaluation and treatment of the patient with persistent symptoms following hip arthroscopy. Select cases are shown to highlight effective use of clinical experience and MRI diagnostics in the revision setting. Given the challenges that range from diagnostic and technical limitations to insurance coverage challenges, revision hip arthroscopic surgery should be indicated with caution.

J.J. Christoforetti, MD (✉)
Department of Orthopedic Surgery, Sports Medicine Division, Allegheny Health Network, West Penn Hospital, Pittsburgh, PA, USA
e-mail: John.christoforetti@gmail.com

M.J. Palmer, MD
88th Medical Group, Surgical Operations Squadron, Wright Patterson Air Force Base, Wright Patterson AFB, OH, USA
e-mail: Michael.palmer.30@us.af.mil

B. Zoric, MD
Sports Medicine North, Peabody, MA, USA
e-mail: Bzoric7@gmail.com

M.J. Philippon, MD
The Steadman Clinic and Steadman Philippon Research Institute, Vail, CO, USA
e-mail: drphilippon@sprivail.org

Current Evidence for Revision Hip Arthroscopy

Open and arthroscopic surgery for non-arthritic hip pain can fail to render the patients symptom free and leave treating physicians and patients seeking further treatment. Published evidence to inform the diagnostic process is limited. In all published evidence, modest improvements have been noted in appropriately selected cases.

Evidence exists to support improvement in revision of arthroscopic procedures with additional arthroscopic procedures. The senior author (MJP) has shown results for revision of failed arthroscopic procedures [8]. In this retrospective review of 37 cases of revision arthroscopic hip surgery, 36/37 patients demonstrated unaddressed or inadequately addressed features of femoroacetabular impingement. Thirty-four patients reported hip pain that was unresolved after their prior surgery. Twelve patients had gradually worsening pain, 8 had an acute onset of pain without trauma, and 17 had acute worsening of pain with a traumatic event. The geographic location (lateral, posterior, and groin) of the pain did not correlate to treatment at the time of revision surgery. In another retrospective review of 24 cases in 23 patients, Heyworth et al. identified that 100 % of the patients presented with groin pain that worsened with activity [9]. Thirteen patients reported no improvement of symptoms at all after their prior arthroscopic hip surgery. The average time to recurrence of symptoms was 6.1 months (0–39 months) from their index procedure. They identified 19 cases of unaddressed or incompletely addressed bony impingement. Failed labral repair in the form of a re-torn labrum or loose suture anchor was found in eight cases. Psoas impingement was identified and addressed in seven cases. A variety of concomitant intra-articular/extra-articular pathologies were identified and addressed during revision surgery in patients from both series. Pathologic findings included cam and pincer lesions, synovitis, adhesions, labral fraying/tears, chondral defects, capsular laxity, psoas impingement,

Table 35.1 Authors' tips for patient selection in revision hip arthroscopy (Evidence-Based Medicine Level of Evidence: 5)

Strong potential for success	Relative potential for success
Persistent hip joint pain as confirmed by history/exam/intra-articular injection	Index procedure included implantation of nonabsorbable implants
Under- or unaddressed FAI	MRI signs of failure to heal at prior intended repair
Minimal degenerative hip disease	New onset of different pain in previously untreated area
Intact labrum without prior repair or healed prior repair	
Reasonable expectations	Persistent capsular insufficiency (iatrogenic)
No narcotic medication requirement	Persistent feeling of instability
Absence of major dysplastic or extra-articular impingement morphology	Thickened capsule or adhesions visible on MRI
	Persistent painful psoas snap
	Persistent mechanical symptoms

Table 35.2 Authors' experience with poor indications for revision hip arthroscopy (Evidence-Based Medicine Level of Evidence: 5)

Objective	Subjective
Progressive and severe degenerative joint changes	Pain in a location inconsistent with hip pathology
Severe hip dysplasia	Incomplete or no response to prior treatment performed
Absence of abnormal hip findings on exam or radiographs	Without complication and without surgical implants
Severe bone deformity in areas inaccessible to arthroscopic exposure	Lack of definably different surgical goals in the setting of persistent hip area pain
	Surgeon's experience

ligamentum teres tears, loose bodies, recurrent PVNS, snapping IT band, and trochanteric bursitis.

Evidence also exists that modest gains can be made with revision hip arthroscopy following open hip preserving surgery [10]. Retrospective review of patient reported outcomes in the setting of hip arthroscopy performed, following open hip preserving surgery has shown modest but significant improvements. Once again, the most common finding in successful treatments was treatable residual femoroacetabular impingement (present in 66 % of cases). Treatable segmental labral defects and symptomatic heterotopic bone were also predictors of improved outcome.

Likewise, recent evidence shows that open hip preserving surgery can be effective in improving disappointing outcomes following index hip arthroscopy procedures. Severe extra-articular impingement, posteriorly located intra-articular impingement features, and moderate to severe hip dysplasia have all shown to be common features in failed index hip arthroscopy during salvage open surgery efforts. Periacetabular osteotomy for correction of untreated moderate to severe dysplasia has been shown to be an effective salvage of failed arthroscopy [11].

Given the small numbers of patients present in all studies available for review today [12, 13], selection for arthroscopy of the hip following failed index procedures remains largely a clinical decision. The efforts to ascertain reasons for failure in hip preserving surgery from a research perspective always demonstrate significant observation bias. As knowledge of new and potentially impactful diagnoses grows, investigators

will undoubtedly identify reasons for failure that currently are not under investigation.

Table 35.1 shares the authors' tips for patient selection in revision hip arthroscopy (Evidence-Based Medicine level of Evidence: 5), and Table 35.2 shows the authors' experience with poor indications for revision hip arthroscopy (Evidence-Based Medicine level of Evidence: 5).

Clinical Evaluation of Patients with Persistent Dysfunction After Hip Arthroscopy

When evaluating a patient who has failed arthroscopic hip surgery, it is important to take a detailed history. It is important to identify the characteristics of pain that led to the first surgery and chronologic detail of the pain after that surgery. It is important to tease out if the pain is different in quality or intensity, whether there was a new trauma to the hip, or if the pain ever went away. Understanding the patients and their expectations and insight into their problem is an art that comes with experience but is vital in counseling and educating patients.

Physical exam should include a comprehensive evaluation of all possible causes of hip pain. This includes multi-positional musculoskeletal exam to evaluate gait, stance, core strength, lumbosacral spine pathology, pinpoint areas of maximal tenderness, hip range of motion, provocative maneuvers, weakness, and abnormal sensation or reflexes. It should also include a basic abdominal exam to rule out non-musculoskeletal causes of hip pain. We defer female pelvic exams, but if there is any question of a genitourinary cause of hip or groin pain, a referral to the gynecologist is initiated. Comprehensive review of the history and physical exam in this patient group are beyond the scope of this text, yet it is the opinion of the authors that these considerations are the best guides for selecting appropriate treatment for this patient group.

Imaging of Postoperative Hip

Postoperative changes can complicate the interpretation of imaging studies. Retained implants can cause distortion of MRI imaging decreasing the quality of the study. It is also challenging to identify clinically significant new findings in the postoperative hip.

Standard radiographic studies should include an AP pelvis, AP hip, and a lateral view of the hip (frog leg or cross table) [14]. These images should be scrutinized for pathology including cam and pincer impingement, hip arthritis, fracture, dysplasia, SI joint arthritis, and lumbar stenosis. Original imaging from before the initial surgery should be available for comparison.

MRI arthrogram should be the study of choice when evaluating for intra-articular soft tissue pathology in the postoperative hip. Blankenbaker et al. performed a retrospective review of 20 patients who had undergone revision arthroscopic hip surgery for recurrent labral tear after initially undergoing a labral debridement [15]. Original and postoperative MRI arthrograms, as well as surgical documentation of the revision procedure, were available for evaluation. All MRI arthrograms were obtained at the same institution using the same protocol. Two fellowship trained musculoskeletal radiologists reviewed the images retrospectively. Nineteen patients were diagnosed with recurrent labral tear intraoperatively. Fourteen tears were identified by consensus retrospective review on MRI arthrogram (12 based on high intensity line to the labral surface, two based on labral distortion and paralabral cyst formation). The other five patients were found to have only labral shortening. They concluded that a recurrent labral tear can be diagnosed on MRI arthrogram by the presence of a new high intensity line to the labral surface, an enlarged or distorted labrum, or a new paralabral cyst.

McCarthy and Glassner have shown the useful correlations between arthrography and arthroscopy in the revision setting [16]. We currently use a combination of MRI and MRI arthrogram to evaluate patients after hip arthroscopy when standard plain radiographs do not reveal the complete diagnosis. Figure 35.1 provides a summary of our most common uses for both studies.

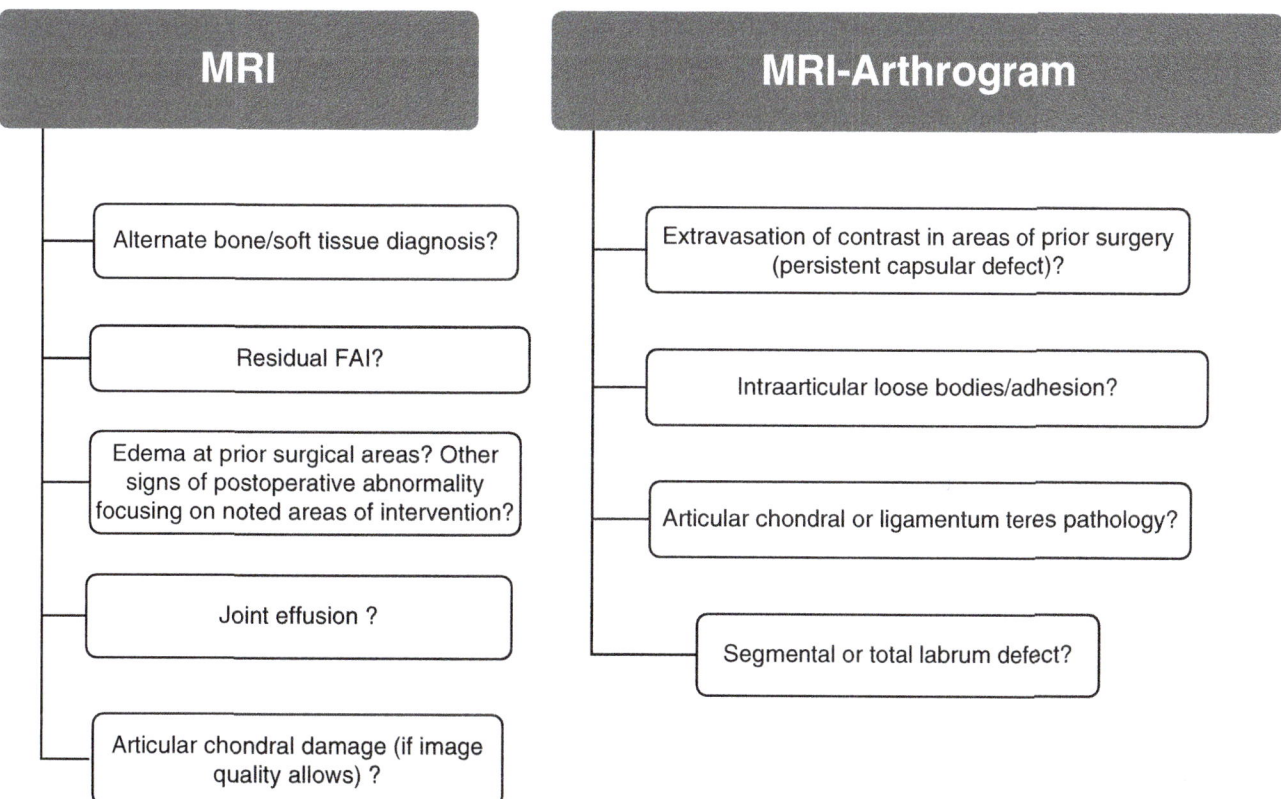

Fig. 35.1 Surgical considerations for review of MRI and MRI arthrogram of the hip in the revision setting

Cases

Case 1: Postoperative Adhesions

History, Clinical Presentation, and Exam

A 32-year-old female presents for second opinion when she failed to have any significant relief after arthroscopic labral debridement and microfracture of a chondral defect 8 months prior. The operative note indicated that minimal labrum debridement in the anterior acetabulum was performed along with a femoral head microfracture procedure. The patient expressed that her initial complaint prior to index surgery was groin pain during and after physical activity for 6 months.

Her only period of significant relief after her first surgery was from an intra-articular steroid injection. Her rehabilitation protocol following the index procedure included crutch protection for 6 weeks. Physical therapeutic exercise was initiated at 8 weeks.

On physical exam, she had pain with flexion adduction internal rotation. She also had a decrease in arc of motion compared to her uninjured side. FABER testing and off the table extension testing reproduced pain. There was tenderness over the anterior hip capsule with no signs of infection and well-healed incisions.

Imaging

Plain radiographs showed no signs of residual femoroacetabular impingement or arthritic change. MRI arthrogram was obtained which demonstrated postoperative adhesions and loss of normal capsulolabral architecture and lacked any significant alternate pathology (see Fig. 35.2).

Treatment

After discussion of risks and benefits, the patient elected for revision hip arthroscopy. During arthroscopy, the labrum was found to be healed in the area of prior debridement, and no segmental loss was present. The supraacetabular space was obliterated with adhesions along the anterior labrum (Fig. 35.3). The area of prior capsulotomy scarred directly to the femoral head region of microfracture (Fig. 35.4). Operative treatment included mechanical and thermal lysis of adhesions and closure of the prior capsulotomy defect.

Postoperative care instructed the patient to use a hip orthosis for 2 weeks. Crutch protection with 20 lb. foot-flat weight bearing was initiated immediately. Continuous passive motion machine was used 6 h daily for 2 weeks, and home caregiver administered passive circumduction exercises were performed.

At 1 year post-revision, the patient had returned to her pre-injury level of activity including outdoor running and fitness class participation.

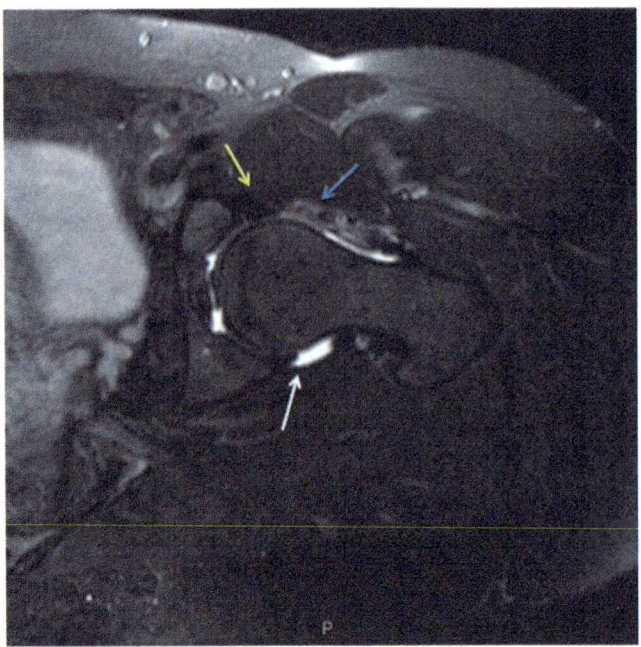

Fig. 35.2 Axial T2-weighted MRI arthrogram image demonstrating low signal interruption of the intra-articular contrast at the area of prior surgical exposure (*blue arrow*). Anteriorly, there is loss of the normal supraacetabular recess as evidenced by lack of contrast fill between the labrum and capsule (*yellow arrow*). Posteriorly, the normal supraacetabular recess contrast fill is demonstrated in the area distant from the prior surgical field (*white arrow*)

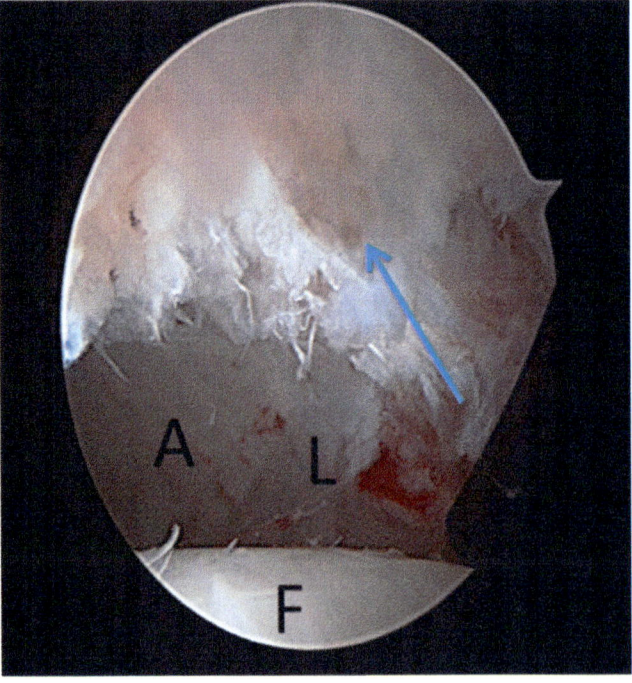

Fig. 35.3 Arthroscopic image corresponding with MRI arthrogram shown in Fig. 35.2 at the level of the acetabular rim. Adhesions obliterating supraacetabular recess (*blue arrow*) in postoperative zone. *A* acetabulum, *F* femoral head, and *L* labrum

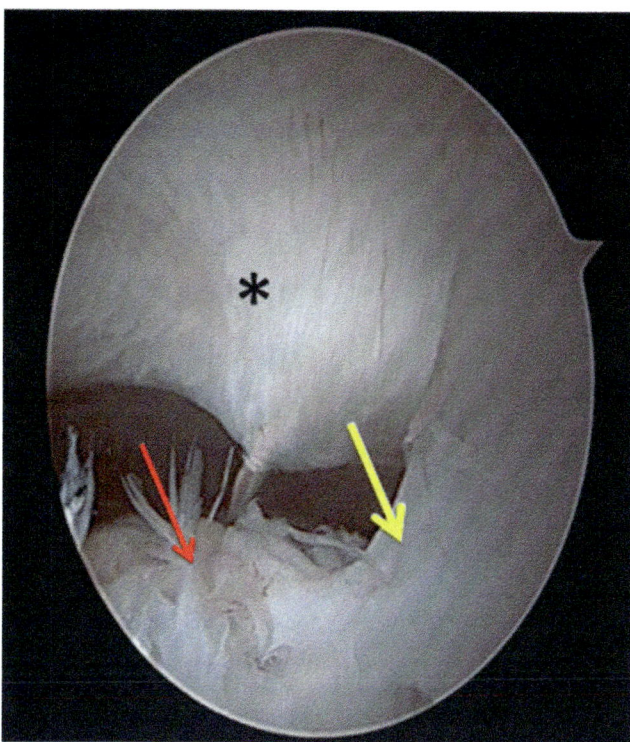

Fig. 35.4 Arthroscopic image in the peripheral space corresponding with MRI arthrogram shown at the level of the capsule-femoral head adhesion. Normal capsule (*asterisk*); adhesion (*yellow area*) sweeping from prior capsulotomy to femoral head at the area of prior microfracture (*red arrow*)

Discussion

The most basic form of appropriate revision hip arthroscopy is shown in this case. Development of untoward effects of appropriate operative care in the form of excessive adhesions can occur, and correction has the potential to help. Particularly, when the index procedure is performed by another center, attention to the potential existence of postoperative adhesions helps to provide an option for salvage.

There are some common features in the clinical presentation that can raise suspicion for this clinical scenario. Delayed rehabilitation in the setting of procedures that stimulate the healing response such as osteochondroplasty or microfracture can predispose to adhesion. Operative steps, such as complete capsulectomy, that allow communication between raw bone surfaces and the soft tissues of the flexor can also contribute. Patients without overt signs of missed structural pathology at the index procedure who seem to demonstrate good response to intra-articular injection and suffer from limited active motion also raise suspicions for involvement of adhesions in the absence of plain radiographic arthritic progression [17].

As in the case shown, the MRI arthrogram confirms the clinical suspicion by first eliminating alternate diagnoses such as avascular necrosis or stress fracture. Secondly, the

use of arthrogram allows appreciation for the loss of normal joint recesses in the area of operative treatment. These are frequently the key signs of potential for successful revision through simple lysis of adhesion.

It is unknown to what degree that the lysis of adhesions component of all revision procedures contributes to overall recovery as no trial exists comparing the simple performance of lysis of adhesions to advanced revision techniques.

Case 2: Postoperative Capsular Defects and Microinstability

History, Clinical Presentation, and Exam

A 22-year-old female Division I rower presented to us with persistent right hip pain for 2 years following arthroscopic labral repair and osteochondroplasty at an outside institution.

The index procedure was performed as an attempt to alleviate rowing-related groin pain and snapping and also included a transcapsular psoas recession, yet capsular management was not noted in the operative report.

Despite early initiation of rehabilitation and good progress, she felt that after 6 weeks postoperatively, she began to suffer recurrence of anterior hip pain. As training intensity increased, her pain increased monthly. She was unable to return to her preoperative level of activity due to the pain and even reported a sense of popping that she felt was new since the procedure.

On physical exam, she had pain with flexion adduction internal rotation but was otherwise comparable to the opposite hip in range of motion and strength. She reported pain upon resisted straight leg raise testing at 30° flexion and pain with FABER testing. Core strength and balance were reduced on the operative side but within normal limits on the asymptomatic side.

Imaging

Plain radiographs showed no signs of residual impingement, heterotopic bone, or dysplasia.

An MRI arthrogram was ordered which revealed extravasation of fluid into the anterior soft tissues, without evidence of recurrent labral tear or residual impingement (Fig. 35.5).

Treatment

Revision hip arthroscopy was performed, which revealed healed labrum tissue in the area of prior repair; there were no signs of recurrent or residual impingement and normal articular cartilage of the femoral head and acetabulum. A persistent 2×2 cm capsulotomy defect was present, through which the muscular psoas was visible (Fig. 35.6) in the area corresponding to the MRI arthrogram identified capsular dye extravasation.

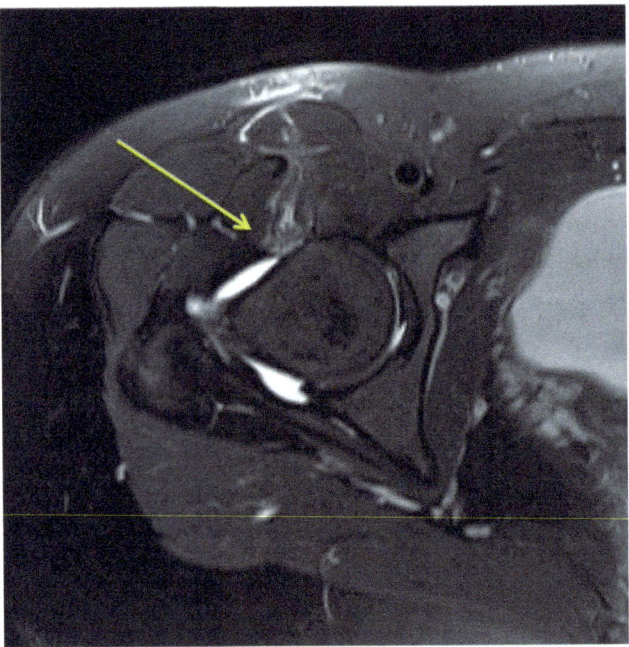

Fig. 35.5 Axial T2-weighted MRI arthrogram demonstrating extravasation of contrast dye into the soft tissues anteriorly

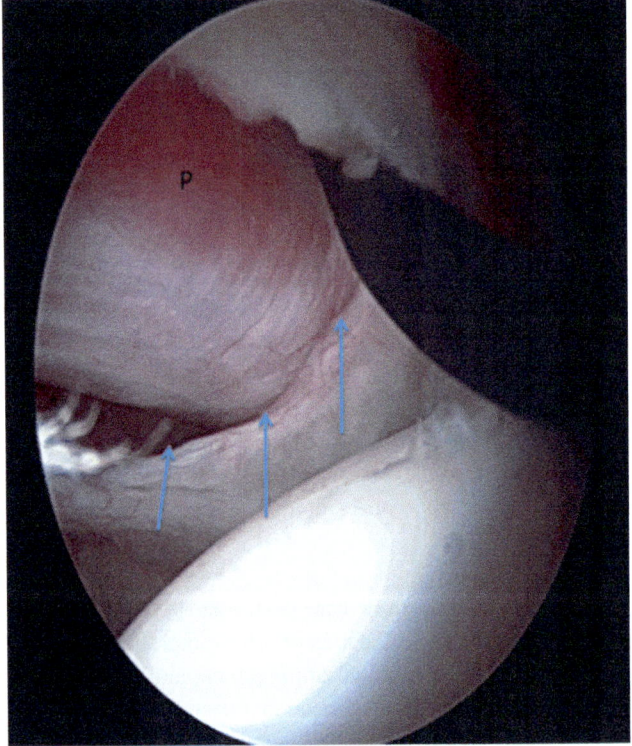

Fig. 35.6 Arthroscopic image of the persistent capsular defect in the anterior hip corresponding to the site of MRI arthrogram leakage. Through the capsule defect (*arrows*), the exposed psoas (P) is visible

Arthroscopic suturing techniques were used to close the capsular defect, restoring the normal anatomy of the anterior capsule. Postoperatively, she was placed in a specific rehabilitation protocol focused on early motion and protection of extreme ranges of extension and abduction or external rotation.

By 8 weeks postoperatively, she reported complete relief of pain. At final 2-year follow-up, she remained pain free and active in recreational sports but had not resumed competitive rowing.

Discussion

This case illustrates an increased complexity of considerations in the revision setting. Unlike in the first case presented, the MRI arthrogram demonstrated increased signal in the anterior soft tissues in the region of prior surgical intervention. Rather than adhesions eliminating expected spaces, the capsule has an absent appearance.

Matching the MRI findings with the understanding of the technical aspects of psoas recession performed in the index procedure, the complaint of anterior hip pain with activity could be understood. With over 2 years of failed postsurgical therapy, revision surgery to assess the healing of the labrum and address the deficiency in the capsule identified on MRI was effective in the absence of new or revision bone correction.

Technical considerations for this case are more advanced than in a simple lysis of adhesions. Appreciation of this pathology requires understanding of the normal appearance of the proximal hip capsule as well as deficiencies when present [18]. Facility with advanced arthroscopic suturing techniques and capsular management strategies are required to avoid overtightening or further damage. Finally, careful rehabilitation to avoid re-tear of the capsule and allow improved outcome is required.

Case 3: Unaddressed FAI and Segmental Labrum Defect

History, Clinical Presentation, and Exam

Thirty-three-year-old male presented with acute onset right hip and groin pain while performing a box-jump plyometric exercise. Four years prior to this event, the patient had undergone an arthroscopic labral debridement without osteoplasty at an outside facility. An MR arthrogram revealed a recurrent tear of the anterior superior labrum with thinning of the articular cartilage adjacent to the tear. He had temporary relief with an intra-articular depomedrol injection, nonsteroidal anti-inflammatory medications, and physical therapy. The patient continued to have persistent hip and groin pain, particularly with climbing ladders/sitting or putting shoes on. Examination showed pain with flexion, adduction, and internal rotation (FADIR) testing.

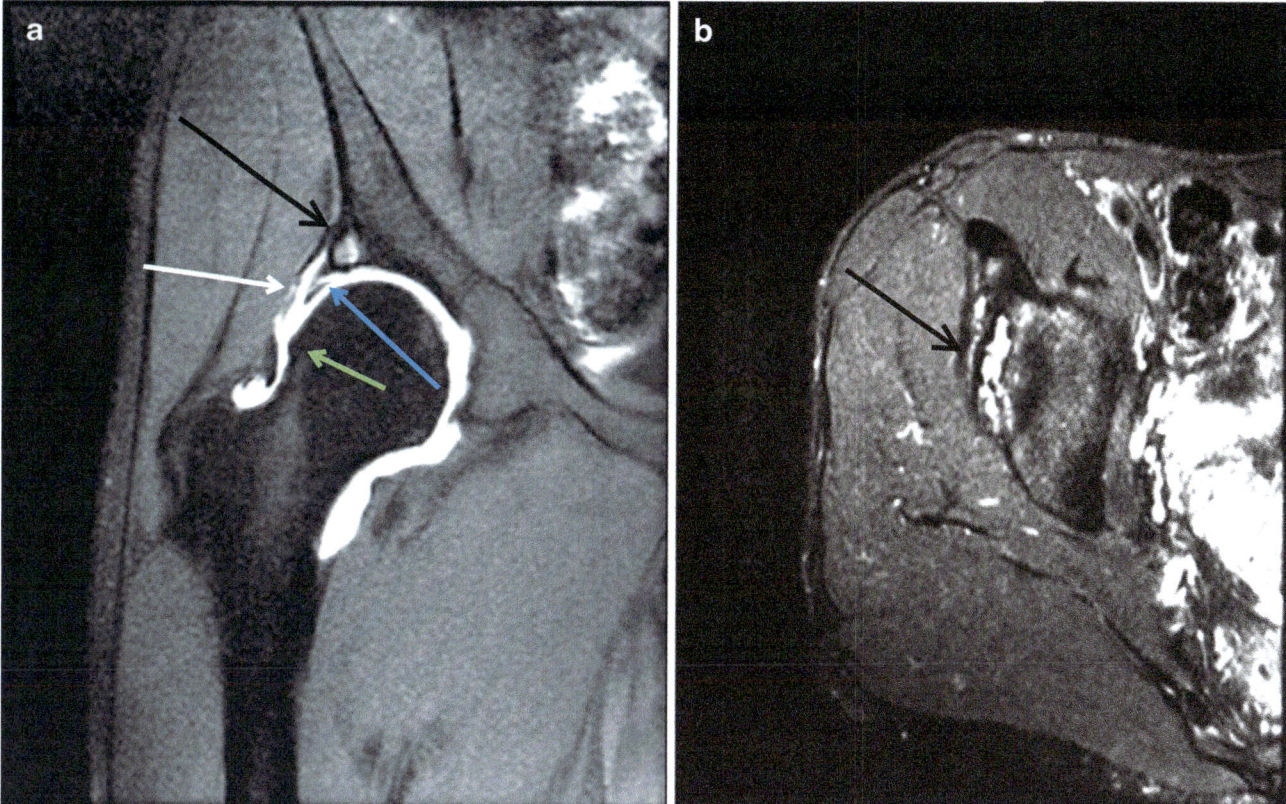

Fig. 35.7 MRI arthrogram of affected hip showing T2-weighted coronal image (**a**) and axial image (**b**). Supraacetabular cyst (*black arrow*); persistent capsular deficiency (*white arrow*); labrum tear; acetabular chondral lesion (*blue arrow*); and femoral head cam lesion (*green arrow*)

Imaging

Plain radiographs (not shown) demonstrated large Cam deformity, supraacetabular intraosseous cyst, and preserved joint space.

MRI arthrogram revealed persistent capsular defect, supraacetabular cyst, labrum tearing, and persistent Cam lesion (Fig. 35.7a, b).

Treatment

Revision hip arthroscopy included lysis of adhesions, capsular closure, femoral osteochondroplasty, and reconstruction of the labrum using semitendinosis allograft. See Fig. 35.8a, b. Postoperative recovery followed a specific protocol for arthroscopic impingement correction. At 1 year postoperatively, the patient continued to report anterior hip pain following vigorous athletics but greatly improved symptoms with daily activities.

Discussion

This case builds further upon the first two cases presented and includes the need for treatment of unaddressed pathology (femoroacetabular impingement) and salvage of iatrogenic tissue damage (labrum reconstruction, capsular closure, and lysis of adhesions). The MRI arthrogram revealed the presence of moderate arthritic damage in the regions of unaddressed impingement as well as the suggestion of persistent labrum and capsule abnormality. Formal discussion of the technical and radiographic parameters of impingement correction is beyond the scope of this chapter. This final case serves as a typical example of the most effective revision steps published to date and reminds the reader that unaddressed impingement is the most common indication for revision hip arthroscopy.

Summary

Revision hip arthroscopy is a difficult task for the treating surgeon and an undesirable need for the suffering patient. Meticulous attention to clinical and radiographic parameters can lead to appropriate patient selection. MRI and MRI arthrogram remain essential to our assessment of the bone and soft tissues of the postoperative hip in this setting. The technical demands of revision hip arthroscopy can range from basic to the most advanced, and surgeons must assess their own capabilities prior to performing these procedures.

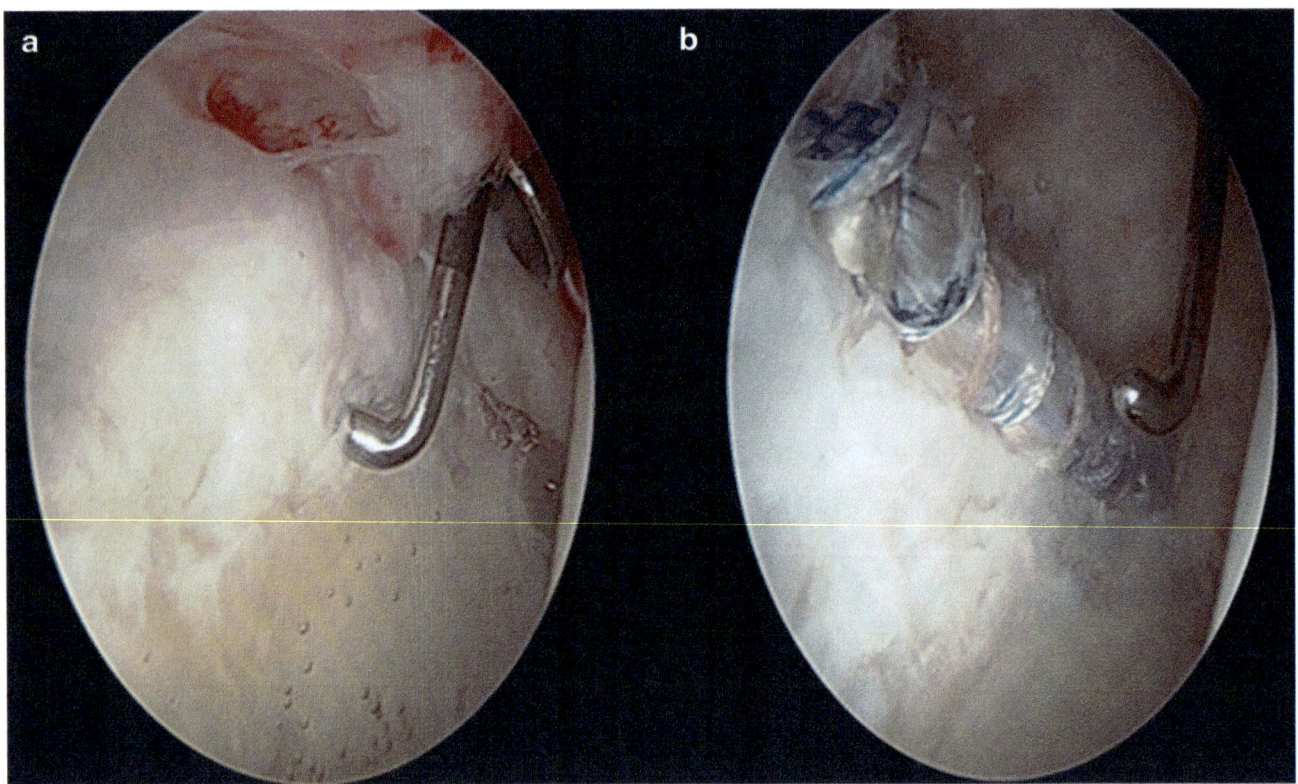

Fig. 35.8 Arthroscopic images showing anterior labrum deficiency and acetabular articular chondral damage corresponding to the zone of unaddressed impingement (**a**) and post-revision labrum reconstruction (**b**)

References

1. McCarthy JC, Lee J. Hip arthroscopy: indications, outcomes and complications. Instr Course Lect. 2006;55:301–8.
2. Smart LR, Oetgen M, Noonan B, Medvecky M. Beginning hip arthroscopy: indications, positioning, portals, basic techniques, and complications. Arthroscopy. 2007;23:1348–53.
3. Chen AF, Wright V. Hip arthroscopy: current indications and setup. Oper Tech Orthop. 2010;20:212–6.
4. Kelly BT, Williams RJ, Philippon MJ. Hip arthroscopy: current indications, treatment options, and management issues. Am J Sports Med. 2003;31:1020–37.
5. McCarthy JC, Jibodh SR, Lee J-A. The role of arthroscopy in evaluation of painful hip arthroplasty. Clin Orthop Relat Res. 2009; 467:174–80.
6. Colivin AC, Harrast J, Harner C. Trends in hip arthroscopy. J Bone Joint Surg Am. 2012;94(4):e23.
7. Bogunovic L, Gottlieb M, Pashos G, Baca G, Clohisy JC. Why do hip arthroscopy procedures fail? Clin Orthop Relat Res. 2013; 471:2523–9.
8. Philippon MJ, Schenker MK, Briggs KK, Kupersmith DA, Maxwell RB, Stubbs AJ. Revision hip arthroscopy. Am J Sports Med. 2007; 35:1918–21.
9. Heyworth BE, Shindle MK, Voos JE, Rudzki JR, Kelly BT. Radiologic and intraoperative findings in revision hip arthroscopy. Arthroscopy. 2007;23:1295–302.
10. Domb BG, Stake CE, Lindner D, El-Bitar Y, Jackson TJ. Revision hip preservation surgery with hip arthroscopy: clinical outcomes. Arthroscopy. 2014;30(5):581–7.
11. Ross JR, Clohisy JC, et al. Patient and disease characteristics associated with hip arthroscopy failure in acetabular dysplasia. J Arthroplasty. 2014;29(9 Suppl):160–3.
12. Aprato A, Jayasekera N, Villar RN. Revision hip arthroscopic surgery: outcome at three years. Knee Surg Sports Traumatol Arthrosc. 2014;22(4):932–7. Available from http://www.ncbi.nlm.nih.gov/pubmed/23328987.
13. Ward JP, Rogers P, Youm T. Failed hip arthroscopy: causes and treatment options. Orthopedics. 2012;35:612–7. Available from http://www.ncbi.nlm.nih.gov/pubmed/22784891.
14. Clohisy JC, Carlisle JC, Beaule PE, Kime Y-J, Trousdale RT, Sierra RJ. A systematic approach to plain radiographic evaluation of the young adult hip. J Bone Joint Surg. 2008;90 Suppl 4:47–66.
15. Blankenbaker DG, Keene JS, DeSmet AA. MR arthrographic appearance of the postoperative acetabular labrum in patients with suspected recurrent labral tears. Am J Roentgenol. 2011;197: 1118–22.
16. McCarthy JC, Glassner PJ. Correlation of magnetic resonance arthrography with revision hip arthroscopy. Clin Orthop Relat Res. 2013;471(12):4006–11. Available from http://www.ncbi.nlm.nih.gov/pubmed/23637056.
17. Byrd JWT, Jones KS. Adhesive capsulitis of the hip. Arthroscopy. 2006;22:89–94.
18. McCormick F, Slikker W, Harris JD, Gupta AK, Abrams GD, Frank J, et al. Evidence of capsular defect following hip arthroscopy. Knee Surg Sports Traumatol Arthrosc. 2014;22(4):902–5. Available from http://www.ncbi.nlm.nih.gov/pubmed/23851921.

Index

The manufacturer's authorised representative in the EU is Springer
Nature Customer Service Centre GmbH, Europaplatz 3, 69115 Heidelberg,
Germany. If you have any concerns regarding our products, please
contact ProductSafety@springernature.com

Printed and bound by CPI Group (UK) Ltd, Croydon, CR0 4YY

23/04/2026

02095656-0001